Litt's

DRUG ERUPTION & REACTION MANUAL

32nd EDITION

Litt's Drug Eruption & Reaction Manual is a succinct reference to give clinicians the essential information for an informed decision about patient management.

The full database from which the manual is derived – Litt's Drug Eruption & Reaction database; www.drugeruptiondata.com – currently holds over 1840 drug profiles with over 74,500 documented drug reactions, as evidenced by over 161,700 references on PubMed, and is internationally relied upon by medical practitioners for its unparalleled focus on adverse effects and cutaneous reactions.

This edition:

✓ Provides documentation of adverse reactions to the 1500 most consulted drug and herbal profiles
✓ Offers clinicians a one-stop reference for the essential information about a drug's safety profile before prescription
✓ Gives clinicians managing patients with many different medications a route to making an informed decision about problematic reactions

Litt's DRUG ERUPTION & REACTION MANUAL

32nd EDITION

2026

Neil H. Shear, MD, FRCPC, FACP
Professor Emeritus
Medicine, Clinical Pharmacology & Therapeutics, and Dermatology
University of Toronto, Canada

CRC Press
Taylor & Francis Group
Boca Raton London New York

CRC Press is an imprint of the
Taylor & Francis Group, an informa business

Designed cover image: Shutterstock

Thirty Second edition published 2026
by CRC Press
2385 NW Executive Center Drive, Suite 320, Boca Raton FL 33431

and by CRC Press
4 Park Square, Milton Park, Abingdon, Oxon, OX14 4RN

CRC Press is an imprint of Taylor & Francis Group, LLC

ISBN: 9781041202295 (hbk)
ISBN: 9781041202288 (pbk)
ISBN: 9781003715672 (ebk)

DOI: 10.1201/9781003715672

CONTENTS

A Note from the Editor

All of us involved with Litt's 32nd Edition are acutely aware of the growing need for timely access to accurate and comprehensive drug safety data. This demand is now more and more highlighted by interest across the globe in what we used to call Drug Safety Clinics. That term might be changing from country to country but more and more specialists in drug safety are now working together to ensure that patients, relatives, allergists, dermatologists, and other specialties can base their guidance on current and future risks of reactions. As we look to understand and integrate changes in risk management we can see that the data in the Litt database, manual, and safety tables are informative for such clinicians and their patients.

Neil H. Shear, MD, FRCPC, FACP

Litt's Drug Eruption & Reaction Manual – at a glance

This 32nd edition has been revised and updated throughout to present a quick clinical reference guide to adverse drug reactions (ADRs), side effects, drug interactions and other safety information for prescription and over-the-counter medications.

There are also tables of material on reactions caused by classes of drugs, enabling you to see at a glance whether a reaction is common to all the drugs in that particular class, or to a majority of them, or only to a significant few.

In addition, Trevor Champagne has kindly updated his note on the implications of Artificial Intelligence for drug safety; and Elizabeth J. Phillips has also kindly updated a table of reported genetic associations with cutaneous adverse drug reactions and other immune-mediated reactions.

The aims of this edition remain:

1. To help medical practitioners make informed and safe decisions when diagnosing and prescribing, and also when generally seeking information.
2. To help healthcare professionals remain pharmacovigilant.
3. To provide all physicians, lecturers, educators, and pharmacists with an easy-to-use and reliable quick reference tool.

Space in the manual is, unfortunately, constrained. The full and comprehensive picture for all drugs – from which our information derives – can be found in the **Litt database** (www.drugeruptiondata.com), which is updated continually. The Litt database was originated by Jerome Z. Litt; and now edited by Neil H. Shear, with advice and input by Rupert Purchase, DPhil, CChem, FRSC.

Drug eruptions and Artificial Intelligence in 2026: AI now . . .

Trevor Champagne[1]

2026 brings increasing polarization to the topic of artificial intelligence - it is increasingly difficult to find a moderate position. However, despite the hype and multitudes of unsupported claims the fundamental properties of the technology have remained exactly the same as they were a year ago. In most modern use cases, there is an outcome of interest, a mathematical/statistical model such as a neural network, and input data used for training and prediction. Traditional statistics exist to demonstrate the strength of a proposed association, but the training of most AI algorithms starts by assuming the relationship exists and *forcing* the model to output the best predictive nonlinear relationship it can possibly find. Should the model not perform well in further prospective tests, it is not possible to differentiate between a poor model, poor quality data, or that the input simply cannot factually predict the output.

Consider HLA-A*24:02, found rigorously to be statistically associated with carbamazepine-associated Stevens-Johnson Syndrome. The AI equivalent might be to plug the entire sequenced major histocompatibility complex of carbamazepine-prescribed patients who have had SJS and a control into an appropriately constructed model. The result would be an algorithm when given a patient's MHC sequence would be to predict which patients given carbamazepine are at risk of SJS. We would not be able to explain why or how it works; therefore, we say: intelligent? We could also ask it to associate the proteins found in a patient's breakfast foods with SJS and it's quite possible a model could find a path to that association. Clinical correlation is required.

Where to deploy it? Modern electronic medical record systems can already compare potential complications. Prescribe a patient acitretin while they are on methotrexate and the warning will flash on screen: "these medications together may impact the liver". By extension, the above MHC scanning algorithm could be integrated and when carbamazepine is prescribed could output to the user: "this patient may be at risk for SJS" - presuming of course the algorithm has been granted appropriate access to the input data itself. Such algorithms en masse may have the potential to identify true risk, with the obvious caveat there is a risk of many false positives when there are few true positives.

Large language models such as ChatGPT, Claude or Llama are based on the popular generative pre-trained transformer and trained on millions to billions of texts. They have a single role: given a series of input words, what word is statistically likely to come next? Feed the sequence forward and sentences and paragraphs emerge. The novelty of the text is controlled by the randomization setting known as temperature - too hot and it outputs spectacular factual errors; too cold and it pseudo-plagaristically outputs its training set. They are quite capable of producing total nonsense. Hallucinations notwithstanding, we are starting to see a powerful value in the ability of LLMs to convert unstructured, messy data (such as heterogeneous medical records) into structured data which can then be used in a more predictable and deterministic way - for example, as entry points into other statistical AI algorithms (such as the system evaluated by Khemani et al.). It's still not true intelligence, but it's closer.

[1]Clinical Assistant Professor, Department of Dermatology and Skin Science, University of British Columbia, Vancouver, Canada; Adjunct Assistant Professor, Department of Medicine, Division of Dermatology, University of Toronto, Toronto, Canada

Bibliography

Dave T *et al*. ChatGPT in medicine: an overview of its applications, advantages, limitations, future prospects, and ethical considerations. *Frontiers in Artificial Intelligence* 2023;6:1169595.

Khemani DB *et al*. AI-driven pharmacovigilance: Enhancing adverse drug reaction detection with deep learning and NLP. *MethodsX*. 2025;23;15:103460.

McDermott MBA *et al*. Reproducibility in machine learning for health research: Still a ways to go. *Science Translational Med* 2021;13:586: eabb1655.

Roosan D *et al*. Artificial intelligent context-aware machine-learning tool to detect adverse drug events from social media platforms. *J Med Toxicol* 2022;18.4:311-320.

Shi YW *et al*. HLA-A* 24: 02 as a common risk factor for antiepileptic drug-induced cutaneous adverse reactions. *Neurol* 2017;88.23:2183-2191.

Vaswani A *et al*. Attention is all you need. *Advances in Neural Information Processing Systems* 2017;30.

A note on ADRs

The incidence and severity of ADRs are influenced by a number of factors:

1. Patient-related factors:

- Age – geriatric, pediatric, adolescent . . . older patients are taking more medications-hence more of a possibility of developing reactions; pediatric patients have more delicate skins; hormonal changes occur in adolescents . . . All these factors play roles in the development of possible adverse reactions.
- Gender – male or female – and if the latter, then pregnant/breast-feeding/menopausal . . .
- Disease – not only the disease being treated, but also other pre-existing health conditions and comorbid diseases. For example, atopic patients are at increased risk for serious allergic reactions; also, there would be an increased risk for hypersensitivity drug reactions if the patient has asthma or lupus erythematosus.
- Genetics – a patient could have abnormal drug metabolism due to inheriting abnormal alleles (see further the Genetic Associations Table).
- Geography – patients living in sunny climes could develop phototoxicities from photosensitizing drugs more readily than those who inhabit cooler, less sunny climates.

2. Drug-related factors:

- Type/class of drug – for example, there is a heightened risk of angioedema with the use of ACE inhibitors (see further the section of tables of class reactions).
- Duration of therapy – the longer a patient maintains the therapy, the more possible it becomes that he/she could develop a reaction due to their changes in drug metabolism (e.g. renal insufficiency) or drug interactions.
- Dosage – the greater the dosage, the more likely an adverse side effect.
- Bioavailability – the extent to and rate at which the drug enters systemic circulation, thereby accessing the site of action.
- Interactions with other drugs – for example, synergistic QT prolongation can occur when two QT prolonging agents, such as erythromycin + ritonavir, are used together.
- Route of administration – intramuscular, intravenous, subcutaneous, and topical administrations are more likely to cause hypersensitivity reactions; oral medications are less likely to result in drug hypersensitivity.

The terms "drug allergy," "drug hypersensitivity," and "drug reaction" are often used interchangeably. "Drug allergy" specifically refers to a reaction mediated by IgE; "drug hypersensitivity" is an immune-mediated response to a drug agent in a sensitized patient; and "drug reactions" comprise all adverse events related to drug administration, regardless of etiology.

Vigilance at point of care:

While the possibilities for adverse drug reactions seem endless, we must be on the lookout for any new medication(s) the patient might be taking. A thorough, detailed history of all medications must be made in order to elicit any remote possibility that the drug in question might be the culprit for the side effect. People do not often realize that the common over-the-counter analgesics – aspirin, Tylenol, Advil, Motrin, Naprosyn, and others – are actually medications. Herbals and supplements such as St. John's wort, ginkgo biloba, and echinacea can be responsible for various hypersensitivity reactions. For example, St. John's wort, in particular, interacts adversely with SSRIs and tricyclic antidepressants.

Contents of the book, and how to use them

1. **The A–Z**

   The major portion of the manual lists in alphabetical order the 1500 most consulted and most important generic drugs, biologics, and supplements, and the adverse reactions that can arise from their use. If you do not find a drug in the main A–Z listing under the name you know it by, you can turn to the concordance of synonyms and trade names to find the generic name it will be listed under.

   Trade (brand) name(s) are listed alphabetically. When there are many trade names, the ten (or so) most commonly recognized ones are listed.

   Following the trade names is – in parentheses – the latest name of the pharmaceutical company that markets the drug.

   Many of the names of companies have changed from earlier editions of this manual because of acquisitions, mergers, and other factors in the pharmaceutical industry.

   Next appear the Indication(s), the Class in which the drug belongs, and the Half-life of each drug, where known.

   Drug interactions: many severe, hazardous drug–drug interactions are recorded. Only clinically significant drug interactions that have been reported to trigger potential harm and that could be life threatening have been included here in the profile. These interactions are predictable and well documented in controlled studies; they should be avoided.

   Pregnancy category: for new drugs approved on or after 30 June 2015 this field gives (where available) a brief summary of the full statement reflecting the risk for pregnant women as given in the prescribing guidelines; health care providers are advised to check the individual label where necessary. An explanation of the categories for older drugs (A, B, C, D, and X) can be found on our website – www.drugeruptiondata.com.

   Any "Black box" Warning required by the FDA or Notes on use then follow.

   Adverse Drug Reactions: under each drug profile is a list of related ADRs. These adverse events have been classified under the following categories: Skin, Hair, Nails, Mucosal; Cardiovascular, Central Nervous System, Endocrine/Metabolic, Gastrointestinal/Hepatic, Genitourinary, Hematologic, Local, Neuromuscular/Skeletal, Ocular, Otic, Renal, Respiratory, Other.

   Within each category, the reactions are listed alphabetically. Thus, the order of listing does not reflect severity or frequency in any way.

   The terminology used to list reaction patterns has been simplified as far as possible by eliminating, for the most part, tags such as "like" (as in "-Psoriasis-like"), "-reactivation," "-syndrome," "-dissemination," "-iform," etc.

   The number of reports is given for each reaction in square brackets. The incidence of the most important reactions is given in parentheses where indicated (usually from the full prescribing information for the relevant drug). For example, the profile for Ampicillin/Sulbactam begins:

   Skin

   Anaphylactoid reactions / anaphylaxis (includes anaphylactic shock) [2]
   Linear IgA bullous dermatosis [3]
   Rash (<10%) [2]

   This means that we have 2 journal articles referring to occurrence of anaphylaxis); 3 articles for the occurrence of bullous dermatosis; and 3 articles for rash, as reactions to Ampicillin within the Skin category. All these articles appear on our website – www.drugeruptiondata.com – together with links to the article abstracts on PubMed®. Additionally, the incidence of rash as a reaction has been reported as up to 10%.

   On some occasions, there are very few adverse reactions to a specific drug. These drugs are still included in the manual as there is a positive significance in knowing there are no adverse reports.

2. **Important eruptions / reactions**

i) This section of the manual includes a listing of descriptions of important eruption and reaction patterns. Over 40 eruptions/reactions are described here in alphabetical order, from Acanthosis nigricans to Xerostomia. (Descriptions of several other reactions, and lists of drugs associated with these reactions, can be found on our website – www.drugeruptiondata.com.)

ii) We follow this with a list of the most common drugs that cause these important eruptions and reaction patterns, as a quick reference guide.

iii) We then have a list of the main classes of drugs, from 5-HT1 agonists to Xanthine alkaloids, as a quick reference guide.

iv) There follows a section of tables of class reactions, enabling you to see at a glance whether a reaction is common to all the drugs in that particular class, or to a majority of them, or only to a significant few.

v) Next comes a table of reported genetic associations with cutaneous adverse drug reactions.

3. **The Concordance**

The final part of the manual is a concordance to match synonyms (noted in italic) and trade names with the generic drug name. If you know only the synonym or trade name, you can use this list to find the corresponding generic name to look up in the main A–Z listing section of the book.

Being a drug reaction sleuth!

Neil H Shear

I'll start off with a real referral sent to me a few years ago (I expect it will sound familiar to all dermatologists):

"*Dear Neil,*
I am just seeing a patient at the hospital.
The patient took ***amoxicillin*** *and* ***clarithromycin*** *1 week before &* ***ceftriaxone*** *45 min before getting a* ***rash****.*
I think it very unlikely that ceftriaxone is the cause. As far as I know he never had it before.
The reason for this note is that our Respiratory Physician feels strongly that ceftriaxone is the cause.
What do you think?"

What I do like about this is the fact that this is a written (email) request, so any reply I give has some demonstrable existence, as against a phone call or hall chat relying on memory only.

However, a common mistake would be to answer the question "What do you think?" There is very limited information about this patient whom I did not see and will never see. The first step in a proper consultation is DIAGNOSIS of the possible drug reaction. There are 3 key components for making a diagnosis:
– Appearance of the rash
– Systemic issues
– Histology
My mnemonic is Remember: Appearance, Systemic, Histology (RASH).

Thinking back on the referral sent to me I have very little information to help make a diagnosis. What was the "rash" and were there systemic symptoms and signs? I don't know. So I will need to ask for more detailed information if this consultation continues.

The second step is to determine CAUSALITY. Note the referral is focused on an assumption that I will pick a single drug that caused the "rash". Unfortunately, that is not how life works. There are at a minimum 3 possible causes that we know of from the history of drugs given. We don't know if the patient was on other drugs or has a drug allergy history. In this case I will have to assume there are NO systemic features and that the "rash" is a "simple exanthem".

Causality assessments demand:
– A quantitative approach (numbers matter)
– Using a Bayesian type of approach we can generate probabilities that each drug we know of might have caused a reaction.

So now I need to see what the baseline rate of "exanthem" is for each drug. This is where Litt comes in . . .

Amoxicillin

Looking at the Amoxicillin listing in the database (Fig. 1) or the Amoxicillin summary in the manual I can see that there are 33 reports of exanthem and that the background rate is estimated at >5%. This is not the final step, but it gives me some evidence to demonstrate that, although each of these drugs could cause exanthem, one is much more likely than the others.

Exanthems >5%
(2016): Santos-Alarcon S+, *Semergen* (Spanish) **42(7)**, e136
(2015): Farshchian M+, *Clin Cosmet Investig Dermatol* **8**, 53
(2015): Qayoom S+, *Arch Iran Med* **18(4)**, 228 (1 case)
(2015): Sharma R+, *Indian Dermatol Online J* **6(3)**, 168
(2014): Lisi P+, *G Ital Dermatol Venereol* **149(2)**, 237
(2011): Huang HY+, *Clin Exp Dermatol* **36(2)**, 135
(2011): Seitz CS+, *Allergol Immunopathol (Madr)* **39(4)**, 193 (8 cases)
(2010): Ben Fredj N+, *Br J Clin Pharmacol* **70(2)**, 273
(2007): Jappe U, *Allergy* **62(12)**, 1474
(2006): Hernandez-Salazar A+, *Arch Med Res* **37(7)**, 899
(2005): Reig Rincon de Arellano I+, *Allergol Immunopathol (Madr)* **33(5)**, 282
(2003): Leung AK+, *Int J Dermatol* **42(7)**, 553
(2003): Zhang YM+, *Zhonghua Er Ke Za Zhi* **41(2)**, 135 (2 cases)
(2002): Renn CN+, *Br J Dermatol* **147(6)**, 1166 (4 cases) (all with infectious mononucleosis)
(1999): Wakelin SH+, *Clin Exp Dermatol* **24**, 71 (flexural)
(1997): Barbaud AM+, *Arch Dermatol* **133**, 481
(1995): Romano A+, *Allergy* **50**, 113
(1995): Wolkenstein P+, *Arch Dermatol* **131**, 544
(1993): Fellner MJ, *Int J Dermatol* **32**, 308
(1993): Romano A+, *J Invest Allergol Clin Immunol* **3**, 53
(1990): Pauszek ME, *Indiana Med* **83**, 330
(1989): Battegay M+, *Lancet* **2**, 1100
(1989): Chopra R+, *CMAJ* **140(8)**, 921
(1989): Kennedy C+, *Contact Dermatitis* **20**, 313
(1986): Bigby M+, *JAMA* **256**, 3358 5%
(1986): de Haan P+, *Allergy* **41**, 75
(1986): Sonntag MR+, *Schweiz Med Wochenschr* (German) **116(5)**, 142 7%
(1985): Levine LR, *Pediatr Infect Dis* **4**, 358
(1981): Odegaard OR, *Tidsskr Nor Laegeforen* (Norwegian) **101**, 1973
(1977): Taylor B+, *BMJ* **2**, 552 4%
(1975): Brogden RN+, *Drugs* **9**, 88
(1974): Wise PJ+, *J Infect Dis* **129(0)**, S266
(1973): Dubb S, *S Afr Med J* **47(28)**, 1218

Figure 1

After we have the background rate from Litt we can think of data that might modify the background rate. Nothing is as helpful as knowing the timing of drug exposure to onset of a rash. In this instance we know that aminopenicillin rashes come on around day 8 to 10 after exposure. That is very powerful additional information.

Ceftriaxone

There are comparatively few (7) reports and lower reported background rates (none in the package insert information) for this reaction in the database (Fig. 2) and manual for a drug that is widely used. Clearly exanthems are not a major clinical issue, and the figures here are reassuringly low – not nearly as high as Amoxicillin, although not impossible.

Exanthems
(2003): Zhang YM+, *Zhonghua Er Ke Za Zhi* **41(2)**, 135 (2 cases)
(1990): Schaad UB+, *N Engl J Med* **322**, 141 4%
(1988): Brogden RN+, *Drugs* **35(6)**, 604
(1985): Judson FN+, *JAMA* **253**, 1417 1%
(1984): Moskowitz BL, *Am J Med* **77 (Suppl 4C)**, 84 2%
(1984): Richards DM+, *Drugs* **27**, 469 1% [REVIEW]
(1983): Eron LJ+, *J Antimicrob Chemother* **12**, 65 6%

Figure 2

Clarithromycin

Figure 3 shows the very few (3) reports from the database and manual of this drug causing a rash; the lack of any reported background rate supports the conclusion it is not a major clinical issue.

Exanthems
(2018): Ito T, *Oxf Med Case Reports* **2018(9)** (1 case)
(2017): Moreira C+, *An Bras Dermatol* **92(4)**, 587
(2011): Seitz CS+, *Allergol Immunopathol (Madr)* **39(4)**, 193 (1 case)

Figure 3

We have to come to some conclusion and all possibilities need to be represented. Based on Amoxicillin being a common cause of an exanthem (AND on the timing), we have to give it a big lead. Then we think of "I don't know" and "I will never know", which I always mark down as 15% each. We now know the other antibiotics have a much small risk. So 30% for the unknowns, 5% or so for the drugs that were unlikely, leaves the remainder for Amoxicillin.

The numbers are approximations based on the data to hand. Having other unknowns reflects real life: maybe it was due to some contrast media? Or a comorbid risk? Or dozens of other possibilities. And truly sometimes we never know.

Now I am ready (and armed with data I can defend rationally) to send my report back to the referring doctor:

"Dear colleague
Thank you for sending information about your patient. I have not seen the patient and some key information is missing. My report is based on what information I have but clearly that could change with more data.
Assuming the patient had a simple exanthem and no fever etc., the estimated likelihood of what caused the rash is as follows:
Amoxicillin: 65%
Ceftriaxone: 4%
Clarithromycin: 1%
Other unknown exposures or risks: 15%
We will never know: 15%"

CONCLUSIONS

LESSON 1: Look for good quality clinical data.
LESSON 2: Give opinions in text, not conversation.
LESSON 3: Use a structured summary that is uniform, every time, to increase the impact and be on target.
LESSON 4: Be quantitative; it is clear and respected.

I hope this enhances your search for quality information and enhanced patient safety.

ABACAVIR

Trade names: Epzicom (ViiV), Triumeq (ViiV), Trizivir (ViiV), Ziagen (ViiV)
Indications: HIV infections in combination with other antiretrovirals
Class: Nucleoside analog reverse transcriptase inhibitor
Half-life: 1.5 hours
Clinically important, potentially hazardous interactions with: alcohol, arbutamine, argatroban, arsenic, darunavir, ganciclovir, lopinavir, methadone, phenobarbital, phenytoin, protease inhibitors, ribavirin, rifampin, tipranavir, valganciclovir
Important contra-indications noted in the prescribing guidelines for: nursing mothers
Note: Check for presence of HLA B*57:01
Epzicom is abacavir and lamivudine; Triumeq is abacavir, dolutegravir and lamivudine; Trizivir is abacavir, lamivudine and zidovudine.
Warning: HYPERSENSITIVITY REACTIONS, LACTIC ACIDOSIS and SEVERE HEPATOMEGALY, and EXACERBATIONS OF HEPATITIS B

Skin
Anaphylactoid reactions / anaphylaxis (includes anaphylactic shock) (3%) [3]
Exanthems [2]
Hypersensitivity (8–9%) [69]
Lipoatrophy [2]
Rash (5–7%) [18]
Stevens-Johnson syndrome and toxic epidermal necrolysis (SJS/TEN) [4]

Cardiovascular
Myocardial infarction [10]

Central Nervous System
Abnormal dreams (10%) [2]
Anxiety (5%)
Chills (6%)
Depression (6%)
Fever (pyrexia) (includes hyperpyrexia) (6%) [2]
Headache (7–13%) [4]
Insomnia [2]
Migraine (7%)
Neuropsychiatric / neuropsychological adverse effect [4]
Sleep-related disorder (10%)
Vertigo / dizziness (6%) [3]

Endocrine/Metabolic
ALT increased (6%)
AST increased (6%)
Hyperamylasemia (2–4%)
Hypertriglyceridemia (includes triglycerides increased) (2–6%)

Gastrointestinal/Hepatic
Abdominal pain (6%)
Diarrhea (7%) [4]
Gastritis / pangastritis / gastric irritation (6%)
Hepatotoxicity / liver injury / acute liver injury / drug-induced liver injury (DILI) [4]
Nausea (7–19%) [6]
Vomiting (2–10%)

Hematologic
Agranulocytosis / severe selective neutropenia [3]
Neutropenia (neutrophils decreased) (2–5%)

Neuromuscular/Skeletal
Asthenia / fatigue (7–12%) [2]
Bone pain / joint pain (5–6%)
Myalgia/Myopathy (5–6%) [2]

Renal
Fanconi syndrome (proximal tubular dysfunction) [2]

Respiratory
Bronchitis (4%)
Cough [2]
Pneumonia (4%)
Upper respiratory tract infection [2]

Other
Adverse effects / adverse reactions [4]
Infection (5%)

ABALOPARATIDE

Trade name: Tymlos (Radius Health)
Indications: Osteoporosis in postmenopausal women
Class: Parathyroid hormone analog
Half-life: <2 hours
Clinically important, potentially hazardous interactions with: none known
Pregnancy category: Not indicated for use in females of reproductive potential
Important contra-indications noted in the prescribing guidelines for: pediatric patients
Warning: RISK OF OSTEOSARCOMA

Cardiovascular
Orthostatic hypotension (<4%)
Palpitation (5%)
Tachycardia (2%) [2]

Central Nervous System
Headache (8%)
Vertigo / dizziness (2–10%)

Endocrine/Metabolic
Hypercalcemia (3%) [3]
Hyperuricemia (25%)

Gastrointestinal/Hepatic
Abdominal pain (3%)
Nausea (8%)

Genitourinary
Hypercalciuria (11%)
Urolithiasis / ureteral stones / urinary calculi (2%)

Local
Injection-site edema (10%)
Injection-site erythema (58%)
Injection-site pain (9%)

Neuromuscular/Skeletal
Asthenia / fatigue (3%)

Other
Adverse effects / adverse reactions [2]

ABAMETAPIR

Trade name: Xeglyze (Dr Reddy's Laboratories)
Indications: Topical treatment of head lice infestation
Class: Metalloproteinase inhibitor, Pediculocide
Half-life: 71 ± 40 hours (data for a metabolite)
Clinically important, potentially hazardous interactions with: CYP3A4, CYP2B6, CYP1A2 substrates
Pregnancy category: No available data
Note: Abametapir is formulated with benzyl alcohol. Systemic exposure to benzyl alcohol has been associated with serious adverse reactions and death in neonates and low birth-weight infants. Use of the formulated product is not recommended in pediatric patients under 6 months of age because of the potential for increased systemic absorption.

Skin
Burning / skin burning sensation (3%)
Contact dermatitis (2%)
Erythema (4%)
Rash (3%) [2]

Gastrointestinal/Hepatic
Vomiting (2%)

Ocular
Ocular irritation (1%–2%)

ABARELIX

Trade name: Plenaxis (Praecis)
Indications: Prostate cancer (advanced)
Class: Gonadotropin-releasing hormone (GnRH) antagonist
Half-life: 13.2 days
Clinically important, potentially hazardous interactions with: amiodarone, procainamide, quinidine, sotalol
Important contra-indications noted in the prescribing guidelines for: pediatric patients

---

Skin
Hot flashes / hot flushes (79%)
Peripheral edema (15%)

Central Nervous System
Headache (12%)
Pain (31%)
Vertigo / dizziness (12%)

Endocrine/Metabolic
Gynecomastia (30%)
Mastodynia (20%)

Neuromuscular/Skeletal
Asthenia / fatigue (10%)
Back pain (31%)

Respiratory
Upper respiratory tract infection (12%)

Other
Allergic reactions [2]

ABATACEPT

Trade name: Orencia (Bristol-Myers Squibb)
Indications: Rheumatoid arthritis, juvenile idiopathic arthritis in pediatric patients 6 years of age and older
Class: Biologic, Biologic disease-modifying antirheumatic drug (bDMARD), Disease-modifying antirheumatic drug (DMARD), T-cell co-stimulation modulator
Half-life: 12–23 days
Clinically important, potentially hazardous interactions with: adalimumab, anakinra, certolizumab, denosumab, echinacea, etanercept, golimumab, infliximab, lenalidomide, live vaccines, natalizumab, pimecrolimus, sipuleucel-T, tacrolimus, TNF antagonists, trastuzumab
Important contra-indications noted in the prescribing guidelines for: nursing mothers; pediatric patients

---

Skin
Basal cell carcinoma [3]
Eczema / eczematous reaction / eczematous eruption [2]
Herpes simplex (<5%) [3]
Herpes zoster [3]

DOI: 10.1201/9781003715672-1

Hypersensitivity [2]
Psoriasis [14]
Rash (4%) [6]
Squamous cell carcinoma [5]
Vasculitis (angiitis) / cutaneous vasculitis (angiitis) [2]

Mucosal
Sjögren's syndrome (see also sicca syndrome) [4]
Stomatitis (oral mucositis) [3]

Cardiovascular
Hypertension (7%) [4]
Hypotension [2]

Central Nervous System
Fever (pyrexia) (includes hyperpyrexia) (5%) [2]
Headache (5–18%) [6]
Vertigo / dizziness (9%) [3]

Gastrointestinal/Hepatic
Abdominal pain (5%)
Diarrhea (5%) [3]
Dyspepsia / functional dyspepsia (indigestion) (see also gastroparesis) (6%)
Gastroenteritis [5]
Nausea (5%) [2]
Vomiting [2]

Genitourinary
Urinary tract infection (5–13%) [10]

Local
Infusion-related reactions [4]
Infusion-site reactions (9%) [5]
Injection-site erythema [3]
Injection-site hematoma [2]
Injection-site pain [3]
Injection-site pruritus [2]
Injection-site reaction (3%) [8]

Neuromuscular/Skeletal
Asthenia / fatigue [2]
Back pain (7%) [2]
Pain in extremities (3%)

Respiratory
Bronchitis (<13%) [4]
Cough (5–8%)
Influenza (5–13%) [2]
Nasopharyngitis (12%) [6]
Pharyngitis (sore throat) [3]
Pneumonia (<5%) [7]
Pulmonary toxicity [2]
Rhinitis / rhinosinusitis (see also sinusitis) (<5%) [2]
Sinusitis (see also rhinitis / rhinosinusitis) (5–13%) [3]
Tuberculosis [2]
Upper respiratory tract infection (>10%) [9]

Other
Adverse effects / adverse reactions [27]
Death [2]
Infection (36–54%) [25]
Malignancies [10]

ABCIXIMAB

Synonym: C7E3
Trade name: ReoPro (Janssen Biotech)
Indications: Thrombotic arterial disease
Class: Antiplatelet (antithrombotic), Glycoprotein IIb/IIIa inhibitor, Monoclonal antibody
Half-life: 10–30 minutes – given intravenously
Clinically important, potentially hazardous interactions with: anticoagulants, antiplatelets, collagenase, dasatinib, dextran, drotrecogin alfa, fondaparinux, glucosamine, herbals with anticoagulant properties, lepirudin, monoclonal antibodies, NSAIDs, omega-3 fatty acids, pentosan, pentoxifylline, prostacyclin analogues, reteplase, salicylates, thrombolytic agents, tositumomab & iodine131, trastuzumab
Important contra-indications noted in the prescribing guidelines for: nursing mothers; pediatric patients

---

Skin
Anaphylactoid reactions / anaphylaxis (includes anaphylactic shock) [3]
Peripheral edema (2%)

Cardiovascular
Bradycardia / sinus bradycardia (5%)
Chest pain (9%)
Hypotension (15%)
Myocardial infarction [4]

Central Nervous System
Headache (6%)
Pain (5%)

Gastrointestinal/Hepatic
Nausea (12%)
Vomiting (7%)

Hematologic
Bleeding [2]
Thrombocytopenia / platelets decreased [15]

Local
Injection-site reaction (4%)

Neuromuscular/Skeletal
Back pain (17%)

Other
Death [3]

ABEMACICLIB

Trade name: Verzenio (Lilly)
Indications: Hormone receptor-positive, human epidermal growth factor 2-negative advanced or metastatic breast cancer, either as monotherapy or in combination with fulvestrant, or as inital endocrine-based therapy with an aromatase inhibitor
Class: Cyclin-dependent kinase (CDK) 4/6 inhibitor
Half-life: 18 hours
Clinically important, potentially hazardous interactions with: grapefruit juice, ketoconazole, strong CYP3A4 inducers or inhibitors
Pregnancy category: Can cause fetal harm
Important contra-indications noted in the prescribing guidelines for: nursing mothers; pediatric patients

---

Hair
Alopecia / hair loss (12%)

Mucosal
Stomatitis (oral mucositis) (14%)
Xerostomia (dry mouth) (17%)

Central Nervous System
Anorexia [3]
Dysgeusia (taste perversion) (12%)
Fever (pyrexia) (includes hyperpyrexia) (11%)
Headache (20%)
Vertigo / dizziness (11%)

Endocrine/Metabolic
ALT increased (31%)
Appetite decreased (45%) [3]
AST increased (30%)
Dehydration (10%)
Serum creatinine increased (13%) [4]
Weight loss (14%) [2]

Gastrointestinal/Hepatic
Abdominal pain (39%) [2]
Constipation (17%)
Diarrhea (90%) [13]
Hepatotoxicity / liver injury / acute liver injury / drug-induced liver injury (DILI) [2]
Nausea (64%) [9]
Vomiting (35%) [4]

Hematologic
Anemia (25%) [3]
Leukocytopenia (leukopenia) / leukocytes (white blood cells) decreased (17%) [5]
Neutropenia (neutrophils decreased) (37%) [10]
Thrombocytopenia / platelets decreased (20%) [3]

Neuromuscular/Skeletal
Arthralgia (15%)
Asthenia / fatigue (65%) [9]

Respiratory
Cough (19%)
Interstitial lung disease / interstitial pneumonitis / interstitial pneumonia (cryptogenic organizing pneumonia) / drug-induced interstitial lung disease [3]
Pneumonitis [2]

Other
Infection (31%)

ABIRATERONE

Trade name: Zytiga (Janssen Biotech)
Indications: Metastatic castration-resistant prostate cancer (in combination with prednisone)
Class: CYP17 inhibitor, Enzyme inhibitor
Half-life: 12 hours
Clinically important, potentially hazardous interactions with: atazanavir, carbamazepine, clarithromycin, CYP3A4 inducers or inhibitors, indinavir, itraconazole, ketoconazole, nefazodone, nelfinavir, phenobarbital, phenytoin, rifabutin, rifampin, rifapentine, ritonavir, saquinavir, telithromycin, thioridazine, voriconazole
Important contra-indications noted in the prescribing guidelines for: nursing mothers; pediatric patients
Note: Contra-indicated in women who are or may become pregnant.

Skin
Edema / fluid retention (27%) [21]
Hot flashes / hot flushes (19%) [4]

Cardiovascular
Arrhythmias (7%)
Atrial fibrillation [3]
Cardiac failure (2%)
Cardiotoxicity [6]
Chest pain (4%)
Hypertension (9%) [27]
Tachycardia [4]

Central Nervous System
Headache [2]

Endocrine/Metabolic
Adrenal insufficiency (hypoadrenalism) / Addisonian crisis (includes Addison's disease) [2]
ALT increased (11%) [8]
AST increased (31%) [4]

Hypercholesterolemia [2]
Hyperglycemia (includes glucose increased) [2]
Hypertriglyceridemia (includes triglycerides increased) (63%)
Hypokalemia [29]
Mineralocorticoid excess / apparent mineralocorticoid excess [2]

Gastrointestinal/Hepatic
Constipation [8]
Diarrhea (18%) [6]
Dyspepsia / functional dyspepsia (indigestion) (see also gastroparesis) (6%)
Hepatic (liver) disorder / hepatobiliary disorder / hepatic (liver) dysfunction [2]
Hepatitis [2]
Hepatotoxicity / liver injury / acute liver injury / drug-induced liver injury (DILI) (2%) [13]
Nausea [9]
Vomiting [2]

Genitourinary
Nocturia (6%)
Urinary frequency (7%)
Urinary tract infection (12%) [3]

Hematologic
Anemia [7]
Febrile neutropenia [2]
Neutropenia (neutrophils decreased) [2]
Thrombocytopenia / platelets decreased [3]

Neuromuscular/Skeletal
Arthralgia [6]
Asthenia / fatigue [14]
Back pain [6]
Bone pain / joint pain (30%) [9]
Myalgia/Myopathy (26%)
Pain in extremities [3]
Rhabdomyolysis [3]

Respiratory
Cough (11%)
Dyspnea / shortness of breath [3]
Nasopharyngitis [2]
Upper respiratory tract infection (5%) [2]

Other
Adverse effects / adverse reactions [8]
Death [2]

ABROCITINIB

Trade name: Cibinqo (Pfizer)
Indications: Atopic dermatitis
Class: Janus kinase (JAK) inhibitor, Kinase inhibitor
Half-life: 3 to 5 hours
Clinically important, potentially hazardous interactions with: CYP2C19 inducers, CYP2C19 inhibitors, CYP2C9 inducers, CYP2C9 inhibitors
Pregnancy category: Insufficient data to establish a drug-associated risk for major birth defects, miscarriage, or other adverse maternal or fetal outcomes.
Warning: INCREASED RISK OF SERIOUS BACTERIAL, FUNGAL, VIRAL AND OPPORTUNISTIC INFECTIONS LEADING TO HOSPITALIZATION OR DEATH, INCLUDING TUBERCULOSIS (TB). DISCONTINUE TREATMENT WITH ABROCITINIB IF SERIOUS OR OPPORTUNISTIC INFECTION OCCURS. TEST FOR LATENT TB BEFORE AND DURING THERAPY; TREAT LATENT TB PRIOR TO USE. MONITOR ALL PATIENTS FOR ACTIVE TB DURING TREATMENT, EVEN PATIENTS WITH INITIAL NEGATIVE LATENT TB TEST.
HIGHER RATE OF ALL-CAUSE MORTALITY, INCLUDING SUDDEN CARDIOVASCULAR DEATH, WITH ANOTHER JAK INHIBITOR VS. TNF BLOCKERS IN RHEUMATOID ARTHRITIS (RA) PATIENTS. ABROCITINIB IS NOT APPROVED FOR USE IN RA PATIENTS.
MALIGNANCIES HAVE OCCURRED WITH ABROCITINIB. HIGHER RATE OF LYMPHOMAS AND LUNG CANCERS WITH ANOTHER JAK INHIBITOR VS. TNF BLOCKERS IN RA PATIENTS.
MACE HAS OCCURRED WITH ABROCITINIB. HIGHER RATE OF MACE (DEFINED AS CARDIOVASCULAR DEATH, MYOCARDIAL INFARCTION, AND STROKE) WITH ANOTHER JAK INHIBITOR VS. TNF BLOCKERS IN RA PATIENTS.
THROMBOSIS HAS OCCURRED WITH ABROCITINIB. INCREASED INCIDENCE OF PULMONARY EMBOLISM, VENOUS AND ARTERIAL THROMBOSIS WITH ANOTHER JAK INHIBITOR VS. TNF BLOCKERS.

Skin
Acne (unspecified) (2–5%) [3]
Herpes simplex (3–4%)
Impetigo (1–2%)

Central Nervous System
Headache (6–8%) [2]
Vertigo / dizziness (2–3%)

Endocrine/Metabolic
Creatine phosphokinase (CPK) / creatine kinase increased (hyperCKemia) (2–3%)

Gastrointestinal/Hepatic
Abdominal pain (1–2%)
Nausea (6–15%) [2]
Vomiting (2–3%)

Genitourinary
Urinary tract infection (2%) [2]

Hematologic
Thrombocytopenia / platelets decreased (2%)

Neuromuscular/Skeletal
Asthenia / fatigue (1–2%)

Respiratory
Nasopharyngitis (9–12%) [2]
Upper respiratory tract infection [2]

ACALABRUTINIB

Trade name: Calquence (AstraZeneca)
Indications: Treatment of adult patients with mantle cell lymphoma (MCL) who have received at least one prior therapy
Class: Bruton's tyrosine kinase (BTK) inhibitor
Half-life: <3 hours
Clinically important, potentially hazardous interactions with: antacids, famotidine, H2-receptor antagonists, itraconazole, proton pump inhibitors, ranitidine, rifampin, strong CYP3A inducers, strong or moderate CYP3A inhibitors
Pregnancy category: May cause fetal toxicity based on findings in animal studies
Important contra-indications noted in the prescribing guidelines for: nursing mothers; pediatric patients

---

Skin
Bruise / bruising / contusion / ecchymosis (ecchymoses) (21%) [2]
Hematoma / cutaneous hematoma (8%)
Petechiae (21%)
Rash (18%)

Mucosal
Epistaxis (nosebleed) (6%)

Cardiovascular
Atrial fibrillation (3%)
Atrial flutter (3%)
Hypertension [2]

Central Nervous System
Fever (pyrexia) (includes hyperpyrexia) [2]
Headache (39%) [7]

Endocrine/Metabolic
Weight gain [4]

Gastrointestinal/Hepatic
Abdominal pain (15%)
Constipation (15%)
Diarrhea (31%) [6]
Nausea (19%) [2]
Vomiting (13%)

Hematologic
Anemia (46%)
Hemorrhage (8%)
Neutropenia (neutrophils decreased) (36%)
Thrombocytopenia / platelets decreased (44%)

Neuromuscular/Skeletal
Arthralgia [2]
Asthenia / fatigue (28%) [3]
Myalgia/Myopathy (21%) [2]

Respiratory
Pneumonia [3]
Upper respiratory tract infection [2]

Other
Malignancies (11%)

ACAMPROSATE

Trade name: Campral (Forest) (Lipha)
Indications: Alcohol dependence
Class: Amino acid (synthetic)
Half-life: 20–33 hours
Clinically important, potentially hazardous interactions with: none known
Important contra-indications noted in the prescribing guidelines for: nursing mothers; pediatric patients
Note: Contra-indicated in patients with severe renal impairment.

Skin
Diaphoresis (2%)
Peripheral edema (<10%)
Pruritus (itching) (4%) [2]

Mucosal
Xerostomia (dry mouth) (2%)

Cardiovascular
Chest pain (<10%)
Hypertension (<10%)
Palpitation (<10%)
Vasodilation (1–10%)

Central Nervous System
Amnesia (<10%)
Anorexia (2–5%)
Anxiety (5–8%) [2]
Chills (<10%)
Depression (4–8%)
Headache (<10%) [2]

Insomnia (6–9%)
Pain (2–4%)
Paresthesias (2–3%)
Somnolence (drowsiness) (<10%)
Suicidal ideation (1–10%)
Syncope / fainting (<10%)
Tremor (<10%)
Vertigo / dizziness (3–4%)

Endocrine/Metabolic
Appetite increased (<10%)
Libido decreased (<10%)
Weight gain (<10%)

Gastrointestinal/Hepatic
Abdominal pain (<10%)
Constipation (<10%)
Diarrhea (16%) [6]
Dyspepsia / functional dyspepsia (indigestion) (see also gastroparesis) (<10%)
Flatulence (<4%) [2]
Nausea (3–4%) [2]
Vomiting (<10%) [2]

Genitourinary
Impotence (<10%)

Neuromuscular/Skeletal
Arthralgia (<10%)
Asthenia / fatigue (5–7%)
Back pain (<10%)
Myalgia/Myopathy (<10%)

Ocular
Abnormal vision (<10%)

Respiratory
Bronchitis (<10%)
Cough (<10%)
Dyspnea / shortness of breath (<10%)
Influenza- ('flu)-like syndrome (<10%)
Pharyngitis (sore throat) (<10%)
Rhinitis / rhinosinusitis (see also sinusitis) (<10%)

Other
Adverse effects / adverse reactions [3]
Infection (<10%)

ACARBOSE

Trade names: Glucobay (Bayer), Precose (Bayer)
Indications: Non-insulin dependent diabetes Type II
Class: Alpha-glucosidase inhibitor, Antidiabetic, Hypoglycemic (antihyperglycemic) agent
Half-life: 2 hours
Clinically important, potentially hazardous interactions with: alcohol, anabolic steroids, beta blockers, cholestyramine, corticosteroids, diazoxide, digoxin, diuretics, estrogens, hypoglycemic agents, MAO inhibitors, neomycin, orlistat, pancreatin, pegvisomant, pramlintide, progestogens, somatropin, testosterone
Important contra-indications noted in the prescribing guidelines for: nursing mothers; pediatric patients
Note: Contra-indicated in patients with diabetic ketoacidosis or cirrhosis; also in patients with inflammatory bowel disease, colonic ulceration, partial intestinal obstruction or in patients predisposed to intestinal obstruction.

Skin
AGEP [2]

Gastrointestinal/Hepatic
Abdominal distension [2]
Abdominal pain (19%)
Diarrhea (31%)
Flatulence (74%) [3]
Hepatitis [2]
Hepatotoxicity / liver injury / acute liver injury / drug-induced liver injury (DILI) [3]
Pneumatosis intestinalis / pneumatosis cystoides intestinalis [9]

Other
Adverse effects / adverse reactions [5]

ACEBUTOLOL

Trade name: Sectral (Sanofi-Aventis)
Indications: Hypertension, angina, ventricular arrhythmias
Class: Antiarrhythmic class II, Beta adrenergic blocker, Beta blocker
Half-life: 3–7 hours
Clinically important, potentially hazardous interactions with: ACE inhibitors, adrenergic neurone blockers, alcohol, aldesleukin, alpha blockers, alprostadil, amiodarone, angiotensin II receptor antagonists, antiarrhythmics, antidiabetics, anxiolytics and hypnotics, baclofen, calcium channel blockers, cardiac glycosides, clonidine, corticosteroids, diazoxide, diltiazem, disopyramide, diuretics, ergotamine, estrogens, flecainide, general anesthetics, hydralazine, insulin, levodopa, MAO inhibitors, mefloquine, methyldopa, methysergide, minoxidil, moxisylyte, moxonidine, nifedipine, nitrates, nitroprusside, NSAIDs, phenothiazines, pilocarpine, prazosin, tizanidine, verapamil
Important contra-indications noted in the prescribing guidelines for: nursing mothers; pediatric patients
Note: Contraindicated in persistently severe bradycardia, second- and third-degree heart block, overt cardiac failure, and cardiogenic shock. Cutaneous side effects of beta-receptor blockers are clinically polymorphous. They apparently appear after several months of continuous therapy.

Skin
Edema / fluid retention (2%)
Exanthems (4%)
Lichenoid eruption / lichenoid reaction [2]
Lupus erythematosus (subacute cutaneous lupus erythematosus (SCLE)) [14]
Pruritus (itching) (<2%)
Psoriasis [2]
Rash (2%)
Raynaud's phenomenon [2]
Urticaria / hives [2]
Vasculitis (angiitis) / cutaneous vasculitis (angiitis) [2]

Cardiovascular
Bradycardia / sinus bradycardia (<2%)
Cardiac failure (<2%)
Chest pain (2%)
Hypotension (<2%)

Central Nervous System
Abnormal dreams (3%)
Anxiety (<2%)
Depression (2%)
Headache (6%)
Hyperesthesia (<2%)
Hypoesthesia / hypesthesia (numbness) (<2%)
Insomnia (3%)
Vertigo / dizziness (6%)

Gastrointestinal/Hepatic
Abdominal pain (<2%)
Constipation (4%)
Diarrhea (4%)
Dyspepsia / functional dyspepsia (indigestion) (see also gastroparesis) (4%)
Flatulence (3%)
Nausea (4%)
Vomiting (<2%)

Genitourinary
Dysuria (<2%)
Impotence (<2%)
Nocturia (<2%)
Urinary frequency (3%)

Neuromuscular/Skeletal
Arthralgia (2%)
Asthenia / fatigue (11%)
Back pain (<2%)
Bone pain / joint pain (<2%)
Myalgia/Myopathy (2%)

Ocular
Abnormal vision (2%)
Conjunctivitis (conjunctival inflammation) (<2%)
Ocular pain (<2%)
Xerophthalmia (dry eyes) (<2%)

Respiratory
Dyspnea / shortness of breath (4%)
Pharyngitis (sore throat) (<2%)
Rhinitis / rhinosinusitis (see also sinusitis) (2%)
Wheezing (<2%)

ACECLOFENAC

Trade name: Preservex (UCB Pharma)
Indications: Ankylosing spondylitis, osteoarthritis, inflammatory disease of the joints
Class: Analgesic, Non-steroidal anti-inflammatory (NSAID)
Half-life: 4 hours
Clinically important, potentially hazardous interactions with: lithium
Important contra-indications noted in the prescribing guidelines for: nursing mothers; pediatric patients
Note: NSAIDs may cause an increased risk of serious cardiovascular and gastrointestinal adverse events, which can be fatal. This risk may increase with duration of use.

Skin
Anaphylactoid reactions / anaphylaxis (includes anaphylactic shock) [2]
Contact dermatitis [2]
Fixed eruption / fixed drug eruption [2]
Photosensitivity [2]
Vasculitis (angiitis) / cutaneous vasculitis (angiitis) [3]

Gastrointestinal/Hepatic
Hepatotoxicity / liver injury / acute liver injury / drug-induced liver injury (DILI) [7]

Renal
Nephrotoxicity / kidney injury / acute kidney injury (AKI) / drug-induced kidney injury [2]

ACEMETACIN

Synonyms: acemetacine; acemetacinum
Trade name: Emflex (Merck)
Indications: Osteoarthritis, rheumatoid arthritis, lower back pain, post-operative pain, inflammation, musculoskeletal disorders, psychoses
Class: Non-steroidal anti-inflammatory (NSAID)
Half-life: <1.1 hours
Clinically important, potentially hazardous interactions with: ACE inhibitors, anti-coagulants, aspirin, beta blockers, beta-carotene, diflunisal, furosemide, haloperidol, lithium, methotrexate, potassium sparing diuretics, probenecid, salicylates, thiazide diuretics, triamterene, warfarin
Pregnancy category: Contra-indicated in the third trimester of pregnancy
Important contra-indications noted in the prescribing guidelines for: nursing mothers
Note: Inhibition of platelet aggregation may occur. Aggravation of psychiatric disorders, epilepsy or Parkinsonism may occur. Patients receiving long-term treatment should be periodically screened for renal and hepatic function and blood counts.

Other
Adverse effects / adverse reactions [4]
Side effects [2]

ACENOCOUMAROL

Trade names: Sinthrome (Alliance), Sintrom (Alliance)
Indications: Thromboembolic diseases
Class: Anticoagulant (antithrombotic)
Half-life: 8–11 hours
Clinically important, potentially hazardous interactions with: allopurinol, amiodarone, aspirin, cimetidine, danazol, disulfiram, econazole, heparin, lepirudin, nandrolone
Important contra-indications noted in the prescribing guidelines for: nursing mothers

---

Skin
Calcinosis cutis / calcification (includes calciphylaxis) [3]
Necrosis (skin necrosis) [4]
Vasculitis (angiitis) / cutaneous vasculitis (angiitis) [4]

Central Nervous System
Fever (pyrexia) (includes hyperpyrexia) [2]

Hematologic
Prothrombin time (INR) increased [3]

Respiratory
Dyspnea / shortness of breath [2]

ACETAMINOPHEN

Synonyms: APAP; paracetamol
Trade names: Anacin-3 (Wyeth), Darvocet-N (aaiPharma), Excedrin (Bristol-Myers Squibb), Lorcet (Forest), Panadol (GSK), Percocet (Endo), Tylenol (Ortho-McNeil), Vicodin (AbbVie)
Indications: Pain, fever
Class: Analgesic; non-narcotic
Half-life: <3 hours
Clinically important, potentially hazardous interactions with: alcohol, anticonvulsants, barbiturates, busulfan, carbamazepine, cholestyramine, conivaptan, coumarins, didanosine, dong quai, exenatide, imatinib, isoniazid, liraglutide, melatonin, metoclopramide, metyrapone, PEG-interferon, pramlintide, probenecid, St John's wort
Important contra-indications noted in the prescribing guidelines for: nursing mothers
Note: Acetaminophen is the active metabolite of phenacetin. [IV] = intravenous. As a general point most reactions listed are those that have developed following the normal prescribing doses for acetaminophen and the overdosing, poisoning, and other toxicities that have been reported have been excluded.

Skin
AGEP [10]
Anaphylactoid reactions / anaphylaxis (includes anaphylactic shock) [19]
Angioedema (formerly named angioneurotic edema) [8]
Baboon syndrome / symmetrical drug-related intertriginous and flexural exanthema (SDRIFE) [4]
Dermatitis [3]
Erythema [3]
Erythema multiforme [3]
Exanthems [7]
Exfoliative dermatitis [2]
Fixed eruption / fixed drug eruption [43]
Hyperhidrosis [2]
Hypersensitivity [12]
Neutrophilic eccrine hidradenitis [2]
Pemphigus [2]
Pruritus (itching) [5]
Purpura [6]
Rash [IV] [3]
Stevens-Johnson syndrome and toxic epidermal necrolysis (SJS/TEN) [19]
Urticaria / hives [17]
Vasculitis (angiitis) / cutaneous vasculitis (angiitis) [4]

Mucosal
Xerostomia (dry mouth) [3]

Cardiovascular
Hypertension [IV] [3]
Hypotension [5]

Central Nervous System
Agitation [IV] (>5%)
Fever (pyrexia) (includes hyperpyrexia) [IV] (5%)
Headache [IV] (10%) [5]
Insomnia [IV] (7%)
Somnolence (drowsiness) [8]
Vertigo / dizziness [15]

Endocrine/Metabolic
Acidosis (includes lactic acidosis) [3]

Gastrointestinal/Hepatic
Abdominal distension [2]
Abdominal pain [IV] [3]
Constipation [IV] (>5%) [7]
Diarrhea [IV] [2]
Hepatotoxicity / liver injury / acute liver injury / drug-induced liver injury (DILI) [75]
Nausea [IV] (34%) [18]
Pancreatitis / acute pancreatitis [6]
Vomiting (15%) [16]

Hematologic
Thrombocytopenia / platelets decreased [2]

Neuromuscular/Skeletal
Rhabdomyolysis [4]

Renal
Nephritis / interstitial nephritis / tubulointerstitial nephritis [3]
Nephrotoxicity / kidney injury / acute kidney injury (AKI) / drug-induced kidney injury [9]
Renal failure [3]

Respiratory
Asthma [3]
Pulmonary toxicity [IV] (>5%)

Other
Adverse effects / adverse reactions [18]
Death [6]

ACETAZOLAMIDE

Trade name: Diamox (Duramed)
Indications: Epilepsy, glaucoma
Class: Carbonic anhydrase inhibitor, Diuretic
Half-life: 2–6 hours
Clinically important, potentially hazardous interactions with: arsenic, aspirin, ephedra, indacaterol, lisdexamfetamine, lithium, metformin, mivacurium, triamcinolone
Important contra-indications noted in the prescribing guidelines for: the elderly; nursing mothers; pediatric patients
Note: Acetazolamide is a sulfonamide and can be absorbed systemically. Sulfonamides can produce severe, possibly fatal, reactions such as toxic epidermal necrolysis and Stevens-Johnson syndrome.

Skin
AGEP [2]
Anaphylactoid reactions / anaphylaxis (includes anaphylactic shock) [4]
Exanthems [2]
Pemphigus [2]
Stevens-Johnson syndrome and toxic epidermal necrolysis (SJS/TEN) [8]

Central Nervous System
Depression [2]
Dysgeusia (taste perversion) (>10%) [8]
Paresthesias [6]

Endocrine/Metabolic
Acidosis (includes lactic acidosis) [3]
Libido decreased [2]
Weight loss [2]

Gastrointestinal/Hepatic
Diarrhea [2]
Dyspepsia / functional dyspepsia (indigestion) (see also gastroparesis) [2]
Nausea [2]
Vomiting [2]

Neuromuscular/Skeletal
Asthenia / fatigue [4]

Ocular
Choroidal detachment [2]
Corneal edema [2]

Glaucoma (includes acute angle-closure glaucoma) [5]
Myopia [2]

Renal

Nephrolithiasis (kidney stones / renal calculi) [3]

Respiratory

Pulmonary edema (cardiogenic / non-cardiogenic) [8]

ACETOHEXAMIDE

Trade name: Dymelor (Barr)
Indications: Non-insulin dependent diabetes Type II
Class: Antidiabetic, Hypoglycemic (antihyperglycemic) agent, Sulfonylurea
Half-life: 1–6 hours
Clinically important, potentially hazardous interactions with: phenylbutazones
Important contra-indications noted in the prescribing guidelines for: nursing mothers
Note: Acetohexamide is a sulfonamide and can be absorbed systemically. Sulfonamides can produce severe, possibly fatal, reactions such as toxic epidermal necrolysis and Stevens-Johnson syndrome.

Skin

Photosensitivity (<10%)
Rash (<10%)
Urticaria / hives (<10%)

Endocrine/Metabolic

Hypoglycemia [2]

ACETYLCHOLINE

Trade name: Miochol (Novartis)
Indications: Cataract surgery, in penetrating keratoplasty, iridectomy and other anterior segment surgery where rapid miosis may be required
Class: Ophthalmic agent, miotic, Parasympathomimetic
Half-life: N/A
Clinically important, potentially hazardous interactions with: none known
Important contra-indications noted in the prescribing guidelines for: pediatric patients

---

Cardiovascular

Bradycardia / sinus bradycardia [7]
Hypotension [8]

Ocular

Intraocular pressure increased [5]

Respiratory

Bronchospasm [2]

ACETYLCYSTEINE

Synonyms: N-acetylcysteine; L-Cysteine; NAC
Indications: Emphysema, bronchitis, tuberculosis, bronchiectasis, tracheostomy care, antidote for acetaminophen toxicity
Class: Antidote, Antioxidant
Half-life: N/A
Clinically important, potentially hazardous interactions with: carbamazepine, nitroglycerin
Note: As an antidote, it is difficult to differentiate side effects due to the drug from those due to the effects of the poison.

Skin

Anaphylactoid reactions / anaphylaxis (includes anaphylactic shock) (8–18%) [14]
Angioedema (formerly named angioneurotic edema) [6]
Flushing / rubefaction (<8%) [2]
Pruritus (itching) (<4%) [3]
Rash (2–4%) [4]
Urticaria / hives (6–8%)

Cardiovascular

Tachycardia (<4%)

Central Nervous System

Seizures [2]

Gastrointestinal/Hepatic

Diarrhea [2]
Nausea (<6%) [3]
Vomiting (2–10%) [2]

Other

Adverse effects / adverse reactions [2]
Death [2]

ACITRETIN

Trade names: Neotigason (Actavis), Soriatane (Stiefel)
Indications: Psoriasis
Class: Antipsoriatic agent, Retinoid
Half-life: 49 hours
Clinically important, potentially hazardous interactions with: alcohol, bexarotene, chloroquine, cholestyramine, corticosteroids, coumarins, danazol, demeclocycline, doxycycline, ethanolamine, isotretinoin, lithium, lymecycline, medroxyprogesterone, methotrexate, minocycline, oxytetracycline, phenytoin, progestins, sarecycline, St John's wort, tetracycline, tigecycline, vitamin A
Important contra-indications noted in the prescribing guidelines for: nursing mothers; pediatric patients
Note: Oral retinoids can cause birth defects, and women should avoid acitretin when pregnant or trying to conceive.
Used for the treatment of Darier disease (keratosis follicularis).
Warning: CONTRA-INDICATED IN PREGNANCY

Skin

Angioedema (formerly named angioneurotic edema) [2]
Atrophy / Skin atrophy (10–25%)
Bromhidrosis (<10%)
Bullous dermatosis (<10%)
Clammy skin (<10%)
Cutaneous toxicity / skin toxicity [3]
Dermatitis (<10%)
Diaphoresis (<10%) [2]
Edema / fluid retention (<10%)
Erythema (18%)
Erythroderma [3]
Exanthems (10–25%) [2]
Exfoliative dermatitis (25–50%) [3]
Fissures (<10%)
Hot flashes / hot flushes (<10%)
Hyperhidrosis (<10%) [2]
Palmar–plantar desquamation (20–80%) [7]
Photosensitivity [3]
Pigmentation (Skin) (includes hyperpigmentation) [3]
Pruritus (itching) (10–50%) [10]
Psoriasis (aggravated) (<10%)
Purpura (<10%)
Rash (>10%)
Seborrhea (<10%)
Stickiness (3–50%) [7]
Sunburn (<10%)
Ulcerations (<10%)
Xerosis / xeroderma (25–50%) [14]

Hair

Alopecia / hair loss (10–75%) [21]
Curly hair [3]
Hair changes (<10%)
Hair pigmentation [3]

Nails

Brittle nails [3]
Nail changes (25–50%)
Paronychia (10–25%) [6]
Pyogenic granuloma (<10%) [4]

Mucosal

Cheilitis (inflammation of the lips) (>75%) [14]
Dry mucous membranes [4]
Epistaxis (nosebleed) (10–25%) [2]
Gingival bleeding (<10%)
Gingivitis (<10%)
Mucocutaneous reactions [3]
Sialorrhea (ptyalism; hypersalivation) (<10%)
Stomatitis (oral mucositis) (<10%) [2]
Tongue (lingua / lingual) disorder (<10%)
Ulcerative stomatitis (<10%)
Xerostomia (dry mouth) (10–60%) [7]

Cardiovascular

Capillary leak syndrome [3]

Central Nervous System

Anorexia (<10%)
Depression (<10%) [4]
Dysgeusia (taste perversion) (<10%)
Headache (<10%) [2]
Hyperesthesia (10–25%)
Insomnia (<10%)
Neurotoxicity [3]
Pain (<10%)
Paralysis / paraplegia (facial) (<10%)
Paresthesias (10–25%) [2]
Pseudotumor cerebri [5]
Rigors (10–25%) [2]
Somnolence (drowsiness) (<10%)
Stroke / cerebrovascular accident [2]
Suicidal ideation [2]

Endocrine/Metabolic

GGT increased [2]
Hyperbilirubinemia [2]
Hypercholesterolemia (25–50%) [3]
Hyperlipidemia / lipids elevated [5]
Hypertriglyceridemia (includes triglycerides increased) (50–75%) [4]

Gastrointestinal/Hepatic

Abdominal pain (<10%)
Diarrhea (<10%) [2]
Hepatitis [5]
Hepatotoxicity / liver injury / acute liver injury / drug-induced liver injury (DILI) [8]
Nausea (<10%) [2]
Pancreatitis / acute pancreatitis [3]
Vomiting [2]

Genitourinary

Vulvovaginal candidiasis [2]

Neuromuscular/Skeletal

Arthralgia (10–25%) [2]
Asthenia / fatigue (<10%) [3]
Back pain (<10%)
Bone pain / joint pain [2]

Hyperostosis [11]
Myalgia/Myopathy [4]
Osteoporosis [2]

Ocular
Blepharitis (<10%)
Cataract (<10%)
Conjunctivitis (conjunctival inflammation) (<10%) [2]
Diplopia (double vision) (<10%)
Night blindness (<10%) [2]
Ocular adverse effect [2]
Ocular itching / ocular pruritus [2]
Ocular pain (<10%)
Photophobia (<10%) [2]
Vision blurred (<10%)
Xerophthalmia (dry eyes) (10–25%) [3]

Otic
Ear pain (<10%)
Tinnitus (<10%)

Respiratory
Laryngitis [2]
Rhinitis / rhinosinusitis (see also sinusitis) (25–50%) [2]
Sinusitis (see also rhinitis / rhinosinusitis) (<10%)

Other
Adverse effects / adverse reactions [9]
Dipsia (thirst) / polydipsia (<10%)
Infection [2]
Side effects [4]
Teratogenicity [7]

ACLIDINIUM

Trade name: Tudorza Pressair (Forest)
Indications: Long-term maintenance treatment of bronchospasm associated with chronic obstructive pulmonary disease, including chronic bronchitis and emphysema
Class: Anticholinergic, Muscarinic antagonist
Half-life: 5–8 hours
Clinically important, potentially hazardous interactions with: anticholinergics
Important contra-indications noted in the prescribing guidelines for: nursing mothers; pediatric patients

---

Mucosal
Xerostomia (dry mouth) [2]

Central Nervous System
Headache (7%)

Gastrointestinal/Hepatic
Diarrhea (3%)

Respiratory
Cough (3%)
Nasopharyngitis (6%)
Rhinitis / rhinosinusitis (see also sinusitis) (2%)
Sinusitis (see also rhinitis / rhinosinusitis) (2%)

Other
Adverse effects / adverse reactions [5]

ACYCLOVIR

Synonyms: aciclovir; ACV; acycloguanosine
Trade names: Sitavig (Cipher), Zovirax (GSK)
Indications: Herpes simplex, herpes zoster
Class: Antiviral, Antiviral; topical, Guanine nucleoside analog
Half-life: 3 hours (adults)
Clinically important, potentially hazardous interactions with: cobicistat/elvitegravir/emtricitabine/tenofovir alafenamide, cobicistat/elvitegravir/emtricitabine/tenofovir disoproxil, meperidine, tenofovir disoproxil
Important contra-indications noted in the prescribing guidelines for: nursing mothers

---

Skin
Acneiform eruption / acneiform dermatitis / acneiform rash (<3%)
Dermatitis [12]
Exanthems (<5%) [5]
Facial edema (3–5%)
Peripheral edema [2]
Pruritus (itching) (<10%)
Radiation recall dermatitis [2]
Rash (<3%) [3]
Urticaria / hives (<5%) [4]

Hair
Alopecia / hair loss (<3%)

Central Nervous System
Hallucinations, visual [2]
Headache (2%) [4]
Neurotoxicity [11]

Gastrointestinal/Hepatic
Diarrhea (2–3%)
Nausea (2–5%) [3]
Vomiting (3%)

Hematologic
Thrombocytopenia / platelets decreased [5]

Local
Injection-site inflammation (>10%)
Injection-site thrombophlebitis (9%)

Neuromuscular/Skeletal
Asthenia / fatigue (12%)

Ocular
Periorbital edema (3–5%)

Renal
Nephrotoxicity / kidney injury / acute kidney injury (AKI) / drug-induced kidney injury [18]
Renal failure [4]

Other
Adverse effects / adverse reactions [2]

ADALIMUMAB

Trade names: Amgevita (Amgen), Amjevita (Amgen), Humira (AbbVie), Hyrimoz (Sandoz), Idacio (Fresenius Kabi USA) (adalimumab-aacf), Imraldi (Biogen), Yuflyma (Celltrion)
Indications: Rheumatoid arthritis, polyarticular juvenile idiopathic arthritis, psoriatic arthritis, ankylosing spondylitis, Crohn's disease, ulcerative colitis, psoriasis
Class: Anti-Tumor Necrosis Factor-alpha (TNF-α antagonist), Antipsoriatic agent, Biologic, Biologic disease-modifying antirheumatic drug (bDMARD), Cytokine inhibitor, Disease-modifying antirheumatic drug (DMARD), Monoclonal antibody
Half-life: 10–20 days
Clinically important, potentially hazardous interactions with: abatacept, anakinra, live vaccines
Important contra-indications noted in the prescribing guidelines for: nursing mothers
Note: TNF inhibitors should be used in patients with heart failure only after consideration of other treatment options. TNF inhibitors are contra-indicated in patients with a personal or family history of multiple sclerosis or demyelinating disease. TNF inhibitors should not be administered to patients with moderate to severe heart failure (New York Heart Association Functional Class III/IV). Adalimumab-atto (Amjevita) is biosimilar to Adalimumab (Humira). Approved 09/23/2016 Adalimumab-adbm (Cyltezo) is biosimilar to Adalimumab (Humira). Approved 08/25/2017 Adalimumab-adaz (Hyrimoz) is biosimilar to Adalimumab (Humira). Approved 10/30/2018 Adalimumab-bwwd (Hadlima) is biosimilar to Adalimumab (Humira). Approved 07/23/2019 Adalimumab-afzb (Abrilada) is biosimilar to Adalimumab (Humira). Approved 11/15/2019 Adalimumab-fkjp (Hulio) is biosimilar to Adalimumab (Humira). Approved 07/06/2020 Adalimumab-aqvh (Yusimry) is biosimilar to Adalimumab (Humira). Approved 12/17/2021 AAdalimumab-aacf (Idacio) is biosimilar to Adalimumab (Humira). Approved 12/13/2022 Adalimumab-ryvk (Simlandi) is biosimilar to Adalimumab (Humira). Approved 02/23/2024 Adalimumab-aaty (Yuflyma) is biosimilar to Adalimumab (Humira). Approved 05/23/2023.
Warning: SERIOUS INFECTIONS AND MALIGNANCY

Skin
Acneiform eruption / acneiform dermatitis / acneiform rash [3]
Anaphylactoid reactions / anaphylaxis (includes anaphylactic shock) [2]
Angioedema (formerly named angioneurotic edema) [4]
Bullous pemphigoid / pemphigoid [8]
Carcinoma [2]
Cellulitis and pseudocellulitis (<5%) [2]
Dermatomyositis [5]
Eczema / eczematous reaction / eczematous eruption [2]
Eosinophilic cellulitis / Wells' syndrome [2]
Erysipelas (<5%)
Erythema multiforme [4]
Granulomatous reaction [6]
Henoch-Schönlein purpura / IgA vasculitis / immunoglobulin A vasculitis [3]

Herpes zoster [10]
Hidradenitis suppurativa (acne inversa) [6]
Hypersensitivity [3]
Lesions (includes skin lesions) [2]
Lichenoid eruption / lichenoid reaction [5]
Lupus erythematosus (subacute cutaneous lupus erythematosus (SCLE)) [18]
Lupus syndrome / drug-induced lupus (DIL) [5]
Lymphoma [8]
Melanoma [6]
Palmoplantar pustulosis [6]
Peripheral edema (<5%)
Pityriasis lichenoides / pityriasis lichenoides chronica / pityriasis lichenoides et varioliformis acuta [2]
Pruritus (itching) [6]
Psoriasiform dermatitis [2]
Psoriasis [47]
Pyoderma gangrenosum [4]
Rash (12%) [6]
Sarcoidosis / sarcoid-like reaction (cutaneous sarcoidosis) [9]
Squamous cell carcinoma [5]
Stevens-Johnson syndrome and toxic epidermal necrolysis (SJS/TEN) [2]
Sweet's syndrome [4]
Urticaria / hives [5]
Vasculitis (angiitis) / cutaneous vasculitis (angiitis) [9]
Vitiligo [10]

Hair

Alopecia / hair loss [10]
Alopecia areata [7]
Alopecia universalis [4]
Pityriasis amiantacea [2]
Scalp psoriasis [3]

Cardiovascular

Arrhythmias (<5%)
Cardiac arrest (<5%)
Chest pain (<5%)
Congestive heart failure (<5%) [2]
Hypertension (<5%)
Myocardial infarction (<5%)
Palpitation [2]
Pericarditis (<5%)
Tachycardia (<5%)
Thromboembolism [2]

Central Nervous System

Aseptic meningitis [2]
Confusion (<5%)
Depression [2]
Encephalitis [2]
Fever (pyrexia) (includes hyperpyrexia) (<5%) [3]
Guillain-Barré syndrome / acute inflammatory demyelinating polyradiculoneuropathy / acute motor axonal neuropathy [5]
Headache (12%) [9]
Leukoencephalopathy / posterior reversible encephalopathy syndrome (PRES) [3]
Mania [2]
Multiple sclerosis (<5%) [3]
Neurotoxicity [3]
Paresthesias (<5%) [2]
Syncope / fainting (<5%)
Tremor (<5%)
Vertigo / dizziness [2]

Endocrine/Metabolic

Creatine phosphokinase (CPK) / creatine kinase increased (hyperCKemia) (<5%)
Hypercholesterolemia (6%)
Weight gain [2]

Gastrointestinal/Hepatic

Abdominal pain (7%) [2]
Cholecystitis (calculous / acalculous) (<5%)
Colitis [2]
Esophagitis (<5%)
Gastroenteritis (<5%)
Hepatitis [7]
Hepatotoxicity / liver injury / acute liver injury / drug-induced liver injury (DILI) [12]
Nausea (9%) [2]
Vomiting (<5%)

Genitourinary

Cystitis (includes interstitial cystitis / bladder pain syndrome) (<5%)
Hematuria (5%)
Pelvic pain (<5%)
Urinary tract infection (8%) [2]

Hematologic

Agranulocytosis / severe selective neutropenia (<5%)
Eosinophilia / eosinophils increased [3]
Hemolytic anemia [4]
Hemophilia [3]
Leukocytopenia (leukopenia) / leukocytes (white blood cells) decreased (<5%)
Pancytopenia (includes bicytopenia) [2]
Sepsis [2]
Thrombocytopenia / platelets decreased [2]

Local

Infusion-related reactions [2]
Injection-site edema (15%) [2]
Injection-site erythema (15%) [3]
Injection-site pain (12%) [3]
Injection-site reaction [30]

Neuromuscular/Skeletal

Arthralgia (<5%) [6]
Asthenia / fatigue [2]
Back pain (6%) [3]
Tuberculous arthritis [2]

Ocular

Cataract (<5%)
Optic neuritis / papillitis [6]
Uveitis / anterior uveitis / posterior uveitis / panuveitis [5]

Renal

Nephrotoxicity / kidney injury / acute kidney injury (AKI) / drug-induced kidney injury [3]

Respiratory

Asthma (<5%)
Bronchitis [3]
Bronchospasm (<5%)
Dyspnea / shortness of breath (<5%)
Influenza- ('flu)-like syndrome (7%)
Nasopharyngitis [8]
Pleural effusion (<5%)
Pneumonia (<5%) [6]
Pneumonitis [3]
Pulmonary fibrosis [3]
Pulmonary toxicity [7]
Sinusitis (see also rhinitis / rhinosinusitis) (11%) [4]
Tonsillitis [2]
Tuberculosis [11]
Upper respiratory tract infection (17%) [14]

Other

Adverse effects / adverse reactions [51]
Allergic reactions [2]
Death [9]
Infection (5%) [81]
Malignancies [7]
Neoplasms [2]
Side effects [2]

ADAPALENE

Trade names: Differin (Galderma), Epiduo (Galderma)
Indications: Acne vulgaris
Class: Retinoid
Half-life: N/A
Clinically important, potentially hazardous interactions with: resorcinol, salicylates
Important contra-indications noted in the prescribing guidelines for: nursing mothers; pediatric patients
Note: Epiduo is adapalene and benzoyl peroxide.

Skin

Burning / skin burning sensation (38%) [7]
Erythema (38%) [9]
Pruritus (itching) (>10%) [11]
Scaling (44%) [6]
Stinging (38%) [3]
Xerosis / xeroderma (45%) [10]

Other

Adverse effects / adverse reactions [3]

ADEFOVIR

Trade name: Hepsera (Gilead)
Indications: HIV infection, hepatitis B infection
Class: Antiretroviral, Nucleotide analog reverse transcriptase inhibitor
Half-life: 16–18 hours
Clinically important, potentially hazardous interactions with: amikacin, amphotericin B, cobicistat/elvitegravir/emtricitabine/tenofovir disoproxil, delavirdine, drugs causing kidney toxicity, foscarnet, gentamicin, hydroxyurea, pentamidine, tenofovir disoproxil, tobramycin
Important contra-indications noted in the prescribing guidelines for: the elderly; nursing mothers; pediatric patients
Warning: SEVERE ACUTE EXACERBATIONS OF HEPATITIS, NEPHROTOXICITY, HIV RESISTANCE, LACTIC ACIDOSIS AND SEVERE HEPATOMEGALY WITH STEATOSIS

Skin

Pruritus (itching) (<10%)
Rash (<10%)
Stevens-Johnson syndrome and toxic epidermal necrolysis (SJS/TEN) [2]

Central Nervous System

Headache (9%) [2]
Pain [2]

Endocrine/Metabolic

Hypophosphatemia [6]

Gastrointestinal/Hepatic

Abdominal pain (9%)
Diarrhea (3%)
Dyspepsia / functional dyspepsia (indigestion) (see also gastroparesis) (3%)
Flatulence (4%)
Hepatotoxicity / liver injury / acute liver injury / drug-induced liver injury (DILI) (<25%)
Nausea (5%)
Vomiting (<10%)

Genitourinary

Hematuria (11%)

Neuromuscular/Skeletal

Asthenia / fatigue (13%) [3]
Back pain (<10%)

Fractures [2]
Osteomalacia [9]

Renal
Fanconi syndrome (proximal tubular dysfunction) [13]
Nephrotoxicity / kidney injury / acute kidney injury (AKI) / drug-induced kidney injury [14]

Respiratory
Cough (6–8%)
Rhinitis / rhinosinusitis (see also sinusitis) (<5%)

ADENOSINE

Synonym: ATP
Trade names: Adenocard (Astellas), Adenocur (Sanofi-Aventis)
Indications: Paroxysmal supraventricular tachycardia, varicose vein complications with stasis dermatitis
Class: Antiarrhythmic class IV, Neurotransmitter
Half-life: <10 seconds
Clinically important, potentially hazardous interactions with: aminophylline, antiarrhythmics, beta blockers, bupivacaine, carbamazepine, dipyridamole, inotersen, levobupivacaine, nicotine, prilocaine, QT prolonging agents, ropivacaine
Important contra-indications noted in the prescribing guidelines for: pediatric patients

---

Skin
Flushing / rubefaction (18–44%)

Cardiovascular
Arrhythmias [2]
Atrial fibrillation [7]
Chest pain [5]
Coronary vasospasm [2]
Torsades de pointes [2]

Central Nervous System
Headache (2–18%) [2]
Vertigo / dizziness (2–12%)

Gastrointestinal/Hepatic
Abdominal pain (13%)

Neuromuscular/Skeletal
Jaw pain (<15%)

Respiratory
Cough (6–8%)
Dyspnea / shortness of breath [3]
Respiratory distress (11%)

Other
Adverse effects / adverse reactions [3]

AFATINIB

Trade name: Gilotrif (Boehringer Ingelheim)
Indications: Metastatic non-small cell lung cancer in patients whose tumors have epidermal growth factor receptor exon 19 deletions or exon 21 (L858R) substitution mutations, metastatic squamous non-small cell lung cancer progressing following platinium-based chemotherapy
Class: Epidermal growth factor receptor (EGFR) inhibitor / antagonist, Tyrosine kinase inhibitor
Half-life: 37 hours
Clinically important, potentially hazardous interactions with: amiodarone, carbamazepine, cyclosporine, erythromycin, itraconazole, ketoconazole, nelfinavir, P-glycoprotein inhibitors, phenobarbital, phenytoin, quinidine, rifampin, ritonavir, saquinavir, St John's wort, tacrolimus, verapamil
Important contra-indications noted in the prescribing guidelines for: nursing mothers; pediatric patients

---

Skin
Acneiform eruption / acneiform dermatitis / acneiform rash [30]
Cutaneous toxicity / skin toxicity [3]
Erosive pustular dermatosis [2]
Fissures [2]
Hand–foot syndrome (palmar–plantar erythrodysesthesia) [2]
Pruritus (itching) [3]
Rash [54]
Stevens-Johnson syndrome and toxic epidermal necrolysis (SJS/TEN) [8]
Xerosis / xeroderma [8]

Nails
Nail changes [2]
Paronychia (58%) [18]

Mucosal
Epistaxis (nosebleed) [3]
Mucosal inflammation [7]
Mucositis [10]
Rhinorrhea (11%)
Stomatitis (oral mucositis) (71%) [23]

Central Nervous System
Anorexia [3]
Fever (pyrexia) (includes hyperpyrexia) (12%)

Endocrine/Metabolic
ALT increased [2]
Appetite decreased (29%) [5]
Dehydration [3]
Hypokalemia [2]

Gastrointestinal/Hepatic
Diarrhea (96%) [73]
Dysphagia [2]
Hepatotoxicity / liver injury / acute liver injury / drug-induced liver injury (DILI) (10%) [5]
Nausea [16]
Vomiting [10]

Hematologic
Anemia [3]
Febrile neutropenia [2]
Leukocytopenia (leukopenia) / leukocytes (white blood cells) decreased [2]
Neutropenia (neutrophils decreased) [6]
Thrombocytopenia / platelets decreased [2]

Neuromuscular/Skeletal
Asthenia / fatigue [18]

Respiratory
Dyspnea / shortness of breath [3]
Pneumonitis [2]
Pulmonary toxicity [5]

Other
Adverse effects / adverse reactions [7]
Death [4]

AFLIBERCEPT

Synonym: ziv-aflibercept
Trade names: Eylea (Regeneron), Zaltrap (Sanofi-Aventis)
Indications: Neovascular (wet) age-related macular degeneration (Eylea), metastatic colorectal cancer (Zaltrap) in combination with FOLFIRI (fluorouracil, leucovorin and irinotecan)
Class: Angiogenesis inhibitor / antiangiogenic agent, Fusion protein
Half-life: terminal 5–6 days
Clinically important, potentially hazardous interactions with: none known
Important contra-indications noted in the prescribing guidelines for: nursing mothers; pediatric patients
Note: Eylea: Contra-indicated in patients with ocular or periocular infection or active intraocular inflammation. Aflibercept-jbvf (Yesafili) is biosimilar to Aflibercept (Eylea). Approved 05/20/2024 Aflibercept-yszy (Opuviz) is biosimilar to Aflibercept (Eylea). Approved 05/20/2024 Aflibercept-mrbb (Ahzantive) is biosimilar to Aflibercept (Eylea). Approved 06/28/2024.
Warning: Zaltrap: HEMORRHAGE, GASTROINTESTINAL PERFORATION, COMPROMISED WOUND HEALING

Mucosal
Epistaxis (nosebleed) [3]
Stomatitis (oral mucositis) [6]

Cardiovascular
Hypertension [16]
Myocardial infarction (<2%)
Venous thromboembolism [2]

Central Nervous System
Anorexia [2]
Headache [2]
Stroke / cerebrovascular accident (<2%)

Endocrine/Metabolic
Weight loss [2]

Gastrointestinal/Hepatic
Diarrhea [8]
Gastrointestinal perforation / perforated colon / gastric perforation [5]
Nausea [2]

Hematologic
Hemorrhage [3]
Neutropenia (neutrophils decreased) [13]

Local
Injection-site pain (3%)

Neuromuscular/Skeletal
Asthenia / fatigue [7]

Ocular
Cataract (7%) [3]
Conjunctival hemorrhage (25%) [3]
Conjunctival hyperemia / conjunctival injection (4%)
Conjunctivitis (conjunctival inflammation) [3]
Corneal erosion (4%)
Endophthalmitis [4]
Intraocular pressure increased (5%) [2]
Lacrimation (3%)
Ocular adverse effect [7]
Ocular pain (3–9%)
Vision blurred (2%)
Vitreous detachment (6%)
Vitreous floaters / floaters / myodesopsia / myiodesopsia / muscae volitantes (6%)

Renal
Proteinuria [11]

Respiratory
Dysphonia (includes voice disorders / voice changes) [5]
Dyspnea / shortness of breath [2]
Pulmonary embolism [2]

Other
Adverse effects / adverse reactions [6]
Death [3]
Infection [3]

ALBENDAZOLE

Trade name: Albenza (GSK)
Indications: Nematode infections, hydatid cyst disease
Class: Anthelmintic
Half-life: 8–12 hours
Clinically important, potentially hazardous interactions with: antimalarials, conivaptan, dexamethasone, high fat foods
Important contra-indications noted in the prescribing guidelines for: nursing mothers

---

Skin
Fixed eruption / fixed drug eruption [2]
Pruritus (itching) [4]
Urticaria / hives [2]

Hair
Alopecia / hair loss (reversible) (<2%) [8]

Central Nervous System
Fever (pyrexia) (includes hyperpyrexia) (<2%) [3]
Headache (<11%) [10]
Intracranial pressure increased (intracranial hypertension) (<2%)
Psychosis [2]
Somnolence (drowsiness) [2]
Vertigo / dizziness (<2%) [6]

Gastrointestinal/Hepatic
Abdominal pain (<7%) [10]
Hepatitis [7]
Nausea (4–6%) [6]
Vomiting (4–6%) [3]

Hematologic
Pancytopenia (includes bicytopenia) [6]

Neuromuscular/Skeletal
Asthenia / fatigue [3]
Dystonia [3]

Other
Adverse effects / adverse reactions [6]
Death [3]

ALBIGLUTIDE

Trade name: Tanzeum (GSK)
Indications: To improve glycemic control in adults with Type II diabetes mellitus
Class: Antidiabetic, Glucagon-like peptide-1 (GLP-1) receptor agonist
Half-life: 5 days
Clinically important, potentially hazardous interactions with: none known
Important contra-indications noted in the prescribing guidelines for: nursing mothers; pediatric patients
Note: Contra-indicated in patients with a personal or family history of medullary thyroid carcinoma or in patients with multiple endocrine neoplasia syndrome Type 2.
Warning: RISK OF THYROID C-CELL TUMORS

Central Nervous System
Headache [4]
Vertigo / dizziness [2]

Endocrine/Metabolic
GGT increased (2%)
Hypoglycemia (2%) [5]

Gastrointestinal/Hepatic
Constipation [2]
Diarrhea (13%) [15]
Dyspepsia / functional dyspepsia (indigestion) (see also gastroparesis) (3%)
Gastroesophageal reflux (4%)
Nausea (11%) [20]
Pancreatitis / acute pancreatitis [4]
Vomiting (4%) [15]

Local
Injection-site hematoma (2%)
Injection-site reaction (11%) [16]

Neuromuscular/Skeletal
Arthralgia (7%)
Back pain (7%) [2]

Respiratory
Cough (7%)
Influenza (5%)
Nasopharyngitis [3]
Pneumonia (2%)
Sinusitis (see also rhinitis / rhinosinusitis) (6%)
Upper respiratory tract infection (14%) [4]

Other
Adverse effects / adverse reactions [4]

ALBUTEROL

Synonym: salbutamol
Trade names: AccuNeb (Mylan Specialty), Combivent (Boehringer Ingelheim), Duoneb (Mylan Specialty), Proventil (Schering), Ventolin (GSK), Volmax (Muro)
Indications: Bronchospasm associated with asthma
Class: Beta-2 adrenergic agonist, Bronchodilator, Tocolytic
Half-life: 3–6 hours
Clinically important, potentially hazardous interactions with: atomoxetine, epinephrine, insulin degludec, insulin detemir, insulin glargine, insulin glulisine
Important contra-indications noted in the prescribing guidelines for: nursing mothers
Note: Combivent is albuterol and ipratropium.

Skin
Dermatitis [2]
Diaphoresis (<10%)
Erythema (palmar) (with infusion) [2]
Flushing / rubefaction (<10%)

Mucosal
Xerostomia (dry mouth) (<10%)

Cardiovascular
Atrial fibrillation [2]
Hypertension [2]
Myocardial infarction [2]
Palpitation [3]
QT interval prolonged / QT prolongation [3]
Tachyarrhythmia [2]
Tachycardia [3]

Central Nervous System
Dysgeusia (taste perversion) (<10%)
Tremor [2]

Endocrine/Metabolic
Acidosis (includes lactic acidosis) [10]

Respiratory
Dyspnea / shortness of breath [2]

Other
Adverse effects / adverse reactions [3]

ALCAFTADINE

Trade name: Lastacaft (Allergan)
Indications: Prevention of itching associated with allergic conjunctivitis
Class: Histamine H1 receptor antagonist
Half-life: 2 hours
Clinically important, potentially hazardous interactions with: none known
Important contra-indications noted in the prescribing guidelines for: pediatric patients

---

Central Nervous System
Headache (3%)

Ocular
Ocular burning (4%)
Ocular erythema (4%)
Ocular stinging (4%)

Respiratory
Influenza (3%)
Nasopharyngitis (3%)

ALCLOMETASONE

Trade names: Aclovate (GSK), Modrasone (Pliva)
Indications: Dermatoses
Class: Corticosteroid / Glucocorticoid, Corticosteroid, topical
Half-life: N/A
Clinically important, potentially hazardous interactions with: licorice, live vaccines

---

Skin
Dermatitis [3]

ALDESLEUKIN

Synonyms: IL-2; interleukin-2
Trade name: Proleukin (Chiron)
Indications: Metastatic renal cell carcinoma and metastatic melanoma
Class: Biologic, Immunomodulator, Interleukin-2
Half-life: 6–85 minutes
Clinically important, potentially hazardous interactions with: acebutolol, alfuzosin, altretamine, amikacin, aminoglycosides, antineoplastics, betamethasone, bleomycin, busulfan, captopril, carboplatin, carmustine, chlorambucil, ciclesonide, cilazapril, cisplatin, corticosteroids, cyclophosphamide, cytarabine, dacarbazine, dactinomycin, daunorubicin, docetaxel, doxorubicin, enalapril, estramustine, etoposide, fludarabine, fluorouracil, fosinopril, gemcitabine, gentamicin, hydroxyurea, idarubicin, ifosfamide, indomethacin, interferon alfa, irbesartan, kanamycin, levamisole, lisinopril, lomustine, mechlorethamine, melphalan, mercaptopurine, methotrexate, mitomycin, mitotane, mitoxantrone, neomycin, olmesartan, PEG-interferon, pentostatin, plicamycin, procarbazine, quinapril, ramipril, streptomycin, streptozocin, thioguanine, thiotepa, tobramycin,

trandolapril, tretinoin, triamcinolone, uracil, vinblastine, vincristine, vinorelbine
Important contra-indications noted in the prescribing guidelines for: nursing mothers; pediatric patients
Note: Contra-indicated in patients with significant cardiac, pulmonary, renal, hepatic, or CNS impairment.
Warning: CAPILLARY LEAK SYNDROME

Skin
Angioedema (formerly named angioneurotic edema) [2]
Cutaneous toxicity / skin toxicity [6]
Dermatitis [2]
Edema / fluid retention (47%) [3]
Erythema (41%) [5]
Erythema nodosum [3]
Erythroderma [4]
Exanthems [5]
Exfoliative dermatitis (18%)
Linear IgA bullous dermatosis [4]
Necrosis (skin necrosis) [2]
Pemphigus [2]
Peripheral edema (28%)
Petechiae (4%)
Pruritus (itching) (24%) [7]
Psoriasis [4]
Purpura (4%)
Rash (42%) [2]
Scleroderma [2]
Stevens-Johnson syndrome and toxic epidermal necrolysis (SJS/TEN) [2]
Urticaria / hives (2%) [3]
Vitiligo [3]
Xerosis / xeroderma (15%)

Hair
Alopecia / hair loss [2]

Mucosal
Oral mucosal eruption [2]
Stomatitis (oral mucositis) (22%)

Cardiovascular
Arrhythmias (10%)
Capillary leak syndrome [12]
Cardiotoxicity (11%) [2]
Hypotension (71%) [6]
Supraventricular tachycardia (12%)
Tachycardia (23%)
Vascular leak syndrome [6]
Vasodilation (13%)

Central Nervous System
Anorexia (20%)
Anxiety (12%)
Chills (52%)
Confusion (34%)
Depression [3]
Dysgeusia (taste perversion) (7%)
Fever (pyrexia) (includes hyperpyrexia) (29%) [8]
Neurotoxicity [3]
Pain (12%)
Rigors [3]
Somnolence (drowsiness) (22%)
Vertigo / dizziness (11%)

Endocrine/Metabolic
Acidosis (includes lactic acidosis) (12%)
ALP increased (10%)
AST increased (23%)
Creatine phosphokinase (CPK) / creatine kinase increased (hyperCKemia) (33%) [2]
Hypocalcemia (11%)
Hypomagnesemia [2]
Hypophosphatemia [2]
Weight gain (16%)
Weight loss [2]

Gastrointestinal/Hepatic
Abdominal pain (11%)
Diarrhea (67%) [3]
Hepatotoxicity / liver injury / acute liver injury / drug-induced liver injury (DILI) [2]
Nausea (35%) [9]
Vomiting (50%) [6]

Genitourinary
Oliguria (63%)

Hematologic
Anemia (29%)
Leukocytopenia (leukopenia) / leukocytes (white blood cells) decreased (16%) [2]
Sepsis [3]
Thrombocytopenia / platelets decreased (37%) [2]

Local
Injection-site inflammation [2]
Injection-site nodules [2]
Injection-site reaction (3%) [2]

Neuromuscular/Skeletal
Asthenia / fatigue (23–27%)
Myalgia/Myopathy (6%)
Myasthenia gravis [2]

Renal
Nephrotoxicity / kidney injury / acute kidney injury (AKI) / drug-induced kidney injury [4]

Respiratory
Cough (11%)
Dyspnea / shortness of breath (43%)
Pulmonary toxicity (11–24%) [2]
Rhinitis / rhinosinusitis (see also sinusitis) (10%)

Other
Adverse effects / adverse reactions [3]
Death [5]
Infection (13%) [2]

ALECTINIB

Trade name: Alecensa (Genentech)
Indications: Anaplastic lymphoma kinase-positive, metastatic non-small cell lung cancer in patients who have progressed on, or are intolerant to, crizotinib
Class: Anaplastic lymphoma kinase (ALK) inhibitor, Kinase inhibitor
Half-life: 33 hours
Clinically important, potentially hazardous interactions with: none known
Pregnancy category: Can cause fetal harm
Important contra-indications noted in the prescribing guidelines for: nursing mothers; pediatric patients

---

Skin
Edema / fluid retention (30%)
Peripheral edema [7]
Photosensitivity (10%) [3]
Rash (18%) [5]

Hair
Alopecia / hair loss [2]

Central Nervous System
Dysgeusia (taste perversion) [3]
Headache (17%) [3]

Endocrine/Metabolic
ALP increased (47%) [3]
ALT increased (34%) [6]
AST increased (51%) [7]
Creatine phosphokinase (CPK) / creatine kinase increased (hyperCKemia) (43%) [8]
GGT increased [2]
Hyperbilirubinemia (39%) [6]
Hyperglycemia (includes glucose increased) (36%)
Hypocalcemia (32%)
Hypokalemia (29%)
Hyponatremia (20%)
Hypophosphatemia (21%)
Serum creatinine increased (28%)
Weight gain (11%)

Gastrointestinal/Hepatic
Constipation (34%) [10]
Diarrhea (16%) [3]
Gastrointestinal perforation / perforated colon / gastric perforation [2]
Hepatic (liver) disorder / hepatobiliary disorder / hepatic (liver) dysfunction [3]
Nausea (18%) [5]
Vomiting (12%) [3]

Hematologic
Anemia (56%) [4]
Hemolytic anemia [5]
Lymphopenia (lymphocytopenia) / lymphocytes decreased (22%)
Neutropenia (neutrophils decreased) [7]

Neuromuscular/Skeletal
Asthenia / fatigue (41%) [6]
Back pain (12%)
Myalgia/Myopathy (29%) [8]

Ocular
Visual disturbances (10%)

Renal
Nephrotoxicity / kidney injury / acute kidney injury (AKI) / drug-induced kidney injury [2]
Renal failure [2]

Respiratory
Cough (19%)
Dyspnea / shortness of breath (16%)
Interstitial lung disease / interstitial pneumonitis / interstitial pneumonia (cryptogenic organizing pneumonia) / drug-induced interstitial lung disease [4]
Pulmonary toxicity [5]

Other
Adverse effects / adverse reactions [2]

ALEFACEPT

Trade name: Amevive (Astellas)
Indications: Chronic plaque psoriasis (in adults)
Class: Immunosuppressant
Half-life: 270 hours
Clinically important, potentially hazardous interactions with: alcohol, BCG vaccine, echinacea, leflunomide, live vaccines, natalizumab, pimecrolimus, sipuleucel-T, tacrolimus, trastuzumab
Important contra-indications noted in the prescribing guidelines for: nursing mothers; pediatric patients
Note: Contra-indicated in patients with HIV.

Skin
Lymphoma (3 cases)
Pruritus (itching) (2–5%) [2]

Central Nervous System
Chills (transient) (6%) [2]
Headache [6]
Vertigo / dizziness (<2%)

Gastrointestinal/Hepatic
Nausea (2–5%)
Hematologic
Lymphopenia (lymphocytopenia) / lymphocytes decreased (1–10%)
Local
Injection-site bleeding (4%)
Injection-site edema (2%)
Injection-site inflammation (4%)
Injection-site pain (7%)
Neuromuscular/Skeletal
Asthenia / fatigue [2]
Myalgia/Myopathy (2–5%)
Respiratory
Cough (2–5%) [2]
Influenza- ('flu)-like syndrome [2]
Pharyngitis (sore throat) (2–5%)
Upper respiratory tract infection [4]
Other
Adverse effects / adverse reactions (2%) [4]
Infection (2%) [3]

ALEMTUZUMAB

Trade names: Campath (Bayer), MabCampath (Schering)
Indications: B-cell chronic lymphcyotic leukemia, non-Hodgkin's lymphoma
Class: Biologic, Immunosuppressant, Monoclonal antibody
Half-life: 12 days
Clinically important, potentially hazardous interactions with: ponesimod
Note: Prophylactic therapy against PCP pneumonia and herpes viral infections is recommended upon initiation of therapy and for at least 2 months following last dose.
Warning: CYTOPENIAS, INFUSION REACTIONS, and INFECTIONS

Skin
Carcinoma [2]
Erythema (4%)
Flushing / rubefaction [2]
Herpes [2]
Herpes simplex [2]
Herpes zoster [3]
Lymphoma [2]
Lymphoproliferative disease / lymphoproliferative disorder (64–70%)
Peripheral edema (13%)
Pruritus (itching) (14–24%)
Purpura (8%)
Rash (13–40%) [5]
Thrombocytopenic purpura [11]
Urticaria / hives (16–30%) [2]
Vitiligo [2]
Hair
Alopecia areata [3]
Alopecia universalis [2]
Mucosal
Stomatitis (oral mucositis) (14%)
Cardiovascular
Hypertension (11–15%)
Hypotension (15–32%) [2]
Tachycardia (10%)
Central Nervous System
Anorexia (20%)
Anxiety (8%)
Chills (53%)
Depression (7%)
Dysesthesia (15%)
Fever (pyrexia) (includes hyperpyrexia) (69–85%) [6]
Guillain-Barré syndrome / acute inflammatory demyelinating polyradiculoneuropathy / acute motor axonal neuropathy [3]
Headache (13–24%) [3]
Insomnia (10%)
Intracranial hemorrhage [2]
Leukoencephalopathy / posterior reversible encephalopathy syndrome (PRES) [5]
Rigors (87%)
Tremor (3%)
Vertigo / dizziness (12%)
Endocrine/Metabolic
Graves' disease [5]
Hyperthyroidism (includes 'thyroid storm') [2]
Hypothyroidism [2]
Thyroid dysfunction [19]
Gastrointestinal/Hepatic
Abdominal pain (11%)
Diarrhea (10–22%) [2]
Nausea (47–54%) [4]
Vomiting (33–41%) [2]
Genitourinary
Cystitis (includes interstitial cystitis / bladder pain syndrome) [2]
Hematologic
Anemia (76%) [4]
Cytopenia [2]
Hemolytic anemia [6]
Hemophagocytic lymphohistiocytosis / hemophagocytic syndrome [2]
Hemotoxicity [4]
Leukocytopenia (leukopenia) / leukocytes (white blood cells) decreased [4]
Lymphopenia (lymphocytopenia) / lymphocytes decreased (97%) [2]
Neutropenia (neutrophils decreased) (77%) [10]
Sepsis [2]
Thrombocytopenia / platelets decreased (71%) [13]
Local
Application-site reactions [2]
Infusion-related reactions [14]
Infusion-site reactions [5]
Injection-site pruritus (30–40%)
Injection-site reaction (90%) [5]
Neuromuscular/Skeletal
Asthenia / fatigue (22–34%)
Bone pain / joint pain (24%)
Myalgia/Myopathy (11%)
Ocular
Ocular adverse effect [3]
Renal
Nephrotoxicity / kidney injury / acute kidney injury (AKI) / drug-induced kidney injury [4]
Respiratory
Acute respiratory distress syndrome [2]
Alveolar hemorrhage (pulmonary) [3]
Dyspnea / shortness of breath (14–26%)
Influenza- ('flu)-like syndrome [2]
Pharyngitis (sore throat) (12%)
Pneumonia (16%) [3]
Pneumonitis [5]
Respiratory tract infection [2]
Tuberculosis [2]
Other
Adverse effects / adverse reactions [8]
Death [13]
Infection (43–74%) [52]

ALENDRONATE

Trade names: Binosto (Mission), Fosamax (Merck)
Indications: Osteoporosis in postmenopausal women, Paget's disease
Class: Bisphosphonate
Half-life: >10 years
Clinically important, potentially hazardous interactions with: none known
Important contra-indications noted in the prescribing guidelines for: nursing mothers; pediatric patients

Skin
Angioedema (formerly named angioneurotic edema) [2]
Erythema multiforme [2]
Hypersensitivity [3]
Rash [5]
Mucosal
Oral ulceration [9]
Central Nervous System
Headache [2]
Endocrine/Metabolic
Hypocalcemia (18%) [5]
Gastrointestinal/Hepatic
Abdominal pain (<7%) [8]
Dyspepsia / functional dyspepsia (indigestion) (see also gastroparesis) [8]
Dysphagia [4]
Esophageal perforation [2]
Esophagitis [13]
Hepatotoxicity / liver injury / acute liver injury / drug-induced liver injury (DILI) [7]
Nausea [7]
Vomiting [4]
Neuromuscular/Skeletal
Arthralgia [6]
Bone pain / joint pain (<6%) [5]
Fractures [21]
Osteonecrosis / avascular necrosis (includes steroid-induced osteonecrosis of the femoral head) [13]
Ocular
Conjunctivitis (conjunctival inflammation) [2]
Ocular adverse effect [2]
Ocular inflammation [3]
Scleritis [3]
Uveitis / anterior uveitis / posterior uveitis / panuveitis [6]
Renal
Nephrotoxicity / kidney injury / acute kidney injury (AKI) / drug-induced kidney injury [2]
Renal failure [2]
Other
Adverse effects / adverse reactions [5]

ALFENTANIL

Trade name: Alfenta (Akorn)
Indications: General anesthesia, post-operative pain
Class: Analgesic; opioid, Anesthetic
Half-life: 83–97 minutes (adults)
Clinically important, potentially hazardous interactions with: ceritinib, crizotinib, dasatinib, eluxadoline, enzalutamide, erythromycin,

itraconazole, letermovir, ranitidine, ribociclib, rifapentine, ritonavir, telithromycin, viloxazine, voriconazole

Cardiovascular
Arrhythmias (>10%)
Bradycardia / sinus bradycardia (>10%) [2]
Hypotension (>10%)
Vasodilation (peripheral) (>10%)

Central Nervous System
Confusion (1–10%)
Depression (1–10%)
Intracranial pressure increased (intracranial hypertension) (>10%)
Shivering (3–9%)
Somnolence (drowsiness) (>10%)

ALFUZOSIN

Trade names: Uroxatral (Concordia), Xatral (Sanofi-Aventis)
Indications: Benign prostatic hyperplasia
Class: Adrenergic alpha-receptor antagonist
Half-life: 10 hours
Clinically important, potentially hazardous interactions with: ACE inhibitors, adrenergic neurone blockers, alcohol, aldesleukin, alprostadil, amitriptyline, angiotensin II receptor antagonists, antipsychotics, anxiolytics and hypnotics, arsenic, atazanavir, atenolol, baclofen, beta blockers, boceprevir, calcium channel blockers, cimetidine, citalopram, clonidine, conivaptan, corticosteroids, CYP3A4 inducers or inhibitors, darunavir, dasatinib, deferasirox, degarelix, delavirdine, diazoxide, diltiazem, diuretics, dolasetron, estrogens, food, general anesthetics, hydralazine, indinavir, itraconazole, ketoconazole, lapatinib, levodopa, levofloxacin, lopinavir, MAO inhibitors, methyldopa, minoxidil, moxifloxacin, moxisylyte, moxonidine, nelfinavir, nitrates, nitroprusside, NSAIDs, ombitasvir/paritaprevir/ritonavir and dasabuvir, pazopanib, phosphodiesterase 5 inhibitors, protease inhibitors, QT prolonging agents, ritonavir, sildenafil, St John's wort, tadalafil, telaprevir, telavancin, telithromycin, tipranavir, tizanidine, vardenafil, voriconazole, vorinostat, ziprasidone
Important contra-indications noted in the prescribing guidelines for: pediatric patients

Cardiovascular
Hypotension [2]
Orthostatic hypotension [3]
QT interval prolonged / QT prolongation [2]

Central Nervous System
Headache (3%)
Pain (<2%)
Vertigo / dizziness (6%) [19]

Gastrointestinal/Hepatic
Abdominal pain (<2%)
Hepatotoxicity / liver injury / acute liver injury / drug-induced liver injury (DILI) [2]

Genitourinary
Ejaculatory dysfunction [3]
Erectile dysfunction [2]

Hematologic
Thrombocytopenia / platelets decreased [3]

Neuromuscular/Skeletal
Asthenia / fatigue (3%)

Ocular
Floppy iris syndrome [4]

Respiratory
Bronchitis (<2%)
Pharyngitis (sore throat) (<2%)
Sinusitis (see also rhinitis / rhinosinusitis) (<2%)
Upper respiratory tract infection (3%)

Other
Adverse effects / adverse reactions [2]

ALGLUCOSIDASE ALFA

Trade name: Myozyme (Genzyme)
Indications: Pompe disease (glycogen storage disease type II), GAA deficiency
Class: Alfa-glucosidase, Enzyme
Half-life: 2–3 hours
Clinically important, potentially hazardous interactions with: none known

Skin
Anaphylactoid reactions / anaphylaxis (includes anaphylactic shock) (5–8%) [2]
Flushing / rubefaction (21%)
Rash (54%)
Urticaria / hives (21%)

Mucosal
Oral candidiasis (31%)

Cardiovascular
Bradycardia / sinus bradycardia (21%)
Hypertension (5–8%)
Tachycardia (23%)

Central Nervous System
Fever (pyrexia) (includes hyperpyrexia) (97%)
Pain (15–26%)

Gastrointestinal/Hepatic
Constipation (10–23%)
Diarrhea (62%)
Vomiting (22–49%)

Hematologic
Anemia (31%)

Local
Catheter-related infection (28%)

Neuromuscular/Skeletal
Myalgia/Myopathy (37%)

Otic
Otitis (otitis externa, otitis media, otitis interna) (44%)

Respiratory
Cough (46%)
Nasopharyngitis (23%)
Pneumonia (46%)
Upper respiratory tract infection (44%)

ALIROCUMAB

Trade name: Praluent (Regeneron)
Indications: Adjunct to diet and statin therapy in hypercholesterolemia or clinical atherosclerotic cardiovascular disease where additional lowering of low density lipoprotein cholesterol is required
Class: Monoclonal antibody, Proprotein convertase subtilisin kexin type 9 (PCSK9) inhibitor
Half-life: 17–20 days
Clinically important, potentially hazardous interactions with: none known
Pregnancy category: No data available but likely to cross the placenta in second and third trimester
Important contra-indications noted in the prescribing guidelines for: pediatric patients

Skin
Hematoma / cutaneous hematoma (2%)

Cardiovascular
Cardiotoxicity [3]
Myocardial infarction [3]

Central Nervous System
Cognitive impairment [2]
Headache [5]
Neurotoxicity [4]
Stroke / cerebrovascular accident [2]
Vertigo / dizziness [6]

Endocrine/Metabolic
ALT increased [3]
Creatine phosphokinase (CPK) / creatine kinase increased (hyperCKemia) [3]

Gastrointestinal/Hepatic
Diarrhea (5%) [3]
Gastrointestinal disorder / discomfort [2]
Hepatotoxicity / liver injury / acute liver injury / drug-induced liver injury (DILI) (3%)
Nausea [2]

Genitourinary
Urinary tract infection (5%)

Local
Injection-site pain [2]
Injection-site reaction (7%) [23]

Neuromuscular/Skeletal
Arthralgia [6]
Asthenia / fatigue [3]
Back pain [6]
Bone pain / joint pain (2%) [2]
Muscle spasm (3%)
Myalgia/Myopathy (4%) [11]

Ocular
Ocular adverse effect [2]

Respiratory
Bronchitis (4%)
Cough (3%)
Influenza (6%) [5]
Nasopharyngitis (11%) [11]
Sinusitis (see also rhinitis / rhinosinusitis) (3%) [2]
Upper respiratory tract infection [8]

Other
Adverse effects / adverse reactions [12]
Allergic reactions (9%)
Death [2]

ALISKIREN

Trade names: Rasilez (Novartis), Tekamlo (Novartis), Tekturna (Novartis), Tekturna HCT (Novartis), Valturna (Novartis)
Indications: Hypertension
Class: Antihypertensive, Renin inhibitor
Half-life: 24 hours
Clinically important, potentially hazardous interactions with: ACE inhibitors, aldosterone antagonists, atorvastatin, candesartan, celecoxib, cyclosporine, diclofenac, furosemide, heparin, irbesartan, itraconazole, ketoconazole, losartan, meloxicam, moexipril, NSAIDs, olmesartan, potassium salts, potassium-sparing diuretics, sacubitril/valsartan, tinzaparin, trandolapril, verapamil

Pregnancy category: category C in first trimester; category D in second and third trimesters
Important contra-indications noted in the prescribing guidelines for: nursing mothers; pediatric patients
Note: Tekamlo is aliskiren and amlodipine; Tekturna HCT is aliskiren and hydrochlorothiazide; Valturna is aliskiren and valsartan. Hydrochlorothiazide is a sulfonamide and can be absorbed systemically. Sulfonamides can produce severe, possibly fatal, reactions such as toxic epidermal necrolysis and Stevens-Johnson syndrome.
Contra-indicated for concomitant use with angiotensin receptor blockers or angiotensin-converting enzyme (ACE) inhibitors in patients with diabetes.
Warning: FETAL TOXICITY

Skin
Angioedema (formerly named angioneurotic edema) [4]
Peripheral edema [4]

Central Nervous System
Headache [12]
Vertigo / dizziness [8]

Endocrine/Metabolic
Hyperkalemia [3]

Gastrointestinal/Hepatic
Diarrhea (2%) [5]

Neuromuscular/Skeletal
Asthenia / fatigue [7]

Respiratory
Cough [4]
Nasopharyngitis [7]

Other
Adverse effects / adverse reactions [11]

ALITRETINOIN

Trade name: Panretin (Ligand)
Indications: Kaposi's sarcoma cutaneous lesions
Class: Retinoid
Half-life: N/A
Clinically important, potentially hazardous interactions with: ketoconazole, simvastatin, St John's wort, St John's wort, vitamin A
Important contra-indications noted in the prescribing guidelines for: the elderly; pediatric patients
Note: Oral alitretinoin (Toctino) is not available in the USA.

Skin
Edema / fluid retention (3–8%)
Erythema [2]
Exfoliative dermatitis (3–9%)
Flushing / rubefaction [2]
Pigmentation (Skin) (includes hyperpigmentation) (3%)
Pruritus (itching) (8–11%)
Rash (25–77%)
Ulcerations (2%)
Xerosis / xeroderma (10%)

Hair
Curly hair [2]

Mucosal
Mucocutaneous reactions [2]

Central Nervous System
Depression [2]
Headache [8]
Paresthesias (3–22%)

Endocrine/Metabolic
Creatine phosphokinase (CPK) / creatine kinase increased (hyperCKemia) [2]
Dyslipidemia [2]
Hypertriglyceridemia (includes triglycerides increased) [2]

Gastrointestinal/Hepatic
Nausea [2]

ALLOPURINOL

Trade names: Duzallo (AstraZeneca), Zyloprim (Prometheus)
Indications: Gouty arthritis
Class: Purine analog, Uricosuric, Xanthine oxidase inhibitor
Half-life: <3 hours
Clinically important, potentially hazardous interactions with: acenocoumarol, amoxicillin, ampicillin, ampicillin/sulbactam, azathioprine, benazepril, capecitabine, captopril, cilazapril, cyclopenthiazide, dicumarol, enalapril, fosinopril, imidapril, lisinopril, mercaptopurine, pantoprazole, quinapril, ramipril, trandolapril, uracil/tegafur, vidarabine, zofenopril
Note: HLA-B*5801 confers a risk of allopurinol-induced serious skin reactions like SJS/TEN and DRESS. Should be seriously considered in patients of south Asian ancestry.
Duzallo is allopurinol and lesinurad (see separate entry).

Skin
AGEP [6]
Cutaneous adverse reaction (includes severe cutaneous adverse drug reaction (SCAR)) [12]
Cutaneous toxicity / skin toxicity [2]
DRESS syndrome (Drug-induced hypersensitivity syndrome) [55]
Eosinophilic pustular folliculitis [2]
Erythema multiforme [7]
Exanthems (<5%) [20]
Exfoliative dermatitis (>10%) [15]
Fixed eruption / fixed drug eruption [11]
Granuloma annulare (disseminated) [2]
Hypersensitivity [49]
Lupus erythematosus (subacute cutaneous lupus erythematosus (SCLE)) [3]
Pityriasis rosea [2]
Pruritus (itching) [7]
Purpura (>10%) [2]
Rash (>10%) [11]
Stevens-Johnson syndrome and toxic epidermal necrolysis (SJS/TEN) (>10%) [96]
Toxic pustuloderma [3]
Urticaria / hives (>10%) [6]
Vasculitis (angiitis) / cutaneous vasculitis (angiitis) [7]

Hair
Alopecia / hair loss (<10%) [2]

Mucosal
Oral ulceration [3]
Stomatitis (oral mucositis) [2]

Cardiovascular
Polyarteritis nodosa [3]

Central Nervous System
Chills (<10%)
Fever (pyrexia) (includes hyperpyrexia) [2]
Headache [3]
Vertigo / dizziness [3]

Endocrine/Metabolic
ALT increased [2]
AST increased [3]

Gastrointestinal/Hepatic
Diarrhea [5]
Hepatotoxicity / liver injury / acute liver injury / drug-induced liver injury (DILI) [10]
Nausea [3]

Neuromuscular/Skeletal
Arthralgia [3]
Asthenia / fatigue [2]
Back pain [2]
Bone pain / joint pain [2]
Joint disorder [2]
Myalgia/Myopathy [3]

Renal
Nephrotoxicity / kidney injury / acute kidney injury (AKI) / drug-induced kidney injury [4]
Renal failure [2]

Respiratory
Nasopharyngitis [2]
Upper respiratory tract infection [4]

Other
Adverse effects / adverse reactions [13]
Allergic reactions (severe) [2]
Death [9]

ALMOTRIPTAN

Trade names: Almogran (Almirall), Axert (Ortho-McNeil)
Indications: Migraine headaches
Class: 5-HT1 agonist, Serotonin receptor agonist, Triptan
Half-life: 3–4 hours
Clinically important, potentially hazardous interactions with: conivaptan, darunavir, delavirdine, dihydroergotamine, ergotamine, indinavir, ketoconazole, methysergide, SNRIs, SSRIs, telithromycin, triptans, voriconazole
Important contra-indications noted in the prescribing guidelines for: pediatric patients
Note: Contra-indicated in patients with history, symptoms, or signs of ischemic cardiac, cerebrovascular, or peripheral vascular syndromes, or with uncontrolled hypertension.

Cardiovascular
Chest pain [3]

Central Nervous System
Headache [2]
Neurotoxicity [2]
Paresthesias [4]
Somnolence (drowsiness) [5]
Vertigo / dizziness [6]

Gastrointestinal/Hepatic
Nausea [6]
Vomiting [3]

Neuromuscular/Skeletal
Asthenia / fatigue [4]

Respiratory
Influenza- ('flu)-like syndrome (12%)
Upper respiratory tract infection (20%)

Other
Adverse effects / adverse reactions [10]

ALOE VERA (GEL, JUICE, LEAF)

Family: Liliaceae
Scientific names: *Aloë africana, Aloë barbadensis, Aloë ferox, Aloë spicata*
Indications: Oral: anesthetic, antiseptic, antipyretic, antipruritic, vasodilator, anti-inflammatory, vermifuge, antifungal. antiulcer, diabetes, asthma
Topical: promote healing, cold sores, ulceration, radiations injuries, psoriasis, frostbite. Also used in cosmetics and for its moisturizing and emollient properties
Class: Anthroquinone glycoside, Anti-inflammatory
Half-life: N/A
Clinically important, potentially hazardous interactions with: arsenic
Note: One blade of aloe can be used for weeks. The severed end of the blade is self healing.
I have perfumed my bed with myrrh, aloes and cinnamon (Proverbs 7:17).
Cleopatra regarded the gel as a fountain of youth and used it to preserve her skin against the ravages of the Egyptian sun.

Skin
- Contact dermatitis [2]
- Henoch-Schönlein purpura / IgA vasculitis / immunoglobulin A vasculitis [2]
- Hypersensitivity [2]

Endocrine/Metabolic
- Hypokalemia [2]

Gastrointestinal/Hepatic
- Diarrhea [2]
- Hepatitis [6]

Other
- Allergic reactions [2]

ALOGLIPTIN

Trade name: Nesina (Takeda)
Indications: Type II diabetes mellitus
Class: Antidiabetic, Dipeptidyl peptidase-4 (DPP-4) (gliptin) inhibitor
Half-life: 21 hours
Clinically important, potentially hazardous interactions with: none known
Important contra-indications noted in the prescribing guidelines for: nursing mothers; pediatric patients

---

Skin
- Bullous pemphigoid / pemphigoid [2]
- Hypersensitivity [2]
- Pruritus (itching) [2]

Central Nervous System
- Headache (4%) [8]
- Vertigo / dizziness [3]

Endocrine/Metabolic
- Hypoglycemia [14]

Gastrointestinal/Hepatic
- Constipation [2]
- Diarrhea [2]
- Pancreatitis / acute pancreatitis [3]

Neuromuscular/Skeletal
- Arthralgia [2]

Respiratory
- Nasopharyngitis (4%) [8]
- Upper respiratory tract infection (4%) [6]

Other
- Adverse effects / adverse reactions [6]
- Infection [3]

ALOSETRON

Trade name: Lotronex (GSK)
Indications: Irritable bowel syndrome
Class: 5-HT3 antagonist, Serotonin type 3 receptor antagonist
Half-life: 1.5 hours
Clinically important, potentially hazardous interactions with: apomorphine, conivaptan, CYP1A2 inhibitors, CYP3A4 inhibitors, darunavir, delavirdine, eluxadoline, fluvoxamine, indinavir, telithromycin, teriflunomide, viloxazine, voriconazole
Important contra-indications noted in the prescribing guidelines for: the elderly; nursing mothers; pediatric patients
Note: Alosetron was approved in 2000 for use in women with diarrhea-predominant irritable bowel syndrome (IBS-D), however infrequent serious adverse events (including ischemic colitis and serious complications of constipation, resulting in hospitalization, blood transfusion, surgery and death) prompted alosetron's voluntary withdrawal from the US market in November 2000. Public request prompted its reintroduction in 2002 under a Risk Management Plan, including a more restricted indication and a Prescribing Program for Lotronex. Only licensed for use in female patients. Contra-indicated in patients with constipation or a history of chronic or severe constipation or sequelae from constipation; intestinal obstruction, stricture, toxic megacolon, gastrointestinal perforation, and/or adhesions; ischemic colitis; impaired intestinal circulation, thrombophlebitis, or hypercoagulable state; Crohn's disease or ulcerative colitis; diverticulitis; severe hepatic impairment.
Warning: SERIOUS GASTROINTESTINAL ADVERSE REACTIONS

Gastrointestinal/Hepatic
- Abdominal distension (2%)
- Abdominal pain (<7%) [3]
- Colitis [12]
- Constipation (9–29%) [14]
- Diarrhea (2–3%)
- Flatulence (<3%)
- Gastroenteritis (>3%)
- Gastroesophageal reflux (2%)
- Hemorrhoids (<3%)
- Nausea (6%)
- Vomiting (<3%)

Genitourinary
- Urinary tract infection (>3%)

Neuromuscular/Skeletal
- Asthenia / fatigue (3%)
- Muscle spasm (3%)

Respiratory
- Cough (>3%)
- Nasopharyngitis (>3%)
- Sinusitis (see also rhinitis / rhinosinusitis) (>3%)
- Upper respiratory tract infection (>3%)

Other
- Adverse effects / adverse reactions [5]

ALPELISIB

Trade name: Piqray (Novartis)
Indications: Postmenopausal women, and men, with hormone receptor (HR)-positive, human epidermal growth factor receptor 2 (HER2)-negative, PIK3CA mutated, advanced or metastatic breast cancer as detected by an FDA-approved test following progression on or after an endocrine-based regimen
Class: Kinase inhibitor, Phosphoinositide 3-kinase (Phosphatidylinositol 3-kinase) (PI3K) inhibitor
Half-life: 8–9 hours
Clinically important, potentially hazardous interactions with: breast cancer resistance protein inhibitors, CYP2C9 substrates, CYP3A4 inducers
Pregnancy category: Based on animal data and mechanism of action can cause fetal harm when administered to a pregnant woman. There are no available data in pregnant women to inform the drug associated risk. When used in combination with fulvestrant, refer to the prescribing information of fulvestrant for pregnancy information.

Skin
- Dry skin (<1% grade 3) (with fulvestrant) (18%)
- Edema / fluid retention (with fulvestrant) (15%)
- Maculopapular rash / morbilliform rash [4]
- Pruritus (itching) (<1% grade 3) (with fulvestrant) (18%)
- Rash (20% grade 3) (with fulvestrant) (52%) [4]

Hair
- Alopecia / hair loss (with fulvestrant) (20%)

Mucosal
- Mucosal dryness (<1% grade 3) (with fulvestrant) (12%)
- Mucosal inflammation (2% grade 3) (with fulvestrant) (19%)
- Stomatitis (oral mucositis) (3% grade 3) (with fulvestrant) (30%)

Central Nervous System
- Dysgeusia (taste perversion) (<1% grade 3) (with fulvestrant) (18%)
- Fever (pyrexia) (includes hyperpyrexia) (<1% grade 3–4) (with fulvestrant) (14%)
- Headache (<1% grade 3) (with fulvestrant) (18%)

Endocrine/Metabolic
- ALT increased (4% grade 3–4) (with fulvestrant) (44%)
- Appetite decreased (<1% grade 3) (with fulvestrant) (36%) [2]
- Diabetic ketoacidosis [5]
- GGT increased (11% grade 3–4) (with fulvestrant) (52%)
- Hyperglycemia (includes glucose increased) (39% grade 3–4) (with fulvestrant) (79%) [11]
- Hyperlipasemia (7% grade 3–4) (with fulvestrant) (42%)
- Hypoalbuminemia / albumin decreased (with fulvestrant) (14%)
- Hypocalcemia (2% grade 3–4) (with fulvestrant) (27%)
- Hypoglycemia (<1% grade 3–4) (with fulvestrant) (26%)

Hypokalemia (6% grade 3–4) (with fulvestrant) (14%)
Hypomagnesemia (<1% grade 3–4) (with fulvestrant) (11%)
Serum creatinine increased (3% grade 3) (with fulvestrant) (67%)
Weight loss (4% grade 3) (with fulvestrant) (27%)

Gastrointestinal/Hepatic
Abdominal pain (1% grade 3) (with fulvestrant) (17%)
Diarrhea (7% grade 3) (with fulvestrant) (58%) [5]
Dyspepsia / functional dyspepsia (indigestion) (see also gastroparesis) (with fulvestrant) (11%)
Nausea (3% grade 3) (with fulvestrant) (45%) [2]
Vomiting (<1% grade 3) (with fulvestrant) (27%) [2]

Genitourinary
Urinary tract infection (<1% grade 3) (with fulvestrant) (10%)

Hematologic
Hemoglobin decreased (4% grade 3) (with fulvestrant) (42%)
Lymphopenia (lymphocytopenia) / lymphocytes decreased (8% grade 3–4) (with fulvestrant) (52%)
Partial thromboplastin time increased (<1% grade 3) (with fulvestrant) (21%)
Thrombocytopenia / platelets decreased (1% grade 3–4) (with fulvestrant) (14%)

Neuromuscular/Skeletal
Asthenia / fatigue (5% grade 3) (with fulvestrant) (42%) [2]
Osteonecrosis / avascular necrosis (includes steroid-induced osteonecrosis of the femoral head) (with fulvestrant) (4%)

ALPHA-LIPOIC ACID

Synonym: ALA
Indications: Diabetic neuropathy, vasodilation, photoaging
Class: Dietary supplement
Half-life: N/A
Clinically important, potentially hazardous interactions with: none known

---

Skin
Rash [2]

Central Nervous System
Vertigo / dizziness [2]

Endocrine/Metabolic
Insulin autoimmune syndrome / insulin autoimmune hypoglycemia / Hirata's disease [4]

ALPRAZOLAM

Trade name: Xanax (Pfizer)
Indications: Anxiety, depression, panic attacks
Class: Benzodiazepine
Half-life: 11–16 hours
Clinically important, potentially hazardous interactions with: alcohol, amprenavir, aprepitant, boceprevir, clarithromycin, CNS depressants, darunavir, delavirdine, digoxin, efavirenz, fluconazole, fluoxetine, fluvoxamine, grapefruit juice, indinavir, itraconazole, ivermectin, kava, ketoconazole, posaconazole, propoxyphene, ritonavir, saquinavir, St John's wort, telaprevir, tipranavir
Important contra-indications noted in the prescribing guidelines for: the elderly; nursing mothers; pediatric patients

---

Skin
Dermatitis (4%) [5]
Diaphoresis (16%)
Edema / fluid retention (5%)
Photosensitivity [4]
Pruritus (itching) (<10%) [2]
Rash (11%) [4]

Mucosal
Sialopenia (33%)
Sialorrhea (ptyalism; hypersalivation) (4%)
Xerostomia (dry mouth) (15%) [6]

Cardiovascular
Hypotension (<10%)

Central Nervous System
Cognitive impairment (>10%)
Coma [2]
Depression (>10%)
Dysarthria (>10%)
Incoordination (<10%)
Memory loss/memory impaired [2]
Neuroleptic malignant syndrome [2]
Neurotoxicity [2]
Paresthesias (2%)
Restlessness [2]
Sedation [2]
Seizures (<10%) [2]
Somnolence (drowsiness) (>10%)

Endocrine/Metabolic
Galactorrhea [2]

Genitourinary
Micturition difficulty (>10%)

Neuromuscular/Skeletal
Asthenia / fatigue (>10%) [2]

ALPROSTADIL

Synonyms: PGE; prostaglandin E_1
Trade names: Caverject (Pfizer), Edex (Schwarz), Muse (Vivus), Prostin VR (Pfizer)
Indications: Impotence, to maintain patent ductus arteriosus
Class: Prostaglandin
Half-life: 5–10 minutes
Clinically important, potentially hazardous interactions with: acebutolol, alfuzosin, captopril, cilazapril, enalapril, fosinopril, irbesartan, lisinopril, olmesartan, quinapril, ramipril
Pregnancy category: not indicated for use in women
Important contra-indications noted in the prescribing guidelines for: pediatric patients
Warning: APNEA (in neonates with congenital heart defects)

Skin
Edema / fluid retention (<10%)
Flushing / rubefaction (>10%)

Mucosal
Nasal congestion (<10%)

Cardiovascular
Bradycardia / sinus bradycardia (<10%)
Hypertension (<10%)
Hypotension (<10%)
Tachycardia (<10%)

Central Nervous System
Fever (pyrexia) (includes hyperpyrexia) (>10%)
Headache (>10%)
Pain (>10%)
Vertigo / dizziness (>10%)

Gastrointestinal/Hepatic
Diarrhea (<10%)

Genitourinary
Erectile dysfunction (prolonged erection / >4 hours) (4%)
Penile pain (>10%)
Penile rash (<10%)
Priapism (4%) [8]
Urethral burning (>10%) [2]

Local
Application-site burning [3]
Application-site erythema [3]
Application-site pain [2]
Application-site pruritus [2]
Injection-site ecchymoses (<10%)
Injection-site hematoma (3%)
Injection-site pain (2%)

Neuromuscular/Skeletal
Back pain (<10%)

Respiratory
Apnea (>10%)
Cough (<10%)
Influenza- ('flu)-like syndrome (<10%)
Sinusitis (see also rhinitis / rhinosinusitis) (<10%)

ALTEPLASE

Synonym: tPA
Trade name: Activase (Genentech)
Indications: Acute myocardial infarction, acute pulmonary embolism
Class: Fibrinolytic, Plasminogen activator
Half-life: 30–45 minutes
Clinically important, potentially hazardous interactions with: defibrotide, nitroglycerin, ticlopidine
Important contra-indications noted in the prescribing guidelines for: the elderly; nursing mothers

---

Skin
Anaphylactoid reactions / anaphylaxis (includes anaphylactic shock) [5]
Angioedema (formerly named angioneurotic edema) [12]
Bruise / bruising / contusion / ecchymosis (ecchymoses) (<10%)
Purpura (<10%)

Central Nervous System
Fever (pyrexia) (includes hyperpyrexia) (<10%)
Intracranial hemorrhage [8]

Gastrointestinal/Hepatic
Hemorrhagic colitis (5%)

Hematologic
Bleeding [3]
Hemorrhage (4%)

Other
Death [4]

ALTRETAMINE

Synonym: hexamethylmelamine
Trade name: Hexalen (Eisai)
Indications: Palliative treatment of recurrent ovarian cancer
Class: Alkylating agent
Half-life: 13 hours
Clinically important, potentially hazardous interactions with: aldesleukin, amitriptyline, linezolid
Important contra-indications noted in the prescribing guidelines for: nursing mothers; pediatric patients

---

Central Nervous System
Neurotoxicity [5]
Paresthesias [2]
Peripheral neuropathy (31%)

Gastrointestinal/Hepatic
Abdominal pain [2]
Nausea (33%)
Vomiting (33%) [2]

Hematologic
Anemia (33%)
Leukocytopenia (leukopenia) / leukocytes (white blood cells) decreased (5%)
Neutropenia (neutrophils decreased) [2]
Thrombocytopenia / platelets decreased (9%)

Neuromuscular/Skeletal
Asthenia / fatigue [3]

ALVIMOPAN

Trade name: Entereg (Adolor)
Indications: Postoperative ileus
Class: Opioid antagonist, Opioid receptor antagonist
Half-life: 10–18 hours
Clinically important, potentially hazardous interactions with: hydromorphone, opioid receptor antagonist (for longer than 7 days), tapentadol
Important contra-indications noted in the prescribing guidelines for: nursing mothers; pediatric patients
Warning: FOR SHORT-TERM HOSPITAL USE ONLY

Cardiovascular
Hypotension [2]
Myocardial infarction [3]

Endocrine/Metabolic
Hypokalemia (7–10%)

Gastrointestinal/Hepatic
Abdominal pain [4]
Constipation (4–10%)
Diarrhea [4]
Dyspepsia / functional dyspepsia (indigestion) (see also gastroparesis) (6–7%)
Flatulence (3–9%) [2]
Nausea [6]
Vomiting [3]

Genitourinary
Urinary retention (3–4%)

Hematologic
Anemia (5%)

Neuromuscular/Skeletal
Back pain (3%)

AMANTADINE

Trade names: Gocovri (Adamas Pharma), Symmetrel (Endo)
Indications: Parkinsonism, influenza A viral infection
Class: Adamantane, Antiviral
Half-life: 10–28 hours
Clinically important, potentially hazardous interactions with: cyclopenthiazide, fesoterodine, levomepromazine, memantine, quinine, risperidone, tetrabenazine, trimethoprim, zuclopenthixol
Important contra-indications noted in the prescribing guidelines for: nursing mothers; pediatric patients
Note: Amantadine should be prescribed with caution to patients with a history of myocardial disease.

Skin
Dermatitis [20]
Edema / fluid retention [3]
Livedo reticularis / livedo racemosa (50–90%) [25]
Peripheral edema (<10%) [10]
Photosensitivity [2]

Mucosal
Xerostomia (dry mouth) (<10%) [12]

Cardiovascular
Cardiac arrest [3]
Cardiac failure [2]
Hypotension (<10%)
Orthostatic hypotension [3]
QT interval prolonged / QT prolongation [4]

Central Nervous System
Abnormal dreams (<10%)
Agitation (<10%)
Anorexia (<10%)
Anxiety (<10%)
Confusion (<10%) [2]
Delirium (<10%) [4]
Depression (<10%)
Gait instability / postural instability [3]
Hallucinations [10]
Hallucinations, visual [6]
Headache (<10%)
Insomnia (<10%) [4]
Psychosis [7]
Somnolence (drowsiness) (<10%)
Vertigo / dizziness (<10%) [4]

Endocrine/Metabolic
Hyponatremia [2]

Gastrointestinal/Hepatic
Constipation (<10%) [9]
Diarrhea (<10%)
Nausea [3]

Neuromuscular/Skeletal
Asthenia / fatigue (<10%)
Ataxia (<10%)
Myoclonus (see also hypnic jerk) [4]

Ocular
Corneal edema [8]
Vision blurred [2]

AMBRISENTAN

Trade names: Letairis (Gilead), Volibris (GSK)
Indications: Pulmonary arterial hypertension
Class: Antihypertensive, Endothelin receptor (ETR) antagonist, Vasodilator
Half-life: 9 hours
Clinically important, potentially hazardous interactions with: conivaptan, cyclosporine, CYP2C19 inducers or inhibitors, CYP3A4 inducers or inhibitors, dasatinib, deferasirox, grapefruit juice, St John's wort
Important contra-indications noted in the prescribing guidelines for: nursing mothers; pediatric patients
Note: Also contra-indicated in patients with idiopathic pulmonary fibrosis.
Warning: CONTRA-INDICATED IN PREGNANCY

Skin
Edema / fluid retention [5]
Flushing / rubefaction (4%)
Peripheral edema (17%) [9]

Mucosal
Nasal congestion (6%) [2]

Cardiovascular
Palpitation (5%)

Central Nervous System
Headache (15%) [5]

Gastrointestinal/Hepatic
Abdominal pain (3%)
Constipation (4%)
Hepatotoxicity / liver injury / acute liver injury / drug-induced liver injury (DILI) [3]

Hematologic
Anemia [5]

Respiratory
Dyspnea / shortness of breath (4%)
Nasopharyngitis (3%)
Sinusitis (see also rhinitis / rhinosinusitis) (3%)

AMIFOSTINE

Synonyms: ethiofos; gammaphos
Trade name: Ethyol (Medimmune)
Indications: Nephrotoxicity prophylaxis
Class: Thiophosphate cytoprotective
Half-life: 9 minutes
Clinically important, potentially hazardous interactions with: benazepril, captopril, clevidipine, enalapril, fosinopril, irbesartan, lisinopril, olmesartan, quinapril, ramipril
Important contra-indications noted in the prescribing guidelines for: the elderly; nursing mothers; pediatric patients

---

Skin
Anaphylactoid reactions / anaphylaxis (includes anaphylactic shock) [3]
Dermatitis [3]
Flushing / rubefaction (>10%) [4]
Rash [6]
Stevens-Johnson syndrome and toxic epidermal necrolysis (SJS/TEN) [4]

Mucosal
Mucositis [4]
Xerostomia (dry mouth) [7]

Cardiovascular
Hypotension (15–61%) [5]

Central Nervous System
Chills (>10%)
Dysgeusia (taste perversion) [2]
Fever (pyrexia) (includes hyperpyrexia) [3]

Endocrine/Metabolic
Hypocalcemia [2]

Gastrointestinal/Hepatic
Nausea (53–96%) [2]
Vomiting (53–96%) [2]

Respiratory
Dyspnea / shortness of breath (4%)

Other
Allergic reactions [2]

AMIKACIN

Trade name: Amikacin sulfate (Bedford)
Indications: Short-term treatment of serious infections due to gram-negative bacteria
Class: Antibiotic, Antibiotic; aminoglycoside, Antimicrobial, Drug-resistant antituberculosis agent
Half-life: 1.5–2.5 hours (adults)
Clinically important, potentially hazardous interactions with: adefovir, aldesleukin, aminoglycosides, atracurium, bumetanide, cephalexin, doxacurium, ethacrynic acid, furosemide, succinylcholine, teicoplanin, torsemide
Important contra-indications noted in the prescribing guidelines for: nursing mothers; pediatric patients
Note: Aminoglycosides may cause neurotoxicity and/or nephrotoxicity.

Skin
Dermatitis [3]
DRESS syndrome (Drug-induced hypersensitivity syndrome) [2]
Exanthems [2]

Central Nervous System
Neurotoxicity (<10%)

Ocular
Macular infarction [3]

Otic
Hearing loss (hypoacusis) [6]
Ototoxicity (<10%) [9]
Tinnitus [3]

Renal
Nephrotoxicity / kidney injury / acute kidney injury (AKI) / drug-induced kidney injury (<10%) [11]

AMILORIDE

Trade names: Midamor (Merck), Moduretic (Merck)
Indications: Prevention of hypokalemia associated with kaliuretic diuretics, management of edema in hypertension
Class: Diuretic, potassium-sparing
Half-life: 6–9 hours
Clinically important, potentially hazardous interactions with: ACE inhibitors, benazepril, captopril, cyclosporine, enalapril, fosinopril, lisinopril, magnesium, metformin, moexipril, potassium salts, quinapril, quinidine, ramipril, spironolactone, trandolapril, zofenopril
Note: Moduretic is amiloride and hydrochlorothiazide. Hydrochlorothiazide is a sulfonamide and can be absorbed systemically. Sulfonamides can produce severe, possibly fatal, reactions such as toxic epidermal necrolysis and Stevens-Johnson syndrome.

Skin
Photosensitivity [4]

Central Nervous System
Headache (<10%)
Vertigo / dizziness (<10%)

Endocrine/Metabolic
Gynecomastia (<10%)
Hyperkalemia [2]

Genitourinary
Impotence (<10%)

Neuromuscular/Skeletal
Asthenia / fatigue (<10%)
Myalgia/Myopathy (<10%)

Respiratory
Cough (<10%)
Dyspnea / shortness of breath (<10%)

AMINOCAPROIC ACID

Trade name: Amicar (Xanodyne)
Indications: To provide hemostasis in the treatment of fibrinolysis
Class: Antifibrinolytic
Half-life: 1–2 hours
Clinically important, potentially hazardous interactions with: none known
Important contra-indications noted in the prescribing guidelines for: nursing mothers; pediatric patients

---

Skin
Dermatitis [4]
Purpura [2]
Rash (<10%)

Neuromuscular/Skeletal
Myalgia/Myopathy (<10%)
Rhabdomyolysis [11]

Renal
Nephrotoxicity / kidney injury / acute kidney injury (AKI) / drug-induced kidney injury [2]

AMINO-GLUTETHIMIDE

Trade name: Cytadren (Novartis)
Indications: Suppression of adrenal function, metastatic carcinoma
Class: Aromatase inhibitor
Half-life: 7–15 hours
Clinically important, potentially hazardous interactions with: betamethasone, dexamethasone, doxercalciferol, oxtriphylline, triamcinolone
Important contra-indications noted in the prescribing guidelines for: the elderly; nursing mothers; pediatric patients

---

Skin
Exanthems [8]
Lupus erythematosus (subacute cutaneous lupus erythematosus (SCLE)) (>10%)
Pruritus (itching) (5%)
Rash (>10%)

Hair
Hirsutism (<10%)

Mucosal
Oral mucosal eruption [2]

Neuromuscular/Skeletal
Myalgia/Myopathy (3%)

AMINOLEVULINIC ACID

Synonym: 5-Aminolevulinic acid
Trade names: Ameluz (Biofrontera), Levulan Kerastick (Dusa)
Indications: Non-hyperkeratotic actinic keratoses of face and scalp
Class: Photosensitizer, Protoporphyrin IX (PpIX) (wakefulness promoting agent)
Half-life: 20–40 hours
Clinically important, potentially hazardous interactions with: none known
Important contra-indications noted in the prescribing guidelines for: nursing mothers; pediatric patients
Note: In photodynamic therapy: to be used in conjunction with the relevant illuminator as approved by the manufacturer.

Skin
Burning / skin burning sensation (>50%) [6]
Crusting (64–71%) [2]
Dermatitis [2]
Desquamation [2]
Edema / fluid retention (35%) [9]
Erosions (14%) [2]
Erythema (99%) [14]
Exfoliative dermatitis (from topical treatment) [3]
Hypomelanosis (22%)
Photosensitivity [4]
Pigmentation (Skin) (includes hyperpigmentation) (from topical treatment) (22%) [7]
Pruritus (itching) (25%) [2]
Pustules / pustular eruption (<4%)
Scaling (64–71%)
Stinging (>50%) [2]
Ulcerations (4%)
Vesiculation (4%) [2]

Cardiovascular
Hypotension [4]

Central Nervous System
Dysesthesia (2%)
Pain [12]

AMINOPHYLLINE

Synonym: theophylline ethylenediamine
Trade names: Elixophyllin (Forest), Phyllocontin (Napp), Quibron (Monarch)
Indications: Prevention or treatment of reversible bronchospasm
Class: Xanthine alkaloid
Half-life: 3–15 hours (in adult nonsmokers)
Clinically important, potentially hazardous interactions with: adenosine, anagrelide, arformoterol, azithromycin, BCG vaccine, caffeine, capsicum, carbimazole, cimetidine, ciprofloxacin, clorazepate, cocoa, erythromycin, eucalyptus, febuxostat, fluvoxamine, halothane, indacaterol, influenza vaccine, levofloxacin, mebendazole, methylprednisolone, moxifloxacin, nilutamide, norfloxacin, obeticholic acid, ofloxacin, oral contraceptives, prednisolone, prednisone, propranolol, rasagiline, raspberry leaf, roflumilast, ropivacaine, roxithromycin, St John's wort, torasemide, torsemide, triamcinolone, zafirlukast

Important contra-indications noted in the prescribing guidelines for: the elderly; nursing mothers

Skin
Dermatitis [7]
Exanthems [5]
Exfoliative dermatitis [6]
Hypersensitivity [6]
Pruritus (itching) [3]
Stevens-Johnson syndrome and toxic epidermal necrolysis (SJS/TEN) [3]
Urticaria / hives [6]

Cardiovascular
Arrhythmias [2]
Palpitation [3]
Tachycardia [2]

Central Nervous System
Insomnia [2]
Seizures [11]
Tremor [2]

Endocrine/Metabolic
SIADH [2]

Gastrointestinal/Hepatic
Abdominal pain [2]
Nausea [5]
Vomiting [2]

Neuromuscular/Skeletal
Rhabdomyolysis [5]

Other
Adverse effects / adverse reactions [3]
Allergic reactions [5]
Death [2]

AMINOSALICYLATE SODIUM

Synonyms: PAS; para-aminosalicylate sodium
Trade name: Paser Granules (Jacobus)
Indications: Tuberculosis
Class: Antibiotic, Antimicrobial, Antimycobacterial (including antitubercular), Salicylate
Half-life: 45–60 minutes
Clinically important, potentially hazardous interactions with: none known
Important contra-indications noted in the prescribing guidelines for: nursing mothers

Skin
Angioedema (formerly named angioneurotic edema) [2]
Bullous dermatosis [2]
DRESS syndrome (Drug-induced hypersensitivity syndrome) [2]
Exanthems [10]
Exfoliative dermatitis [6]
Fixed eruption / fixed drug eruption [6]
Hypersensitivity [2]
Lichenoid eruption / lichenoid reaction [3]
Lupus erythematosus (subacute cutaneous lupus erythematosus (SCLE)) [4]
Photosensitivity [3]
Pruritus (itching) [3]
Purpura [4]
Stevens-Johnson syndrome and toxic epidermal necrolysis (SJS/TEN) [2]
Urticaria / hives [5]

Hair
Alopecia / hair loss [4]

Mucosal
Oral mucosal eruption [2]

Endocrine/Metabolic
Hypothyroidism [2]

Renal
Nephrotoxicity / kidney injury / acute kidney injury (AKI) / drug-induced kidney injury [2]

Other
Adverse effects / adverse reactions [4]

AMIODARONE

Trade names: Cordarone (Wyeth), Pacerone (Upsher-Smith)
Indications: Ventricular fibrillation, ventricular tachycardia
Class: Antiarrhythmic, Antiarrhythmic class III, CYP1A2 inhibitor, CYP3A4 inhibitor
Half-life: 26–107 days
Clinically important, potentially hazardous interactions with: abarelix, acebutolol, acenocoumarol, afatinib, amisulpride, amitriptyline, amprenavir, anisindione, anticoagulants, arsenic, artemether/lumefantrine, asenapine, astemizole, atazanavir, atorvastatin, azoles, betrixaban, boceprevir, bosentan, carbimazole, celiprolol, cholestyramine, cimetidine, ciprofloxacin, clopidogrel, cobicistat/elvitegravir/emtricitabine/tenofovir alafenamide, cobicistat/elvitegravir/emtricitabine/tenofovir disoproxil, colchicine, cyclosporine, dabigatran, daclatasvir, darunavir, degarelix, delavirdine, dextromethorphan, dicumarol, digoxin, diltiazem, disopyramide, dronedarone, droperidol, echinacea, enoxacin, fentanyl, finerenone, flecainide, fosamprenavir, gatifloxacin, grapefruit juice, indinavir, ledipasvir & sofosbuvir, lesinurad, letermovir, levofloxacin, levomepromazine, lidocaine, lomefloxacin, lopinavir, loratadine, macrolide antibiotics, methotrexate, moxifloxacin, naldemedine, nelfinavir, nevirapine, nilotinib, norfloxacin, ofloxacin, orlistat, oxprenolol, pentamidine, phenytoin, pimavanserin, ponesimod, procainamide, propranolol, quinidine, quinine, quinolones, ribociclib, rifabutin, rifampin, rifapentine, ritonavir, ropivacaine, rosuvastatin, simvastatin, sofosbuvir & velpatasvir, sofosbuvir/velpatasvir/voxilaprevir, sotalol, sparfloxacin, St John's wort, sulpiride / levosulpiride, tacrolimus, talazoparib, telaprevir, tetrabenazine, thalidomide, tipranavir, trazodone, vandetanib, venetoclax, verapamil, warfarin, zuclopenthixol
Important contra-indications noted in the prescribing guidelines for: the elderly; nursing mothers; pediatric patients
Note: Amiodarone induced pulmonary toxicity has an incidence of about 5%-10%, and it is considered the most serious adverse effect with mortalities reaching up to 10% of the patients.
Warning: PULMONARY TOXICITY

Skin
Anaphylactoid reactions / anaphylaxis (includes anaphylactic shock) [3]
Angioedema (formerly named angioneurotic edema) [2]
Cutaneous toxicity / skin toxicity [5]
Diaphoresis [2]
Edema / fluid retention (<10%)
Erythema nodosum [2]
Exanthems [5]
Facial erythema (3%) [2]
Flushing / rubefaction (<10%)
Iododerma [2]
Linear IgA bullous dermatosis [6]
Lupus erythematosus (subacute cutaneous lupus erythematosus (SCLE)) [5]
Myxedema [2]
Photosensitivity (10–75%) [42]
Phototoxicity [4]
Pigmentation (Skin) (includes hyperpigmentation) (blue) (<10%) [70]
Pruritus (itching) (<5%) [2]
Psoriasis [2]
Purpura (2%)
Stevens-Johnson syndrome and toxic epidermal necrolysis (SJS/TEN) [2]
Vasculitis (angiitis) / cutaneous vasculitis (angiitis) [6]

Hair
Alopecia / hair loss [5]

Mucosal
Sialorrhea (ptyalism; hypersalivation) (<10%)

Cardiovascular
Arrhythmias (<3%) [3]
Atrial fibrillation (paroxysmal) [3]
Atrioventricular block [3]
Bradycardia / sinus bradycardia [19]
Cardiomyopathy [2]
Cardiotoxicity [4]
Hypotension (16%) [4]
QT interval prolonged / QT prolongation [25]
Tachycardia [2]
Thrombophlebitis [2]
Torsades de pointes [38]
Ventricular arrhythmia [2]

Central Nervous System
Anorexia (10–33%)
Dysgeusia (taste perversion) (<10%)
Headache (3–40%)
Insomnia (3–40%)
Neuromyopathy [5]
Neurotoxicity [6]
Paresthesias (4–9%)
Parkinsonism [4]
Parosmia (<10%)
Peripheral neuropathy [4]
Syncope / fainting [2]
Tremor (3–40%) [5]
Vertigo / dizziness (3–40%)

Endocrine/Metabolic
Hyperthyroidism (includes 'thyroid storm') (<3%) [10]
Hypertransaminasemia (hepatic transaminitis) / elevated transaminases [3]
Hyponatremia [7]
Hypothyroidism (<3%) [21]
Myxedema coma / myxedema crisis [10]
SIADH [13]
Thyroid dysfunction [28]
Thyroiditis [2]
Thyrotoxicosis [29]

Gastrointestinal/Hepatic
Abdominal pain (<10%)
Constipation (10–33%)
Hepatic failure [6]
Hepatic steatosis [2]
Hepatitis (<3%) [3]
Hepatotoxicity / liver injury / acute liver injury / drug-induced liver injury (DILI) [36]
Nausea (10–33%)
Pancreatitis / acute pancreatitis [5]

Vomiting (10–33%)

Genitourinary
Epididymitis [4]

Hematologic
Neutropenia (neutrophils decreased) [2]

Local
Injection-site phlebitis [4]

Neuromuscular/Skeletal
Ataxia [7]
Myoclonus (see also hypnic jerk) [3]
Rhabdomyolysis [7]

Ocular
Corneal deposits (>90%) [2]
Keratopathy [6]
Ocular adverse effect [5]
Ocular toxicity [3]
Optic neuropathy [8]
Visual disturbances (2–9%)

Otic
Vestibular disorder / vestibulopathy [3]

Renal
Renal failure [3]
Renal phospholipidosis [2]

Respiratory
Acute respiratory distress syndrome [5]
Alveolar hemorrhage (pulmonary) [2]
Cough [2]
Eosinophilic pneumonia [2]
Interstitial lung disease / interstitial pneumonitis / interstitial pneumonia (cryptogenic organizing pneumonia) / drug-induced interstitial lung disease [5]
Pneumonia [4]
Pneumonitis [5]
Pulmonary fibrosis [2]
Pulmonary toxicity [32]

Other
Adverse effects / adverse reactions [5]
Death [13]
Side effects (12%) [4]

AMISULPRIDE

Trade names: Barhemsys (Acacia Pharma), Deniban (Sanofi-Aventis), Solian (Sanofi-Aventis)
Indications: Prevention of postoperative nausea and vomiting (lower doses). Psychoses, schizophrenia (higher doses)
Class: Antiemetic, Antipsychotic, Antipsychotic, atypical, Dopamine receptor antagonist
Half-life: 4–5 hours (following intravenous infusion)
Clinically important, potentially hazardous interactions with: amiodarone, bepridil, cisapride, disopyramide, droperidol, erythromycin, flecainide, levodopa, ondansetron, pentamidine, procainamide, quinidine, sotalol, sparfloxacin, terfenadine, thioridazine
Pregnancy category: Insufficient data to establish a drug associated risk of major birth defects, miscarriage or adverse maternal or fetal outcomes.
Important contra-indications noted in the prescribing guidelines for: nursing mothers
Note: Approved by FDA for prevention of postoperative nausea and vomiting, February 2020. Avoid use in patients with congenital long QT syndrome and in patients taking droperidol.

Cardiovascular
Bradycardia / sinus bradycardia [5]
Hypertension [2]
Hypotension (3%) [2]
QT interval prolonged / QT prolongation [10]
Torsades de pointes [5]

Central Nervous System
Agitation [2]
Akathisia [2]
Chills (4%)
Extrapyramidal symptoms [3]
Insomnia [4]
Mania [4]
Neuroleptic malignant syndrome [5]
Rabbit syndrome (oral vertical dyskinesia) [2]
Sedation [3]
Seizures [2]
Somnolence (drowsiness) [2]
Tardive syndrome / tardive dyskinesia [3]
Tic disorder [2]
Tremor [2]

Endocrine/Metabolic
ALT increased [2]
Creatine phosphokinase (CPK) / creatine kinase increased (hyperCKemia) [2]
Galactorrhea [4]
Hyperprolactinemia (5%) [8]
Hypokalemia (4%)
Lactate dehydrogenase levels increased [2]
Weight gain [10]

Gastrointestinal/Hepatic
Abdominal distension (2%)

Local
Infusion-site pain (6%)

Neuromuscular/Skeletal
Asthenia / fatigue [2]
Dystonia [5]

Ocular
Oculogyric crisis / oculogyric dystonic reaction [2]

AMITRIPTYLINE

Trade names: Elavil (AstraZeneca), Limbitrol (Valeant)
Indications: Depression
Class: Antidepressant; tricyclic, Muscarinic antagonist
Half-life: 10–25 hours
Clinically important, potentially hazardous interactions with: adrenergic neurone blockers, alcohol, alfuzosin, altretamine, amiodarone, amphetamines, amprenavir, anticholinergics, antiepileptics, antihistamines, antimuscarinics, antipsychotics, apraclonidine, arsenic, artemether/lumefantrine, aspirin, atomoxetine, baclofen, barbiturates, brimonidine, bupropion, cannabis extract, carbamazepine, cimetidine, cinacalcet, ciprofloxacin, cisapride, clonidine, clozapine, cobicistat/elvitegravir/emtricitabine/tenofovir alafenamide, cobicistat/elvitegravir/emtricitabine/tenofovir disoproxil, conivaptan, coumarins, CYP2D6 inhibitors, desmopressin, dexmethylphenidate, diltiazem, disopyramide, disulfiram, diuretics, dronedarone, droperidol, duloxetine, entacapone, ephedra, epinephrine, estrogens, eucalyptus, flecainide, gadobutrol, general anesthetics, gotu kola, grapefruit juice, guanethidine, histamine, interferon alfa, iobenguane, isocarboxazid, isoproterenol, kava, linezolid, lithium, MAO inhibitors, methylphenidate, metoclopramide, moclobemide, moxifloxacin, moxonidine, nefopam, nicorandil, nilotinib, nitrates, NSAIDs, opioid analgesics, paroxetine hydrochloride, pentamidine, phenelzine, phenothiazines, phenytoin, pimozide, pramlintide, primidone, propafenone, propoxyphene, protease inhibitors, QT interval prolonging agents, quinidine, quinine, quinolones, rasagiline, ritonavir, saquinavir, selegiline, sibutramine, sodium oxybate, sotalol, sparfloxacin, SSRIs, St John's wort, sulfonylureas, terbinafine, tetrabenazine, thioridazine, thyroid hormones, tramadol, tranylcypromine, valerian, valproic acid, verapamil, vitamin K antagonists, yohimbine, ziprasidone
Important contra-indications noted in the prescribing guidelines for: the elderly; nursing mothers; pediatric patients
Note: Limbitrol is amitriptyline and chlordiazepoxide.
Warning: SUICIDALITY AND ANTIDEPRESSANT DRUGS

Skin
Diaphoresis (<10%)
DRESS syndrome (Drug-induced hypersensitivity syndrome) [2]
Erythema annulare centrifugum [2]
Photosensitivity [3]
Pigmentation (Skin) (includes hyperpigmentation) [4]
Pruritus (itching) [3]
Pseudolymphoma / cutaneous pseudolymphoma [2]
Purpura [2]

Mucosal
Xerostomia (dry mouth) (>10%) [17]

Cardiovascular
Brugada syndrome [4]
Myocardial infarction [2]
Postural hypotension [2]
QT interval prolonged / QT prolongation [2]

Central Nervous System
Delirium [2]
Depression [2]
Dysgeusia (taste perversion) (>10%) [2]
Hallucinations [3]
Hallucinations, visual [2]
Headache [2]
Restless legs syndrome / Willis-Ekbom disease (includes restless arms syndrome variant) [2]
Sedation [3]
Seizures [7]
Serotonin syndrome [4]
Somnolence (drowsiness) [8]
Vertigo / dizziness [6]

Endocrine/Metabolic
SIADH [5]
Weight gain [7]

Gastrointestinal/Hepatic
Cholestasis / cholestatic jaundice [2]
Constipation [5]
Nausea [2]

Neuromuscular/Skeletal
Asthenia / fatigue [4]
Rhabdomyolysis [2]

Ocular
Vision blurred [2]

Otic
Tinnitus [3]

Other
Adverse effects / adverse reactions [5]
Death [3]

AMLEXANOX

Trade names: Aphthasol (Discus), Aphtheal (Straken), OraDisc (Access), Solfa (Takeda)
Indications: Aphthous ulcers, canker sores
Class: Anti-inflammatory
Half-life: ~3.5 hours
Clinically important, potentially hazardous interactions with: none known
Important contra-indications noted in the prescribing guidelines for: the elderly; nursing mothers; pediatric patients

---

Skin
Dermatitis [3]

AMLODIPINE

Synonyms: Levamlodipine (levoamlodipine); (S)-amlodipine
Trade names: Caduet (Pfizer), Exforge (Novartis), Istin (Pfizer), Lotrel (Novartis), Norvasc (Pfizer), Prestalia (Symplmed), Tekamlo (Novartis)
Indications: Hypertension, angina

Class: Antiarrhythmic class IV, Calcium channel blocker
Half-life: 30–50 hours
Clinically important, potentially hazardous interactions with: amprenavir, carbamazepine, cobicistat/elvitegravir/emtricitabine/tenofovir alafenamide, cobicistat/elvitegravir/emtricitabine/tenofovir disoproxil, conivaptan, delavirdine, epirubicin, imatinib, phenytoin, primidone, sildenafil, simvastatin, St John's wort, tadalafil, telaprevir
Important contra-indications noted in the prescribing guidelines for: the elderly; nursing mothers; pediatric patients
Note: Caduet is amlodipine and atorvastatin; Exforge is amlodipine and valsartan; Lotrel is amlodipine and benazepril; Prestalia is amlodipine and perindopril; Tekamlo is amlodipine and aliskiren.

Skin
Angioedema (formerly named angioneurotic edema) [6]
Cutaneous toxicity / skin toxicity [2]
Dermatitis (<10%)
Eczema / eczematous reaction / eczematous eruption [2]
Edema / fluid retention (5–14%) [22]
Erythema multiforme [2]
Exanthems (2–4%) [2]
Flushing / rubefaction (<10%) [5]
Peripheral edema (>10%) [47]
Pigmentation (Skin) (includes hyperpigmentation) [2]
Pruritus (itching) (2–4%) [3]
Purpura [2]
Rash (<10%)
Stevens-Johnson syndrome and toxic epidermal necrolysis (SJS/TEN) [2]
Telangiectasia [6]
Vasculitis (angiitis) / cutaneous vasculitis (angiitis) [2]

Mucosal
Gingival hyperplasia / gingival hypertrophy / gingival enlargement / gingival overgrowth [44]
Oral pigmentation [2]

Cardiovascular
Bradycardia / sinus bradycardia [2]
Hypotension [9]
Orthostatic hypotension [2]

Central Nervous System
Headache [14]
Parkinsonism [2]
Syncope / fainting [2]
Vertigo / dizziness [18]

Endocrine/Metabolic
Hyponatremia [2]

Gastrointestinal/Hepatic
Diarrhea [3]
Gastritis / pangastritis / gastric irritation [2]
Hepatotoxicity / liver injury / acute liver injury / drug-induced liver injury (DILI) [3]
Nausea [5]
Vomiting [2]

Neuromuscular/Skeletal
Asthenia / fatigue [5]
Rhabdomyolysis [2]

Respiratory
Bronchitis [2]
Cough [3]
Upper respiratory tract infection [5]

Other
Adverse effects / adverse reactions [8]

AMOBARBITAL

Indications: Insomnia, sedation
Class: Barbiturate
Half-life: initial: 40 minutes; terminal: 20 hours
Clinically important, potentially hazardous interactions with: alcohol, dicumarol, ethanolamine, warfarin
Important contra-indications noted in the prescribing guidelines for: nursing mothers; pediatric patients

---

Local
Injection-site pain (>10%)

AMODIAQUINE

Trade names: Camoquin (Pfizer), Flavoquin (Sanofi-Aventis)
Indications: Malaria
Class: Anti-inflammatory, Antimalarial
Half-life: 15.7–19.5 hours
Clinically important, potentially hazardous interactions with: none known
Important contra-indications noted in the prescribing guidelines for: pediatric patients

---

Skin
Pruritus (itching) [4]

Central Nervous System
Extrapyramidal symptoms [4]

Gastrointestinal/Hepatic
Abdominal pain [3]
Diarrhea [3]
Hepatotoxicity / liver injury / acute liver injury / drug-induced liver injury (DILI) [3]
Vomiting [9]

Hematologic
Neutropenia (neutrophils decreased) [2]

Neuromuscular/Skeletal
Asthenia / fatigue [5]

Other
Adverse effects / adverse reactions [3]
Death [2]

AMOXAPINE

Trade name: Amoxapine (Watson)
Indications: Depression
Class: Antidepressant; tricyclic, Muscarinic antagonist
Half-life: 11–30 hours
Clinically important, potentially hazardous interactions with: amprenavir, artemether/lumefantrine, clonidine, dronedarone, epinephrine, fluoxetine, guanethidine, iobenguane, isocarboxazid, linezolid, MAO inhibitors, nilotinib, phenelzine, pimozide, quetiapine, quinine, quinolones, sparfloxacin, tetrabenazine, thioridazine, toremifene, tranylcypromine, vandetanib, vemurafenib, ziprasidone
Important contra-indications noted in the prescribing guidelines for: the elderly; nursing mothers; pediatric patients
Warning: SUICIDALITY AND ANTIDEPRESSANT DRUGS

Skin
AGEP [3]
Diaphoresis (<10%)
Edema / fluid retention (<10%)
Exanthems [2]
Rash (<10%)
Stevens-Johnson syndrome and toxic epidermal necrolysis (SJS/TEN) [2]

Mucosal
Xerostomia (dry mouth) (14%)

Central Nervous System
Dysgeusia (taste perversion) (>10%)
Headache (<10%)
Insomnia (<10%)
Neuroleptic malignant syndrome [2]
Seizures [2]
Somnolence (drowsiness) (14%)
Vertigo / dizziness (<10%)

Endocrine/Metabolic
Galactorrhea [2]

Gastrointestinal/Hepatic
Constipation (12%)
Nausea (<10%)

Neuromuscular/Skeletal
Asthenia / fatigue (<10%)

Ocular
Vision blurred (7%)

Other
Side effects (5%)

AMOXICILLIN

Synonym: amoxycillin
Trade names: Amoxil (GSK), Augmentin (GSK), Clavulin (GSK), Prevpac (TAP), Trimox (Bristol-Myers Squibb)
Indications: Infections of the respiratory tract, skin and urinary tract
Class: Antibiotic, Antibiotic; beta-lactam, Antibiotic; penicillin, Antimicrobial
Half-life: 0.7–1.4 hours
Clinically important, potentially hazardous interactions with: allopurinol, bromelain, chloramphenicol, demeclocycline, doxycycline,

erythromycin, imipenem/cilastatin, methotrexate, minocycline, omeprazole, oxytetracycline, sulfonamides, tetracycline

Note: Augmentin and Clavulin are trade names for a combination of amoxicillin and clavulanic acid. The International Nonproprietary Name for this combination is amoxicillin/clavulanic acid, and co-amoxiclav the British Approved Name.

Skin
- AGEP [30]
- Anaphylactoid reactions / anaphylaxis (includes anaphylactic shock) [17]
- Angioedema (formerly named angioneurotic edema) (<10%) [5]
- Baboon syndrome / symmetrical drug-related intertriginous and flexural exanthema (SDRIFE) [16]
- Bullous pemphigoid / pemphigoid [2]
- Dermatitis [4]
- DRESS syndrome (Drug-induced hypersensitivity syndrome) [12]
- Edema / fluid retention [2]
- Erythema multiforme [18]
- Exanthems (>5%) [33]
- Exfoliative dermatitis [2]
- Fixed eruption / fixed drug eruption [10]
- Hypersensitivity [5]
- Jarisch–Herxheimer reaction [2]
- Linear IgA bullous dermatosis [5]
- Pemphigus [4]
- Pruritus (itching) [7]
- Pustules / pustular eruption [8]
- Rash (<10%) [14]
- Serum sickness-like reaction (<10%) [6]
- Stevens-Johnson syndrome and toxic epidermal necrolysis (SJS/TEN) [23]
- Sweet's syndrome [2]
- Toxic pustuloderma [2]
- Urticaria / hives (<5%) [16]

Mucosal
- Black tongue / black hairy tongue (lingua villosa nigra) [2]
- Stomatitis (oral mucositis) [2]

Cardiovascular
- Kounis syndrome / allergic angina syndrome / allergic myocardial infarction [8]

Central Nervous System
- Anorexia [2]
- Aseptic meningitis [17]
- Dysgeusia (taste perversion) [6]
- Hallucinations [3]
- Headache [5]
- Psychosis [3]
- Somnolence (drowsiness) [3]
- Vertigo / dizziness [5]

Gastrointestinal/Hepatic
- Abdominal distension [2]
- Abdominal pain [7]
- Diarrhea [20]
- Dyspepsia / functional dyspepsia (indigestion) (see also gastroparesis) [2]
- Enterocolitis [4]
- Gut microbiome / gut microbiota / gastrointestinal microbiota changes / disturbance [2]
- Hepatotoxicity / liver injury / acute liver injury / drug-induced liver injury (DILI) [39]
- Nausea [13]
- Pancreatitis / acute pancreatitis [2]
- Vomiting [9]

Genitourinary
- Vaginitis (includes vulvitis) [3]

Hematologic
- Neutropenia (neutrophils decreased) [2]

Neuromuscular/Skeletal
- Asthenia / fatigue [3]
- Rhabdomyolysis [2]

Renal
- Nephropathy [3]
- Nephrotoxicity / kidney injury / acute kidney injury (AKI) / drug-induced kidney injury [2]

Other
- Adverse effects / adverse reactions [20]
- Side effects [4]
- Tooth fluorosis / dental fluorosis [2]
- Tooth pigmentation / discoloration [2]

AMPHOTERICIN B

Trade names: Abelcet (Sigma-Tau), AmBisome (Astellas), Amphocin (Pfizer), Amphotec (Alkopharma)

Indications: Potentially life-threatening fungal infections

Class: Antifungal / antimycotic, Antimicrobial

Half-life: initial: 15–48 hours; terminal: 15 days

Clinically important, potentially hazardous interactions with: adefovir, aminoglycosides, arsenic, astemizole, betamethasone, cephalothin, cidofovir, cyclosporine, digoxin, ethoxzolamide, fluconazole, flucytosine, ganciclovir, griseofulvin, hydrocortisone, itraconazole, ketoconazole, micafungin, pentamidine, probenecid, sulpiride / levosulpiride, terbinafine, triamcinolone, voriconazole

Important contra-indications noted in the prescribing guidelines for: nursing mothers

---

Skin
- Anaphylactoid reactions / anaphylaxis (includes anaphylactic shock) [4]
- Cutaneous toxicity / skin toxicity [2]
- Diaphoresis (7%)
- Exanthems [4]
- Flushing / rubefaction (<10%) [2]
- Peripheral edema (15%)
- Pruritus (itching) (11%) [2]
- Purpura [3]
- Rash (25%) [2]
- Urticaria / hives [2]

Mucosal
- Epistaxis (nosebleed) (15%)

Cardiovascular
- Chest pain (12%)
- Hypertension (8%) [4]
- Hypotension (14%)
- Tachycardia (13%)
- Thrombophlebitis (<10%)

Central Nervous System
- Anorexia (>10%)
- Anxiety (14%)
- Chills (48%) [6]
- Confusion (11%)
- Delirium (>10%)
- Fever (pyrexia) (includes hyperpyrexia) (>10%) [6]
- Headache (20%)
- Insomnia (17%)
- Leukoencephalopathy / posterior reversible encephalopathy syndrome (PRES) [4]
- Pain (14%)
- Paresthesias (<10%)
- Parkinsonism [2]
- Rigors [2]

Endocrine/Metabolic
- ALP increased (22%)
- ALT increased (15%)
- AST increased (13%)
- Creatine phosphokinase (CPK) / creatine kinase increased (hyperCKemia) (22%)
- Hyperglycemia (includes glucose increased) (23%)
- Hypernatremia (4%)
- Hypervolemia (fluid overload) (12%)
- Hypocalcemia (18%)
- Hypokalemia [5]
- Hypomagnesemia (20%)

Gastrointestinal/Hepatic
- Abdominal pain (20%)
- Diarrhea (30%)
- Gastrointestinal bleeding (10%)
- Hepatotoxicity / liver injury / acute liver injury / drug-induced liver injury (DILI) [6]
- Nausea (40%)
- Vomiting (32%)

Genitourinary
- Hematuria (14%)
- Urinary retention (<10%)

Hematologic
- Anemia (>10%) [4]
- Leukocytosis (elevated white blood cell (WBC) count) (<10%)
- Pancytopenia (includes bicytopenia) [3]
- Sepsis (14%)
- Thrombocytopenia / platelets decreased [3]

Local
- Infusion-related reactions [6]
- Infusion-site reactions [2]
- Injection-site pain (>10%)
- Injection-site phlebitis [2]
- Injection-site reaction [5]

Neuromuscular/Skeletal
- Asthenia / fatigue (13%)
- Back pain (12%)

Otic
- Ototoxicity [3]

Renal
- Nephrotoxicity / kidney injury / acute kidney injury (AKI) / drug-induced kidney injury [57]

Respiratory
- Bronchospasm [2]
- Cough (18%)
- Dyspnea / shortness of breath (23%)
- Hypoxia (8%)
- Pleural effusion (13%)
- Pulmonary toxicity (18%)
- Rhinitis / rhinosinusitis (see also sinusitis) (11%)
- Tachypnea / respiratory rate increased (>10%)

Other
- Adverse effects / adverse reactions [6]
- Death [5]
- Infection (11%)

AMPICILLIN

Trade name: Totacillin (GSK)
Indications: Susceptible strains of gram-negative and gram-positive bacterial infections
Class: Antibiotic, Antibiotic; beta-lactam, Antibiotic; penicillin, Antimicrobial
Half-life: 1–1.5 hours
Clinically important, potentially hazardous interactions with: allopurinol, anticoagulants, chloramphenicol, cyclosporine, demeclocycline, doxycycline, erythromycin, imipenem/cilastatin, levodopa, methotrexate, minocycline, oxytetracycline, sulfonamides, tetracycline
Important contra-indications noted in the prescribing guidelines for: nursing mothers
Note: Five to 10% of people taking ampicillin develop eruptions between the 5th and 14th day following initiation of therapy. Also, there is a 95% incidence of exanthematous eruptions in patients who are treated for infectious mononucleosis with ampicillin. The allergenicity of ampicillin appears to be enhanced by allopurinol or by hyperuricemia. Ampicillin is clearly the more allergenic of the two drugs when given alone.
Used in combination with sulbactam (as Unasyn).

Skin
- AGEP [9]
- Anaphylactoid reactions / anaphylaxis (includes anaphylactic shock) [10]
- Angioedema (formerly named angioneurotic edema) [2]
- Baboon syndrome / symmetrical drug-related intertriginous and flexural exanthema (SDRIFE) [3]
- Dermatitis [8]
- Erythema multiforme [11]
- Exanthems (>10%) [84]
- Exfoliative dermatitis [3]
- Fixed eruption / fixed drug eruption [10]
- Hypersensitivity [5]
- Linear IgA bullous dermatosis [4]
- Pemphigus [6]
- Pruritus (itching) (<5%) [5]
- Psoriasis [5]
- Purpura [6]
- Pustules / pustular eruption [4]
- Rash (<10%)
- Stevens-Johnson syndrome and toxic epidermal necrolysis (SJS/TEN) [23]
- Urticaria / hives [16]
- Vasculitis (angiitis) / cutaneous vasculitis (angiitis) [4]

Hematologic
- Thrombocytopenia / platelets decreased [2]

Local
- Injection-site pain (>10%)

Other
- Allergic reactions (<10%) [3]

AMPICILLIN/ SULBACTAM

Trade name: Unasyn (Pfizer)
Indications: Various infections caused by susceptible organisms
Class: Antibiotic, Antibiotic; beta-lactam, Antibiotic; penicillin, Antimicrobial
Half-life: 1 hour
Clinically important, potentially hazardous interactions with: allopurinol, probenecid
Important contra-indications noted in the prescribing guidelines for: nursing mothers
Note: Serious and occasionally fatal hypersensitivity (anaphylactic) reactions have been reported in patients on penicillin therapy. Contra-indicated in patients with a history of hypersensitivity reactions to any of the penicillins.

Skin
- Anaphylactoid reactions / anaphylaxis (includes anaphylactic shock) [2]
- Linear IgA bullous dermatosis [3]
- Rash (<10%) [2]

Gastrointestinal/Hepatic
- Diarrhea (<10%)
- Hepatotoxicity / liver injury / acute liver injury / drug-induced liver injury (DILI) [2]

Local
- Injection-site pain (16%)

Renal
- Nephrotoxicity / kidney injury / acute kidney injury (AKI) / drug-induced kidney injury [2]

AMPRENAVIR

Trade name: Agenerase (GSK)
Indications: HIV infection
Class: Antiretroviral, HIV-1 protease inhibitor
Half-life: 7–11 hours
Clinically important, potentially hazardous interactions with: alprazolam, amiodarone, amitriptyline, amlodipine, amoxapine, antacids, atorvastatin, avanafil, benzodiazepines, bepridil, bosentan, carbamazepine, cisapride, clomipramine, clonazepam, clorazepate, cyclosporine, delavirdine, desipramine, dexamethasone, diazepam, didanosine, dihydroergotamine, diltiazem, doxepin, efavirenz, ergotamine, estradiol, felodipine, fentanyl, flibanserin, flurazepam, fluticasone propionate, imipramine, indinavir, isradipine, itraconazole, ixabepilone, ketoconazole, lidocaine, lopinavir, lorazepam, lovastatin, lumateperone, methadone, methylergonovine, methysergide, midazolam, mifepristone, nelfinavir, nevirapine, nicardipine, nifedipine, nimodipine, nisoldipine, nortriptyline, olaparib, oral contraceptives, oxazepam, phenobarbital, phenytoin, pimozide, protriptyline, quazepam, quinidine, rapamycin, rifabutin, rifampin, ritonavir, saquinavir, sildenafil, simvastatin, St John's wort, tacrolimus, temazepam, trazodone, triazolam, tricyclic antidepressants, trimipramine, verapamil, vitamin E, warfarin
Important contra-indications noted in the prescribing guidelines for: nursing mothers; pediatric patients

---

Skin
- Rash (20–27%) [6]
- Stevens-Johnson syndrome and toxic epidermal necrolysis (SJS/TEN) (4%)

Central Nervous System
- Depression (9–16%)
- Dysgeusia (taste perversion) (10%)
- Mood changes (includes mood disorder) (9–16%)
- Paresthesias (perioral) (26–31%) [4]

Gastrointestinal/Hepatic
- Diarrhea (39–60%)
- Loose stools / soft feces (39–60%)
- Nausea (43–74%)
- Vomiting (24–34%)

AMYL NITRITE

Indications: Angina pectoris
Class: Nitrate, Vasodilator
Half-life: N/A
Clinically important, potentially hazardous interactions with: furosemide, sildenafil, tadalafil, vardenafil
Important contra-indications noted in the prescribing guidelines for: nursing mothers; pediatric patients

---

Skin
- Dermatitis [3]
- Flushing / rubefaction (<10%)

ANAGRELIDE

Trade names: Agrylin (Shire), Xagrid (Shire)
Indications: Essential thrombocytopenia, to reduce elevated platelet count and the risk of thrombosis
Class: Phospholipase A2 inhibitor
Half-life: 1.3 hours
Clinically important, potentially hazardous interactions with: aminophylline, aspirin, cilostazol, enoximone, fluvoxamine, fondaparinux, inamrinone, milrinone, olprinone, sucralfate
Important contra-indications noted in the prescribing guidelines for: nursing mothers
Note: Contraindicated in patients with severe hepatic impairment.

Skin
- Bruise / bruising / contusion / ecchymosis (ecchymoses) (<5%)
- Edema / fluid retention (21%) [10]
- Peripheral edema (7%)
- Photosensitivity (<5%)
- Pruritus (itching) (<5%)
- Rash (8%)
- Urticaria / hives (8%)

Hair
- Alopecia / hair loss (<5%)

Mucosal
- Aphthous stomatitis / aphthous ulcer / aphtha (aphthae) (<5%)

Cardiovascular
- Arrhythmias [5]
- Cardiomyopathy [2]
- Myocardial toxicity [2]
- Palpitation (26%) [4]
- Pericardial effusion [2]
- Tachycardia [5]

Central Nervous System
- Chills (<5%)
- Depression (<5%)

Headache (44%) [12]
Pain (15%)
Paresthesias (7%)
Vertigo / dizziness (15%)

Gastrointestinal/Hepatic
Abdominal pain [3]

Genitourinary
Erectile dysfunction [2]

Hematologic
Anemia [2]

Neuromuscular/Skeletal
Arthralgia (<5%)
Asthenia / fatigue (23%)
Back pain (6%)
Leg cramps (<5%)
Myalgia/Myopathy (<5%)

Otic
Tinnitus (<5%)

Respiratory
Dyspnea / shortness of breath (12%)
Influenza- ('flu)-like syndrome (<5%)

Other
Adverse effects / adverse reactions (<5%)

ANAKINRA

Trade name: Kineret (Amgen)
Indications: Rheumatoid arthritis, neonatal-onset multisystem inflammatory disease
Class: Biologic, Biologic disease-modifying antirheumatic drug (bDMARD), Covid-19 putative drug, Disease-modifying antirheumatic drug (DMARD), Interleukin-1 receptor antagonist (IL-IRa)
Half-life: 4–6 hours
Clinically important, potentially hazardous interactions with: abatacept, adalimumab, certolizumab, etanercept, golimumab, infliximab, lenalidomide, live vaccines
Important contra-indications noted in the prescribing guidelines for: nursing mothers

---

Central Nervous System
Fever (pyrexia) (includes hyperpyrexia) (12%)
Headache (12–14%) [2]

Gastrointestinal/Hepatic
Abdominal pain (5%)
Diarrhea (8%)
Nausea (8%)
Vomiting (14%)

Local
Injection-site edema [2]
Injection-site erythema [3]
Injection-site inflammation [2]
Injection-site pain [4]
Injection-site reaction (71%) [32]

Neuromuscular/Skeletal
Arthralgia (6–12%)

Respiratory
Influenza- ('flu)-like syndrome (6%)
Nasopharyngitis (12%)
Sinusitis (see also rhinitis / rhinosinusitis) (7%)
Upper respiratory tract infection (4%) [2]

Other
Adverse effects / adverse reactions [6]
Death [2]
Infection (40%) [11]

ANASTROZOLE

Trade name: Arimidex (AstraZeneca)
Indications: Breast carcinoma (localized &#x2013, advanced or metastatic)
Class: Antineoplastic / anticancer agent (see also Immune checkpoint inhibitor), Aromatase inhibitor
Half-life: 50 hours
Clinically important, potentially hazardous interactions with: estradiol, estrogens, tamoxifen
Pregnancy category: Contra-indicated in women of premenopausal endocrine status, including pregnant women
Important contra-indications noted in the prescribing guidelines for: nursing mothers
Note: The efficacy of anastrozole in the treatment of pubertal gynecomastia in adolescent boys and in the treatment of precocious puberty in girls with McCune-Albright syndrome has not been demonstrated.

Skin
Flushing / rubefaction (>5%)
Hot flashes / hot flushes (12–36%) [13]
Lupus erythematosus (subacute cutaneous lupus erythematosus (SCLE)) [3]
Peripheral edema (10%)
Pruritus (itching) (2–5%)
Rash (6–11%) [2]
Vasculitis (angiitis) / cutaneous vasculitis (angiitis) [2]

Hair
Alopecia / hair loss (2–5%)

Cardiovascular
Angina (2%)
Hypertension (2–13%)
Thrombophlebitis (2–5%)

Central Nervous System
Carpal tunnel syndrome [2]
Depression (5–13%)
Headache (9–13%) [2]
Pain (14%)
Tumor pain (>5%)

Endocrine/Metabolic
Mastodynia (2–5%)

Gastrointestinal/Hepatic
Diarrhea [2]
Hepatitis [2]
Hepatotoxicity / liver injury / acute liver injury / drug-induced liver injury (DILI) [6]
Nausea (11–19%)
Vomiting (8–13%)

Genitourinary
Vaginal dryness (2%) [3]

Neuromuscular/Skeletal
Arthralgia (2–5%) [8]
Asthenia / fatigue (19%) [7]
Back pain (12%) [2]
Bone pain / joint pain (6–11%) [2]
Joint disorder [3]
Myalgia/Myopathy (2–5%) [2]
Osteoporosis (11%)

Respiratory
Cough (11%)
Influenza- ('flu)-like syndrome (7%)
Pharyngitis (sore throat) (6–14%)

Other
Infection (2–5%)

ANDROSTENEDIONE

Synonym: N/A
Other common trade names: Andro, Androstene
Indications: Enhanced athletic performance, increased energy, to keep red blood cells healthy
Class: Aromatase inhibitor
Half-life: N/A
Clinically important, potentially hazardous interactions with: none known
Note: Protease inhibitors cause dyslipidemia which includes elevated triglycerides and cholesterol and redistribution of body fat centrally to produce the so-called 'protease paunch', breast enlargement, facial atrophy, and 'buffalo hump'
In 2004 the FDA requested companies to stop distributing products containing androstenedione. Studies have shown that it does not increase muscle mass and that it poses the same kind of health risks as anabolic steroids, including abnormal elevations in serum estrogen, increased risk of prostate, pancreatic and endometrial cancers, and increased cardiovascular disease risk.

Skin
Acneiform eruption / acneiform dermatitis / acneiform rash [2]

Other
Adverse effects / adverse reactions [6]

ANIDULAFUNGIN

Trade names: Ecalta (Pfizer), Eraxis (Pfizer)
Indications: Candidemia, candidal esophagitis
Class: Antimycobacterial; echinocandin
Half-life: 40–50 hours
Clinically important, potentially hazardous interactions with: none known
Important contra-indications noted in the prescribing guidelines for: nursing mothers; pediatric patients

---

Skin
Angioedema (formerly named angioneurotic edema) (<2%)
Erythema (<2%)
Flushing / rubefaction (<2%) [2]
Hot flashes / hot flushes (<2%)
Hyperhidrosis (<2%)
Peripheral edema (11%)
Pruritus (itching) (<2%)
Ulcerations (5%)
Urticaria / hives (<2%)

Mucosal
Oral candidiasis (5%)

Cardiovascular
Atrial fibrillation (<2%)
Bundle branch block (<2%)
Chest pain (5%)
Hypertension (12%)
Hypotension (15%)
Phlebitis [2]
Thrombophlebitis (<2%)
Venous thromboembolism (10%)

Central Nervous System
Confusion (8%)
Depression (6%)

Fever (pyrexia) (includes hyperpyrexia) (9–18%) [4]
Headache (8%) [5]
Insomnia (15%)
Rigors (<2%)
Seizures (<2%)
Vertigo / dizziness (<2%)

Endocrine/Metabolic
ALP increased (12%)
ALT increased (2%)
Creatine phosphokinase (CPK) / creatine kinase increased (hyperCKemia) (5%)
Dehydration (6%)
Hyperglycemia (includes glucose increased) (6%)
Hyperkalemia (6%)
Hypoglycemia (7%)
Hypokalemia (5–15%)
Hypomagnesemia (12%)

Gastrointestinal/Hepatic
Abdominal pain (6%)
Cholestasis / cholestatic jaundice (<2%)
Constipation (8%)
Diarrhea (9–18%) [3]
Dyspepsia / functional dyspepsia (indigestion) (see also gastroparesis) (aggravated) (7%)
Hepatotoxicity / liver injury / acute liver injury / drug-induced liver injury (DILI) [4]
Nausea (7–24%) [5]
Vomiting (7–18%) [6]

Genitourinary
Urinary tract infection (15%)

Hematologic
Anemia (8–9%)
Coagulopathy / coagulation dysfunction / clotting factor deficiency (includes disseminated intravascular coagulation / DIC) (<2%)
Leukocytosis (elevated white blood cell (WBC) count) (5%)
Sepsis (7%)
Thrombocythemia (thrombocytosis) / platelets increased (6%)
Thrombocytopenia / platelets decreased (<2%)

Local
Infusion-related reactions [2]

Neuromuscular/Skeletal
Back pain (5%)

Ocular
Ocular pain (<2%)
Vision blurred (<2%)
Visual disturbances (<2%)

Respiratory
Cough (7%)
Dyspnea / shortness of breath (12%)
Pleural effusion (10%)
Pneumonia (6%)
Respiratory distress (6%)

Other
Adverse effects / adverse reactions [4]
Infection (63%)

ANIFROLUMAB

Trade name: Saphnelo (AstraZeneca)
Indications: Systemic lupus erythematosus
Class: Interferon receptor antagonist, Monoclonal antibody
Half-life: not available
Clinically important, potentially hazardous interactions with: none known
Note: Serious hypersensitivity reactions (including anaphylaxis) have been reported following anifrolumab administration.
The efficacy of anifrolumab has not been evaluated in patients with severe active lupus nephritis or severe active central nervous system lupus. Use of anifrolumab is not recommended in these situations.

Skin
Herpes zoster (6%) [2]
Hypersensitivity (3%)

Local
Infusion-related reactions (9%)

Respiratory
Bronchitis (11%) [2]
Cough (5%)
Nasopharyngitis [2]
Respiratory tract infection (3%)
Upper respiratory tract infection (34%) [2]

Other
Adverse effects / adverse reactions [3]

ANISINDIONE

Trade name: Miradon (Schering)
Indications: Adjunct in treatment of coronary occlusion, atrial fibrillation
Class: Anticoagulant (antithrombotic), Indanedione
Half-life: 3–5 days
Clinically important, potentially hazardous interactions with: amiodarone, anabolic steroids, antithyroid agents, barbiturates, bivalirudin, cimetidine, clofibrate, clopidogrel, cyclosporine, delavirdine, dextrothyroxine, disulfiram, fluconazole, glutethimide, imatinib, itraconazole, ketoconazole, metronidazole, miconazole, nandrolone, penicillins, phenylbutazones, piperacillin, quinidine, quinine, rifabutin, rifampin, rifapentine, rofecoxib, salicylates, sulfinpyrazone, sulfonamides, testosterone, thyroid, zileuton
Important contra-indications noted in the prescribing guidelines for: nursing mothers

ANISTREPLASE

Indications: Acute myocardial infarction
Class: Fibrinolytic
Half-life: 70–120 minutes
Clinically important, potentially hazardous interactions with: none known
Important contra-indications noted in the prescribing guidelines for: nursing mothers

---

Skin
Anaphylactoid reactions / anaphylaxis (includes anaphylactic shock) (<10%) [2]
Vasculitis (angiitis) / cutaneous vasculitis (angiitis) [5]

ANTHRAX VACCINE

Trade name: BioThrax (Emergent BioSolutions)
Indications: Anthrax prophylaxis
Class: Vaccine
Half-life: Requires 1 month to achieve immunity (92.5% efficient)
Clinically important, potentially hazardous interactions with: corticosteroids, immunosuppressive therapies, other vaccines
Important contra-indications noted in the prescribing guidelines for: the elderly; nursing mothers; pediatric patients
Note: Dr. Sue Bailey, Assistant Secretary for Health Affairs, released a statement on June 29, 1999 that 'almost one million shots given, the anthrax immunization is proving to be one of the safest vaccination programs on record.' The ADRs reported occurred for '50 service members at one installation alone.' Note that no number of military personnel was mentioned at this installation, nor did it give any percentages for the reactions reported.

Skin
Diaphoresis [2]
Edema / fluid retention (3%) [2]
Hypersensitivity [5]
Lupus erythematosus (subacute cutaneous lupus erythematosus (SCLE)) [2]
Pruritus (itching) (<10%) [2]
Rash [2]
Stevens-Johnson syndrome and toxic epidermal necrolysis (SJS/TEN) [2]
Urticaria / hives [2]

Central Nervous System
Chills [2]
Fever (pyrexia) (includes hyperpyrexia) [3]
Guillain-Barré syndrome / acute inflammatory demyelinating polyradiculoneuropathy / acute motor axonal neuropathy [2]
Headache (4–64%) [2]

Gastrointestinal/Hepatic
Diarrhea (6–8%)
Nausea (6%)

Genitourinary
Dysmenorrhea (7%)

Local
Injection-site edema [4]
Injection-site nodules [2]
Injection-site pain [4]
Injection-site pruritus [2]
Injection-site reaction [6]

Neuromuscular/Skeletal
Arthralgia [3]
Asthenia / fatigue (5–62%)
Myalgia/Myopathy (2–72%) [3]

Respiratory
Influenza- ('flu)-like syndrome [3]
Nasopharyngitis (12–15%)

Other
Allergic reactions [2]

ANTI-THYMOCYTE GLOBULIN (EQUINE)

Trade name: Atgam (Pfizer)
Indications: Management of allograft rejection in renal transplant patients, prophylaxis of moderate to severe aplastic anemia in patients who are unsuitable for bone marrow transplantation
Class: Immunosuppressant
Half-life: 3–9 days
Clinically important, potentially hazardous interactions with: none known
Important contra-indications noted in the prescribing guidelines for: nursing mothers
Note: Contraindicated in patients who have had a severe systemic reaction during prior administration of any equine gamma globulin preparation.

Skin
- Lymphadenopathy [2]
- Serum sickness [6]

Central Nervous System
- Fever (pyrexia) (includes hyperpyrexia) [2]

Genitourinary
- Hematuria [2]

Hematologic
- Anemia (70%)
- Leukocytopenia (leukopenia) / leukocytes (white blood cells) decreased (47%)
- Lymphopenia (lymphocytopenia) / lymphocytes decreased (41%)

Neuromuscular/Skeletal
- Arthralgia (16%) [3]
- Asthenia / fatigue (39%) [5]
- Back pain [2]
- Fractures (12%)
- Pain in extremities [2]

APALUTAMIDE

Trade name: Erleada (Janssen Biotech)
Indications: Non-metastatic castration-resistant prostate cancer
Class: Androgen antagonist
Clinically important, potentially hazardous interactions with: none known
Pregnancy category: Can cause fetal harm and potential loss of pregnancy

---

Skin
- Cutaneous adverse reaction (includes severe cutaneous adverse drug reaction (SCAR)) [4]
- DRESS syndrome (Drug-induced hypersensitivity syndrome) [2]
- Exanthems (24%)
- Hot flashes / hot flushes (14%) [2]
- Maculopapular rash / morbilliform rash [5]
- Peripheral edema (11%)
- Pruritus (itching) (6%)
- Rash (24%) [7]
- Stevens-Johnson syndrome and toxic epidermal necrolysis (SJS/TEN) [6]

Cardiovascular
- Cardiac failure (2%)
- Hypertension (25%) [2]
- Myocardial ischemia (4%)

Central Nervous System
- Gait instability / postural instability (16%)

Endocrine/Metabolic
- Appetite decreased (12%)
- Hypercholesterolemia (76%)
- Hyperglycemia (includes glucose increased) (70%)
- Hyperkalemia (32%)
- Hypertriglyceridemia (includes triglycerides increased) (67%)
- Hypothyroidism (8%) [3]
- Weight loss (16%) [3]

Gastrointestinal/Hepatic
- Abdominal pain [3]
- Constipation [2]
- Diarrhea (20%) [4]
- Nausea (18%) [4]

APIXABAN

Trade name: Eliquis (Bristol-Myers Squibb)
Indications: Reduce the risk of stroke and systemic embolism in patients with nonvalvular atrial fibrillation
Class: Anticoagulant (antithrombotic), Direct factor Xa inhibitor
Half-life: 5–12 hours
Clinically important, potentially hazardous interactions with: carbamazepine, darunavir, phenytoin, rifampin, St John's wort, tipranavir, voriconazole
Important contra-indications noted in the prescribing guidelines for: nursing mothers; pediatric patients
Note: Contra-indicated in patients with active pathological bleeding.
Warning: DISCONTINUING ELIQUIS IN PATIENTS WITHOUT ADEQUATE CONTINUOUS ANTICOAGULATION INCREASES RISK OF STROKE

Skin
- Pruritic rash [2]

Cardiovascular
- Cardiac tamponade / pericardial tamponade [5]
- Pericardial effusion [3]

Gastrointestinal/Hepatic
- Esophagitis [2]
- Hepatotoxicity / liver injury / acute liver injury / drug-induced liver injury (DILI) [2]

Hematologic
- Hemorrhage [15]

Neuromuscular/Skeletal
- Spinal epidural hematoma [2]

Respiratory
- Interstitial lung disease / interstitial pneumonitis / interstitial pneumonia (cryptogenic organizing pneumonia) / drug-induced interstitial lung disease [3]

Other
- Adverse effects / adverse reactions [5]

APOMORPHINE

Trade names: Apokyn (Ipsen), Uprima (AbbVie)
Indications: Parkinsonism, erectile dysfunction
Class: Dopamine receptor agonist
Half-life: 40 minutes
Clinically important, potentially hazardous interactions with: 5HT3 antagonists, alcohol, alosetron, antihypertensives, dolasetron, granisetron, levomepromazine, ondansetron, palonosetron, risperidone, vasodilators, zuclopenthixol
Important contra-indications noted in the prescribing guidelines for: the elderly; nursing mothers
Note: Apomorphine contains sodium metabisulfite which is capable of causing anaphylactoid reactions in patients with sulfite allergy.

Skin
- Bruise / bruising / contusion / ecchymosis (ecchymoses) (>5%)
- Diaphoresis (1–10%)
- Edema / fluid retention (10%)
- Nodular eruption [5]
- Panniculitis [2]
- Peripheral edema (10%)

Mucosal
- Rhinorrhea (20%)

Cardiovascular
- Angina (15%)
- Chest pain (15%)
- Congestive heart failure (>5%)

Central Nervous System
- Confusion (10%)
- Depression (>5%)
- Dysgeusia (taste perversion) [2]
- Dyskinesia (24–35%) [2]
- Hallucinations (10%) [2]
- Headache (>5%) [4]
- Impulse control disorder / impulsivity / drug-induced impulsivity [2]
- Psychosis [2]
- Somnolence (drowsiness) (35%) [2]
- Syncope / fainting (2%)
- Vertigo / dizziness (20%) [5]
- Yawning (40%) [2]

Gastrointestinal/Hepatic
- Nausea (30%) [6]
- Vomiting (30%) [2]

Local
- Infusion-site granuloma (4%)
- Injection-site pruritus (2%)
- Injection-site reaction (26%) [3]

Neuromuscular/Skeletal
- Arthralgia (>5%)
- Asthenia / fatigue (>5%)
- Back pain (>5%)

APRACLONIDINE

Trade name: Iopidine (Alcon)
Indications: Post-surgical intraocular pressure elevation
Class: Adrenergic alpha2-receptor agonist
Half-life: 8 hours
Clinically important, potentially hazardous interactions with: amitriptyline
Important contra-indications noted in the prescribing guidelines for: nursing mothers; pediatric patients

---

Skin
- Dermatitis [3]
- Pruritus (itching) (10%)

Mucosal
- Xerostomia (dry mouth) (<10%)

Central Nervous System
- Dysgeusia (taste perversion) (3%)

Ocular
- Conjunctivitis (conjunctival inflammation) (<5%)
- Eyelid edema / palpebral edema / blepharedema (<3%)
- Ocular itching / ocular pruritus (5–15%)
- Xerophthalmia (dry eyes) (<5%)

Other
- Allergic reactions [5]

APREMILAST

Trade name: Otezla (Celgene)
Indications: Psoriatic arthritis, plaque psoriasis
Class: Antipsoriatic agent, Phosphodiesterase inhibitor, Phosphodiesterase type 4 (PDE4) inhibitor
Half-life: 6–9 hours
Clinically important, potentially hazardous interactions with: carbamazepine, phenobarbital, phenytoin, rifampin
Important contra-indications noted in the prescribing guidelines for: nursing mothers; pediatric patients

---

Central Nervous System
- Depression [4]
- Headache (5–6%) [35]

Endocrine/Metabolic
- ALT increased [2]
- Appetite decreased [2]
- Weight loss (10–12%) [8]

Gastrointestinal/Hepatic
- Abdominal pain (<2%) [5]
- Diarrhea (8–9%) [43]
- Dyspepsia / functional dyspepsia (indigestion) (see also gastroparesis) [2]
- Gastrointestinal disorder / discomfort [3]
- Loose stools / soft feces [2]
- Nausea (7–9%) [42]
- Vomiting (<3%) [11]

Neuromuscular/Skeletal
- Arthralgia [2]
- Asthenia / fatigue [5]

Respiratory
- Nasopharyngitis (<3%) [23]
- Upper respiratory tract infection (<4%) [17]

Other
- Adverse effects / adverse reactions [6]
- Infection [2]

APREPITANT

Trade name: Emend (Merck)
Indications: Prevention of postoperative and chemotherapy induced nausea and vomiting
Class: Antiemetic, CYP3A4 inhibitor, Neurokinin 1 receptor antagonist
Half-life: 9–13 hours
Clinically important, potentially hazardous interactions with: alprazolam, antifungal agents, astemizole, avanafil, betamethasone, carbamazepine, cisapride, clarithromycin, colchicine, conivaptan, corticosteroids, CYP2C9 substrates, CYP3A4 inducers or inhibitors, dasatinib, deferasirox, dexamethasone, diltiazem, docetaxel, eplerenone, estrogens, everolimus, fentanyl, grapefruit juice, halofantrine, ifosfamide, imatinib, irinotecan, itraconazole, ketoconazole, lumateperone, methylprednisolone, midazolam, mifepristone, naldemedine, nefazodone, neratinib, olaparib, oral contraceptives, paroxetine hydrochloride, phenobarbital, phenytoin, pimecrolimus, pimozide, progestins, ranolazine, rifampin, rifamycin derivatives, rifapentine, ritonavir, salmeterol, saxagliptin, St John's wort, telithromycin, terfenadine, tolbutamide, tolvaptan, trabectedin, triamcinolone, troleandomycin, vinblastine, vincristine, voriconazole, warfarin
Pregnancy category: Insufficient evidence to inform drug-associated risk
Important contra-indications noted in the prescribing guidelines for: nursing mothers; pediatric patients
Note: Fosaprepitant is a prodrug of aprepitant for injection. Aprepitant treatment is given along with a 5-HT3-receptor antagonist and dexamethasone.

Skin
- Pruritus (itching) (8%)

Hair
- Alopecia / hair loss (12%)

Mucosal
- Mucocutaneous reactions (3%)
- Stomatitis (oral mucositis) (3%)

Cardiovascular
- Hypertension (2%)
- Hypotension (6%)

Central Nervous System
- Anorexia (6–10%) [4]
- Encephalopathy (includes hepatic encephalopathy) [2]
- Fever (pyrexia) (includes hyperpyrexia) (3–6%)
- Headache (5–9%) [6]
- Insomnia (2–3%)
- Somnolence (drowsiness) [2]
- Vertigo / dizziness (3–7%) [3]

Endocrine/Metabolic
- ALT increased (6%)
- AST increased (3%)
- Creatine phosphokinase (CPK) / creatine kinase increased (hyperCKemia) (4%)
- Dehydration (6%)

Gastrointestinal/Hepatic
- Abdominal pain (5%) [3]
- Constipation (9–10%) [10]
- Diarrhea (<10%) [3]
- Dyspepsia / functional dyspepsia (indigestion) (see also gastroparesis) (5–6%)
- Flatulence (4%)
- Gastritis / pangastritis / gastric irritation (4%)
- Nausea (6–13%) [2]
- Vomiting (3–8%)

Genitourinary
- Urinary tract infection (2%)

Hematologic
- Anemia (3%)
- Febrile neutropenia [3]
- Neutropenia (neutrophils decreased) (3–6%) [4]

Local
- Infusion-related reactions [2]
- Infusion-site pain [2]

Neuromuscular/Skeletal
- Asthenia / fatigue (5–18%) [11]

Otic
- Tinnitus (4%)

Renal
- Proteinuria (7%)

Other
- Hiccups / singultus (11%) [9]
- Infection [3]

APROBARBITAL

Trade name: Alurate (Roche)
Indications: Short-term sedation, sleep induction
Class: Barbiturate
Half-life: 14–34 hours
Clinically important, potentially hazardous interactions with: alcohol, brompheniramine, buclizine, dicumarol, ethanolamine, warfarin
Important contra-indications noted in the prescribing guidelines for: the elderly; nursing mothers; pediatric patients

APROTININ

Trade name: Trasylol (Bayer)
Indications: For prophylactic use to reduce blood loss in patients undergoing coronary artery bypass surgery
Class: Antifibrinolytic, Serine protease inhibitor
Half-life: 150 minutes
Clinically important, potentially hazardous interactions with: captopril, enalapril, lisinopril, quinapril
Important contra-indications noted in the prescribing guidelines for: nursing mothers; pediatric patients
Warning: ANAPHYLACTIC OR ANAPHYLACTOID REACTIONS

Skin
- Anaphylactoid reactions / anaphylaxis (includes anaphylactic shock) [26]
- Hypersensitivity [4]
- Lipohypertrophy [2]
- Peripheral edema (5%)
- Rash (2%)

Cardiovascular
- Arrhythmias (3–4%)
- Atrial fibrillation (21%)
- Atrial flutter (6%)
- Cardiac failure (5%)
- Chest pain (2%)
- Extrasystoles (6%)
- Hypertension (4%)
- Hypotension (8%)
- Myocardial infarction (6%)
- Pericarditis (5%)
- Phlebitis (1–10%)
- Supraventricular tachycardia (4%)
- Tachycardia (6%)
- Ventricular tachycardia (5%)

Central Nervous System
- Confusion (4%)
- Fever (pyrexia) (includes hyperpyrexia) (15%)
- Insomnia (3%)

Endocrine/Metabolic
- Creatine phosphokinase (CPK) / creatine kinase increased (hyperCKemia) (2%)

Gastrointestinal/Hepatic
- Constipation (4%)
- Diarrhea (3%)
- Nausea (11%)
- Vomiting (3%)

Genitourinary
- Urinary retention (3%)
- Urinary tract infection (2%)

Hematologic
- Anemia (2%)
- Thrombosis (<2%)

Neuromuscular/Skeletal
- Asthenia / fatigue (2%)

Renal
- Nephrotoxicity / kidney injury / acute kidney injury (AKI) / drug-induced kidney injury [2]
- Renal failure (<2%)
- Renal function abnormal / renal dysfunction (3%)

Respiratory
- Asthma (2%)
- Dyspnea / shortness of breath (4%)
- Hypoxia (2%)
- Pleural effusion (7%)
- Pneumothorax (4–5%)
- Pulmonary edema (cardiogenic / non-cardiogenic) (<2%)
- Pulmonary toxicity (8%)

Other
- Allergic reactions [2]
- Death [2]
- Infection (6%)

ARBUTAMINE

Trade name: GenESA (Sicor)
Indications: Diagnostic aid for coronary artery disease
Class: Adrenergic beta-receptor agonist
Half-life: 1.8 hours
Clinically important, potentially hazardous interactions with: abacavir, clidinium, clomipramine, desipramine, dicyclomine, digoxin, doxepin, flavoxate, glycopyrrolate, hyoscyamine, imipramine, mepenzolate, methantheline, nortriptyline, oxybutynin, procyclidine, propantheline, protriptyline, scopolamine, trihexyphenidyl, trimipramine
Important contra-indications noted in the prescribing guidelines for: pediatric patients

---

Skin
- Diaphoresis (2%)
- Flushing / rubefaction (3%)
- Hot flashes / hot flushes (3%)

Central Nervous System
- Pain (2%)
- Paresthesias (2%)
- Tremor (15%)

ARFORMOTEROL

Trade name: Brovana (Sunovion)
Indications: Chronic obstructive pulmonary disease including chronic bronchitis and emphysema
Class: Beta-2 adrenergic agonist, Bronchodilator
Half-life: 26 hours
Clinically important, potentially hazardous interactions with: aminophylline, beta blockers, MAO inhibitors, tricyclic antidepressants
Important contra-indications noted in the prescribing guidelines for: nursing mothers; pediatric patients
Note: Studies in asthma patients showed that long-acting beta$_2$-adrenergic agonists may increase the risk of asthma-related death. Contra-indicated in patients with asthma without use of a long-term asthma control medication.
Warning: ASTHMA-RELATED DEATH

Skin
- Abscess (<2%)
- Edema / fluid retention (<2%)
- Herpes simplex (<2%)
- Herpes zoster (<2%)
- Peripheral edema (3%)
- Pigmentation (Skin) (includes hyperpigmentation) (<2%)
- Rash (4%)
- Xerosis / xeroderma (<2%)

Mucosal
- Oral candidiasis (<2%)

Cardiovascular
- Arteriosclerosis (<2%)
- Atrioventricular block (<2%)
- Chest pain (7%) [2]
- Digitalis intoxication (<2%)
- QT interval prolonged / QT prolongation (<2%)
- Supraventricular tachycardia (<2%)

Central Nervous System
- Agitation (<2%)
- Fever (pyrexia) (includes hyperpyrexia) (<2%)
- Headache [2]
- Hypokinesia (<2%)
- Insomnia [2]
- Nervousness [3]
- Pain (8%)
- Paresthesias (<2%)
- Somnolence (drowsiness) (<2%)
- Tremor (<2%) [3]

Gastrointestinal/Hepatic
- Nausea [2]

Genitourinary
- Cystitis (includes interstitial cystitis / bladder pain syndrome) (<2%)
- Nocturia (<2%)

Local
- Injection-site pain (<2%)

Neuromuscular/Skeletal
- Arthralgia (<2%)
- Back pain (6%)
- Leg cramps (4%)
- Neck rigidity (<2%)

Ocular
- Glaucoma (includes acute angle-closure glaucoma) (<2%)
- Visual disturbances (<2%)

Respiratory
- Bronchitis [3]
- COPD (exacerbation) [3]
- Dysphonia (includes voice disorders / voice changes) (<2%)
- Dyspnea / shortness of breath (4%)
- Influenza- ('flu)-like syndrome (3%)
- Nasopharyngitis [3]
- Sinusitis (see also rhinitis / rhinosinusitis) (4%) [2]

Other
- Adverse effects / adverse reactions [2]
- Allergic reactions (<2%)
- Neoplasms (<2%)

ARGATROBAN

Trade name: Acova (GSK)
Indications: Heparin-induced thrombocytopenia
Class: Anticoagulant (antithrombotic), Thrombin inhibitor
Half-life: 40–50 minutes
Clinically important, potentially hazardous interactions with: abacavir, anticoagulants, antiplatelet agents, butabarbital, collagen (bovine)collagenase, dasatinib, ibritumomab, NSAIDs, pentosan, prostacyclin analogs, salicylates, throbolytic agents, tositumomab & iodine^{131}
Important contra-indications noted in the prescribing guidelines for: nursing mothers; pediatric patients
Note: Contraindicated in patients with overt major bleeding.

Cardiovascular
- Atrial fibrillation (3%)
- Bradycardia / sinus bradycardia (5%)
- Cardiac arrest (6%)
- Chest pain (15%)
- Hypotension (7–11%)
- Myocardial infarction (4%)
- Ventricular tachycardia (5%)

Central Nervous System
- Fever (pyrexia) (includes hyperpyrexia) (4–7%)
- Headache (5%)
- Neurotoxicity (2%)
- Pain (5%)

Gastrointestinal/Hepatic
- Abdominal pain (3–4%)
- Diarrhea (6%)
- Gastrointestinal bleeding (2%)
- Hematemesis (3%)
- Nausea (5–7%)
- Vomiting (4–6%)

Genitourinary
- Hematuria (2–12%)
- Urinary tract infection (5%)

Hematologic
- Bleeding (5%) [3]
- Sepsis (6%)
- Thrombosis [2]

Local
- Injection-site bleeding (2–5%)

Neuromuscular/Skeletal
- Back pain (8%)

Renal
- Renal function abnormal / renal dysfunction (3%)

Respiratory
- Cough (3%)
- Dyspnea / shortness of breath (8%)
- Hemoptysis (<3%)
- Pneumonia (3%)

Other
- Infection (4%)

ARIPIPRAZOLE

Trade names: Abilify (Bristol-Myers Squibb), Aristada (Alkermes)
Indications: Schizophrenia, bipolar I disorder, major depressive disorder, irritability associated with autistic disorder
Class: Antipsychotic, Antipsychotic, atypical, Mood stabilizer
Half-life: 75–94 hours
Clinically important, potentially hazardous interactions with: alcohol, atazanavir, carbamazepine, CYP3A4 inhibitors, efavirenz, itraconazole, ketoconazole, lopinavir, nelfinavir, paroxetine hydrochloride, quinidine
Important contra-indications noted in the prescribing guidelines for: the elderly; pediatric patients
Warning: INCREASED MORTALITY IN ELDERLY PATIENTS WITH DEMENTIA-RELATED PSYCHOSIS
SUICIDALITY AND ANTIDEPRESSANT DRUGS

Skin
Rash (6%) [2]
Stevens-Johnson syndrome and toxic epidermal necrolysis (SJS/TEN) [2]

Mucosal
Sialorrhea (ptyalism; hypersalivation) (4–9%) [5]
Xerostomia (dry mouth) (5%) [7]

Cardiovascular
Arrhythmias [2]
Hypertension [3]
Palpitation [2]
QT interval prolonged / QT prolongation [2]

Central Nervous System
Agitation (19%) [5]
Akathisia (8–13%) [40]
Anxiety (17%) [11]
Compulsions / obsessive-compulsive symptoms / obsessive-compulsive disorder [4]
Dyskinesia [3]
Extrapyramidal symptoms [12]
Fever (pyrexia) (includes hyperpyrexia) (2%)
Headache (27%) [15]
Hypersexuality [2]
Hypothermia [3]
Impulse control disorder / impulsivity / drug-induced impulsivity [6]
Insomnia (18%) [23]
Irritability [5]
Mania [2]
Neuroleptic malignant syndrome [17]
Neurotoxicity [2]
Parkinsonism [14]
Psychosis [2]
Rabbit syndrome (oral vertical dyskinesia) [4]
Restlessness [11]
Schizophrenia (exacerbation) [2]
Sedation [12]
Somnolence (drowsiness) (5–11%) [15]
Stroke / cerebrovascular accident [2]
Suicidal ideation [6]
Tardive syndrome / tardive dyskinesia [8]
Tic disorder [3]
Tremor (3%) [10]
Vertigo / dizziness [8]

Endocrine/Metabolic
Appetite increased [5]
Diabetes mellitus [2]
Galactorrhea [2]
Hyperprolactinemia [2]
SIADH [2]
Weight gain (2–30%) [37]

Gastrointestinal/Hepatic
Constipation (11%) [6]
Dyspepsia / functional dyspepsia (indigestion) (see also gastroparesis) (9%)
Hepatotoxicity / liver injury / acute liver injury / drug-induced liver injury (DILI) [2]
Nausea (15%) [14]
Vomiting (11%) [6]

Genitourinary
Enuresis (urinary incontinence) [3]
Priapism [5]
Urinary retention [2]
Vaginitis (includes vulvitis) [2]

Hematologic
Neutropenia (neutrophils decreased) [5]

Local
Injection-site pain [10]

Neuromuscular/Skeletal
Asthenia / fatigue [6]
Ataxia [4]
Dystonia [14]
Pisa syndrome (pleurothotonus) [2]
Rhabdomyolysis [4]

Ocular
Oculogyric crisis / oculogyric dystonic reaction [7]
Vision blurred (3–8%)

Respiratory
Cough (3%)
Nasopharyngitis [2]
Upper respiratory tract infection [3]

Other
Adverse effects / adverse reactions [6]
Death [3]
Hiccups / singultus [6]
Toothache (odontalgia) [2]

ARISTOLOCHIA

Family: Aristolochiaceae
Scientific names: *Aristolochia clematitis, Aristolochia serpentaria*
Indications: Aphrodisiac, anti-allergy, anticonvulsant, promotes menstruation
Class: Immunomodulator
Half-life: N/A
Clinically important, potentially hazardous interactions with: none known
Note: Aristolochia has been reported to cause severe kidney damage or 'Chinese herb nephropathy'. Eighteen patients developed carcinomas of the bladder, ureter and/or renal pelvis.
Aristolochia is banned in the European Union and Japan.

Skin
Carcinoma [2]
Cutaneous toxicity / skin toxicity [2]

Renal
Nephrotoxicity / kidney injury / acute kidney injury (AKI) / drug-induced kidney injury [9]

ARNICA

Family: Asteraceae; Compositae
Scientific names: *Arnica fulgens, Arnica montana, Arnica sororia*
Indications: Bruising, aches and sprains, insect bites, superficial phlebitis, diuretic, flavoring agent, found in hair tonic and shampoo
Class: Immunomodulator
Half-life: N/A
Clinically important, potentially hazardous interactions with: none known

---

Skin
Dermatitis [5]

ARSENIC

Synonyms: Arsenic trioxide (Trisenox); Potassium arsenite solution (Fowler's solution)
Trade name: Trisenox (Cephalon)
Indications: Acute promyelocytic leukemia, psoriasis (in the early 1900s), devitalization of pulp in dental procedures
Class: Antineoplastic / anticancer agent (see also Immune checkpoint inhibitor), Trace element
Half-life: 10–14 hours
Clinically important, potentially hazardous interactions with: abacavir, acetazolamide, alfuzosin, aloe vera (gel, juice, leaf), amiodarone, amitriptyline, amphotericin B, artemether/lumefantrine, bretylium, chloroquine, chlorpromazine, ciprofloxacin, clomipramine, clozapine, disopyramide, diuretics, dronedarone, droperidol, enoxacin, erythromycin, fluphenazine, gadobutrol, garlic, gatifloxacin, ginger, ginseng, haloperidol, indacaterol, levofloxacin, levomepromazine, lithium, lomefloxacin, mesoridazine, moxifloxacin, nilotinib, norfloxacin, ofloxacin, phenothiazines, pimozide, procainamide, prochlorperazine, promethazine, QT prolonging antipsychotics, quetiapine, quinidine, quinine, quinolones, sotalol, sparfloxacin, tetrabenazine, thioridazine, toremifene, trifluoperazine, vandetanib, vemurafenib, ziprasidone, zuclopenthixol
Important contra-indications noted in the prescribing guidelines for: nursing mothers; pediatric patients
Warning: APL DIFFERENTIATION SYNDROME and ECG ABNORMALITIES

Skin
Basal cell carcinoma [5]
Bruise / bruising / contusion / ecchymosis (ecchymoses) (20%)
Bullous dermatosis [4]
Carcinoma [20]
Dermatitis (43%) [6]
Edema / fluid retention (40%) [2]
Erythema (13%)
Erythema multiforme [4]
Exanthems [5]
Exfoliative dermatitis (5%) [7]
Facial edema (8%)
Fixed eruption / fixed drug eruption [2]
Flushing / rubefaction (10%)
Gangrene [2]
Herpes simplex (13%)
Herpes zoster (8%) [4]
Hyperhidrosis (13%)
Hyperkeratosis (palms and soles) (40%) [5]

Hypersensitivity (5%)
Keratoses [20]
Leukomelanosis [7]
Lymphadenopathy (8%)
Melanoma [5]
Melanosis / melanocytosis [6]
Merkel cell carcinoma [4]
Pallor (10%)
Palmar–plantar desquamation [16]
Palmar–plantar hyperhidrosis [2]
Palmar–plantar hyperkeratosis [20]
Palmar–plantar punctate keratoses [2]
Petechiae (8%)
Pigmentation (Skin) (includes hyperpigmentation) (8%) [15]
Pityriasis rosea (from organic arsenic) [2]
Pruritus (itching) (33%)
Purpura (20%)
Squamous cell carcinoma [15]
Squamous cell carcinoma in situ (Bowen disease) [6]
Stevens-Johnson syndrome and toxic epidermal necrolysis (SJS/TEN) [4]
Urticaria / hives (8%)
Xerosis / xeroderma (15%)

Hair

Alopecia / hair loss [4]

Nails

Leukonychia striata (Mees' lines) [3]
Nail pigmentation [2]

Mucosal

Epistaxis (nosebleed) (25%)
Oral candidiasis (5%)
Oral mucosal eruption (8%) [3]
Xerostomia (dry mouth) (8%)

Cardiovascular

Arrhythmias [2]
Chest pain (25%)
Hypertension (10%)
Hypotension (25%)
Palpitation (10%)
QT interval prolonged / QT prolongation (40%) [10]
Tachycardia (55%)
Torsades de pointes [3]

Central Nervous System

Agitation (5%)
Anorexia (23%)
Anxiety (30%)
Coma (5%)
Confusion (5%)
Depression (20%)
Fever (pyrexia) (includes hyperpyrexia) (63%)
Headache (60%)
Insomnia (43%)
Neurotoxicity [2]
Pain (15%)
Paresthesias (33%)
Pseudotumor cerebri [2]
Rigors (38%)
Seizures (8%)
Somnolence (drowsiness) (8%)
Tremor (13%)
Vertigo / dizziness (23%)

Endocrine/Metabolic

Acidosis (includes lactic acidosis) (5%)
ALT increased (20%)
Appetite decreased (15%)
AST increased (13%)
Hyperglycemia (includes glucose increased) (45%)
Hyperkalemia (18%)
Hypocalcemia (10%)
Hypoglycemia (8%)
Hypokalemia (50%)
Hypomagnesemia (45%)
Weight gain (13%)
Weight loss (8%)

Gastrointestinal/Hepatic

Abdominal distension (8%)
Abdominal pain (58%)
Black stools / melena (8%)
Constipation (28%) [2]
Diarrhea (53%)
Dyspepsia / functional dyspepsia (indigestion) (see also gastroparesis) (10%)
Fecal incontinence (8%)
Gastrointestinal bleeding (8%)
Hepatotoxicity / liver injury / acute liver injury / drug-induced liver injury (DILI) [3]
Loose stools / soft feces (10%)
Nausea (75%) [2]
Pancreatitis / acute pancreatitis [2]
Vomiting (58%) [2]

Genitourinary

Enuresis (urinary incontinence) (5%)
Oliguria (5%)
Vaginal bleeding (13%)

Hematologic

Anemia (20%)
Bleeding (8%)
Febrile neutropenia (13%)
Leukocytosis (elevated white blood cell (WBC) count) (50%)
Neutropenia (neutrophils decreased) (10%) [2]
Sepsis (5%)
Thrombocytopenia / platelets decreased (18%)

Local

Injection-site edema (10%)
Injection-site erythema (13%)
Injection-site pain (20%)

Neuromuscular/Skeletal

Arthralgia (33%)
Asthenia / fatigue (63%)
Back pain (18%)
Bone pain / joint pain (23%)
Myalgia/Myopathy (25%)
Neck pain (13%)
Osteonecrosis / avascular necrosis (includes steroid-induced osteonecrosis of the femoral head) [8]
Pain in extremities (13%)

Ocular

Eyelid edema / palpebral edema / blepharedema (5%)
Ocular itching / ocular pruritus (10%)
Vision blurred (10%)
Xerophthalmia (dry eyes) (8%)

Otic

Ear pain (8%)
Tinnitus (5%)

Renal

Renal failure (8%)

Respiratory

Cough (65%)
Dyspnea / shortness of breath (53%)
Hemoptysis (8%)
Hypoxia (23%)
Nasopharyngitis (5%)
Pharyngolaryngeal pain (35%)
Pleural effusion (20%)
Rhonchi (8%)
Sinusitis (see also rhinitis / rhinosinusitis) (20%)
Tachypnea / respiratory rate increased (8%)
Upper respiratory tract infection (13%)
Wheezing (13%)

Other

Death [3]

ARTEMETHER/LUMEFANTRINE

Trade name: Coartem (Novartis)
Indications: Acute, uncomplicated malaria infections due to *Plasmodium falciparum* in patients of 5kg bodyweight and above
Class: Antimalarial
Half-life: ~2 hours (artemether); 3–6 days (lumefantrine)
Clinically important, potentially hazardous interactions with: amiodarone, amitriptyline, amoxapine, antimalarials, antiretrovirals, arsenic, astemizole, atazanavir, atovaquone/proguanil, azithromycin, carbamazepine, ciprofloxacin, citalopram, clomipramine, conivaptan, CYP2D6 substrates, CYP3A4 inducers, inhibitors or substrates, darunavir, dasatinib, degarelix, delavirdine, disopyramide, dolasetron, duloxetine, flecainide, halofantrine, hormonal contraceptives, imipramine, indinavir, itraconazole, lapatinib, levofloxacin, levomepromazine, lopinavir, mefloquine, moxifloxacin, nelfinavir, norfloxacin, ofloxacin, paroxetine hydrochloride, pazopanib, phenytoin, pimozide, procainamide, quinidine, quinine, rifampin, risperidone, sotalol, St John's wort, telavancin, telithromycin, terfenadine, tipranavir, venlafaxine, voriconazole, vorinostat, ziprasidone, zuclopenthixol
Important contra-indications noted in the prescribing guidelines for: nursing mothers; pediatric patients
Note: Artemether/Lumefantrine tablets should not be used to treat severe malaria or to prevent malaria.

Skin

Abscess (<3%)
Impetigo (<3%)
Inflammation [3]
Pruritus (itching) (4%) [2]
Rash (3%) [6]
Urticaria / hives (<3%) [2]

Cardiovascular

Palpitation (18%) [2]

Central Nervous System

Agitation (<3%)
Anorexia (40%) [6]
Chills (23%)
Fever (pyrexia) (includes hyperpyrexia) (25–29%) [6]
Gait instability / postural instability (<3%)
Headache (56%) [9]
Hypoesthesia / hypesthesia (numbness) (<3%)
Insomnia (5%) [2]
Mood changes (includes mood disorder) (<3%)
Seizures [2]
Sleep disturbances (22%)
Sleep-related disorder [2]
Tremor (<3%)
Vertigo / dizziness (39%) [9]

Endocrine/Metabolic
ALT increased (<3%)
AST increased (<3%)
Hypokalemia (<3%)

Gastrointestinal/Hepatic
Abdominal pain (17%) [12]
Constipation (<3%)
Diarrhea (8%) [12]
Dyspepsia / functional dyspepsia (indigestion) (see also gastroparesis) (<3%)
Dysphagia (<3%)
Gastroenteritis (<3%)
Hepatomegaly (6–9%)
Nausea [8]
Peptic ulceration (includes duodenal ulcer, esophageal ulcer) (<3%)
Vomiting [17]

Genitourinary
Hematuria (<3%)
Urinary tract infection (<3%)

Hematologic
Anemia (4–9%) [4]
Eosinophilia / eosinophils increased (<3%)
Hemolytic anemia [2]
Neutropenia (neutrophils decreased) [2]
Thrombocytopenia / platelets decreased (<3%)

Neuromuscular/Skeletal
Arthralgia (34%)
Asthenia / fatigue (38%) [10]
Ataxia (<3%)
Back pain (<3%)
Myalgia/Myopathy (32%)

Ocular
Conjunctivitis (conjunctival inflammation) (<3%)
Nystagmus (<3%)

Otic
Ear infection (<3%)
Hearing impairment [2]
Tinnitus (<3%)

Renal
Proteinuria (<3%)

Respiratory
Asthma (<3%)
Bronchitis (<3%)
Cough (6–23%) [3]
Influenza (<3%)
Nasopharyngitis (4%)
Pharyngolaryngeal pain (<3%)
Pneumonia (<3%)
Rhinitis / rhinosinusitis (see also sinusitis) (4%)
Upper respiratory tract infection (<3%)

Other
Adverse effects / adverse reactions [5]
Death [2]
Infection (<3%)

ARTEMISIA

Family: Asteraceae
Scientific names: *Artemisia annua, Benflumetol, Co-artemether, Coartem, Riamet (Novartis)*
Indications: Fever, multidrug-resistant malaria, parasitemia, leukemia, colon cancer, diarrhea, schistosomiasis, worms, insect bites (topical)
Class: Antimalarial
Half-life: 10 hours
Clinically important, potentially hazardous interactions with: none known
Note: This drug profile only refers to *Artemisia annua*, NOT *Artemisia absinthium*. The latter, the main constituent of absinthe, has serious side effects, including seizures, hallucinations, and death.
Derivatives of *Artemisia annua* are often used in combination with piperaquine, or mefloquine in treatment of malaria. Benflumetol, Coartem and Co-artemether are a combination of artemether-lumefantrine (see separate profile).

Skin
Pruritus (itching) [2]
Rash [2]

Central Nervous System
Headache [2]

Local
Injection-site pain [2]

ARTESUNATE

Trade name: Rtsun (Wiscon)
Indications: *Plasmodium falciparum* malaria
Class: Antimalarial
Half-life: 0.5 hours
Clinically important, potentially hazardous interactions with: efavirenz
Pregnancy category: Use carefully in first three trimesters of pregnancy
Note: Artesunate therapy should be combined with other antimalarials (e.g. mefloquine) if given for less than 5 days.

Skin
Pruritus (itching) [4]

Cardiovascular
QT interval prolonged / QT prolongation [2]

Central Nervous System
Anorexia [3]
Extrapyramidal symptoms [3]
Fever (pyrexia) (includes hyperpyrexia) [4]
Headache [8]
Insomnia [2]
Vertigo / dizziness [12]

Gastrointestinal/Hepatic
Abdominal pain [5]
Diarrhea [6]
Hepatotoxicity / liver injury / acute liver injury / drug-induced liver injury (DILI) [2]
Nausea [6]
Vomiting [16]

Hematologic
Anemia [5]
Hemolysis [7]
Hemolytic anemia [2]
Neutropenia (neutrophils decreased) [2]

Neuromuscular/Skeletal
Asthenia / fatigue [7]
Myalgia/Myopathy [2]

Respiratory
Cough [4]

Other
Adverse effects / adverse reactions [5]

ARTICAINE

Trade names: Orabloc (Pierrel), Septanest (Septodont), Septocaine (Septodont)
Indications: Local, infiltrative, or conductive anesthesia in both simple and complex dental procedures
Class: Anesthetic; local
Half-life: 44 minutes
Clinically important, potentially hazardous interactions with: beta adrenergic blockers, MAO inhibitors, tricyclic antidepressants
Important contra-indications noted in the prescribing guidelines for: pediatric patients
Note: Contra-indicated in patients with a known hypersensitivity to sulfite. All named products above are articaine and epinephrine.

Skin
Facial edema [2]

Cardiovascular
Hypotension [2]

Central Nervous System
Headache [2]
Paresthesias [6]
Somnolence (drowsiness) [2]
Vertigo / dizziness [2]

Gastrointestinal/Hepatic
Nausea [3]

Local
Injection-site pain [3]

Other
Adverse effects / adverse reactions [2]

ARTICHOKE

Family: Asteraceae; Compositae
Scientific names: *Cynara cardunculus, Cynara scolymus*
Indications: Dyspepsia, hyperlipidemia, nausea, hangover, irritable bowel syndrome (IBS), liver dysfunction, hypoglycemia. Flavoring, sweetener, prebiotic
Class: Antiemetic, Carminative
Half-life: N/A
Clinically important, potentially hazardous interactions with: none known
Note: Jerusalem artichoke (*Helianthus tuberosus*) is a completely different plant.

Skin
Dermatitis [3]

ASCIMINIB

Trade name: Scemblix (Novartis)
Indications: Philadelphia chromosome-positive chronic myeloid leukemia in chronic phase, previously treated with two or more tyrosine kinase inhibitors.

Class: Kinase inhibitor, Tyrosine kinase inhibitor
Half-life: 6–9 hours
Clinically important, potentially hazardous interactions with: CYP3A inhibitors, imatinib, itraconazole oral solution containing hydroxypropyl-β-cyclodextrin
Pregnancy category: Based on findings from animal studies, asciminib can cause fetal harm when administered to a pregnant woman. Females of reproductive potential should use

effective contraception during treatment with asciminib and for one week after the last dose.

Skin
Rash (17%) [2]

Mucosal
Oropharyngeal pain [2]

Cardiovascular
Hypertension (6% grade 3 or 4) (13%) [2]

Central Nervous System
Fever (pyrexia) (includes hyperpyrexia) [2]
Headache (2% grade 3 or 4) (19%) [2]
Insomnia [2]
Vertigo / dizziness [2]

Endocrine/Metabolic
ALT increased (23%)
Appetite decreased [3]
AST increased (2% grade 3 or 4) (19%)
Creatine phosphokinase (CPK) / creatine kinase increased (hyperCKemia) (3% grade 3 or 4) (27%)
Hyperamylasemia (12%) [2]
Hyperbilirubinemia (12%)
Hypercholesterolemia (11%)
Hyperlipasemia (4% grade 3 or 4) (14%) [2]
Hypertriglyceridemia (includes triglycerides increased) (5% grade 3 or 4) (44%)
Hyperuricemia (6% grade 3 or 4) (19%)
Hypocalcemia (14%)
Hypokalemia (10%)
Hypophosphatemia (6% grade 3 or 4) (17%)
Serum creatinine increased (14%)

Gastrointestinal/Hepatic
Abdominal pain (10%) [2]
Constipation [2]
Diarrhea (12%) [2]
Nausea (12%) [2]
Vomiting [2]

Hematologic
Anemia [3]
Hemoglobin decreased (2% grade 3 or 4) (35%)
Lymphopenia (lymphocytopenia) / lymphocytes decreased (2% grade 3 or 4) (18%)
Neutropenia (neutrophils decreased) (17% grade 3 or 4) (39%) [3]
Thrombocytopenia / platelets decreased [4]

Neuromuscular/Skeletal
Arthralgia (12%) [2]
Asthenia / fatigue (17%) [3]
Musculoskeletal pain (3% grade 3 or 4) (22%)

Respiratory
Cough [2]
Dyspnea / shortness of breath [2]
Upper respiratory tract infection (26%) [2]

Other
Adverse effects / adverse reactions [2]

ASCORBIC ACID

Synonym: Vitamin C
Indications: Prevention of scurvy
Class: Covid-19 putative drug, Vitamin
Half-life: N/A
Clinically important, potentially hazardous interactions with: deferoxamine, estradiol, penicillamine
Pregnancy category: the pregnancy category will be C if used in doses above the RDA

Genitourinary
Hyperoxaluria [2]

Renal
Oxalate nephropathy [8]

Other
Side effects [2]

ASENAPINE

Trade name: Saphris (Merck)
Indications: Schizophrenia, bipolar disorder
Class: Antipsychotic, Antipsychotic, atypical
Half-life: 24 hours
Clinically important, potentially hazardous interactions with: alcohol, amiodarone, chlorpromazine, CYP2D6 substrates and inhibitors, fluvoxamine, gatifloxacin, moxifloxacin, paroxetine hydrochloride, procainamide, QT prolonging drugs, quinidine, sotalol, thioridazine, ziprasidone
Important contra-indications noted in the prescribing guidelines for: the elderly; nursing mothers; pediatric patients
Warning: INCREASED MORTALITY IN ELDERLY PATIENTS WITH DEMENTIA-RELATED PSYCHOSIS

Skin
Peripheral edema (3%)

Mucosal
Oral numbness [4]
Salivary hypersecretion (2%)
Xerostomia (dry mouth) (2–3%)

Cardiovascular
Hypertension (2–3%) [2]

Central Nervous System
Akathisia (4–6%) [10]
Anxiety (4%)
Depression (2%) [3]
Dysgeusia (taste perversion) (3%) [4]
Extrapyramidal symptoms (6–10%) [11]
Headache (12%) [3]
Hypersomnia [2]
Hypoesthesia / hypesthesia (numbness) (4–5%) [7]
Insomnia (6–15%) [3]
Irritability (2%)
Sedation [9]
Somnolence (drowsiness) (13–24%) [15]
Tardive syndrome / tardive dyskinesia [2]
Vertigo / dizziness (4–11%) [5]

Endocrine/Metabolic
Appetite increased (2–4%)
Weight gain (3–5%) [12]

Gastrointestinal/Hepatic
Abdominal pain [2]
Constipation (5%)
Dyspepsia / functional dyspepsia (indigestion) (see also gastroparesis) (3–4%)
Vomiting (5%)

Neuromuscular/Skeletal
Arthralgia (3%)
Asthenia / fatigue (3–4%)
Dystonia [3]
Pain in extremities (2%)

Other
Adverse effects / adverse reactions [4]

ASPARAGINASE

Synonym: L-asparaginase
Trade names: Elspar (Merck), Kidrolase (EUSA Pharma)
Indications: Acute lymphoblastic leukemia, lymphoma
Class: Antineoplastic / anticancer agent (see also Immune checkpoint inhibitor), Enzyme
Half-life: 8–30 hours (intravenous); 34–49 hours (intramuscular)
Clinically important, potentially hazardous interactions with: none known
Important contra-indications noted in the prescribing guidelines for: nursing mothers

Skin
Anaphylactoid reactions / anaphylaxis (includes anaphylactic shock) (3–40%) [4]
Angioedema (formerly named angioneurotic edema) [3]
Cutaneous toxicity / skin toxicity [2]
Hypersensitivity (6–40%) [16]
Stevens-Johnson syndrome and toxic epidermal necrolysis (SJS/TEN) [2]
Urticaria / hives (<15%) [5]

Mucosal
Aphthous stomatitis / aphthous ulcer / aphtha (aphthae) (<10%)
Oral lesions (26%)
Parotitis [5]
Stomatitis (oral mucositis) (<10%)

Central Nervous System
Chills (>10%)
Coma (25%)
Depression (>10%)
Encephalopathy (includes hepatic encephalopathy) [2]
Fever (pyrexia) (includes hyperpyrexia) (>10%)
Leukoencephalopathy / posterior reversible encephalopathy syndrome (PRES) [3]
Neurotoxicity [4]
Seizures (10–60%) [2]
Somnolence (drowsiness) (>10%)
Stroke / cerebrovascular accident [3]

Endocrine/Metabolic
Hyperglycemia (includes glucose increased) [4]
Hyperlipidemia / lipids elevated [2]
Hypertriglyceridemia (includes triglycerides increased) [4]

Gastrointestinal/Hepatic
Abdominal pain (70%)
Hepatotoxicity / liver injury / acute liver injury / drug-induced liver injury (DILI) [4]
Pancreatitis / acute pancreatitis (15%) [28]
Vomiting (50–60%)

Genitourinary
Azotemia (66%)

Hematologic
Sepsis [2]
Thrombosis [10]

Other
Adverse effects / adverse reactions [2]
Allergic reactions (15–35%) [2]

ASPARTAME

Class: Sweetening agent
Half-life: N/A
Clinically important, potentially hazardous interactions with: none known
Pregnancy category: the pregnancy category will be C for women with phenylketonuria
Note: Upon ingestion, aspartame is metabolized to formaldehyde in the body and has been reportedly associated with systemic contact dermatitis in patients exquisitely sensitive to formaldehyde.
Aspartame can be found in instant breakfasts, breath mints, cereals, sugar-free chewing gum, cocoa mixes, coffee beverages, frozen desserts, gelatin desserts, juice beverages, laxatives, multivitamins, milk drinks, pharmaceuticals and supplements, shake mixes, soft drinks, tabletop sweeteners, tea beverages, instant teas and coffees, topping mixes, wine coolers, yogurt.

Skin
Angioedema (formerly named angioneurotic edema) [2]
Panniculitis [3]
Urticaria / hives [4]

Other
Allergic reactions [2]

ASPIRIN

Synonyms: acetylsalicylic acid; ASA
Trade names: Aggrenox (Boehringer Ingelheim), Anacin (Wyeth), Ascriptin (Novartis) (Wallace), Darvon Compound (aaiPharma), Durlaza (New Haven), Ecotrin (GSK), Equagesic (Women First), Excedrin (Bristol-Myers Squibb), Fiorinal (Watson), Norgesic (3M), Soma Compound (MedPointe), Talwin Compound (Sanofi-Aventis), Yosprala (Aralez)
Indications: Pain, fever, inflammation
Class: Antiplatelet (antithrombotic), Non-steroidal anti-inflammatory (NSAID), Salicylate
Half-life: 15–20 minutes
Clinically important, potentially hazardous interactions with: acemetacin, acenocoumarol, acetazolamide, amitriptyline, anagrelide, anticoagulants, azficel-t, bismuth, calcium hydroxylapatite, capsicum, celecoxib, cholestyramine, cilazapril, citalopram, desvenlafaxine, devil's claw, dexamethasone, dexibuprofen, dichlorphenamide, diclofenac, dicumarol, duloxetine, enoxaparin, etodolac, evening primrose, flunisolide, flurbiprofen, ginkgo biloba, ginseng, heparin, ibuprofen, iloprost, indomethacin, inotersen, ketoprofen, ketorolac, lumiracoxib, meloxicam, methotrexate, methyl salicylate, methylprednisolone, milnacipran, nilutamide, NSAIDs, paroxetine hydrochloride, phellodendron, piroxicam, prednisone, resveratrol, reteplase, rivaroxaban, sermorelin, sulfites, tinzaparin, tirofiban, tolmetin, triamcinolone, urokinase, valdecoxib, valproic acid, venlafaxine, verapamil, vilazodone, warfarin, zafirlukast
Important contra-indications noted in the prescribing guidelines for: nursing mothers; pediatric patients
Note: NSAIDs may cause an increased risk of serious cardiovascular and gastrointestinal adverse events, which can be fatal. This risk may increase with duration of use.
Aggrenox is aspirin and dipyridamole; Yosprala is aspirin and omeprazole.

Skin
Anaphylactoid reactions / anaphylaxis (includes anaphylactic shock) (<10%) [8]
Angioedema (formerly named angioneurotic edema) (<5%) [32]
Bullous dermatosis [4]
DRESS syndrome (Drug-induced hypersensitivity syndrome) [2]
Erythema multiforme [9]
Erythema nodosum [9]
Erythroderma [2]
Exanthems [11]
Fixed eruption / fixed drug eruption [22]
Hypersensitivity [5]
Lichenoid eruption / lichenoid reaction [2]
Linear IgA bullous dermatosis [2]
Pityriasis rosea [3]
Pruritus (itching) [6]
Psoriasis [3]
Purpura [8]
Rash (<10%)
Stevens-Johnson syndrome and toxic epidermal necrolysis (SJS/TEN) [14]
Urticaria / hives (<10%) [72]
Vasculitis (angiitis) / cutaneous vasculitis (angiitis) [2]

Mucosal
Aphthous stomatitis / aphthous ulcer / aphtha (aphthae) [3]
Epistaxis (nosebleed) [2]
Nasal polyp [4]
Oral mucosal eruption [3]
Oral ulceration [4]

Cardiovascular
Kounis syndrome / allergic angina syndrome / allergic myocardial infarction [2]

Central Nervous System
Stroke / cerebrovascular accident [2]

Gastrointestinal/Hepatic
Black stools / melena [3]
Gastritis / pangastritis / gastric irritation [2]
Gastrointestinal bleeding [10]
Gastrointestinal ulceration [7]
Hepatotoxicity / liver injury / acute liver injury / drug-induced liver injury (DILI) [5]
Pancreatitis / acute pancreatitis [2]

Hematologic
Bleeding [17]

Neuromuscular/Skeletal
Spinal epidural hematoma [5]

Ocular
Periorbital edema [3]

Otic
Tinnitus [17]

Renal
Fanconi syndrome (proximal tubular dysfunction) [2]

Respiratory
Asthma [10]
Pulmonary toxicity [2]
Rhinitis / rhinosinusitis (see also sinusitis) [3]
Sinusitis (see also rhinitis / rhinosinusitis) [2]

Other
Adverse effects / adverse reactions [9]
Allergic reactions [2]

ASTEMIZOLE

Trade name: Histeamen (Janssen)
Indications: Urticaria, pruritus, allergic rhinitis
Class: Histamine H1 receptor antagonist
Half-life: 20 hours
Clinically important, potentially hazardous interactions with: amiodarone, amphotericin B, aprepitant, artemether/lumefantrine, azithromycin, bepredil, bosentan, bretylium, cisapride, clarithromycin, darunavir, dasatinib, delavirdine, disopyramide, erythromycin, erythromycin fluconazole, fluoxetine, fluvoxamine, grapefruit juice, indinavir, itraconazole, ketoconazole, metronidazole, miconazole, nefazodone, nilotinib, paroxetine hydrochloride, pimozide, probucol, procainamide, quinidine, quinine, ritonavir, saquinavir, sertindole, sertraline, sotalol, SSRIs, terfenadine, troleandomycin, voriconazole, zileuton, ziprasidone
Note: Hismanal has been withdrawn in the USA as of 1999.

Skin
Urticaria / hives [2]

Mucosal
Xerostomia (dry mouth) [4]

Cardiovascular
Arrhythmias [2]
QT interval prolonged / QT prolongation [10]
Torsades de pointes [10]

Central Nervous System
Paresthesias [3]
Somnolence (drowsiness) [3]

ASTRAGALUS ROOT

Family: Fabaceae; Leguminosae
Scientific names: *Astragalus membranaceus, Astragalus mongholicus*
Indications: Arrhythmia, colds, upper respiratory infections, chronic fatigue syndrome, colitis, diabetes, hepatitis, hypotension, herpes simplex keratitis
Class: Antioxidant, Immune stimulant, Vasodilator
Half-life: N/A
Clinically important, potentially hazardous interactions with: none known

ATAZANAVIR

Trade names: Evotaz (Bristol-Myers Squibb), Reyataz (Bristol-Myers Squibb)
Indications: HIV infection
Class: Antiretroviral, HIV-1 protease inhibitor
Half-life: 7 hours
Clinically important, potentially hazardous interactions with: abiraterone, alfuzosin, amiodarone, antacids, aripiprazole, artemether/lumefantrine, atorvastatin, avanafil, bepridil, bosentan, buprenorphine, cabazitaxel, cabozantinib, calcifediol, cisapride, clarithromycin, colchicine, crizotinib, cyclosporine, darifenacin, dasatinib, dexlansoprazole, diltiazem, dofetilide, efavirenz, elbasvir & grazoprevir, eluxadoline, ergot derivatives, erlotinib, estrogens, etravirine, everolimus, famotidine, felodipine, fentanyl,

fesoterodine, flibanserin, fluticasone propionate, garlic, glecaprevir & pibrentasvir, indinavir, irinotecan, itraconazole, ixabepilone, ketoconazole, lapatinib, lidocaine, lopinavir, lovastatin, maraviroc, marihuana, midazolam, mifepristone, naldemedine, nevirapine, nicardipine, nifedipine, olaparib, ombitasvir/paritaprevir/ritonavir, omeprazole, oral contraceptives, paclitaxel, pantoprazole, pazopanib, pimozide, posaconazole, proton-pump inhibitors, quetiapine, quinidine, quinine, rabeprazole, raltegravir, ranolazine, rifabutin, rifampin, rilpivirine, ritonavir, rivaroxaban, romidepsin, rosuvastatin, salmeterol, saquinavir, sildenafil, simeprevir, simvastatin, sirolimus, sofosbuvir/velpatasvir/voxilaprevir, solifenacin, sonidegib, St John's wort, sunitinib, tacrolimus, tadalafil, telaprevir, telithromycin, temsirolimus, tenofovir disoproxil, ticagrelor, tipranavir, trazodone, triazolam, tricyclic antidepressants, vardenafil, vemurafenib, verapamil, voriconazole, warfarin
Important contra-indications noted in the prescribing guidelines for: the elderly; nursing mothers; pediatric patients
Note: Evotaz is atazanavir and cobicistat.

Skin
Jaundice (see also cholestasis / cholestatic jaundice) (5–7%) [11]
Rash (3–20%) [7]

Cardiovascular
QT interval prolonged / QT prolongation [2]
Torsades de pointes [2]

Central Nervous System
Depression (2%)
Fever (pyrexia) (includes hyperpyrexia) (2%)
Headache (<6%) [3]
Insomnia (3%)
Neurotoxicity [2]
Pain (3%)
Vertigo / dizziness (3%)

Endocrine/Metabolic
ALT increased (3%)
AST increased (3%)
Creatine phosphokinase (CPK) / creatine kinase increased (hyperCKemia) (8%)
Hyperbilirubinemia [8]

Gastrointestinal/Hepatic
Abdominal pain (4%)
Cholelithiasis (gallstones in the gall bladder or the bile duct) [4]
Diarrhea (2%) [3]
Hepatotoxicity / liver injury / acute liver injury / drug-induced liver injury (DILI) [3]
Nausea (6–14%) [4]
Vomiting (3–4%)

Genitourinary
Urolithiasis / ureteral stones / urinary calculi [5]

Hematologic
Neutropenia (neutrophils decreased) (5%)

Neuromuscular/Skeletal
Asthenia / fatigue (2%)
Back pain (2%)
Myalgia/Myopathy (4%)

Renal
Nephrolithiasis (kidney stones / renal calculi) [5]
Nephrotoxicity / kidney injury / acute kidney injury (AKI) / drug-induced kidney injury [7]

Respiratory
Upper respiratory tract infection [2]

Other
Adverse effects / adverse reactions [5]
Infection (~50%)

ATENOLOL

Trade names: Beta-Adalat (Bayer), Kalten (BPC), Tenif (AstraZeneca), Tenoret 50 (AstraZeneca), Tenoretic (AstraZeneca), Tenormin (AstraZeneca)
Indications: Angina, hypertension, acute myocardial infarction
Class: Antiarrhythmic class II, Beta adrenergic blocker, Beta blocker
Half-life: 6–7 hours (adults)
Clinically important, potentially hazardous interactions with: alfuzosin, calcium channel blockers, cisplatin, clonidine, digitalis glycosides, diltiazem, disopyramide, epinephrine, indomethacin, reserpine, verapamil
Important contra-indications noted in the prescribing guidelines for: the elderly; nursing mothers; pediatric patients
Note: Contra-indicated in patients with sinus bradycardia, heart block greater than first degree, cardiogenic shock, or overt cardiac failure. Beta-Adalat and Tenif are atenolol and nifedipine. Kalten, Tenoret 50 and Tenoretic are atenolol and chlorthalidone. Chlorthalidone is a sulfonamide and can be absorbed systemically. Sulfonamides can produce severe, possibly fatal, reactions such as toxic epidermal necrolysis and Stevens-Johnson syndrome.
Warning: CESSATION OF THERAPY

Skin
Anaphylactoid reactions / anaphylaxis (includes anaphylactic shock) [2]
Lupus erythematosus (subacute cutaneous lupus erythematosus (SCLE)) [2]
Necrosis (skin necrosis) [3]
Pruritus (itching) (<5%)
Psoriasis [7]
Raynaud's phenomenon [2]
Urticaria / hives [2]

Cardiovascular
Atrial fibrillation (5%) [2]
Atrial flutter (2%)
Bradycardia / sinus bradycardia (3–18%) [8]
Cardiac arrest (2%)
Cardiac failure (19%)
Heart block (5%)
Hypotension (25%) [2]
Postural hypotension (12%)
Supraventricular tachycardia (12%)
Ventricular tachycardia (16%)

Central Nervous System
Depression (12%)
Somnolence (drowsiness) (2%)
Stroke / cerebrovascular accident [2]
Syncope / fainting [2]
Vertigo / dizziness (15%)

Gastrointestinal/Hepatic
Diarrhea (3%)
Nausea (3%)

Neuromuscular/Skeletal
Asthenia / fatigue (26%)
Leg pain (3%)

Respiratory
Dyspnea / shortness of breath (6%)
Wheezing (3%)

Other
Adverse effects / adverse reactions [5]

ATEZOLIZUMAB

Trade name: Tecentriq (Genentech)
Indications: Locally advanced or metastatic urothelial carcinoma in patients having disease progression following platinum-containing chemotherapy, bladder cancer, non-small cell lung cancer
Class: Antineoplastic / anticancer agent (see also Immune checkpoint inhibitor), Immune checkpoint inhibitor (incl. programmed death receptor-1 (PD-1) inhibitor), Monoclonal antibody, Programmed death-ligand (PD-L1) inhibitor
Half-life: 27 days
Clinically important, potentially hazardous interactions with: none known
Pregnancy category: Can cause fetal harm
Important contra-indications noted in the prescribing guidelines for: nursing mothers; pediatric patients

---

Skin
Anaphylactoid reactions / anaphylaxis (includes anaphylactic shock) [4]
Lichenoid dermatitis [2]
Peripheral edema (18%) [2]
Pruritus (itching) (13%) [6]
Psoriasis [6]
Rash (15%) [7]
Sarcoidosis / sarcoid-like reaction (cutaneous sarcoidosis) [2]

Mucosal
Sjögren's syndrome (see also sicca syndrome) [2]

Cardiovascular
Hypertension [4]
Myocarditis [4]
Venous thromboembolism (>2%)

Central Nervous System
Aseptic meningitis [3]
Encephalitis [14]
Fever (pyrexia) (includes hyperpyrexia) (21%) [4]
Meningoencephalitis [2]

Endocrine/Metabolic
ALP increased (4%)
ALT increased (2%) [3]
Appetite decreased (26%) [8]
AST increased (2%) [7]
Dehydration (>2%)
Diabetes mellitus [4]
Diabetic ketoacidosis [4]
Hyperglycemia (includes glucose increased) (5%)
Hyperthyroidism (includes 'thyroid storm') (2%)
Hyponatremia (10%) [2]
Hypothyroidism (6%) [4]
Serum creatinine increased (3%)

Gastrointestinal/Hepatic
Abdominal pain (17%)
Cholangitis / sclerosing cholangitis [2]
Colitis [6]
Constipation (21%) [2]
Diarrhea (18%) [4]
Gastrointestinal obstruction / gastrointestinal stricture (>2%)

Hepatitis [3]
Hepatotoxicity / liver injury / acute liver injury / drug-induced liver injury (DILI) [2]
Nausea (25%) [6]
Vomiting (17%)

Genitourinary
Hematuria (14%)
Urinary tract infection (22%)

Hematologic
Anemia (8%) [4]
Hemolytic anemia [3]
Lymphopenia (lymphocytopenia) / lymphocytes decreased (10%)
Pure red cell aplasia [2]
Sepsis (>2%)
Thrombocytopenia / platelets decreased [4]

Local
Infusion-related reactions (3%)

Neuromuscular/Skeletal
Arthralgia (14%) [2]
Asthenia / fatigue (52%) [13]
Ataxia [4]
Back pain (15%)
Lambert-Eaton myasthenic syndrome [2]
Myalgia/Myopathy [7]
Myasthenia gravis [2]
Neck pain (15%)

Ocular
Keratitis (ocular keratitis) / corneal inflammation) [2]
Uveitis / anterior uveitis / posterior uveitis / panuveitis [2]

Renal
Glomerulonephritis (includes membranous nephropathy) [3]
Nephrotoxicity / kidney injury / acute kidney injury (AKI) / drug-induced kidney injury (>2%)

Respiratory
Cough (14%) [4]
Dyspnea / shortness of breath (16%) [6]
Hypoxia [2]
Interstitial lung disease / interstitial pneumonitis / interstitial pneumonia (cryptogenic organizing pneumonia) / drug-induced interstitial lung disease [2]
Pneumonia (>2%) [2]
Pneumonitis (3%) [5]
Pneumothorax [2]

Other
Adverse effects / adverse reactions [9]
Death [2]
Infection (38%)

ATOGEPANT

Trade name: Qulipta (AbbVie)
Indications: Treatment of episodic migraine in adults
Class: Calcitonin gene-related peptide (CGRP) receptor antagonist
Half-life: approximately 11 hours
Clinically important, potentially hazardous interactions with: cimetidine, ciprofloxacin, cyclosporine, CYP3A4 inducers, CYP3A4 inhibitors, esomeprazole, fluconazole, grapefruit juice, itraconazole, quinidine, rifampin
Pregnancy category: No adequate data on the developmental risk associated with the use of atogepant in pregnant women.

Endocrine/Metabolic
Appetite decreased (2%)

Gastrointestinal/Hepatic
Constipation (6%) [2]
Nausea (9%) [2]

Neuromuscular/Skeletal
Asthenia / fatigue (6%)

ATOMOXETINE

Trade name: Strattera (Lilly)
Indications: Attention deficit hyperactivity disorder
Class: Anti-attention deficit hyperactivity disorder (anti-ADHD), Norepinephrine reuptake inhibitor
Half-life: 5 hours
Clinically important, potentially hazardous interactions with: albuterol, amitriptyline, cinacalcet, citalopram, delavirdine, droperidol, duloxetine, levalbuterol, levomepromazine, linezolid, lisdexamfetamine, MAO inhibitors, moxifloxacin, paroxetine hydrochloride, sotalol, terbinafine, terbutaline, tipranavir, venlafaxine, viloxazine, zuclopenthixol
Important contra-indications noted in the prescribing guidelines for: nursing mothers; pediatric patients
Warning: SUICIDAL IDEATION IN CHILDREN AND ADOLESCENTS

Skin
Pruritus (itching) (>2%)

Mucosal
Xerostomia (dry mouth) (>5%) [9]

Cardiovascular
Cardiotoxicity [3]
Tachycardia [2]

Central Nervous System
Aggression (includes anger) [3]
Anorexia [5]
Depression (>2%) [3]
Headache [9]
Hypomania [2]
Insomnia [7]
Irritability [8]
Mania [2]
Mood changes (includes mood disorder) [5]
Nervousness [3]
Seizures [2]
Somnolence (drowsiness) [11]
Suicidal ideation [6]
Tic disorder [7]
Tremor (>2%) [2]
Vertigo / dizziness (>5%) [10]

Endocrine/Metabolic
Appetite decreased [27]
Weight loss [5]

Gastrointestinal/Hepatic
Abdominal pain [12]
Constipation [2]
Dyspepsia / functional dyspepsia (indigestion) (see also gastroparesis) [3]
Hepatotoxicity / liver injury / acute liver injury / drug-induced liver injury (DILI) [12]
Nausea [18]
Vomiting [10]

Genitourinary
Erectile dysfunction [4]
Urinary hesitancy [2]

Neuromuscular/Skeletal
Asthenia / fatigue [11]

Other
Adverse effects / adverse reactions [10]
Bruxism (teeth grinding) [2]

ATORVASTATIN

Trade names: Caduet (Pfizer), Lipitor (Pfizer), Liptruzet (Merck Sharpe & Dohme)
Indications: Hypercholesterolemia
Class: HMG-CoA reductase inhibitor / statin
Half-life: 14 hours
Clinically important, potentially hazardous interactions with: alcohol, aliskiren, amiodarone, amprenavir, antifungals, atazanavir, azithromycin, bexarotene, boceprevir, bosentan, ciprofibrate, clarithromycin, clopidogrel, cobicistat/elvitegravir/emtricitabine/tenofovir alafenamide, cobicistat/elvitegravir/emtricitabine/tenofovir disoproxil, colchicine, conivaptan, cyclosporine, CYP3A4 inhibitors, dabigatran, danazol, daptomycin, darunavir, dasatinib, delavirdine, digoxin, diltiazem, dronedarone, efavirenz, elbasvir & grazoprevir, eltrombopag, erythromycin, estradiol, etravirine, everolimus, fenofibrate, fenofibric acid, fibrates, fluconazole, fosamprenavir, fusidic acid, gemfibrozil, glecaprevir & pibrentasvir, grapefruit juice, imatinib, imidazoles, indinavir, itraconazole, letermovir, liraglutide, lonafarnib, lopinavir, macrolide antibiotics, midazolam, nefazodone, nelfinavir, niacin, niacinamide, norethisterone, oral contraceptives, P-glycoprotein inhibitors, posaconazole, protease inhibitors, quinine, red rice yeast, rifampin, ritonavir, rivaroxaban, saquinavir, silodosin, St John's wort, telaprevir, telithromycin, tipranavir, topotecan, trabectedin, verapamil, voriconazole, warfarin
Important contra-indications noted in the prescribing guidelines for: the elderly; nursing mothers; pediatric patients
Note: Caduet is atorvastatin and amlodipine; Liptruzet is atorvastatin and ezetimibe.

Skin
Acneiform eruption / acneiform dermatitis / acneiform rash (<2%)
Angioedema (formerly named angioneurotic edema) [4]
Bruise / bruising / contusion / ecchymosis (ecchymoses) (<2%)
Cutaneous toxicity / skin toxicity [2]
Dermatitis (<2%)
Dermatomyositis [4]
Diaphoresis (<2%)
Eczema / eczematous reaction / eczematous eruption (<2%)
Edema / fluid retention (<2%)
Facial edema (<2%)
Jaundice (see also cholestasis / cholestatic jaundice) [2]
Leukocytoclastic vasculitis (angiitis) [2]
Lupus erythematosus (subacute cutaneous lupus erythematosus (SCLE)) [3]
Lymphocytic infiltration / Jessner lymphocytic infiltration [2]
Petechiae (<2%)
Photosensitivity (<2%)
Pruritus (itching) (<2%)
Rash (>3%) [2]
Seborrhea (<2%)

Stevens-Johnson syndrome and toxic epidermal necrolysis (SJS/TEN) [2]
Ulcerations (<2%)
Urticaria / hives (<2%)
Xerosis / xeroderma (<2%)

Hair
Alopecia / hair loss (<2%)

Mucosal
Cheilitis (inflammation of the lips) (<2%)
Glossitis (inflammation of the tongue) (<2%)
Oral ulceration (<2%)
Stomatitis (oral mucositis) (<2%)

Cardiovascular
Hypotension [2]
Myocarditis [2]

Central Nervous System
Ageusia (taste loss) / taste disorder (<2%)
Cognitive impairment [2]
Depression [3]
Dysgeusia (taste perversion) (<2%)
Headache [5]
Neurotoxicity [2]
Paresthesias (<2%)
Parosmia (<2%)
Vertigo / dizziness [2]

Endocrine/Metabolic
ALT increased [3]
Creatine phosphokinase (CPK) / creatine kinase increased (hyperCKemia) [5]
Diabetes mellitus [2]
Gynecomastia (<2%)

Gastrointestinal/Hepatic
Cholelithiasis (gallstones in the gall bladder or the bile duct) [2]
Diarrhea (5–14%)
Hepatitis [3]
Hepatotoxicity / liver injury / acute liver injury / drug-induced liver injury (DILI) [12]
Nausea (4–7%)
Pancreatitis / acute pancreatitis [8]

Genitourinary
Urinary tract infection (4–8%)

Neuromuscular/Skeletal
Arthralgia (4–12%)
Asthenia / fatigue [5]
Back pain [3]
Muscle spasm [2]
Myalgia/Myopathy (3–8%) [40]
Necrotizing myopathy / immune-mediated necrotizing myopathy [22]
Pain in extremities (6%)
Rhabdomyolysis [44]
Tendinopathy/Tendon rupture [2]

Otic
Hearing loss (hypoacusis) [2]

Renal
Nephrotoxicity / kidney injury / acute kidney injury (AKI) / drug-induced kidney injury [5]

Respiratory
Cough [2]
Nasopharyngitis (4–13%)

Other
Adverse effects / adverse reactions [11]
Allergic reactions (<2%)
Death [7]
Multiorgan failure [2]

ATOVAQUONE

Trade names: Mepron (GSK), Wellvone (GSK)
Indications: *Pneumocystis carinii* infection
Class: Antimalarial, Antimicrobial, Antiprotozoal
Half-life: 1.5–4 days
Clinically important, potentially hazardous interactions with: efavirenz, etoposide, histamine, hypoglycemic agents, indinavir, lopinavir, metoclopramide, rifabutin, rifampin, rifapentine, ritonavir, tetracycline, zidovudine
Important contra-indications noted in the prescribing guidelines for: the elderly; nursing mothers; pediatric patients

---

Skin
Diaphoresis (10%)
Pruritus (itching) (11%) [2]
Rash (23%) [4]
Stevens-Johnson syndrome and toxic epidermal necrolysis (SJS/TEN) [2]

Mucosal
Oral candidiasis (<10%)

Central Nervous System
Depression (>10%)
Dysgeusia (taste perversion) (3%)
Fever (pyrexia) (includes hyperpyrexia) (14–40%)
Headache (16–31%)
Insomnia (10–19%)
Pain (>10%)

Gastrointestinal/Hepatic
Abdominal pain (4–21%)
Diarrhea (9–42%) [3]
Nausea (21–32%) [4]
Vomiting (14–22%) [2]

Neuromuscular/Skeletal
Asthenia / fatigue (8–31%)
Myalgia/Myopathy (>10%)

Respiratory
Cough (increased) (14–25%)
Dyspnea / shortness of breath (21–25%)
Influenza- ('flu)-like syndrome (>10%)
Rhinitis / rhinosinusitis (see also sinusitis) (5–24%)
Sinusitis (see also rhinitis / rhinosinusitis) (7–10%)

Other
Adverse effects / adverse reactions [3]
Infection (18–22%)

ATOVAQUONE/ PROGUANIL

Trade name: Malarone (GSK)
Indications: Malaria prophylaxis and treatment
Class: Antimalarial
Half-life: 24 hours
Clinically important, potentially hazardous interactions with: artemether/lumefantrine, dapsone, etoposide, hypoglycemic agents, indinavir, metoclopramide, phenothiazines, rifabutin, rifampin, ritonavir, tetracycline, typhoid vaccine
Important contra-indications noted in the prescribing guidelines for: the elderly; nursing mothers

---

Skin
Erythema multiforme [2]
Pruritus (itching) (<10%)

Mucosal
Oral ulceration (6%) [3]

Central Nervous System
Abnormal dreams (7%)
Anorexia (5%)
Headache (10%) [4]
Insomnia (3%)
Vertigo / dizziness (5%) [3]

Gastrointestinal/Hepatic
Abdominal pain (17%) [5]
Diarrhea (8%)
Dyspepsia / functional dyspepsia (indigestion) (see also gastroparesis) (2%)
Gastritis / pangastritis / gastric irritation (3%)
Hepatotoxicity / liver injury / acute liver injury / drug-induced liver injury (DILI) [2]
Nausea (12%)
Vomiting (12%) [2]

Neuromuscular/Skeletal
Asthenia / fatigue (8%)

Ocular
Vision impaired (2%)

Respiratory
Cough [3]

Other
Adverse effects / adverse reactions [3]

ATRACURIUM

Trade name: Tracrium (AbbVie)
Indications: Neuromuscular blockade, endotracheal intubation
Class: Non-depolarizing neuromuscular blocker
Half-life: 20 minutes
Clinically important, potentially hazardous interactions with: amikacin, aminoglycosides, anesthetics, antibiotics, gentamicin, halothane, kanamycin, neomycin, piperacillin, streptomycin, tobramycin
Important contra-indications noted in the prescribing guidelines for: nursing mothers

---

Skin
Anaphylactoid reactions / anaphylaxis (includes anaphylactic shock) [12]
Flushing / rubefaction (<10%) [2]
Rash [2]

Cardiovascular
Hypotension [4]

Ocular
Periorbital edema [2]

Other
Adverse effects / adverse reactions [2]
Allergic reactions [2]

ATROPINE SULFATE

Trade name: Lomotil (Pfizer)
Indications: Salivation, sinus bradycardia, uveitis, peptic ulcer
Class: Muscarinic antagonist
Half-life: 2–3 hours
Clinically important, potentially hazardous interactions with: anticholinergics, zuclopenthixol
Note: Many of the trade name drugs for atropine sulfate contain phenobarbital, scopolamine, hyoscyamine, hydrocodone, methenamine, etc.

Skin
Anaphylactoid reactions / anaphylaxis (includes anaphylactic shock) [3]
Dermatitis [3]
Erythema multiforme [2]
Photosensitivity (<10%)

Mucosal
Xerostomia (dry mouth) (>10%) [4]

Cardiovascular
Arrhythmias [2]
Atrial fibrillation [2]
Bradycardia / sinus bradycardia [3]
Tachycardia [5]

Central Nervous System
Confusion [2]
Hallucinations, visual [3]

Local
Injection-site irritation (>10%)

Ocular
Amblyopia [5]
Dilated pupils [2]
Periocular dermatitis [4]
Photophobia [2]
Vision blurred [3]

Other
Allergic reactions [3]
Central anticholinergic syndrome [2]

AVANAFIL

Trade name: Stendra (Vivus)
Indications: Erectile dysfunction
Class: Phosphodiesterase type 5 (PDE5) inhibitor
Half-life: 5 hours
Clinically important, potentially hazardous interactions with: alcohol, alpha blockers, amprenavir, antihypertensives, aprepitant, atazanavir, clarithromycin, diltiazem, erythromycin, fluconazole, fosamprenavir, indinavir, itraconazole, ketoconazole, nefazodone, nelfinavir, nitrates, ritonavir, saquinavir, strong CYP3A4 inhibitors, telithromycin, verapamil, viloxazine
Pregnancy category: Not indicated for use in women
Important contra-indications noted in the prescribing guidelines for: pediatric patients
Note: Contra-indicated in patients using any form of nitrates.

Skin
Facial flushing [2]
Flushing / rubefaction (3–10%) [11]
Rash (<2%)

Mucosal
Nasal congestion (<3%) [7]

Cardiovascular
Hypertension (<2%)

Central Nervous System
Headache (5–12%) [10]
Vertigo / dizziness (<2%) [3]

Gastrointestinal/Hepatic
Constipation (<2%)
Diarrhea (<2%)
Dyspepsia / functional dyspepsia (indigestion) (see also gastroparesis) (<2%) [5]
Nausea (<2%)

Neuromuscular/Skeletal
Arthralgia (<2%)
Asthenia / fatigue [2]
Back pain (<3%) [3]

Respiratory
Bronchitis (<2%)
Influenza (<2%)
Nasopharyngitis (<5%) [5]
Sinusitis (see also rhinitis / rhinosinusitis) (<2%) [2]
Upper respiratory tract infection (<3%)

Other
Adverse effects / adverse reactions [5]

AVAPRITINIB

Trade name: Ayvakit (Blueprint Medicines)
Indications: Treatment of adults with unresectable or metastatic gastrointestinal stromal tumor harboring a platelet-derived growth factor receptor alpha (PDGFRA) exon 18 mutation, including PDGFRA D842V mutations
Class: Tyrosine kinase inhibitor
Half-life: 32–57 hours
Clinically important, potentially hazardous interactions with: CYP3A inducer, CYP3A inhibitor, efavirenz, fluconazole, itraconazole
Pregnancy category: Can cause fetal harm. Advise females of reproductive potential of the potential risk to a fetus and to use effective contraception.
Note: Intracranial Hemorrhage: Withhold avapritinib for grade 1 or 2 reactions (subdural hematoma, intracranial hemorrhage, and cerebral hemorrhage) until resolution and then resume at a reduced dose. Permanently discontinue for recurrent grade 1 or 2 reactions or first occurrence of grade 3 or 4 reactions.

Skin
Edema / fluid retention (2% ≥ grade 3) (72%)
Rash (2% ≥ grade 3) (23%)

Hair
Alopecia / hair loss (13%)
Hair color changes (<1% ≥ grade 3) (21%)

Cardiovascular
Hypertension (8%)

Central Nervous System
Cognitive impairment (5% ≥ grade 3) (48%) [2]
Dysgeusia (taste perversion) (15%)
Fever (pyrexia) (includes hyperpyrexia) (<1% ≥ grade 3) (14%)
Headache (<1% ≥ grade 3) (17%)
Mood changes (includes mood disorder) (1% ≥ grade 3) (13%)
Sleep-related disorder (16%)
Vertigo / dizziness (<1% ≥ grade 3) (22%)

Endocrine/Metabolic
ALP increased (1% ≥ grade 3) (14%)
ALT increased (<1% ≥ grade 3) (19%)
Appetite decreased (3% ≥ grade 3) (38%)
AST increased (2% ≥ grade 3) (51%)
Hyperbilirubinemia (9% ≥ grade 3) (69%)
Hypoalbuminemia / albumin decreased (2% ≥ grade 3) (31%)
Hypokalemia (6% ≥ grade 3) (34%)
Hypomagnesemia (1% ≥ grade 3) (29%)
Hyponatremia (7% ≥ grade 3) (28%)
Hypophosphatemia (13% ≥ grade 3) (49%)
Serum creatinine increased (29%)
Thyroid disorder (3%)
Weight loss (1% ≥ grade 3) (13%)

Gastrointestinal/Hepatic
Abdominal pain (6% ≥ grade 3) (31%)
Constipation (2% ≥ grade 3) (23%)
Diarrhea (5% ≥ grade 3) (37%) [3]
Dyspepsia / functional dyspepsia (indigestion) (see also gastroparesis) (16%)
Nausea (3% ≥ grade 3) (64%) [3]
Vomiting (5% ≥ grade 3) (38%)

Hematologic
Anemia [5]
Hemoglobin decreased (28% ≥ grade 3) (81%)
Leukocytopenia (leukopenia) / leukocytes (white blood cells) decreased (5% ≥ grade 3) (62%)
Neutropenia (neutrophils decreased) (6% ≥ grade 3) (43%) [3]
Partial thromboplastin time increased (13%)
Prothrombin time (INR) increased (<1% ≥ grade 3) (24%)
Thrombocytopenia / platelets decreased (<1% ≥ grade 3) (27%)

Neuromuscular/Skeletal
Asthenia / fatigue (9% ≥ grade 3) (61%)

Ocular
Lacrimation (33%)
Periorbital edema [3]

Respiratory
Dyspnea / shortness of breath (3% ≥ grade 3) (17%)
Pleural effusion (2% ≥ grade 3) (12%)

AVATROMBOPAG

Trade name: Doptelet (Akarx Inc)
Indications: treatment of thrombocytopenia in adult patients with chronic liver disease who are scheduled to undergo a procedure
Class: Thrombopoietin receptor (TPO) agonist
Half-life: ~19 hours
Clinically important, potentially hazardous interactions with: none known
Pregnancy category: may cause fetal harm
Important contra-indications noted in the prescribing guidelines for: nursing mothers

---

Skin
Peripheral edema (3%)

Central Nervous System
Fever (pyrexia) (includes hyperpyrexia) (10%)
Headache (6%) [4]

Gastrointestinal/Hepatic
Abdominal pain (7%)
Nausea (7%)

Hematologic
Thrombocythemia (thrombocytosis) / platelets increased [2]

Neuromuscular/Skeletal
Asthenia / fatigue (4%) [2]

AVELUMAB

Trade name: Bavencio (Merck Serono)
Indications: Metastatic Merkel cell carcinoma
Class: Antineoplastic / anticancer agent (see also Immune checkpoint inhibitor), Immune checkpoint inhibitor (incl. programmed death receptor-1 (PD-1) inhibitor), Monoclonal antibody, Programmed death-ligand (PD-L1) inhibitor
Half-life: 6 days
Clinically important, potentially hazardous interactions with: none known
Pregnancy category: Can cause fetal harm
Important contra-indications noted in the prescribing guidelines for: nursing mothers; pediatric patients

---

Skin
Peripheral edema (20%)
Pruritus (itching) (10%)
Rash (22%)

Cardiovascular
Hypertension (13%)

Central Nervous System
Chills [2]
Fever (pyrexia) (includes hyperpyrexia) [2]
Headache (10%)
Vertigo / dizziness (14%)

Endocrine/Metabolic
ALT increased (20%) [2]
Appetite decreased (20%)
AST increased (34%) [3]
Creatine phosphokinase (CPK) / creatine kinase increased (hyperCKemia) [3]
Hyperamylasemia (8%)
Hyperbilirubinemia (6%)
Hyperglycemia (includes glucose increased) (>10%)
Hyperlipasemia (14%)
Thyroid dysfunction (6%)
Weight loss (15%)

Gastrointestinal/Hepatic
Abdominal pain (16%)
Colitis (2%)
Constipation (17%)
Diarrhea (23%) [3]
Nausea (22%) [3]
Vomiting (13%)

Hematologic
Anemia (35%)
Lymphopenia (lymphocytopenia) / lymphocytes decreased (49%)
Neutropenia (neutrophils decreased) (6%)
Thrombocytopenia / platelets decreased (27%)

Local
Infusion-related reactions (22%) [7]

Neuromuscular/Skeletal
Arthralgia (16%)
Asthenia / fatigue (50%) [5]
Bone pain / joint pain (32%)

Respiratory
Cough (18%)
Dyspnea / shortness of breath (11%)

Other
Adverse effects / adverse reactions [5]
Death [2]
Immune-related adverse effect [2]

AXITINIB

Trade name: Inlyta (Pfizer)
Indications: Advanced renal cell carcinoma (after failure of one prior systemic therapy)
Class: Angiogenesis inhibitor / antiangiogenic agent, Tyrosine kinase inhibitor, Vascular endothelial growth factor (VEGF) inhibitor / antagonist
Half-life: 2–6 hours
Clinically important, potentially hazardous interactions with: ketoconazole, rifampin
Important contra-indications noted in the prescribing guidelines for: nursing mothers; pediatric patients

---

Skin
Cutaneous collagenous vasculopathy [2]
Erythema (2%)
Hand–foot syndrome (palmar–plantar erythrodysesthesia) (27%) [20]
Pruritus (itching) (7%)
Rash (13%) [3]
Xerosis / xeroderma (10%)

Hair
Alopecia / hair loss (4%) [2]

Mucosal
Mucosal inflammation (15%) [2]
Stomatitis (oral mucositis) (15%) [3]

Cardiovascular
Hypertension (40%) [41]
Takotsubo syndrome [2]

Central Nervous System
Anorexia [5]
Dysgeusia (taste perversion) (11%)
Headache (14%) [4]
Leukoencephalopathy / posterior reversible encephalopathy syndrome (PRES) [2]

Endocrine/Metabolic
ALT increased (22%) [3]
Appetite decreased (34%) [9]
AST increased [2]
Dehydration [2]
Hyperthyroidism (includes 'thyroid storm') [2]
Hyponatremia [2]
Hypothyroidism (19%) [8]
Serum creatinine increased [2]
Thyroid dysfunction [2]
Weight loss (25%) [3]

Gastrointestinal/Hepatic
Abdominal pain (14%)
Constipation (20%) [2]
Diarrhea (55%) [27]
Dyspepsia / functional dyspepsia (indigestion) (see also gastroparesis) (10%)
Gastrointestinal disorder / discomfort [3]
Hepatotoxicity / liver injury / acute liver injury / drug-induced liver injury (DILI) [2]
Nausea (32%) [10]
Vomiting (24%) [6]

Hematologic
Anemia [2]
Hemorrhage (16%)
Neutropenia (neutrophils decreased) [2]
Thrombocytopenia / platelets decreased [2]
Thrombotic complications (3%)

Neuromuscular/Skeletal
Arthralgia (15%) [2]
Asthenia / fatigue (39%) [31]
Pain in extremities (13%)

Renal
Proteinuria (11%) [5]

Respiratory
Cough (15%) [3]
Dysphonia (includes voice disorders / voice changes) (>20%) [13]
Dyspnea / shortness of breath (15%) [4]

Other
Adverse effects / adverse reactions [5]
Death [2]

AZACITIDINE

Synonym: Azacytidine
Trade name: Vidaza (Celgene)
Indications: Myelodysplastic syndromes, refractory anemia
Class: Antimetabolite, Antineoplastic / anticancer agent (see also Immune checkpoint inhibitor), Cytosine analog
Half-life: 40–56 minutes
Clinically important, potentially hazardous interactions with: BCG vaccine, denosumab, echinacea, leflunomide, natalizumab, pimecrolimus, sipuleucel-T, tacrolimus, trastuzumab, vaccines
Important contra-indications noted in the prescribing guidelines for: nursing mothers; pediatric patients
Note: Contra-indicated in patients with advanced malignant hepatic tumors.

Skin
Anaphylactoid reactions / anaphylaxis (includes anaphylactic shock) (<5%)
Bruise / bruising / contusion / ecchymosis (ecchymoses) (31%)
Cellulitis and pseudocellulitis (8%)
Cutaneous toxicity / skin toxicity [2]
Diaphoresis (11%)
Edema / fluid retention (14%)
Erythema (7–17%)
Hematoma / cutaneous hematoma (9%)
Herpes simplex (9%)
Hypersensitivity (<5%)
Induration (<5%)
Lymphoproliferative disease / lymphoproliferative disorder [2]
Nodular eruption (5%)
Pallor (16%)
Peripheral edema (19%)
Petechiae (11–24%)
Pruritus (itching) (12%)
Pyoderma gangrenosum (<5%) [2]
Rash (10–14%) [4]
Sweet's syndrome [10]
Urticaria / hives (6%)
Xerosis / xeroderma (5%)

Mucosal
Gingival bleeding (10%)
Oral bleeding (5%)
Stomatitis (oral mucositis) (8%)
Tongue ulceration (5%)

Cardiovascular
Arrhythmias [2]
Atrial fibrillation (<5%)
Cardiac failure (<5%)
Cardiomyopathy (<5%)
Cardiotoxicity [3]
Chest pain (5–16%) [4]
Congestive heart failure (<5%)
Hypertension (9%)
Hypotension (7%) [2]

Orthostatic hypotension (<5%)
Pericardial effusion [3]
Pericarditis [2]
QT interval prolonged / QT prolongation [2]
Tachycardia [3]

Central Nervous System
Anorexia (21%)
Anxiety (5–13%)
Cerebral hemorrhage (<5%)
Depression (12%)
Fever (pyrexia) (includes hyperpyrexia) (30–52%) [4]
Headache (22%)
Insomnia (9–11%)
Intracranial hemorrhage (<5%)
Pain (11%)
Seizures (<5%)
Syncope / fainting [2]
Vertigo / dizziness (19%)

Endocrine/Metabolic
Dehydration (<5%)
Hyperglycemia (includes glucose increased) [2]
Hypokalemia (6%)
Weight loss (8%)

Gastrointestinal/Hepatic
Abdominal pain (12–13%)
Black stools / melena (<5%)
Cholecystitis (calculous / acalculous) (<5%)
Constipation (34–50%) [4]
Diarrhea (36%) [4]
Dyspepsia / functional dyspepsia (indigestion) (see also gastroparesis) (6%)
Dysphagia (5%)
Gastrointestinal bleeding (<5%)
Loose stools / soft feces (6%)
Nausea (48–71%) [7]
Vomiting (27–54%) [4]

Genitourinary
Hematuria (6%)
Urinary tract infection (9%)

Hematologic
Agranulocytosis / severe selective neutropenia (<5%)
Anemia (51–70%) [5]
Bleeding [3]
Cytopenia [4]
Febrile neutropenia (14–16%) [8]
Leukocytopenia (leukopenia) / leukocytes (white blood cells) decreased (18–48%) [2]
Myelosuppression / bone marrow suppression / myelotoxicity [3]
Neutropenia (neutrophils decreased) (32–66%) [12]
Pancytopenia (includes bicytopenia) (<5%)
Splenomegaly (<5%)
Thrombocytopenia / platelets decreased (66–70%) [8]

Local
Injection-site bruising (5–14%)
Injection-site edema (5%)
Injection-site erythema (35–43%)
Injection-site hematoma (6%)
Injection-site pain (19–23%)
Injection-site pigmentation / injection-site discoloration (5%)
Injection-site pruritus (7%)
Injection-site purpura (14%)
Injection-site reaction (14–29%) [7]

Neuromuscular/Skeletal
Arthralgia (22%) [2]
Asthenia / fatigue (7–36%) [5]
Back pain (19%)
Bone pain / joint pain (<5%)
Myalgia/Myopathy (16%)
Neck pain (<5%)

Ocular
Ocular hemorrhage (<5%)

Renal
Renal failure (<5%)

Respiratory
Cough (30%)
Dyspnea / shortness of breath (14–29%) [2]
Hemoptysis (<5%)
Lung injury [2]
Nasopharyngitis (15%)
Pharyngolaryngeal pain (6%)
Pneumonia (11%) [2]
Pneumonitis (<5%) [7]
Pulmonary toxicity [2]
Respiratory distress (<5%)
Rhinitis / rhinosinusitis (see also sinusitis) (6%)
Upper respiratory tract infection (9–13%)

Other
Adverse effects / adverse reactions [6]
Death [5]
Infection (<5%) [9]
Neoplasms (<5%)

AZATADINE

Trade names: Optimine (Schering), Trinalin (Schering)
Indications: Allergic rhinitis, urticaria
Class: Histamine H1 receptor antagonist
Half-life: 9 hours
Clinically important, potentially hazardous interactions with: barbiturates, chloral hydrate, paraldehyde, phenylthiazines, zolpidem
Important contra-indications noted in the prescribing guidelines for: nursing mothers; pediatric patients

---

Mucosal
Xerostomia (dry mouth) (<10%)

AZATHIOPRINE

Trade names: Azasan (aaiPharma), Imuran (Prometheus)
Indications: Lupus nephritis, psoriatic arthritis, rheumatoid arthritis, autoimmune diseases, as an adjunct for the prevention of rejection in kidney transplant patients
Class: Antimetabolite, Disease-modifying antirheumatic drug (DMARD), Immunosuppressant, Purine analog
Half-life: 12 minutes
Clinically important, potentially hazardous interactions with: allopurinol, aminosalicylates, balsalazide, benazepril, captopril, chlorambucil, co-trimoxazole, cyclophosphamide, cyclosporine, enalapril, febuxostat, fosinopril, Hemophilus B vaccine, imidapril, lisinopril, mesalamine, mycophenolate, natalizumab, olsalazine, quinapril, ramipril, ribavirin, sulfamethoxazole, tofacitinib, trimethoprim, typhoid vaccine, vaccines, warfarin, yellow fever vaccine
Important contra-indications noted in the prescribing guidelines for: nursing mothers; pediatric patients
Note: Patients receiving immunosuppressants, including azathioprine, are at increased risk of developing lymphoma and other malignancies, particularly of the skin.
Warning: MALIGNANCY

Skin
Acanthosis nigricans [2]
Acneiform eruption / acneiform dermatitis / acneiform rash [2]
AGEP [2]
Angioedema (formerly named angioneurotic edema) [2]
Basal cell carcinoma [2]
Carcinoma [3]
Cutaneous toxicity / skin toxicity [3]
Dermatitis [4]
Erythema gyratum repens [2]
Erythema multiforme [2]
Erythema nodosum [5]
Exanthems [10]
Fixed eruption / fixed drug eruption [2]
Herpes simplex [3]
Herpes zoster [8]
Hypersensitivity [29]
Kaposi's sarcoma [14]
Lymphoproliferative disease / lymphoproliferative disorder [4]
Neutrophilic dermatosis [4]
Nevi (naevi) [3]
Pellagra [2]
Porokeratosis [4]
Rash (<10%) [11]
Scabies [5]
Squamous cell carcinoma [11]
Stevens-Johnson syndrome and toxic epidermal necrolysis (SJS/TEN) [2]
Sweet's syndrome [19]
Tinea [3]
Tumors [8]
Urticaria / hives [5]
Vasculitis (angiitis) / cutaneous vasculitis (angiitis) [5]
Verrucae vulgaris / warts / verrucae [3]

Hair
Alopecia / hair loss [14]
Anagen effluvium [2]

Nails
Onychomycosis [2]

Mucosal
Oral ulceration [2]
Sialadenitis [3]
Stomatitis (oral mucositis) [3]

Cardiovascular
Atrial fibrillation [3]

Central Nervous System
Aseptic meningitis [2]
Chills (>10%)
Encephalopathy (includes hepatic encephalopathy) [2]
Fever (pyrexia) (includes hyperpyrexia) [8]
Headache [3]
Leukoencephalopathy / posterior reversible encephalopathy syndrome (PRES) [2]

Gastrointestinal/Hepatic
Abdominal pain [2]
Hepatitis [5]
Hepatotoxicity / liver injury / acute liver injury / drug-induced liver injury (DILI) [29]
Nausea [8]
Pancreatitis / acute pancreatitis [50]
Vomiting [4]

Hematologic
Agranulocytosis / severe selective neutropenia [2]

Anemia [2]
Leukocytopenia (leukopenia) / leukocytes (white blood cells) decreased [19]
Myelosuppression / bone marrow suppression / myelotoxicity [18]
Neutropenia (neutrophils decreased) [2]
Pancytopenia (includes bicytopenia) [7]
Pure red cell aplasia [3]
Thrombocytopenia / platelets decreased [6]

Neuromuscular/Skeletal
Arthralgia [5]
Asthenia / fatigue [7]
Myalgia/Myopathy [2]

Respiratory
Influenza- ('flu)-like syndrome [2]
Pneumonitis [2]
Pulmonary toxicity [3]

Other
Adverse effects / adverse reactions [12]
Allergic reactions [5]
Death [2]
Infection [9]
Malignancies [2]
Neoplasms [2]

AZELASTINE

Trade names: Astelin (MedPointe), Optivar (MedPointe)
Indications: Allergic rhinitis
Class: Histamine H1 receptor antagonist
Half-life: 22 hours
Clinically important, potentially hazardous interactions with: barbiturates, chloral hydrate, paraldehyde, phenothiazines, zolpidem
Important contra-indications noted in the prescribing guidelines for: nursing mothers

---

Skin
Dermatitis (<2%)
Eczema / eczematous reaction / eczematous eruption (<2%)
Flushing / rubefaction (<2%)
Folliculitis (<2%)
Furunculosis (<2%)
Herpes simplex (<2%)

Mucosal
Aphthous stomatitis / aphthous ulcer / aphtha (aphthae) (<2%)
Glossitis (inflammation of the tongue) (<2%)
Stomatitis (oral mucositis) (ulcerative) (<2%)
Xerostomia (dry mouth) [2]

Central Nervous System
Ageusia (taste loss) / taste disorder (<2%)
Dysgeusia (taste perversion) [10]
Hyperesthesia (<2%)

Endocrine/Metabolic
Mastodynia (<2%)

Neuromuscular/Skeletal
Myalgia/Myopathy (2%)

Other
Allergic reactions (<2%)

AZFICEL-T

Trade name: laViv (Fibrocell)
Indications: Correction of moderate to severe nasolabial folds
Class: Dermal filler
Half-life: N/A
Clinically important, potentially hazardous interactions with: aniticoagulants, aspirin, NSAIDs
Important contra-indications noted in the prescribing guidelines for: pediatric patients

---

Local
Injection-site ecchymoses (11%)
Injection-site edema (4–14%)
Injection-site erythema (16%)
Injection-site pain (6%)

AZILSARTAN

Trade name: Edarbi (Takeda)
Indications: Hypertension
Class: Angiotensin receptor antagonist (blocker), Antihypertensive
Half-life: 11 hours
Clinically important, potentially hazardous interactions with: NSAIDs
Pregnancy category: category C in first trimester; category D in second and third trimesters
Important contra-indications noted in the prescribing guidelines for: nursing mothers; pediatric patients
Warning: FETAL TOXICITY

Cardiovascular
Hypotension [3]

Central Nervous System
Headache [10]
Vertigo / dizziness [11]

Endocrine/Metabolic
Creatine phosphokinase (CPK) / creatine kinase increased (hyperCKemia) [2]
Dyslipidemia [3]
Serum creatinine increased [3]

Gastrointestinal/Hepatic
Diarrhea [3]

Neuromuscular/Skeletal
Asthenia / fatigue [3]
Back pain [2]

Renal
Nephrotoxicity / kidney injury / acute kidney injury (AKI) / drug-induced kidney injury [2]

Respiratory
Nasopharyngitis [3]
Upper respiratory tract infection [2]

AZITHROMYCIN

Trade names: AzaSite (Merck), Zithromax (Pfizer)
Indications: Infections of the upper and lower respiratory tract, skin infections, sexually transmitted diseases, conjunctivitis (ophthalmic preparations only)
Class: Antibiotic, Antibiotic; macrolide, Antimicrobial, Covid-19 putative drug
Half-life: 68 hours
Clinically important, potentially hazardous interactions with: aminophylline, antacids, artemether/lumefantrine, astemizole, atorvastatin, betrixaban, bromocriptine, cabergoline, colchicine, coumarins, cyclosporine, digoxin, droperidol, ergotamine, fluvastatin, lovastatin, methysergide, mizolastine, oral typhoid vaccine, pimozide, pravastatin, quetiapine, reboxetine, rifabutin, ritonavir, simvastatin, venetoclax, warfarin
Important contra-indications noted in the prescribing guidelines for: nursing mothers; pediatric patients
Note: AzaSite is for topical ophthalmic use only (see reactions noted [Ophth] below).

Skin
AGEP [3]
Anaphylactoid reactions / anaphylaxis (includes anaphylactic shock) [2]
Churg-Strauss syndrome [2]
DRESS syndrome (Drug-induced hypersensitivity syndrome) [4]
Erythema [2]
Exanthems [3]
Fixed eruption / fixed drug eruption [5]
Hypersensitivity [3]
Jarisch-Herxheimer reaction [2]
Linear IgA bullous dermatosis [2]
Pruritus (itching) [5]
Rash [Ophth] (2–10%) [7]
Stevens-Johnson syndrome and toxic epidermal necrolysis (SJS/TEN) [9]
Urticaria / hives [Ophth] [2]

Cardiovascular
Bradycardia / sinus bradycardia [2]
Cardiotoxicity [8]
QT interval prolonged / QT prolongation [12]
Torsades de pointes [5]

Central Nervous System
Anorexia (2–10%)
Headache [3]
Vertigo / dizziness [2]

Gastrointestinal/Hepatic
Abdominal pain (2–10%) [4]
Cholestasis / cholestatic jaundice [4]
Diarrhea (4–9%) [19]
Gastrointestinal disorder / discomfort [3]
Hepatotoxicity / liver injury / acute liver injury / drug-induced liver injury (DILI) [8]
Nausea (7%) [9]
Vomiting (2–10%) [6]

Genitourinary
Vaginitis (includes vulvitis) (2–10%)

Local
Injection-site erythema (2–10%)
Injection-site pain (2–10%) [3]

Neuromuscular/Skeletal
Rhabdomyolysis [5]

Ocular
Keratitis (ocular keratitis) / corneal inflammation) [2]

Otic
Hearing loss (hypoacusis) [4]
Tinnitus [2]

Other
Adverse effects / adverse reactions [15]
Death [2]
Hiccups / singultus [2]
Side effects [2]

AZTREONAM

Trade names: Azactam (Bristol-Myers Squibb), Cayston (Gilead)
Indications: Aerobic gram-negative bacillary infections, improve respiratory symptoms in cystic fibrosis patients
Class: Antibiotic, Antibiotic; beta-lactam, Antimicrobial
Half-life: 1.4–2.2 hours
Clinically important, potentially hazardous interactions with: none known
Important contra-indications noted in the prescribing guidelines for: pediatric patients
Note: Safety and effectiveness have not been established in pediatric patients <7 years of age, patients with FEV1 <25% or >75% predicted, or patients colonized with *Burkholderia cepacia*.

Skin
Exanthems [4]
Hypersensitivity [2]
Pruritus (itching) [5]
Purpura [2]
Rash (<10%)
Stevens-Johnson syndrome and toxic epidermal necrolysis (SJS/TEN) [2]
Urticaria / hives [5]

Mucosal
Nasal congestion [2]

Cardiovascular
Thrombophlebitis (<10%)

Central Nervous System
Headache [3]

Gastrointestinal/Hepatic
Diarrhea [3]
Nausea [2]

Local
Injection-site pain (<10%)
Injection-site phlebitis (<10%)

Respiratory
Cough [3]
Dyspnea / shortness of breath [2]
Wheezing [2]

BACAMPICILLIN

Synonym: carampicillin
Indications: Respiratory tract infections, urinary tract infections, gonorrhea
Class: Antibiotic, Antibiotic; beta-lactam, Antibiotic; penicillin, Antimicrobial
Half-life: 65 minutes
Clinically important, potentially hazardous interactions with: anticoagulants, cyclosporine, demeclocycline, doxycycline, imipenem/cilastatin, methotrexate, minocycline, oxytetracycline, tetracycline
Important contra-indications noted in the prescribing guidelines for: nursing mothers

---

Skin
Exanthems [3]

BACITRACIN

Trade names: Baciguent (Pharmacia & Upjohn), Baciim (X-Gen), Cortisporin (Monarch), Neosporin (Johnson & Johnson)
Indications: Bacterial infections
Class: Antibiotic, Antimicrobial
Half-life: N/A
Clinically important, potentially hazardous interactions with: clioquinol, colistin, kanamycin, neomycin, pyridostigmine, rocuronium, streptomycin
Note: Bacitracin is supplied in many forms and vehicles: intramuscular; topical, ophthalmic, otic, aerosols, for irrigations. Many bacitracin ointments are combinations with neomycin and polymyxin B.

Skin
Anaphylactoid reactions / anaphylaxis (includes anaphylactic shock) [21]
Contact dermatitis [11]
Facial edema (<10%)
Pruritus (itching) (<10%)
Rash (<10%)

Mucosal
Rectal itch (<10%)

Cardiovascular
Chest pain (<10%)
Hypotension (<10%)

Central Nervous System
Anorexia (<10%)
Pain (<10%)

Gastrointestinal/Hepatic
Nausea (<10%)
Vomiting (<10%)

Renal
Nephrotoxicity / kidney injury / acute kidney injury (AKI) / drug-induced kidney injury (from intramuscular injections) (<10%)

BACLOFEN

Trade names: Baclofen (Watson), Gablofen (Mallinckrodt), Lioresal (Medtronic)
Indications: Spasticity resulting from multiple sclerosis
Class: GABA receptor agonist, Skeletal muscle relaxant
Half-life: 2.5–4 hours
Clinically important, potentially hazardous interactions with: acebutolol, alcohol, alfuzosin, amitriptyline, captopril, cilazapril, diclofenac, enalapril, fosinopril, irbesartan, levodopa, lisinopril, meloxicam, olmesartan, quinapril, ramipril, trandolapril
Important contra-indications noted in the prescribing guidelines for: pediatric patients
Note: Children appear to be at higher risk for complications than adults when using intrathecal baclofen (ITB). ITB therapy is a safe and effective treatment for severe spasticity in the pediatric population, but does have a 31% rate of complications requiring surgical management over a 3-year treatment period.
Warning: DO NOT DISCONTINUE ABRUPTLY

Skin
Cutaneous toxicity / skin toxicity [2]
Exanthems [2]
Rash (<10%)

Cardiovascular
Bradycardia / sinus bradycardia [2]
Hypertension [2]
Hypotension [3]

Central Nervous System
Coma [4]
Confusion (<10%)
Dyskinesia [2]
Encephalopathy (includes hepatic encephalopathy) [6]
Hallucinations [4]
Headache (<10%)
Insomnia (>10%) [2]
Psychosis [4]
Seizures [11]
Sleep apnea [4]
Slurred speech (>10%)
Somnolence (drowsiness) (>10%) [8]
Vertigo / dizziness (>10%) [7]

Gastrointestinal/Hepatic
Constipation (<10%)
Intestinal pseudo-obstruction (Ogilvie syndrome) [2]
Nausea (<10%)

Genitourinary
Polyuria (includes polyuric syndrome) (<10%)

Neuromuscular/Skeletal
Asthenia / fatigue (>10%) [8]
Myoclonus (see also hypnic jerk) [2]

Other
Adverse effects / adverse reactions [2]
Infection [2]
Side effects (<2%)

BALOXAVIR MARBOXIL

Trade name: Xofluza (Shionogi)
Indications: Indicated for the treatment of acute uncomplicated influenza in patients 12 years of age and older who have been symptomatic for no more than 48 hours
Class: Polymerase acidic (PA) endonuclease inhibitor
Half-life: 79.1 hours
Clinically important, potentially hazardous interactions with: calcium hydroxylapatite, selenium, zinc
Pregnancy category: no available data

Gastrointestinal/Hepatic
Diarrhea (3%) [3]
Vomiting [4]

Respiratory
Bronchitis (2%)

Other
Adverse effects / adverse reactions [4]

BALSALAZIDE

Trade names: Colazal (Salix), Colazide (Almirall)
Indications: Mild to moderately active ulcerative colitis
Class: Aminosalicylate
Half-life: N/A
Clinically important, potentially hazardous interactions with: azathioprine, cardiac glycosides, folic acid, heparin, low molecular weight heparins, mercaptopurine, thiopurine analogs, varicella virus-containing vaccines
Important contra-indications noted in the prescribing guidelines for: nursing mothers; pediatric patients

---

Skin
- Hypersensitivity [2]

Mucosal
- Stomatitis (oral mucositis) (3%)

Central Nervous System
- Anorexia (2%)
- Fever (pyrexia) (includes hyperpyrexia) (2–6%)
- Headache (15%)
- Insomnia (2%)

Gastrointestinal/Hepatic
- Abdominal pain (6–13%)
- Colitis (ulcerative, exacerbation) (6%)
- Diarrhea (5–9%)
- Dyspepsia / functional dyspepsia (indigestion) (see also gastroparesis) (2%)
- Flatulence (2%)
- Nausea (4%)
- Vomiting (10%)

Genitourinary
- Dysmenorrhea (3%)

Neuromuscular/Skeletal
- Arthralgia (4%)
- Asthenia / fatigue (2%)

Respiratory
- Cough (2–3%)
- Influenza- ('flu)-like syndrome (<4%)
- Nasopharyngitis (6%)
- Pharyngitis (sore throat) (2%)
- Pharyngolaryngeal pain (3%)
- Rhinitis / rhinosinusitis (see also sinusitis) (2%)

BARICITINIB

Trade name: Olumiant (Eli Lilly and Co)
Indications: Treatment of adult patients with moderately to severely active rheumatoid arthritis who have had an inadequate response to one or more TNF antagonist therapies. Treatment of atopic dermatitis
Class: Covid-19 putative drug, Janus kinase (JAK) inhibitor
Half-life: ~12 hours
Clinically important, potentially hazardous interactions with: none known
Pregnancy category: Insufficient data to inform a drug-associated risk for major birth defects or miscarriage
Warning: ◆ INCREASED RISK OF SERIOUS BACTERIAL, FUNGAL, VIRAL AND OPPORTUNISTIC INFECTIONS LEADING TO HOSPITALIZATION OR DEATH, INCLUDING TUBERCULOSIS (TB). INTERRUPT TREATMENT WITH BARICITINIB IF SERIOUS INFECTION OCCURS UNTIL THE INFECTION IS CONTROLLED. TEST FOR LATENT TB BEFORE AND DURING THERAPY; TREAT LATENT TB PRIOR TO USE. MONITOR ALL PATIENTS FOR ACTIVE TB DURING TREATMENT, EVEN PATIENTS WITH INITIAL NEGATIVE, LATENT TB TEST.
◆ HIGHER RATE OF ALL-CAUSE MORTALITY, INCLUDING SUDDEN CARDIOVASCULAR DEATH WITH ANOTHER JANUS KINASE INHIBITOR (JAK) VS. TNF BLOCKERS IN RHEUMATOID ARTHRITIS (RA) PATIENTS.
◆ MALIGNANCIES HAVE OCCURRED IN PATIENTS TREATED WITH BARICITINIB. HIGHER RATE OF LYMPHOMAS AND LUNG CANCERS WITH ANOTHER JAK INHIBITOR VS. TNF BLOCKERS IN RA PATIENTS.
◆ HIGHER RATE OF MACE (DEFINED AS CARDIOVASCULAR DEATH, MYOCARDIAL INFARCTION, AND STROKE) WITH ANOTHER JAK INHIBITOR VS. TNF BLOCKERS IN RA PATIENTS.
◆ THROMBOSIS HAS OCCURRED IN PATIENTS TREATED WITH BARICITINIB. INCREASED INCIDENCE OF PULMONARY EMBOLISM, VENOUS AND ARTERIAL THROMBOSIS WITH ANOTHER JAK INHIBITOR VS. TNF

Skin
- Herpes simplex (1–2%)

Endocrine/Metabolic
- Hypercholesterolemia [2]
- Serum creatinine increased [2]

Gastrointestinal/Hepatic
- Nausea (3%)

Hematologic
- Neutropenia (neutrophils decreased) [2]

Respiratory
- Upper respiratory tract infection (15–16%) [3]

Other
- Adverse effects / adverse reactions [5]
- Cytomegalovirus infection [2]
- Death [2]
- Infection [6]

BASILIXIMAB

Trade name: Simulect (Novartis)
Indications: Prophylaxis of organ rejection in renal transplantation
Class: Interleukin-2 receptor antagonist, Monoclonal antibody
Half-life: 7.2 days
Clinically important, potentially hazardous interactions with: cyclosporine, Hemophilus B vaccine, mycophenolate
Important contra-indications noted in the prescribing guidelines for: nursing mothers

---

Skin
- Acneiform eruption / acneiform dermatitis / acneiform rash (>10%)
- Candidiasis / candidosis (3–10%)
- Cyst / pseudocyst (3–10%)
- Edema / fluid retention (generalized) (3–10%)
- Facial edema (3–10%)
- Genital edema (3–10%)
- Hematoma / cutaneous hematoma (3–10%)
- Herpes simplex (3–10%)
- Herpes zoster (3–10%)
- Peripheral edema (>10%)
- Pruritus (itching) (3–10%)
- Rash (3–10%)
- Ulcerations (3–10%)
- Wound complications (>10%)

Hair
- Hypertrichosis (3–10%)

Mucosal
- Gingival hyperplasia / gingival hypertrophy / gingival enlargement / gingival overgrowth (3–10%)
- Stomatitis (oral mucositis) (3–10%)
- Ulcerative stomatitis (3–10%)

Cardiovascular
- Angina (3–10%)
- Arrhythmias (3–10%)
- Atrial fibrillation (3–10%)
- Cardiac failure (3–10%)
- Chest pain (3–10%)
- Hypertension (>10%)
- Hypotension (3–10%)
- Tachycardia (3–10%)

Central Nervous System
- Agitation (3–10%)
- Anxiety (3–10%)
- Depression (3–10%)
- Fever (pyrexia) (includes hyperpyrexia) (>10%)
- Headache (>10%)
- Hypoesthesia / hypesthesia (numbness) (3–10%)
- Insomnia (>10%)
- Pain (>10%)
- Paresthesias (3–10%)
- Rigors (3–10%)
- Tremor (>10%)
- Vertigo / dizziness (3–10%)

Endocrine/Metabolic
- Acidosis (includes lactic acidosis) (3–10%)
- Dehydration (3–10%)
- Diabetes mellitus (3–10%)
- Hypercalcemia (3–10%)
- Hypercholesterolemia (>10%)
- Hyperglycemia (includes glucose increased) (>10%)
- Hyperkalemia (>10%)
- Hyperlipidemia / lipids elevated (3–10%)
- Hypertriglyceridemia (includes triglycerides increased) (3–10%)
- Hyperuricemia (>10%)
- Hypocalcemia (3–10%)
- Hypoglycemia (3–10%)
- Hypokalemia (>10%)
- Hypophosphatemia (>10%)
- Weight gain (3–10%)

Gastrointestinal/Hepatic
- Abdominal distension (3–10%)
- Abdominal pain (>10%)
- Black stools / melena (3–10%)
- Constipation (>10%)
- Diarrhea (>10%)
- Dyspepsia / functional dyspepsia (indigestion) (see also gastroparesis) (>10%)
- Esophagitis (3–10%)
- Flatulence (3–10%)
- Gastroenteritis (3–10%)
- Gastrointestinal bleeding (3–10%)
- Gastrointestinal disorder / discomfort (69%)
- Hernia (3–10%)
- Nausea (>10%)
- Vomiting (>10%)

Genitourinary
Albuminuria (3–10%)
Dysuria (3–10%)
Hematuria (3–10%)
Impotence (3–10%)
Oliguria (3–10%)
Urinary frequency (3–10%)
Urinary retention (3–10%)
Urinary tract infection (>10%)

Hematologic
Anemia (>10%)
Hemorrhage (3–10%)
Leukocytopenia (leukopenia) / leukocytes (white blood cells) decreased (3–10%)
Polycythemia / erythrocytosis (3–10%)
Sepsis (3–10%)
Thrombocytopenia / platelets decreased (3–10%)
Thrombosis (3–10%)

Neuromuscular/Skeletal
Arthralgia (3–10%)
Asthenia / fatigue (3–10%)
Back pain (3–10%)
Cramps (3–10%)
Fractures (3–10%)
Leg pain (3–10%)
Myalgia/Myopathy (3–10%)

Ocular
Abnormal vision (3–10%)
Cataract (3–10%)
Conjunctivitis (conjunctival inflammation) (3–10%)

Renal
Renal tubular necrosis (3–10%)

Respiratory
Bronchitis (3–10%)
Bronchospasm (3–10%)
Cough (3–10%)
Dyspnea / shortness of breath (>10%)
Pharyngitis (sore throat) (3–10%)
Pneumonia (3–10%)
Pulmonary edema (cardiogenic / non-cardiogenic) (3–10%)
Rhinitis / rhinosinusitis (see also sinusitis) (3–10%)
Sinusitis (see also rhinitis / rhinosinusitis) (3–10%)
Upper respiratory tract infection (>10%)

Other
Infection (viral) (>10%)

BCG VACCINE

Synonym: Bacille Calmette-Guerin
Trade names: Mycobax (Sanofi-Aventis), TICE BCG (Organon)
Indications: Immunization against tuberculosis
Class: Vaccine
Half-life: N/A
Clinically important, potentially hazardous interactions with: alefacept, aminophylline, azacitidine, betamethasone, cabazitaxel, cefazolin, cefixime, ceftaroline fosamil, ceftobiprole, ciprofloxacin, demeclocycline, denileukin, docetaxel, doripenem, doxycycline, fingolimod, gefitinib, gemifloxacin, leflunomide, levofloxacin, minocycline, monosodium glutamate, moxifloxacin, ofloxacin, oxaliplatin, pazopanib, pralatrexate, rifaximin, rifaximin, sulfadiazine, telavancin, telithromycin, temsirolimus

---

Skin
Abscess [16]
Anaphylactoid reactions / anaphylaxis (includes anaphylactic shock) [5]
Churg-Strauss syndrome [15]
Dermatitis [2]
Erythema [3]
Fixed eruption / fixed drug eruption [2]
Hypersensitivity [2]
Keloid [4]
Lupus vulgaris [22]
Lymphadenitis [9]
Lymphadenopathy [92]
Papular lesions [6]
Sarcoidosis / sarcoid-like reaction (cutaneous sarcoidosis) [4]
Scar [8]
Scrofuloderma [5]
Sweet's syndrome [2]
Ulcerations [6]
Vasculitis (angiitis) / cutaneous vasculitis (angiitis) [2]

Mucosal
Mucocutaneous lymph node syndrome (Kawaski syndrom) [2]

Central Nervous System
Fever (pyrexia) (includes hyperpyrexia) [6]
Neurotoxicity [2]

Gastrointestinal/Hepatic
Hepatitis [3]
Hepatotoxicity / liver injury / acute liver injury / drug-induced liver injury (DILI) [2]

Genitourinary
Balanitis (glans penile inflammation) [3]
Balanoposthitis [2]
Bladder disorder [2]
Cystitis (includes interstitial cystitis / bladder pain syndrome) [2]
Hematuria [2]

Hematologic
Sepsis [3]

Local
Injection-site abscess [3]
Injection-site reaction [3]
Injection-site ulceration [4]

Neuromuscular/Skeletal
Arthralgia [7]
Asthenia / fatigue [4]
Osteomyelitis [35]
Reiter's syndrome (reactive arthritis) [3]

Ocular
Optic neuritis / papillitis [2]
Uveitis / anterior uveitis / posterior uveitis / panuveitis [4]

Other
Adverse effects / adverse reactions [5]
Cancer [3]
Death [14]
Infection [3]
Systemic reactions [2]

BECAPLERMIN

Trade names: PDGF (Novartis), Regranex (Janssen) (Cilag AG)
Indications: Diabetic ulcers $\leq$ 5 cm^2
Class: Platelet derived growth factor-BB
Half-life: N/A
Clinically important, potentially hazardous interactions with: none known
Important contra-indications noted in the prescribing guidelines for: nursing mothers; pediatric patients
Warning: INCREASED RATE OF MORTALITY SECONDARY TO MALIGNANCY

Skin
Cellulitis and pseudocellulitis (>10%)
Ulcerations (>10%)

BECLOMETHASONE

Trade names: Beconase AQ (GSK), Qnasl (Teva), Qvar (3M), Vanceril (Schering)
Indications: Allergic rhinitis, asthma
Class: Corticosteroid / Glucocorticoid, Corticosteroid, inhaled
Half-life: N/A
Clinically important, potentially hazardous interactions with: diuretics, estrogens, ketoconazole, live vaccines, oral contraceptives, phenytoin, rifampin, warfarin
Important contra-indications noted in the prescribing guidelines for: nursing mothers; pediatric patients

---

Skin
Bruise / bruising / contusion / ecchymosis (ecchymoses) [3]
Candidiasis / candidosis [2]

Mucosal
Epistaxis (nosebleed) (with nasally-inhaled formulation) (2%)
Nasal discomfort (5%)
Oral candidiasis [4]

Central Nervous System
Headache (2%) [2]

Neuromuscular/Skeletal
Osteoporosis [5]

Ocular
Cataract [4]
Glaucoma (includes acute angle-closure glaucoma) [3]

Respiratory
Upper respiratory tract infection [2]

Other
Adverse effects / adverse reactions [10]

BEDAQUILINE

Trade name: Sirturo (Janssen)
Indications: Pulmonary multi-drug resistant tuberculosis
Class: Antimycobacterial (including antitubercular), Diarylquinoline
Half-life: 5.5 months
Clinically important, potentially hazardous interactions with: ketoconazole, rifabutin, rifampin, rifapentine, strong CYP3A4 inducers or inhibitors
Important contra-indications noted in the prescribing guidelines for: nursing mothers; pediatric patients
Warning: INCREASED RISK OF DEATH / QT PROLONGATION

Skin
Rash (8%)

Cardiovascular
Chest pain (11%) [2]

QT interval prolonged / QT prolongation [10]

Central Nervous System
Anorexia (9%)
Headache (28%) [3]
Vertigo / dizziness [2]

Endocrine/Metabolic
ALT increased (<10%)
AST increased (<10%)
Hyperuricemia [2]

Gastrointestinal/Hepatic
Diarrhea [2]
Hepatotoxicity / liver injury / acute liver injury / drug-induced liver injury (DILI) [4]
Nausea (38%) [5]
Vomiting [3]

Neuromuscular/Skeletal
Arthralgia (33%) [2]
Pain in extremities [2]

Otic
Hearing loss (hypoacusis) [2]

Respiratory
Hemoptysis (18%)

Other
Adverse effects / adverse reactions [6]
Infection [3]

BELATACEPT

Trade name: Nulojix (Bristol-Myers Squibb)
Indications: Prophylaxis of organ rejection in kidney transplantation
Class: Immunosuppressant, T-cell co-stimulation blocker
Half-life: 7–10 days
Clinically important, potentially hazardous interactions with: live vaccines, mycophenolate
Important contra-indications noted in the prescribing guidelines for: nursing mothers; pediatric patients
Note: Contra-indicated in patients without immunity to Epstein-Barr virus.
Warning: POST-TRANSPLANT LYMPHOPROLIFERATIVE DISORDER, OTHER MALIGNANCIES, AND SERIOUS INFECTIONS

Skin
Acneiform eruption / acneiform dermatitis / acneiform rash (8%)
Hematoma / cutaneous hematoma (<10%)
Hyperhidrosis (<10%)
Lymphoproliferative disease / lymphoproliferative disorder (post-transplant) [7]
Peripheral edema (34%)

Hair
Alopecia / hair loss (<10%)

Mucosal
Aphthous stomatitis / aphthous ulcer / aphtha (aphthae) (<10%)
Stomatitis (oral mucositis) (<10%)

Cardiovascular
Atrial fibrillation (<10%)
Hypertension (32%)
Hypotension (18%)

Central Nervous System
Anxiety (10%)
Fever (pyrexia) (includes hyperpyrexia) (28%)
Guillain-Barré syndrome / acute inflammatory demyelinating polyradiculoneuropathy / acute motor axonal neuropathy (<10%)
Headache (21%)
Insomnia (15%)
Tremor (8%)
Vertigo / dizziness (9%)

Endocrine/Metabolic
Creatine phosphokinase (CPK) / creatine kinase increased (hyperCKemia) (15%)
Dyslipidemia (19%)
Hypercholesterolemia (11%)
Hyperglycemia (includes glucose increased) (19%)
Hyperkalemia (20%)
Hyperuricemia (5%)
Hypocalcemia (13%)
Hypokalemia (21%)
Hypomagnesemia (7%)
Hypophosphatemia (19%)

Gastrointestinal/Hepatic
Abdominal pain (9–19%)
Constipation (33%)
Diarrhea (39%)
Nausea (24%)
Vomiting (22%)

Genitourinary
Dysuria (11%)
Enuresis (urinary incontinence) (<10%)
Hematuria (16%)
Urinary tract infection (37%) [2]

Hematologic
Anemia (45%)
Leukocytopenia (leukopenia) / leukocytes (white blood cells) decreased (20%)
Neutropenia (neutrophils decreased) (<10%) [2]

Neuromuscular/Skeletal
Arthralgia (17%)
Back pain (13%)
Bone pain / joint pain (<10%)

Renal
Proteinuria (16%)
Renal failure (<10%)
Renal tubular necrosis (9%)

Respiratory
Bronchitis (10%)
Cough (24%)
Dyspnea / shortness of breath (12%)
Influenza (11%)
Nasopharyngitis (13%)
Upper respiratory tract infection (15%)

Other
Graft dysfunction (25%)
Infection (<10%) [7]
Malignancies [3]

BELIMUMAB

Trade name: Benlysta (GSK)
Indications: Systemic lupus erythematosus
Class: Immunosuppressant, Monoclonal antibody
Half-life: 19.4 days
Clinically important, potentially hazardous interactions with: biologic therapies, cyclophosphamide, denileukin, live vaccines, typhoid vaccine, yellow fever vaccine
Important contra-indications noted in the prescribing guidelines for: the elderly; nursing mothers
Note: Contra-indicated in patients who have had anaphylaxis with belimumab.

Skin
Hypersensitivity (13%) [2]

Central Nervous System
Anxiety (4%)
Depression (5%)
Fever (pyrexia) (includes hyperpyrexia) (10%)
Headache [3]
Insomnia (7%)
Leukoencephalopathy / posterior reversible encephalopathy syndrome (PRES) [2]
Migraine (5%)

Gastrointestinal/Hepatic
Diarrhea (12%)
Gastroenteritis (3%)
Nausea (15%) [2]

Genitourinary
Cystitis (includes interstitial cystitis / bladder pain syndrome) (4%)

Local
Infusion-related reactions [3]

Neuromuscular/Skeletal
Asthenia / fatigue [2]
Pain in extremities (6%)

Respiratory
Bronchitis (9%)
Nasopharyngitis (9%)
Pharyngitis (sore throat) (5%)
Upper respiratory tract infection [2]

Other
Adverse effects / adverse reactions [3]
Death [2]
Infection [4]

BELINOSTAT

Trade name: Beleodaq (Spectrum)
Indications: Peripheral T-cell lymphoma
Class: Histone deacetylase (HDAC) inhibitor
Half-life: 1 hour
Clinically important, potentially hazardous interactions with: strong UGT1A1 inhibitors
Important contra-indications noted in the prescribing guidelines for: nursing mothers; pediatric patients

---

Skin
Peripheral edema (20%) [2]
Pruritus (itching) (16%)
Rash (20%)

Hair
Alopecia / hair loss [2]

Cardiovascular
Hypotension (10%)
Phlebitis (10%)
QT interval prolonged / QT prolongation (11%) [2]

Central Nervous System
Anorexia [2]
Chills (16%)
Fever (pyrexia) (includes hyperpyrexia) (35%) [2]
Headache (15%) [3]
Peripheral neuropathy [2]
Vertigo / dizziness (10%) [2]

Endocrine/Metabolic
Appetite decreased (15%)
Creatine phosphokinase (CPK) / creatine kinase increased (hyperCKemia) (>2%)
Hypokalemia (12%)

Gastrointestinal/Hepatic
Abdominal pain (11%)
Constipation (23%) [5]
Diarrhea (23%) [6]
Nausea (42%) [11]
Vomiting (29%) [11]

Hematologic
Anemia (32%) [5]
Leukocytopenia (leukopenia) / leukocytes (white blood cells) decreased [2]
Lymphopenia (lymphocytopenia) / lymphocytes decreased [2]
Neutropenia (neutrophils decreased) [4]
Thrombocytopenia / platelets decreased (16%) [3]
Thrombosis [2]

Local
Infusion-site pain (14%)
Injection-site reaction [2]

Neuromuscular/Skeletal
Asthenia / fatigue (37%) [12]
Myalgia/Myopathy [2]

Respiratory
Cough (19%)
Dyspnea / shortness of breath (22%) [4]
Pneumonia (>2%)
Pneumonitis [2]

Other
Allergic reactions [2]
Hiccups / singultus [2]
Multiorgan failure (>2%)

BEMPEDOIC ACID

Trade name: Nexletol (Esperion Therapeutics)
Indications: An adjunct to diet and maximally tolerated statin therapy for the treatment of adults with heterozygous familial hypercholesterolemia or established atherosclerotic cardiovascular disease who require additional lowering of LDL-C
Class: Adenosine triphosphate-citrate lyase inhibitor
Half-life: ~21 hours
Clinically important, potentially hazardous interactions with: pravastatin, simvastatin
Pregnancy category: Discontinue bempedoic acid when pregnancy is recognized unless the benefits of therapy outweigh the potential risks to the fetus. Breastfeeding is not recommended.
Important contra-indications noted in the prescribing guidelines for: nursing mothers
Note: Hyperuricemia: Elevations in serum uric acid have occurred. Assess uric acid levels periodically as clinically indicated. Monitor for signs and symptoms of hyperuricemia, and initiate treatment with urate-lowering drugs as appropriate. Bempedoic acid is associated with an increased risk of tendon rupture or injury. Discontinue treatment immediately if a patient experiences rupture of a tendon.

Cardiovascular
Atrial fibrillation (with statin +/- other lipid lowering therapies) (2%)

Endocrine/Metabolic
Hypertransaminasemia (hepatic transaminitis) / elevated transaminases (with statin +/- other lipid lowering therapies) (2%)
Hyperuricemia (with statin +/- other lipid lowering therapies) (4%) [2]
Serum creatinine increased (with statin +/- other lipid lowering therapies) (2%)
Uremia (with statin +/- other lipid lowering therapies) (4%)

Gastrointestinal/Hepatic
Abdominal pain (with statin +/- other lipid lowering therapies) (3%)
Cholelithiasis (gallstones in the gall bladder or the bile duct) [2]

Hematologic
Anemia (with statin +/- other lipid lowering therapies) (3%)
Hemoglobin decreased (with statin +/- other lipid lowering therapies) (5%)
Leukocytopenia (leukopenia) / leukocytes (white blood cells) decreased (with statin +/- other lipid lowering therapies) (~ 9%)
Thrombocythemia (thrombocytosis) / platelets increased (with statin +/- other lipid lowering therapies) (10%)

Neuromuscular/Skeletal
Back pain (with statin +/- other lipid lowering therapies) (3%)
Gout (with statin +/- other lipid lowering therapies) (2%) [4]
Muscle spasm (with statin +/- other lipid lowering therapies) (4%)
Myalgia/Myopathy [3]
Pain in extremities (with statin +/- other lipid lowering therapies) (3%)

Respiratory
Bronchitis (with statin +/- other lipid lowering therapies) (3%)
Upper respiratory tract infection (with statin +/- other lipid lowering therapies) (5%)

Other
Adverse effects / adverse reactions [4]

BENAZEPRIL

Trade names: Lotensin (Novartis), Lotensin HCT (Novartis), Lotrel (Novartis)
Indications: Hypertension
Class: Angiotensin-converting enzyme (ACE) inhibitor, Antihypertensive, Vasodilator
Half-life: 10–11 hours
Clinically important, potentially hazardous interactions with: allopurinol, amifostine, amiloride, angiotensin II receptor blockers, antacids, antidiabetics, antihypertensives, azathioprine, cyclosporine, diazoxide, diuretics, eplerenone, everolimus, gold & gold compounds, herbals, lithium, MAO inhibitors, methylphenidate, NSAIDs, pentoxifylline, phosphodiesterase 5 inhibitors, potassium salts, prostacyclin analogues, rituximab, sirolimus, spironolactone, temsirolimus, tizanidine, tolvaptan, triamterene, trimethoprim, yohimbine
Important contra-indications noted in the prescribing guidelines for: pediatric patients
Note: Lotrel is benazepril and amlodipine. Lotensin-HCT is benazepril and hydrochlorothiazide. Hydrochlorothiazide is a sulfonamide and can be absorbed systemically. Sulfonamides can produce severe, possibly fatal, reactions such as toxic epidermal necrolysis and Stevens-Johnson syndrome.
Contra-indicated in patients with a history of angioedema with or without previous ACE inhibitor treatment.
Warning: FETAL TOXICITY

Skin
Angioedema (formerly named angioneurotic edema) [8]
Peripheral edema [3]

Central Nervous System
Headache (6%)
Vertigo / dizziness (4%)

Respiratory
Cough [10]

BENDAMUSTINE

Trade names: Ribomustin (Mundipharma), Treanda (Cephalon)
Indications: Chronic lymphatic leukemia, non-Hodgkin's lymphoma
Class: Alkylating agent
Half-life: 40 minutes
Clinically important, potentially hazardous interactions with: ciprofloxacin, fluvoxamine, nicotine, ofloxacin, omeprazole
Important contra-indications noted in the prescribing guidelines for: nursing mothers; pediatric patients

---

Skin
Herpes simplex (3%)
Herpes zoster (10%)
Hyperhidrosis (5%)
Hypersensitivity (5%)
Peripheral edema (13%)
Pruritus (itching) (5–6%)
Rash (8–16%) [6]
Stevens-Johnson syndrome and toxic epidermal necrolysis (SJS/TEN) [4]
Xerosis / xeroderma (5%)

Mucosal
Nasal congestion (5%)
Oral candidiasis (6%)
Stomatitis (oral mucositis) (15%)
Xerostomia (dry mouth) (9%) [4]

Cardiovascular
Cardiotoxicity [3]
Chest pain (6%)
Hypotension (6%) [2]
Tachycardia (7%)

Central Nervous System
Anorexia (23%) [5]
Anxiety (8%)
Chills (6–14%) [2]
Depression (6%)
Dysgeusia (taste perversion) (7%)
Fever (pyrexia) (includes hyperpyrexia) (24–34%) [10]
Headache (21%)
Insomnia (13%)
Leukoencephalopathy / posterior reversible encephalopathy syndrome (PRES) [3]
Neurotoxicity [3]
Pain (6%)
Vertigo / dizziness (14%)

Endocrine/Metabolic
Appetite decreased (13%)
Dehydration (14%)
Hyperuricemia (7%)
Hypokalemia (9%)
Weight loss (7–18%) [2]

Gastrointestinal/Hepatic
Abdominal distension (5%)
Abdominal pain (13%)
Constipation (29%) [3]
Diarrhea (9–37%) [3]

Dyspepsia / functional dyspepsia (indigestion) (see also gastroparesis) (11%)
Gastroesophageal reflux (10%)
Hepatotoxicity / liver injury / acute liver injury / drug-induced liver injury (DILI) [2]
Nausea (20–75%) [10]
Vomiting (16–40%) [5]

Genitourinary
Urinary tract infection (10%)

Hematologic
Anemia [11]
Febrile neutropenia (6%) [10]
Hemotoxicity [2]
Leukocytopenia (leukopenia) / leukocytes (white blood cells) decreased [3]
Lymphopenia (lymphocytopenia) / lymphocytes decreased [5]
Myelosuppression / bone marrow suppression / myelotoxicity [2]
Neutropenia (neutrophils decreased) [23]
Sepsis [2]
Thrombocytopenia / platelets decreased [24]

Local
Infusion-related reactions [4]
Infusion-site pain (6%)

Neuromuscular/Skeletal
Arthralgia (6%)
Asthenia / fatigue (8–11%) [14]
Back pain (14%)
Bone pain / joint pain (5%)
Pain in extremities (5%)

Renal
Nephrogenic diabetes insipidus / arginine vasopressin resistance [3]
Nephrotoxicity / kidney injury / acute kidney injury (AKI) / drug-induced kidney injury [2]
Tumor lysis syndrome (TLS) [3]

Respiratory
Cough (4–22%) [2]
Dyspnea / shortness of breath (16%) [2]
Nasopharyngitis (6–7%)
Pneumonia (8%)
Sinusitis (see also rhinitis / rhinosinusitis) (9%)
Upper respiratory tract infection (10%)
Wheezing (5%)

Other
Adverse effects / adverse reactions [3]
Allergic reactions [3]
Death [3]
Infection (6%) [24]

BENDROFLUME-THIAZIDE

Trade names: Corzide (Monarch), Naturetin (Bristol-Myers Squibb)
Indications: Edema, diabetes insipidus, hypertension
Class: Diuretic, thiazide
Half-life: 8.5 hours
Clinically important, potentially hazardous interactions with: digoxin, lithium, tadalafil
Important contra-indications noted in the prescribing guidelines for: the elderly; nursing mothers
Note: Bendroflumethiazide is a sulfonamide and can be absorbed systemically. Sulfonamides can produce severe, possibly fatal, reactions such as toxic epidermal necrolysis and Stevens-Johnson syndrome.
Corzide is bendroflumethiazide and nadolol.

Skin
Phototoxicity [2]

BENRALIZUMAB

Trade name: Fasenra (AstraZeneca)
Indications: Add-on maintenance treatment of patients with severe asthma with an eosinophilic phenotype
Class: Interleukin-5 antagonist, Monoclonal antibody
Half-life: 15 days
Clinically important, potentially hazardous interactions with: none known
Pregnancy category: Insufficient evidence to inform on drug-associated risk
Important contra-indications noted in the prescribing guidelines for: nursing mothers; pediatric patients

---

Skin
Hypersensitivity (3%)
Rash (3%)
Urticaria / hives (3%) [2]

Central Nervous System
Fever (pyrexia) (includes hyperpyrexia) (3%) [2]
Headache (8%) [4]
Vertigo / dizziness [2]

Local
Infusion-site erythema (2%)
Infusion-site pain (2%)
Injection-site papules and nodules (2%)
Injection-site pruritus (2%)
Injection-site reaction [2]

Respiratory
Asthma [8]
Bronchitis [4]
Nasopharyngitis [8]
Pharyngitis (sore throat) (5%)
Sinusitis (see also rhinitis / rhinosinusitis) [2]
Upper respiratory tract infection [5]

BENZALKONIUM

Trade name: Zephrex (Sanofi-Aventis)
Indications: Antisepsis, preoperative skin preparation, wound treatment, vaginal douche
Class: Antiseptic
Half-life: N/A
Clinically important, potentially hazardous interactions with: none known

---

Skin
Anaphylactoid reactions / anaphylaxis (includes anaphylactic shock) [4]
Dermatitis [13]

Ocular
Ocular adverse effect [3]

Other
Allergic reactions [2]

BENZNIDAZOLE

Indications: Chagas disease (trypanosomiasis) in pediatric patients aged 2–12 years
Class: Antibiotic, Antibiotic; nitroimidazole, Antimicrobial
Half-life: 13 hours
Clinically important, potentially hazardous interactions with: disulfiram
Pregnancy category: Can cause fetal harm
Important contra-indications noted in the prescribing guidelines for: nursing mothers
Note: Has the potential for genotoxicity and carcinogenicity.

Skin
DRESS syndrome (Drug-induced hypersensitivity syndrome) [2]
Edema / fluid retention [4]
Hypersensitivity [3]
Pigmentation (Skin) (includes hyperpigmentation) [2]
Pruritus (itching) [5]
Rash [7]
Stevens-Johnson syndrome and toxic epidermal necrolysis (SJS/TEN) [2]
Urticaria / hives [2]

Central Nervous System
Anorexia (<5%)
Fever (pyrexia) (includes hyperpyrexia) [6]
Headache (<5%) [5]
Neurotoxicity [3]
Peripheral neuropathy (2%) [2]
Tremor (2%)
Vertigo / dizziness (4%)

Gastrointestinal/Hepatic
Abdominal distension [2]
Abdominal pain (25%) [4]
Diarrhea [2]
Dyspepsia / functional dyspepsia (indigestion) (see also gastroparesis) [2]
Hepatotoxicity / liver injury / acute liver injury / drug-induced liver injury (DILI) (5%) [2]
Nausea [4]
Vomiting [2]

Hematologic
Eosinophilia / eosinophils increased [2]
Neutropenia (neutrophils decreased) [2]

Neuromuscular/Skeletal
Arthralgia (<5%) [5]
Asthenia / fatigue [5]
Myalgia/Myopathy [3]

Other
Adverse effects / adverse reactions [8]
Allergic reactions [2]

BENZONATATE

Trade name: Tessalon (Forest)
Indications: Symptomatic relief of cough
Class: Antitussive
Half-life: duration: 3–8 hours
Clinically important, potentially hazardous interactions with: none known
Important contra-indications noted in the prescribing guidelines for: nursing mothers; pediatric patients
Note: Benzonatate is related to tetracaine and other anesthetics of the para-aminobenzoic acid class.

Skin
Rash (<10%)

Central Nervous System
Seizures [2]

Ocular
Ocular burning (<10%)

Other
Death [3]

BENZPHETAMINE

Trade name: Didrex (Pfizer)
Indications: Adjunct to diet plan to reduce weight
Class: Amphetamine
Half-life: N/A
Clinically important, potentially hazardous interactions with: furazolidone, guanethidine, MAO inhibitors, SSRIs
Important contra-indications noted in the prescribing guidelines for: the elderly; nursing mothers; pediatric patients

---

Mucosal
Xerostomia (dry mouth) [2]

Central Nervous System
Insomnia [3]
Nervousness [2]
Restlessness [2]
Vertigo / dizziness [2]

BENZTHIAZIDE

Indications: Hypertension
Class: Diuretic, thiazide
Half-life: N/A
Clinically important, potentially hazardous interactions with: digoxin, lithium
Note: Benzthiazide is a sulfonamide and can be absorbed systemically. Sulfonamides can produce severe, possibly fatal, reactions such as toxic epidermal necrolysis and Stevens-Johnson syndrome.

BENZTROPINE

Trade name: Cogentin (Merck)
Indications: Parkinsonism
Class: Anticholinergic, Muscarinic antagonist
Half-life: 6–48 hours
Clinically important, potentially hazardous interactions with: haloperidol, other anticholinergics
Important contra-indications noted in the prescribing guidelines for: nursing mothers; pediatric patients

---

Skin
Photosensitivity (<10%)
Xerosis / xeroderma (>10%)

Mucosal
Xerostomia (dry mouth) (>10%) [3]

Other
Death [2]

BENZYDAMINE

Trade name: Difflam (Meda)
Indications: Musculoskeletal pain
Class: Non-steroidal anti-inflammatory (NSAID)
Half-life: 24 hours
Clinically important, potentially hazardous interactions with: none known
Note: NSAIDs may cause an increased risk of serious cardiovascular and gastrointestinal adverse events, which can be fatal. This risk may increase with duration of use.
Benzdyamine has been used in Brazil as a rave, or club, drug.

Skin
Contact dermatitis [5]
Photocontact dermatitis [8]
Rash [2]

BEPOTASTINE

Synonym: bepotastine besilate
Trade name: Bepreve (ISTA Pharma)
Indications: Allergic conjunctivitis
Class: Histamine H1 receptor antagonist
Half-life: 2.4 hours
Clinically important, potentially hazardous interactions with: none known
Important contra-indications noted in the prescribing guidelines for: nursing mothers; pediatric patients

---

Central Nervous System
Headache (2–5%)

Ocular
Ocular stinging (2–5%)

Respiratory
Nasopharyngitis (2–5%)

BEPRIDIL

Indications: Angina pectoris
Class: Antiarrhythmic, Antiarrhythmic class IV, Calcium channel blocker
Half-life: 24 hours
Clinically important, potentially hazardous interactions with: amisulpride, amprenavir, atazanavir, boceprevir, celiprolol, ciprofloxacin, cobicistat/elvitegravir/emtricitabine/tenofovir alafenamide, cobicistat/elvitegravir/emtricitabine/tenofovir disoproxil, delavirdine, efavirenz, enoxacin, epirubicin, fosamprenavir, gatifloxacin, indinavir, lomefloxacin, lopinavir, mistletoe, moxifloxacin, nilotinib, norfloxacin, ofloxacin, quinolones, ribociclib, ritonavir, sotalol, sparfloxacin, telaprevir, tipranavir
Important contra-indications noted in the prescribing guidelines for: nursing mothers; pediatric patients

---

Skin
Diaphoresis (<2%)
Edema / fluid retention (<10%)
Rash (<2%)

Mucosal
Xerostomia (dry mouth) (<10%) [2]

Cardiovascular
Bradycardia / sinus bradycardia [3]
QT interval prolonged / QT prolongation [5]
Torsades de pointes [11]

Central Nervous System
Paresthesias (2%)
Tremor (<9%)
Vertigo / dizziness [2]

Neuromuscular/Skeletal
Asthenia / fatigue [2]

Respiratory
Pneumonia [5]

BERACTANT

Trade name: Survanta (AbbVie)
Indications: Respiratory distress syndrome (RDS), hyaline membrane disease
Class: Pulmonary surfactant
Half-life: N/A
Clinically important, potentially hazardous interactions with: none known

---

Respiratory
Apnea (65%)

BERGAMOT

Family: Rutaceae
Scientific name: *Citrus aurantium ssp bergamia*
Indications: Headache, bronchitis, vitiligo, mycosis fungoides, psoriasis (in conjunction with UVA), insecticide, essential oil in perfumery, cosmetics, flavoring
Class: Stimulant, mild
Half-life: N/A
Clinically important, potentially hazardous interactions with: none known
Note: Two distinct species are known by the common name of bergamot. This profile does not refer to *Monarda didyma*.
Oil of bergamot possesses photosensitive and melanogenic properties because of the presence of furocoumarins, primarily bergapten (5-methoxypsoralen [5-MOP]).
Its use is restricted or banned in many countries.

Skin
Dermatitis [2]
Photosensitivity [3]
Phototoxicity [8]
Phytophotodermatitis / berloque dermatitis [2]

Other
Adverse effects / adverse reactions [2]

BEROTRALSTAT

Trade name: Orladeyo (BioCryst)
Indications: A prophylactic for the prevention of attacks of hereditary angioedema.

Class: Kallikrein inhibitor
Half-life: ~ 93 hours
Clinically important, potentially hazardous interactions with: cyclosporine, P-gp inhibitors, P-gp inducers, bcrp inhibitors, rifampin, St John's wort
Pregnancy category: Insufficient data in pregnant women available to inform drug-related risks with use in pregnancy.
Note: Berotralstat should not be used for treatment of acute attacks of hereditary angioedema. Additional doses or doses of berotralstat higher than 150 mg once daily are not recommended. An increase in QT was observed at dosages higher than the recommended 150 mg once daily dosage and was concentration dependent.

Central Nervous System
Headache (9%)

Gastrointestinal/Hepatic
Abdominal pain (16%)

Diarrhea (12%)
Flatulence (6%)
Gastroesophageal reflux (7%)
Gastrointestinal disorder / discomfort [2]
Vomiting (12%)

Neuromuscular/Skeletal
Asthenia / fatigue (6%)
Back pain (6%)

BESIFLOXACIN

Trade name: Besivance (Bausch & Lomb)
Indications: Conjunctivitis
Class: Antibiotic, Antibiotic; fluoroquinolone, Antimicrobial
Half-life: 7 hours
Clinically important, potentially hazardous interactions with: none known
Important contra-indications noted in the prescribing guidelines for: nursing mothers; pediatric patients
Note: Fluoroquinolones are associated with an increased risk of tendinitis and tendon rupture in all ages. This risk is further increased in older patients usually over 60 years of age, in patients taking corticosteroid drugs, and in patients with kidney, heart or lung transplants.
Fluoroquinolones may exacerbate muscle weakness in persons with myasthenia gravis.

Central Nervous System
Headache (<2%) [2]

Ocular
Conjunctival erythema (2%)
Conjunctivitis (conjunctival inflammation) [3]
Ocular itching / ocular pruritus (<2%) [2]
Ocular pain (<2%) [3]
Ocular stinging (<2%)
Vision blurred (<2%) [3]

BETA-CAROTENE

Trade name: Solatene (Merck)
Indications: Photosensitivity reactions
Class: Vitamin
Half-life: N/A
Clinically important, potentially hazardous interactions with: acemetacin, bexarotene

---

Skin
Carotenemia (>10%)

BETAMETHASONE

Trade names: Beta-Val (Teva), Betatrex (Savage), Celestone (Schering), Diprolene (Schering), Luxiq (Connetics), Sernivo (Promius), Soluspan (Schering)
Indications: Arthralgia, dermatoses, rhinitis
Class: Corticosteroid / Glucocorticoid
Half-life: N/A
Clinically important, potentially hazardous interactions with: alcohol, aldesleukin, aminoglutethimide, amphotericin B, antacids, antidiabetics, antifungals, aprepitant, barbiturates, BCG vaccine, bile acid sequestrants, calcitriol, calcium channel blockers, clotrimazole, corticorelin, denosumab, diuretics, echinacea, estrogens, fluconazole, isoniazid, leflunomide, mitotane, natalizumab, NSAIDs, phenobarbital, pimecrolimus, primidone, quinolones, rifampin, salicylates, sipuleucel-T, tacrolimus, tetracycline, trastuzumab, vaccines, vecuronium, warfarin
Important contra-indications noted in the prescribing guidelines for: nursing mothers; pediatric patients
Note: Topical [T].

Skin
Acneiform eruption / acneiform dermatitis / acneiform rash [2]
Anaphylactoid reactions / anaphylaxis (includes anaphylactic shock) [2]
Atrophy / Skin atrophy [2]
Dermatitis [4]
Facial edema [2]
Pruritus (itching) [T] [3]
Psoriasis [T] [3]
Striae [T] [2]

Cardiovascular
Cardiomyopathy [6]

Central Nervous System
Headache [2]

Endocrine/Metabolic
Cushing's syndrome [5]

Gastrointestinal/Hepatic
Diarrhea [2]
Pancreatitis / acute pancreatitis [2]

Local
Application-site pain [3]
Application-site pruritus [2]
Injection-site atrophy [2]
Injection-site ulceration [2]

Ocular
Glaucoma (includes acute angle-closure glaucoma) [T] [2]

Respiratory
Nasopharyngitis [4]

Other
Adverse effects / adverse reactions [5]
Allergic reactions [2]

BETAXOLOL

Trade names: Betoptic [Ophthalmic] (Alcon), Kerlone (Pfizer)
Indications: Open-angle glaucoma, hypertension
Class: Adrenergic beta-receptor antagonist
Half-life: 14–22 hours
Clinically important, potentially hazardous interactions with: clonidine, verapamil
Important contra-indications noted in the prescribing guidelines for: nursing mothers; pediatric patients
Note: Cutaneous side effects of beta-receptor blockers are clinically polymorphous. They apparently appear after several months of continuous therapy.

Skin
Cold extremities (2%)
Dermatitis [3]
Diaphoresis (<2%)
Eczema / eczematous reaction / eczematous eruption (<2%)
Edema / fluid retention (<2%)
Erythema (<2%)
Flushing / rubefaction (<2%)
Lymphadenopathy (<2%)
Pruritus (itching) (<2%)
Purpura (<2%)
Rash (<2%) [3]

Hair
Alopecia / hair loss (<2%)
Hypertrichosis (<2%)

Mucosal
Epistaxis (nosebleed) (<2%)
Oral ulceration (<2%)
Sialorrhea (ptyalism; hypersalivation) (<2%)
Xerostomia (dry mouth) (<2%)

Cardiovascular
Angina (<2%)
Arrhythmias (<2%)
Atrioventricular block (<2%)
Bradycardia / sinus bradycardia (6–8%)
Cardiac failure (<2%)
Chest pain (2–7%)
Hypertension (<2%)
Hypotension (<2%)
Myocardial infarction (<2%)
Palpitation (2%)
Peripheral ischemia (<2%)

Central Nervous System
Ageusia (taste loss) / taste disorder (<2%)
Amnesia (<2%)
Anorexia (<2%)
Confusion (<2%)
Dysgeusia (taste perversion) (<2%)
Emotional lability (<2%)
Fever (pyrexia) (includes hyperpyrexia) (<2%)
Hallucinations (<2%)
Headache (7–15%)
Insomnia (<5%)
Myokymia / twitching / fasciculation (<2%)
Pain (<2%)
Paresthesias (2%)
Rigors (<2%)
Stupor (<2%)
Syncope / fainting (<2%)
Tremor (<2%)
Vertigo / dizziness (5–15%)

Endocrine/Metabolic
Acidosis (includes lactic acidosis) (<2%)
ALT increased (<2%)
Appetite increased (<2%)
AST increased (<2%)
Diabetes mellitus (<2%)
Gynecomastia (<2%)
Hypercholesterolemia (<2%)
Hyperglycemia (includes glucose increased) (<2%)
Hyperkalemia (<2%)
Hyperuricemia (<2%)
Hypokalemia (<2%)
Libido decreased (<2%)
Mastodynia (<2%)
Menstrual irregularities (<2%)
Weight gain (<2%)
Weight loss (<2%)

Gastrointestinal/Hepatic
Constipation (<2%)
Diarrhea (2%)
Dyspepsia / functional dyspepsia (indigestion) (see also gastroparesis) (4–5%)
Dysphagia (<2%)
Nausea (2–6%)
Vomiting (<2%)

Genitourinary
Cystitis (includes interstitial cystitis / bladder pain syndrome) (<2%)
Dysuria (<2%)
Oliguria (<2%)
Peyronie's disease (<2%)
Prostatitis (<2%)

Hematologic
Anemia (<2%)
Lymphocytosis / lymphocytes increased (<2%)
Thrombocytopenia / platelets decreased (<2%)
Thrombosis (<2%)

Neuromuscular/Skeletal
Arthralgia (3%)
Asthenia / fatigue (3–10%)
Ataxia (<2%)
Bone pain / joint pain (5%)
Leg cramps (<2%)
Myalgia/Myopathy (3%)
Neck pain (<2%)
Tendinitis (<2%)

Ocular
Abnormal vision (<2%)
Blepharitis (<2%)
Cataract (<2%)
Conjunctivitis (conjunctival inflammation) (<2%)
Iritis (<2%)
Lacrimation (<2%)
Ocular hemorrhage (<2%)
Scotoma (<2%)
Xerophthalmia (dry eyes) (<2%)

Otic
Ear pain (<2%)
Hearing loss (hypoacusis) (<2%)
Tinnitus (<2%)

Renal
Proteinuria (<2%)
Renal function abnormal / renal dysfunction (<2%)

Respiratory
Bronchitis (<2%)
Bronchospasm (<2%)
Cough (<2%)
Dysphonia (includes voice disorders / voice changes) (<2%)
Dyspnea / shortness of breath (2%)
Influenza (<2%)
Pharyngitis (sore throat) (2%)
Pneumonia (<2%)
Sinusitis (see also rhinitis / rhinosinusitis) (<2%)
Upper respiratory tract infection (3%)

Other
Allergic reactions (<2%)
Dipsia (thirst) / polydipsia (<2%)

BETRIXABAN

Trade name: Bevyxxa (Portola)
Indications: Prophylaxis of venous thromboembolism in adult patients hospitalized for an acute medical illness who are at risk for thromboembolic complications
Class: Direct factor Xa inhibitor
Half-life: 19–27 hours
Clinically important, potentially hazardous interactions with: amiodarone, anticoagulants, antiplatelet drugs and thrombolytics, azithromycin, clarithromycin, ketoconazole, verapamil
Pregnancy category: Likely to increase the risk of hemorrhage during pregnancy and delivery
Important contra-indications noted in the prescribing guidelines for: nursing mothers; pediatric patients
Note: Contra-indicated in patients with active pathological bleeding.
Warning: SPINAL/EPIDURAL HEMATOMA

Mucosal
Epistaxis (nosebleed) (2%)

Cardiovascular
Hypertension (2%)

Central Nervous System
Headache (2%)

Endocrine/Metabolic
Hypokalemia (3%)

Gastrointestinal/Hepatic
Constipation (3%)
Diarrhea (2%)
Nausea (2%)

Genitourinary
Hematuria (2%)
Urinary tract infection (3%)

Hematologic
Bleeding (<2%) [4]

BEVACIZUMAB

Trade name: Avastin (Genentech)
Indications: Colon cancer, lung cancer, glioblastoma, renal-cell carcinoma
Class: Angiogenesis inhibitor / antiangiogenic agent, Biologic, Covid-19 putative drug, Monoclonal antibody, Vascular endothelial growth factor (VEGF) inhibitor / antagonist
Half-life: ~ 20 days
Clinically important, potentially hazardous interactions with: antineoplastics, irinotecan, sorafenib, sunitinib
Important contra-indications noted in the prescribing guidelines for: the elderly; nursing mothers; pediatric patients
Note: Bevacizumab-awwb (Mvasi) is biosimilar to Bevacizumab (Avastin). Approved 09/14/2017 Bevacizumab-bvzr (Zirabev) is biosimilar to Bevacizumab (Avastin). Approved 06/27/2019 Bevacizumab-maly (Alymsys) is a biosimilar to Bevacizumab (Avastin). Approved 04/13/2022 Bevacizumab-adcd (Vegzelma) is a biosimilar to Bevacizumab (Avastin). Approved 09/27/2022 Bevacizumab-tnjn (Avzivi) is a biosimilar to Bevacizumab (Avastin). Approved 12/06/2023.
Warning: GASTROINTESTINAL PERFORATIONS, SURGERY AND WOUND HEALING COMPLICATIONS, and HEMORRHAGE

Skin
Acneiform eruption / acneiform dermatitis / acneiform rash [6]
Cutaneous toxicity / skin toxicity [9]
Edema / fluid retention [2]
Hand–foot syndrome (palmar–plantar erythrodysesthesia) [13]
Necrosis (skin necrosis) [2]
Rash [18]
Thrombocytopenic purpura [2]
Ulcerations [3]
Wound complications [11]

Hair
Alopecia / hair loss [5]

Nails
Paronychia [2]

Mucosal
Epistaxis (nosebleed) [6]
Mucosal inflammation [2]
Mucositis [14]
Nasal septal perforation [8]
Oral ulceration [2]
Stomatitis (oral mucositis) [8]

Cardiovascular
Aortic dissection [3]
Cardiac failure [2]
Cardiotoxicity [6]
Hypertension (23–67%) [113]
Hypotension (7–15%)
Thromboembolism (<21%) [16]
Venous thromboembolism [7]

Central Nervous System
Anorexia [17]
Cerebral hemorrhage [7]
Encephalitis [4]
Hallucinations, visual [2]
Headache [8]
Intracranial hemorrhage [2]
Leukoencephalopathy / posterior reversible encephalopathy syndrome (PRES) [20]
Neurotoxicity [13]
Pain [3]
Peripheral neuropathy [11]
Seizures [2]

Endocrine/Metabolic
ALT increased [3]
AST increased [3]
Creatine phosphokinase (CPK) / creatine kinase increased (hyperCKemia) [2]
Hyperglycemia (includes glucose increased) [2]
Hypokalemia [3]
Hypomagnesemia [2]

Gastrointestinal/Hepatic
Abdominal pain [4]
Colitis [3]
Constipation [3]
Diarrhea [46]
Gastrointestinal bleeding [5]
Gastrointestinal fistula [6]
Gastrointestinal perforation / perforated colon / gastric perforation [29]
Hepatotoxicity / liver injury / acute liver injury / drug-induced liver injury (DILI) [5]
Nausea [20]
Pneumatosis intestinalis / pneumatosis cystoides intestinalis [2]
Vomiting [12]

Hematologic
Anemia [21]
Bleeding [16]
Evans' syndrome [2]
Febrile neutropenia [16]
Hemolytic anemia [2]
Hemorrhage [13]
Hemotoxicity [2]
Leukocytopenia (leukopenia) / leukocytes (white blood cells) decreased [21]
Lymphopenia (lymphocytopenia) / lymphocytes decreased [6]
Neutropenia (neutrophils decreased) [56]
Thrombocytopenia / platelets decreased [29]
Thrombosis [19]
Thrombotic complications [4]
Thrombotic microangiopathy [5]

Neuromuscular/Skeletal
Arthralgia [2]

Asthenia / fatigue [46]
Osteonecrosis / avascular necrosis (includes steroid-induced osteonecrosis of the femoral head) [6]

Ocular
Intraocular pressure increased [3]
Iritis [2]
Ocular adverse effect [3]
Uveitis / anterior uveitis / posterior uveitis / panuveitis [2]

Renal
Glomerulonephritis (includes membranous nephropathy) [2]
Nephrotoxicity / kidney injury / acute kidney injury (AKI) / drug-induced kidney injury [2]
Proteinuria [49]

Respiratory
Hemoptysis [5]
Interstitial lung disease / interstitial pneumonitis / interstitial pneumonia (cryptogenic organizing pneumonia) / drug-induced interstitial lung disease [2]
Pneumothorax [12]
Pulmonary embolism [5]
Pulmonary toxicity [2]

Other
Adverse effects / adverse reactions [29]
Allergic reactions [3]
Death [21]
Hiccups / singultus [2]
Infection [11]

BEXAROTENE

Trade name: Targretin (Eisai)
Indications: Cutaneous T-cell lymphoma, mycosis fungoides
Class: Antineoplastic / anticancer agent (see also Immune checkpoint inhibitor), Retinoid
Half-life: 7 hours
Clinically important, potentially hazardous interactions with: acitretin, atorvastatin, beta-carotene, carboplatin, conivaptan, dexamethasone, dong quai, gemfibrozil, grapefruit juice, isotretinoin, oral contraceptives, paclitaxel, saxagliptin, St John's wort, tamoxifen, tetracyclines, tretinoin, vitamin A
Important contra-indications noted in the prescribing guidelines for: nursing mothers; pediatric patients
Note: Retinoids can cause birth defects, and women should avoid bexarotene when pregnant or trying to conceive.
Warning: AVOID IN PREGNANCY

Skin
Acneiform eruption / acneiform dermatitis / acneiform rash (<10%)
Bacterial infection (<13%)
Dermatitis [2]
Erythema [2]
Exanthems (<10%)
Exfoliative dermatitis (10–28%)
Necrosis (skin necrosis) [2]
Nodular eruption (<10%)
Peripheral edema (13%)
Pruritus (itching) (20–30%) [5]
Rash (17%) [3]
Ulcerations (<10%)
Vesiculobullous eruption (<10%)
Xerosis / xeroderma (11%) [2]

Hair
Alopecia / hair loss (4–11%)

Mucosal
Cheilitis (inflammation of the lips) (<10%)
Gingivitis (<10%)
Mucositis [2]
Xerostomia (dry mouth) (<10%)

Central Nervous System
Chills (10%)
Hyperesthesia (<10%)

Endocrine/Metabolic
Hypercholesterolemia [5]
Hyperlipidemia / lipids elevated [4]
Hypertriglyceridemia (includes triglycerides increased) [10]
Hypothyroidism [11]
Mastodynia (<10%)

Hematologic
Anemia [4]
Leukocytopenia (leukopenia) / leukocytes (white blood cells) decreased [5]
Lymphopenia (lymphocytopenia) / lymphocytes decreased [2]
Neutropenia (neutrophils decreased) [9]

Neuromuscular/Skeletal
Arthralgia [2]
Asthenia / fatigue [2]
Myalgia/Myopathy (<10%) [2]

Respiratory
Influenza- ('flu)-like syndrome (4–13%)

Other
Adverse effects / adverse reactions [3]

BEZAFIBRATE

Trade name: Bezalip (Roche)
Indications: Hypercholesterolemia, hyperlipidemia, Type II diabetes
Class: Antilipemic, Fibrate
Half-life: 1–2 hours
Clinically important, potentially hazardous interactions with: cholestyramine, cyclosporine, HMG-CoA reductase inhibitors, MAO inhibitors, warfarin
Important contra-indications noted in the prescribing guidelines for: the elderly; nursing mothers; pediatric patients
Note: This drug is not available in the USA; Israel withdrew bezafibrate in 2006. The Committee for Medicinal Products for Human Use (CHMP) of the European Medicines Agency (EMA) has concluded that the benefits of bezafibrate outweigh the risks in the treatment of patients with blood lipid disorders. However, bezafibrate should not be prescribed for newly-diagnosed patients as first-line treatment, except for those with severe hypertriglyceridemia or patients who cannot take statins.

Skin
Anaphylactoid reactions / anaphylaxis (includes anaphylactic shock) [2]
Pruritus (itching) (3%)

Central Nervous System
Headache [2]
Vertigo / dizziness (2%)

Neuromuscular/Skeletal
Myalgia/Myopathy [9]
Rhabdomyolysis [12]

Renal
Renal failure [5]

BICALUTAMIDE

Trade name: Casodex (AstraZeneca)
Indications: Metastatic prostatic carcinoma
Class: Androgen antagonist
Half-life: up to 10 days
Clinically important, potentially hazardous interactions with: CYP3A4 substrates
Pregnancy category: not indicated for use in women
Important contra-indications noted in the prescribing guidelines for: pediatric patients

Skin
Diaphoresis (6%)
Edema / fluid retention (2–5%)
Hot flashes / hot flushes (49%) [9]
Peripheral edema (8%)
Pruritus (itching) (2–5%)
Rash (6%)
Xerosis / xeroderma (2–5%)

Hair
Alopecia / hair loss (2–5%)

Mucosal
Xerostomia (dry mouth) (2–5%)

Central Nervous System
Paresthesias (6%)

Endocrine/Metabolic
Gynecomastia (38%) [34]
Mastodynia (39%) [16]

Gastrointestinal/Hepatic
Constipation [2]
Hepatotoxicity / liver injury / acute liver injury / drug-induced liver injury (DILI) [5]

Local
Injection-site reaction (2–5%)

Neuromuscular/Skeletal
Asthenia / fatigue [4]
Myalgia/Myopathy (2–5%)

Respiratory
Dyspnea / shortness of breath [2]

Other
Death [2]

BICTEGRAVIR/EMTRICITABINE/TENOFOVIR ALAFENAMIDE

Trade name: Biktarvy (Gilead)
Indications: HIV-1 infection
Class: Antiretroviral, Hepatitis B virus necleoside analog reverse transcriptase inhibitor (tenofovir alafenamide), Integrase strand transfer inhibitor (bictegravir), Nucleoside analog reverse transcriptase inhibitor (emtricitabine)
Half-life: 17 hours (bictegravir); 10 hours (emtricitabine); <1 hour (tenofovir alafenamide)
Clinically important, potentially hazardous interactions with: carbamazepine, dofetilide, metformin, other antiretroviral drugs, oxcarbazepine, phenobarbital, phenytoin, rifabutin, rifampin, rifapentine, St John's wort
Pregnancy category: Insufficient evidence to inform drug-associated risk
Important contra-indications noted in the prescribing guidelines for: nursing mothers; pediatric patients
Warning: POST-TREATMENT ACUTE EXACERBATION OF HEPATITIS B

Skin
Rash (<2%)
Central Nervous System
Abnormal dreams (<3%)
Depression (<2%)
Headache (4–5%)
Insomnia (2%)
Vertigo / dizziness (2%)
Endocrine/Metabolic
ALT increased (<2%)
AST increased (<2%)
Creatine phosphokinase (CPK) / creatine kinase increased (hyperCKemia) (4%)
Hyperamylasemia (2%)
Hyperbilirubinemia (12%)
Hypercholesterolemia (2–3%)
Gastrointestinal/Hepatic
Abdominal pain (<2%)
Diarrhea (3–6%)
Dyspepsia / functional dyspepsia (indigestion) (see also gastroparesis) (<2%)
Flatulence (<2%)
Nausea (3–5%) [2]
Vomiting (<2%)
Hematologic
Neutropenia (neutrophils decreased) (2%)
Neuromuscular/Skeletal
Asthenia / fatigue (2–3%)
Other
Adverse effects / adverse reactions [3]

BIFIDOBACTERIA

Family: Actinomycetaceae
Scientific names: *Bifidobacterium adolescentis, Bifidobacterium animalis, Bifidobacterium bifidum, Bifidobacterium breve, Bifidobacterium infantis, Bifidobacterium lactis, Bifidobacterium longum*
Indications: Diarrhea, atopic eczema, candidiasis, colds and flu, hepatitis, hypercholesterolemia, lactose intolerance, ulcerative colitis, pouchitis, irritable bowel syndrome
Class: Immunomodulator, Probiotic
Half-life: N/A
Clinically important, potentially hazardous interactions with: none known
Note: Immune-deficient subjects or those with mucosal disease may experience serious adverse effects.
Bifidobacterium is often combined with *Lactobacillus, Saccharomyces* or *Streptococcus thermophilus*.

BIMATOPROST

Trade names: Latisse (Allergan), Lumigan (Allergan)
Indications: Reduction of elevated intraocular pressure in open-angle glaucoma or ocular hypertension, hypotrichosis of the eyelashes
Class: Prostaglandin analog, Prostaglandin receptor agonist
Half-life: 45 minutes
Clinically important, potentially hazardous interactions with: none known
Important contra-indications noted in the prescribing guidelines for: nursing mothers; pediatric patients

Skin
Pigmentation (Skin) (includes hyperpigmentation) [2]
Hair
Hirsutism (<5%)
Hypertrichosis [2]
Central Nervous System
Headache (<5%)
Neuromuscular/Skeletal
Asthenia / fatigue (<5%)
Ocular
Asthenopia (<10%)
Blepharitis (<10%)
Cataract (<10%)
Choroidal detachment [2]
Conjunctival edema (<10%)
Conjunctival hemorrhage (<10%)
Conjunctival hyperemia / conjunctival injection (25–45%) [43]
Conjunctivitis (conjunctival inflammation) (<10%)
Deepening of upper lid sulcus [9]
Eyelashes – hypertrichosis (eyelash megalotrichosis) (>10%) [13]
Eyelashes – pigmentation (<10%) [3]
Eyelid erythema (3–10%) [2]
Eyelid irritation (3–10%)
Eyelid pain (3–10%)
Eyelid pigmentation (3–10%) [6]
Eyelid xerosis (3–10%)
Foreign body sensation (<10%)
Iris pigmentation (<10%) [4]
Keratitis (ocular keratitis) / corneal inflammation) [2]
Lacrimation (<10%)
Macular edema [2]
Ocular adverse effect [12]
Ocular burning (<10%)
Ocular discharge (<10%)
Ocular hyperemia [4]
Ocular itching / ocular pruritus (<10%) [5]
Ocular pain [2]
Ocular pigmentation (<3%) [5]
Periorbital pigmentation (<10%) [3]
Photophobia (<10%)
Punctate keratitis (<10%) [2]
Uveitis / anterior uveitis / posterior uveitis / panuveitis [3]
Respiratory
Nasopharyngitis [2]
Upper respiratory tract infection (10%)

BIPERIDEN

Trade name: Akineton (Par)
Indications: Parkinsonism
Class: Anticholinergic, Muscarinic antagonist
Half-life: 18–24 hours
Clinically important, potentially hazardous interactions with: anticholinergics, cyclopenthiazide
Important contra-indications noted in the prescribing guidelines for: nursing mothers; pediatric patients

Central Nervous System
Delirium [2]

BISACODYL

Trade name: Dulcolax (Boehringer Ingelheim)
Indications: Constipation
Class: Stimulant laxative
Half-life: N/A
Clinically important, potentially hazardous interactions with: adreno-corticosteroids, antibiotics, cardiac glycosides, digoxin, diuretics
Important contra-indications noted in the prescribing guidelines for: pediatric patients

Central Nervous System
Headache [3]
Somnolence (drowsiness) [2]
Gastrointestinal/Hepatic
Abdominal pain (<10%) [4]
Diarrhea (<10%)

BISMUTH

Trade names: Helidac (Prometheus), Pepto-Bismol (Procter & Gamble)
Indications: As part of 'triple therapy' (antibiotics + bismuth) for eradication of *H. pylori*. Bismuth subgallate initiates clotting via activation of factor XII, and is used for bleeding during tonsillectomy and adenoidectomy. BIPP impregnated ribbon gauze is used for packing following ear surgery. Bismuth subsalicylate is in OTC products for gastrointestinal complaints and peptic ulcer disease
Class: Disinfectant, Heavy metal
Half-life: 21–72 days
Clinically important, potentially hazardous interactions with: aspirin, ciprofloxacin, demeclocycline, doxycycline, hypoglycemics, lomefloxacin, lymecycline, methotrexate, minocycline, tetracycline, warfarin
Pregnancy category: category C in first and second trimesters; category D in third trimester

Skin
Dermatitis [2]
Hypersensitivity [2]
Pigmentation (Skin) (includes hyperpigmentation) [5]
Pruritus (itching) (triple therapy) [2]
Rash [4]
Mucosal
Oral pigmentation [3]
Stomatitis (oral mucositis) [4]
Tongue pigmentation (>10%) [3]
Xerostomia (dry mouth) (triple therapy) (41%)
Central Nervous System
Dysgeusia (taste perversion) (triple therapy) (46%) [9]
Encephalopathy (includes hepatic encephalopathy) [4]
Pain (triple therapy) (10%)
Tremor [2]
Vertigo / dizziness [2]
Gastrointestinal/Hepatic
Diarrhea [5]
Nausea [4]
Vomiting [2]
Neuromuscular/Skeletal
Arthralgia [10]
Asthenia / fatigue [2]

Other
Adverse effects / adverse reactions (triple therapy) [52]
Allergic reactions [2]
Death [10]

BISOPROLOL

Trade names: Cardicor (Merck Serono), Concor (Merck Serono), Emcor (Merck Serono), Zebeta (Barr), Ziac (Barr)
Indications: Hypertension
Class: Beta adrenergic blocker, Beta blocker
Half-life: 9–12 hours
Clinically important, potentially hazardous interactions with: diltiazem, disopyramide, guanethidine, reserpine, rifampin, verapamil
Important contra-indications noted in the prescribing guidelines for: nursing mothers; pediatric patients
Note: Ziac is bisoprolol and hydrochlorothiazide. Hydrochlorothiazide is a sulfonamide and can be absorbed systemically. Sulfonamides can produce severe, possibly fatal, reactions such as toxic epidermal necrolysis and Stevens-Johnson syndrome.
Contra-indicated in patients with cardiogenic shock, overt cardiac failure, second or third degree AV block, and marked sinus bradycardia.

Skin
Edema / fluid retention (3%)
Peripheral edema (<10%)
Rash (<10%)
Raynaud's phenomenon (<10%)

Cardiovascular
Bradycardia / sinus bradycardia [7]
Hypotension [4]

Central Nervous System
Headache [2]
Hyperesthesia (2%)
Vertigo / dizziness [3]

Neuromuscular/Skeletal
Asthenia / fatigue [2]
Myalgia/Myopathy (<10%)

Other
Adverse effects / adverse reactions [4]

BIVALIRUDIN

Trade name: Angiomax (The Medicines Company)
Indications: Angioplasty adjunct
Class: Thrombin inhibitor
Half-life: 25 minutes
Clinically important, potentially hazardous interactions with: anisindione, dicumarol, heparin, reteplase, streptokinase, tenecteplase, urokinase, warfarin

---

Central Nervous System
Pain (15%)

Hematologic
Bleeding [6]
Thrombosis [3]

Local
Injection-site pain (8%)

Neuromuscular/Skeletal
Back pain (42%)

BLACK COHOSH

Family: Ranunculaceae
Scientific names: *Actaea macrotys, Actaea racemosa, Cimicifuga racemosa*
Indications: Anxiety, arthritis, asthma, cardiovascular and circulatory problems, climacteric, menstrual and premenstrual disorders, colds, cough, constipation, depression, kidney disorders, malaria, sore throat, tinnitus
Class: Phytoestrogen
Half-life: N/A
Clinically important, potentially hazardous interactions with: clevidipine, salicylates
Note: In 2001, the American College of Obstetricians and Gynecologists stated that black cohosh might be helpful in the short term (6 months or less) for women with vasomotor symptoms of menopause.

Skin
Diaphoresis [2]
Rash [2]

Central Nervous System
Seizures [3]
Vertigo / dizziness [2]

Gastrointestinal/Hepatic
Hepatic failure [2]
Hepatitis [3]
Hepatotoxicity / liver injury / acute liver injury / drug-induced liver injury (DILI) [6]

Other
Adverse effects / adverse reactions [5]

BLEOMYCIN

Synonyms: bleo; BLM
Trade name: Blenoxane (Mead Johnson)
Indications: Melanomas, sarcomas, lymphomas, testicular carcinoma
Class: Antibiotic, Antibiotic; anthracycline, Antimicrobial
Half-life: 1.3–9 hours
Clinically important, potentially hazardous interactions with: aldesleukin, brentuximab vedotin
Important contra-indications noted in the prescribing guidelines for: nursing mothers; pediatric patients

---

Skin
Acral erythema [2]
Acral necrosis [2]
Bullous dermatosis (<5%)
Calcinosis cutis / calcification (includes calciphylaxis) [2]
Cutaneous toxicity / skin toxicity [2]
Erythema [6]
Exanthems [3]
Flagellate dermatitis [13]
Flagellate erythema/pigmentation [46]
Gangrene (digital) [3]
Hand–foot syndrome (palmar–plantar erythrodysesthesia) [2]
Hyperkeratosis (palms and soles) [3]
Hypersensitivity (<10%) [5]
Linear streaking [4]
Lipodystrophy / acquired generalized lipodystrophy [2]
Neutrophilic eccrine hidradenitis [2]
Pigmentation (Skin) (includes hyperpigmentation) (~50%) [21]
Pruritus (itching) (>5%) [7]
Raynaud's phenomenon (>10%) [35]
Scleroderma [16]
Stevens-Johnson syndrome and toxic epidermal necrolysis (SJS/TEN) [2]

Hair
Alopecia / hair loss (~50%) [8]

Nails
Melanonychia [2]
Nail changes [2]
Nail growth reduced [2]
Nail loss [3]
Nail pigmentation (banding) [2]
Onychodystrophy [2]
Onycholysis [3]

Mucosal
Oral ulceration [2]
Stomatitis (oral mucositis) (>10%) [8]

Central Nervous System
Chills (>10%)
Fever (pyrexia) (includes hyperpyrexia) [4]

Endocrine/Metabolic
SIADH [2]

Hematologic
Hemolytic uremic syndrome [8]
Thrombotic microangiopathy [2]

Local
Injection-site phlebitis (<10%)

Neuromuscular/Skeletal
Digital necrosis [3]

Respiratory
Pneumonitis [3]
Pulmonary fibrosis [3]
Pulmonary toxicity [7]

Other
Adverse effects / adverse reactions [2]
Allergic reactions [2]
Death [3]

BLOODROOT

Family: Papaveraceae
Scientific name: *Sanguinaria canadensis*
Indications: Oral: emetic, cathartic, expectorant. **Topical:** debriding agent, bronchitis, asthma, croup, laryngitis, pharyngitis, scabies, eczema, athlete's foot, nasal polyps, rheumatism, fever, anemia
Class: Anti-inflammatory
Half-life: N/A
Clinically important, potentially hazardous interactions with: none known

---

Mucosal
Leukoplakia [2]

BLUE COHOSH

Family: Berberidaceae
Scientific name: *Caulophyllum thalictroides*
Indications: Rheumatism, dropsy, epilepsy, hysteria, uterine inflammation, thrush, menopause, headache, sexual debility, aphthous stomatitis, laxative, colic, sore throat, hiccups
Class: Diuretic, Oxytocic
Half-life: N/A
Clinically important, potentially hazardous interactions with: cardioactive drugs, clevidipine
Note: Cohosh is from the Algonquin word 'rough', referring to the appearance of the roots.

It is a toxic herb and should not be confused with the safer, unrelated herb, black cohosh.

Other
Adverse effects / adverse reactions [2]

BOCEPREVIR

Trade name: Victrelis (Merck)
Indications: Chronic hepatitis C
Class: CYP3A4 inhibitor, Direct-acting antiviral, Hepatitis C virus NS3/4A protease inhibitor
Half-life: 3 hours
Clinically important, potentially hazardous interactions with: alfuzosin, alprazolam, amiodarone, atorvastatin, bepridil, bosentan, brigatinib, budesonide, buprenorphine, cabozantinib, carbamazepine, cisapride, clarithromycin, colchicine, copanlisib, cyclosporine, dasatinib, desipramine, dexamethasone, digoxin, dihydroergotamine, drospirenone, efavirenz, ergonovine, ergotamine, estradiol, felodipine, flecainide, flibanserin, fluticasone propionate, gefitinib, itraconazole, ketoconazole, lomitapide, lovastatin, methadone, methylergonovine, midazolam, midostaurin, mifepristone, neratinib, nicardipine, nifedipine, olaparib, pazopanib, phenobarbital, phenytoin, pimozide, ponatinib, posaconazole, propafenone, quinidine, ribociclib, rifabutin, rifampin, ritonavir, ruxolitinib, salmeterol, sildenafil, simvastatin, sirolimus, St John's wort, tacrolimus, tadalafil, trazodone, triazolam, vardenafil, vorapaxar, voriconazole, warfarin
Pregnancy category: boceprevir is pregnancy category B but must not be used in monotherapy
Important contra-indications noted in the prescribing guidelines for: nursing mothers; pediatric patients
Note: Must be used in combination with PEG-interferon and ribavirin (see separate entries) Combination treatment is contra-indicated in pregnant women and men whose female partners are pregnant because of the risks for birth defects and fetal death associated with ribavirin, or in coadministration with drugs that are highly dependent on CYP3A4/5 for clearance, or with potent CYP3A4/5 inducers.

Skin
Pruritus (itching) [3]
Rash [3]

Central Nervous System
Dysgeusia (taste perversion) [6]

Gastrointestinal/Hepatic
Hepatotoxicity / liver injury / acute liver injury / drug-induced liver injury (DILI) [2]

Hematologic
Anemia [24]
Neutropenia (neutrophils decreased) [8]
Thrombocytopenia / platelets decreased [8]

Other
Adverse effects / adverse reactions [6]
Infection [2]

BORTEZOMIB

Trade name: Velcade (Millennium)
Indications: Multiple myeloma, mantle cell lymphoma
Class: Biologic, Proteasome inhibitor
Half-life: 9–15 hours
Clinically important, potentially hazardous interactions with: conivaptan, darunavir, delavirdine, efavirenz, indinavir, strong CYP3A4 inducers or inhibitors, telithromycin, thalidomide, voriconazole
Important contra-indications noted in the prescribing guidelines for: nursing mothers; pediatric patients
Note: Contra-indicated in patients with hypersensitivity to boron or mannitol.

Skin
Cutaneous toxicity / skin toxicity [5]
DRESS syndrome (Drug-induced hypersensitivity syndrome) [2]
Edema / fluid retention (23%)
Erythema [2]
Folliculitis [2]
Herpes zoster (12%) [13]
Peripheral edema [6]
Pruritus (itching) (11%)
Purpura [2]
Rash (18%) [11]
Stevens-Johnson syndrome and toxic epidermal necrolysis (SJS/TEN) [3]
Sweet's syndrome [12]
Vasculitis (angiitis) / cutaneous vasculitis (angiitis) [5]

Mucosal
Mucositis [2]

Cardiovascular
Arrhythmias [2]
Cardiac failure [4]
Cardiotoxicity [4]
Congestive heart failure [4]
Hypertension [3]
Hypotension (13%) [4]
QT interval prolonged / QT prolongation [2]

Central Nervous System
Anorexia [2]
Anxiety (10%)
Dysesthesia (23%)
Dysgeusia (taste perversion) (13%)
Encephalopathy (includes hepatic encephalopathy) [3]
Fever (pyrexia) (includes hyperpyrexia) (34%) [9]
Guillain-Barré syndrome / acute inflammatory demyelinating polyradiculoneuropathy / acute motor axonal neuropathy [2]
Headache [3]
Hypoesthesia / hypesthesia (numbness) [2]
Insomnia (20%) [2]
Neuropathy [2]
Neurotoxicity [27]
Pain [2]
Paresthesias (22%) [3]
Peripheral neuropathy (39%) [74]
Vertigo / dizziness (17%)

Endocrine/Metabolic
Appetite decreased (36%)
Dehydration (10%) [2]
Hypocalcemia [2]
Hypokalemia [3]
Serum creatinine increased [2]
SIADH [2]
Weight loss [2]

Gastrointestinal/Hepatic
Abdominal distension [2]
Abdominal pain [4]
Colitis [2]
Constipation (41%) [7]
Diarrhea (52%) [26]
Gastrointestinal disorder / discomfort [3]
Hepatitis [3]
Hepatotoxicity / liver injury / acute liver injury / drug-induced liver injury (DILI) [5]
Ileus / adynamic ileus / paralytic ileus [9]
Nausea (55%) [11]
Pancreatitis / acute pancreatitis [6]
Vomiting (33%) [5]

Hematologic
Anemia (29%) [19]
Febrile neutropenia [6]
Hemotoxicity [5]
Leukocytopenia (leukopenia) / leukocytes (white blood cells) decreased [10]
Lymphopenia (lymphocytopenia) / lymphocytes decreased [12]
Myelosuppression / bone marrow suppression / myelotoxicity [2]
Neutropenia (neutrophils decreased) (17%) [37]
Sepsis [4]
Thrombocytopenia / platelets decreased (36%) [59]
Thrombotic microangiopathy [2]

Local
Infusion-related reactions [2]
Injection-site irritation (5%)
Injection-site reaction [4]

Neuromuscular/Skeletal
Arthralgia (17%) [2]
Asthenia / fatigue (64%) [43]
Back pain (13%)
Bone pain / joint pain (14%) [3]
Cramps (11%)
Myalgia/Myopathy (12%)

Renal
Nephrotoxicity / kidney injury / acute kidney injury (AKI) / drug-induced kidney injury [2]
Tumor lysis syndrome (TLS) [3]

Respiratory
Cough (20%) [2]
Dyspnea / shortness of breath (21%) [6]
Nasopharyngitis (12%)
Pneumonia (12%) [9]
Pneumonitis [4]
Pulmonary toxicity [7]
Upper respiratory tract infection (12%) [3]

Other
Adverse effects / adverse reactions [13]
Death [9]
Infection [12]

BOSENTAN

Trade name: Tracleer (Actelion)
Indications: Pulmonary arterial hypertension
Class: Antihypertensive, Endothelin receptor (ETR) antagonist, Vasodilator
Half-life: ~5 hours
Clinically important, potentially hazardous interactions with: amiodarone, amprenavir, astemizole, atazanavir, atorvastatin, boceprevir, cobicistat/elvitegravir/emtricitabine/tenofovir alafenamide, cobicistat/elvitegravir/emtricitabine/

tenofovir disoproxil, cyclosporine, diltiazem, elbasvir & grazoprevir, enzalutamide, erythromycin, fluconazole, fluvastatin, glibenclamide, glyburide, ibrexafungerp, indinavir, itraconazole, ketoconazole, lemborexant, levonorgestrel, lopinavir, lovastatin, neratinib, olaparib, oral contraceptives, palbociclib, progestogens, reboxetine, rifampin, ritonavir, sildenafil, simvastatin, St John's wort, tacrolimus, tadalafil, telaprevir, tipranavir, ulipristal, vardenafil, venetoclax, voriconazole, warfarin
Important contra-indications noted in the prescribing guidelines for: nursing mothers; pediatric patients
Warning: RISKS OF HEPATOTOXICITY and TERATOGENICITY

Skin
- Edema / fluid retention (8%) [4]
- Flushing / rubefaction (9%) [2]
- Peripheral edema (8%) [5]
- Pruritus (itching) (4%)

Central Nervous System
- Headache [3]
- Syncope / fainting [2]

Endocrine/Metabolic
- AST increased [2]

Gastrointestinal/Hepatic
- Diarrhea [2]
- Hepatic (liver) disorder / hepatobiliary disorder / hepatic (liver) dysfunction [3]
- Hepatotoxicity / liver injury / acute liver injury / drug-induced liver injury (DILI) [18]
- Nausea [2]

Hematologic
- Anemia [5]

Respiratory
- Bronchitis [2]

Other
- Adverse effects / adverse reactions [7]

BOSUTINIB

Trade name: Bosulif (Wyeth)
Indications: Chronic, accelerated, or blast phase Ph+ chronic myelogenous leukemia in adult patients with resistance or intolerance to prior therapy
Class: Bcr-Abl tyrosine kinase inhibitor / (Breakpoint cluster region Abelson (Bcr-Abl) tyrosine kinase inhibitor, Tyrosine kinase inhibitor
Half-life: 23 hours
Clinically important, potentially hazardous interactions with: CYP3A inhibitors (strong or moderate), digoxin, ketoconazole, lansoprazole, P-glycoprotein inhibitors, proton pump inhibitors
Important contra-indications noted in the prescribing guidelines for: nursing mothers; pediatric patients

---

Skin
- Acneiform eruption / acneiform dermatitis / acneiform rash (<10%)
- Edema / fluid retention (14%)
- Hypersensitivity (<10%)
- Pruritus (itching) (10%) [2]
- Rash (35%) [9]
- Urticaria / hives (<10%)

Cardiovascular
- Atrial fibrillation [2]
- Chest pain (<10%)
- Pericardial effusion (<10%)
- QT interval prolonged / QT prolongation [2]

Central Nervous System
- Dysgeusia (taste perversion) (<10%)
- Fever (pyrexia) (includes hyperpyrexia) (26%) [2]
- Headache (20%) [4]
- Pain (<10%)
- Vertigo / dizziness (10%)

Endocrine/Metabolic
- ALT increased (17%) [8]
- Appetite decreased (13%)
- AST increased (14%) [6]
- Creatine phosphokinase (CPK) / creatine kinase increased (hyperCKemia) (<10%) [2]
- Dehydration (<10%)
- Hyperkalemia (<10%)
- Hypophosphatemia [2]

Gastrointestinal/Hepatic
- Abdominal pain (37%) [2]
- Constipation [2]
- Diarrhea (82%) [17]
- Gastritis / pangastritis / gastric irritation (<10%)
- Hepatotoxicity / liver injury / acute liver injury / drug-induced liver injury (DILI) (<10%) [5]
- Nausea (46%) [10]
- Vomiting (39%) [9]

Hematologic
- Anemia (27%) [2]
- Febrile neutropenia (<10%)
- Myelosuppression / bone marrow suppression / myelotoxicity [2]
- Neutropenia (neutrophils decreased) (17%) [3]
- Thrombocytopenia / platelets decreased (41%) [5]

Neuromuscular/Skeletal
- Arthralgia (14%)
- Asthenia / fatigue (11–24%) [4]
- Back pain (11%)
- Myalgia/Myopathy (<10%)

Renal
- Renal failure (<10%)

Respiratory
- Bronchitis (<10%)
- Cough (20%)
- Dyspnea / shortness of breath (12%)
- Influenza (<10%)
- Nasopharyngitis (10%)
- Pleural effusion (<10%) [5]
- Pneumonia (<10%)
- Respiratory tract infection (12%)

Other
- Adverse effects / adverse reactions [4]

BOSWELLIA

Family: Burseraceae
Scientific names: *Boswellia carterii, Boswellia commiphora, Boswellia ovalifoliolata, Boswellia serrata*
Indications: Allergic rhinitis, arthritis, asthma, atherosclerosis, chronic colitis, ulcerative colitis, Crohn's disease, peritumoral brain edema, rheumatism, trypanosomiasis, ulcers
Class: Anti-inflammatory, Diuretic
Half-life: N/A
Clinically important, potentially hazardous interactions with: none known

---

Other
- Adverse effects / adverse reactions [2]

BOTULINUM TOXIN (A & B)

Synonym: OnabotulinumtoxinA
Trade names: Azzalure (Galderma), Bocouture (Merz), Botox (Allergan), Dysport (Ipsen), Myobloc (Solstice), Neurobloc (Eisai), Vistabel (Allergan), Xeomin (Merz)
Indications: Blepharospasm, hemifacial spasm, spasmodic torticollis, sialorrhea, hyperhidrosis, strabismus, oromandibular dystonia, cervical dystonia, spasmodic dysphonia, chronic migraine, urinary incontinence in people with neurologic conditions such as spinal cord injury and multiple sclerosis who have overactivity of the bladder, cosmetic application for wrinkles
Class: Acetylcholine inhibitor, Neuromuscular blocker, Ophthalmic agent, toxin
Half-life: 3–6 months
Clinically important, potentially hazardous interactions with: aminoglycosides, anticholinergics, fesoterodine, tiotropium, trospium
Important contra-indications noted in the prescribing guidelines for: nursing mothers; pediatric patients
Note: Distant spread of toxin effect - postmarketing reports indicate that all botulinum toxin products may spread from the area of injection to produce symptoms consistent with botulinum toxin effects. These may include asthenia, generalized muscle weakness, diplopia, ptosis, dysphagia, dysphonia, dysarthria, urinary incontinence and breathing diffculties. These symptoms have been reported hours to weeks after injection.
An antitoxin is available in the event of overdose or misinjection.
Warning: DISTANT SPREAD OF TOXIN EFFECT

Skin
- Anaphylactoid reactions / anaphylaxis (includes anaphylactic shock) [4]
- Bruise / bruising / contusion / ecchymosis (ecchymoses) [4]
- Erythema [2]
- Granulomas [2]
- Hematoma / cutaneous hematoma [3]
- Peripheral edema (<10%)
- Pruritus (itching) (<10%)
- Purpura (<10%)
- Rash [2]

Mucosal
- Epistaxis (nosebleed) [2]
- Parotitis [3]
- Stomatitis (oral mucositis) (<10%)
- Xerostomia (dry mouth) (3–34%) [13]

Central Nervous System
- Dysgeusia (taste perversion) (<10%)
- Gait instability / postural instability [2]
- Headache [8]
- Hyperesthesia (<10%)
- Neurotoxicity [3]
- Pain (6–13%) [4]
- Seizures [2]
- Tremor (<10%)
- Vertigo / dizziness [2]

Gastrointestinal/Hepatic
Constipation [3]
Diarrhea [3]
Dysphagia [21]

Genitourinary
Dysuria [2]
Enuresis (urinary incontinence) [3]
Hematuria [5]
Urinary retention [15]
Urinary tract infection [17]
Vulvovaginal candidiasis (<10%)

Local
Injection-site bruising [4]
Injection-site ecchymoses [2]
Injection-site edema [8]
Injection-site erythema [4]
Injection-site pain (2–10%) [22]
Injection-site paralysis [2]
Injection-site reaction [6]

Neuromuscular/Skeletal
Arthralgia (<7%)
Asthenia / fatigue [16]
Myasthenia gravis [2]
Neck pain [4]

Ocular
Conjunctivitis (conjunctival inflammation) [2]
Diplopia (double vision) [11]
Epiphora [2]
Eyebrow ptosis / brow ptosis [2]
Eyelid edema / palpebral edema / blepharedema [4]
Eyelid ptosis / blepharoptosis [30]
Ocular adverse effect [2]
Xerophthalmia (dry eyes) (6%) [2]

Otic
Tinnitus (<10%)

Respiratory
Dysphonia (includes voice disorders / voice changes) [2]
Dyspnea / shortness of breath [2]
Influenza- ('flu)-like syndrome (2–10%) [8]
Nasopharyngitis [2]
Pulmonary toxicity [3]

Other
Adverse effects / adverse reactions [25]
Death [4]
Infection (13–19%)
Side effects [3]

BREMELANOTIDE

Trade name: Vyleesi (AMAG Pharmaceuticals)
Indications: Treatment of premenopausal women with acquired, generalized hypoactive sexual desire disorder
Class: Melanocortin receptor agonist
Half-life: ~2.7 hours
Clinically important, potentially hazardous interactions with: naltrexone
Pregnancy category: Advise patients to discontinue treatment if pregnancy is suspected.

Skin
Flushing / rubefaction (20%) [4]
Hot flashes / hot flushes (3%)
Pigmentation (Skin) (includes hyperpigmentation) (<2%)

Mucosal
Nasal congestion (2%)
Rhinorrhea (<2%)

Cardiovascular
Blood pressure variations (<2%)

Central Nervous System
Headache (11%) [3]
Pain (<2%)
Paresthesias (3%)
Restless legs syndrome / Willis-Ekbom disease (includes restless arms syndrome variant) (<2%)
Vertigo / dizziness (2%)

Endocrine/Metabolic
Creatine phosphokinase (CPK) / creatine kinase increased (hyperCKemia) (<2%)

Gastrointestinal/Hepatic
Abdominal pain (<2%)
Diarrhea (<2%)
Nausea (40%) [4]
Vomiting (5%)

Local
Injection-site reaction (13%)

Neuromuscular/Skeletal
Arthralgia (<2%)
Asthenia / fatigue (3%)
Myalgia/Myopathy (<2%)
Pain in extremities (<2%)

Respiratory
Cough (3%)

BRENTUXIMAB VEDOTIN

Trade name: Adcetris (Seattle Genetics)
Indications: Hodgkin's lymphoma, systemic anaplastic large cell lymphoma
Class: Antibody-drug conjugate (ADC), CD30-directed antibody-drug conjugate, Monoclonal antibody
Half-life: 4–6 days
Clinically important, potentially hazardous interactions with: bleomycin, efavirenz, ketoconazole, rifampin, strong CYP3A4 inhibitors
Important contra-indications noted in the prescribing guidelines for: the elderly; nursing mothers; pediatric patients
Warning: PROGRESSIVE MULTIFOCAL LEUKOENCEPHALOPATHY

Skin
Diaphoresis (12%)
Lymphadenopathy (11%)
Peripheral edema (4–16%)
Pruritus (itching) (19%)
Rash (31%)
Xerosis / xeroderma (10%)

Hair
Alopecia / hair loss (14%)

Central Nervous System
Anxiety (11%)
Chills (13%)
Fever (pyrexia) (includes hyperpyrexia) (29–38%) [4]
Headache (19%)
Insomnia (16%)
Neurotoxicity [2]
Pain (7–28%)
Peripheral neuropathy (68%) [19]
Vertigo / dizziness (11–16%)

Endocrine/Metabolic
Appetite decreased (16%)
Weight loss (6–12%)

Gastrointestinal/Hepatic
Abdominal pain (9–25%)
Constipation (19%)
Diarrhea (36%) [6]
Nausea (42%) [4]
Vomiting (22%)

Hematologic
Anemia (33–52%) [2]
Lymphopenia (lymphocytopenia) / lymphocytes decreased [2]
Neutropenia (neutrophils decreased) (55%) [12]
Thrombocytopenia / platelets decreased (16–28%) [2]

Neuromuscular/Skeletal
Arthralgia (9–19%)
Asthenia / fatigue (41–49%) [4]
Back pain (14%)
Muscle spasm (10%)
Myalgia/Myopathy (17%)
Pain in extremities (10%)

Ocular
Uveitis / anterior uveitis / posterior uveitis / panuveitis [2]

Renal
Tumor lysis syndrome (TLS) [2]

Respiratory
Cough (17–25%)
Dyspnea / shortness of breath (13–19%)
Interstitial lung disease / interstitial pneumonitis / interstitial pneumonia (cryptogenic organizing pneumonia) / drug-induced interstitial lung disease [4]
Pneumonia [2]
Pulmonary toxicity [4]
Upper respiratory tract infection (12–47%)

Other
Adverse effects / adverse reactions [5]
Death [2]

BRETYLIUM

Indications: Ventricular tachycardia and fibrillation
Class: Antiarrhythmic class III
Half-life: 4–17 hours
Clinically important, potentially hazardous interactions with: arsenic, astemizole, ciprofloxacin, enoxacin, gatifloxacin, lomefloxacin, moxifloxacin, norfloxacin, ofloxacin, quinolones, sparfloxacin
Important contra-indications noted in the prescribing guidelines for: the elderly; pediatric patients

---

Cardiovascular
Hypotension [7]

BREWER'S YEAST

Family: Saccharomycetaceae
Scientific names: *Saccharomyces boulardii, Saccharomyces cerevisiae*
Indications: Diarrhea, rotaviral diarrhea, irritable bowel syndrome, Crohn's disease, ulcerative colitis, urinary tract infections, vaginal infections, acne, premenstrual syndrome, furunculosis
Class: Immunomodulator, Probiotic
Half-life: N/A
Clinically important, potentially hazardous interactions with: MAO inhibitors
Note: Immune-deficient subjects or those with mucosal disease may experience serious adverse effects.

BREXANOLONE

Synonym: Zulresso
Trade name: Zulresso (Sage Therapeutics)
Indications: Indicated for the treatment of postpartum depression (PPD) in adults
Class: GABA A receptor positive modulator
Half-life: ~ 9 hours
Clinically important, potentially hazardous interactions with: antidepressants, CNS depressants
Pregnancy category: Based on findings from animal studies of other drugs that enhance GABAergic inhibition, ZULRESSO may cause fetal harm. There are no available data on ZULRESSO use in pregnant women to determine a drug-associated risk of major birth defects, miscarriage, or adverse maternal or fetal outcomes.
Note: Pregnancy: May cause fetal harm. Avoid use in patients with end stage renal disease.
Warning: PATIENTS ARE AT RISK OF EXCESSIVE SEDATION OR SUDDEN LOSS OF CONSCIOUSNESS DURING ADMINISTRATION OF ZULRESSO (BREXANOLONE). BECAUSE OF THE RISK OF SERIOUS HARM, PATIENTS MUST BE MONITORED FOR EXCESSIVE SEDATION AND SUDDEN LOSS OF CONSCIOUSNESS AND HAVE CONTINUOUS PULSE OXIMETRY MONITORING. PATIENTS MUST BE ACCOMPANIED DURING INTERACTIONS WITH THEIR CHILD(REN). ZULRESSO IS AVAILABLE ONLY THROUGH A RESTRICTED PROGRAM CALLED THE ZULRESSO REMS.

Skin
Flushing / rubefaction (≥5%)
Hot flashes / hot flushes (≥5%)

Mucosal
Oropharyngeal pain (≥2%)
Xerostomia (dry mouth) (≥5%)

Cardiovascular
Sinus tachycardia (≥2%)

Central Nervous System
Loss of consciousness (≥5%)
Psychiatric adverse effect [2]
Sedation (≥5%)
Somnolence (drowsiness) (≥5%) [2]
Syncope / fainting (≥2%)
Vertigo / dizziness (13%) [2]

Gastrointestinal/Hepatic
Diarrhea (≥2%)
Dyspepsia / functional dyspepsia (indigestion) (see also gastroparesis) (≥2%)

BREXPIPRAZOLE

Trade name: Rexulti (Otsuka)
Indications: Schizophrenia, major depressive disorder (with antidepressants)
Class: Antipsychotic, Antipsychotic, atypical
Half-life: 86–91 hours
Clinically important, potentially hazardous interactions with: strong or moderate CYP2D6 inhibitors, strong or moderate CYP3A4 inducers or inhibitors
Pregnancy category: Neonatal risk in third trimester exposure
Important contra-indications noted in the prescribing guidelines for: the elderly; nursing mothers; pediatric patients
Warning: INCREASED MORTALITY IN ELDERLY PATIENTS WITH DEMENTIA-RELATED PSYCHOSIS and SUICIDAL THOUGHTS AND BEHAVIORS

Central Nervous System
Agitation [3]
Akathisia (6–9%) [16]
Anxiety (3%) [3]
Headache (7%) [12]
Insomnia [8]
Psychosis [2]
Restlessness (3%) [2]
Schizophrenia [4]
Sedation (2%) [2]
Somnolence (drowsiness) (5%) [7]
Tremor (3–4%)
Vertigo / dizziness (3%) [2]

Endocrine/Metabolic
Appetite increased (3%) [3]
Creatine phosphokinase (CPK) / creatine kinase increased (hyperCKemia) (2%)
Hyperprolactinemia [2]
Weight gain (4–7%) [17]
Weight loss (10%)

Gastrointestinal/Hepatic
Constipation (2%)
Diarrhea (3%) [3]
Dyspepsia / functional dyspepsia (indigestion) (see also gastroparesis) (3%)
Nausea [6]

Hematologic
Hemotoxicity (2%)

Neuromuscular/Skeletal
Asthenia / fatigue (3%) [4]

Respiratory
Nasopharyngitis (4%) [2]

BRIGATINIB

Trade name: Alunbrig (Ariad)
Indications: Anaplastic lymphoma kinase-positive metastatic non-small cell lung cancer in patients who have progressed on, or are intolerant to, crizotinib
Class: Anaplastic lymphoma kinase (ALK) inhibitor, Tyrosine kinase inhibitor
Half-life: 25 hours
Clinically important, potentially hazardous interactions with: boceprevir, carbamazepine, clarithromycin, cobicistat, conivaptan, CYP3A substrates and strong CYP3A inducers or inhibitors, grapefruit juice, hormonal contraceptives, indinavir, itraconazole, ketoconazole, lopinavir, nelfinavir, phenytoin, posaconazole, rifampin, ritonavir, saquinavir, St John's wort, voriconazole
Pregnancy category: May cause fetal toxicity based on findings in animal studies
Important contra-indications noted in the prescribing guidelines for: nursing mothers; pediatric patients

---

Skin
Photosensitivity [2]
Rash (15–24%)

Cardiovascular
Bradycardia / sinus bradycardia (6–8%)
Hypertension (11–21%) [4]

Central Nervous System
Fever (pyrexia) (includes hyperpyrexia) (6–14%)
Headache (27–28%) [2]
Insomnia (7–11%)
Peripheral neuropathy (13%)

Endocrine/Metabolic
ALT increased (34–40%) [2]
Appetite decreased (15–22%)
AST increased (38–65%)
Creatine phosphokinase (CPK) / creatine kinase increased (hyperCKemia) (27–48%) [5]
Hyperglycemia (includes glucose increased) (38–49%)
Hyperlipasemia (21–45%) [4]
Hypophosphatemia (15–23%)

Gastrointestinal/Hepatic
Abdominal pain (10–17%)
Constipation (15–19%)
Diarrhea (19–38%) [6]
Nausea (33–40%) [5]
Vomiting (23–24%)

Hematologic
Anemia (23–40%)
Lymphopenia (lymphocytopenia) / lymphocytes decreased (19–27%)
Prothrombin time (INR) increased (20–22%)

Neuromuscular/Skeletal
Arthralgia (14%)
Asthenia / fatigue (29–36%) [2]
Back pain (10–15%)
Muscle spasm (12–17%)
Myalgia/Myopathy (9–15%)
Pain in extremities (4–11%)

Ocular
Visual disturbances (7–10%)

Respiratory
Cough (18–34%) [4]
Dyspnea / shortness of breath (21–27%) [5]
Hypoxia (<3%) [4]
Pneumonia (5–10%) [4]
Pneumonitis (4–9%)
Pulmonary hypertension [2]
Pulmonary toxicity [3]

Other
Death [3]

BRIMONIDINE

Trade names: Alphagan P (Allergan), Mirvaso (Galderma)
Indications: Open-angle glaucoma, ocular hypertension, topical application for rosacea
Class: Adrenergic alpha2-receptor agonist
Half-life: 12 hours
Clinically important, potentially hazardous interactions with: amitriptyline, MAO inhibitors, tricyclic antidepressants
Important contra-indications noted in the prescribing guidelines for: nursing mothers; pediatric patients
Note: [T] = Topical.

Skin
Burning / skin burning sensation [T] (2%) [4]
Contact dermatitis [T] [2]
Dermatitis [2]
Erythema [T] (4%) [7]
Flushing / rubefaction [T] (3%) [3]
Hypersensitivity [3]

Irritation (skin) [3]
Pruritus (itching) [4]
Rosacea [2]
Xerosis / xeroderma [2]

Mucosal
Xerostomia (dry mouth) (5–20%) [12]

Cardiovascular
Hypertension (5–20%)

Central Nervous System
Dysgeusia (taste perversion) (<10%) [4]
Somnolence (drowsiness) [2]

Neuromuscular/Skeletal
Asthenia / fatigue [4]

Ocular
Blepharitis (<10%) [3]
Conjunctival hyperemia / conjunctival injection (5–20%) [7]
Conjunctivitis (conjunctival inflammation) (5–20%) [8]
Eyelid crusting (<10%)
Eyelid edema / palpebral edema / blepharedema (<10%)
Eyelid erythema (<10%)
Intraocular pressure increased [2]
Ocular adverse effect [4]
Ocular allergy (4%) [8]
Ocular burning (<10%) [7]
Ocular hyperemia [5]
Ocular itching / ocular pruritus [5]
Ocular pain [3]
Ocular stinging (<10%) [6]
Periocular dermatitis [2]
Uveitis / anterior uveitis / posterior uveitis / panuveitis [11]
Vision blurred [T] [3]
Visual disturbances (5–20%)
Xerophthalmia (dry eyes) [3]

Respiratory
Upper respiratory tract infection (<10%)

Other
Adverse effects / adverse reactions [4]
Allergic reactions [2]

BRINZOLAMIDE

Trade name: Azopt (Alcon)
Indications: Open-angle glaucoma, ocular hypertension
Class: Carbonic anhydrase inhibitor, Diuretic
Half-life: 111 days
Clinically important, potentially hazardous interactions with: conivaptan, darunavir, delavirdine, indinavir, salicylates, telithromycin, voriconazole
Important contra-indications noted in the prescribing guidelines for: nursing mothers
Note: Brinzolamide is a sulfonamide and can be absorbed systemically. Sulfonamides can produce severe, possibly fatal, reactions such as toxic epidermal necrolysis and Stevens-Johnson syndrome.

Skin
Dermatitis (<5%)

Mucosal
Xerostomia (dry mouth) [4]

Central Nervous System
Dysgeusia (taste perversion) (5–10%) [15]
Headache (<5%)

Endocrine/Metabolic
Acidosis (includes lactic acidosis) [2]

Neuromuscular/Skeletal
Asthenia / fatigue [3]

Ocular
Blepharitis (<5%) [2]
Conjunctival hyperemia / conjunctival injection [10]
Conjunctivitis (conjunctival inflammation) [5]
Corneal abnormalities [3]
Foreign body sensation (<5%)
Keratitis (ocular keratitis) / corneal inflammation) (<5%)
Lacrimation [3]
Ocular adverse effect [3]
Ocular allergy [2]
Ocular burning [4]
Ocular discharge (<5%)
Ocular hyperemia [5]
Ocular itching / ocular pruritus [8]
Ocular pain (<5%) [6]
Ocular stinging [4]
Vision blurred (5–10%) [16]
Xerophthalmia (dry eyes) (<5%) [5]

Respiratory
Rhinitis / rhinosinusitis (see also sinusitis) (<5%)

Other
Adverse effects / adverse reactions [3]

BRIVARACETAM

Trade name: Briviact (UCB)
Indications: Epilepsy adjunct therapy
Class: Anticonvulsant (see also antiepileptic (anti-seizure)), Antiepileptic (anti-seizure)
Half-life: 9 hours
Clinically important, potentially hazardous interactions with: carbamazepine, phenytoin, rifampin
Important contra-indications noted in the prescribing guidelines for: the elderly; nursing mothers; pediatric patients

---

Central Nervous System
Aggression (includes anger) [5]
Agitation [2]
Anxiety [2]
Balance disorder (3%)
Behavioral disturbances / personality changes [2]
Depression [6]
Dysgeusia (taste perversion) (<3%)
Euphoria / elation (<3%)
Headache [13]
Impaired concentration [2]
Insomnia [2]
Irritability (3%) [8]
Neurotoxicity (13%)
Psychosis [2]
Sedation (16%)
Seizures [3]
Somnolence (drowsiness) (16%) [30]
Vertigo / dizziness (12%) [26]

Gastrointestinal/Hepatic
Constipation (2%)
Nausea (5%) [6]
Vomiting (5%) [3]

Genitourinary
Urinary tract infection [2]

Hematologic
Leukocytopenia (leukopenia) / leukocytes (white blood cells) decreased (2%)

Local
Infusion-site pain (<3%)

Neuromuscular/Skeletal
Asthenia / fatigue (9%) [20]
Back pain [2]
Convulsions [2]

Respiratory
Nasopharyngitis [8]

Other
Adverse effects / adverse reactions [6]

BRODALUMAB

Trade name: Siliq (Valeant)
Indications: Moderate-to-severe plaque psoriasis
Class: Interleukin-17 (IL-17) antagonist / interleukin-17 inhibitor, Monoclonal antibody
Half-life: N/A
Clinically important, potentially hazardous interactions with: cyP450 substrates, live vaccines
Pregnancy category: Insufficient evidence to inform drug-associated risk
Important contra-indications noted in the prescribing guidelines for: nursing mothers; pediatric patients
Note: Contra-indicated in patients with Crohn's disease.
Warning: SUICIDAL IDEATION AND BEHAVIOR

Skin
Candidiasis / candidosis [5]
Contact dermatitis [3]
Eczema / eczematous reaction / eczematous eruption [4]
Folliculitis [3]
Rash [2]
Tinea (pedis, versicolor, cruris) [2]

Mucosal
Oral candidiasis [2]
Oropharyngeal pain (2%)

Central Nervous System
Headache (4%) [9]
Suicidal ideation [5]

Gastrointestinal/Hepatic
Diarrhea (2%) [5]
Nausea (2%) [3]

Hematologic
Neutropenia (neutrophils decreased) [5]

Local
Injection-site bleeding (<2%)
Injection-site bruising (<2%)
Injection-site erythema (<2%) [4]
Injection-site pain (<2%)
Injection-site pruritus (<2%)
Injection-site reaction (2%) [2]

Neuromuscular/Skeletal
Arthralgia (5%) [10]
Asthenia / fatigue (3%) [2]
Back pain [2]
Myalgia/Myopathy (2%)

Respiratory
Influenza [2]
Nasopharyngitis [16]
Upper respiratory tract infection [16]

Other
Adverse effects / adverse reactions [3]
Infection (25%) [2]

BROMELAIN

Family: Bromeliaceae
Scientific names: *Ananas comosus, Ananas duckei, Ananas sativus, Bromelia ananas, Bromelia comosa*
Indications: Oral: inflammation, mild ulcerative colitis, osteoarthritis, sinusitis, sprains. **Topical:** burn debridement
Class: Analgesic, Anti-inflammatory
Half-life: N/A
Clinically important, potentially hazardous interactions with: amoxicillin, fluorouracil, tetracycline, vincristine
Note: Phlogenzym is rutoside, bromelain and trypsin.

Skin
Contact dermatitis [2]
Central Nervous System
Headache [2]
Respiratory
Asthma (occupational / inhalation) [3]
Other
Adverse effects / adverse reactions [8]

BROMFENAC

Trade names: BromSite (Sun Pharma), Prolensa (Bausch & Lomb)
Indications: Postoperative ophthalmic inflammation and prevention of ocular pain in cataract surgery
Class: Non-steroidal anti-inflammatory (NSAID)
Half-life: N/A
Clinically important, potentially hazardous interactions with: NSAIDs
Important contra-indications noted in the prescribing guidelines for: nursing mothers; pediatric patients
Note: NSAIDs may cause an increased risk of serious cardiovascular and gastrointestinal adverse events, which can be fatal. This risk may increase with duration of use.
Prolensa and Xibrom preparations contain sodium sulfite, which may cause hypersensitivity in sensitive individuals.

Skin
Stevens-Johnson syndrome and toxic epidermal necrolysis (SJS/TEN) [2]
Central Nervous System
Headache (2–7%)
Ocular
Conjunctival hyperemia / conjunctival injection (2–7%) [2]
Corneal melting (see also corneal ulceration) [3]
Foreign body sensation [2]
Iritis (2–7%)
Ocular burning (2–7%)
Ocular erythema (2–7%)
Ocular itching / ocular pruritus (2–7%)
Ocular pain (2–7%) [2]
Ocular stinging (2–7%)

BROMOCRIPTINE

Trade name: Parlodel (Novartis)
Indications: Amenorrhea, Parkinsonism, infertility, acromegaly, type 2 diabetes
Class: Dopamine receptor agonist
Half-life: initial: 6–8 hours; terminal: 50 hours
Clinically important, potentially hazardous interactions with: alcohol, antipsychotics, azithromycin, domperidone, erythromycin, isometheptene, lanreotide, levomepromazine, macrolides, memantine, methyldopa, metoclopramide, octreotide, pasireotide, pseudoephedrine, risperidone, sympathomimetics, zuclopenthixol
Pregnancy category: Contra-indicated in women who become pregnant or in the postpartum period
Important contra-indications noted in the prescribing guidelines for: nursing mothers; pediatric patients
Note: Cycloset (bromocriptine mesylate), quick-release bromocriptine (bromocriptine-QR), was approved for the treatment of type 2 diabetes, either as an adjunctive therapy or as monotherapy, in 2009.

Skin
Erythromelalgia / erythermalgia [5]
Flushing / rubefaction [2]
Livedo reticularis / livedo racemosa [3]
Raynaud's phenomenon (<10%) [8]
Scleroderma [2]
Hair
Alopecia / hair loss [2]
Mucosal
Cerebrospinal fluid rhinorrhea [2]
Nasal congestion (3–4%)
Xerostomia (dry mouth) (4–10%) [3]
Cardiovascular
Cardiotoxicity [2]
Coronary spasm [2]
Orthostatic hypotension (6%)
Postural hypotension (6%)
Central Nervous System
Anorexia (4%)
Hallucinations [4]
Headache (<19%) [4]
Seizures (in postpartum patients) [3]
Somnolence (drowsiness) (3%)
Syncope / fainting (<2%)
Vertigo / dizziness (17%)
Gastrointestinal/Hepatic
Abdominal pain (4%)
Constipation (3–14%) [2]
Diarrhea (3%)
Dyspepsia / functional dyspepsia (indigestion) (see also gastroparesis) (4%)
Gastrointestinal bleeding (<2%)
Nausea (18–49%) [8]
Vomiting (2–5%) [4]
Neuromuscular/Skeletal
Asthenia / fatigue (3–7%) [2]
Respiratory
Pleural effusion [2]
Pulmonary fibrosis [2]
Other
Adverse effects / adverse reactions [2]

BROMPHENIRAMINE

Trade names: Bromfed (Muro), Rondec (Biovail)
Indications: Allergic rhinitis, urticaria
Class: Histamine H1 receptor antagonist
Half-life: 12–48 hours
Clinically important, potentially hazardous interactions with: aprobarbital, butabarbital, chloral hydrate, ethchlorvynol, mephobarbital, pentobarbital, phenobarbital, phenothiazines, primidone, secobarbital, zolpidem
Important contra-indications noted in the prescribing guidelines for: pediatric patients

---

Mucosal
Xerostomia (dry mouth) (<10%)

BUCILLAMINE

Trade name: Rimatil (Santen)
Indications: Rheumatoid arthritis
Class: Disease-modifying antirheumatic drug (DMARD)
Half-life: N/A
Clinically important, potentially hazardous interactions with: none known

---

Skin
Pemphigus [3]
Rash [2]
Nails
Yellow nail syndrome [6]
Central Nervous System
Fever (pyrexia) (includes hyperpyrexia) [4]
Endocrine/Metabolic
Breast hypertropy / gigantomastia / macromastia [2]
Neuromuscular/Skeletal
Myasthenia gravis [2]
Renal
Nephrotoxicity / kidney injury / acute kidney injury (AKI) / drug-induced kidney injury [4]
Proteinuria [2]
Respiratory
Cough [4]
Other
Adverse effects / adverse reactions [2]

BUCLIZINE

Indications: Motion sickness, nausea/vomiting
Class: Histamine H1 receptor antagonist
Half-life: N/A
Clinically important, potentially hazardous interactions with: aprobarbital, butabarbital, chloral hydrate, ethchlorvynol, mephobarbital, pentobarbital, phenobarbital, phenothiazines, primidone, secobarbital, zolpidem
Important contra-indications noted in the prescribing guidelines for: pediatric patients

BUDESONIDE

Trade names: Pulmicort Turbuhaler (AstraZeneca), Rhinocort (AstraZeneca), Symbicort (AstraZeneca)
Indications: Asthma, rhinitis
Class: Corticosteroid / Glucocorticoid, Corticosteroid, inhaled
Half-life: N/A
Clinically important, potentially hazardous interactions with: boceprevir, efavirenz, itraconazole, ketoconazole, live vaccines, oral contraceptives, telaprevir
Important contra-indications noted in the prescribing guidelines for: nursing mothers; pediatric patients
Note: Budesonide–MMX is an oral formulation of budesonide that uses Multi-Matrix System (MMX) technology to extend release to the colon. Symbicort is budesonide and formoterol.

Skin
Acneiform eruption / acneiform dermatitis / acneiform rash [3]
Dermatitis [8]
Exanthems [2]
Moon face [2]
Pruritus (itching) [2]
Rash [2]

Mucosal
Oral candidiasis [2]

Central Nervous System
Fever (pyrexia) (includes hyperpyrexia) [2]
Headache [3]
Insomnia [2]
Mood changes (includes mood disorder) [2]

Endocrine/Metabolic
Adrenal insufficiency (hypoadrenalism) / Addisonian crisis (includes Addison's disease) [3]
Cushing's syndrome [2]

Ocular
Cataract [2]

Respiratory
Asthma (exacerbation) [4]
Cough [2]
Nasopharyngitis [2]

Other
Adverse effects / adverse reactions [14]
Allergic reactions [3]
Infection [2]
Systemic reactions [2]

BUMETANIDE

Trade name: Bumex (Roche)
Indications: Edema associated with congestive heart failure
Class: Diuretic, loop, Sulfonamide
Half-life: 1–1.5 hours
Clinically important, potentially hazardous interactions with: amikacin, aminoglycosides, digoxin, gentamicin, kanamycin, neomycin, streptomycin, tobramycin
Important contra-indications noted in the prescribing guidelines for: the elderly; nursing mothers; pediatric patients
Note: Bumetanide is a sulfonamide and can be absorbed systemically. Sulfonamides can produce severe, possibly fatal, reactions such as toxic epidermal necrolysis and Stevens-Johnson syndrome.

Skin
Pruritus (itching) [2]

BUPIVACAINE

Trade names: Exparel (Pacira), Marcaine (AstraZeneca), Sensorcaine (AstraZeneca)
Indications: Local or regional anesthesia or analgesia
Class: Anesthetic; local
Half-life: N/A
Clinically important, potentially hazardous interactions with: adenosine, antiarrhythmics, beta blockers, conivaptan, dronedarone, MAO inhibitors, PEG-interferon, propranolol, tricyclic antidepressants
Important contra-indications noted in the prescribing guidelines for: the elderly; nursing mothers; pediatric patients

---

Skin
Pruritus (itching) [4]

Cardiovascular
Bradycardia / sinus bradycardia [2]
Cardiac arrest [5]
Hypotension [4]

Central Nervous System
Headache [2]
Sedation [2]
Seizures [3]
Vertigo / dizziness [2]

Gastrointestinal/Hepatic
Constipation [2]
Nausea [5]
Vomiting [5]

Other
Adverse effects / adverse reactions [2]
Death [3]

BUPRENORPHINE

Trade names: Probuphine (Braeburn), Suboxone (Reckitt Benckiser), Subutex (Reckitt Benckiser), Transtec (Napp)
Indications: Opioid dependence, moderate to severe pain
Class: Analgesic, Mixed opioid agonist/antagonist, Narcotic
Half-life: 37 hours
Clinically important, potentially hazardous interactions with: antihistamines, atazanavir, azole antifungals, benzodiazepines, boceprevir, carbamazepine, cimetidine, cobicistat/elvitegravir/emtricitabine/tenofovir alafenamide, cobicistat/elvitegravir/emtricitabine/tenofovir disoproxil, delavirdine, diazepam, efavirenz, erythromycin, HIV protease inhibitors, hydrocodone, hydromorphone, ketoconazole, ketorolac, linezolid, macrolide antibiotics, morphine, neuroleptics, oliceridine, oxymorphone, phenobarbital, phenytoin, rifampin, ritonavir, tapentadol, tipranavir
Important contra-indications noted in the prescribing guidelines for: nursing mothers; pediatric patients
Note: Suboxone is buprenorphine and naloxone. Probuphine is an implant for subdermal administration.
Warning: ABUSE POTENTIAL, LIFE-THREATENING RESPIRATORY DEPRESSION, and ACCIDENTAL EXPOSURE
Probuphine: IMPLANT MIGRATION, PROTRUSION, EXPULSION, and NERVE DAMAGE ASSOCIATED WITH INSERTION and REMOVAL

Skin
Abscess (2%)
Dermatitis [2]
Diaphoresis (12–14%)
Erythema [4]
Hyperhidrosis [4]
Pruritus (itching) [11]

Mucosal
Xerostomia (dry mouth) [3]

Cardiovascular
Bradycardia / sinus bradycardia [3]
Hypotension [4]
QT interval prolonged / QT prolongation [2]
Vasodilation (9%)

Central Nervous System
Anxiety (12%)
Chills (6–8%)
Depression (11%)
Fever (pyrexia) (includes hyperpyrexia) (3%)
Headache (30–36%) [6]
Insomnia (14–25%)
Nervousness (6%)
Neurotoxicity [2]
Pain (22–24%)
Seizures [3]
Somnolence (drowsiness) (5%) [4]
Vertigo / dizziness (4%) [14]

Gastrointestinal/Hepatic
Abdominal pain (11%) [2]
Constipation (11–12%) [12]
Diarrhea (4–5%) [2]
Dyspepsia / functional dyspepsia (indigestion) (see also gastroparesis) (3%)
Hepatotoxicity / liver injury / acute liver injury / drug-induced liver injury (DILI) [6]
Nausea (10–15%) [15]
Vomiting (5–8%) [12]

Local
Application-site reactions [3]

Neuromuscular/Skeletal
Asthenia / fatigue (7–14%) [4]
Back pain (4–14%)
Myalgia/Myopathy [2]

Ocular
Lacrimation (5%)

Respiratory
Cough (4%)
Influenza- ('flu)-like syndrome (6%)
Pharyngitis (sore throat) (4%)
Pulmonary edema (cardiogenic / non-cardiogenic) [2]
Respiratory depression [3]
Rhinitis / rhinosinusitis (see also sinusitis) (5–11%)

Other
Adverse effects / adverse reactions [4]
Death [9]
Infection (6–20%)

BUPROPION

Trade names: Wellbutrin (GSK), Zyban (GSK)
Indications: Depression, aid to smoking cessation.
Adjunct for the treatment of obesity and for weight loss management in defined populations and health conditions.

Class: Anti-obesity / weight loss pharmacotherapy, Antidepressant, Dopamine reuptake inhibitor
Half-life: 14 hours
Clinically important, potentially hazardous interactions with: amitriptyline, citalopram, cobicistat/elvitegravir/emtricitabine/tenofovir alafenamide, cobicistat/elvitegravir/emtricitabine/tenofovir disoproxil, cyclosporine, deutetrabenazine, efavirenz, eluxadoline, erythromycin, escitalopram, isocarboxazid, levodopa, linezolid, lopinavir, lorcaserin, methylphenidate, mifepristone, oliceridine, phenelzine, ritonavir, tranylcypromine, trimipramine, vortioxetine
Important contra-indications noted in the prescribing guidelines for: nursing mothers; pediatric patients
Note: Contrave, a combination of naltrexone and bupropion, has been approved by the FDA for chronic weight management.
Warning: NEUROPSYCHIATRIC REACTIONS; AND SUICIDAL THOUGHTS AND BEHAVIORS

Skin
- Acneiform eruption / acneiform dermatitis / acneiform rash (<10%)
- AGEP [3]
- Anaphylactoid reactions / anaphylaxis (includes anaphylactic shock) [2]
- Angioedema (formerly named angioneurotic edema) [3]
- Diaphoresis (5%) [4]
- Erythema multiforme [4]
- Exanthems [2]
- Flushing / rubefaction (4%)
- Hypersensitivity [6]
- Lupus erythematosus (subacute cutaneous lupus erythematosus (SCLE)) [2]
- Peripheral edema [2]
- Pruritus (itching) (4%) [3]
- Psoriasis [3]
- Rash (4%) [3]
- Serum sickness [3]
- Serum sickness-like reaction [10]
- Stevens-Johnson syndrome and toxic epidermal necrolysis (SJS/TEN) [2]
- Thrombocytopenic purpura [2]
- Urticaria / hives [9]
- Xerosis / xeroderma (<10%)

Hair
- Hirsutism (<10%)

Mucosal
- Tongue edema [2]
- Xerostomia (dry mouth) (<64%) [20]

Cardiovascular
- Arrhythmias [2]
- Hypertension [3]
- Myocardial ischemia [2]
- Palpitation [2]
- Tachycardia [3]

Central Nervous System
- Aggression (includes anger) [2]
- Agitation [5]
- Anxiety [5]
- Delirium [2]
- Depression [4]
- Dysgeusia (taste perversion) (4%)
- Dyskinesia [2]
- Hallucinations [7]
- Hallucinations, visual [3]
- Headache [8]
- Insomnia [9]
- Irritability [2]
- Mania [3]
- Myokymia / twitching / fasciculation (2%)
- Nightmares [2]
- Paresthesias (2%)
- Parkinsonism [4]
- Psychosis [7]
- Seizures [40]
- Serotonin syndrome [2]
- Sleep-related disorder [2]
- Somnolence (drowsiness) [5]
- Stuttering (dysphemia) / stammering [2]
- Suicidal ideation [5]
- Tremor (>10%) [7]
- Vertigo / dizziness [7]

Gastrointestinal/Hepatic
- Constipation [5]
- Diarrhea [2]
- Hepatotoxicity / liver injury / acute liver injury / drug-induced liver injury (DILI) [3]
- Nausea [17]
- Vomiting [6]

Genitourinary
- Priapism [2]

Neuromuscular/Skeletal
- Arthralgia [3]
- Asthenia / fatigue [3]
- Dystonia [11]
- Myalgia/Myopathy (6%) [2]
- Rhabdomyolysis [3]

Respiratory
- Upper respiratory tract infection [2]

Other
- Adverse effects / adverse reactions [2]
- Congenital malformations [2]
- Death [5]

BUSPIRONE

Trade name: BuSpar (Bristol-Myers Squibb)
Indications: Anxiety
Class: Anxiolytic, Serotonin antagonist
Half-life: 2–3 hours
Clinically important, potentially hazardous interactions with: citalopram, cobicistat/elvitegravir/emtricitabine/tenofovir alafenamide, cobicistat/elvitegravir/emtricitabine/tenofovir disoproxil, desipramine, grapefruit juice, itraconazole, linezolid, nefazodone, paclitaxel, rifapentine, ritonavir, St John's wort, telithromycin, vilazodone, voriconazole

---

Hair
- Alopecia / hair loss [2]

Mucosal
- Xerostomia (dry mouth) (3%)

Central Nervous System
- Serotonin syndrome [4]

BUSULFAN

Trade name: Myleran (GSK)
Indications: Chronic myelogenous leukemia, bone marrow disorders
Class: Alkylating agent
Half-life: 3.4 hours (after first dose)
Clinically important, potentially hazardous interactions with: acetaminophen, aldesleukin, itraconazole, metronidazole, voriconazole
Warning: LEUKEMOGENESIS and PANCYTOPENIA

Skin
- Erythema (macular) (>10%)
- Erythema multiforme [5]
- Erythema nodosum [3]
- Exanthems [2]
- Pigmentation (Skin) (includes hyperpigmentation) ('busulfan tan') (<10%) [13]
- Urticaria / hives (>10%) [5]
- Vasculitis (angiitis) / cutaneous vasculitis (angiitis) [3]

Hair
- Alopecia / hair loss (>10%) [7]

Mucosal
- Mucositis [4]
- Stomatitis (oral mucositis) [4]

Central Nervous System
- Neurotoxicity [3]
- Seizures [5]

Endocrine/Metabolic
- Gynecomastia [3]
- Porphyria cutanea tarda [2]

Gastrointestinal/Hepatic
- Hepatotoxicity / liver injury / acute liver injury / drug-induced liver injury (DILI) [4]

Hematologic
- Febrile neutropenia [3]

Respiratory
- Pulmonary toxicity [3]

Other
- Death [4]
- Infection [3]

BUTABARBITAL

Trade name: Butisol (MedPointe)
Indications: Sedation
Class: Barbiturate
Half-life: 40–140 hours
Clinically important, potentially hazardous interactions with: alcohol, antihistamines, ardeparin, argatroban, brompheniramine, buclizine, chlorpheniramine, dalteparin, danaparoid, dicumarol, enoxaparin, ethanolamine, heparin, imatinib, tinzaparin, warfarin

---

Skin
- Lupus erythematosus (subacute cutaneous lupus erythematosus (SCLE)) [2]

BUTALBITAL

Trade names: Esgic (Forest), Fioricet (Watson), Fiorinal (Watson)
Indications: Tension headaches
Class: Barbiturate
Half-life: 35 hours
Clinically important, potentially hazardous interactions with: alcohol, dicumarol, pizotifen
Pregnancy category: the pregnancy category will be D if used in high doses or for prolonged periods

Skin
Anaphylactoid reactions / anaphylaxis (includes anaphylactic shock) (<10%)
Erythema multiforme [2]
Lupus erythematosus (subacute cutaneous lupus erythematosus (SCLE)) [2]
Rash (<10%)

BUTORPHANOL

Trade name: Stadol (Bristol-Myers Squibb)
Indications: Pain, migraine
Class: Opiate agonist-antagonist
Half-life: 2.5–4 hours
Clinically important, potentially hazardous interactions with: cimetidine, hydrocodone, hydromorphone, oliceridine, oxymorphone, tapentadol

Skin
Diaphoresis (<10%)
Flushing / rubefaction (<10%)
Pruritus (itching) (<10%) [2]
Mucosal
Xerostomia (dry mouth) (3–9%)
Central Nervous System
Dysgeusia (taste perversion) (3–9%)
Vertigo / dizziness [5]

BUTTERBUR

Family: Asteraceae; Compositae
Scientific names: *Petasites hybridus, Petasites officinalis*
Indications: Allergic rhinitis, asthma, bronchitis, chills, cough, dysmenorrhea, hay fever, headache, heart tonic, migraine, peptic ulcer, appetite stimulant, irritable bladder, poultice for wounds or skin ulcers
Class: Anti-inflammatory
Half-life: N/A
Clinically important, potentially hazardous interactions with: none known
Pregnancy category: Contraindicated in pregnancy
Important contra-indications noted in the prescribing guidelines for: nursing mothers
Note: Petadolex formulation has had the potentially carcinogenic pyrrolizidine alkaloids removed.

Skin
Edema / fluid retention [2]
Erythema [2]
Hypersensitivity [2]
Rash [2]
Gastrointestinal/Hepatic
Eructation (belching) [3]
Other
Adverse effects / adverse reactions [2]

C1-ESTERASE INHIBITOR

Trade names: Berinert (CSL Behring), Cinryze (Viropharma)
Indications: Hereditary angioedema type I and II
Class: C1 inhibitor
Half-life: 36.1 hours
Clinically important, potentially hazardous interactions with: none known

CABAZITAXEL

Trade name: Jevtana (Sanofi-Aventis)
Indications: Hormone-refractory metastatic prostate cancer (in combination with prednisone)
Class: Antineoplastic / anticancer agent (see also Immune checkpoint inhibitor), Microtubule inhibitor
Half-life: α-, β-, and γ-half-lives of 4 minutes, 2 hours, and 95 hours, respectively
Clinically important, potentially hazardous interactions with: antineoplastics, atazanavir, BCG vaccine, carbamazepine, cardiac glycosides, clarithromycin, clozapine, conivaptan, CYP3A4 inhibitors and inducers, dasatinib, deferasirox, denosumab, doxorubicin, echinacea, grapefruit juice, indinavir, itraconazole, ketoconazole, leflunomide, natalizumab, nelfinavir, phenobarbital, phenytoin, pimecrolimus, rifabutin, rifampin, ritonavir, saquinavir, sipuleucel-T, St John's wort, tacrolimus, telithromycin, trastuzumab, vaccines, vitamin K antagonists, voriconazole
Important contra-indications noted in the prescribing guidelines for: nursing mothers; pediatric patients
Warning: NEUTROPENIC DEATH and SEVERE HYPERSENSITIVITY

Skin
Cutaneous toxicity / skin toxicity [3]
Hypersensitivity [2]
Peripheral edema (9%)
Hair
Alopecia / hair loss (10%)
Mucosal
Mucosal inflammation (6%)
Cardiovascular
Arrhythmias (5%)
Hypotension (5%)
Central Nervous System
Anorexia (16%)
Dysgeusia (taste perversion) (11%)
Fever (pyrexia) (includes hyperpyrexia) (12%) [2]
Headache (8%)
Neurotoxicity [5]
Pain (5%) [2]
Peripheral neuropathy (13%) [2]
Vertigo / dizziness (8%)
Endocrine/Metabolic
Dehydration (5%)
Weight loss (9%)
Gastrointestinal/Hepatic
Abdominal pain (17%)
Constipation (20%)
Diarrhea (47%) [17]
Dyspepsia / functional dyspepsia (indigestion) (see also gastroparesis) (10%)
Nausea (34%) [4]
Vomiting (22%) [4]
Genitourinary
Dysuria (7%)
Hematuria (17%) [4]
Urinary tract infection (8%)
Hematologic
Anemia (98%) [9]
Febrile neutropenia (7%) [19]
Leukocytopenia (leukopenia) / leukocytes (white blood cells) decreased (96%) [3]
Myelosuppression / bone marrow suppression / myelotoxicity [2]
Neutropenia (neutrophils decreased) (94%) [22]
Thrombocytopenia / platelets decreased (48%) [7]
Neuromuscular/Skeletal
Arthralgia (11%) [2]
Asthenia / fatigue (20–37%) [9]
Back pain [2]
Muscle spasm (7%)
Respiratory
Cough (11%)
Dyspnea / shortness of breath (12%) [2]
Other
Death [2]

CABERGOLINE

Trade name: Dostinex (Pfizer)
Indications: Hyperprolactinemia, Parkinsonism
Class: Dopamine receptor agonist
Half-life: 63–69 hours
Clinically important, potentially hazardous interactions with: azithromycin, levomepromazine, risperidone, zuclopenthixol
Important contra-indications noted in the prescribing guidelines for: the elderly; nursing mothers; pediatric patients

Skin
Edema / fluid retention [2]
Hot flashes / hot flushes (3%)
Mucosal
Cerebrospinal fluid rhinorrhea [4]
Xerostomia (dry mouth) (2%)
Cardiovascular
Cardiac failure [2]
Hypotension [5]
Myocardial toxicity [3]
Pericarditis [4]
Valve regurgitation [2]
Valvulopathy [9]
Central Nervous System
Dyskinesia [2]
Headache (26%) [7]
Mania [3]
Neurotoxicity [3]
Paresthesias (5%) [2]
Psychosis [3]
Somnolence (drowsiness) (<5%)
Vertigo / dizziness (15–17%) [7]
Endocrine/Metabolic
Mastodynia (2%)
Gastrointestinal/Hepatic
Abdominal pain (5%)
Constipation (7–10%)
Nausea (28%) [4]

Neuromuscular/Skeletal
Asthenia / fatigue (6%) [5]

Ocular
Ocular adverse effect [2]

CABOZANTINIB

Trade names: Carbometyx (Exelixis), Cometriq (Exelixis)
Indications: Metastatic medullary thyroid cancer (Cometriq), advanced renal cell carcinoma (Cabometyx)
Class: Angiogenesis inhibitor / antiangiogenic agent, MET (mesenchymal-epithelial transition) inhibitor / MET tyrosine kinase inhibitor, RET (Rearranged during Transfection) kinase inhibitor, Tyrosine kinase inhibitor, Vascular endothelial growth factor (VEGF) inhibitor / antagonist
Half-life: 55 hours (Cometriq); 99 hours (Cabometyx)
Clinically important, potentially hazardous interactions with: atazanavir, boceprevir, carbamazepine, clarithromycin, conivaptan, grapefruit juice, indinavir, itraconazole, ketoconazole, lopinavir, nefazodone, nelfinavir, phenobarbital, phenytoin, posaconazole, rifabutin, rifampin, rifapentine, ritonavir, saquinavir, St John's wort, telithromycin, voriconazole
Important contra-indications noted in the prescribing guidelines for: the elderly; nursing mothers; pediatric patients
Warning: PERFORATIONS AND FISTULAS, and HEMORRHAGE

Skin
Cutaneous toxicity / skin toxicity [3]
Erythema (11%)
Hand–foot syndrome (palmar–plantar erythrodysesthesia) (50%) [25]
Hyperkeratosis (7%)
Jaundice (see also cholestasis / cholestatic jaundice) (25%)
Rash (19%) [2]
Wound complications [2]
Xerosis / xeroderma (19%)

Hair
Alopecia / hair loss (16%)
Hair changes (34%)
Hair pigmentation (34%) [2]

Mucosal
Mucosal inflammation [3]
Stomatitis (oral mucositis) (51%) [5]

Cardiovascular
Cardiomyopathy [2]
Chest pain (9%)
Hypertension (33%) [21]
Hypotension (7%)
Systolic dysfunction / ejection fraction reduced [2]

Central Nervous System
Anorexia [3]
Anxiety (9%)
Dysgeusia (taste perversion) (34%) [3]
Headache (18%) [2]
Paresthesias (7%)
Peripheral neuropathy (5%)
Vertigo / dizziness (14%)

Endocrine/Metabolic
ALP increased (52%)
ALT increased (86%) [3]
Appetite decreased (46%) [6]
AST increased (86%) [3]
Creatine phosphokinase (CPK) / creatine kinase increased (hyperCKemia) [2]
Dehydration (7%)
GGT increased (27%)
Hypoalbuminemia / albumin decreased (36%)
Hypocalcemia (52%)
Hypokalemia (18%)
Hypomagnesemia (19%)
Hyponatremia (10%)
Hypophosphatemia (28%)
Hypothyroidism [6]
Serum creatinine increased (58%)
Weight loss (48%) [9]

Gastrointestinal/Hepatic
Abdominal pain (27%)
Constipation (27%) [2]
Diarrhea (63%) [26]
Dyspepsia / functional dyspepsia (indigestion) (see also gastroparesis) (11%)
Dysphagia (13%)
Gastrointestinal perforation / perforated colon / gastric perforation (3%)
Hemorrhoids (9%)
Hepatic (liver) disorder / hepatobiliary disorder / hepatic (liver) dysfunction [2]
Nausea (43%) [11]
Vomiting (24%) [5]

Hematologic
Anemia [3]
Hemorrhage [2]
Lymphopenia (lymphocytopenia) / lymphocytes decreased (53%)
Neutropenia (neutrophils decreased) (35%) [2]
Thrombocytopenia / platelets decreased (35%) [3]
Thrombosis [2]

Neuromuscular/Skeletal
Arthralgia (14%)
Asthenia / fatigue (21–41%) [29]
Muscle spasm (12%)
Osteonecrosis / avascular necrosis (includes steroid-induced osteonecrosis of the femoral head) (jaw) [4]
Pain in extremities (14%)

Renal
Proteinuria (2%) [2]

Respiratory
Cough (18%)
Dysphonia (includes voice disorders / voice changes) (20%)
Dyspnea / shortness of breath (19%)
Pulmonary embolism [2]

Other
Adverse effects / adverse reactions [8]
Death (6%) [7]

CAFFEINE

Family: Rubiales
Scientific names: *Cafcit (Bedford), Coffea arabica, Coffea canephora, Coffea robusta, Cola acuminata, Thea sinensis, Theobroma cacao*
Indications: With ergotamine for migraine, with NSAIDs in analgesics, headache, respiratory depression in neonates, postprandial hypotension, enhances seizure duration in electroconvulsive therapy, ingredient in cough and cold remedies
Class: Diuretic, Xanthine alkaloid
Half-life: 2–7 hours
Clinically important, potentially hazardous interactions with: aminophylline, carbamazepine, cimetidine, clozapine, cocoa, ephedra, ferrous sulfate, fluorides, ginseng, guarana, idrocilamide, ketoconazole, ketoprofen, levomepromazine, linezolid, methoxsalen, mexiletine, norfloxacin, phenobarbital, phenylpropanolamine, phenytoin, regadenoson, terbinafine, teriflunomide, zonisamide
Important contra-indications noted in the prescribing guidelines for: nursing mothers
Note: Caffeine is an addictive psychoactive substance. Spontaneous abortion and low birthweight babies have occurred in pregnant women consuming 150 mg caffeine per day. Abuse can lead to cardiac damage or death. See also separate profile for guarana.
Common symptoms of caffeine withdrawal are headache; drowsiness; yawning, impaired concentration; lassitude; irritability; decreased contentedness, well-being and self-confidence; decreased sociability; flu-like symptoms; muscle aches and stiffness; hot or cold spells; nausea or vomiting; and blurred vision. Cafcit is caffeine citrate.

Skin
Anaphylactoid reactions / anaphylaxis (includes anaphylactic shock) [3]
Hypersensitivity [2]
Urticaria / hives [5]

Cardiovascular
Arrhythmias [4]
Atrial fibrillation [2]
Hypertension [2]
Palpitation [2]

Central Nervous System
Anxiety [2]
Depression [2]
Headache [2]
Insomnia [2]
Psychosis [3]
Restlessness [2]
Seizures [6]
Tremor [4]

Gastrointestinal/Hepatic
Gastrointestinal disorder / discomfort [2]

Neuromuscular/Skeletal
Rhabdomyolysis [6]

Other
Adverse effects / adverse reactions [4]
Death (from abuse / overdose) [21]

CALCIFEDIOL

Synonym: calcidiol
Trade name: Rayaldee (Opko)
Indications: Hyperparathyroidism in stage 3 or 4 chronic kidney disease
Class: Vitamin D analog
Half-life: 11 days
Clinically important, potentially hazardous interactions with: anticonvulsants, atazanavir, cholestyramine, clarithromycin, indinavir, itraconazole, ketoconazole, nefazodone, nelfinavir, phenobarbital, ritonavir, saquinavir, telithromycin, thiazides, voriconazole
Important contra-indications noted in the prescribing guidelines for: nursing mothers; pediatric patients

---

Skin
Hematoma / cutaneous hematoma (2%)
Cardiovascular
Congestive heart failure (4%)
Endocrine/Metabolic
Hyperkalemia (3%)
Hyperuricemia (2%)
Serum creatinine increased (5%)
Gastrointestinal/Hepatic
Constipation (3%)
Hematologic
Anemia (5%)
Neuromuscular/Skeletal
Arthralgia (2%)
Respiratory
Bronchitis (3%)
Cough (4%)
Dyspnea / shortness of breath (4%)
Nasopharyngitis (5%)

CALCIPOTRIOL

Synonym: calcipotriene
Trade name: Dovonex (Leo Pharma)
Indications: Psoriasis
Class: Antipsoriatic agent, Vitamin D analog
Half-life: ~30 minutes
Clinically important, potentially hazardous interactions with: none known
Important contra-indications noted in the prescribing guidelines for: nursing mothers; pediatric patients
Note: Contra-indicated in patients with acute psoriatic eruptions, hypercalcemia or vitamin D toxicity.

Skin
Burning / skin burning sensation (23%)
Contact dermatitis [8]
Erythema (<10%)
Pigmentation (Skin) (includes hyperpigmentation) [3]
Pruritus (itching) (>10%) [6]
Psoriasis (<10%) [3]
Rash (11%)
Xerosis / xeroderma (<5%)
Endocrine/Metabolic
Hypercalcemia [3]
Local
Application-site pain [3]
Application-site pruritus [2]
Application-site reactions [2]
Respiratory
Nasopharyngitis [4]
Other
Adverse effects / adverse reactions [3]

CALCITONIN

Trade names: Calcimar (Sanofi-Aventis), Miacalcin (Novartis)
Indications: Paget's disease of bone
Class: Parathyroid hormone antagonist
Half-life: 70–90 minutes
Clinically important, potentially hazardous interactions with: none known

---

Skin
Flushing / rubefaction (>10%) [5]
Gastrointestinal/Hepatic
Diarrhea [2]
Nausea [2]
Local
Injection-site edema (>10%)
Injection-site inflammation (>10%) [2]
Injection-site reaction (10%)
Respiratory
Rhinitis / rhinosinusitis (see also sinusitis) (12%)

CALCIUM HYDROXYLAPATITE

Trade name: Radiesse (Merz)
Indications: Correction of facial wrinkles and folds
Class: Dermal filler
Half-life: N/A
Clinically important, potentially hazardous interactions with: anticoagulants, antiplatelet drugs, aspirin, baloxavir marboxil

---

Skin
Bruise / bruising / contusion / ecchymosis (ecchymoses) [2]
Granulomas [6]
Necrosis (skin necrosis) [2]
Nodular eruption [3]
Mucosal
Oral lesions [3]

CANAGLIFLOZIN

Trade names: Invokamet (Janssen), Invokana (Janssen)
Indications: Type II diabetes mellitus
Class: Antidiabetic, Sodium-glucose co-transporter 2 (SGLT2) inhibitor ('gliflozin')
Half-life: 11–13 hours
Clinically important, potentially hazardous interactions with: digoxin, rifampin
Important contra-indications noted in the prescribing guidelines for: nursing mothers; pediatric patients
Note: Contra-indicated in patients with severe renal impairment, end stage renal disease, or on dialysis. Invokamet is canagliflozin and metformin.

Skin
Pruritus (itching) [2]
Cardiovascular
Postural hypotension [2]
Central Nervous System
Headache [3]
Vertigo / dizziness [3]
Endocrine/Metabolic
Dehydration [3]
Diabetic ketoacidosis [2]
Hypoglycemia [8]
Gastrointestinal/Hepatic
Abdominal pain (2%) [3]
Constipation (2%) [3]
Diarrhea [2]
Nausea (2%) [4]
Pancreatitis / acute pancreatitis [3]
Genitourinary
Genital mycotic infection (4–11%) [29]
Pollakiuria [8]
Polyuria (includes polyuric syndrome) [2]
Urinary frequency (5%) [6]
Urinary tract infection (4–6%) [24]
Vulvovaginal candidiasis [2]
Vulvovaginal pruritus (2–3%) [3]
Neuromuscular/Skeletal
Arthralgia [2]
Asthenia / fatigue (2%)
Back pain [2]
Renal
Nephrotoxicity / kidney injury / acute kidney injury (AKI) / drug-induced kidney injury [2]
Respiratory
Nasopharyngitis [2]
Upper respiratory tract infection [2]
Other
Adverse effects / adverse reactions [5]
Death [2]
Dipsia (thirst) / polydipsia (2–3%) [4]
Infection [2]

CANAKINUMAB

Trade name: Ilaris (Novartis)
Indications: Periodic fever syndromes, systemic juvenile idiopathic arthritis
Class: Interleukin-1 inhibitor, Monoclonal antibody
Half-life: 26 days
Clinically important, potentially hazardous interactions with: cytochrome P450, IL-1 blockers, lenalidomide, TNF-blockers
Important contra-indications noted in the prescribing guidelines for: nursing mothers; pediatric patients
Note: Interleukin-1 blockade may interfere with immune response to infections. Treatment with medications that work through inhibition of IL-1 has been associated with an increased risk of serious infections.

Central Nervous System
Headache [2]
Vertigo / dizziness (11%) [2]
Endocrine/Metabolic
Weight gain (11%)
Gastrointestinal/Hepatic
Gastroenteritis (11%) [2]
Nausea (14%)
Genitourinary
Urinary tract infection [2]
Hematologic
Macrophage activation syndrome [3]
Neutropenia (neutrophils decreased) [2]

Local
Injection-site reaction [4]

Neuromuscular/Skeletal
Myalgia/Myopathy (11%)

Respiratory
Bronchitis (11%)
Influenza- ('flu)-like syndrome (20%)
Nasopharyngitis (34%) [3]
Pharyngitis (sore throat) (11%)
Pneumonia [2]
Rhinitis / rhinosinusitis (see also sinusitis) (17%)
Upper respiratory tract infection [4]

Other
Adverse effects / adverse reactions [8]
Infection [14]

CANDESARTAN

Trade name: Atacand (AstraZeneca)
Indications: Hypertension and heart failure
Class: Angiotensin receptor antagonist (blocker), Antihypertensive
Half-life: 9 hours
Clinically important, potentially hazardous interactions with: aliskiren
Important contra-indications noted in the prescribing guidelines for: nursing mothers; pediatric patients
Warning: FETAL TOXICITY

Skin
Angioedema (formerly named angioneurotic edema) [3]

Cardiovascular
Hypotension [5]

Central Nervous System
Dysgeusia (taste perversion) [2]
Headache [5]
Vertigo / dizziness (4%) [6]

Endocrine/Metabolic
Hyperkalemia (2%)

Gastrointestinal/Hepatic
Gastroenteritis [2]

Hematologic
Neutropenia (neutrophils decreased) [2]

Neuromuscular/Skeletal
Back pain (3%) [3]

Renal
Renal failure [3]

Respiratory
Pharyngitis (sore throat) (2%)
Rhinitis / rhinosinusitis (see also sinusitis) (2%)
Upper respiratory tract infection (6%) [3]

Other
Adverse effects / adverse reactions [4]
Fetotoxicity [2]

CANGRELOR

Trade name: Kengreal (Medicines Co)
Indications: Adjunct to percutaneous coronary intervention for reducing the risk of periprocedural myocardial infarction, repeat coronary revascularization and stent thrombosis
Class: Antiplatelet (antithrombotic), Antiplatelet; cyclopentyl triazolo-pyrimidine (CPTP)
Half-life: 3–6 minutes
Clinically important, potentially hazardous interactions with: clopidogrel, prasugrel
Important contra-indications noted in the prescribing guidelines for: nursing mothers; pediatric patients
Note: Contra-indicated in patients with significant active bleeding.

Hematologic
Bleeding (<15%) [7]

Renal
Nephrotoxicity / kidney injury / acute kidney injury (AKI) / drug-induced kidney injury (3%)

Respiratory
Dyspnea / shortness of breath [5]

CAPECITABINE

Trade name: Xeloda (Roche)
Indications: Metastatic breast or colorectal cancer, adjuvant colon cancer
Class: Antimetabolite, Antineoplastic / anticancer agent (see also Immune checkpoint inhibitor), Fluoropyrimidine
Half-life: 0.5–1 hour
Clinically important, potentially hazardous interactions with: allopurinol, anticoagulants, CYP2C9 substrates, erlotinib, leucovorin, phenprocoumon, phenytoin, tegafur/gimeracil/oteracil, tegafur/gimeracil/oteracil, warfarin
Important contra-indications noted in the prescribing guidelines for: nursing mothers
Note: Patients receiving concomitant capecitabine and oral coumarin-derivative anticoagulants such as warfarin and phenprocoumon should have their anticoagulant response (INR or prothrombin time) monitored frequently in order to adjust the anticoagulant dose accordingly. Altered coagulation parameters and/or bleeding, including death, have been reported during concomitant use.
Contra-indicated in patients with severe renal impairment or with known hypersensitivity to fluorouracil. Capecitabine is a prodrug of 5-fluorouracil. CapeOX (also called XELOX) is a combination of capecitabine and oxaliplatin.
Warning: XELODA - WARFARIN INTERACTION

Skin
Acneiform eruption / acneiform dermatitis / acneiform rash [3]
Actinic keratoses [3]
Adermatoglyphia (fingerprint loss) [3]
Cutaneous toxicity / skin toxicity [4]
Dermatitis (37%) [10]
Edema / fluid retention (9%) [3]
Exfoliative dermatitis (31–37%)
Hand–foot syndrome (palmar–plantar erythrodysesthesia) (7–58%) [185]
Jaundice (see also cholestasis / cholestatic jaundice) [3]
Lupus erythematosus (subacute cutaneous lupus erythematosus (SCLE)) [4]
Photosensitivity [2]
Pigmentation (Skin) (includes hyperpigmentation) [10]
Pruritus (itching) [2]
Radiation recall dermatitis [6]
Rash [14]
Stevens-Johnson syndrome and toxic epidermal necrolysis (SJS/TEN) [3]
Vitiligo [2]
Xerosis / xeroderma [2]

Hair
Alopecia / hair loss [10]

Nails
Nail changes (7%)
Onycholysis [3]
Onychomadesis [3]
Paronychia [2]
Pyogenic granuloma [2]

Mucosal
Mucosal inflammation [2]
Mucositis [17]
Oral pigmentation [2]
Stomatitis (oral mucositis) (24%) [19]

Cardiovascular
Angina [6]
Cardiotoxicity [7]
Chest pain [3]
Coronary vasospasm [7]
Hypertension [6]
Myocardial infarction [4]
QT interval prolonged / QT prolongation [2]
Takotsubo syndrome [2]
Thromboembolism [2]
Ventricular fibrillation [2]

Central Nervous System
Anorexia [13]
Cranial neuropathy (includes types of palsy) [2]
Fever (pyrexia) (includes hyperpyrexia) [2]
Headache [2]
Leukoencephalopathy / posterior reversible encephalopathy syndrome (PRES) [6]
Neurotoxicity [14]
Pain [4]
Paresthesias (21%)
Peripheral neuropathy [12]
Vertigo / dizziness [3]

Endocrine/Metabolic
ALT increased [5]
Appetite decreased [2]
AST increased [5]
Hyperammonemia [2]
Hyperbilirubinemia [4]
Hyperglycemia (includes glucose increased) [6]
Hypertriglyceridemia (includes triglycerides increased) [5]
Hypokalemia [2]
Hypophosphatemia [2]

Gastrointestinal/Hepatic
Abdominal pain [9]
Colitis [2]
Constipation [3]
Diarrhea [78]
Enteritis [2]
Enterocolitis [4]
Hepatotoxicity / liver injury / acute liver injury / drug-induced liver injury (DILI) [8]
Ileitis [7]

Ileus / adynamic ileus / paralytic ileus [2]
Nausea [41]
Pancreatitis / acute pancreatitis [2]
Vomiting [30]

Hematologic
Anemia [28]
Febrile neutropenia [4]
Hemotoxicity [2]
Leukocytopenia (leukopenia) / leukocytes (white blood cells) decreased [19]
Lymphopenia (lymphocytopenia) / lymphocytes decreased [2]
Neutropenia (neutrophils decreased) [52]
Thrombocytopenia / platelets decreased [24]
Thrombosis [2]

Neuromuscular/Skeletal
Asthenia / fatigue [54]
Ataxia [2]
Myalgia/Myopathy (9%) [3]
Pain in extremities [2]

Respiratory
Nasopharyngitis [2]

Other
Adverse effects / adverse reactions [7]
Allergic reactions [2]
Death [7]
Infection [2]

CAPMATINIB

Synonym: Capmatinib hydrochloride
Trade name: Tabrecta (Novartis)
Indications: Metastatic non-small cell lung cancer in adult patients.
NOTE: (2020) FDA approved under accelerated approval based on overall response rate and duration of response. Continued approval may be contingent upon verification and description of clinical benefit in confirmatory trial(s).

Class: Kinase inhibitor, MET (mesenchymal-epithelial transition) inhibitor / MET tyrosine kinase inhibitor
Half-life: 6.5 hours
Clinically important, potentially hazardous interactions with: CYP3A inducers, CYP3A inhibitors, itraconazole, rabeprazole, rifampin
Pregnancy category: Can cause fetal harm. Advise patients of the potential risk to a fetus and to use effective contraception.

Skin
Peripheral edema (52%) [2]

Cardiovascular
Chest pain (15%)

Central Nervous System
Fever (pyrexia) (includes hyperpyrexia) (14%)

Endocrine/Metabolic
ALP increased (32%)
ALT increased (37%)
Appetite decreased (21%)
AST increased (25%)
GGT increased (29%)
Hyperamylasemia (31%)
Hyperkalemia (23%)
Hyperlipasemia (26%)
Hypoalbuminemia / albumin decreased (68%)
Hypoglycemia (21%)
Hyponatremia (23%)
Hypophosphatemia (23%)
Serum creatinine increased (62%)
Weight loss (10%)

Gastrointestinal/Hepatic
Constipation (18%)
Diarrhea (18%)
Hepatotoxicity / liver injury / acute liver injury / drug-induced liver injury (DILI) [2]
Nausea (44%) [4]
Vomiting (28%)

Hematologic
Hemoglobin decreased (24%)
Leukocytopenia (leukopenia) / leukocytes (white blood cells) decreased (23%)
Lymphopenia (lymphocytopenia) / lymphocytes decreased (44%)

Neuromuscular/Skeletal
Asthenia / fatigue (32%)

Respiratory
Cough (16%)
Dyspnea / shortness of breath (24%)
Interstitial lung disease / interstitial pneumonitis / interstitial pneumonia (cryptogenic organizing pneumonia) / drug-induced interstitial lung disease [2]

CAPREOMYCIN

Trade name: Capastat (King)
Indications: Tuberculosis
Class: Antibiotic, Antimicrobial, Drug-resistant antituberculosis agent
Half-life: 12 hours
Clinically important, potentially hazardous interactions with: aminoglycosides, non-depolarizing neuromuscular blocking agents, oxaliplatin

---

Endocrine/Metabolic
Hypocalcemia [2]
Hypokalemia [3]
Hypomagnesemia [2]

CAPSICUM

Family: Solanaceae
Scientific names: *Capsicum annuum, Capsicum baccatum, Capsicum chinense, Capsicum frutescens, Capsicum pubscens*
Indications: Nausea, neuropathic pain, osteoarthritis, fibromyalgia, anticarcinogen, rheumatoid arthritis, diabetic neuropathy, postherpetic neuralgia (shingles), psoriasis, pruritus, vitiligo, dyspepsia, flatulence, ulcers, stomach cramps, hypertension, improved circulation, weight-loss
Class: Rubefacient
Half-life: N/A
Clinically important, potentially hazardous interactions with: ACE inhibitors, aminophylline, antiplatelet drugs, aspirin, latex, salicylic acid
Note: Pepper spray or gas contains 5% oleoresin capsicum (OC). It is used by police and in personal defense sprays.

Skin
Burning / skin burning sensation [5]
Dermatitis [3]
Erythema [3]
Hypersensitivity [2]
Pruritus (itching) [2]
Urticaria / hives [2]

Cardiovascular
Hypertension [2]

Central Nervous System
Hyperalgesia [2]
Pain [5]

Ocular
Conjunctivitis (conjunctival inflammation) [3]

Other
Adverse effects / adverse reactions [6]
Allergic reactions [3]
Death [5]

CAPTOPRIL

Trade names: Capoten (Par), Capozide (Par)
Indications: Hypertension, congestive heart failure, to improve survival following myocardial infarction in clinically stable patients with left ventricular dysfunction, diabetic nephropathy in patients with Type I insulin-dependent diabetes mellitus and retinopathy
Class: Angiotensin-converting enzyme (ACE) inhibitor, Antihypertensive, Vasodilator
Half-life: <3 hours
Clinically important, potentially hazardous interactions with: alcohol, aldesleukin, allopurinol, alpha blockers, alprostadil, amifostine, amiloride, angiotensin II receptor antagonists, antacids, antidiabetics, antihypertensives, antipsychotics, anxiolytics and hypnotics, aprotinin, azathioprine, baclofen, beta blockers, calcium channel blockers, clonidine, cyclosporine, CYP2D6 inhibitors, darunavir, diazoxide, digoxin, diuretics, eplerenone, estrogens, everolimus, general anesthetics, gold & gold compounds, heparins, herbals, hydralazine, hypotensives, insulin, interferon alfa, levodopa, lithium, MAO inhibitors, metformin, methyldopa, methylphenidate, minoxidil, moxisylyte, moxonidine, naldemedine, nitrates, nitroprusside, NSAIDs, pentoxifylline, phosphodiesterase 5 inhibitors, potassium salts, probenecid, prostacyclin analogues, rituximab, salicylates, sirolimus, spironolactone, sulfonylureas, temsirolimus, tizanidine, tolvaptan, triamterene, trimethoprim, venetoclax, yohimbine
Pregnancy category: category C in first trimester; category D in second and third trimesters
Important contra-indications noted in the prescribing guidelines for: nursing mothers; pediatric patients
Note: Capozide is captopril and hydrochlorothiazide. Hydrochlorothiazide is a sulfonamide and can be absorbed systemically. Sulfonamides can produce severe, possibly fatal, reactions such as toxic epidermal necrolysis and Stevens-Johnson syndrome.
Warning: FETAL TOXICITY

Skin
Angioedema (formerly named angioneurotic edema) (<15%) [45]
Bullous pemphigoid / pemphigoid [2]
Dermatitis [3]
DRESS syndrome (Drug-induced hypersensitivity syndrome) [2]
Erythroderma [2]
Exanthems (4–7%) [19]
Exfoliative dermatitis (<2%) [4]
Flushing / rubefaction [2]
Kaposi's sarcoma [2]

Lichen planus pemphigoides [2]
Lichenoid eruption / lichenoid reaction [12]
Linear IgA bullous dermatosis [5]
Lupus erythematosus (subacute cutaneous lupus erythematosus (SCLE)) [8]
Mycosis fungoides [2]
Pemphigus (<2%) [24]
Pemphigus foliaceus [2]
Photosensitivity [3]
Phototoxicity (<2%)
Pigmentation (Skin) (includes hyperpigmentation) [2]
Pityriasis rosea (<2%) [6]
Pruritus (itching) (<7%) [8]
Pseudolymphoma / cutaneous pseudolymphoma [2]
Psoriasis [8]
Rash (4–7%) [12]
Stevens-Johnson syndrome and toxic epidermal necrolysis (SJS/TEN) [4]
Urticaria / hives [9]
Vasculitis (angiitis) / cutaneous vasculitis (angiitis) [7]

Hair
Alopecia / hair loss (<2%) [4]

Nails
Nail dystrophy [2]
Onycholysis [2]

Mucosal
Aphthous stomatitis / aphthous ulcer / aphtha (aphthae) (<2%) [5]
Burning Mouth Syndrome / glossodynia / glossalgia / glossopyrosis (also includes stomatodynia / oral dysesthesia / stomatopyrosis) [2]
Glossitis (inflammation of the tongue) [3]
Oral mucosal eruption [3]
Oral ulceration [4]
Sialadenitis [2]
Tongue ulceration [3]
Xerostomia (dry mouth) (<2%)

Central Nervous System
Ageusia (taste loss) / taste disorder (2–4%) [11]
Dysgeusia (taste perversion) (metallic or salty taste) (2–4%) [14]
Hallucinations [2]
Paresthesias (<2%)

Endocrine/Metabolic
Gynecomastia [3]

Gastrointestinal/Hepatic
Hepatotoxicity / liver injury / acute liver injury / drug-induced liver injury (DILI) [3]
Nausea [2]

Genitourinary
Penile ulceration [2]

Renal
Nephrotoxicity / kidney injury / acute kidney injury (AKI) / drug-induced kidney injury [2]

Respiratory
Cough [19]

Other
Adverse effects / adverse reactions [4]
Allergic reactions [2]

CARAWAY

Family: Apiaceae Umbelliferae
Scientific names: *Apium carvi, Carum carvi*
Indications: Hypotensive, dyspepsia, hysteria, tonic, stomachic, flatulent indigestion, flatulent colic of infants, fragrance, flavoring in foods, toothpaste, and cosmetics
Class: Anti-inflammatory, Carminative
Half-life: N/A
Clinically important, potentially hazardous interactions with: none known

Other
Adverse effects / adverse reactions [4]

CARBACHOL

Trade name: Carbastat Ophthalmic (Novartis)
Indications: Glaucoma
Class: Miotic, Muscarinic cholinergic agonist
Half-life: N/A
Clinically important, potentially hazardous interactions with: none known

CARBAMAZEPINE

Trade names: Epitol (Teva), Tegretol (Novartis)
Indications: Epilepsy, pain or trigeminal neuralgia
Class: Anticonvulsant (see also antiepileptic (anti-seizure)), Antipsychotic, CYP1A2 inducer, CYP3A4 inducer, Gabapentinoid, Mood stabilizer
Half-life: 18–55 hours
Clinically important, potentially hazardous interactions with: abiraterone, acetaminophen, acetylcysteine, adenosine, afatinib, amitriptyline, amlodipine, amprenavir, apixaban, apremilast, aprepitant, aripiprazole, artemether/lumefantrine, bictegravir/emtricitabine/tenofovir alafenamide, boceprevir, brigatinib, brivaracetam, buprenorphine, cabazitaxel, cabozantinib, caffeine, caspofungin, cefixime, cenobamate, ceritinib, charcoal, citalopram, clarithromycin, clobazam, clopidogrel, clorazepate, clozapine, cobicistat/elvitegravir/emtricitabine/tenofovir disoproxil, cobimetinib, copanlisib, crizotinib, dabigatran, daclatasvir, darunavir, dasatinib, deflazacort, delavirdine, dexamethasone, diltiazem, doravirine, doravirine/lamiduvine/tenofovir disoproxil, doxacurium, doxycycline, dronedarone, efavirenz, elbasvir & grazoprevir, eliglustat, emtricitabine/rilpivirine/tenofovir alafenamide, enzalutamide, erlotinib, erlotinib, erythromycin, eslicarbazepine, estradiol, ethosuximide, etravirine, ezogabine, felodipine, fesoterodine, flibanserin, fosamprenavir, fostemsavir, gefitinib, glecaprevir & pibrentasvir, ibrexafungerp, ibrutinib, idelalisib, imatinib, indinavir, influenza vaccine, isavuconazonium sulfate, isotretinoin, itraconazole, ixabepilone, ixazomib, lacosamide, lapatinib, ledipasvir & sofosbuvir, lemborexant, lesinurad, levetiracetam, levomepromazine, levonorgestrel, linezolid, lopinavir, lumateperone, methylprednisolone, midazolam, midostaurin, mifepristone, naldemedine, nelfinavir, neratinib, nevirapine, nifedipine, nilotinib, nintedanib, olanzapine, olaparib, oliceridine, ombitasvir/paritaprevir/ritonavir, ombitasvir/paritaprevir/ritonavir and dasabuvir, ondansetron, osilodrostat, osimertinib, oxcarbazepine, oxtriphylline, paclitaxel, palbociclib, paliperidone, perampanel, pimavanserin, piracetam, ponatinib, ponesimod, prednisolone, propoxyphene, regorafenib, rilpivirine, riociguat, risperidone, ritonavir, rivaroxaban, roflumilast, romidepsin, rufinamide, simeprevir, simvastatin, sodium picosulfate, sofosbuvir, sofosbuvir & velpatasvir, sofosbuvir/velpatasvir/voxilaprevir, solifenacin, sonidegib, sorafenib, St John's wort, sunitinib, telaprevir, telithromycin, temsirolimus, tenofovir alafenamide, terbinafine, tezacaftor/ivacaftor, thalidomide, tiagabine, ticagrelor, tipranavir, tolvaptan, tramadol, triamcinolone, troleandomycin, ulipristal, valbenazine, vandetanib, vemurafenib, venetoclax, verapamil, vorapaxar, voriconazole, vortioxetine, ziprasidone, zuclopenthixol
Note: Carbamazepine is the main cause of Stevens-Johnson syndrome (SJS), toxic epidermal necrolysis (TEN), and the hypersensitivity syndrome in Han Chinese, and in peoples of other Southeast Asian countries, as a result of a strong pharmacogenetic association that has been reported in these patients between the human leukocyte antigen (HLA)-B*1502 and carbamazepine.
Warning: SERIOUS DERMATOLOGIC REACTIONS AND HLA-B*1502 ALLELE; APLASTIC ANEMIA AND AGRANULOCYTOSIS

Skin
AGEP [7]
Angioedema (formerly named angioneurotic edema) [5]
Bullous dermatosis [4]
Cutaneous adverse reaction (includes severe cutaneous adverse drug reaction (SCAR)) [8]
Cutaneous toxicity / skin toxicity [2]
Dermatitis [7]
Diaphoresis (<10%)
DRESS syndrome (Drug-induced hypersensitivity syndrome) [82]
Eczema / eczematous reaction / eczematous eruption [2]
Erythema multiforme [17]
Erythroderma [12]
Exanthems (>5%) [36]
Exfoliative dermatitis [24]
Facial edema [2]
Fixed eruption / fixed drug eruption [10]
Hypersensitivity [72]
Lichen planus (includes hypertrophic lichen planus) [2]
Lichenoid eruption / lichenoid reaction [8]
Lupus erythematosus (subacute cutaneous lupus erythematosus (SCLE)) [35]
Lymphadenopathy [2]
Lymphoma [2]
Lymphoproliferative disease / lymphoproliferative disorder [5]
Mycosis fungoides [3]
Pemphigus [3]
Photosensitivity [9]
Pruritus (itching) [7]
Pseudolymphoma / cutaneous pseudolymphoma [17]
Purpura [8]
Pustules / pustular eruption [5]
Rash (>10%) [32]
Serum sickness [2]
Stevens-Johnson syndrome and toxic epidermal necrolysis (SJS/TEN) (<10%) [155]
Toxic pustuloderma [3]

Urticaria / hives [14]
Vasculitis (angiitis) / cutaneous vasculitis (angiitis) [7]

Hair
Alopecia / hair loss [7]

Nails
Onychomadesis [2]

Mucosal
Mucocutaneous eruption (includes fixed eruption) [4]
Mucocutaneous lymph node syndrome (Kawasaki syndrome) [2]
Oral lichenoid eruption [3]
Oral ulceration [2]
Tongue ulceration [2]

Cardiovascular
Bradycardia / sinus bradycardia [3]
Hypertension [2]
Myocarditis [4]

Central Nervous System
Ageusia (taste loss) / taste disorder [3]
Coma [3]
Dysgeusia (taste perversion) [2]
Fever (pyrexia) (includes hyperpyrexia) [2]
Hallucinations, auditory [2]
Headache [5]
Memory loss/memory impaired [2]
Seizures [14]
Somnolence (drowsiness) [9]
Tic disorder [4]
Vertigo / dizziness [9]

Endocrine/Metabolic
Acute intermittent porphyria [5]
Hyponatremia [6]
SIADH [17]
Weight gain [5]

Gastrointestinal/Hepatic
Diarrhea [3]
Hepatotoxicity / liver injury / acute liver injury / drug-induced liver injury (DILI) [12]
Nausea [6]
Pancreatitis / acute pancreatitis [4]
Vanishing bile duct syndrome / ductopenia [4]
Vomiting [3]

Hematologic
Agranulocytosis / severe selective neutropenia [4]
Aplastic anemia [3]
Eosinophilia / eosinophils increased [2]
Hypogammaglobulinemia [5]
Leukocytopenia (leukopenia) / leukocytes (white blood cells) decreased [3]
Leukocytosis (elevated white blood cell (WBC) count) [3]
Thrombocytopenia / platelets decreased [4]

Neuromuscular/Skeletal
Asthenia / fatigue [3]
Ataxia [5]
Myasthenia gravis [2]
Osteoporosis [2]

Ocular
Diplopia (double vision) [2]
Oculogyric crisis / oculogyric dystonic reaction [2]

Renal
Nephrotoxicity / kidney injury / acute kidney injury (AKI) / drug-induced kidney injury [2]

Respiratory
Respiratory depression [2]

Other
Adverse effects / adverse reactions [10]
Allergic reactions [9]
Death [8]
Side effects [3]
Teratogenicity [12]

CARBENICILLIN

Trade name: Geocillin (Pfizer)
Indications: Urinary tract infections
Class: Antibiotic, Antibiotic; beta-lactam, Antibiotic; penicillin, Antimicrobial
Half-life: 1.0–1.5 hours
Clinically important, potentially hazardous interactions with: anticoagulants, ceftobiprole, cyclosporine, demeclocycline, doxycycline, gentamicin, imipenem/cilastatin, methotrexate, minocycline, oxytetracycline, tetracycline

---

Skin
Purpura [2]

Mucosal
Glossitis (inflammation of the tongue) (<10%)

Central Nervous System
Dysgeusia (taste perversion) (<10%)
Seizures [2]

CARBETOCIN

Trade name: Pabal (Ferring)
Indications: Prevention of uterine atony following delivery of an infant by cesarean section under epidural or spinal anaesthesia
Class: Oxytocic
Half-life: 40 minutes
Clinically important, potentially hazardous interactions with: cyclopropane, halothane, methylergometrine, prostaglandins, vasoconstrictors

---

Skin
Flushing / rubefaction (>10%) [3]
Pruritus (itching) (<10%)

Cardiovascular
Chest pain (<10%)
Hypotension (>10%) [4]

Central Nervous System
Chills (<10%)
Headache (>10%) [2]
Tremor (>10%)
Vertigo / dizziness (<10%)

Gastrointestinal/Hepatic
Abdominal pain (>10%)
Nausea (>10%) [2]
Vomiting (<10%)

Hematologic
Anemia (<10%)

Neuromuscular/Skeletal
Back pain (<10%)

Respiratory
Dyspnea / shortness of breath (<10%)

CARBIMAZOLE

Trade name: NeoMercazole (Amdipharm)
Indications: Hyperthyroidism
Class: Antithyroid, Imidazole antithyroid agent
Half-life: 6–8 hours
Clinically important, potentially hazardous interactions with: aminophylline, amiodarone, digoxin, prednisolone
Note: Carbimazole is a prodrug of methimazole (see separate entry).

Skin
Hypersensitivity [3]
Vasculitis (angiitis) / cutaneous vasculitis (angiitis) [2]

Gastrointestinal/Hepatic
Hepatotoxicity / liver injury / acute liver injury / drug-induced liver injury (DILI) [10]

Hematologic
Agranulocytosis / severe selective neutropenia [8]
Neutropenia (neutrophils decreased) [2]

Neuromuscular/Skeletal
Myalgia/Myopathy [4]

Renal
Nephrotoxicity / kidney injury / acute kidney injury (AKI) / drug-induced kidney injury [2]

Respiratory
Pleural effusion [2]

Other
Teratogenicity [2]

CARBINOXAMINE

Trade name: Histex (TEAMM)
Indications: Allergic rhinitis
Class: Histamine H1 receptor antagonist
Half-life: 10–20 hours
Clinically important, potentially hazardous interactions with: none known

CARBOPLATIN

Trade name: Paraplatin (Bristol-Myers Squibb)
Indications: Various carcinomas and sarcomas
Class: Alkylating agent, Antineoplastic / anticancer agent (see also Immune checkpoint inhibitor), Platinum-based antineoplastic
Half-life: terminal: 22–40 hours
Clinically important, potentially hazardous interactions with: aldesleukin, bexarotene
Important contra-indications noted in the prescribing guidelines for: the elderly; nursing mothers; pediatric patients

---

Skin
Anaphylactoid reactions / anaphylaxis (includes anaphylactic shock) [5]
Cutaneous toxicity / skin toxicity [6]
Erythema (2%) [2]
Exanthems [3]
Flushing / rubefaction [3]
Hand–foot syndrome (palmar–plantar erythrodysesthesia) [5]
Hypersensitivity (2%) [27]
Pigmentation (Skin) (includes hyperpigmentation) [2]
Pruritus (itching) (2%) [2]
Radiation recall dermatitis [2]
Rash (2%) [10]

Scleroderma [2]
Stevens-Johnson syndrome and toxic epidermal necrolysis (SJS/TEN) [2]
Urticaria / hives (2%) [4]

Hair
Alopecia / hair loss (3%) [19]
Alopecia areata [2]

Mucosal
Epistaxis (nosebleed) [2]
Mucositis [5]
Stomatitis (oral mucositis) (>10%) [2]

Cardiovascular
Hypertension [10]

Central Nervous System
Anorexia [8]
Fever (pyrexia) (includes hyperpyrexia) [2]
Headache [2]
Leukoencephalopathy / posterior reversible encephalopathy syndrome (PRES) [2]
Neurotoxicity [16]
Pain [2]
Paresthesias [2]
Peripheral neuropathy [9]
Vertigo / dizziness [2]

Endocrine/Metabolic
ALT increased [4]
AST increased [3]
Hyperbilirubinemia [2]
Hyperglycemia (includes glucose increased) [5]
Hyponatremia [3]
SIADH [3]

Gastrointestinal/Hepatic
Constipation [3]
Diarrhea [16]
Dyspepsia / functional dyspepsia (indigestion) (see also gastroparesis) [2]
Gastrointestinal perforation / perforated colon / gastric perforation [2]
Hepatotoxicity / liver injury / acute liver injury / drug-induced liver injury (DILI) [4]
Nausea [18]
Pancreatitis / acute pancreatitis [2]
Vomiting [18]

Genitourinary
Hematuria [3]

Hematologic
Anemia [31]
Febrile neutropenia [23]
Hemolytic anemia [2]
Hemorrhage [2]
Hemotoxicity [8]
Leukocytopenia (leukopenia) / leukocytes (white blood cells) decreased [15]
Lymphopenia (lymphocytopenia) / lymphocytes decreased [3]
Myelosuppression / bone marrow suppression / myelotoxicity [5]
Neutropenia (neutrophils decreased) [59]
Pancytopenia (includes bicytopenia) [2]
Thrombocytopenia / platelets decreased [41]

Local
Injection-site pain (>10%)

Neuromuscular/Skeletal
Asthenia / fatigue [27]
Myalgia/Myopathy [3]

Otic
Hearing loss (hypoacusis) [2]
Ototoxicity [7]
Tinnitus [3]

Renal
Nephrotoxicity / kidney injury / acute kidney injury (AKI) / drug-induced kidney injury [9]
Proteinuria [3]

Respiratory
Cough [2]
Hemoptysis [3]
Pneumonia [3]
Pulmonary toxicity [3]

Other
Adverse effects / adverse reactions [3]
Allergic reactions [4]
Death [7]
Infection [5]

CARIPRAZINE

Trade name: Vraylar (Forest)
Indications: Schizophrenia, manic or mixed episodes associated with bipolar I disorder
Class: Antipsychotic, Antipsychotic, atypical
Half-life: 2–4 days
Clinically important, potentially hazardous interactions with: CYP3A4 inducers
Pregnancy category: Neonatal risk in third trimester exposure
Important contra-indications noted in the prescribing guidelines for: the elderly; nursing mothers; pediatric patients
Warning: INCREASED MORTALITY IN ELDERLY PATIENTS WITH DEMENTIA-RELATED PSYCHOSIS

Skin
Rash (<2%)

Mucosal
Oropharyngeal pain (<3%)
Xerostomia (dry mouth) (<3%)

Cardiovascular
Hypertension (2–6%)
Tachycardia (<3%)

Central Nervous System
Agitation (3–5%)
Akathisia (20–21%) [28]
Anxiety (3–6%) [3]
Extrapyramidal symptoms (15–29%) [20]
Fever (pyrexia) (includes hyperpyrexia) (<4%) [4]
Headache (9–18%) [12]
Insomnia (8–13%) [15]
Mania (worsening) [2]
Parkinsonism (13–26%) [6]
Restlessness (4–7%) [9]
Schizophrenia (worsening) [3]
Sedation [9]
Somnolence (drowsiness) (5–10%) [5]
Tremor [11]
Vertigo / dizziness (3–7%) [8]

Endocrine/Metabolic
Appetite decreased (<4%)
Creatine phosphokinase (CPK) / creatine kinase increased (hyperCKemia) (<3%)
Weight gain (2–3%) [7]

Gastrointestinal/Hepatic
Abdominal pain (3–8%) [2]
Constipation (6–11%) [11]
Diarrhea (<5%) [5]
Dyspepsia / functional dyspepsia (indigestion) (see also gastroparesis) (4–9%) [6]
Hepatotoxicity / liver injury / acute liver injury / drug-induced liver injury (DILI) (<3%)
Nausea (5–13%) [14]
Vomiting (4–10%) [9]

Genitourinary
Urinary tract infection (<2%)

Neuromuscular/Skeletal
Arthralgia (<2%)
Asthenia / fatigue (<5%) [2]
Back pain (<3%)
Dystonia (2–5%) [3]
Pain in extremities [2]

Ocular
Vision blurred (4%) [4]

Respiratory
Cough (<4%)
Nasopharyngitis (<2%)

Other
Adverse effects / adverse reactions [3]
Toothache (odontalgia) (3–6%) [2]

CARISOPRODOL

Trade name: Soma (MedPointe)
Indications: Painful musculoskeletal disorders
Class: Central muscle relaxant
Half-life: 4–6 hours
Clinically important, potentially hazardous interactions with: CNS depressants, eucalyptus, meprobamate
Important contra-indications noted in the prescribing guidelines for: the elderly; nursing mothers; pediatric patients
Note: Contra-indicated in patients with acute intermittent porphyria.

Skin
Angioedema (formerly named angioneurotic edema) (<10%)
Fixed eruption / fixed drug eruption [2]
Flushing / rubefaction (<10%)
Urticaria / hives [2]

Central Nervous System
Amnesia [2]
Trembling (<10%)

Other
Death [2]

CARMUSTINE

Trade names: BiCNU (Bristol-Myers Squibb), Gliadel Wafer (Guilford)
Indications: Brain tumors, Hodgkin's disease, multiple myeloma
Class: Alkylating agent, Nitrosourea
Half-life: initial: 1.4 minutes; secondary: 20 minutes
Clinically important, potentially hazardous interactions with: aldesleukin, cimetidine, clorazepate
Important contra-indications noted in the prescribing guidelines for: nursing mothers; pediatric patients

---

Skin
Dermatitis [3]
Flushing / rubefaction (<10%) [2]
Pigmentation (Skin) (includes hyperpigmentation) (on accidental contact) [2]
Telangiectasia [2]

Hair
Alopecia / hair loss (<10%)

Central Nervous System
Intracranial hemorrhage [2]
Meningococcal infection [2]
Seizures [2]

Gastrointestinal/Hepatic
Nausea [2]
Vomiting [2]

Hematologic
Leukocytopenia (leukopenia) / leukocytes (white blood cells) decreased [3]
Thrombocytopenia / platelets decreased [2]

Local
Injection-site burning (>10%)

Neuromuscular/Skeletal
Asthenia / fatigue [2]

CARTEOLOL

Trade name: Ocupress (ophthalmic) (Novartis)
Indications: Glaucoma, hypertension
Class: Adrenergic beta-receptor antagonist
Half-life: 6 hours
Clinically important, potentially hazardous interactions with: clonidine, epinephrine, verapamil
Pregnancy category: category C in first trimester; category D in second and third trimesters
Note: Cutaneous side effects of beta-receptor blockers are clinically polymorphous. They apparently appear after several months of continuous therapy.

Skin
Dermatitis (eyedrops) [3]
Rash (2%) [2]

Central Nervous System
Paresthesias (2%)

Ocular
Blepharitis [2]

CARVEDILOL

Trade name: Coreg (GSK)
Indications: Hypertension
Class: Adrenergic beta-receptor antagonist
Half-life: 7–10 hours
Clinically important, potentially hazardous interactions with: cinacalcet, delavirdine, efavirenz, irbesartan, leflunomide, propafenone, talazoparib, trimethoprim, venetoclax, voriconazole, zafirlukast
Important contra-indications noted in the prescribing guidelines for: nursing mothers; pediatric patients

---

Skin
Diaphoresis (3%)
Edema / fluid retention (generalized) (5–6%) [2]
Peripheral edema (<7%)
Pruritus (itching) [2]
Purpura (<3%)

Cardiovascular
Angina (2–6%)
Atrial fibrillation [2]
Atrioventricular block (<3%)
Bradycardia / sinus bradycardia (2–10%) [7]
Cardiac failure [2]
Congestive heart failure [2]
Extrasystoles [2]
Hypertension (<3%)
Hypotension (9–14%) [8]
Palpitation (<3%)
Postural hypotension (<3%)

Central Nervous System
Fever (pyrexia) (includes hyperpyrexia) (<3%)
Headache (5–8%) [2]
Pain (9%)
Paresthesias (2%)
Somnolence (drowsiness) (<3%)
Syncope / fainting (3–8%)
Vertigo / dizziness (24–32%) [5]

Endocrine/Metabolic
ALP increased (<3%) [2]
Creatine phosphokinase (CPK) / creatine kinase increased (hyperCKemia) (<3%) [3]
Diabetes mellitus (<3%)
GGT increased (<3%)
Hypercholesterolemia (<4%)
Hyperglycemia (includes glucose increased) (5–12%)
Hyperkalemia (<3%) [2]
Hyperuricemia (<3%)
Hypervolemia (fluid overload) (<3%)
Hypoglycemia (<3%)
Hyponatremia (<3%)
Hypovolemia (<3%)
Weight gain (10–12%)
Weight loss (<3%)

Gastrointestinal/Hepatic
Black stools / melena (<3%)
Diarrhea (2–12%)
Hepatotoxicity / liver injury / acute liver injury / drug-induced liver injury (DILI) [3]
Nausea (4–9%)
Vomiting (<6%)

Genitourinary
Albuminuria (<3%)
Hematuria (<3%)
Impotence (<3%)

Hematologic
Anemia [2]
Prothrombin time decreased (<3%)
Thrombocytopenia / platelets decreased (<3%)

Neuromuscular/Skeletal
Arthralgia (<6%)
Asthenia / fatigue (7–24%) [2]
Muscle spasm (<3%)
Myalgia/Myopathy (3%)

Ocular
Abnormal vision (5%)
Vision blurred (<3%)

Respiratory
Cough (5–8%)
Dyspnea / shortness of breath [4]
Stridor [2]

Other
Adverse effects / adverse reactions [8]
Infection (2%)

CASCARA

Family: Rhamnaceae
Scientific names: *Frangula purshianus, Rhamnus purshiana*
Indications: Atonic constipation, dyspepsia, colitis, diverticulitis, dyspepsia, gallstones, gout, hemorrhoids, hypertension, indigestion, insomnia, jaundice, liver disease, nervous disorders, parasites, stomach disorders
Class: Stimulant laxative
Half-life: N/A
Clinically important, potentially hazardous interactions with: antiarrhythmics, cardiac glycosides, corticosteroids, licorice, thiazide diuretics

---

Gastrointestinal/Hepatic
Hepatotoxicity / liver injury / acute liver injury / drug-induced liver injury (DILI) [2]

CASPOFUNGIN

Trade name: Cancidas (Merck)
Indications: Invasive *Aspergillus* and *Candida* infections
Class: Antifungal / antimycotic, Antimicrobial, Antimycobacterial; echinocandin
Half-life: beta phase: 9–11 hours; terminal: 40–50 hours
Clinically important, potentially hazardous interactions with: carbamazepine, cyclosporine, dexamethasone, efavirenz, nevirapine, phenytoin, rifampin, tacrolimus
Important contra-indications noted in the prescribing guidelines for: nursing mothers; pediatric patients

---

Skin
Anaphylactoid reactions / anaphylaxis (includes anaphylactic shock) (<2%)
Edema / fluid retention (~3%)
Erythema (<4%)
Facial edema (3%)
Flushing / rubefaction (3%)
Jaundice (see also cholestasis / cholestatic jaundice) (<5%)
Peripheral edema (11%)
Petechiae (<5%)
Pruritus (itching) (2–7%)
Rash (4–16%) [5]
Septic-toxic shock (11–13%)
Ulcerations (3%)
Urticaria / hives (<5%)
Vasculitis (angiitis) / cutaneous vasculitis (angiitis) (2%)

Mucosal
Epistaxis (nosebleed) (<5%)
Mucosal inflammation (6–10%)

Cardiovascular
Arrhythmias (<5%)
Atrial fibrillation (<5%)
Bradycardia / sinus bradycardia (<5%)
Cardiac arrest (<5%)
Hypertension (5–10%)
Hypotension (6–12%)
Myocardial infarction (<5%)
Phlebitis (18%) [3]
Tachycardia (4–7%)
Thrombophlebitis [2]

Central Nervous System
Anxiety (<5%)

Chills (9–23%)
Confusion (<5%)
Depression (<5%)
Fever (pyrexia) (includes hyperpyrexia) (6–29%) [8]
Headache (5–15%) [3]
Insomnia (<5%)
Pain (<5%)
Paresthesias (<3%)
Seizures (<5%)
Tremor (<2%)
Vertigo / dizziness (<5%)

Endocrine/Metabolic
ALP increased (12–23%) [4]
ALT increased (4–18%) [4]
Appetite decreased (<5%)
AST increased (6–16%) [5]
Hypercalcemia (<5%)
Hyperglycemia (includes glucose increased) (<5%)
Hypokalemia (6–8%) [4]
Hypomagnesemia (<5%)

Gastrointestinal/Hepatic
Abdominal distension (<5%)
Abdominal pain (7–9%)
Constipation (<5%)
Diarrhea (6–27%)
Dyspepsia / functional dyspepsia (indigestion) (see also gastroparesis) (<5%)
Hepatic failure (<5%)
Hepatotoxicity / liver injury / acute liver injury / drug-induced liver injury (DILI) (<5%) [8]
Nausea (5–15%) [2]
Vomiting (9–17%) [2]

Genitourinary
Hematuria (<5%)
Urinary tract infection (<5%)

Hematologic
Anemia (2–11%)
Coagulopathy / coagulation dysfunction / clotting factor deficiency (includes disseminated intravascular coagulation / DIC) (<5%)
Eosinophilia / eosinophils increased [2]
Febrile neutropenia (<5%)
Neutropenia (neutrophils decreased) (<5%)
Sepsis (5%)
Thrombocytopenia / platelets decreased (<5%) [2]

Local
Infusion-related reactions [4]
Infusion-site pain (<5%)
Infusion-site reactions (<5%) [2]
Injection-site induration (~3%)
Injection-site reaction (2–12%) [4]

Neuromuscular/Skeletal
Arthralgia (<5%)
Asthenia / fatigue (<5%)
Back pain (<5%)
Myalgia/Myopathy (~3%)
Pain in extremities (<5%)

Renal
Nephrotoxicity / kidney injury / acute kidney injury (AKI) / drug-induced kidney injury [5]
Renal failure (<5%)

Respiratory
Cough (6–11%)
Dyspnea / shortness of breath (9%)
Hypoxia (<5%)
Influenza- ('flu)-like syndrome (3%)
Pleural effusion (9%)
Pneumonia (4–11%)
Respiratory distress (8%)
Respiratory failure (6–11%)
Tachypnea / respiratory rate increased (8%)

Other
Adverse effects / adverse reactions [8]

CEFACLOR

Trade name: Ceclor (Lilly)
Indications: Various infections caused by susceptible organisms
Class: Antibiotic, Antimicrobial, Cephalosporin, Cephalosporin; 2nd generation
Half-life: 0.6–0.9 hours
Clinically important, potentially hazardous interactions with: none known
Important contra-indications noted in the prescribing guidelines for: the elderly; nursing mothers; pediatric patients
Note: Penicillin and cephalosporins share a common beta-lactam structure. People who are allergic to penicillin are approximately 4 times more likely to develop an allergic reaction to a cephalosporin than those people who have no penicillin allergy (from 5–16% of patients allergic to penicillin develop reactions to cephalosporins).

Skin
AGEP [2]
Anaphylactoid reactions / anaphylaxis (includes anaphylactic shock) [6]
Erythema multiforme [6]
Exanthems [9]
Fixed eruption / fixed drug eruption [2]
Hypersensitivity [2]
Pruritus (itching) [4]
Purpura [2]
Rash (<2%) [2]
Serum sickness [7]
Serum sickness-like reaction [23]
Stevens-Johnson syndrome and toxic epidermal necrolysis (SJS/TEN) [2]
Urticaria / hives [5]

Gastrointestinal/Hepatic
Diarrhea [2]

Other
Adverse effects / adverse reactions [3]

CEFADROXIL

Trade name: Duricef (Warner Chilcott)
Indications: Various infections caused by susceptible organisms
Class: Antibiotic, Antimicrobial, Cephalosporin, Cephalosporin; 1st generation
Half-life: 1.2–1.5 hours
Clinically important, potentially hazardous interactions with: none known
Important contra-indications noted in the prescribing guidelines for: nursing mothers
Note: Penicillin and cephalosporins share a common beta-lactam structure. People who are allergic to penicillin are approximately 4 times more likely to develop an allergic reaction to a cephalosporin than those people who have no penicillin allergy (from 5–16% of patients allergic to penicillin develop reactions to cephalosporins).

Skin
Baboon syndrome / symmetrical drug-related intertriginous and flexural exanthema (SDRIFE) [2]
Urticaria / hives [2]

Gastrointestinal/Hepatic
Diarrhea [2]
Nausea [2]

Other
Adverse effects / adverse reactions [3]

CEFAMANDOLE

Indications: Various infections caused by susceptible organisms
Class: Antibiotic, Antimicrobial, Cephalosporin, Cephalosporin; 2nd generation
Half-life: 0.5–1.0 hours
Clinically important, potentially hazardous interactions with: none known
Note: Penicillin and cephalosporins share a common beta-lactam structure. People who are allergic to penicillin are approximately 4 times more likely to develop an allergic reaction to a cephalosporin than those people who have no penicillin allergy (from 5–16% of patients allergic to penicillin develop reactions to cephalosporins).

Skin
Exanthems [2]
Linear IgA bullous dermatosis [2]
Stevens-Johnson syndrome and toxic epidermal necrolysis (SJS/TEN) [2]

Local
Injection-site thrombophlebitis (1–10%)

CEFAZOLIN

Trade name: Ancef (GSK)
Indications: Various infections caused by susceptible organisms
Class: Antibiotic, Antimicrobial, Cephalosporin, Cephalosporin; 1st generation
Half-life: 1.4–1.8 hours
Clinically important, potentially hazardous interactions with: BCG vaccine, phenytoin, probenecid, vitamin K antagonists
Important contra-indications noted in the prescribing guidelines for: nursing mothers; pediatric patients
Note: Safety and effectiveness in premature infants and neonates have not been established. Penicillin and cephalosporins share a common beta-lactam structure. People who are allergic to penicillin are approximately 4 times more likely to develop an allergic reaction to a cephalosporin than those people who have no penicillin allergy (from 5–16% of patients allergic to penicillin develop reactions to cephalosporins).

Skin
AGEP [2]
Anaphylactoid reactions / anaphylaxis (includes anaphylactic shock) [7]
Exanthems [3]
Hypersensitivity [3]
Pruritus (itching) [3]
Pustules / pustular eruption [3]
Radiation recall dermatitis [2]
Serum sickness-like reaction [2]
Stevens-Johnson syndrome and toxic epidermal necrolysis (SJS/TEN) [2]

Gastrointestinal/Hepatic
Hepatotoxicity / liver injury / acute liver injury / drug-induced liver injury (DILI) [4]

Hematologic
Coagulopathy / coagulation dysfunction / clotting factor deficiency (includes disseminated intravascular coagulation / DIC) [2]
Hemolytic anemia [3]
Hypoprothrombinemia [4]
Neutropenia (neutrophils decreased) [2]

Other
Adverse effects / adverse reactions [2]
Allergic reactions [2]

CEFDINIR

Trade name: Omnicef (Medicis)
Indications: Community-acquired pneumonia and various infections caused by susceptible organisms
Class: Antibiotic, Antimicrobial, Cephalosporin, Cephalosporin; 3rd generation
Half-life: 1–2 hours
Clinically important, potentially hazardous interactions with: none known
Important contra-indications noted in the prescribing guidelines for: pediatric patients
Note: Penicillin and cephalosporins share a common beta-lactam structure. People who are allergic to penicillin are approximately 4 times more likely to develop an allergic reaction to a cephalosporin than those people who have no penicillin allergy (from 5–16% of patients allergic to penicillin develop reactions to cephalosporins).

Skin
Rash (3%)

Gastrointestinal/Hepatic
Red stools / hematochezia [2]

Genitourinary
Vulvovaginal candidiasis (5%)

Other
Adverse effects / adverse reactions [2]

CEFDITOREN

Trade name: Spectracef (Meiji)
Indications: Various infections caused by susceptible organisms
Class: Antibiotic, Antimicrobial, Cephalosporin, Cephalosporin; 3rd generation
Half-life: ~1.6 hours
Clinically important, potentially hazardous interactions with: antacids, famotidine, H_2 antagonists, high-fat foods, pantoprazole, probenecid, proton pump inhibitors, vitamin K antagonists
Important contra-indications noted in the prescribing guidelines for: nursing mothers; pediatric patients
Note: Contraindicated in patients with carnitine deficiency or inborn errors of metabolism that may result in clinically significant carnitine deficiency. Penicillin and cephalosporins share a common beta-lactam structure. People who are allergic to penicillin are approximately 4 times more likely to develop an allergic reaction to a cephalosporin than those people who have no penicillin allergy (from 5–16% of patients allergic to penicillin develop reactions to cephalosporins).

Central Nervous System
Headache (2–3%) [3]

Gastrointestinal/Hepatic
Abdominal pain (2%)
Diarrhea (11–15%)
Dyspepsia / functional dyspepsia (indigestion) (see also gastroparesis) (1–2%)
Nausea (4–6%) [2]

Genitourinary
Vulvovaginal candidiasis (3–6%)

CEFEPIME

Trade name: Maxipime (Elan)
Indications: Various infections caused by susceptible organisms
Class: Antibiotic, Antimicrobial, Cephalosporin, Cephalosporin; 4th generation
Half-life: 2–2.3 hours
Clinically important, potentially hazardous interactions with: none known
Important contra-indications noted in the prescribing guidelines for: the elderly; nursing mothers
Note: Penicillin and cephalosporins share a common beta-lactam structure. People who are allergic to penicillin are approximately 4 times more likely to develop an allergic reaction to a cephalosporin than those people who have no penicillin allergy (from 5–16% of patients allergic to penicillin develop reactions to cephalosporins).

Skin
Exanthems (2%)
Hypersensitivity [2]
Lupus erythematosus (subacute cutaneous lupus erythematosus (SCLE)) [2]
Pruritus (itching) [3]
Rash (51%) [12]
Stevens-Johnson syndrome and toxic epidermal necrolysis (SJS/TEN) [2]

Central Nervous System
Encephalopathy (includes hepatic encephalopathy) [15]
Headache [3]
Neurotoxicity [27]
Seizures [17]
Status epilepticus [7]

Hematologic
Agranulocytosis / severe selective neutropenia [2]
Neutropenia (neutrophils decreased) [5]
Thrombocytopenia / platelets decreased [5]

Local
Injection-site reaction (3%) [2]

Neuromuscular/Skeletal
Myoclonus (see also hypnic jerk) [2]

Renal
Nephritis / interstitial nephritis / tubulointerstitial nephritis [2]

Other
Adverse effects / adverse reactions [3]

CEFIDEROCOL

Trade name: Fetroja (Shionogi)
Indications: Treatment of patients 18 years of age or older who have limited or no alternative treatment options, for the treatment of complicated urinary tract infections, including pyelonephritis, caused by susceptible Gram-negative microorganisms
Class: Antibiotic, Antibiotic; beta-lactam, Antimicrobial, Cephalosporin, Cephalosporin; 4th generation
Half-life: 2–3 hours
Clinically important, potentially hazardous interactions with: none known
Pregnancy category: There are no available data on cefiderocol use in pregnant women to evaluate for a drug-associated risk of major birth defects, miscarriage or adverse maternal or fetal outcomes.

Skin
Bacterial infection (<2%)
Candidiasis / candidosis (2%)
Hypersensitivity (<2%)
Peripheral edema (<2%)
Pruritus (itching) (<2%)
Rash (3%) [2]

Mucosal
Stomatitis (oral mucositis) (<2%)
Xerostomia (dry mouth) (<2%)

Cardiovascular
Atrial fibrillation (<2%)
Bradycardia / sinus bradycardia (<2%)
Congestive heart failure (<2%)

Central Nervous System
Dysgeusia (taste perversion) (<2%)
Fever (pyrexia) (includes hyperpyrexia) (<2%)
Headache (2%)
Insomnia (<2%)
Restlessness (<2%)
Seizures (<2%)

Endocrine/Metabolic
Appetite decreased (<2%)
Creatine phosphokinase (CPK) / creatine kinase increased (hyperCKemia) (<2%)
Hypertransaminasemia (hepatic transaminitis) / elevated transaminases (2%)
Hypocalcemia (<2%)
Hypokalemia (2%)

Gastrointestinal/Hepatic
Abdominal pain (<2%)
Cholecystitis (calculous / acalculous) (<2%)
Cholelithiasis (gallstones in the gall bladder or the bile duct) (<2%)
Constipation (3%)
Diarrhea (4%) [2]
Nausea (2%)
Vomiting (2%)

Genitourinary
Hematuria (<2%)

Hematologic
Prothrombin time (INR) increased (<2%)
Thrombocythemia (thrombocytosis) / platelets increased (<2%)

Local
Infusion-site reactions (4%)

Respiratory
Cough (2%)

Dyspnea / shortness of breath (<2%)
Pleural effusion (,2%)

CEFIXIME

Trade name: Suprax (Lupin)
Indications: Various infections caused by susceptible organisms
Class: Antibiotic, Antimicrobial, Cephalosporin, Cephalosporin; 3rd generation
Half-life: 3–4 hours
Clinically important, potentially hazardous interactions with: aminoglycosides, anticoagulants, BCG vaccine, carbamazepine, probenecid, typhoid vaccine, warfarin
Important contra-indications noted in the prescribing guidelines for: nursing mothers; pediatric patients
Note: Penicillin and cephalosporins share a common beta-lactam structure. People who are allergic to penicillin are approximately 4 times more likely to develop an allergic reaction to a cephalosporin than those people who have no penicillin allergy (from 5–16% of patients allergic to penicillin develop reactions to cephalosporins).

Skin
Anaphylactoid reactions / anaphylaxis (includes anaphylactic shock) (<2%)
Angioedema (formerly named angioneurotic edema) (<2%)
Erythema multiforme (<2%)
Facial edema (<2%)
Jaundice (see also cholestasis / cholestatic jaundice) (<2%)
Linear IgA bullous dermatosis [2]
Pruritus (itching) (<2%)
Pruritus ani et vulvae (<2%)
Rash (<2%) [2]
Serum sickness-like reaction (<2%)
Stevens-Johnson syndrome and toxic epidermal necrolysis (SJS/TEN) (<2%) [5]
Urticaria / hives (<2%) [2]

Central Nervous System
Fever (pyrexia) (includes hyperpyrexia) (<2%)

Endocrine/Metabolic
ALP increased (<2%)
Creatine phosphokinase (CPK) / creatine kinase increased (hyperCKemia) (<2%)

Gastrointestinal/Hepatic
Abdominal pain (3%)
Diarrhea (16%)
Dyspepsia / functional dyspepsia (indigestion) (see also gastroparesis) (3%)
Flatulence (4%)
Hepatitis (<2%)
Loose stools / soft feces (6%)
Nausea (7%)
Pseudomembranous colitis (<2%)

Genitourinary
Vaginitis (includes vulvitis) (<2%)
Vulvovaginal candidiasis (<2%)

Renal
Renal failure (<2%)

CEFMETAZOLE

Indications: Various infections caused by susceptible organisms
Class: Antibiotic, Antimicrobial, Cephalosporin, Cephalosporin; 2nd generation
Half-life: 72 minutes
Clinically important, potentially hazardous interactions with: none known
Note: Penicillin and cephalosporins share a common beta-lactam structure. People who are allergic to penicillin are approximately 4 times more likely to develop an allergic reaction to a cephalosporin than those people who have no penicillin allergy (from 5–16% of patients allergic to penicillin develop reactions to cephalosporins).

Skin
Rash (1–10%)

Hematologic
Hypoprothrombinemia [3]

CEFOPERAZONE

Trade name: Cefobid (Pfizer)
Indications: Various infections caused by susceptible organisms
Class: Antibiotic, Antimicrobial, Cephalosporin, Cephalosporin; 3rd generation
Half-life: 1.6–2.6 hours
Clinically important, potentially hazardous interactions with: none known
Note: Penicillin and cephalosporins share a common beta-lactam structure. People who are allergic to penicillin are approximately 4 times more likely to develop an allergic reaction to a cephalosporin than those people who have no penicillin allergy (from 5–16% of patients allergic to penicillin develop reactions to cephalosporins). Used in combination with sulbactam (as Cefina-SB).

Skin
Anaphylactoid reactions / anaphylaxis (includes anaphylactic shock) [2]
Hypersensitivity (>2%)
Rash (2%)

Central Nervous System
Disulfiram-like reaction [2]

Gastrointestinal/Hepatic
Gastrointestinal bleeding [2]

Hematologic
Coagulopathy / coagulation dysfunction / clotting factor deficiency (includes disseminated intravascular coagulation / DIC) [10]
Hemolytic anemia [2]
Hypoprothrombinemia [3]

CEFOTAXIME

Trade name: Claforan (Sanofi-Aventis)
Indications: Various infections caused by susceptible organisms
Class: Antibiotic, Antimicrobial, Cephalosporin, Cephalosporin; 3rd generation
Half-life: 1 hour (adults)
Clinically important, potentially hazardous interactions with: none known
Important contra-indications noted in the prescribing guidelines for: nursing mothers
Note: Penicillin and cephalosporins share a common beta-lactam structure. People who are allergic to penicillin are approximately 4 times more likely to develop an allergic reaction to a cephalosporin than those people who have no penicillin allergy (from 5–16% of patients allergic to penicillin develop reactions to cephalosporins).

Skin
Anaphylactoid reactions / anaphylaxis (includes anaphylactic shock) (2%)
DRESS syndrome (Drug-induced hypersensitivity syndrome) [5]
Erythema multiforme [2]
Exanthems [3]
Hypersensitivity [2]
Pruritus (itching) (2%) [3]
Rash (2%) [3]
Stevens-Johnson syndrome and toxic epidermal necrolysis (SJS/TEN) [3]
Urticaria / hives (2%)

Local
Injection-site inflammation (4%)
Injection-site pain (<10%)

Renal
Nephritis / interstitial nephritis / tubulointerstitial nephritis [2]

Other
Adverse effects / adverse reactions [2]

CEFPODOXIME

Trade name: Vantin (Pfizer)
Indications: Various infections caused by susceptible organisms
Class: Antibiotic, Antimicrobial, Cephalosporin, Cephalosporin; 3rd generation
Half-life: 2.1–2.8 hours
Clinically important, potentially hazardous interactions with: none known
Important contra-indications noted in the prescribing guidelines for: nursing mothers; pediatric patients
Note: Penicillin and cephalosporins share a common beta-lactam structure. People who are allergic to penicillin are approximately 4 times more likely to develop an allergic reaction to a cephalosporin than those people who have no penicillin allergy (from 5–16% of patients allergic to penicillin develop reactions to cephalosporins).

Skin
Diaper rash (12%)
Rash [3]

Gastrointestinal/Hepatic
Abdominal pain (2%)
Diarrhea [3]
Nausea (4%)

Genitourinary
Vulvovaginal candidiasis (3%)

Other
Adverse effects / adverse reactions [6]

CEFTAROLINE FOSAMIL

Trade name: Teflaro (Forest)
Indications: Acute bacterial skin and skin structure infections, community-acquired bacterial pneumonia
Class: Antibiotic, Antimicrobial, Cephalosporin, Cephalosporin; 5th generation
Half-life: 3 hours
Clinically important, potentially hazardous interactions with: BCG vaccine, probenecid, typhoid vaccine
Important contra-indications noted in the prescribing guidelines for: the elderly; nursing mothers; pediatric patients
Note: Ceftaroline fosamil is a prodrug of ceftaroline. Penicillin and cephalosporins share a common beta-lactam structure. People who are allergic to penicillin are approximately 4 times more likely to develop an allergic reaction to a cephalosporin than those people who have no penicillin allergy (from 5–16% of patients allergic to penicillin develop reactions to cephalosporins).

Skin
- Anaphylactoid reactions / anaphylaxis (includes anaphylactic shock) (<2%)
- Hypersensitivity (<2%) [2]
- Pruritus (itching) [7]
- Rash (3%) [10]
- Urticaria / hives (<2%)

Cardiovascular
- Bradycardia / sinus bradycardia (<2%)
- Hypertension [2]
- Palpitation (<2%)
- Phlebitis (2%) [3]

Central Nervous System
- Fever (pyrexia) (includes hyperpyrexia) (<2%)
- Headache [9]
- Insomnia [5]
- Seizures (<2%)
- Vertigo / dizziness (<2%)

Endocrine/Metabolic
- ALT increased (2%)
- Hyperglycemia (includes glucose increased) (<2%)
- Hyperkalemia (<2%)
- Hypokalemia (2%) [2]

Gastrointestinal/Hepatic
- Abdominal pain (<2%)
- Colitis (<2%)
- Constipation (2%)
- Diarrhea (5%) [10]
- Hepatotoxicity / liver injury / acute liver injury / drug-induced liver injury (DILI) (<2%)
- Nausea (4%) [9]
- Vomiting (2%)

Hematologic
- Anemia (<2%)
- Eosinophilia / eosinophils increased (<2%) [2]
- Neutropenia (neutrophils decreased) (<2%) [4]
- Thrombocytopenia / platelets decreased (<2%) [4]

Renal
- Renal failure (<2%)

Respiratory
- Eosinophilic pneumonia [4]

Other
- Adverse effects / adverse reactions [4]
- Infection [2]

CEFTAZIDIME

Trade names: Ceptaz (GSK), Fortaz (Concordia), Tazicef (Hospira)
Indications: Various infections caused by susceptible organisms
Class: Antibiotic, Antimicrobial, Cephalosporin, Cephalosporin; 3rd generation
Half-life: 1–2 hours
Clinically important, potentially hazardous interactions with: none known
Important contra-indications noted in the prescribing guidelines for: the elderly; nursing mothers
Note: Penicillin and cephalosporins share a common beta-lactam structure. People who are allergic to penicillin are approximately 4 times more likely to develop an allergic reaction to a cephalosporin than those people who have no penicillin allergy (from 5–16% of patients allergic to penicillin develop reactions to cephalosporins). See also separate profile for Ceftazidime & Avibactam.

Skin
- Anaphylactoid reactions / anaphylaxis (includes anaphylactic shock) (2%) [3]
- Angioedema (formerly named angioneurotic edema) (2%)
- DRESS syndrome (Drug-induced hypersensitivity syndrome) [2]
- Erythema multiforme (2%)
- Hypersensitivity (2%)
- Pemphigus erythematodes (pemphigus erythematosus) (Senear-Usher syndrome) [2]
- Pruritus (itching) (2%) [3]
- Rash (2%) [5]
- Stevens-Johnson syndrome and toxic epidermal necrolysis (SJS/TEN) (2%)

Central Nervous System
- Encephalopathy (includes hepatic encephalopathy) [7]
- Seizures [3]

Gastrointestinal/Hepatic
- Hepatotoxicity / liver injury / acute liver injury / drug-induced liver injury (DILI) [2]

Genitourinary
- Urolithiasis / ureteral stones / urinary calculi [2]

Hematologic
- Thrombocytopenia / platelets decreased [2]

Local
- Injection-site inflammation (2%)
- Injection-site reaction [2]
- Injection-site thrombophlebitis (2%)

Neuromuscular/Skeletal
- Myoclonus (see also hypnic jerk) [2]

Renal
- Nephrotoxicity / kidney injury / acute kidney injury (AKI) / drug-induced kidney injury [2]

Other
- Adverse effects / adverse reactions [3]
- Death [2]

CEFTAZIDIME & AVIBACTAM

Trade name: Avycaz (Cerexa)
Indications: Various infections caused by susceptible organisms
Class: Antibiotic, Antibiotic; beta-lactam (avibactam), Antimicrobial, Cephalosporin, Cephalosporin; 3rd generation (ceftazidime)
Half-life: <3 hours
Clinically important, potentially hazardous interactions with: probenecid
Important contra-indications noted in the prescribing guidelines for: the elderly; nursing mothers; pediatric patients
Note: See also separate entry for ceftazidime.

Skin
- Rash (<5%)

Central Nervous System
- Anxiety (10%) [3]
- Fever (pyrexia) (includes hyperpyrexia) [4]
- Headache [4]
- Vertigo / dizziness (6%)

Endocrine/Metabolic
- ALP increased (3%)
- ALT increased (3%) [4]
- AST increased [3]
- GGT increased (<5%)

Gastrointestinal/Hepatic
- Abdominal pain (7%) [5]
- Constipation (10%) [2]
- Diarrhea [6]
- Hepatotoxicity / liver injury / acute liver injury / drug-induced liver injury (DILI) [5]
- Nausea (2%) [6]
- Vomiting [5]

Hematologic
- Eosinophilia / eosinophils increased (<5%)
- Prothrombin time (INR) increased (<5%)
- Thrombocytopenia / platelets decreased (<5%)

Local
- Injection-site reaction [4]

Renal
- Nephrotoxicity / kidney injury / acute kidney injury (AKI) / drug-induced kidney injury (<5%)
- Renal failure (<5%) [4]

Other
- Adverse effects / adverse reactions [3]

CEFTIBUTEN

Trade name: Cedax (Shionogi)
Indications: Various infections caused by susceptible organisms
Class: Antibiotic, Antimicrobial, Cephalosporin, Cephalosporin; 3rd generation
Half-life: 2 hours
Clinically important, potentially hazardous interactions with: none known
Note: Penicillin and cephalosporins share a common beta-lactam structure. People who are allergic to penicillin are approximately 4 times more likely to develop an allergic reaction to a cephalosporin than those people who have no penicillin allergy (from 5–16% of patients allergic to penicillin develop reactions to cephalosporins).

CEFTIZOXIME

Trade name: Cefizox (Astellas)
Indications: Various infections caused by susceptible organisms
Class: Antibiotic, Antimicrobial, Cephalosporin, Cephalosporin; 3rd generation
Half-life: 1.6 hours
Clinically important, potentially hazardous interactions with: none known
Important contra-indications noted in the prescribing guidelines for: nursing mothers
Note: Penicillin and cephalosporins share a common beta-lactam structure. People who are allergic to penicillin are approximately 4 times more likely to develop an allergic reaction to a cephalosporin than those people who have no penicillin allergy (from 5–16% of patients allergic to penicillin develop reactions to cephalosporins).

Skin
Pruritus (itching) (<5%)
Rash (<5%)

Central Nervous System
Paresthesias (<5%)

Hematologic
Hemolytic anemia [3]

Local
Injection-site pain (<5%)
Injection-site phlebitis (<5%)

CEFTOBIPROLE

Trade names: BAL5788 (Basilea) (Cilag AG), Zeftera (Janssen)
Indications: Bacterial infections, MRSA
Class: Antibiotic, Antimicrobial, Cephalosporin, Cephalosporin; 5th generation
Half-life: 3 hours
Clinically important, potentially hazardous interactions with: alcohol, anticoagulants, BCG vaccine, carbenicillin, dipyridamole, heparin, pentoxifylline, plicamycin, sulfinpyrazone, ticarcillin, typhoid vaccine, valproic acid
Pregnancy category: not recommended in pregnancy
Important contra-indications noted in the prescribing guidelines for: nursing mothers; pediatric patients
Note: Ceftobiprole medocaril (sodium salt) is a prodrug. Penicillin and cephalosporins share a common beta-lactam structure. People who are allergic to penicillin are approximately 4 times more likely to develop an allergic reaction to a cephalosporin than those people who have no penicillin allergy (from 5–16% of patients allergic to penicillin develop reactions to cephalosporins).

Skin
Erythema (9%)
Pruritus (itching) (9%)

Central Nervous System
Dysgeusia (taste perversion) (8%) [3]
Headache [2]

Endocrine/Metabolic
Hyponatremia [2]

Gastrointestinal/Hepatic
Abdominal pain [2]
Diarrhea [4]
Nausea [6]
Vomiting [4]

Local
Infusion-site reactions [2]

Other
Adverse effects / adverse reactions [4]

CEFTOLOZANE & TAZOBACTAM

Trade name: Zerbaxa (Cubist)
Indications: Various infections caused by susceptible organisms
Class: Antibiotic, Antibiotic; beta-lactam, Antimicrobial, Cephalosporin, Cephalosporin; 5th generation
Half-life: <3 hours
Clinically important, potentially hazardous interactions with: none known
Important contra-indications noted in the prescribing guidelines for: the elderly; nursing mothers; pediatric patients

---

Cardiovascular
Hypertension [3]

Central Nervous System
Fever (pyrexia) (includes hyperpyrexia) (2%) [5]
Headache (3%) [8]
Insomnia [2]
Somnolence (drowsiness) [2]

Endocrine/Metabolic
ALT increased (2%) [2]
AST increased (2%)
Hypokalemia [2]

Gastrointestinal/Hepatic
Constipation (4%) [4]
Diarrhea (2%) [11]
Nausea (3%) [11]
Vomiting [3]

Hematologic
Anemia [2]

Local
Infusion-site reactions [2]

Neuromuscular/Skeletal
Myalgia/Myopathy [2]

CEFTRIAXONE

Trade name: Rocephin (Roche)
Indications: Various infections caused by susceptible organisms
Class: Antibiotic, Antimicrobial, Antimicrobial, Cephalosporin, Cephalosporin; 3rd generation
Half-life: 5–9 hours
Clinically important, potentially hazardous interactions with: aminoglycosides, coumarins, histamine H_2 antagonists, oral typhoid vaccine, probenecid
Important contra-indications noted in the prescribing guidelines for: nursing mothers; pediatric patients
Note: Penicillin and cephalosporins share a common beta-lactam structure. People who are allergic to penicillin are approximately 4 times more likely to develop an allergic reaction to a cephalosporin than those people who have no penicillin allergy (from 5–16% of patients allergic to penicillin develop reactions to cephalosporins).

Skin
AGEP [9]
Anaphylactoid reactions / anaphylaxis (includes anaphylactic shock) [15]
Angioedema (formerly named angioneurotic edema) [3]
Candidiasis / candidosis (5%) [3]
Dermatitis [2]
DRESS syndrome (Drug-induced hypersensitivity syndrome) [4]
Erythroderma [2]
Exanthems [7]
Fixed eruption / fixed drug eruption [3]
Flushing / rubefaction [2]
Hypersensitivity [4]
Linear IgA bullous dermatosis [2]
Pruritus (itching) [2]
Rash (2%) [5]
Serum sickness-like reaction [2]
Stevens-Johnson syndrome and toxic epidermal necrolysis (SJS/TEN) [3]
Urticaria / hives [4]

Mucosal
Glossitis (inflammation of the tongue) [2]

Cardiovascular
Asystole [2]
Hypotension [2]
Kounis syndrome / allergic angina syndrome / allergic myocardial infarction [2]
Phlebitis [2]

Central Nervous System
Encephalopathy (includes hepatic encephalopathy) [12]
Fever (pyrexia) (includes hyperpyrexia) [2]

Gastrointestinal/Hepatic
Cholecystitis (calculous / acalculous) [2]
Cholelithiasis (gallstones in the gall bladder or the bile duct) [5]
Cholestatic liver injury / cholestatic hepatitis [2]
Diarrhea [7]
Hepatotoxicity / liver injury / acute liver injury / drug-induced liver injury (DILI) [10]
Nausea [4]
Pancreatitis / acute pancreatitis [2]
Pseudolithiasis / biliary pseudolithiasis [16]
Vomiting [2]

Hematologic
Agranulocytosis / severe selective neutropenia [5]
Eosinophilia / eosinophils increased [2]
Hemolysis [11]
Hemolytic anemia [20]
Neutropenia (neutrophils decreased) [7]
Thrombocytopenia / platelets decreased [10]

Local
Injection-site pain (<10%) [3]
Injection-site phlebitis [2]

Renal
Nephrolithiasis (kidney stones / renal calculi) [3]
Nephrotoxicity / kidney injury / acute kidney injury (AKI) / drug-induced kidney injury [5]
Renal failure [3]

Respiratory
Dyspnea / shortness of breath [2]

Other
Adverse effects / adverse reactions [7]
Death [12]
Side effects (3%) [2]

CEFUROXIME

Trade names: Ceftin (GSK), Zinacef (Concordia)
Indications: Various infections caused by susceptible organisms
Class: Antibiotic, Antimicrobial, Cephalosporin, Cephalosporin; 2nd generation
Half-life: 1–2 hours
Clinically important, potentially hazardous interactions with: none known
Important contra-indications noted in the prescribing guidelines for: nursing mothers
Note: Penicillin and cephalosporins share a common beta-lactam structure. People who are allergic to penicillin are approximately 4 times more likely to develop an allergic reaction to a cephalosporin than those people who have no penicillin allergy (from 5–16% of patients allergic to penicillin develop reactions to cephalosporins).

Skin
AGEP [2]
Anaphylactoid reactions / anaphylaxis (includes anaphylactic shock) [9]
Baboon syndrome / symmetrical drug-related intertriginous and flexural exanthema (SDRIFE) [2]
Exanthems [2]
Hypersensitivity [4]
Serum sickness-like reaction [2]
Stevens-Johnson syndrome and toxic epidermal necrolysis (SJS/TEN) [2]
Urticaria / hives [2]

Cardiovascular
Kounis syndrome / allergic angina syndrome / allergic myocardial infarction [3]
Thrombophlebitis (<10%)

Gastrointestinal/Hepatic
Nausea [2]

Ocular
Ocular toxicity [2]

Other
Adverse effects / adverse reactions [2]

CELECOXIB

Trade name: Celebrex (Pfizer)
Indications: Osteoarthritis, rheumatoid arthritis (adults and juveniles aged 2 years and over), ankylosing spondylitis, acute pain, primary dysmenorrhea
Class: COX-2 inhibitor, Non-steroidal anti-inflammatory (NSAID), Sulfonamide
Half-life: 11 hours
Clinically important, potentially hazardous interactions with: ACE inhibitors, aliskiren, angiotensin II receptor antagonists, aspirin, dexibuprofen, fluconazole, furosemide, lithium, NSAIDs, warfarin
Pregnancy category: pregnancy category C prior to 30 weeks gestation; category D starting at 30 weeks gestation
Important contra-indications noted in the prescribing guidelines for: the elderly; nursing mothers; pediatric patients
Note: Celecoxib is a sulfonamide and can be absorbed systemically. Sulfonamides can produce severe, possibly fatal, reactions such as toxic epidermal necrolysis and Stevens-Johnson syndrome. NSAIDs may cause an increased risk of serious cardiovascular and gastrointestinal adverse events, which can be fatal. This risk may increase with duration of use.
Contra-indicated in patients with known hypersensitivity to celecoxib, aspirin, or other NSAIDs; in patients who have demonstrated allergic-type reactions to sulfonamides; in patients who have experienced asthma, urticaria, or allergic-type reactions after taking aspirin or other NSAIDs; and for the treatment of peri-operative pain in the setting of coronary artery bypass graft surgery.
Warning: CARDIOVASCULAR AND GASTROINTESTINAL RISKS

Skin
AGEP [8]
Anaphylactoid reactions / anaphylaxis (includes anaphylactic shock) [8]
Angioedema (formerly named angioneurotic edema) [9]
Bacterial infection (<2%)
Candidiasis / candidosis (<2%)
Dermatitis (<2%) [2]
Diaphoresis (<2%)
Edema / fluid retention (<2%) [5]
Erythema [2]
Erythema multiforme [3]
Exanthems (<2%) [7]
Facial edema (<2%)
Fixed eruption / fixed drug eruption [2]
Herpes simplex (<2%)
Herpes zoster (<2%)
Hot flashes / hot flushes (<2%)
Hypersensitivity [9]
Nodular eruption (<2%)
Peripheral edema (2%) [2]
Photosensitivity (<2%)
Pruritus (itching) (<2%) [6]
Rash (2%) [11]
Stevens-Johnson syndrome and toxic epidermal necrolysis (SJS/TEN) [7]
Sweet's syndrome [4]
Urticaria / hives (<2%) [11]
Vasculitis (angiitis) / cutaneous vasculitis (angiitis) [4]
Xerosis / xeroderma (<2%)

Hair
Alopecia / hair loss (<2%) [3]

Nails
Nail changes (<2%)

Mucosal
Stomatitis (oral mucositis) (<2%) [4]
Xerostomia (dry mouth) (<2%)

Cardiovascular
Cardiotoxicity [2]
Hypertension [2]
Myocardial infarction [4]

Central Nervous System
Anorexia [3]
Aseptic meningitis [2]
Depression [2]
Dysgeusia (taste perversion) (<2%) [2]
Fever (pyrexia) (includes hyperpyrexia) [2]
Headache [3]
Paresthesias (<2%)
Stroke / cerebrovascular accident [4]
Vertigo / dizziness [3]

Endocrine/Metabolic
Dehydration [2]
Mastodynia (<2%)

Gastrointestinal/Hepatic
Abdominal pain [11]
Constipation [5]
Diarrhea [12]
Dyspepsia / functional dyspepsia (indigestion) (see also gastroparesis) [10]
Flatulence [2]
Gastrointestinal bleeding [4]
Hepatotoxicity / liver injury / acute liver injury / drug-induced liver injury (DILI) [3]
Nausea [16]
Vomiting [10]

Genitourinary
Vaginitis (includes vulvitis) (<2%)
Vulvovaginal candidiasis (<2%)

Hematologic
Anemia [2]
Neutropenia (neutrophils decreased) [4]

Local
Application-site cellulitis (<2%)
Application-site reactions (<2%)

Neuromuscular/Skeletal
Asthenia / fatigue [6]
Myalgia/Myopathy (<2%)
Tendinopathy/Tendon rupture (<2%)

Ocular
Visual disturbances [3]

Renal
Nephrotoxicity / kidney injury / acute kidney injury (AKI) / drug-induced kidney injury [4]

Other
Adverse effects / adverse reactions [17]
Allergic reactions (<2%) [2]
Death [4]
Infection (<2%)
Tooth disorder (<2%)

CELIPROLOL

Trade names: Celectol (Winthrop), Celol (Pacific), Selectol (Sanofi-Aventis)
Indications: Hypertension, angina pectoris
Class: Beta blocker
Half-life: 5–6 hours
Clinically important, potentially hazardous interactions with: amiodarone, bepridil, diltiazem, disopyramide, floctafenine, quinidine, theophylline, verapamil
Important contra-indications noted in the prescribing guidelines for: nursing mothers

---

Central Nervous System
Headache [2]
Vertigo / dizziness [2]

Neuromuscular/Skeletal
Asthenia / fatigue [3]

CEMIPLIMAB

Trade names: Libtayo (Regeneron), REGN2810 (Regeneron)
Indications: Metastatic (or locally advanced) cutaneous squamous cell carcinoma
Class: Antineoplastic / anticancer agent (see also Immune checkpoint inhibitor), Immune checkpoint inhibitor (incl. programmed death receptor-1 (PD-1) inhibitor), Monoclonal antibody, Programmed death-ligand (PD-L1) inhibitor
Half-life: 19 days
Clinically important, potentially hazardous interactions with: none known
Pregnancy category: Based on its mechanism of action, cemiplimab cause fetal harm when

administered to a pregnant woman. There are no available data on the use of cemiplimab-rwlc in pregnant women.
Important contra-indications noted in the prescribing guidelines for: nursing mothers
Note: Because of the potential for serious adverse reactions in breastfed children, advise women not to breastfeed during treatment and for at least 4 months after the last dose of cemiplimab.
Cemiplimab-Rwlc is a biosimilar to Cemiplimab.

Skin
- Bullous pemphigoid / pemphigoid [2]
- Pruritus (itching) (15%)
- Rash (1% grade 3–4) (25%)
- Skin (dermatological) reaction (immune-mediated) (2%)

Endocrine/Metabolic
- Appetite decreased (10%)
- AST increased (3%)
- Hyperthyroidism (includes 'thyroid storm') (immune-mediated) (2%)
- Hyponatremia (3%)
- Hypophosphatemia (4%)
- Hypothyroidism (immune-mediated) (6%)

Gastrointestinal/Hepatic
- Constipation (12%)
- Diarrhea (22%)
- Hepatitis (immune-mediated) (2%)
- Nausea (19%) [2]

Hematologic
- Anemia (2%)
- Lymphopenia (lymphocytopenia) / lymphocytes decreased (7%)
- Prothrombin time (INR) increased (2%)

Neuromuscular/Skeletal
- Asthenia / fatigue (2% grade 3–4) (29%) [3]
- Musculoskeletal pain (3% grade 3–4) (17%)
- Myasthenia gravis [2]

Respiratory
- Pneumonitis (immune-mediated) (2%)

Other
- Adverse effects / adverse reactions [2]
- Cytokine release syndrome / cytokine storm [2]
- Death [2]
- Vogt-Koyanagi-Harada syndrome [2]

CENOBAMATE

Trade name: Xcopri (SK Life Science)
Indications: Partial-onset seizures in adults
Class: Anticonvulsant (see also antiepileptic (anti-seizure)), Antiepileptic (anti-seizure), GABA A receptor positive modulator
Half-life: 50–60 hours
Clinically important, potentially hazardous interactions with: carbamazepine, clobazam, CYP2B6 substrates, CYP3A substrates, CYP2C19 substrates, lamotrigine, oral contraceptives, phenobarbital, phenytoin
Pregnancy category: Based on animal data, may cause fetal harm. Women of reproductive potential concomitantly using oral contraceptives should use additional or alternative non-hormonal birth control.
Note: Often used as an adjunctive therapy with other anticonvulsant (antiseizure) medication.

Skin
- Maculopapular rash / morbilliform rash (2%)
- Pruritus (itching) (2%)

Mucosal
- Xerostomia (dry mouth) (3%)

Cardiovascular
- Chest pain (2%)
- Palpitation (2%)

Central Nervous System
- Aphasia (4%)
- Balance disorder (9%)
- Confusion (3%)
- Dysarthria (7%)
- Dysgeusia (taste perversion) (2%)
- Euphoria / elation (2%)
- Gait instability / postural instability (8%) [2]
- Headache (12%) [2]
- Irritability (2%)
- Memory loss/memory impaired (2%)
- Migraine (2%)
- Sedation (2%)
- Somnolence (drowsiness) (37%) [6]
- Suicidal ideation (2%)
- Tremor (3%)
- Vertigo / dizziness (33%) [6]

Endocrine/Metabolic
- ALT increased (4%)
- Appetite decreased (5%)
- AST increased (3%)
- Weight loss (2%)

Gastrointestinal/Hepatic
- Abdominal pain (2%)
- Constipation (8%)
- Diarrhea (5%)
- Dyspepsia / functional dyspepsia (indigestion) (see also gastroparesis) (2%)
- Nausea (9%)
- Vomiting (5%)

Genitourinary
- Dysmenorrhea (2%)
- Urinary tract infection (5%)

Neuromuscular/Skeletal
- Asthenia / fatigue (24%) [3]
- Ataxia (6%) [2]
- Back pain (5%)

Ocular
- Diplopia (double vision) (15%)
- Nystagmus (7%)
- Vision blurred (4%)

Respiratory
- Dyspnea / shortness of breath (3%)
- Nasopharyngitis (5%)
- Pharyngitis (sore throat) (2%)
- Upper respiratory tract infection [2]

Other
- Adverse effects / adverse reactions [3]

CEPHALEXIN

Synonym: cefalexin
Trade names: Keflex (Advancis), Keftab (Biovail)
Indications: Various infections caused by susceptible organisms
Class: Antibiotic, Antimicrobial, Cephalosporin, Cephalosporin; 1st generation
Half-life: 0.9–1.2 hours
Clinically important, potentially hazardous interactions with: amikacin, gentamicin, metformin
Important contra-indications noted in the prescribing guidelines for: the elderly; nursing mothers
Note: Penicillin and cephalosporins share a common beta-lactam structure. People who are allergic to penicillin are approximately 4 times more likely to develop an allergic reaction to a cephalosporin than those people who have no penicillin allergy (from 5–16% of patients allergic to penicillin develop reactions to cephalosporins).

Skin
- AGEP [5]
- Anaphylactoid reactions / anaphylaxis (includes anaphylactic shock) [4]
- Angioedema (formerly named angioneurotic edema) [2]
- Bullous pemphigoid / pemphigoid [3]
- Erythema multiforme [3]
- Exanthems [3]
- Pemphigus [2]
- Pruritus (itching) [3]
- Pustules / pustular eruption [2]
- Stevens-Johnson syndrome and toxic epidermal necrolysis (SJS/TEN) [7]
- Urticaria / hives [2]

Hematologic
- Hemolytic anemia [5]

Renal
- Nephritis / interstitial nephritis / tubulointerstitial nephritis [2]

Other
- Adverse effects / adverse reactions [2]
- Side effects (2%) [2]

CEPHALOTHIN

Indications: Various infections caused by susceptible organisms
Class: Antibiotic, Antimicrobial, Cephalosporin, Cephalosporin; 1st generation
Half-life: 30–50 minutes
Clinically important, potentially hazardous interactions with: amphotericin B, colistin, gentamicin
Note: Penicillin and cephalosporins share a common beta-lactam structure. People who are allergic to penicillin are approximately 4 times more likely to develop an allergic reaction to a cephalosporin than those people who have no penicillin allergy (from 5–16% of patients allergic to penicillin develop reactions to cephalosporins).

Skin
- Anaphylactoid reactions / anaphylaxis (includes anaphylactic shock) [4]
- Exanthems (<5%) [5]
- Purpura [2]
- Urticaria / hives [4]

Cardiovascular
- Phlebitis [5]

Hematologic
- Hemolytic anemia [3]

Other
- Allergic reactions [2]

CEPHAPIRIN

Indications: Various infections caused by susceptible organisms
Class: Antibiotic, Antimicrobial, Cephalosporin, Cephalosporin; 1st generation
Half-life: 36–60 minutes
Clinically important, potentially hazardous interactions with: none known
Note: Penicillin and cephalosporins share a common beta-lactam structure. People who are allergic to penicillin are approximately 4 times more likely to develop an allergic reaction to a cephalosporin than those people who have no penicillin allergy (from 5–16% of patients allergic to penicillin develop reactions to cephalosporins).

Skin
Pruritus (itching) (<5%)
Rash (<5%)

Cardiovascular
Phlebitis [6]

Central Nervous System
Fever (pyrexia) (includes hyperpyrexia) [2]
Paresthesias (<5%)

Local
Injection-site pain (<5%)
Injection-site phlebitis (<5%)

CEPHRADINE

Synonym: cefradine
Trade name: Velosef (Bristol-Myers Squibb)
Indications: Various infections caused by susceptible organisms
Class: Antibiotic, Antimicrobial, Cephalosporin, Cephalosporin; 1st generation
Half-life: 1–2 hours
Clinically important, potentially hazardous interactions with: none known
Note: Penicillin and cephalosporins share a common beta-lactam structure. People who are allergic to penicillin are approximately 4 times more likely to develop an allergic reaction to a cephalosporin than those people who have no penicillin allergy (from 5–16% of patients allergic to penicillin develop reactions to cephalosporins).

Skin
Stevens-Johnson syndrome and toxic epidermal necrolysis (SJS/TEN) [2]

CERITINIB

Trade name: Zykadia (Novartis)
Indications: Anaplastic lymphoma kinase-positive metastatic non-small cell lung cancer
Class: Anaplastic lymphoma kinase (ALK) inhibitor
Half-life: 41 hours
Clinically important, potentially hazardous interactions with: alfentanil, carbamazepine, cyclosporine, CYP3A and CYP2C9 substrates, dihydroergotamine, ergotamine, fentanyl, grapefruit juice, ketoconazole, nefazodone, phenytoin, pimozide, quinidine, rifampin, ritonavir, sirolimus, St John's wort, strong CYP3A inhibitors and inducers, tacrolimus, telithromycin, warfarin
Important contra-indications noted in the prescribing guidelines for: nursing mothers; pediatric patients

---

Skin
Acneiform eruption / acneiform dermatitis / acneiform rash (16%)
Exanthems (16%)
Rash (16%)

Cardiovascular
Bradycardia / sinus bradycardia (3%)
QT interval prolonged / QT prolongation (4%)

Central Nervous System
Anorexia [2]
Dysesthesia (>2%)
Gait instability / postural instability (>2%)
Hypoesthesia / hypesthesia (numbness) (>2%)
Neurotoxicity (17%)
Paresthesias (>2%)
Peripheral neuropathy (>2%)

Endocrine/Metabolic
ALT increased (80%) [7]
Appetite decreased (34%)
AST increased (75%) [5]
Dehydration [2]
Hyperglycemia (includes glucose increased) (49%)
Hypophosphatemia (36%)
Serum creatinine increased (58%) [2]

Gastrointestinal/Hepatic
Abdominal pain (54%) [3]
Constipation (29%)
Diarrhea (86%) [16]
Dyspepsia / functional dyspepsia (indigestion) (see also gastroparesis) (16%)
Dysphagia (16%)
Gastroesophageal reflux (16%)
Gastrointestinal disorder / discomfort [2]
Hepatotoxicity / liver injury / acute liver injury / drug-induced liver injury (DILI) [2]
Nausea (80%) [12]
Vomiting (60%) [11]

Neuromuscular/Skeletal
Asthenia / fatigue (52%) [4]
Hypotonia (>2%)

Ocular
Accommodation disorder (>2%)
Ocular adverse effect (9%)
Photopsia (>2%)
Reduced visual acuity (>2%)
Vision blurred (>2%)
Vision impaired (>2%)

Respiratory
Pneumonitis (4%)
Pulmonary toxicity [2]

Other
Adverse effects / adverse reactions [3]

CERTOLIZUMAB

Synonym: Certolizumab pegol
Trade name: Cimzia (Celltech) (UCB)
Indications: Crohn's disease, rheumatoid arthritis
Class: Anti-Tumor Necrosis Factor-alpha (TNF-α antagonist), Biologic, Disease-modifying antirheumatic drug (DMARD), Monoclonal antibody
Half-life: 14 days
Clinically important, potentially hazardous interactions with: abatacept, anakinra, lenalidomide, live vaccines, natalizumab, rituximab
Pregnancy category: Limited evidence insufficient to inform drug-associated risk
Important contra-indications noted in the prescribing guidelines for: nursing mothers; pediatric patients
Note: TNF inhibitors should be used in patients with heart failure only after consideration of other treatment options. TNF inhibitors are contra-indicated in patients with a personal or family history of multiple sclerosis or demyelinating disease. TNF inhibitors should not be administered to patients with moderate to severe heart failure (New York Heart Association Functional Class III/IV).
Warning: SERIOUS INFECTIONS AND MALIGNANCY

Skin
Herpes zoster [3]
Psoriasis [7]
Rash [2]

Cardiovascular
Hypertension [2]

Central Nervous System
Fever (pyrexia) (includes hyperpyrexia) (5%) [2]
Headache (7–18%) [5]
Vertigo / dizziness (~6%)

Endocrine/Metabolic
Creatine phosphokinase (CPK) / creatine kinase increased (hyperCKemia) [2]

Gastrointestinal/Hepatic
Nausea [2]

Genitourinary
Urinary tract infection (~8%) [8]

Local
Injection-site pain [3]
Injection-site reaction (~7%) [4]

Neuromuscular/Skeletal
Arthralgia (6–7%) [4]
Back pain [3]

Ocular
Optic neuritis / papillitis [2]

Respiratory
Nasopharyngitis (4–13%) [8]
Pneumonia [2]
Pulmonary toxicity [4]
Sinusitis (see also rhinitis / rhinosinusitis) [2]
Tuberculosis [2]
Upper respiratory tract infection (20%) [11]

Other
Adverse effects / adverse reactions [16]
Death [4]
Infection (14–38%) [19]
Neoplasms [2]

CETIRIZINE

Trade name: Zyrtec (Pfizer)
Indications: Allergic rhinitis, urticaria
Class: Histamine H1 receptor antagonist
Half-life: 8–11 hours
Clinically important, potentially hazardous interactions with: alcohol, CNS depressants, pilsicainide
Important contra-indications noted in the prescribing guidelines for: nursing mothers

---

Skin
- Acneiform eruption / acneiform dermatitis / acneiform rash (<2%)
- AGEP [2]
- Anaphylactoid reactions / anaphylaxis (includes anaphylactic shock) (<2%) [2]
- Angioedema (formerly named angioneurotic edema) (<2%)
- Bullous dermatosis (<2%)
- Dermatitis (<2%)
- Diaphoresis (<2%)
- Exanthems (<2%)
- Fixed eruption / fixed drug eruption [7]
- Flushing / rubefaction (<2%)
- Furunculosis (<2%)
- Hyperkeratosis (<2%)
- Photosensitivity (<2%)
- Phototoxicity (<2%)
- Pruritus (itching) (<2%)
- Purpura (<2%)
- Rash (<2%)
- Seborrhea (<2%)
- Urticaria / hives (<2%) [9]
- Xerosis / xeroderma (<2%)

Hair
- Alopecia / hair loss (<2%)
- Hypertrichosis (<2%)

Mucosal
- Sialorrhea (ptyalism; hypersalivation) (<2%)
- Stomatitis (oral mucositis) (<2%)
- Tongue edema (<2%)
- Tongue pigmentation (<2%)
- Xerostomia (dry mouth) (6%) [2]

Cardiovascular
- QT interval prolonged / QT prolongation [2]

Central Nervous System
- Ageusia (taste loss) / taste disorder (<2%)
- Dysgeusia (taste perversion) (<2%)
- Headache [2]
- Hyperesthesia (<2%)
- Insomnia [2]
- Paresthesias (<2%)
- Parosmia (<2%)
- Somnolence (drowsiness) [5]

Endocrine/Metabolic
- Mastodynia (<2%)

Genitourinary
- Vaginitis (includes vulvitis) (<2%)

Neuromuscular/Skeletal
- Asthenia / fatigue [3]
- Dystonia [7]
- Myalgia/Myopathy (<2%)

Ocular
- Oculogyric crisis / oculogyric dystonic reaction [2]

Other
- Adverse effects / adverse reactions [4]

CETUXIMAB

Trade name: Erbitux (Bristol-Myers Squibb)
Indications: Metastatic colorectal cancer, squamous cell carcinoma of the head and neck
Class: Antineoplastic / anticancer agent (see also Immune checkpoint inhibitor), Biologic, Epidermal growth factor receptor (EGFR) inhibitor / antagonist, Monoclonal antibody
Half-life: 75–188 hours
Clinically important, potentially hazardous interactions with: none known
Important contra-indications noted in the prescribing guidelines for: nursing mothers; pediatric patients
Warning: SERIOUS INFUSION REACTIONS and CARDIOPULMONARY ARREST

Skin
- Acneiform eruption / acneiform dermatitis / acneiform rash (88%) [69]
- Anaphylactoid reactions / anaphylaxis (includes anaphylactic shock) [7]
- Cutaneous toxicity / skin toxicity [22]
- Dermatitis [4]
- Desquamation (89%) [3]
- Erythema [3]
- Exanthems [5]
- Fissures [4]
- Flushing / rubefaction [2]
- Folliculitis [13]
- Hand–foot syndrome (palmar–plantar erythrodysesthesia) [5]
- Hypersensitivity [9]
- Papulopustular eruption [7]
- Peripheral edema (10%)
- Pruritus (itching) (40%) [9]
- Pustules / pustular eruption [2]
- Radiation recall dermatitis [4]
- Rash (89%) [53]
- Stevens-Johnson syndrome and toxic epidermal necrolysis (SJS/TEN) [4]
- Xerosis / xeroderma (49%) [15]

Hair
- Abnormal hair growth [2]
- Alopecia / hair loss (5%) [2]
- Hair changes [3]
- Hypertrichosis [5]

Nails
- Nail changes (21%)
- Nail disorder [3]
- Paronychia [19]

Mucosal
- Mucositis [11]
- Stomatitis (oral mucositis) (25%) [7]
- Xerostomia (dry mouth) (11%)

Cardiovascular
- Cardiotoxicity [3]
- Chest pain [2]
- Thromboembolism [2]

Central Nervous System
- Anorexia [2]
- Anxiety (14%)
- Aseptic meningitis [6]
- Chills (13%) [2]
- Confusion (15%)
- Depression (13%)
- Fever (pyrexia) (includes hyperpyrexia) (30%) [5]
- Headache (33%)
- Insomnia (30%)
- Pain (51%)
- Peripheral neuropathy [3]
- Rigors (13%)
- Seizures [2]

Endocrine/Metabolic
- Hypokalemia [6]
- Hypomagnesemia [21]
- Hyponatremia [5]

Gastrointestinal/Hepatic
- Abdominal pain (59%)
- Constipation (46%)
- Diarrhea (39%) [22]
- Dysphagia [2]
- Gastrointestinal bleeding [2]
- Gastrointestinal obstruction / gastrointestinal stricture [2]
- Hepatotoxicity / liver injury / acute liver injury / drug-induced liver injury (DILI) [4]
- Nausea [12]
- Pneumatosis intestinalis / pneumatosis cystoides intestinalis [2]
- Vomiting (37%) [8]

Hematologic
- Anemia [8]
- Febrile neutropenia [7]
- Leukocytopenia (leukopenia) / leukocytes (white blood cells) decreased [11]
- Myelosuppression / bone marrow suppression / myelotoxicity [2]
- Neutropenia (neutrophils decreased) [26]
- Sepsis (<4%)
- Thrombocytopenia / platelets decreased [5]
- Thrombosis [3]

Local
- Application-site reactions (~3%)
- Infusion-related reactions [8]
- Infusion-site reactions (15–21%) [10]

Neuromuscular/Skeletal
- Asthenia / fatigue (89%) [31]
- Back pain (11%)
- Bone pain / joint pain (15%)

Ocular
- Blepharitis [3]
- Conjunctivitis (conjunctival inflammation) (7%) [2]
- Ectropion / cicatricial ectropion [2]
- Eyelashes – hypertrichosis (eyelash megalotrichosis) [3]
- Trichomegaly [14]

Respiratory
- Cough (29%)
- Dyspnea / shortness of breath (48%) [6]
- Interstitial lung disease / interstitial pneumonitis / interstitial pneumonia (cryptogenic organizing pneumonia) / drug-induced interstitial lung disease [11]
- Pneumonia [2]
- Pneumonitis [3]
- Pulmonary toxicity [5]

Other
- Adverse effects / adverse reactions [9]
- Allergic reactions [5]
- Death [12]
- Infection (13–35%) [3]

CHAMOMILE

Family: Asteraceae; Compositae
Scientific names: *Chamomilla recutita, Matricaria chamomilla, Matricaria recutita*
Indications: Flatulence, travel sickness, nervous diarrhea, restlessness, menstrual cramps, hemorrhoids, mastitis, leg ulcers, inflammation of the respiratory tract. Used in flavoring, cosmetics, soaps and mouthwashes
Class: Sedative
Half-life: N/A
Clinically important, potentially hazardous interactions with: none known

---

Skin
Anaphylactoid reactions / anaphylaxis (includes anaphylactic shock) [2]
Dermatitis [5]

Ocular
Ocular adverse effect [2]

Other
Adverse effects / adverse reactions [3]
Allergic reactions (to those allergic to ragweed, marigolds, daisies) [2]

CHARCOAL

Synonyms: activated carbon; activated charcoal; liquid antidote
Trade names: Actidose-Aqua (Cambridge), Carbomix (Meadow)
Indications: Emergency treatment in poisoning
Class: Antidote, Antimotility
Half-life: N/A
Clinically important, potentially hazardous interactions with: carbamazepine, ursodiol
Note: As an antidote, it is difficult to differentiate side effects due to the drug from those due to the effects of the poison.

CHASTEBERRY

Family: Verbenaceae
Scientific name: *Vitex agnus-castus*
Indications: Premenstrual syndrome, abnormal uterine bleeding, mastodynia
Class: Hormone modulator
Half-life: N/A
Clinically important, potentially hazardous interactions with: dopamine-receptor antagonists
Important contra-indications noted in the prescribing guidelines for: nursing mothers
Note: Chasteberry is not a phytoestrogen; it appears to stimulate progesterone production. The Catholic Church once placed it in the pockets of neophyte monks to help them to maintain their vow of chastity.

Skin
Abscess [2]
Acneiform eruption / acneiform dermatitis / acneiform rash [4]
Erythema [2]
Pruritus (itching) [2]
Urticaria / hives [3]

Mucosal
Xerostomia (dry mouth) [3]

Central Nervous System
Headache [5]

Endocrine/Metabolic
Menstrual irregularities [3]

Gastrointestinal/Hepatic
Hepatotoxicity / liver injury / acute liver injury / drug-induced liver injury (DILI) [4]
Nausea [4]

Neuromuscular/Skeletal
Asthenia / fatigue [3]

Other
Adverse effects / adverse reactions [4]

CHICORY

Family: Compositae
Scientific name: *Cichorium intybus*
Indications: Coffee substitute, jaundice, liver enlargement, gout, rheumatism, skin eruptions connected with gout, inflammation. **Topical:** leaves used for swelling and inflammation. Culinary spice, flavoring
Class: Diuretic
Half-life: N/A
Clinically important, potentially hazardous interactions with: none known

---

Skin
Dermatitis [2]

Other
Allergic reactions [3]

CHLORAL HYDRATE

Indications: Insomnia, sedation
Class: Anesthetic; general, Hypnotic
Half-life: 8–11 hours
Clinically important, potentially hazardous interactions with: antihistamines, azatadine, azelastine, brompheniramine, buclizine, chlorpheniramine, clemastine, dexchlorpheniramine, diphenhydramine, meclizine, tripelennamine
Important contra-indications noted in the prescribing guidelines for: nursing mothers

---

Skin
Acneiform eruption / acneiform dermatitis / acneiform rash [2]
Angioedema (formerly named angioneurotic edema) [2]
Dermatitis [2]
Erythema multiforme [2]
Exanthems [3]
Fixed eruption / fixed drug eruption [5]
Pruritus (itching) [2]
Purpura [2]
Rash (<10%)
Urticaria / hives (<10%) [2]

Mucosal
Oral lesions [2]

Cardiovascular
Hypotension [2]

Central Nervous System
Agitation [3]
Sedation (prolonged) [3]

Gastrointestinal/Hepatic
Vomiting [5]

Respiratory
Apnea [2]

Other
Adverse effects / adverse reactions [4]
Death [3]

CHLORAMBUCIL

Trade name: Leukeran (GSK)
Indications: Chronic lymphocytic leukemia, lymphomas, carcinomas
Class: Alkylating agent
Half-life: 1.5 hours
Clinically important, potentially hazardous interactions with: aldesleukin, antineoplastics, azathioprine, bone marrow suppressants, prednisone, vaccines

---

Skin
Exanthems [7]
Exfoliative dermatitis [2]
Herpes simplex [2]
Herpes zoster [3]
Hypersensitivity [2]
Pruritus (itching) [2]
Rash (<10%)
Stevens-Johnson syndrome and toxic epidermal necrolysis (SJS/TEN) [5]
Urticaria / hives [4]

Hair
Alopecia / hair loss [4]

Mucosal
Oral ulceration [2]

Hematologic
Neutropenia (neutrophils decreased) [5]
Thrombocytopenia / platelets decreased [2]

Local
Infusion-related reactions [3]

Ocular
Periorbital edema [3]

Other
Infection [2]

CHLORAMPHENICOL

Indications: Various infections caused by susceptible organisms
Class: Antibiotic, Antimicrobial, CYP3A4 inhibitor
Half-life: 1.5–3.5 hours
Clinically important, potentially hazardous interactions with: amoxicillin, ampicillin, clopidogrel, clozapine, ethotoin, fosphenytoin, gliclazide, levodopa, mephenytoin, phenytoin, propyphenazone, voriconazole
Important contra-indications noted in the prescribing guidelines for: nursing mothers

---

Skin
AGEP [2]
Dermatitis [18]
Erythema multiforme [6]
Exanthems (<5%) [5]
Hypersensitivity [2]
Purpura [2]
Pustules / pustular eruption [2]
Sensitization [2]
Stevens-Johnson syndrome and toxic epidermal necrolysis (SJS/TEN) [3]
Urticaria / hives [3]

Nails
Photo-onycholysis [3]

CHLORDIAZEPOXIDE

Trade names: Libritabs (Valeant), Librium (Valeant), Limbitrol (Valeant)
Indications: Anxiety
Class: Benzodiazepine
Half-life: 6–25 hours
Clinically important, potentially hazardous interactions with: chlorpheniramine, clarithromycin, efavirenz, esomeprazole, imatinib, indinavir, ketoconazole, nelfinavir, nilutamide, ritonavir
Important contra-indications noted in the prescribing guidelines for: the elderly; nursing mothers; pediatric patients
Note: Limbitrol is chlordiazepoxide and amitriptyline.

Skin
Angioedema (formerly named angioneurotic edema) [3]
Dermatitis (<10%)
Diaphoresis (>10%)
Edema / fluid retention (<10%)
Erythema multiforme [5]
Erythema nodosum [2]
Exanthems [3]
Fixed eruption / fixed drug eruption [7]
Lupus erythematosus (subacute cutaneous lupus erythematosus (SCLE)) [3]
Photosensitivity [6]
Purpura [5]
Rash (>10%)
Urticaria / hives [4]
Vasculitis (angiitis) / cutaneous vasculitis (angiitis) [2]

Hair
Alopecia / hair loss [3]

Mucosal
Sialopenia (>10%)
Sialorrhea (ptyalism; hypersalivation) (<10%)
Xerostomia (dry mouth) (>10%)

Endocrine/Metabolic
Galactorrhea [3]

CHLORHEXIDINE

Trade name: Hibiclens (SSL)
Indications: Skin antisepsis, gingivitis
Class: Antiseptic
Half-life: N/A
Clinically important, potentially hazardous interactions with: none known
Important contra-indications noted in the prescribing guidelines for: nursing mothers; pediatric patients

---

Skin
Anaphylactoid reactions / anaphylaxis (includes anaphylactic shock) [29]
Dermatitis [16]
Hypersensitivity [9]
Rash [2]
Urticaria / hives [4]

Mucosal
Gingival pigmentation [2]
Gingivitis [3]
Glossitis (inflammation of the tongue) (<10%)
Mucosal ulceration [2]
Oral burn [2]
Oral mucosal irritation [2]
Tongue irritation (<10%)
Tongue pigmentation (>10%)

Central Nervous System
Dysgeusia (taste perversion) (>10%) [8]

Other
Allergic reactions [6]
Tooth pigmentation / discoloration [6]

CHLOROQUINE

Trade name: Aralen (Sanofi-Aventis)
Indications: Malaria, rheumatoid arthritis, lupus erythematosus
Class: Antimalarial, Antimicrobial, Antiprotozoal, Covid-19 putative drug, Disease-modifying antirheumatic drug (DMARD)
Half-life: 3–5 days
Clinically important, potentially hazardous interactions with: acitretin, antacids, arsenic, cholera vaccine, cholestyramine, citalopram, dapsone, dasatinib, degarelix, dolasetron, droperidol, ethosuximide, furazolidone, halofantrine, hydroxychloroquine, lacosamide, lanthanum, lapatinib, levofloxacin, methotrexate, methoxsalen, mivacurium, moxifloxacin, neostigmine, nilotinib, oxcarbazepine, pazopanib, penicillamine, ribociclib, sulfonamides, telavancin, telithromycin, tiagabine, typhoid vaccine, vandetanib, vigabatrin, voriconazole, vorinostat, ziprasidone
Important contra-indications noted in the prescribing guidelines for: nursing mothers

---

Skin
Cutaneous toxicity / skin toxicity [2]
Dermatitis [2]
Erythema annulare centrifugum [2]
Erythroderma [3]
Exanthems (<5%) [3]
Exfoliative dermatitis [4]
Lichenoid eruption / lichenoid reaction [6]
Photosensitivity [8]
Pigmentation (Skin) (includes hyperpigmentation) [15]
Pruritus (itching) [36]
Psoriasis [19]
Stevens-Johnson syndrome and toxic epidermal necrolysis (SJS/TEN) [9]
Urticaria / hives [5]
Vitiligo [7]

Hair
Hair pigmentation [10]
Poliosis [3]

Nails
Nail pigmentation [2]

Mucosal
Mucosal membrane pigmentation [2]
Oral pigmentation [14]

Cardiovascular
Atrioventricular block [2]
Cardiac failure [3]
Cardiomyopathy [9]
Cardiotoxicity [3]
Cardiovascular adverse effect (includes major adverse cardiovascular events (MACE)) [2]
Congestive heart failure [2]
Myocardial toxicity [2]
QT interval prolonged / QT prolongation [4]
Torsades de pointes [4]
Ventricular arrhythmia [2]

Central Nervous System
Headache [4]
Psychosis [5]
Seizures [2]
Vertigo / dizziness [4]

Endocrine/Metabolic
Porphyria [7]

Gastrointestinal/Hepatic
Diarrhea [2]
Nausea [4]
Vomiting [5]

Neuromuscular/Skeletal
Myalgia/Myopathy [8]
Myasthenia gravis [7]

Ocular
Corneal deposits [2]
Keratopathy [2]
Maculopathy [3]
Ocular adverse effect [2]
Ocular toxicity [4]
Retinopathy [10]
Vision blurred [2]

Other
Adverse effects / adverse reactions [7]
Death [3]

CHLOROTHIAZIDE

Trade names: Aldoclor (Merck), Diuril (Merck)
Indications: Hypertension, edema
Class: Diuretic, thiazide
Half-life: 1–2 hours
Clinically important, potentially hazardous interactions with: cisplatin, digoxin, lithium, zinc
Note: Chlorothiazide is a sulfonamide and can be absorbed systemically. Sulfonamides can produce severe, possibly fatal, reactions such as toxic epidermal necrolysis and Stevens-Johnson syndrome.

Skin
Exanthems [6]
Lichenoid eruption / lichenoid reaction [4]
Photosensitivity [12]
Pruritus (itching) [3]
Purpura [6]
Vasculitis (angiitis) / cutaneous vasculitis (angiitis) [3]

Respiratory
Pulmonary edema (cardiogenic / non-cardiogenic) [3]

CHLORPHENIRAMINE

Synonym: chlorphenamine
Trade names: Chlor-Trimeton (Schering), Triaminic (Novartis)
Indications: Allergic rhinitis, urticaria
Class: Histamine H1 receptor antagonist, Muscarinic antagonist
Half-life: 20–40 hours
Clinically important, potentially hazardous interactions with: alcohol, anticholinergics, barbiturates, benzodiazepines, butabarbital, chloral hydrate, chlordiazepoxide, chlorpromazine, clonazepam, clorazepate, diazepam, ethchlorvynol, fluphenazine, flurazepam, hypnotics, lopinavir, lorazepam, MAO inhibitors, mephobarbital, mesoridazine, midazolam, narcotics, oxazepam, pentobarbital, phenobarbital, phenothiazines, phenylbutazone,

primidone, prochlorperazine, promethazine, quazepam, secobarbital, sedatives, temazepam, thioridazine, tranquilizers, trifluoperazine, zolpidem
Important contra-indications noted in the prescribing guidelines for: the elderly; nursing mothers; pediatric patients

Skin
Anaphylactoid reactions / anaphylaxis (includes anaphylactic shock) [2]
Angioedema (formerly named angioneurotic edema) (<10%)
Dermatitis (<10%) [4]
Photosensitivity (<10%)

Mucosal
Xerostomia (dry mouth) (<10%)

Central Nervous System
Seizures [2]

CHLORPROMAZINE

Trade name: Thorazine (GSK)
Indications: Psychosis, manic-depressive disorders
Class: Antiemetic, Antipsychotic, Muscarinic antagonist, Phenothiazine
Half-life: initial: 2 hours; terminal: 30 hours
Clinically important, potentially hazardous interactions with: alcohol, antihistamines, arsenic, asenapine, chlorpheniramine, dofetilide, epinephrine, evening primrose, guanethidine, lisdexamfetamine, mivacurium, pimavanserin, propranolol, quinolones, sodium picosulfate, sparfloxacin, tetrabenazine, zolpidem
Important contra-indications noted in the prescribing guidelines for: the elderly; nursing mothers; pediatric patients
Note: The prolonged use of chlorpromazine can produce a gray-blue or purplish pigmentation over light-exposed areas. This is a result of either dermal deposits of melanin, a chlorpromazine metabolite, or a combination of both. Chlorpromazine melanosis is seen more often in women.
Warning: INCREASED MORTALITY IN ELDERLY PATIENTS WITH DEMENTIA-RELATED PSYCHOSIS

Skin
Exanthems (>5%) [8]
Lupus erythematosus (subacute cutaneous lupus erythematosus (SCLE)) [12]
Photosensitivity (<10%) [23]
Phototoxicity [6]
Pigmentation (Skin) (includes hyperpigmentation) [16]
Pruritus (itching) (<10%) [2]
Purpura [6]
Rash (<10%)
Seborrheic dermatitis [4]
Stevens-Johnson syndrome and toxic epidermal necrolysis (SJS/TEN) [2]
Urticaria / hives [4]
Vasculitis (angiitis) / cutaneous vasculitis (angiitis) [3]

Nails
Nail pigmentation [4]
Photo-onycholysis [2]

Mucosal
Xerostomia (dry mouth) (<10%)

Cardiovascular
Hypotension [4]
QT interval prolonged / QT prolongation [4]
Tachycardia [2]
Torsades de pointes [2]

Central Nervous System
Extrapyramidal symptoms [2]
Neuroleptic malignant syndrome [8]
Sedation [3]
Seizures [2]
Vertigo / dizziness [2]

Endocrine/Metabolic
Galactorrhea (<10%)
Gynecomastia (<10%)
Mastodynia (<10%)
Weight gain [2]

Genitourinary
Priapism [7]

Ocular
Cataract [2]
Corneal opacity [2]
Eyelid edema / palpebral edema / blepharedema [2]
Retinopathy [2]

Otic
Tinnitus [2]

Other
Adverse effects / adverse reactions [3]

CHLORPROPAMIDE

Trade name: Diabinese (Pfizer)
Indications: Diabetes
Class: Antidiabetic, Hypoglycemic (antihyperglycemic) agent, Sulfonylurea
Half-life: 30–42 hours
Clinically important, potentially hazardous interactions with: alcohol, cortisone, cortisone, garlic, phenylbutazones
Note: Chlorpropamide is a sulfonamide and can be absorbed systemically. Sulfonamides can produce severe, possibly fatal, reactions such as toxic epidermal necrolysis and Stevens-Johnson syndrome.

Skin
Erythema multiforme [7]
Erythema nodosum [2]
Exanthems (<5%) [3]
Exfoliative dermatitis [7]
Flushing / rubefaction [19]
Lichenoid eruption / lichenoid reaction [4]
Photosensitivity (<10%) [3]
Pruritus (itching) (<3%) [2]
Purpura [8]
Rash (<10%)
Stevens-Johnson syndrome and toxic epidermal necrolysis (SJS/TEN) [7]
Urticaria / hives (<10%) [3]
Vasculitis (angiitis) / cutaneous vasculitis (angiitis) [2]

Mucosal
Oral lichenoid eruption [3]

Endocrine/Metabolic
SIADH [4]

Other
Side effects [3]

CHLORTETRACYCLINE

Indications: Various infections due to susceptible organisms
Class: Antibiotic, Antibiotic; tetracycline, Antimicrobial
Half-life: N/A
Clinically important, potentially hazardous interactions with: ACE inhibitors, coumarins, dairy products, ergotamine, kaolin, methysergide, oral iron, oral typhoid vaccine, penicillins, phenindione, quinapril, retinoids, strontium ranelate, sucralfate, sufonylureas, tripotassium dicitratobismuthate, zinc
Important contra-indications noted in the prescribing guidelines for: nursing mothers; pediatric patients
Note: Not available in Canada or the US.

CHLORTHALIDONE

Synonym: chlortalidone
Trade names: Hygroton (Alliance), Tenoretic (AstraZeneca), Thalitone (Monarch)
Indications: Hypertension
Class: Diuretic, thiazide
Half-life: 35–50 hours
Clinically important, potentially hazardous interactions with: digoxin, lithium, zinc
Note: Chlorthalidone is a sulfonamide and can be absorbed systemically. Sulfonamides can produce severe, possibly fatal, reactions such as toxic epidermal necrolysis and Stevens-Johnson syndrome.
Tenoretic is chlorthalidone and atenolol.

Skin
Fixed eruption / fixed drug eruption [2]
Photosensitivity (<10%) [2]

Endocrine/Metabolic
Hypokalemia [4]
Serum creatinine increased [2]

Gastrointestinal/Hepatic
Pancreatitis / acute pancreatitis [2]

Genitourinary
Erectile dysfunction [2]

Ocular
Glaucoma (includes acute angle-closure glaucoma) [2]
Myopia [3]

CHLORZOXAZONE

Trade names: Paraflex (Ortho-McNeil), Parafon Forte DSC (Ortho-McNeil)
Indications: Painful musculoskeletal conditions
Class: Central muscle relaxant
Half-life: 1–2 hours
Clinically important, potentially hazardous interactions with: lemborexant
Important contra-indications noted in the prescribing guidelines for: the elderly

Skin
Angioedema (formerly named angioneurotic edema) (<10%)
Flushing / rubefaction (<10%)

Central Nervous System
Trembling (<10%)

Gastrointestinal/Hepatic
Hepatotoxicity / liver injury / acute liver injury / drug-induced liver injury (DILI) [2]

CHOLERA VACCINE

Trade name: Vaxchora (PaxVax)
Indications: Immunization against cholera for adults traveling to cholera-affected areas
Class: Vaccine
Half-life: N/A
Clinically important, potentially hazardous interactions with: antibiotics, chloroquine
Pregnancy category: Not expected to cause fetal risk
Important contra-indications noted in the prescribing guidelines for: the elderly; pediatric patients

---

Central Nervous System
Headache (29%)

Endocrine/Metabolic
Appetite decreased (17%)

Gastrointestinal/Hepatic
Abdominal pain (19%)
Diarrhea (4%)
Nausea (18%)
Vomiting (18%)

Neuromuscular/Skeletal
Asthenia / fatigue (31%)

CHOLESTYRAMINE

Trade name: Questran (Par)
Indications: Pruritus associated with biliary obstruction, primary hypercholesterolemia
Class: Bile acid sequestrant
Half-life: N/A
Clinically important, potentially hazardous interactions with: acarbose, acetaminophen, acitretin, amiodarone, aspirin, bezafibrate, calcifediol, chloroquine, cyclopenthiazide, cyclosporine, deferasirox, digoxin, doxepin, doxercalciferol, ergocalciferol, ezetimibe, ezetimibe, hydroxychloroquine, isotretinoin, leflunomide, levodopa, lovastatin, meloxicam, mycophenolate, phytonadione, propranolol, raloxifene, sulfasalazine, sulfonylureas, tetracycline, tricyclic antidepressants, troglitazone, ursodiol, valproic acid, vitamin A, vitamin E
Important contra-indications noted in the prescribing guidelines for: nursing mothers; pediatric patients
Note: Contra-indicated in patients with complete biliary obstruction.

Skin
Pruritus (itching) [2]

Hematologic
Hemorrhage [2]

Neuromuscular/Skeletal
Osteomalacia [2]

CHOLIC ACID

Trade name: Cholbam (Asklepion Pharmaceuticals)
Indications: Bile acid synthesis disorders, adjunctive treatment of peroxisomal disorders
Class: Bile acid
Half-life: N/A
Clinically important, potentially hazardous interactions with: cyclosporine
Important contra-indications noted in the prescribing guidelines for: the elderly; nursing mothers

---

Gastrointestinal/Hepatic
Diarrhea (2%)

CHOLINE FENOFIBRATE

Synonym: fenofibric acid
Trade name: Trilipix (AbbVie)
Indications: As adjunctive therapy in hypertriglyceridemia, hypercholesterolemia or mixed dyslipidemia
Class: Fibrate
Half-life: 20 hours
Clinically important, potentially hazardous interactions with: cyclosporine
Important contra-indications noted in the prescribing guidelines for: the elderly; nursing mothers; pediatric patients
Note: Contra-indicated in patients with renal impairment. Fenofibric acid is the active metabolite of fenofibrate (see separate entry).

Central Nervous System
Headache (13%)
Pain (4%)
Vertigo / dizziness (4%)

Endocrine/Metabolic
ALT increased (5%)

Gastrointestinal/Hepatic
Constipation (3%)
Diarrhea (4%)
Dyspepsia / functional dyspepsia (indigestion) (see also gastroparesis) (4%)
Nausea (4%)

Neuromuscular/Skeletal
Arthralgia (4%)
Asthenia / fatigue (2%)
Back pain (6%)
Muscle spasm (2%)
Myalgia/Myopathy (3%)
Pain in extremities (5%)

Respiratory
Nasopharyngitis (4%)
Sinusitis (see also rhinitis / rhinosinusitis) (3%)
Upper respiratory tract infection (5%)

CHONDROITIN

Scientific names: *Chondroitin 4- and 6-sulfate, Chondroitin 4-sulfate, Condrosulf, Structum*
Indications: Osteoarthritis (often with glucosamine), ischemic heart disease, osteoporosis, hyperlipidemia, keratoconjunctivitis, agent in cataract surgery
Class: Amino sugar, Food supplement
Half-life: N/A
Clinically important, potentially hazardous interactions with: warfarin

---

Gastrointestinal/Hepatic
Dyspepsia / functional dyspepsia (indigestion) (see also gastroparesis) [2]
Hepatotoxicity / liver injury / acute liver injury / drug-induced liver injury (DILI) [2]
Nausea [2]

Other
Adverse effects / adverse reactions [2]

CICLESONIDE

Trade names: Alvesco (Nycomed) (Oral inhalation), Omnaris (Nycomed) (Intranasal)
Indications: Allergic rhinitis, asthma
Class: Corticosteroid / Glucocorticoid
Half-life: 5–7 hours
Clinically important, potentially hazardous interactions with: aldesleukin, conivaptan, corticorelin, darunavir, dasatinib, delavirdine, indinavir, itraconazole, ketoconazole, mifepristone, moderate CYP3A4 inhibitors, nelfinavir, ritonavir, telithromycin, voriconazole
Important contra-indications noted in the prescribing guidelines for: nursing mothers

---

Mucosal
Oral candidiasis [2]

CICLOPIROX

Trade names: Loprox (Medicis), Penlac (Sanofi-Aventis)
Indications: Various infections caused by susceptible organisms
Class: Antifungal / antimycotic, Antimicrobial
Half-life: 2 hours
Clinically important, potentially hazardous interactions with: none known
Important contra-indications noted in the prescribing guidelines for: nursing mothers; pediatric patients
Note: For topical use only.

Skin
Burning / skin burning sensation [3]
Contact dermatitis [2]
Erythema [2]
Pruritus (itching) [4]

CIDOFOVIR

Trade name: Vistide (Gilead)
Indications: Cytomegalovirus (CMV) retinitis in patients with acquired immunodeficiency syndrome (AIDS)
Class: Antiviral; nucleotide analog
Half-life: ~2.6 hours
Clinically important, potentially hazardous interactions with: amphotericin B, cobicistat/elvitegravir/emtricitabine/tenofovir alafenamide, cobicistat/elvitegravir/emtricitabine/tenofovir disoproxil, fomivirsen, tenofovir disoproxil
Important contra-indications noted in the prescribing guidelines for: the elderly; nursing mothers; pediatric patients
Warning: RENAL TOXICITY and NEUTROPENIA

Skin
- Acneiform eruption / acneiform dermatitis / acneiform rash (>10%)
- Cutaneous toxicity / skin toxicity [3]
- Diaphoresis (<10%)
- DRESS syndrome (Drug-induced hypersensitivity syndrome) [2]
- Pallor (<10%)
- Pigmentation (Skin) (includes hyperpigmentation) (>10%)
- Pruritus (itching) (<10%) [2]
- Rash (27%) [2]
- Ulcerations [2]
- Urticaria / hives (<10%)

Hair
- Alopecia / hair loss (22%) [2]

Mucosal
- Stomatitis (oral mucositis) (<10%)

Central Nervous System
- Chills (24%)
- Dysgeusia (taste perversion) (<10%)
- Headache [4]
- Paresthesias (>10%)

Local
- Application-site reactions (39%) [4]

Neuromuscular/Skeletal
- Asthenia / fatigue [2]
- Myalgia/Myopathy [2]

Ocular
- Intraocular inflammation [2]
- Iritis [6]
- Ocular hypotension [2]
- Retinal detachment [3]
- Uveitis / anterior uveitis / posterior uveitis / panuveitis [18]
- Vision impaired [3]
- Vision loss [3]

Renal
- Fanconi syndrome (proximal tubular dysfunction) [2]
- Nephrotoxicity / kidney injury / acute kidney injury (AKI) / drug-induced kidney injury [5]

Other
- Allergic reactions (<10%)

CILAZAPRIL

Trade names: Inhibase (Roche), Vascace (Roche)
Indications: Hypertension, chronic heart failure
Class: Angiotensin-converting enzyme (ACE) inhibitor, Antihypertensive, Vasodilator
Half-life: 9 hours
Clinically important, potentially hazardous interactions with: alcohol, aldesleukin, allopurinol, alpha blockers, alprostadil, angiotensin II receptor antagonists, antacids, antidiabetics, antipsychotics, anxiolytics and hypnotics, aspirin, baclofen, beta blockers, calcium channel blockers, clonidine, corticosteroids, cyclosporine, diazoxide, diuretics, estrogens, general anesthetics, gold & gold compounds, heparins, hydralazine, insulin, levodopa, lithium, MAO inhibitors, metformin, methyldopa, minoxidil, moxisylyte, nitrates, nitroprusside, NSAIDs, potassium salts, sulfonylureas, sympathomimetics, tizanidine, trimethoprim
Important contra-indications noted in the prescribing guidelines for: nursing mothers; pediatric patients
Note: Contra-indicated in patients with a history of angioedema with or without previous ACE inhibitor treatment.
Not available in the USA.

Skin
- Angioedema (formerly named angioneurotic edema) [2]
- Pemphigus vulgaris [2]

Central Nervous System
- Headache [3]
- Vertigo / dizziness [2]

Neuromuscular/Skeletal
- Asthenia / fatigue [4]

Respiratory
- Cough [8]

CILOSTAZOL

Trade name: Pletal (Otsuka)
Indications: Peripheral vascular disease, intermittent claudication
Class: Antiplatelet (antithrombotic), Neuroprotectant, Phosphodiesterase inhibitor, Vasodilator, peripheral
Half-life: 11–13 hours
Clinically important, potentially hazardous interactions with: anagrelide, anticoagulants, antifungals, antiplatelet agents, clarithromycin, collagenase, conivaptan, CYP2C19 inhibitors, CYP3A4 inducers or inhibitors, dasatinib, deferasirox, diltiazem, drotrecogin alfa, erythromycin, esomeprazole, fondaparinux, glucosamine, grapefruit juice, high-fat foods, ibritumomab, itraconazole, ketoconazole, macrolide antibiotics, NSAIDs, omeprazole, PEG-interferon, pentosan, pentoxifylline, prostacyclin analogues, salicylates, St John's wort, telithromycin, thrombolytic agents, tositumomab & iodine^{131}, voriconazole
Important contra-indications noted in the prescribing guidelines for: nursing mothers; pediatric patients
Note: Contra-indicated in patients with congestive heart failure or active pathological bleeding.
Warning: CONTRA-INDICATED IN HEART FAILURE PATIENTS

Skin
- Bruise / bruising / contusion / ecchymosis (ecchymoses) (<2%)
- DRESS syndrome (Drug-induced hypersensitivity syndrome) [2]
- Edema / fluid retention (<2%)
- Facial edema (<2%)
- Furunculosis (<2%)
- Hypertrophy (<2%)
- Peripheral edema (7–9%)
- Purpura (<2%)
- Rash (2%) [2]
- Urticaria / hives (<2%)
- Varicosities (<2%)
- Xerosis / xeroderma (<2%)

Mucosal
- Epistaxis (nosebleed) (<2%)
- Gingival bleeding (<2%)
- Perioral abscess (<2%)
- Rectal hemorrhage / rectal bleeding (<2%)
- Tongue edema (<2%)

Cardiovascular
- Arrhythmias (<2%)
- Atrial fibrillation (<2%)
- Atrial flutter (<2%)
- Cardiac arrest (<2%)
- Cardiotoxicity [4]
- Congestive heart failure (<2%)
- Extrasystoles (<2%)
- Hypotension (<2%)
- Myocardial infarction (<2%) [4]
- Myocardial ischemia (<2%)
- Palpitation (5–10%) [8]
- Postural hypotension (<2%)
- Supraventricular tachycardia (<2%)
- Tachycardia (4%) [4]
- Vasodilation (<2%)
- Ventricular tachycardia (<2%)

Central Nervous System
- Anorexia (<2%)
- Anxiety (<2%)
- Cerebral ischemia (<2%)
- Chills (<2%)
- Headache (27–34%) [20]
- Hyperesthesia (2%)
- Insomnia (<2%)
- Neurotoxicity (<2%)
- Paresthesias (2%)
- Syncope / fainting (<2%)
- Vertigo / dizziness (<10%) [4]

Endocrine/Metabolic
- Creatine phosphokinase (CPK) / creatine kinase increased (hyperCKemia) (<2%)
- Diabetes mellitus (<2%)
- GGT increased (<2%)
- Hyperlipidemia / lipids elevated (<2%)
- Hyperuricemia (<2%)

Gastrointestinal/Hepatic
- Abdominal pain (4–5%)
- Black stools / melena (<2%)
- Cholelithiasis (gallstones in the gall bladder or the bile duct) (<2%)
- Colitis (<2%)
- Diarrhea (12–19%) [8]
- Dyspepsia / functional dyspepsia (indigestion) (see also gastroparesis) (6%)
- Esophagitis (<2%)
- Flatulence (2–3%)
- Gastritis / pangastritis / gastric irritation (<2%)

Gastroenteritis (<2%)
Gastrointestinal ulceration (<2%)
Hematemesis (<2%)
Nausea (6–7%) [4]
Peptic ulceration (includes duodenal ulcer, esophageal ulcer) (<2%)
Vomiting (>2%)

Genitourinary
Albuminuria (<2%)
Cystitis (includes interstitial cystitis / bladder pain syndrome) (<2%)
Urinary frequency (<2%)
Vaginal bleeding (<2%)
Vaginitis (includes vulvitis) (<2%)

Hematologic
Anemia (<2%)
Hemorrhage (<2%)
Polycythemia / erythrocytosis (<2%)
Thrombosis [3]

Neuromuscular/Skeletal
Arthralgia (<2%)
Asthenia / fatigue (<2%)
Back pain (6–7%)
Bone pain / joint pain (<2%)
Gouty tophi (<2%)
Myalgia/Myopathy (2–3%)

Ocular
Amblyopia (<2%)
Blindness (<2%)
Conjunctivitis (conjunctival inflammation) (<2%)
Diplopia (double vision) (<2%)
Ocular hemorrhage (<2%)

Otic
Ear pain (<2%)
Tinnitus (<2%)

Renal
Retroperitoneal bleeding (<2%)

Respiratory
Asthma (<2%)
Cough (3–4%) [2]
Hemoptysis (<2%)
Pharyngitis (sore throat) (7–10%)
Pneumonia (<2%)
Rhinitis / rhinosinusitis (see also sinusitis) (7–12%)
Sinusitis (see also rhinitis / rhinosinusitis) (<2%)

Other
Adverse effects / adverse reactions [5]
Death [3]
Infection (10–14%)

CIMETIDINE

Trade name: Tagamet (GSK)
Indications: Duodenal ulcer
Class: CYP1A2 inhibitor, CYP3A4 inhibitor, Histamine H2 receptor antagonist
Half-life: 2 hours
Clinically important, potentially hazardous interactions with: acenocoumarol, alfuzosin, aminophylline, amiodarone, amitriptyline, anisindione, anticoagulants, buprenorphine, butorphanol, caffeine, carmustine, citalopram, clobazam, clopidogrel, clozapine, cocoa, delavirdine, dicumarol, dofetilide, duloxetine, dutasteride, epirubicin, eszopiclone, fentanyl, ferrous sulfate, floxuridine, fluorouracil, galantamine, gliclazide, hydromorphone, itraconazole, ketoconazole, labetalol, levomepromazine, lidocaine, lomustine, meptazinol, metformin, metronidazole, midazolam, mizolastine, moclobemide, morphine, narcotic analgesics, neratinib, oxprenolol, oxtriphylline, oxycodone, oxymorphone, pentazocine, phenytoin, pimecrolimus, posaconazole, prednisone, propranolol, quinine, rilpivirine, risperidone, roflumilast, sertindole, sildenafil, sufentanil, tamsulosin, terbinafine, thalidomide, tolazoline, uracil/tegafur, uracil/tegafur, warfarin, xanthines, zaleplon, zofenopril, zolmitriptan, zolpidem
Important contra-indications noted in the prescribing guidelines for: nursing mothers; pediatric patients

---

Skin
Angioedema (formerly named angioneurotic edema) [3]
Erythema annulare centrifugum [2]
Erythema multiforme [5]
Exanthems [3]
Exfoliative dermatitis [2]
Fixed eruption / fixed drug eruption [2]
Hypersensitivity [4]
Lupus erythematosus (subacute cutaneous lupus erythematosus (SCLE)) [3]
Pruritus (itching) [6]
Pseudolymphoma / cutaneous pseudolymphoma [2]
Psoriasis [6]
Rash (<2%)
Stevens-Johnson syndrome and toxic epidermal necrolysis (SJS/TEN) [5]
Urticaria / hives [6]
Vasculitis (angiitis) / cutaneous vasculitis (angiitis) [3]

Hair
Alopecia / hair loss [4]

Central Nervous System
Hallucinations [3]

Endocrine/Metabolic
Gynecomastia [13]

Neuromuscular/Skeletal
Myalgia/Myopathy [2]

Renal
Nephrotoxicity / kidney injury / acute kidney injury (AKI) / drug-induced kidney injury [3]

CINACALCET

Trade names: Mimpara (Amgen), Sensipar (Amgen)
Indications: Secondary hyperparathyroidism, parathyroid carcinoma
Class: Calcimimetic
Half-life: 30–40 hours
Clinically important, potentially hazardous interactions with: amitriptyline, antifungal agents, atomoxetine, carvedilol, codeine, conivaptan, CYP2D6 substrates, CYP3A4 inhibitors, dasatinib, desipramine, fesoterodine, flecainide, food, itraconazole, ketoconazole, metoprolol, nebivolol, PEG-interferon, tacrolimus, tamoxifen, tetrabenazine, thioridazine, tramadol, tricyclic antidepressants, voriconazole
Important contra-indications noted in the prescribing guidelines for: nursing mothers; pediatric patients
Note: Contra-indicated in patients with hypocalcemia.

Cardiovascular
Chest pain (6%)
Hypertension (7%)

Central Nervous System
Anorexia (6–15%)
Depression (13%)
Headache (13%)
Paresthesias (20%)
Vertigo / dizziness (10%)

Endocrine/Metabolic
Dehydration (15%)
Hypercalcemia (17%) [2]
Hypocalcemia [11]

Gastrointestinal/Hepatic
Constipation (13%)
Diarrhea (21%) [2]
Gastrointestinal disorder / discomfort [3]
Nausea (31–63%) [9]
Vomiting (27–46%) [5]

Genitourinary
Hypercalciuria [2]

Hematologic
Anemia (13%)

Neuromuscular/Skeletal
Arthralgia (13%)
Asthenia / fatigue (7–17%)
Fractures (17%)
Myalgia/Myopathy (15%) [2]
Pain in extremities (11%)

Respiratory
Upper respiratory tract infection (11%)

Other
Adverse effects / adverse reactions [3]
Infection (5%)

CINNARIZINE

Trade names: Stugeron (Janssen), Vertizin (Ram)
Indications: Dizziness, tinnitus, nystagmus, nausea and vomiting, motion sickness
Class: Histamine H1 receptor antagonist, Muscarinic antagonist, Vasodilator, peripheral
Half-life: 4 hours
Clinically important, potentially hazardous interactions with: alcohol, barbiturates, hypnotics, narcotic analgesics, sedatives, tranquilizers, tricyclic antidepressants

---

Skin
Lichen planus (includes hypertrophic lichen planus) [2]
Lichen planus pemphigoides [2]

Central Nervous System
Depression [7]
Headache [2]
Parkinsonism [28]
Tardive syndrome / tardive dyskinesia [4]

Other
Adverse effects / adverse reactions [3]

CIPROFIBRATE

Trade name: Modalim (Sanofi-Aventis)
Indications: Hyperlipidemia
Class: Fibrate, Lipid regulator
Half-life: 1.5 hours
Clinically important, potentially hazardous interactions with: atorvastatin, fluvastatin, ibuprofen, norfloxacin, pravastatin, rosuvastatin, simvastatin

---

Gastrointestinal/Hepatic
Hepatotoxicity / liver injury / acute liver injury / drug-induced liver injury (DILI) [3]
Neuromuscular/Skeletal
Rhabdomyolysis [5]
Renal
Nephrotoxicity / kidney injury / acute kidney injury (AKI) / drug-induced kidney injury [2]

CIPROFLOXACIN

Trade names: Ciloxan Ophthalmic (Alcon), Cipro (Bayer), Ciproxin (Bayer)
Indications: Various infections caused by susceptible organisms, inhalational anthrax (post exposure)
Class: Antibiotic, Antibiotic; fluoroquinolone, Antibiotic; quinolone, Antimicrobial, CYP1A2 inhibitor, CYP3A4 inhibitor
Half-life: 4 hours
Clinically important, potentially hazardous interactions with: agomelatine, aminophylline, amiodarone, amitriptyline, antacids, antineoplastics, arsenic, artemether/lumefantrine, BCG vaccine, bendamustine, bepridil, bismuth, bismuth subsalicylate, bretylium, calcium salts, citalopram, clopidogrel, clozapine, corticosteroids, cyclosporine, dairy products, dasatinib, degarelix, didanosine, disopyramide, dolasetron, duloxetine, dutasteride, eluxadoline, erlotinib, erythromycin, flibanserin, insulin, lanthanum, lapatinib, levofloxacin, lumateperone, magnesium salts, meptazinol, methotrexate, methylxanthines, mifepristone, moxifloxacin, mycophenolate, neratinib, NSAIDs, olanzapine, olaparib, opiod analgesics, oral iron, oxtriphylline, P-glycoprotein inhibitors, pazopanib, pentoxifylline, phenothiazines, phenytoin, pirfenidone, probenecid, procainamide, propranolol, QT prolonging agents, quinapril, quinidine, rasagiline, ropinirole, ropivacaine, sevelamer, sotalol, St John's wort, strontium ranelate, sucralfate, sulfonylureas, telavancin, telithromycin, tizanidine, tricyclic antidepressants, typhoid vaccine, ubrogepant, venetoclax, vitamin K antagonists, voriconazole, vorinostat, warfarin, zinc, ziprasidone, zolmitriptan
Important contra-indications noted in the prescribing guidelines for: the elderly; nursing mothers
Note: Fluoroquinolones are associated with an increased risk of tendinitis and tendon rupture in all ages. This risk is further increased in older patients usually over 60 years of age, in patients taking corticosteroid drugs, and in patients with kidney, heart or lung transplants.
Fluoroquinolones may exacerbate muscle weakness in persons with myasthenia gravis.
Ciprofloxacin is chemically related to nalidixic acid.
Warning: SERIOUS ADVERSE REACTIONS INCLUDING TENDINITIS, TENDON RUPTURE, PERIPHERAL NEUROPATHY, CENTRIAL NERVOUS SYSTEM EFFECTS and EXACERBATION OF MYASTHENIA GRAVIS

Skin
Acneiform eruption / acneiform dermatitis / acneiform rash [3]
AGEP [4]
Anaphylactoid reactions / anaphylaxis (includes anaphylactic shock) [15]
Angioedema (formerly named angioneurotic edema) [8]
Bullae [2]
Candidiasis / candidosis [2]
Cutaneous toxicity / skin toxicity [3]
Diaphoresis [5]
DRESS syndrome (Drug-induced hypersensitivity syndrome) [2]
Erythema multiforme [5]
Exanthems [4]
Facial edema [2]
Fixed eruption / fixed drug eruption [14]
Hypersensitivity [5]
Jaundice (see also cholestasis / cholestatic jaundice) [3]
Leukocytoclastic vasculitis (angiitis) [2]
Linear IgA bullous dermatosis [2]
Photosensitivity [20]
Phototoxicity [5]
Pruritus (itching) [11]
Purpura [4]
Rash (<10%) [14]
Serum sickness-like reaction [2]
Stevens-Johnson syndrome and toxic epidermal necrolysis (SJS/TEN) [20]
Sweet's syndrome [2]
Urticaria / hives [10]
Vasculitis (angiitis) / cutaneous vasculitis (angiitis) [11]
Mucosal
Stomatitis (oral mucositis) [4]
Xerostomia (dry mouth) [3]
Cardiovascular
Palpitation [2]
QT interval prolonged / QT prolongation [11]
Torsades de pointes [8]
Central Nervous System
Delirium [5]
Dysgeusia (taste perversion) [3]
Encephalopathy (includes hepatic encephalopathy) [2]
Fever (pyrexia) (includes hyperpyrexia) [3]
Hallucinations, visual [6]
Headache [6]
Leukoencephalopathy / posterior reversible encephalopathy syndrome (PRES) [2]
Mania [6]
Neuropsychiatric / neuropsychological adverse effect [2]
Peripheral neuropathy [6]
Psychosis [7]
Seizures [5]
Suicidal ideation [2]
Syncope / fainting [2]
Tremor [2]
Vertigo / dizziness [2]
Endocrine/Metabolic
Hypoglycemia [2]
Gastrointestinal/Hepatic
Abdominal pain [2]
Cholestatic liver injury / cholestatic hepatitis [2]
Constipation [2]
Flatulence [2]
Hepatitis [5]
Hepatotoxicity / liver injury / acute liver injury / drug-induced liver injury (DILI) [8]
Nausea (3%) [4]
Pancreatitis / acute pancreatitis [2]
Vomiting [2]
Genitourinary
Vaginitis (includes vulvitis) [2]
Hematologic
Hemolytic anemia [2]
Myelosuppression / bone marrow suppression / myelotoxicity [2]
Thrombocytopenia / platelets decreased [4]
Local
Injection-site pain [2]
Neuromuscular/Skeletal
Arthralgia [2]
Asthenia / fatigue [4]
Myalgia/Myopathy [2]
Myasthenia gravis (exacerbation) [2]
Myoclonus (see also hypnic jerk) [4]
Rhabdomyolysis [4]
Tendinitis [4]
Tendinopathy/Tendon rupture [32]
Ocular
Vision blurred [2]
Otic
Hearing loss (hypoacusis) [2]
Renal
Nephrotoxicity / kidney injury / acute kidney injury (AKI) / drug-induced kidney injury [9]
Renal failure [3]
Other
Adverse effects / adverse reactions [8]
Death [8]

CISATRACURIUM

Trade name: Nimbex (AbbVie)
Indications: Adjunct to general anesthesia, relaxes skeletal muscle
Class: Non-depolarizing neuromuscular blocker
Half-life: 22 minutes
Clinically important, potentially hazardous interactions with: aminoglycosides, clindamycin, cyclopropane, enflurane, halothane, isoflurane, methoxyflurane, piperacillin, rocuronium

---

Skin
Anaphylactoid reactions / anaphylaxis (includes anaphylactic shock) [11]

CISPLATIN

Synonym: CDDP
Trade name: Platinol (Bristol-Myers Squibb)
Indications: Carcinomas, lymphomas
Class: Alkylating agent, Antineoplastic / anticancer agent (see also Immune checkpoint inhibitor), Platinum-based antineoplastic
Half-life: alpha phase: 25–49 minutes; beta phase: 58–73 hours
Clinically important, potentially hazardous interactions with: aldesleukin, atenolol, chlorothiazide, gadobenate, methotrexate, paclitaxel, pentamidine, rituximab, selenium, thalidomide, torsemide, torsemide, trilaciclib, zinc
Important contra-indications noted in the prescribing guidelines for: the elderly; nursing mothers

---

Skin
Acneiform eruption / acneiform dermatitis / acneiform rash [7]
Anaphylactoid reactions / anaphylaxis (includes anaphylactic shock) [10]
Angioedema (formerly named angioneurotic edema) [4]

Cutaneous toxicity / skin toxicity [8]
Edema / fluid retention [3]
Erythema [3]
Exanthems [4]
Flagellate dermatitis [2]
Flushing / rubefaction [5]
Hand–foot syndrome (palmar–plantar erythrodysesthesia) [10]
Hypersensitivity [5]
Necrosis (skin necrosis) [2]
Peripheral edema [2]
Pigmentation (Skin) (includes hyperpigmentation) [5]
Pruritus (itching) [8]
Rash [22]
Raynaud's phenomenon [14]
Recall reaction [2]
Stevens-Johnson syndrome and toxic epidermal necrolysis (SJS/TEN) [2]
Thrombocytopenic purpura [2]
Urticaria / hives [7]
Xerosis / xeroderma [2]

Hair
Alopecia / hair loss (>10%) [26]

Nails
Paronychia [2]

Mucosal
Epistaxis (nosebleed) [3]
Mucosal inflammation [2]
Mucositis [16]
Oral lesions [2]
Stomatitis (oral mucositis) [18]

Cardiovascular
Bradycardia / sinus bradycardia [3]
Cardiotoxicity [3]
Hypertension [9]
Thromboembolism [7]
Venous thromboembolism [4]

Central Nervous System
Anorexia [28]
Dysgeusia (taste perversion) [3]
Encephalopathy (includes hepatic encephalopathy) [4]
Fever (pyrexia) (includes hyperpyrexia) [5]
Headache [4]
Insomnia [4]
Leukoencephalopathy / posterior reversible encephalopathy syndrome (PRES) [10]
Neurotoxicity [17]
Pain [3]
Peripheral neuropathy [9]
Seizures [5]
Stroke / cerebrovascular accident [2]
Vertigo / dizziness [2]

Endocrine/Metabolic
ALP increased [2]
ALT increased [7]
Appetite decreased [7]
AST increased [7]
Dehydration [3]
Hyperbilirubinemia [2]
Hyperglycemia (includes glucose increased) [4]
Hyperkalemia [2]
Hypocalcemia [2]
Hypokalemia [5]
Hypomagnesemia [14]
Hyponatremia [21]
Serum creatinine increased [9]
SIADH [19]
Weight loss [4]

Gastrointestinal/Hepatic
Abdominal pain [4]
Colitis [2]
Constipation [6]
Diarrhea [39]
Esophagitis [2]
Gastrointestinal bleeding [2]
Hepatotoxicity / liver injury / acute liver injury / drug-induced liver injury (DILI) [7]
Nausea [58]
Pancreatitis / acute pancreatitis [2]
Vomiting [42]

Hematologic
Anemia [53]
Coagulopathy / coagulation dysfunction / clotting factor deficiency (includes disseminated intravascular coagulation / DIC) [2]
Febrile neutropenia [42]
Hemolytic uremic syndrome [12]
Hemotoxicity [4]
Leukocytopenia (leukopenia) / leukocytes (white blood cells) decreased [39]
Lymphopenia (lymphocytopenia) / lymphocytes decreased [5]
Myelosuppression / bone marrow suppression / myelotoxicity [11]
Neutropenia (neutrophils decreased) [103]
Sepsis [2]
Thrombocytopenia / platelets decreased [53]
Thrombosis [2]
Thrombotic microangiopathy [2]

Local
Injection-site cellulitis [4]

Neuromuscular/Skeletal
Arthralgia [2]
Asthenia / fatigue [41]
Ataxia [2]
Myalgia/Myopathy [4]
Myasthenia gravis [2]

Ocular
Ocular adverse effect [2]
Retinal artery occlusion [4]

Otic
Hearing loss (hypoacusis) [19]
Ototoxicity [46]
Tinnitus [28]

Renal
Nephrotoxicity / kidney injury / acute kidney injury (AKI) / drug-induced kidney injury [74]
Proteinuria [3]
Renal failure [3]
Renal function abnormal / renal dysfunction [2]

Respiratory
Cough [4]
Dysphonia (includes voice disorders / voice changes) [4]
Dyspnea / shortness of breath [4]
Pneumonia [4]
Pneumonitis [3]
Pulmonary toxicity [5]

Other
Adverse effects / adverse reactions [16]
Death [17]
Hiccups / singultus [6]
Infection [11]

CITALOPRAM

Trade names: Celexa (Forest), Cipramil (Lundbeck)
Indications: Depression, obsessive-compulsive disorder, panic disorder
Class: Antidepressant, Selective serotonin reuptake inhibitor (SSRI)
Half-life: ~35 hours
Clinically important, potentially hazardous interactions with: alcohol, alfuzosin, alpha or beta blockers, antidepressants, antiepileptics, antiplatelet agents, artemether/lumefantrine, aspirin, atomoxetine, barbiturates, bupropion, buspirone, carbamazepine, chloroquine, cimetidine, ciprofloxacin, clozapine, CNS depressants, collagenase, conivaptan, coumarins/anticoagulants, CYP2C19 inhibitors, CYP3A4 inhibitors, cyproheptadine, desmopressin, dexibuprofen, dextromethorphan, dronedarone, drotrecogin alfa, duloxetine, efavirenz, fluconazole, gadobutrol, glucosamine, haloperidol, ibritumomab, iobenguane, isocarboxazid, lithium, macrolide antibiotics, MAO inhibitors, methadone, methylphenidate, metoclopramide, mexiletine, moclobemide, nilotinib, NSAIDs, opioid anagesics, pentoxifylline, phenelzine, phenytoin, pimozide, QT prolonging agents, quinine, rasagiline, risperidone, ritonavir, salicylates, selegiline, serotonin modulators, sibutramine, SSRIs, St John's wort, sumatriptan, tetrabenazine, thioridazine, thrombolytic agents, tositumomab & iodine^{131}, tramadol, tranylcypromine, trazodone, tricyclic antidepressants, tryptophan, vitamin K antagonists, ziprasidone
Important contra-indications noted in the prescribing guidelines for: nursing mothers; pediatric patients
Note: Escitalopram (q.v.) is the (S)-form citalopram.
Warning: SUICIDALITY AND ANTIDEPRESSANT DRUGS

Skin
Diaphoresis (11%) [3]
Hyperhidrosis (11%) [2]
Pigmentation (Skin) (includes hyperpigmentation) [2]
Pruritus (itching) (<10%) [2]
Rash (<10%)

Mucosal
Xerostomia (dry mouth) (20%) [4]

Cardiovascular
Bradycardia / sinus bradycardia [2]
Cardiotoxicity [4]
Chest pain [2]
Palpitation [2]
QT interval prolonged / QT prolongation [22]
Tachycardia [3]
Torsades de pointes [9]

Central Nervous System
Agitation (3%)
Akathisia [2]
Anorexia (4%)
Anxiety (4%) [2]
Fever (pyrexia) (includes hyperpyrexia) (2%)
Hallucinations, auditory [2]
Hallucinations, visual [3]
Headache [5]
Incoordination [2]

Insomnia (15%) [4]
Nightmares [2]
Restless legs syndrome / Willis-Ekbom disease (includes restless arms syndrome variant) [4]
Sedation [2]
Seizures (overdose) [5]
Serotonin syndrome [19]
Somnolence (drowsiness) (18%) [6]
Suicidal ideation [3]
Tremor (8%) [5]
Vertigo / dizziness [5]
Yawning (2%)

Endocrine/Metabolic
Galactorrhea [4]
Hyponatremia [2]
Libido decreased (2%)
SIADH [19]
Weight gain [3]

Gastrointestinal/Hepatic
Abdominal pain (3%)
Constipation [2]
Diarrhea (8%) [2]
Dyspepsia / functional dyspepsia (indigestion) (see also gastroparesis) (5%)
Nausea (21%) [4]
Vomiting (4%) [2]

Genitourinary
Dysmenorrhea (3%)
Ejaculatory dysfunction (6%) [2]
Impotence (3%)
Priapism [4]
Sexual dysfunction [5]
Urinary frequency [2]

Neuromuscular/Skeletal
Arthralgia (2%)
Asthenia / fatigue (5%) [4]
Dystonia [2]
Myalgia/Myopathy (2%)

Ocular
Diplopia (double vision) [2]
Glaucoma (includes acute angle-closure glaucoma) [3]

Respiratory
Rhinitis / rhinosinusitis (see also sinusitis) (5%)
Sinusitis (see also rhinitis / rhinosinusitis) (3%)
Upper respiratory tract infection (5%)

Other
Adverse effects / adverse reactions [2]
Death [8]

CLADRIBINE

Trade name: Leustatin (Janssen Biotech)
Indications: Leukemias
Class: Antimetabolite, Antineoplastic / anticancer agent (see also Immune checkpoint inhibitor), Immunomodulator
Half-life: alpha phase: 25 minutes; beta phase: 7 hours
Clinically important, potentially hazardous interactions with: none known
Important contra-indications noted in the prescribing guidelines for: the elderly; nursing mothers
Note: Licensed for treating relapsing multiple sclerosis in Europe since 2017.

Skin
Diaphoresis (<10%)
Edema / fluid retention (6%)
Erythema (6%)
Exanthems (27–50%) [2]
Herpes zoster [5]
Petechiae (8%)
Pruritus (itching) (6%)
Purpura (10%)
Rash (27%) [3]

Mucosal
Mucositis [2]

Hematologic
Lymphopenia (lymphocytopenia) / lymphocytes decreased [12]
Neutropenia (neutrophils decreased) [8]
Thrombocytopenia / platelets decreased [2]

Local
Injection-site edema (9%)
Injection-site erythema (9%)
Injection-site pain (9%)
Injection-site phlebitis (2%)
Injection-site thrombosis (2%)

Neuromuscular/Skeletal
Asthenia / fatigue [3]
Myalgia/Myopathy (7%)

Other
Adverse effects / adverse reactions [4]
Death [3]
Infection [10]

CLARITHROMYCIN

Trade name: Biaxin (AbbVie)
Indications: Various infections caused by susceptible organisms
Class: Antibiotic, Antibiotic; macrolide, Antimicrobial, CYP3A4 inhibitor
Half-life: 5–7 hours
Clinically important, potentially hazardous interactions with: abiraterone, alprazolam, aprepitant, astemizole, atazanavir, atorvastatin, avanafil, benzodiazepines, betrixaban, boceprevir, brigatinib, cabazitaxel, cabozantinib, calcifediol, carbamazepine, chlordiazepoxide, cilostazol, clonazepam, clorazepate, cobicistat/elvitegravir/emtricitabine/tenofovir alafenamide, cobicistat/elvitegravir/emtricitabine/tenofovir disoproxil, colchicine, conivaptan, copanlisib, crizotinib, cyclosporine, dabigatran, darunavir, dasatinib, deflazacort, delavirdine, diazepam, digoxin, dihydroergotamine, disopyramide, dronedarone, efavirenz, eletriptan, eluxadoline, ergot alkaloids, erlotinib, erlotinib, estradiol, etravirine, everolimus, fesoterodine, flibanserin, fluoxetine, flurazepam, fluticasone propionate, fluvastatin, HMG-CoA reductase inhibitors, ibrutinib, imatinib, indinavir, itraconazole, ivabradine, ivabradine, ixabepilone, lapatinib, lemborexant, lomitapide, lopinavir, lorazepam, lovastatin, lumateperone, maraviroc, methylergonovine, methylprednisolone, methysergide, midazolam, midostaurin, mifepristone, naldemedine, neratinib, nevirapine, nilotinib, olaparib, omeprazole, osilodrostat, oxazepam, oxtriphylline, paclitaxel, palbociclib, paroxetine hydrochloride, pazopanib, pimavanserin, pimozide, ponatinib, pravastatin, prednisone, quazepam, ranolazine, regorafenib, repaglinide, ribociclib, rilpivirine, rimonabant, rivaroxaban, romidepsin, ruxolitinib, sertraline, sildenafil, silodosin, simeprevir, simvastatin, solifenacin, sunitinib, tadalafil, talazoparib, temazepam, temsirolimus, tezacaftor/ivacaftor, ticagrelor, tipranavir, tolvaptan, trabectedin, triazolam, ubrogepant, ulipristal, valbenazine, vandetanib, vemurafenib, venetoclax, voclosporin, vorapaxar, warfarin, zidovudine
Important contra-indications noted in the prescribing guidelines for: the elderly; nursing mothers; pediatric patients

---

Skin
Anaphylactoid reactions / anaphylaxis (includes anaphylactic shock) [2]
Baboon syndrome / symmetrical drug-related intertriginous and flexural exanthema (SDRIFE) [3]
Exanthems [3]
Fixed eruption / fixed drug eruption [3]
Hypersensitivity [3]
Psoriasis [2]
Purpura [3]
Rash (3%) [2]
Serum sickness-like reaction [2]
Stevens-Johnson syndrome and toxic epidermal necrolysis (SJS/TEN) [4]
Vasculitis (angiitis) / cutaneous vasculitis (angiitis) [3]

Mucosal
Stomatitis (oral mucositis) [2]

Cardiovascular
QT interval prolonged / QT prolongation [7]
Torsades de pointes [9]

Central Nervous System
Anorexia [2]
Dysgeusia (taste perversion) (3%) [9]
Hallucinations, visual [5]
Mania [8]
Neurotoxicity [4]
Psychosis [3]

Endocrine/Metabolic
Hypoglycemia [3]

Gastrointestinal/Hepatic
Abdominal distension [2]
Abdominal pain [5]
Diarrhea [10]
Dyspepsia / functional dyspepsia (indigestion) (see also gastroparesis) [2]
Hepatotoxicity / liver injury / acute liver injury / drug-induced liver injury (DILI) [4]
Nausea [5]
Vomiting [3]

Local
Injection-site pain [2]

Neuromuscular/Skeletal
Arthralgia [2]
Rhabdomyolysis [14]

Otic
Hearing loss (hypoacusis) [2]

Renal
Nephrotoxicity / kidney injury / acute kidney injury (AKI) / drug-induced kidney injury [2]

Other
Adverse effects / adverse reactions [11]

CLASCOTERONE

Synonyms: Cortexolone 17α-propionate
Trade name: Winlevi (Cassiopea)
Indications: Topical treatment of acne vulgaris
Class: Androgen receptor inhibitor
Half-life: Excretion of clascoterone has not been fully characterised in humans.
Clinically important, potentially hazardous interactions with: no clinical studies evaluating the drug interaction potential of clascoterone (cream) have been conducted.
Pregnancy category: No available data to assess drug-associated risk of clascoterone in pregnant women.
Note: Formulated as a cream with cetyl alcohol and other excipients. Local skin reactions (edema, erythema/redness, skin atrophy, stinging/burning, striae rubrea, telangiectasia) were observed during a treatment period with clascoterone cream, and occurred in a similar percentage of subjects treated with the vehicle cream.

Other
Adverse effects / adverse reactions [4]

CLEMASTINE

Trade name: Tavist (Novartis)
Indications: Allergic rhinitis, urticaria
Class: Histamine H1 receptor antagonist
Half-life: 4–6 hours
Clinically important, potentially hazardous interactions with: barbiturates, chloral hydrate, ethchlorvynol, phenothiazines, zolpidem
Important contra-indications noted in the prescribing guidelines for: nursing mothers

Mucosal
Xerostomia (dry mouth) (<10%) [2]

CLEVIDIPINE

Trade name: Cleviprex (The Medicines Company)
Indications: Reduction of blood pressure
Class: Calcium channel blocker
Half-life: 1 minute
Clinically important, potentially hazardous interactions with: alpha-1 blockers, amifostine, antihypertensives, black cohosh, blue cohosh, calicium channel blockers (non-dihydropyridine), diazoxide, ephedra, ginger, ginseng, goldenseal, hawthorn (fruit, leaf, flower extract), hypotensives, licorice, magnesium salts, MAO inhibitors, methylphenidate, mistletoe, neuromuscular blocking agents, nitroprusside, pentoxifylline, phosphodiesterase 5 inhibitors, quinidine, quinine, rituximab, yohimbine
Important contra-indications noted in the prescribing guidelines for: nursing mothers; pediatric patients
Note: Contra-indicated in patients with allergies to soy or egg products, with defective lipid metabolism, or severe aortic stenosis.

Cardiovascular
Atrial fibrillation (21%)

Central Nervous System
Headache (6%) [2]

Gastrointestinal/Hepatic
Nausea (5%) [2]
Vomiting (3%)

CLIDINIUM

Trade name: Librax (Valeant)
Indications: Duodenal and gastric ulcers
Class: Muscarinic antagonist
Half-life: N/A
Clinically important, potentially hazardous interactions with: anticholinergics, arbutamine
Note: Librax is clidinium and chlordiazepoxide.

CLINDAMYCIN

Trade names: Benzaclin (Dermik), Cleocin (Pfizer), Cleocin-T (Pfizer), Clindagel (Galderma), Clindets (Stiefel)
Indications: Various serious infections caused by susceptible organisms
Class: Antibiotic, Antibiotic; lincosamide, Antimicrobial
Half-life: 2–3 hours
Clinically important, potentially hazardous interactions with: cisatracurium, erythromycin, kaolin, mivacurium, neostigmine, pyridostigmine, rocuronium, saquinavir
Note: See also separate entry for the combination product clindamycin/tretinoin.

Skin
AGEP [14]
Anaphylactoid reactions / anaphylaxis (includes anaphylactic shock) [5]
Dermatitis (from topical preparations) [7]
DRESS syndrome (Drug-induced hypersensitivity syndrome) [2]
Erythema multiforme [2]
Erythroderma [2]
Exanthems [6]
Hypersensitivity [5]
Rash (<10%) [3]
Stevens-Johnson syndrome and toxic epidermal necrolysis (SJS/TEN) [10]
Sweet's syndrome [3]
Urticaria / hives [3]
Vasculitis (angiitis) / cutaneous vasculitis (angiitis) [2]

Mucosal
Burning Mouth Syndrome / glossodynia / glossalgia / glossopyrosis (also includes stomatodynia / oral dysesthesia / stomatopyrosis) [2]
Xerostomia (dry mouth) [2]

Central Nervous System
Ageusia (taste loss) / taste disorder [2]

Gastrointestinal/Hepatic
Colitis [2]
Diarrhea [4]
Esophagitis [2]
Hepatotoxicity / liver injury / acute liver injury / drug-induced liver injury (DILI) [3]
Pseudomembranous colitis [5]

Hematologic
Myelosuppression / bone marrow suppression / myelotoxicity [2]
Neutropenia (neutrophils decreased) [2]

Local
Application-site erythema [3]

Otic
Tinnitus [2]

Other
Adverse effects / adverse reactions [6]
Death [3]

CLINDAMYCIN/ TRETINOIN

Trade names: Veltin (Astellas) (Stiefel), Ziana (Medicis)
Indications: Acne vulgaris (topical use only)
Class: Antibiotic, Antibiotic; lincosamide, Antimicrobial, Retinoid
Half-life: N/A
Clinically important, potentially hazardous interactions with: erythromycin, neuromuscular blocking agents, other topical medications with a skin drying effect
Important contra-indications noted in the prescribing guidelines for: nursing mothers; pediatric patients
Note: Contra-indicated in patients with regional enteritis, ulcerative colitis, or history of antibiotic-associated colitis. Exposure to sunlight, sunlamps, and weather extremes should be avoided during the use of clindamycin/tretinoin gel. The reactions listed below are specific to the clindamycin/tretinoin combination product. See also profiles of clindamycin and tretinoin for reactions associated with the individual products.

Skin
Erythema [2]
Scaling [2]

Gastrointestinal/Hepatic
Gastrointestinal disorder / discomfort (4%)

Local
Application-site erythema [2]

Other
Adverse effects / adverse reactions [2]

CLIOQUINOL

Synonyms: iodochlorhydroxyquin; chloroiodoquin
Trade name: Vioform (Novartis)
Indications: Athlete's foot, eczema, fungal infections, Parkinsonism
Class: Antifungal / antimycotic, Antimicrobial, Antiprotozoal, Chelator
Half-life: N/A
Clinically important, potentially hazardous interactions with: bacitracin
Important contra-indications noted in the prescribing guidelines for: nursing mothers
Note: Use banned or restricted in some countries.

Skin
Contact dermatitis [4]
Dermatitis [2]

Central Nervous System
Amnesia [3]
Neurotoxicity [9]

Hematologic
Myelosuppression / bone marrow suppression / myelotoxicity [4]

Ocular
Optic neuritis / papillitis [3]

CLOBAZAM

Trade names: Frisium (Sanofi-Aventis), Onfi (Lundbeck)
Indications: Epilepsy adjunct therapy, psychosis
Class: Anticonvulsant (see also antiepileptic (anti-seizure)), Antiepileptic (anti-seizure), Benzodiazepine
Half-life: 36–42 hours
Clinically important, potentially hazardous interactions with: alcohol, cannabidiol, carbamazepine, cenobamate, cimetidine, disulfiram, fluconazole, fluvoxamine, hormonal contraceptives, levodopa, moxonidine, omeprazole, phenytoin, rifampin, sodium oxybate, stiripentol, theophylline, ticlopidine, valproic acid
Important contra-indications noted in the prescribing guidelines for: nursing mothers; pediatric patients

---

Skin
Rash [3]
Stevens-Johnson syndrome and toxic epidermal necrolysis (SJS/TEN) [3]

Central Nervous System
Aggression (includes anger) (8%) [2]
Dysarthria (3%)
Fever (pyrexia) (includes hyperpyrexia) (13%) [2]
Insomnia (5%) [2]
Irritability (7%)
Sedation (5%)
Somnolence (drowsiness) (22%) [4]

Endocrine/Metabolic
Appetite decreased (3%)
Appetite increased (3%)

Gastrointestinal/Hepatic
Constipation (5%)
Dysphagia (2%)
Vomiting (7%)

Genitourinary
Urinary tract infection (4%)

Neuromuscular/Skeletal
Asthenia / fatigue (5–10%) [3]
Ataxia (5%) [3]
Psychomotor hyperactivity (4%)

Respiratory
Bronchitis (2%)
Cough (5%)
Pneumonia (4%) [2]
Upper respiratory tract infection (12%) [3]

Other
Adverse effects / adverse reactions (47%) [2]
Death [2]
Side effects (35%) [2]

CLOFAZIMINE

Trade name: Lamprene (Novartis)
Indications: Leprosy
Class: Anti-inflammatory, Antimycobacterial (including antitubercular)
Half-life: 10 days after a single dose
Clinically important, potentially hazardous interactions with: fludarabine, pentostatin
Important contra-indications noted in the prescribing guidelines for: the elderly; nursing mothers; pediatric patients

---

Skin
Chromhidrosis (red sweat) (<10%) [3]
Ichthyosis (8–28%) [7]
Pigmentation (Skin) (includes hyperpigmentation) (pink to brownish-black) (75–100%) [30]
Pruritus (itching) (<5%)
Rash (<5%) [3]
Xerosis / xeroderma (8–28%) [3]

Nails
Discoloration / nails (dyschromia) [2]

Gastrointestinal/Hepatic
Abdominal pain [5]
Enteropathy [3]
Nausea [2]
Vomiting [2]

Ocular
Corneal deposits [2]
Eyes – keratopathy [2]

Other
Adverse effects / adverse reactions [6]

CLOFIBRATE

Trade name: Atromid-S (Wyeth)
Indications: Type III hyperlipidemia
Class: Fibrate
Half-life: 6–25 hours after a single dose
Clinically important, potentially hazardous interactions with: anisindione, anticoagulants, dicumarol, gliclazide, ursodiol, warfarin

---

Skin
Dermatitis [3]
Exanthems [6]
Photosensitivity [4]

Neuromuscular/Skeletal
Myalgia/Myopathy [3]
Rhabdomyolysis [3]

CLOMIPHENE

Trade names: Clomid (Sanofi-Aventis), Serophene (Merck)
Indications: Ovulatory failure.
Used in the treatment of hypogonadism, especially in men of reproductive age.

Class: Selective estrogen receptor modulator (SERM)
Half-life: 5–7 days
Clinically important, potentially hazardous interactions with: none known
Important contra-indications noted in the prescribing guidelines for: nursing mothers

---

Skin
Exanthems [2]
Flushing / rubefaction (10%)
Hot flashes / hot flushes (>10%)
Melanoma [4]

Hair
Alopecia / hair loss [2]

Cardiovascular
Myocardial infarction [4]

Central Nervous System
Mood changes (includes mood disorder) [2]

Endocrine/Metabolic
Gynecomastia (<10%)
Mastodynia (<10%)

Hematologic
Thrombosis [5]

Ocular
Retinal vein occlusion [3]

CLOMIPRAMINE

Trade name: Anafranil (Mallinckrodt)
Indications: Obsessive-compulsive disorder
Class: Antidepressant; tricyclic, Muscarinic antagonist
Half-life: 21–31 hours
Clinically important, potentially hazardous interactions with: amprenavir, arbutamine, arsenic, artemether/lumefantrine, clonidine, duloxetine, epinephrine, formoterol, guanethidine, isocarboxazid, linezolid, MAO inhibitors, milnacipran, moclobemide, phenelzine, quinolones, sparfloxacin, tranylcypromine
Important contra-indications noted in the prescribing guidelines for: the elderly; nursing mothers; pediatric patients
Warning: SUICIDALITY AND ANTIDEPRESSANT DRUGS

Skin
Acneiform eruption / acneiform dermatitis / acneiform rash (2%)
Cellulitis and pseudocellulitis (2%)
Dermatitis (2%)
Diaphoresis (29%) [2]
Edema / fluid retention (2%)
Flushing / rubefaction (8%)
Hypersensitivity [2]
Photosensitivity [3]
Pruritus (itching) (6%)
Purpura (3%)
Rash (8%)
Xerosis / xeroderma (2%)

Mucosal
Xerostomia (dry mouth) (84%) [6]

Cardiovascular
QT interval prolonged / QT prolongation [4]
Torsades de pointes [2]

Central Nervous System
Dysgeusia (taste perversion) (8%)
Seizures [4]
Serotonin syndrome [4]
Status epilepticus [2]
Vertigo / dizziness [2]

Endocrine/Metabolic
Gynecomastia (2%)
SIADH [3]

Gastrointestinal/Hepatic
Nausea [2]

Genitourinary
Urinary retention [2]
Vaginitis (includes vulvitis) (2%)

Neuromuscular/Skeletal
Myalgia/Myopathy (13%)

Other
Adverse effects / adverse reactions [4]
Allergic reactions (<3%)

CLONAZEPAM

Trade name: Klonopin (Roche)
Indications: Petit mal and myoclonic seizures
Class: Benzodiazepine
Half-life: 18–50 hours
Clinically important, potentially hazardous interactions with: amprenavir, chlorpheniramine, clarithromycin, cobicistat/elvitegravir/emtricitabine/tenofovir disoproxil, efavirenz, esomeprazole, imatinib, indinavir, nelfinavir, nevirapine, oxycodone, piracetam
Important contra-indications noted in the prescribing guidelines for: the elderly; nursing mothers; pediatric patients

---

Skin
Bullous dermatosis [2]
Dermatitis (<10%)
Diaphoresis (>10%)
Lichenoid eruption / lichenoid reaction [2]
Pseudolymphoma / cutaneous pseudolymphoma [2]
Rash (>10%)

Hair
Alopecia / hair loss [2]

Mucosal
Sialopenia (>10%)
Sialorrhea (ptyalism; hypersalivation) (<10%)
Xerostomia (dry mouth) (>10%)

Central Nervous System
Insomnia [2]
Psychosis [2]
Seizures [2]

Other
Adverse effects / adverse reactions [2]
Allergic reactions (<10%)

CLONIDINE

Trade name: Catapres (Boehringer Ingelheim)
Indications: Hypertension
Class: Adrenergic alpha-receptor agonist, Imidazoline receptor agonist
Half-life: 6–24 hours
Clinically important, potentially hazardous interactions with: acebutolol, alfuzosin, amitriptyline, amoxapine, atenolol, betaxolol, captopril, carteolol, cilazapril, clomipramine, desipramine, dexmethylphenidate, diclofenac, doxepin, enalapril, esmolol, fosinopril, imipramine, insulin aspart, insulin degludec, insulin detemir, insulin glargine, insulin glulisine, irbesartan, levodopa, levomepromazine, lisinopril, meloxicam, metoprolol, milnacipran, nadolol, nebivolol, nortriptyline, olmesartan, oxprenolol, penbutolol, pericyazine, pindolol, propranolol, protriptyline, quinapril, ramipril, sotalol, sulpiride / levosulpiride, timolol, trandolapril, triamcinolone, tricyclic antidepressants, trimipramine, verapamil
Important contra-indications noted in the prescribing guidelines for: nursing mothers; pediatric patients

---

Skin
Depigmentation [2]
Dermatitis (from patch) (20%) [23]
Eczema / eczematous reaction / eczematous eruption [2]
Erythema [2]
Lupus erythematosus (subacute cutaneous lupus erythematosus (SCLE)) [5]
Pigmentation (Skin) (includes hyperpigmentation) [2]
Pityriasis rosea [2]
Pruritus (itching) (>5%) [6]
Psoriasis [2]
Rash (<10%) [4]
Ulcerations (<10%)

Mucosal
Xerostomia (dry mouth) (40%) [14]

Cardiovascular
Bradycardia / sinus bradycardia [9]
Hypotension [19]

Central Nervous System
Fever (pyrexia) (includes hyperpyrexia) [2]
Hallucinations [3]
Headache [4]
Hyperesthesia (<10%)
Sedation [2]
Seizures [2]
Somnolence (drowsiness) [7]
Vertigo / dizziness [5]

Gastrointestinal/Hepatic
Nausea [2]

Neuromuscular/Skeletal
Asthenia / fatigue [2]

Other
Adverse effects / adverse reactions [3]

CLOPIDOGREL

Trade name: Plavix (Bristol-Myers Squibb) (Sanofi-Aventis)
Indications: Acute coronary syndrome, recent myocardial infarction, recent stroke, or established peripheral arterial disease
Class: Antiplatelet (antithrombotic), Antiplatelet; thienopyridine
Half-life: 6 hours
Clinically important, potentially hazardous interactions with: amiodarone, anisindione, anticoagulants, atorvastatin, calcium channel blockers, cangrelor, carbamazepine, chloramphenicol, cimetidine, ciprofloxacin, collagenase, dabigatran, dasatinib, delavirdine, dexlansoprazole, diclofenac, dicumarol, dipyridamole, drotrecogin alfa, efavirenz, enoxaparin, erythromycin, esomeprazole, etravirine, fluconazole, fluoxetine, fluvoxamine, fondaparinux, glucosamine, herbals with anticoagulant properties, ibritumomab, iloprost, inotersen, itraconazole, ketoconazole, lansoprazole, lepirudin, macrolide antibiotics, meloxicam, miconazole, moclobemide, NSAIDs, omega-3 fatty acids, omeprazole, oxcarbazepine, pantoprazole, pentosan, pentoxifylline, polysulfate sodium, prasugrel, rabeprazole, rifapentine, rivaroxaban, salicylates, simvastatin, telithromycin, thrombolytic agents, tinzaparin, tositumomab & iodine^{131}, voriconazole, warfarin
Important contra-indications noted in the prescribing guidelines for: nursing mothers; pediatric patients
Note: Contra-indicated in patients with active pathological bleeding.
Warning: DIMINISHED EFFECTIVENESS IN POOR METABOLIZERS

Skin
AGEP [2]
Angioedema (formerly named angioneurotic edema) [4]
Bullous dermatosis (<3%)
Eczema / eczematous reaction / eczematous eruption (<3%)
Edema / fluid retention (3–5%)
Exanthems (<3%) [2]
Hypersensitivity [9]
Pruritus (itching) (3%) [2]
Psoriasis [2]
Purpura [18]
Rash (4%) [5]
Stevens-Johnson syndrome and toxic epidermal necrolysis (SJS/TEN) [2]
Thrombocytopenic purpura [9]
Thrombotic thrombocytopenic purpura [2]
Ulcerations (<3%)
Urticaria / hives (<3%) [3]

Cardiovascular
Acute coronary syndrome [2]
Cardiovascular adverse effect (includes major adverse cardiovascular events (MACE)) [2]
Myocardial infarction [2]

Central Nervous System
Ageusia (taste loss) / taste disorder [3]
Fever (pyrexia) (includes hyperpyrexia) [4]
Hyperesthesia (<3%)
Intracranial hemorrhage [2]
Paresthesias (<3%)

Endocrine/Metabolic
Hypoglycemia [7]
Insulin autoimmune syndrome / insulin autoimmune hypoglycemia / Hirata's disease [6]

Gastrointestinal/Hepatic
Gastrointestinal bleeding [3]
Hepatotoxicity / liver injury / acute liver injury / drug-induced liver injury (DILI) [6]

Hematologic
Bleeding [17]
Hemolytic uremic syndrome [2]
Leukocytopenia (leukopenia) / leukocytes (white blood cells) decreased [2]
Neutropenia (neutrophils decreased) [5]
Thrombocytopenia / platelets decreased [4]
Thrombosis [2]
Thrombotic microangiopathy [3]

Neuromuscular/Skeletal
Arthritis / polyarthritis [17]
Hemarthrosis (articular bleeding) [2]
Rhabdomyolysis [3]
Spinal epidural hematoma [8]

Ocular
Ocular hemorrhage [2]

Respiratory
Dyspnea / shortness of breath [3]
Influenza- ('flu)-like syndrome (8%)

Other
Adverse effects / adverse reactions [3]
Allergic reactions (<3%) [2]

CLORAZEPATE

Trade name: Tranxene (Recordati)
Indications: Anxiety and panic disorders
Class: Benzodiazepine
Half-life: 48–96 hours
Clinically important, potentially hazardous interactions with: aminophylline, amprenavir, antacids, carbamazepine, carmustine, chlorpheniramine, clarithromycin, cobicistat/

elvitegravir/emtricitabine/tenofovir alafenamide, cobicistat/elvitegravir/emtricitabine/tenofovir disoproxil, efavirenz, esomeprazole, imatinib, indinavir, itraconazole, ketoconazole, MAO inhibitors, midazolam, moclobemide, nelfinavir, phenytoin, sucralfate, warfarin
Important contra-indications noted in the prescribing guidelines for: nursing mothers; pediatric patients

---

Skin
- Dermatitis (<10%)
- Diaphoresis (>10%)
- Rash (>10%)

Mucosal
- Sialopenia (>10%)
- Sialorrhea (ptyalism; hypersalivation) (<10%)
- Xerostomia (dry mouth) (>10%)

CLOTRIMAZOLE

Trade names: Canesten (Bayer), Mycelex (Bayer)
Indications: Candidiasis, dermatophyte infections of the skin
Class: Antifungal / antimycotic, Antifungal; imidazole, Antimicrobial
Half-life: N/A
Clinically important, potentially hazardous interactions with: betamethasone, cyproterone, neratinib

---

Skin
- Burning / skin burning sensation [2]
- Dermatitis [9]
- Pruritus (itching) [2]

CLOXACILLIN

Trade name: Cloxapen (GSK)
Indications: Various infections caused by susceptible organisms
Class: Antibiotic, Antibiotic; beta-lactam, Antibiotic; penicillin, Antimicrobial
Half-life: 0.5–1.1 hours
Clinically important, potentially hazardous interactions with: anticoagulants, cyclosporine, demeclocycline, doxycycline, imipenem/cilastatin, methotrexate, minocycline, oxytetracycline, proguanil, tetracycline

---

Skin
- Angioedema (formerly named angioneurotic edema) [2]

Nails
- Nail loss [2]

Hematologic
- Neutropenia (neutrophils decreased) [2]

CLOZAPINE

Trade names: Clozaril (Novartis), Denzapine (Merz), Leponex (Novartis), Zaponex (Teva)
Indications: Treatment-resistant schizophrenia
Class: Antipsychotic, Antipsychotic, atypical
Half-life: 4–12 hours
Clinically important, potentially hazardous interactions with: alcohol, amitriptyline, antimuscarinics, arsenic, benzodiazepines, cabazitaxel, caffeine, carbamazepine, chloramphenicol, cimetidine, ciprofloxacin, citalopram, cocoa, cyclophosphamide, cytotoxics, darifenacin, dasatinib, encainide, epinephrine, erythromycin, everolimus, flecainide, fluoxetine, flupentixol, fluphenazine, fluvoxamine, gefitinib, guarana, haloperidol, insulin degludec, insulin detemir, insulin glargine, insulin glulisine, lapatinib, lithium, lomustine, lorazepam, MAO inhibitors, nilotinib, norfloxacin, ofloxacin, omeprazole, oxaliplatin, oxybutynin, paroxetine hydrochloride, pazopanib, pemetrexed, penicillamine, pipotiazine, propafenone, quinidine, rifampin, risperidone, ritonavir, saquinavir, selenium, sertraline, sorafenib, sulfonamides, sunitinib, telithromycin, temozolomide, temsirolimus, tetrazepam, tricyclic antidepressants, trospium, uracil/tegafur, valproic acid, venlafaxine, viloxazine, zuclopenthixol
Important contra-indications noted in the prescribing guidelines for: the elderly; nursing mothers; pediatric patients
Note: Contra-indicated in patients with myeloproliferative disorders, uncontrolled epilepsy, paralytic ileus, or a history of clozapine-induced agranulocytosis or severe granulocytopenia.
Warning: AGRANULOCYTOSIS / SEIZURES / MYOCARDITIS / OTHER ADVERSE CARDIOVASCULAR AND RESPIRATORY EFFECTS.
INCREASED MORTALITY IN ELDERLY PATIENTS WITH DEMENTIA-RELATED PSYCHOSIS

Skin
- Angioedema (formerly named angioneurotic edema) [2]
- Baboon syndrome / symmetrical drug-related intertriginous and flexural exanthema (SDRIFE) [2]
- Cutaneous toxicity / skin toxicity [5]
- Diaphoresis (6%) [4]
- Exanthems [2]
- Hyperhidrosis [2]
- Lupus erythematosus (subacute cutaneous lupus erythematosus (SCLE)) [4]
- Pityriasis rosea [2]
- Rash (2%) [2]
- Sweet's syndrome [3]

Mucosal
- Parotitis [4]
- Sialorrhea (ptyalism; hypersalivation) (31%) [86]
- Xerostomia (dry mouth) [3]

Cardiovascular
- Atrial fibrillation [2]
- Cardiac tamponade / pericardial tamponade [2]
- Cardiomyopathy [17]
- Cardiotoxicity [3]
- Hypertension (4%) [6]
- Hypotension (9%) [5]
- Myocarditis [58]
- Orthostatic hypotension [4]
- Pericardial effusion [3]
- Pericarditis [13]
- QT interval prolonged / QT prolongation [7]
- Tachycardia (25%) [13]
- Venous thromboembolism [5]

Central Nervous System
- Akathisia [4]
- Anxiety [2]
- Compulsions / obsessive-compulsive symptoms / obsessive-compulsive disorder [18]
- Fever (pyrexia) (includes hyperpyrexia) [14]
- Headache (7%) [2]
- Neuroleptic malignant syndrome [32]
- Neurotoxicity [2]
- Pain [2]
- Parkinsonism [2]
- Restless legs syndrome / Willis-Ekbom disease (includes restless arms syndrome variant) [2]
- Sedation (39%) [13]
- Seizures [28]
- Somnolence (drowsiness) [10]
- Stuttering (dysphemia) / stammering [2]
- Syncope / fainting [2]
- Tardive syndrome / tardive dyskinesia [6]
- Tic disorder [2]
- Tremor (<10%) [2]
- Vertigo / dizziness (19%) [3]

Endocrine/Metabolic
- Diabetes mellitus [7]
- Diabetic ketoacidosis [2]
- Dyslipidemia [3]
- Galactorrhea [2]
- Hyperglycemia (includes glucose increased) [7]
- Hyperlipidemia / lipids elevated [3]
- Metabolic syndrome (includes metabolic disorder) [13]
- Weight gain [30]

Gastrointestinal/Hepatic
- Colitis [2]
- Constipation (14%) [8]
- Diarrhea [4]
- Eosinophilic gastrointestinal disorders (includes eosinophilic esophagitis, eosinophilic gastroenteritis and eosinophilic colitis) [3]
- Gastrointestinal hypomotility [11]
- Gastrointestinal obstruction / gastrointestinal stricture [3]
- Hepatic failure [2]
- Hepatotoxicity / liver injury / acute liver injury / drug-induced liver injury (DILI) [10]
- Ileus / adynamic ileus / paralytic ileus [10]
- Intestinal pseudo-obstruction (Ogilvie syndrome) [5]
- Pancreatitis / acute pancreatitis [8]

Genitourinary
- Enuresis (urinary incontinence) [6]
- Priapism [15]

Hematologic
- Agranulocytosis / severe selective neutropenia [46]
- Eosinophilia / eosinophils increased [17]
- Granulocytopenia [2]
- Hematological adverse effect [3]
- Hemotoxicity [2]
- Leukocytopenia (leukopenia) / leukocytes (white blood cells) decreased [14]
- Neutropenia (neutrophils decreased) [29]
- Neutrophilia / neutrophil leukocytosis / neutrocytosis (neutrophils increased) [2]
- Pancytopenia (includes bicytopenia) [4]
- Pure red cell aplasia [3]
- Thrombosis [2]

Neuromuscular/Skeletal
- Myoclonus (see also hypnic jerk) [2]
- Rhabdomyolysis [8]

Ocular
- Maculopathy [2]

Periorbital edema [2]

Renal

Nephritis / interstitial nephritis / tubulointerstitial nephritis [2]
Nephrotoxicity / kidney injury / acute kidney injury (AKI) / drug-induced kidney injury [2]

Respiratory

Pleural effusion [4]
Pneumonia [6]
Pneumonitis [4]
Pulmonary embolism [7]
Respiratory aspiration [2]

Other

Adverse effects / adverse reactions [16]
Death [21]
Serositis / polyserositis [6]

CO-TRIMOXAZOLE

Synonyms: Cotrimoxazole; sulfamethoxazole-trimethoprim; SMX-TMP; SMZ-TMP; TMP-SMX; TMP-SMZ
Trade names: Bactrim (GSK), Septra (Monarch)
Indications: Various infections caused by susceptible organisms
Class: Antibiotic, Antibiotic; sulfonamide, Antimicrobial
Half-life: 6–10 hours
Clinically important, potentially hazardous interactions with: anticoagulants, azathioprine, cyclosporine, dofetilide, isotretinoin, methotrexate, prilocaine, repaglinide, warfarin
Important contra-indications noted in the prescribing guidelines for: the elderly; nursing mothers; pediatric patients
Note: Co-trimoxazole is a sulfonamide and can be absorbed systemically. Sulfonamides can produce severe, possibly fatal, reactions such as toxic epidermal necrolysis and Stevens-Johnson syndrome.
Co-trimoxazole is sulfamethoxazole and trimethoprim.

Skin

AGEP [4]
Anaphylactoid reactions / anaphylaxis (includes anaphylactic shock) [6]
Angioedema (formerly named angioneurotic edema) [3]
Bullous dermatosis [2]
Cutaneous adverse reaction (includes severe cutaneous adverse drug reaction (SCAR)) [10]
Cutaneous toxicity / skin toxicity [2]
Dermatitis [4]
DRESS syndrome (Drug-induced hypersensitivity syndrome) [16]
Erythema multiforme [19]
Erythema nodosum [2]
Exanthems [35]
Exfoliative dermatitis [5]
Fixed eruption / fixed drug eruption [52]
Hypersensitivity [19]
Jarisch–Herxheimer reaction [2]
Leukocytoclastic vasculitis (angiitis) [4]
Linear IgA bullous dermatosis [5]
Lupus erythematosus (subacute cutaneous lupus erythematosus (SCLE)) [4]
Photosensitivity [4]
Pruritus (itching) [10]
Purpura [3]
Pustules / pustular eruption [6]
Radiation recall dermatitis [3]
Rash (>10%) [14]
Stevens-Johnson syndrome and toxic epidermal necrolysis (SJS/TEN) (<10%) [83]
Sweet's syndrome [12]
Thrombocytopenic purpura [3]
Thrombotic thrombocytopenic purpura [2]
Urticaria / hives [12]
Vasculitis (angiitis) / cutaneous vasculitis (angiitis) [11]

Mucosal

Oral mucosal eruption [2]
Oral ulceration [2]

Cardiovascular

QT interval prolonged / QT prolongation [2]
Torsades de pointes [3]

Central Nervous System

Aseptic meningitis [10]
Fever (pyrexia) (includes hyperpyrexia) [4]
Psychosis [5]
Tremor [4]
Vertigo / dizziness [2]

Endocrine/Metabolic

ALT increased [2]
Hyperkalemia [12]
Hypoglycemia [10]
Hyponatremia [11]
Serum creatinine increased [4]

Gastrointestinal/Hepatic

Hepatotoxicity / liver injury / acute liver injury / drug-induced liver injury (DILI) [9]
Nausea [2]
Pancreatitis / acute pancreatitis [4]
Vomiting [4]

Genitourinary

Urolithiasis / ureteral stones / urinary calculi [2]

Hematologic

Agranulocytosis / severe selective neutropenia [4]
Anemia [3]
Hematological adverse effect [2]
Hemolytic anemia [6]
Hemophagocytic lymphohistiocytosis / hemophagocytic syndrome [3]
Methemoglobinemia [2]
Neutropenia (neutrophils decreased) [7]
Pancytopenia (includes bicytopenia) [4]
Thrombocytopenia / platelets decreased [13]

Neuromuscular/Skeletal

Asthenia / fatigue [2]
Myalgia/Myopathy [2]
Rhabdomyolysis [7]

Ocular

Glaucoma (includes acute angle-closure glaucoma) [2]
Myopia [2]
Ocular adverse effect [2]

Renal

Nephrotoxicity / kidney injury / acute kidney injury (AKI) / drug-induced kidney injury [2]
Renal failure [2]

Respiratory

Acute respiratory distress syndrome [2]
Interstitial lung disease / interstitial pneumonitis / interstitial pneumonia (cryptogenic organizing pneumonia) / drug-induced interstitial lung disease [2]

Other

Adverse effects / adverse reactions [15]
Allergic reactions [2]
Death [4]
Side effects [2]

COAGULATION FACTOR IX (RECOMBINANT)

Trade names: Alprolix (Biogen Idec), BeneFIX (Wyeth), Idelvion (CSL Behring), Rixubis (Baxter)
Indications: Treatment and prophylaxis of bleeding in patients with hemophilia B (congenital factor IX deficiency)
Class: Factor IX stimulant
Half-life: variable e.g. 13–43 hours (Xinity); 26 hours (Rixubis); 90–93 hours (Idelvion)
Clinically important, potentially hazardous interactions with: none known
Important contra-indications noted in the prescribing guidelines for: nursing mothers; pediatric patients

---

Skin

Anaphylactoid reactions / anaphylaxis (includes anaphylactic shock) [2]

Central Nervous System

Dysgeusia (taste perversion) [2]

COBICISTAT/ ELVITEGRAVIR/ EMTRICITABINE/ TENOFOVIR ALAFENAMIDE

Trade name: Genvoya (Gilead)
Indications: HIV-1 infection
Class: Antiretroviral, CYP3A inhibitor (cobicistat), Hepatitis B virus necleoside analog reverse transcriptase inhibitor (tenofovir alafenamide), Integrase strand transfer inhibitor (elvitegravir), Nucleoside analog reverse transcriptase inhibitor (emtricitabine)
Half-life: 3.5 hours (cobicistat); 13 hours (elvitegravir); 10 hours (emtricitabine); <1 hour (tenofovir alafenamide)
Clinically important, potentially hazardous interactions with: acyclovir, aminoglycosides, amiodarone, amitriptyline, amlodipine, antacids, antiarrhythmics, atorvastatin, benzodiazepines, bepridil, beta blockers, bosentan, buprenorphine, bupropion, buspirone, calcium channel blockers, cidofovir, clarithromycin, clorazepate, colchicine, desipramine, dexamethasone, diazepam, digoxin, diltiazem, disopyramide, drugs affecting renal function, estazolam, ethosuximide, felodipine, flecainide, flurazepam, fluticasone furoate, fluticasone propionate, ganciclovir, gentamicin, hormonal contraceptives, imipramine, immunosuppressants, itraconazole, ketoconazole, lidocaine, lorazepam, metoprolol, mexiletine, midazolam, naloxone, neuroleptics, nicardipine, nifedipine, nortriptyline, oxcarbazepine, paroxetine hydrochloride, perphenazine, propafenone, quinidine, rifabutin, rifapentine, risperidone, salmeterol, sildenafil, SSRIs, tadalafil, telithromycin, thioridazine, timolol, trazodone, tricyclic antidepressants, valacyclovir, valganciclovir, vardenafil, verapamil, voriconazole, warfarin, zolpidem

Important contra-indications noted in the prescribing guidelines for: nursing mothers
Note: See also separate profiles for emtricitabine and tenofovir alafenamide.
Warning: LACTIC ACIDOSIS/SEVERE HEPATOMEGALY WITH STEATOSIS and POST TREATMENT ACUTE EXACERBATION OF HEPATITIS B

Central Nervous System
Headache (6%)
Gastrointestinal/Hepatic
Diarrhea (7%)
Nausea (5%) [3]
Neuromuscular/Skeletal
Asthenia / fatigue (5%)
Other
Adverse effects / adverse reactions [2]

COBICISTAT/ ELVITEGRAVIR/ EMTRICITABINE/ TENOFOVIR DISOPROXIL

Trade name: Stribild (Gilead)
Indications: HIV-1 infection
Class: Antiretroviral, CYP3A inhibitor (cobicistat), Integrase strand transfer inhibitor (elvitegravir), Nucleoside analog reverse transcriptase inhibitor (emtricitabine and tenofovir disoproxil)
Half-life: 3.5 hours (cobicistat); 13 hours (elvitegravir); 10 hours (emtricitabine); 12–18 hours (tenofovir disoproxil)
Clinically important, potentially hazardous interactions with: acyclovir, adefovir, amiodarone, amitriptyline, amlodipine, antacids, antirarrhythmics, antiretrovirals, atorvastatin, benzodiazepines, bepridil, beta blockers, bosentan, buprenorphine, bupropion, buspirone, calcium channel blockers, carbamazepine, cidofovir, clarithromycin, clonazepam, clorazepate, colchicine, cyclosporine, desipramine, dexamethasone, diazepam, digoxin, diltiazem, disopyramide, drugs affecting renal function, elbasvir & grazoprevir, emtricitabine, estazolam, ethosuximide, felodipine, flecainide, flurazepam, fluticasone propionate, ganciclovir, hormonal contraceptives, imipramine, immunosuppressants, itraconazole, ketoconazole, lamivudine, ledipasvir & sofosbuvir, lidocaine, metoprolol, mexiletine, midazolam, naloxone, neuroleptics, nicardipine, nifedipine, non-nucleoside reverse transcriptase inhibitors, nortriptyline, oxcarbazepine, paroxetine hydrochloride, perphenazine, phenobarbital, phenytoin, propafenone, protease inhibitors, quinidine, rifabutin, rifapentine, risperidone, ritonavir, salmeterol, sedatives / hypnotics, sildenafil, simeprevir, sirolimus, SSRIs, tacrolimus, tadalafil, telithromycin, tenofovir disoproxil, thioridazine, timolol, trazodone, tricyclic antidepressants, valacyclovir, valganciclovir, vardenafil, verapamil, voriconazole, warfarin, zolpidem
Important contra-indications noted in the prescribing guidelines for: the elderly; nursing mothers; pediatric patients
Note: See also separate profiles for emtricitabine and tenofovir disoproxil.
Warning: LACTIC ACIDOSIS/SEVERE HEPATOMEGALY WITH STEATOSIS and POST TREATMENT ACUTE EXACERBATION OF HEPATITIS B

Skin
Rash (3%) [3]
Central Nervous System
Abnormal dreams (9%) [3]
Headache (7%) [5]
Insomnia (3%) [2]
Vertigo / dizziness (3%) [3]
Endocrine/Metabolic
AST increased (2%)
Serum creatinine increased [2]
Gastrointestinal/Hepatic
Diarrhea (12%) [6]
Flatulence (2%)
Gastrointestinal disorder / discomfort [2]
Hepatotoxicity / liver injury / acute liver injury / drug-induced liver injury (DILI) [2]
Nausea (16%) [8]
Genitourinary
Hematuria (3%)
Neuromuscular/Skeletal
Asthenia / fatigue (5%) [2]
Renal
Nephrotoxicity / kidney injury / acute kidney injury (AKI) / drug-induced kidney injury [2]
Proteinuria (39%)
Respiratory
Upper respiratory tract infection [2]
Other
Adverse effects / adverse reactions [5]

COBIMETINIB

Trade name: Cotellic (Genentech)
Indications: Melanoma (unresectable or metastatic) in patients with BRAF V600E or V600K mutations, in combination with vemurafenib
Class: MEK inhibitor (mitogen-activated protein kinase (MEK1 and MEK2) inhibitor)
Half-life: 23–70 hours
Clinically important, potentially hazardous interactions with: carbamazepine, efavirenz, itraconazole, phenytoin, rifampin, St John's wort, strong or moderate CYP3A4 inducers or inhibitors
Pregnancy category: Can cause fetal harm
Important contra-indications noted in the prescribing guidelines for: nursing mothers; pediatric patients

---

Skin
Acneiform eruption / acneiform dermatitis / acneiform rash (16%) [4]
Basal cell carcinoma (5%)
Erythema (10%) [2]
Hyperkeratosis (11%) [3]
Keratoacanthoma (Grzybowski syndrome) [3]
Photosensitivity (46%) [8]
Rash [7]
Squamous cell carcinoma (6%) [6]
Stevens-Johnson syndrome and toxic epidermal necrolysis (SJS/TEN) [2]
Hair
Alopecia / hair loss (15%) [3]
Mucosal
Stomatitis (oral mucositis) (14%)
Cardiovascular
Hypertension (15%)
Central Nervous System
Chills (10%)
Fever (pyrexia) (includes hyperpyrexia) (28%) [4]
Endocrine/Metabolic
ALP increased (71%) [3]
ALT increased (68%) [3]
AST increased (73%) [3]
Creatine phosphokinase (CPK) / creatine kinase increased (hyperCKemia) (79%) [4]
GGT increased (65%)
Hyperkalemia (26%)
Hypoalbuminemia / albumin decreased (42%)
Hypocalcemia (24%)
Hypokalemia (25%)
Hyponatremia (38%)
Hypophosphatemia (68%)
Serum creatinine increased (100%)
Gastrointestinal/Hepatic
Diarrhea (60%) [9]
Gastrointestinal bleeding (4%)
Hepatotoxicity / liver injury / acute liver injury / drug-induced liver injury (DILI) [5]
Nausea (41%) [8]
Vomiting (24%) [5]
Genitourinary
Hematuria (2%)
Hematologic
Anemia (69%) [3]
Hemorrhage (13%)
Lymphopenia (lymphocytopenia) / lymphocytes decreased (73%)
Thrombocytopenia / platelets decreased (18%)
Neuromuscular/Skeletal
Arthralgia [4]
Asthenia / fatigue [7]
Myalgia/Myopathy [2]
Ocular
Chorioretinopathy (13%) [3]
Ocular adverse effect [2]
Retinal detachment (12%) [2]
Vision impaired (15%)
Respiratory
Pneumonitis (<10%)
Other
Adverse effects / adverse reactions [2]

COCAINE

Indications: Topical anesthesia
Class: Anesthetic; local, CNS stimulant
Half-life: 75 minutes
Clinically important, potentially hazardous interactions with: epinephrine, iobenguane, mazindol, mazindol
Pregnancy category: the pregnancy category is X for non-medicinal use
Note: Drug of abuse. Levamisole is a common adulterant of street cocaine.

Skin
- Angioedema (formerly named angioneurotic edema) [3]
- Diaphoresis [3]
- Hyperkeratosis (fingers and palms) [2]
- Necrosis (skin necrosis) [6]
- Purpura [4]
- Pyoderma gangrenosum [5]
- Raynaud's phenomenon [3]
- Scleroderma (reversible) [3]
- Vasculitis (angiitis) / cutaneous vasculitis (angiitis) [14]

Mucosal
- Nasal septal perforation [6]
- Oronasal midline defect (includes cocaine-induced midline destructive lesions) [7]
- Palatal perforation [7]

Cardiovascular
- Angina [2]
- Brugada syndrome [3]
- Cardiac disorder / cardiac dysfunction [2]
- Chest pain [6]
- Myocardial infarction [7]
- Myocardial ischemia [2]

Central Nervous System
- Ageusia (taste loss) / taste disorder (>10%)
- Anosmia (smell loss) / smell disorder (>10%)
- Compulsions / obsessive-compulsive symptoms / obsessive-compulsive disorder [2]
- Hallucinations [4]
- Hallucinations, auditory [2]
- Hallucinations, visual [3]
- Leukoencephalopathy / posterior reversible encephalopathy syndrome (PRES) [4]
- Psychosis [2]
- Seizures [6]
- Suicidal ideation [2]
- Tic disorder [2]
- Tremor (<10%)

Gastrointestinal/Hepatic
- Mesenteric ischemia / colonic ischemia / intestinal ischemia [4]

Genitourinary
- Priapism [5]

Hematologic
- Agranulocytosis / severe selective neutropenia [2]
- Hemolytic uremic syndrome [2]
- Neutropenia (neutrophils decreased) [6]

Neuromuscular/Skeletal
- Arthralgia [2]
- Rhabdomyolysis [19]

Otic
- Hearing loss (hypoacusis) [5]

Renal
- Glomerulonephritis (includes membranous nephropathy) [2]
- Nephrotoxicity / kidney injury / acute kidney injury (AKI) / drug-induced kidney injury [2]

Other
- Cocaine/Levamisole-Associated Autoimmune Syndrome (see also oronasal midline defect) [2]
- Death [3]

COCOA

Family: Sterculiaceae
Scientific names: *Theobroma cacao, Theobroma sativum*
Indications: Oral: asthma, bronchitis, cardiovascular disease, diarrhea. **Topical:** cosmetics, pharmaceutical preparations, foods. Chocolate is produced from cocoa powder
Class: Food supplement
Half-life: 5 hours
Clinically important, potentially hazardous interactions with: aminophylline, caffeine, cimetidine, clozapine, ephedra

---

Skin
- Prurigo [2]

Central Nervous System
- Headache [4]
- Migraine [4]

CODEINE

Synonym: methylmorphine
Trade names: Halotussin (Watson), Nucofed (Monarch), Robitussin AC (Wyeth), Tussi-Organidin (MedPointe)
Indications: Pain, cough suppressant
Class: Opiate agonist
Half-life: 2.5–4 hours
Clinically important, potentially hazardous interactions with: alcohol, cinacalcet, CNS depressants, delavirdine, MAO inhibitors, mianserin, terbinafine, tipranavir
Important contra-indications noted in the prescribing guidelines for: the elderly; nursing mothers; pediatric patients
Note: September 2022: Codeine with ibuprofen – EMA warning for serious renal and gastrointestinal harms The European Medicine Agency Pharmacovigilance Risk Assessment Committee has recommended a change to the product information for codeine with ibuprofen combination medicines to include a warning of serious harms, including death, particularly when taken for prolonged periods at higher than recommended doses. The recommendation is based on several cases of renal, gastrointestinal and metabolic toxicities that have been reported in association with cases of abuse of and dependence from codeine with ibuprofen combinations, some of which have been fatal. .
Warning: DEATH RELATED TO ULTRA-RAPID METABOLISM OF CODEINE TO MORPHINE

Skin
- Angioedema (formerly named angioneurotic edema) [2]
- Dermatitis [5]
- Erythema multiforme [4]
- Exanthems [6]
- Fixed eruption / fixed drug eruption [6]
- Pruritus (itching) [3]
- Rash (<10%)
- Stevens-Johnson syndrome and toxic epidermal necrolysis (SJS/TEN) [2]
- Urticaria / hives (<10%) [9]

Mucosal
- Xerostomia (dry mouth) (<10%)

Central Nervous System
- Somnolence (drowsiness) [4]
- Vertigo / dizziness [3]

Gastrointestinal/Hepatic
- Constipation [4]
- Nausea [3]
- Pancreatitis / acute pancreatitis [5]
- Vomiting [2]

Local
- Injection-site pain (<10%)

Respiratory
- Respiratory depression [4]

Other
- Death [5]

COENZYME Q-10

Family: None
Scientific names: *Mitoquinone, Ubidecarenone, Ubiquinone*
Indications: Congestive heart failure, angina, diabetes, hypertension, breast cancer, increasing exercise tolerance, muscular dystrophy, chronic fatigue
Class: Food supplement
Half-life: N/A
Clinically important, potentially hazardous interactions with: none known
Note: CoQ-10 was first identified in 1957. It is widely used in Japan where millions of Japanese patients receive CoQ-10 as part of their treatment for congestive heart failure.

COLCHICINE

Indications: Gouty arthritis (in adults), gout, familial Mediterranean fever
Class: Alkaloid, Anti-inflammatory, Covid-19 putative drug
Half-life: 27–31 hours (following multiple doses)
Clinically important, potentially hazardous interactions with: amiodarone, aprepitant, atazanavir, atorvastatin, azithromycin, boceprevir, clarithromycin, cobicistat/elvitegravir/emtricitabine/tenofovir alafenamide, cobicistat/elvitegravir/emtricitabine/tenofovir disoproxil, conivaptan, cyanocobalamin, cyclosporine, darunavir, dasatinib, delavirdine, digoxin, diltiazem, efavirenz, erythromycin, fenofibrate, fibrates, fluvastatin, gemfibrozil, grapefruit juice, HMG-CoA reductase inhibitors, indinavir, itraconazole, ketoconazole, lapatinib, lopinavir, ombitasvir/paritaprevir/ritonavir, P-glycoprotein inhibitors or inducers, pravastatin, protease inhibitors, ritonavir, rosuvastatin, saxagliptin, simvastatin, strong CYP3A4 inhibitors, telithromycin, troleandomycin, verapamil, voriconazole
Important contra-indications noted in the prescribing guidelines for: the elderly
Note: Contra-indicated in patients with renal or hepatic impairment where P-glycoprotein or strong CYP3A4 inhibitors are also prescribed. Low-dose colchicine (0.5 mg daily) has been approved by the FDA for secondary prevention in patients with coronary disease.

Skin
- Pruritus (itching) [2]
- Staphylococcal scalded skin syndrome [2]
- Stevens-Johnson syndrome and toxic epidermal necrolysis (SJS/TEN) [3]

Vasculitis (angiitis) / cutaneous vasculitis (angiitis) [2]

Hair

Alopecia / hair loss (<10%) [6]

Central Nervous System

Headache (2%)
Neurotoxicity [3]

Endocrine/Metabolic

Hypertransaminasemia (hepatic transaminitis) / elevated transaminases [2]

Gastrointestinal/Hepatic

Abdominal pain (<20%) [4]
Diarrhea (23%) [11]
Gastrointestinal adverse reaction [6]
Gastrointestinal disorder / discomfort [2]
Hepatotoxicity / liver injury / acute liver injury / drug-induced liver injury (DILI) [3]
Nausea (<20%) [4]
Vomiting (<20%) [4]

Hematologic

Leukocytopenia (leukopenia) / leukocytes (white blood cells) decreased [2]

Neuromuscular/Skeletal

Asthenia / fatigue (<4%)
Gouty tophi (4%)
Myalgia/Myopathy [22]
Rhabdomyolysis [20]

Respiratory

Pharyngolaryngeal pain (3%)

Other

Adverse effects / adverse reactions [8]
Death [3]
Side effects (14%)

COLESEVELAM

Trade names: Cholestagel (Genzyme), Welchol (Sankyo)
Indications: Hypercholesterolemia, hyperlipidemia, Type II diabetes mellitus
Class: Bile acid sequestrant
Half-life: N/A
Clinically important, potentially hazardous interactions with: cyclosporine, deferasirox, estradiol, glyburide, levothyroxine, olmesartan, phenytoin, warfarin
Important contra-indications noted in the prescribing guidelines for: pediatric patients
Note: Contra-indicated in patients with a history of bowel obstruction, with serum triglyceride concentrations >500 mg/dL or with a history of hypertriglyceridemia-induced pancreatitis.

Cardiovascular

Hypertension (3%)

Central Nervous System

Headache [2]

Endocrine/Metabolic

Hypoglycemia (3%) [3]

Gastrointestinal/Hepatic

Abdominal pain (4%)
Constipation (9–10%) [3]
Diarrhea (3%)
Dyspepsia / functional dyspepsia (indigestion) (see also gastroparesis) (4–6%) [3]
Flatulence (11%)
Gastrointestinal disorder / discomfort [4]
Nausea (3%)

Neuromuscular/Skeletal

Myalgia/Myopathy (2%)

Respiratory

Nasopharyngitis (4%)

Other

Adverse effects / adverse reactions [5]

COLESTIPOL

Trade name: Colestid (Pfizer)
Indications: Primary hypercholesterolemia
Class: Anion exchange resin, Bile acid sequestrant, Lipid regulator
Half-life: N/A
Clinically important, potentially hazardous interactions with: deferasirox, propranolol, tetracycline, ursodiol

COLISTIN

Synonym: Polymyxin E
Trade name: Colomycin (Forest)
Indications: Gram-negative bacterial infections, cystic fibrosis
Class: Antibiotic, Antibiotic; polymyxin, Antimicrobial
Half-life: 8 hours
Clinically important, potentially hazardous interactions with: aminoglycosides, bacitracin, cephalothin, pyridostigmine, teicoplanin
Important contra-indications noted in the prescribing guidelines for: nursing mothers; pediatric patients

---

Skin

Dermatitis [3]

Central Nervous System

Neurotoxicity [6]
Paresthesias [3]
Seizures [3]

Neuromuscular/Skeletal

Ataxia [2]

Renal

Bartter-like syndrome [3]
Nephrotoxicity / kidney injury / acute kidney injury (AKI) / drug-induced kidney injury [33]

Other

Death [2]

COLLAGEN (BOVINE)

Trade names: Bellafill (Suneva), Zyderm (Inamed), Zyplast (Inamed)
Indications: Cataract surgery (collagen shields), depressed cutaneous scars, facial lines, wrinkles, glottic insufficiency, phonosurgey, urinary incontinence
Class: Protein
Half-life: Several months to years
Clinically important, potentially hazardous interactions with: argatroban, avitene
Important contra-indications noted in the prescribing guidelines for: nursing mothers
Note: A reaction to the anesthetic, lidocaine, in liquid collagen injections may occur. Artecoll and Bellafill contain polymethyl-methacrylate microspheres.

Skin

Abscess [2]
Churg-Strauss syndrome [7]
Dermatomyositis [3]
Edema / fluid retention [2]
Erythema [3]
Granulomatous reaction [2]
Hypersensitivity [10]
Induration [3]
Panniculitis [2]

Neuromuscular/Skeletal

Arthralgia [2]
Polymyositis [3]

Other

Adverse effects / adverse reactions [12]
Allergic reactions [7]

COMFREY

Family: Boraginaceae
Scientific names: *Symphytum asperum, Symphytum officinale, Symphytum peregrinum, Symphytum x uplandicum*
Indications: Leaf: Gastric and duodenal ulcer, rheumatic pain, gout, arthritis. **Topical:** poultice for bruises, sprains, athlete's foot, crural ulcers, mastitis, varicose ulcers. **Root**: Gastric and duodenal ulcers, hematemesis, colitis, diarrhea. **Topical:** ulcers, wounds, fractures, hernia
Class: Carminative
Half-life: N/A
Clinically important, potentially hazardous interactions with: eucalyptus
Note: The FDA warns that comfrey contains pyrrolizidine alkaloids that can cause cirrhosis and liver failure when taken orally in high doses. Topical application is safer and more effective; allantoin in comfrey stimulates cell proliferation, accelerating wound healing.
Oral products containing comfrey are banned in the USA, UK, Australia, Canada and Germany.

Skin

Erythema [2]
Pruritus (itching) [2]

Cardiovascular

Veno-occlusive disease [4]

Gastrointestinal/Hepatic

Hepatotoxicity / liver injury / acute liver injury / drug-induced liver injury (DILI) [3]

Local

Application-site reactions [2]

Other

Adverse effects / adverse reactions [2]
Death [2]

CONIVAPTAN

Trade name: Vaprisol (Astellas)
Indications: Hyponatremia, SIADH
Class: CYP3A4 inhibitor, Vasopressin receptor antagonist
Half-life: 5 hours
Clinically important, potentially hazardous interactions with: acetaminophen, albendazole, alfuzosin, almotriptan, alosetron, ambrisentan, amitriptyline, amlodipine, antifungals, aprepitant, artemether/lumefantrine, atorvastatin, bexarotene, bortezomib, brigatinib, brinzolamide, bupivacaine, cabazitaxel, cabozantinib, ciclesonide, cilostazol, cinacalcet, citalopram, clarithromycin, colchicine, copanlisib, cyclobenzaprine, CYP3A4 inhibitors or substrates, darunavir, dasatinib, deferasirox, delavirdine, dienogest, digoxin, docetaxel,

dolasetron, dronedarone, dutasteride, efavirenz, enalapril, eplerenone, estradiol, eszopiclone, everolimus, fentanyl, fesoterodine, fingolimod, flibanserin, gefitinib, guanfacine, halofantrine, indinavir, itraconazole, ixabepilone, ketoconazole, lapatinib, lomitapide, maraviroc, meloxicam, metaxalone, methylprednisolone, micafungin, midazolam, midostaurin, mifepristone, mometasone, neratinib, nilotinib, nisoldipine, oxybutynin, pantoprazole, paricalcitol, pazopanib, pimecrolimus, pioglitazone, ponatinib, prasugrel, ramelteon, ranolazine, ribociclib, ritonavir, rivaroxaban, romidepsin, rosuvastatin, ruxolitinib, salmeterol, saxagliptin, sildenafil, silodosin, simvastatin, sorafenib, St John's wort, tadalafil, tamsulosin, telithromycin, temsirolimus, terbinafine, tiagabine, tiotropium, tipranavir, tolvaptan, trimethoprim, ulipristal, vardenafil, venetoclax, vorapaxar, voriconazole, ziprasidone
Important contra-indications noted in the prescribing guidelines for: nursing mothers; pediatric patients

---

Skin
- Erythema (3%)
- Peripheral edema (3–8%)
- Pruritus (itching) (<5%)

Mucosal
- Oral candidiasis (2%)
- Xerostomia (dry mouth) (4%)

Cardiovascular
- Atrial fibrillation (2–5%)
- Hypertension (6–8%)
- Hypotension (5–8%) [4]
- Orthostatic hypotension (6–14%)
- Phlebitis (32–51%)

Central Nervous System
- Confusion (<5%)
- Fever (pyrexia) (includes hyperpyrexia) (5–11%) [2]
- Headache (8–10%)
- Insomnia (4–5%)

Endocrine/Metabolic
- Hypokalemia (10–22%)
- Hypomagnesemia (2–5%)
- Hyponatremia (6–8%)

Gastrointestinal/Hepatic
- Constipation (6–8%)
- Diarrhea (<7%)
- Nausea (3–5%)
- Vomiting (5–7%)

Genitourinary
- Urinary tract infection (4–5%)

Hematologic
- Anemia (5–6%)

Local
- Infusion-site erythema (<6%)
- Infusion-site pain (<5%)
- Infusion-site reactions (63–73%) [5]

Respiratory
- Pharyngolaryngeal pain (<5%)
- Pneumonia (2–5%)

Other
- Dipsia (thirst) / polydipsia (3–6%) [2]

COPANLISIB

Trade name: Aliqopa (Bayer)
Indications: Relapsed follicular lymphoma in adult patients who have received at least two prior systemic therapies
Class: Kinase inhibitor, Phosphoinositide 3-kinase (Phosphatidylinositol 3-kinase) (PI3K) inhibitor
Half-life: 39 hours
Clinically important, potentially hazardous interactions with: boceprevir, carbamazepine, clarithromycin, cobicistat, conivaptan, danoprevir, diltiazem, elvitegravir, enzalutamide, grapefruit juice, idelalisib, indinavir, itraconazole, ketoconazole, lopinavir, mitotane, nefazodone, nelfinavir, ombitasvir/paritaprevir/ritonavir and dasabuvir, phenytoin, posaconazole, rifampin, ritonavir, saquinavir, St John's wort, strong CYP3A4 inducers or inhibitors, tipranavir, troleandomycin, voriconazole
Pregnancy category: Can cause fetal harm
Important contra-indications noted in the prescribing guidelines for: nursing mothers; pediatric patients

---

Skin
- Rash (15%)

Mucosal
- Mucosal inflammation (8%)
- Stomatitis (oral mucositis) (14%)

Cardiovascular
- Hypertension (26%) [7]

Central Nervous System
- Dysesthesia (7%)
- Paresthesias (7%)

Endocrine/Metabolic
- Hyperglycemia (includes glucose increased) (54%) [9]
- Hyperlipasemia (21%)
- Hypertriglyceridemia (includes triglycerides increased) (58%)
- Hyperuricemia (25%)
- Hypophosphatemia (44%)

Gastrointestinal/Hepatic
- Diarrhea (36%) [5]
- Nausea (26%) [4]
- Vomiting (13%)

Hematologic
- Hemoglobin decreased (78%)
- Leukocytopenia (leukopenia) / leukocytes (white blood cells) decreased (36%)
- Lymphopenia (lymphocytopenia) / lymphocytes decreased (78%)
- Neutropenia (neutrophils decreased) (32%) [4]
- Thrombocytopenia / platelets decreased (22%) [2]

Neuromuscular/Skeletal
- Asthenia / fatigue (36%) [3]

Respiratory
- Pneumonitis (9%)

Other
- Infection (21%)

CORDYCEPS

Family: Ascomycetes; Clavicipitaceae
Scientific name: *Cordyceps sinensis*
Indications: Anemia, arrhythmia, anti-aging, atherosclerosis, bronchitis, cough, dizziness, hyperlipidemia, athletic performance, lethargy, liver disorders, male sexual dysfunction, nocturia, tinnitus
Class: Immunomodulator
Half-life: N/A
Clinically important, potentially hazardous interactions with: none known

CORTISONE

Trade name: Cortone (Merck)
Indications: Arthralgia, dermatoses
Class: Corticosteroid / Glucocorticoid
Half-life: N/A
Clinically important, potentially hazardous interactions with: chlorpropamide, diuretics, ethambutol, live vaccines, pancuronium, rifampin
Important contra-indications noted in the prescribing guidelines for: nursing mothers

---

Neuromuscular/Skeletal
- Osteonecrosis / avascular necrosis (includes steroid-induced osteonecrosis of the femoral head) [15]
- Osteoporosis [10]
- Tendinopathy/Tendon rupture [2]

Ocular
- Cataract [5]
- Glaucoma (includes acute angle-closure glaucoma) [8]

Other
- Adverse effects / adverse reactions [2]

COVID-19 VACCINE, MRNA

Synonyms: Moderna Covid-19 Vaccine, mRNA
Trade name: Spikevax (Moderna Biotech)
Indications: Prevention of coronavirus disease 2019 (Covid-19) caused by severe acute respiratory syndrome coronavirus 2 (SARS-CoV-2)
Class: Covid-19 vaccine, Vaccine
Clinically important, potentially hazardous interactions with: none known
Pregnancy category: Available data on pregnant women are insufficient to inform vaccine-associated risks of Moderna Covid-19 Vaccine, mRNA in pregnancy.
Note: Do not administer Moderna Covid-19 Vaccine, mRNA to individuals with a known history of severe allergic reaction (e.g., anaphylaxis) to any component of this vaccine. Postmarketing data demonstrate increased risks of myocarditis and pericarditis, particularly within 7 days following the second dose of Moderna Covid-19 Vaccine, mRNA. The observed risk is higher among males under 40 years of age than among females and older males. The observed risk is highest in males 18 through 24 years of age. Although some cases required intensive care support, available data from short-term follow-up suggest that most individuals have had resolution of symptoms with conservative management. Information is not yet available about potential

long-term sequelae. The CDC has published considerations related to myocarditis and pericarditis after vaccination, including for vaccination of individuals with a history of myocarditis or pericarditis (https://www.cdc.gov/vaccines/covid-19/clinical-considerations/myocarditis.html).

Skin
Linear IgA bullous dermatosis [2]

Central Nervous System
Chills (In study participants 18 through 64 years of age.) (50%)
Fever (pyrexia) (includes hyperpyrexia) (In study participants 18 through 64 years of age.) (17%)
Headache (In study participants 18 through 64 years of age.) (69%)

Gastrointestinal/Hepatic
Nausea (In study participants 18 through 64 years of age.) (26%)
Vomiting (In study participants 18 through 64 years of age.) (26%)

Local
Injection-site erythema (In study participants 18 through 64 years of age.) (11%)
Injection-site pain (In study participants 18 through 64 years of age.) (93%)
Injection-site swelling (In study participants 18 through 64 years of age.) (15%)

Neuromuscular/Skeletal
Arthralgia (In study participants 18 through 64 years of age.) (49%)
Asthenia / fatigue (In study participants 18 through 64 years of age.) (72%)
Myalgia/Myopathy (In study participants 18 through 64 years of age.) (65%)

Other
Adverse effects / adverse reactions [7]

COVID-19 VACCINE, MRNA

Synonym: Pfizer-BioNTech Covid-19 mRNA Vaccine
Trade names: BNT162b2 (Pfizer-BioNTech), Comirnaty (Pfizer-BioNTech), Comirnaty (Pfizer-BioNTech), Tozinameran (Pfizer-BioNTech)
Indications: Prevention of coronavirus disease 2019 (Covid-19) caused by severe acute respiratory syndrome coronavirus 2 (SARS-CoV-2)
Class: Covid-19 vaccine, Vaccine
Clinically important, potentially hazardous interactions with: none known
Pregnancy category: Insufficient data to inform of vaccine-associated risks in pregnancy.
Note: Increased risks of myocarditis and pericarditis, particularly within 7 days following the second dose. The observed risk is higher among males under 40 years of age than among females and older males. The observed risk is highest in males 12 through 17 years of age. Although some cases required intensive care support, available data from short-term follow-up suggest that most individuals have had resolution of symptoms with conservative management. Information is not yet available about potential long-term sequelae. The Centers for Disease Control and Prevention (CDC) have published considerations related to myocarditis and pericarditis after vaccination, including for vaccination of individuals with a history of myocarditis or pericarditis.

Skin
Baboon syndrome / symmetrical drug-related intertriginous and flexural exanthema (SDRIFE) [2]
Lupus erythematosus (subacute cutaneous lupus erythematosus (SCLE)) [2]
Pernio / chilblain (includes pernio-like lesions) [4]
Pityriasis lichenoides / pityriasis lichenoides chronica / pityriasis lichenoides et varioliformis acuta [2]
Sweet's syndrome [3]
Thrombocytopenic purpura [4]

Cardiovascular
Myocarditis [2]

Central Nervous System
Chills (25–42%)
Fever (pyrexia) (includes hyperpyrexia) (12–18%)
Headache (46–65%)
Parsonage-Turner syndrome (PTS) (brachial plexopathy; neuralgic amyotrophy) [2]

Genitourinary
Vulvar ulceration [3]

Hematologic
Aplastic anemia [5]
Thrombocytopenia / platelets decreased [4]

Local
Injection-site erythema (10%)
Injection-site pain (78–89%) [2]
Injection-site swelling (11–12%)

Neuromuscular/Skeletal
Asthenia / fatigue (57–70%)
Bone pain / joint pain (22–28%)
Musculoskeletal pain (33–46%)
Rhabdomyolysis [4]

Other
Adverse effects / adverse reactions [18]

CRANBERRY

Family: Ericaceae
Scientific name: *Vaccinium oxycoccus*
Indications: Erythema, hyperplasia, thrush, cystitis, prevention of urinary tract infections, tumor inhibition, influenza, common cold, scurvy, pleurisy
Class: Diuretic, Proanthocyanadin
Half-life: N/A
Clinically important, potentially hazardous interactions with: none known
Note: Cranberry juice contains oxalates, a common component of kidney stones, and should be limited in patients with a history of nephrolithiasis.

CREATINE

Scientific names: *N-(aminoiminomethyl)-N methyl glycine, N-amidinosarcosine*
Indications: Improve exercise performance, increase muscle mass, heart failure, neuromuscular disease, cholesterol-lowering, amyotrophic lateral sclerosis, rheumatoid arthritis, cardiac surgery (IV)
Class: Food supplement
Half-life: N/A
Clinically important, potentially hazardous interactions with: none known
Note: Creatine is found primarily in skeletal muscle (95%), also in heart, brain, testes and other tissues. The body synthesizes 1–2 grams of creatine a day.
Creatine use is widespread among amateur and professional athletes. Americans use more than 4 million kilograms of creatine each year.

Gastrointestinal/Hepatic
Hepatotoxicity / liver injury / acute liver injury / drug-induced liver injury (DILI) [3]

Neuromuscular/Skeletal
Myalgia/Myopathy [2]
Rhabdomyolysis [5]

Renal
Nephrotoxicity / kidney injury / acute kidney injury (AKI) / drug-induced kidney injury [2]

Other
Adverse effects / adverse reactions [2]

CRIZOTINIB

Trade name: Xalkori (Pfizer)
Indications: Advanced or metastatic non-small cell lung cancer in ALK-positive patients
Class: Anaplastic lymphoma kinase (ALK) inhibitor, MET (mesenchymal-epithelial transition) inhibitor / MET tyrosine kinase inhibitor, Tyrosine kinase inhibitor
Half-life: 42 hours
Clinically important, potentially hazardous interactions with: alfentanil, atazanavir, carbamazepine, clarithromycin, cyclosporine, CYP3A4 inducers, inhibitors or substrates, dihydroergotamine, efavirenz, ergotamine, fentanyl, grapefruit juice, indinavir, itraconazole, ketoconazole, nefazodone, nelfinavir, neratinib, olaparib, phenobarbital, phenytoin, pimozide, quinidine, rifabutin, rifampin, ritonavir, saquinavir, sirolimus, St John's wort, tacrolimus, telithromycin, troleandomycin, voriconazole
Important contra-indications noted in the prescribing guidelines for: nursing mothers; pediatric patients

---

Skin
Edema / fluid retention (38%) [15]
Peripheral edema [7]
Photosensitivity [3]
Rash (16%) [5]

Mucosal
Rectal perforation [2]
Stomatitis (oral mucositis) (11%)

Cardiovascular
Bradycardia / sinus bradycardia (5%) [7]
Cardiotoxicity [2]
Chest pain (12%)
QT interval prolonged / QT prolongation [9]

Central Nervous System
Dysgeusia (taste perversion) (13%) [7]
Fever (pyrexia) (includes hyperpyrexia) (12%) [2]
Headache (13%)
Insomnia (12%)
Neurotoxicity (23%) [2]
Vertigo / dizziness (24%) [6]

Endocrine/Metabolic
ALT increased (15%) [14]
Appetite decreased (27%) [5]
AST increased (11%) [12]
Dehydration [2]
Hyperbilirubinemia [3]
Hypertransaminasemia (hepatic transaminitis) / elevated transaminases [2]
Hypocalcemia [2]
Hypogonadism (includes androgen deficiency) [6]
Hypophosphatemia [5]

Gastrointestinal/Hepatic
Abdominal pain (16%) [2]
Constipation (38%) [14]
Diarrhea (49%) [30]
Dyspepsia / functional dyspepsia (indigestion) (see also gastroparesis) [3]
Dysphagia [3]
Esophagitis [8]
Gastroesophageal reflux [2]
Hepatitis [5]
Hepatotoxicity / liver injury / acute liver injury / drug-induced liver injury (DILI) [15]
Nausea (57%) [30]
Vomiting (45%) [27]

Hematologic
Anemia [4]
Leukocytopenia (leukopenia) / leukocytes (white blood cells) decreased [2]
Lymphopenia (lymphocytopenia) / lymphocytes decreased (11%) [5]
Neutropenia (neutrophils decreased) (5%) [10]

Neuromuscular/Skeletal
Arthralgia (11%)
Asthenia / fatigue (31%) [16]
Back pain (11%)
Bone pain / joint pain [2]

Ocular
Diplopia (double vision) [2]
Ocular adverse effect (64%) [14]
Photophobia [2]
Photopsia [4]
Reduced visual acuity [2]
Vision blurred [7]
Vision impaired [5]
Visual disturbances [18]
Vitreous floaters / floaters / myodesopsia / myiodesopsia / muscae volitantes [2]

Renal
Nephrotoxicity / kidney injury / acute kidney injury (AKI) / drug-induced kidney injury [10]

Respiratory
Cough (21%)
Dyspnea / shortness of breath (22%) [2]
Pneumonia [3]
Pneumonitis [6]
Pneumothorax [2]
Pulmonary toxicity [11]
Upper respiratory tract infection (20%)

Other
Adverse effects / adverse reactions [5]
Death [4]
Side effects [2]

CROMOLYN

Synonyms: cromolyn sodium; disodium cromoglycate
Trade names: Gastrocrom (Celltech), Intal (Monarch), Nasalcrom (Pfizer), Opticrom (Allergan)
Indications: Allergic rhinitis, asthma, mastocytosis
Class: Mast cell stabilizer
Half-life: 80 minutes
Clinically important, potentially hazardous interactions with: none known

---

Skin
Anaphylactoid reactions / anaphylaxis (includes anaphylactic shock) [5]
Angioedema (formerly named angioneurotic edema) (<10%) [4]
Dermatitis (generalized) [4]
Facial rash [2]
Urticaria / hives [3]

Mucosal
Xerostomia (dry mouth) (<10%)

Central Nervous System
Dysgeusia (taste perversion) (>10%)

CYANOCOBALAMIN

Synonym: Vitamin B_{12}
Trade name: Nascobal (Nastech)
Indications: Vitamin B_{12} deficiency, pernicious anemia
Class: Vitamin
Half-life: 6 days
Clinically important, potentially hazardous interactions with: colchicine

---

Skin
Acneiform eruption / acneiform dermatitis / acneiform rash [8]
Anaphylactoid reactions / anaphylaxis (includes anaphylactic shock) [6]
Dermatitis [2]
Exanthems [3]
Hypersensitivity [2]
Nicolau syndrome [2]
Pruritus (itching) (<10%)
Urticaria / hives [7]

Other
Allergic reactions [3]

CYCLAMATE

Trade name: Sucaryl (AbbVie)
Indications: Sweetening
Class: Sweetening agent
Half-life: N/A
Clinically important, potentially hazardous interactions with: none known
Note: Cyclamate is a sulfonamide and can be absorbed systemically. Sulfonamides can produce severe, possibly fatal, reactions such as toxic epidermal necrolysis and Stevens-Johnson syndrome.

Skin
Photosensitivity [7]
Pruritus (itching) [3]
Urticaria / hives [2]

CYCLOBENZAPRINE

Trade name: Flexeril (McNeil)
Indications: Muscle spasms
Class: Central muscle relaxant
Half-life: 8–37 hours
Clinically important, potentially hazardous interactions with: acetylcholinesterase inhibitors, anticholinergics, barbiturates, cisapride, CNS depressants, conivaptan, CYP1A2 inhibitors, droperidol, levomepromazine, linezolid, MAO inhibitors, phendimetrazine, pramlintide, safinamide
Important contra-indications noted in the prescribing guidelines for: the elderly; nursing mothers; pediatric patients

---

Mucosal
Xerostomia (dry mouth) (7–32%) [7]

Central Nervous System
Confusion (<3%)
Dysgeusia (taste perversion) (<3%)
Headache (5%) [3]
Irritability (<3%)
Nervousness (<3%)
Serotonin syndrome [3]
Somnolence (drowsiness) (29–39%) [8]
Vertigo / dizziness (<11%) [8]

Gastrointestinal/Hepatic
Abdominal pain (<3%)
Constipation (<3%) [3]
Diarrhea (<3%)
Nausea (<3%)

Neuromuscular/Skeletal
Asthenia / fatigue (6%) [3]

Ocular
Vision blurred (<3%)

Respiratory
Pharyngitis (sore throat) (<3%)
Upper respiratory tract infection (<3%)

Other
Adverse effects / adverse reactions [2]

CYCLOPENTHIAZIDE

Trade name: Navidrex (Goldshield)
Indications: Hypertension
Class: Antihypertensive
Clinically important, potentially hazardous interactions with: ACE inhibitors, ACTH, allopurinol, amantadine, amphotericin, atropine, beta blockers, biperiden, calcium antagonists, calcium salts, carbenoxolone, cholestyramine, corticosteroids, cyclophosphamide, diazoxide, digitalis, digoxin, ergocalciferol, guanethidine, indomethacin, lithium, methotrexate, methyldopa, vasodilators

CYCLOPHOSPHAMIDE

Synonyms: CPM; CTX; CYT
Trade names: Cytoxan (Mead Johnson), Neosar (Gensia)
Indications: Lymphomas, minimal change nephrotic syndrome in pediatric patients
Class: Alkylating agent
Half-life: 3–12 hours
Clinically important, potentially hazardous interactions with: aldesleukin, azathioprine, belimumab, clozapine, cyclopenthiazide, cyclosporine, dexamethasone, etanercept, itraconazole, mycophenolate, pentostatin, prednisone, vaccines
Important contra-indications noted in the prescribing guidelines for: nursing mothers
Note: Contra-indicated in patients with urinary outflow obstruction.

Skin
Acral erythema [3]
Anaphylactoid reactions / anaphylaxis (includes anaphylactic shock) [3]
Cutaneous toxicity / skin toxicity [6]
Edema / fluid retention [5]
Exanthems [4]
Flushing / rubefaction (<10%)
Graft-versus-host reaction [2]
Hand–foot syndrome (palmar–plantar erythrodysesthesia) [10]
Herpes zoster [4]
Hypersensitivity [6]
Kaposi's sarcoma [2]
Lupus erythematosus (subacute cutaneous lupus erythematosus (SCLE)) [2]
Lymphoma [4]
Pemphigus [2]
Peripheral edema [2]
Pigmentation (Skin) (includes hyperpigmentation) [16]
Pruritus (itching) [2]
Radiation recall dermatitis [6]
Rash (<10%) [6]
Scleroderma [2]
Squamous cell carcinoma [2]
Stevens-Johnson syndrome and toxic epidermal necrolysis (SJS/TEN) [3]
Urticaria / hives [8]
Vasculitis (angiitis) / cutaneous vasculitis (angiitis) [2]

Hair
Alopecia / hair loss [32]

Nails
Beau's lines (transverse nail bands) [2]
Melanonychia [3]
Muehrcke's lines [4]
Nail pigmentation [17]

Mucosal
Gingival pigmentation [2]
Mucositis [4]
Oral ulceration [2]
Stomatitis (oral mucositis) (10%) [8]

Cardiovascular
Atrial fibrillation [2]
Cardiotoxicity [6]
Hypotension [2]

Central Nervous System
Anorexia [3]
Dysgeusia (taste perversion) [2]
Fever (pyrexia) (includes hyperpyrexia) [3]
Headache [3]
Leukoencephalopathy / posterior reversible encephalopathy syndrome (PRES) [7]
Neurotoxicity [7]
Peripheral neuropathy [8]

Endocrine/Metabolic
Amenorrhea [16]
Diabetes mellitus [2]
Hyperglycemia (includes glucose increased) [2]
Hyponatremia [5]
Menstrual irregularities [2]
SIADH [9]

Gastrointestinal/Hepatic
Abdominal pain [2]
Constipation [2]
Diarrhea [10]
Hepatotoxicity / liver injury / acute liver injury / drug-induced liver injury (DILI) [13]
Nausea [12]
Vomiting [12]

Genitourinary
Cystitis (includes interstitial cystitis / bladder pain syndrome) [11]
Urinary tract infection [2]

Hematologic
Anemia [11]
Cytopenia [2]
Febrile neutropenia [17]
Hemorrhage [2]
Hemotoxicity [10]
Leukocytopenia (leukopenia) / leukocytes (white blood cells) decreased [14]
Lymphopenia (lymphocytopenia) / lymphocytes decreased [3]
Myelosuppression / bone marrow suppression / myelotoxicity [6]
Neutropenia (neutrophils decreased) [38]
Sepsis [2]
Thrombocytopenia / platelets decreased [17]

Local
Infusion-related reactions [2]

Neuromuscular/Skeletal
Arthralgia [2]
Asthenia / fatigue [16]
Myalgia/Myopathy [7]

Respiratory
Pneumonia [4]

Other
Adverse effects / adverse reactions [17]
Allergic reactions [2]
Death [9]
Hiccups / singultus [4]
Infection [23]
Malignancies [2]

CYCLOSERINE

Synonym: D-cycloserine
Trade name: Seromycin (Lilly)
Indications: Tuberculosis
Class: Antibiotic, Antimicrobial, Drug-resistant antituberculosis agent
Half-life: 10 hours
Clinically important, potentially hazardous interactions with: none known
Important contra-indications noted in the prescribing guidelines for: nursing mothers; pediatric patients

---

Skin
Dermatitis [2]
Exanthems [4]
Lichenoid eruption / lichenoid reaction [2]

Mucosal
Gingival hyperplasia / gingival hypertrophy / gingival enlargement / gingival overgrowth [3]

Central Nervous System
Depression [2]
Insomnia [2]
Neuropsychiatric / neuropsychological adverse effect [2]
Neurotoxicity [2]
Psychosis [10]
Seizures [5]
Suicidal ideation [2]

Renal
Nephrotoxicity / kidney injury / acute kidney injury (AKI) / drug-induced kidney injury [2]

Other
Adverse effects / adverse reactions [4]

CYCLOSPORINE

Synonyms: Cyclosporine-A; CsA; CyA
Trade names: Neoral (Novartis), Restasis (Allergan), Sandimmune (Novartis)
Indications: Rheumatoid arthritis, prophylaxis of organ rejection in transplants, psoriasis, Restasis is indicated for patients with moderate-to-severe dry eye syndrome
Class: Antipsoriatic agent, Calcineurin inhibitor, Disease-modifying antirheumatic drug (DMARD), Immunosuppressant
Half-life: 10–27 hours (adults)
Clinically important, potentially hazardous interactions with: afatinib, aliskiren, ambrisentan, amiloride, aminoglycosides, amiodarone, amphotericin B, ampicillin, amprenavir, anisindione, anticoagulants, armodafinil, atazanavir, atorvastatin, azathioprine, azithromycin, bacampicillin, basiliximab, benazepril, berotralstat, bezafibrate, boceprevir, bosentan, bupropion, captopril, carbenicillin, caspofungin, ceritinib, cholestyramine, cholic acid, choline fenofibrate, cilazapril, ciprofloxacin, clarithromycin, cloxacillin, co-trimoxazole, cobicistat/elvitegravir/emtricitabine/tenofovir disoproxil, colchicine, colesevelam, corticosteroids, crizotinib, cyclophosphamide, dabigatran, daclizumab, danazol, daptomycin, darifenacin, darunavir, dasatinib, delavirdine, dichlorphenamide, diclofenac, dicloxacillin, dicumarol, digoxin, diltiazem, disulfiram, docetaxel, doxycycline, dronedarone, echinacea, efavirenz, elbasvir & grazoprevir, eluxadoline, enalapril, enzalutamide, erythromycin, ethotoin, etoposide, etoricoxib, everolimus, ezetimibe, flunisolide, fluoxymesterone, fluvastatin, foscarnet, fosinopril, fosphenytoin, gemfibrozil, glecaprevir & pibrentasvir, grapefruit juice, Hemophilus B vaccine, HMG-CoA reductase inhibitors, imatinib, imipenem/cilastatin, indinavir, influenza vaccine, irbesartan, itraconazole, ketoconazole, lanreotide, letermovir, levofloxacin, lisinopril, lopinavir, lovastatin, lumateperone, meloxicam, mephenytoin, methicillin, methoxsalen, methylphenidate, methylprednisolone, methyltestosterone, mezlocillin, micafungin, mifepristone, mizolastine, moxifloxacin, mycophenolate, nafcillin, naldemedine, natalizumab, nelfinavir, neratinib, nevirapine, nifedipine, nisoldipine, norfloxacin, NSAIDs, ofloxacin, olmesartan, omeprazole,

orlistat, osimertinib, oxacillin, oxcarbazepine, ozanimod, pasireotide, penicillins, phenytoin, pitavastatin, posaconazole, pravastatin, prednisolone, prednisone, pristinamycin, quinapril, rabeprazole, ramipril, ranolazine, revefenacin, ribociclib, rifabutin, rifampin, rifapentine, ritonavir, rosuvastatin, sevelamer, silodosin, simvastatin, sirolimus, sofosbuvir/velpatasvir/voxilaprevir, spironolactone, St John's wort, sulfacetamide, sulfadiazine, sulfamethoxazole, sulfisoxazole, sulfonamides, tacrolimus, telithromycin, temsirolimus, tenoxicam, terbinafine, testosterone, ticarcillin, tinidazole, tipranavir, tofacitinib, tolvaptan, trabectedin, trandolapril, triamterene, trimethoprim, troleandomycin, ubrogepant, ursodiol, vaccines, vecuronium, venetoclax, voriconazole, warfarin, zofenopril

Important contra-indications noted in the prescribing guidelines for: nursing mothers; pediatric patients

Note: Restasis is an ophthalmic emulsion.

Skin
- Acne keloid [2]
- Acneiform eruption / acneiform dermatitis / acneiform rash [7]
- Anaphylactoid reactions / anaphylaxis (includes anaphylactic shock) [8]
- Basal cell carcinoma [4]
- Candidiasis / candidosis [2]
- Cutaneous toxicity / skin toxicity [2]
- Cyst / pseudocyst [5]
- Edema / fluid retention (5–14%)
- Erythromelalgia / erythermalgia [3]
- Fibroadenoma [2]
- Flushing / rubefaction (2–5%) [5]
- Folliculitis [9]
- Herpes simplex [4]
- Herpes zoster [2]
- Hot flashes / hot flushes [2]
- Hypersensitivity [2]
- Kaposi's sarcoma [5]
- Keratoses [3]
- Keratosis pilaris [2]
- Linear IgA bullous dermatosis [3]
- Lymphocytic infiltration / Jessner lymphocytic infiltration [5]
- Lymphoma [12]
- Lymphoproliferative disease / lymphoproliferative disorder [2]
- Mycosis fungoides [2]
- Peripheral edema [3]
- Pruritus (itching) (<2%) [2]
- Pseudolymphoma / cutaneous pseudolymphoma [6]
- Psoriasis [2]
- Purpura (3%) [4]
- Rash (7–12%)
- Raynaud's phenomenon [2]
- Sebaceous hyperplasia [9]
- Squamous cell carcinoma [12]
- Thrombocytopenic purpura [5]
- Urticaria / hives [2]
- Vasculitis (angiitis) / cutaneous vasculitis (angiitis) [3]

Hair
- Alopecia / hair loss (3–4%) [3]
- Alopecia areata [6]
- Hirsutism [12]
- Hypertrichosis (5–19%) [35]
- Pseudofolliculitis barbae [2]

Nails
- Brittle nails (<2%)
- Leukonychia striata (Mees' lines) [2]

Mucosal
- Aphthous stomatitis / aphthous ulcer / aphtha (aphthae) [2]
- Gingival hyperplasia / gingival hypertrophy / gingival enlargement / gingival overgrowth (2–6%) [166]
- Gingivitis (3–4%)
- Oral ulceration [2]
- Rectal hemorrhage / rectal bleeding (<3%)
- Stomatitis (oral mucositis) (5–7%)

Cardiovascular
- Arrhythmias (2–5%)
- Bradycardia / sinus bradycardia [3]
- Capillary leak syndrome [2]
- Chest pain (4–6%)
- Hypertension (8–28%) [28]

Central Nervous System
- Akinetic mutism / mutism [2]
- Anorexia (3%)
- Depression (<6%)
- Dysesthesia [2]
- Encephalopathy (includes hepatic encephalopathy) [4]
- Fever (pyrexia) (includes hyperpyrexia) (3–6%)
- Hallucinations, visual [2]
- Headache (14–25%) [5]
- Insomnia (<4%)
- Leukoencephalopathy / posterior reversible encephalopathy syndrome (PRES) [19]
- Migraine (2–3%)
- Neurotoxicity [12]
- Pain (3–13%)
- Paresthesias (5–11%) [8]
- Parkinsonism [6]
- Pseudotumor cerebri [3]
- Rigors (<3%)
- Seizures [4]
- Tremor (7–13%) [6]
- Vertigo / dizziness (6–8%)

Endocrine/Metabolic
- Diabetes mellitus [2]
- Dyslipidemia [4]
- Gynecomastia (>3%) [3]
- Hypertriglyceridemia (includes triglycerides increased) [2]
- Hypomagnesemia (4–6%)
- Menstrual irregularities (<3%)
- Serum creatinine increased (16–43%) [4]

Gastrointestinal/Hepatic
- Abdominal pain (15%) [3]
- Diarrhea (5–13%) [3]
- Dyspepsia / functional dyspepsia (indigestion) (see also gastroparesis) (2–12%)
- Flatulence (4–5%)
- Gastrointestinal disorder / discomfort (2–4%) [2]
- Hepatotoxicity / liver injury / acute liver injury / drug-induced liver injury (DILI) [10]
- Nausea (6–23%) [2]
- Vomiting (6–9%) [2]

Genitourinary
- Buschke–Lowenstein penile carcinoma [2]
- Urinary frequency (2–4%)
- Urinary tract infection (3%) [2]

Hematologic
- Anemia [4]
- Hemolytic uremic syndrome [17]
- Leukocytopenia (leukopenia) / leukocytes (white blood cells) decreased [2]
- Neutropenia (neutrophils decreased) [3]
- Thrombotic microangiopathy [3]

Neuromuscular/Skeletal
- Arthralgia (<6%)
- Asthenia / fatigue (3–6%) [4]
- Myalgia/Myopathy [11]
- Rhabdomyolysis [13]

Ocular
- Ocular burning (Restasis) (17%)
- Ocular pain [3]
- Papilledema [3]

Renal
- Nephrotoxicity / kidney injury / acute kidney injury (AKI) / drug-induced kidney injury [95]
- Renal function abnormal / renal dysfunction [4]

Respiratory
- Bronchitis (<3%)
- Bronchospasm (5%)
- Cough (3–5%)
- Dyspnea / shortness of breath (<5%) [2]
- Influenza (<10%)
- Pharyngitis (sore throat) (3–4%)
- Pneumonia (<4%)
- Rhinitis / rhinosinusitis (see also sinusitis) (<5%)
- Sinusitis (see also rhinitis / rhinosinusitis) (3–4%)
- Upper respiratory tract infection (8–15%)

Other
- Adverse effects / adverse reactions [22]
- Infection [6]
- Malignancies [2]

CYCLOTHIAZIDE

Indications: Edema, hypertension
Class: Diuretic, thiazide
Half-life: N/A
Clinically important, potentially hazardous interactions with: digoxin
Note: Cyclothiazide is a sulfonamide and can be absorbed systemically. Sulfonamides can produce severe, possibly fatal, reactions such as toxic epidermal necrolysis and Stevens-Johnson syndrome.

CYPROHEPTADINE

Indications: Allergic rhinitis, urticaria
Class: Histamine H1 receptor antagonist
Half-life: 1–4 hours
Clinically important, potentially hazardous interactions with: anticholinergics, citalopram, MAO inhibitors, paroxetine hydrochloride, phenelzine, tranylcypromine
Important contra-indications noted in the prescribing guidelines for: the elderly; nursing mothers; pediatric patients

---

Mucosal
- Xerostomia (dry mouth) (1–10%) [3]

Central Nervous System
- Agitation [2]
- Hallucinations [2]
- Somnolence (drowsiness) [4]

Endocrine/Metabolic
- Weight gain [3]

CYPROTERONE

Trade name: Androcur (Bayer)
Indications: Control of libido in severe hypersexuality and/or sexual deviation in the adult male
Class: Androgen antagonist, Progesterone agonist
Half-life: 1.7 days
Clinically important, potentially hazardous interactions with: alcohol, clotrimazole, fingolimod, itraconazole, ketoconazole, pazopanib, phenytoin, rifampin, ritonavir, St John's wort
Pregnancy category: not indicated for use in women
Important contra-indications noted in the prescribing guidelines for: pediatric patients

---

Skin
Tumors [3]

Cardiovascular
Venous thromboembolism [2]

Gastrointestinal/Hepatic
Hepatotoxicity / liver injury / acute liver injury / drug-induced liver injury (DILI) [24]

Neuromuscular/Skeletal
Osteoporosis [2]

Respiratory
Dyspnea / shortness of breath [4]

CYSTEAMINE

Synonym: mercaptamine
Trade names: Cystagon (Mylan), Procysbi (Raptor Pharma)
Indications: Nephropathic cystinosis
Class: Aminothiol, Anticystine agent
Half-life: N/A
Clinically important, potentially hazardous interactions with: none known
Important contra-indications noted in the prescribing guidelines for: nursing mothers
Note: Contra-indicated in patients with hypersensitivity to penicillamine.

Skin
Lupus erythematosus (subacute cutaneous lupus erythematosus (SCLE)) [3]
Rash (7%)
Urticaria / hives (<5%)

Mucosal
Halitosis [3]

Cardiovascular
Hypertension (<5%)

Central Nervous System
Anorexia (31%)
Confusion (<5%)
Depression (<5%)
Encephalopathy (includes hepatic encephalopathy) (<5%)
Fever (pyrexia) (includes hyperpyrexia) (22%)
Hallucinations (<5%)
Headache (<5%)
Nervousness (<5%)
Neurotoxicity [2]
Seizures (<5%)
Somnolence (drowsiness) (<5%)
Tremor [2]
Vertigo / dizziness (<5%)

Endocrine/Metabolic
Dehydration (<5%)

Gastrointestinal/Hepatic
Constipation (<5%)
Diarrhea (16%)
Duodenitis (<5%)
Dyspepsia / functional dyspepsia (indigestion) (see also gastroparesis) (<5%)
Gastroenteritis (<5%)
Gastrointestinal bleeding (<5%)
Gastrointestinal ulceration (<5%)
Hepatotoxicity / liver injury / acute liver injury / drug-induced liver injury (DILI) (<5%) [2]
Nausea (<5%)
Vomiting (35%)

Hematologic
Anemia (<5%)
Leukocytopenia (leukopenia) / leukocytes (white blood cells) decreased (<5%)

Neuromuscular/Skeletal
Asthenia / fatigue (11%) [2]
Ataxia (<5%)

Otic
Hearing loss (hypoacusis) (<5%)

Renal
Nephrotoxicity / kidney injury / acute kidney injury (AKI) / drug-induced kidney injury (<5%)

CYTARABINE

Synonym: ara-C
Trade names: Cytosar-U (Sicor), DepoCyt (Pacira)
Indications: Leukemias
Class: Antimetabolite, Antineoplastic / anticancer agent (see also Immune checkpoint inhibitor), Antiviral
Half-life: initial: 10–15 minutes
Clinically important, potentially hazardous interactions with: aldesleukin
Important contra-indications noted in the prescribing guidelines for: nursing mothers; pediatric patients
Note: DepoCyt is a liposomal formulation. Vasculitis, a part of the cytarabine syndrome, consists of fever, malaise, myalgia, conjunctivitis, arthralgia and a diffuse erythematous maculopapular eruption that occurs from 6–12 hours following the administration of the drug.
Warning: DepoCyt: CHEMICAL ARACHNOIDITIS ADVERSE REACTIONS

Skin
Acral erythema [16]
Anaphylactoid reactions / anaphylaxis (includes anaphylactic shock) [3]
Cutaneous toxicity / skin toxicity [5]
Desquamation [2]
Ephelides (freckles) (<10%)
Erythema [7]
Exanthems [7]
Hand–foot syndrome (palmar–plantar erythrodysesthesia) [22]
Herpes zoster [2]
Hypersensitivity [2]
Neutrophilic eccrine hidradenitis [11]
Pruritus (itching) (<10%)
Rash (>10%) [4]
Seborrheic keratoses (inflammation of) (Leser–Trélat syndrome) [2]
Stevens-Johnson syndrome and toxic epidermal necrolysis (SJS/TEN) [2]
Toxic erythema of chemotherapy (TEC) [2]
Vasculitis (angiitis) / cutaneous vasculitis (angiitis) [3]

Hair
Alopecia / hair loss (<10%) [5]

Nails
Leukonychia striata (Mees' lines) [3]

Mucosal
Mucositis [3]
Oral lesions [5]
Oral ulceration (>10%)
Perianal ulcerations (>10%)
Stomatitis (oral mucositis) [2]

Cardiovascular
Thrombophlebitis (>10%)

Central Nervous System
Aseptic meningitis [2]
Fever (pyrexia) (includes hyperpyrexia) [3]
Headache [4]
Leukoencephalopathy / posterior reversible encephalopathy syndrome (PRES) [8]
Neurotoxicity [11]
Peripheral neuropathy [3]

Endocrine/Metabolic
Hypokalemia [2]

Gastrointestinal/Hepatic
Diarrhea [5]
Hepatotoxicity / liver injury / acute liver injury / drug-induced liver injury (DILI) [5]
Nausea [4]
Pancreatitis / acute pancreatitis [5]
Vomiting [4]

Hematologic
Anemia [2]
Bleeding [2]
Febrile neutropenia [8]
Hemotoxicity [3]
Leukocytopenia (leukopenia) / leukocytes (white blood cells) decreased [2]
Myelosuppression / bone marrow suppression / myelotoxicity [3]
Neutropenia (neutrophils decreased) [7]
Sepsis [2]
Thrombocytopenia / platelets decreased [6]

Local
Injection-site cellulitis (<10%)

Neuromuscular/Skeletal
Myalgia/Myopathy (<10%)
Rhabdomyolysis [3]

Ocular
Conjunctivitis (conjunctival inflammation) [2]
Ocular adverse effect [3]

Otic
Hearing loss (hypoacusis) [2]

Respiratory
Pneumonia [3]

Other
Adverse effects / adverse reactions [5]
Death [4]
Infection [6]

DABIGATRAN

Trade name: Pradaxa (Boehringer Ingelheim)
Indications: Prevention of venous thromboembolic events, reduce stroke risk
Class: Anticoagulant (antithrombotic), Thrombin inhibitor
Half-life: 2.5 days
Clinically important, potentially hazardous interactions with: amiodarone, antacids, anticoagulants, atorvastatin, carbamazepine, clarithromycin, clopidogrel, collagenase, cyclosporine, daclatasvir, darunavir, dasatinib, deferasirox, desirudin, dextran, diclofenac, dronedarone, fondaparinux, heparin, ibritumomab, itraconazole, ketoconazole, ketorolac, lapatinib, meloxicam, nandrolone, neratinib, NSAIDs, P-glycoprotein inducers and inhibitors, pantoprazole, pentosan, phenytoin, polysulfate sodium, prostacyclin analogues, proton pump inhibitors, quinidine, rifampin, rivaroxaban, salicylates, St John's wort, sulfinpyrazone, tacrolimus, telaprevir, thrombolytic agents, ticlopidine, tipranavir, tositumomab & iodine^{131}, ulipristal, verapamil, vitamin K antagonists
Important contra-indications noted in the prescribing guidelines for: the elderly; nursing mothers; pediatric patients
Note: Contra-indicated in patients with active pathological bleeding or with a mechanical prosthetic heart valve.
Warning: DISCONTINUING PRADAXA IN PATIENTS WITHOUT ADEQUATE CONTINUOUS ANTICOAGULATION INCREASES RISK OF STROKE

Skin
- Bruise / bruising / contusion / ecchymosis (ecchymoses) (<10%)
- Exanthems [2]
- Rash [2]

Mucosal
- Epistaxis (nosebleed) [3]
- Oral ulceration [2]

Cardiovascular
- Myocardial infarction [5]

Central Nervous System
- Headache [2]
- Intracranial hemorrhage [4]
- Subarachnoid hemorrhage [2]

Gastrointestinal/Hepatic
- Abdominal pain [2]
- Dyspepsia / functional dyspepsia (indigestion) (see also gastroparesis) (11%) [8]
- Esophagitis [7]
- Gastritis / pangastritis / gastric irritation [2]
- Gastrointestinal bleeding (6%) [13]

Genitourinary
- Hematuria [2]

Hematologic
- Anemia (<4%)
- Anticoagulation [2]
- Bleeding [3]
- Hemorrhage [9]
- Thrombosis [3]

Renal
- Nephropathy [7]
- Renal failure [4]

Other
- Adverse effects / adverse reactions [6]
- Death [6]

DABRAFENIB

Trade name: Tafinlar (Novartis)
Indications: Melanoma (unresectable or metastatic) in patients with BRAF V600E mutation
Class: BRAF inhibitor, Kinase inhibitor
Half-life: 8 hours
Clinically important, potentially hazardous interactions with: strong CYP3A4 or CYP2C8 inducers or inhibitors inhibitors
Important contra-indications noted in the prescribing guidelines for: nursing mothers; pediatric patients

---

Skin
- Acneiform eruption / acneiform dermatitis / acneiform rash [5]
- Actinic keratoses [3]
- Basal cell carcinoma [4]
- Bullae (<10%)
- Cutaneous toxicity / skin toxicity [5]
- Erythema [2]
- Exanthems [2]
- Hand–foot syndrome (palmar–plantar erythrodysesthesia) (20%) [7]
- Hyperkeratosis (37%) [14]
- Hypersensitivity (<10%)
- Keratoacanthoma (Grzybowski syndrome) (7%) [7]
- Keratosis pilaris [4]
- Lesions (includes skin lesions) [2]
- Malignant melanoma (2%)
- Panniculitis [6]
- Papillomas (27%) [5]
- Peripheral edema [4]
- Photosensitivity [8]
- Pruritus (itching) [4]
- Rash (17%) [8]
- Seborrheic keratoses [2]
- Squamous cell carcinoma (7%) [18]
- Sweet's syndrome [4]
- Transient acantholytic dermatosis (Grover's disease) [4]
- Verrucae vulgaris / warts / verrucae [2]
- Xerosis / xeroderma [5]

Hair
- Alopecia / hair loss (22%) [8]
- Hair changes [2]

Cardiovascular
- Cardiotoxicity [2]
- Chest pain [2]
- Hypertension [4]

Central Nervous System
- Chills [6]
- Fever (pyrexia) (includes hyperpyrexia) (28%) [31]
- Headache (32%) [9]
- Intracranial hemorrhage [3]

Endocrine/Metabolic
- ALP increased (19%) [2]
- ALT increased [4]
- Appetite decreased [3]
- AST increased [6]
- Hyperglycemia (includes glucose increased) (50%)
- Hyponatremia (8%) [2]
- Hypophosphatemia (37%)

Gastrointestinal/Hepatic
- Abdominal pain [2]
- Constipation (11%) [2]
- Diarrhea [8]
- Nausea [11]
- Pancreatitis / acute pancreatitis (<10%)
- Vomiting [10]

Hematologic
- Anemia [5]
- Hemophagocytic lymphohistiocytosis / hemophagocytic syndrome [4]
- Leukocytopenia (leukopenia) / leukocytes (white blood cells) decreased [3]
- Neutropenia (neutrophils decreased) [5]

Neuromuscular/Skeletal
- Arthralgia (27%) [12]
- Asthenia / fatigue [17]
- Back pain (12%)
- Myalgia/Myopathy (11%) [2]
- Rhabdomyolysis [2]

Ocular
- Chorioretinopathy [2]
- Retinopathy [2]
- Uveitis / anterior uveitis / posterior uveitis / panuveitis [3]
- Vision blurred [3]

Renal
- Nephrotoxicity / kidney injury / acute kidney injury (AKI) / drug-induced kidney injury (<10%) [2]

Respiratory
- Cough (12%) [3]
- Nasopharyngitis (10%)

Other
- Adverse effects / adverse reactions [10]

DACARBAZINE

Synonym: DIC
Trade name: DTIC-Dome (Bayer)
Indications: Malignant melanoma, carcinomas
Class: Alkylating agent, Antineoplastic / anticancer agent (see also Immune checkpoint inhibitor)
Half-life: 5 hours
Clinically important, potentially hazardous interactions with: aldesleukin
Important contra-indications noted in the prescribing guidelines for: nursing mothers

---

Skin
- Anaphylactoid reactions / anaphylaxis (includes anaphylactic shock) (<10%)
- Flushing / rubefaction (<10%) [2]
- Hypersensitivity [2]
- Photosensitivity [10]
- Rash (<10%) [2]
- Urticaria / hives [2]

Hair
- Alopecia / hair loss (<10%) [4]

Mucosal
- Stomatitis (oral mucositis) (48%)

Central Nervous System
- Dysgeusia (taste perversion) (<10%)
- Peripheral neuropathy [2]

Endocrine/Metabolic
- ALT increased [2]
- AST increased [2]

Gastrointestinal/Hepatic
- Diarrhea [3]
- Hepatotoxicity / liver injury / acute liver injury / drug-induced liver injury (DILI) [3]
- Nausea [3]

Vomiting [2]

Hematologic

Neutropenia (neutrophils decreased) [5]
Thrombocytopenia / platelets decreased [2]

Local

Injection-site burning (>10%)
Injection-site necrosis (>10%)
Injection-site pain (>10%)

Neuromuscular/Skeletal

Asthenia / fatigue (75%) [4]
Myalgia/Myopathy (<10%)

Respiratory

Influenza- ('flu)-like syndrome [2]
Pulmonary toxicity [2]

Other

Adverse effects / adverse reactions [7]

DACLATASVIR

Trade name: Daklinza (Bristol-Myers Squibb)
Indications: Hepatitis C (in combination with sofosbuvir)
Class: Covid-19 putative drug, Direct-acting antiviral, Hepatitis C virus NS5A inhibitor
Half-life: 12–15 hours
Clinically important, potentially hazardous interactions with: amiodarone, carbamazepine, dabigatran, phenytoin, rifampin, St John's wort
Pregnancy category: No data available
Important contra-indications noted in the prescribing guidelines for: nursing mothers; pediatric patients
Note: See also separate entry for sofosbuvir.

Skin

Pruritus (itching) [4]
Rash [3]

Central Nervous System

Anorexia [2]
Fever (pyrexia) (includes hyperpyrexia) [4]
Headache (14%) [22]
Insomnia [5]
Irritability [2]

Endocrine/Metabolic

ALT increased [10]
AST increased [4]
Hyperbilirubinemia [2]

Gastrointestinal/Hepatic

Abdominal pain [3]
Diarrhea (5%) [12]
Hepatotoxicity / liver injury / acute liver injury / drug-induced liver injury (DILI) [2]
Nausea (8%) [17]
Vomiting [2]

Hematologic

Anemia [8]
Hemoglobin decreased [2]
Lymphopenia (lymphocytopenia) / lymphocytes decreased [2]
Neutropenia (neutrophils decreased) [4]
Thrombocytopenia / platelets decreased [2]

Neuromuscular/Skeletal

Arthralgia [2]
Asthenia / fatigue (14%) [19]

Renal

Renal failure [2]

Respiratory

Dyspnea / shortness of breath [2]
Nasopharyngitis [2]

Other

Adverse effects / adverse reactions [10]

DACLIZUMAB

Trade names: Zenapax (Roche), Zinbryta (Biogen)
Indications: Transplant rejection (Zenapax), relapsing forms of multiple sclerosis (Zinbryta)
Class: Immunosuppressant, Monoclonal antibody
Half-life: 11–38 days
Clinically important, potentially hazardous interactions with: corticosteroids, cyclosporine, Hemophilus B vaccine, methylprednisolone, mycophenolate, prednisolone
Important contra-indications noted in the prescribing guidelines for: the elderly; nursing mothers; pediatric patients
Warning: Zinbryta: HEPATIC INJURY INCLUDING AUTOIMMUNE HEPATITIS and OTHER IMMUNE-MEDIATED DISORDERS

Skin

Acneiform eruption / acneiform dermatitis / acneiform rash (>5%)
Cutaneous toxicity / skin toxicity [2]
Dermatitis [2]
Eczema / eczematous reaction / eczematous eruption [6]
Edema / fluid retention (>5%)
Hypersensitivity [2]
Hypohidrosis (2–5%)
Lymphadenopathy [4]
Peripheral edema (>5%)
Pruritus (itching) (2–5%)
Psoriasis [2]
Rash (2–5%) [8]
Wound complications (>5%)

Hair

Hirsutism (2–5%)

Cardiovascular

Chest pain (>5%)
Hypertension (>5%)
Hypotension (>5%)
Tachycardia (>5%)

Central Nervous System

Anxiety (2–5%)
Depression (2–5%)
Fever (pyrexia) (includes hyperpyrexia) (>5%)
Headache (>5%) [3]
Insomnia (>5%)
Pain (>5%)
Tremor (>5%)
Vertigo / dizziness (>5%)

Endocrine/Metabolic

ALT increased [2]
AST increased [2]
Dehydration (2–5%)
Diabetes mellitus (2–5%)

Gastrointestinal/Hepatic

Abdominal distension (>5%)
Abdominal pain (>5%)
Colitis [2]
Constipation (>5%)
Diarrhea (>5%)
Flatulence (2–5%)
Gastritis / pangastritis / gastric irritation (2–5%)
Hemorrhoids (2–5%)
Hepatotoxicity / liver injury / acute liver injury / drug-induced liver injury (DILI) [5]
Nausea (>5%)
Vomiting (>5%)

Genitourinary

Urinary retention (2–5%)
Urinary tract infection [2]

Hematologic

Hemolytic anemia [2]
Hemorrhage (>5%)
Thrombosis (>5%)

Local

Application-site reactions (2–5%)

Neuromuscular/Skeletal

Arthralgia (2–5%)
Asthenia / fatigue (>5%)
Back pain (>5%)
Bone pain / joint pain (>5%)
Myalgia/Myopathy (2–5%)

Ocular

Vision blurred (2–5%)

Renal

Nephrotoxicity / kidney injury / acute kidney injury (AKI) / drug-induced kidney injury (2–5%)

Respiratory

Cough (>5%)
Dyspnea / shortness of breath (>5%)
Hypoxia (2–5%)
Nasopharyngitis [2]
Pharyngitis (sore throat) (2–5%)
Pleural effusion (2–5%)
Pneumonia [2]
Pulmonary edema (cardiogenic / non-cardiogenic) (>5%)
Rhinitis / rhinosinusitis (see also sinusitis) (2–5%)
Upper respiratory tract infection [3]

Other

Adverse effects / adverse reactions [5]
Infection [7]

DACOMITINIB

Trade name: Vizimpro (Pfizer)
Indications: indicated for the first-line treatment of patients with metastatic non-small cell lung cancer (NSCLC) with epidermal growth factor receptor (EGFR) exon 19 deletion or exon 21 L858R substitution mutations as detected by an FDA-approved test
Class: Epidermal growth factor receptor (EGFR) inhibitor / antagonist, Kinase inhibitor, Tyrosine kinase inhibitor
Half-life: 70 hours
Clinically important, potentially hazardous interactions with: mirtazapine
Pregnancy category: can cause fetal harm

Skin

Acneiform eruption / acneiform dermatitis / acneiform rash [3]
Cutaneous toxicity / skin toxicity [3]
Dermatitis (11%) [6]
Fissures (9%)
Hand–foot syndrome (palmar–plantar erythrodysesthesia) (15%)
Pruritus (itching) (21%)
Rash (69%) [15]
Xerosis / xeroderma (30%) [3]

Hair

Alopecia / hair loss (23%)

Nails
Paronychia (64%) [8]
Mucosal
Mucositis [4]
Nasal discomfort (19%)
Oral ulceration [2]
Orogenital ulceration (12%)
Stomatitis (oral mucositis) (45%) [10]
Cardiovascular
Chest pain (10%)
Central Nervous System
Dysgeusia (taste perversion) (7%)
Insomnia (11%)
Endocrine/Metabolic
Appetite decreased (31%)
Appetite increased (26%)
Gastrointestinal/Hepatic
Constipation (13%)
Diarrhea (87%) [25]
Nausea (19%) [2]
Vomiting (9%)
Neuromuscular/Skeletal
Asthenia / fatigue (13%) [9]
Bone pain / joint pain (12%)
Pain in extremities (14%)
Ocular
Conjunctivitis (conjunctival inflammation) (19%)
Keratitis (ocular keratitis) / corneal inflammation) (2%)
Respiratory
Cough (21%)
Dyspnea / shortness of breath (13%)
Upper respiratory tract infection (12%)
Other
Adverse effects / adverse reactions [6]
Death [2]

DACTINOMYCIN

Synonyms: ACT; actinomycin-D
Trade name: Cosmegen (Merck)
Indications: Melanomas, sarcomas
Class: Antibiotic, Antibiotic; anthracycline, Antimicrobial
Half-life: 36 hours
Clinically important, potentially hazardous interactions with: aldesleukin
Important contra-indications noted in the prescribing guidelines for: the elderly; nursing mothers; pediatric patients
Note: Contra-indicated in patients with chickenpox or herpes zoster infection.

Skin
Acneiform eruption / acneiform dermatitis / acneiform rash (>10%) [6]
Erythema [2]
Folliculitis [2]
Pigmentation (Skin) (includes hyperpigmentation) [4]
Pruritus (itching) [2]
Pustules / pustular eruption [2]
Radiation recall dermatitis (>10%) [4]
Hair
Alopecia / hair loss (>10%)
Mucosal
Oral lesions [3]
Stomatitis (oral mucositis) (ulcerative) (>5%)
Gastrointestinal/Hepatic
Nausea [2]
Hematologic
Febrile neutropenia [2]
Neutropenia (neutrophils decreased) [2]
Thrombocytopenia / platelets decreased [2]
Local
Injection-site extravasation (>10%)
Injection-site necrosis (>10%)
Injection-site phlebitis (>10%)
Other
Death [2]

DALBAVANCIN

Trade name: Dalvance (Durata)
Indications: Skin infections and drug resistant gram-positive coccal infections
Class: Antibiotic, Antibiotic; lipoglycopeptide, Antimicrobial, Cell wall synthesis inhibitor
Half-life: 170–210 hours
Clinically important, potentially hazardous interactions with: none known
Important contra-indications noted in the prescribing guidelines for: nursing mothers; pediatric patients

---

Skin
Anaphylactoid reactions / anaphylaxis (includes anaphylactic shock) (<2%) [3]
Flushing / rubefaction (<2%)
Hematoma / cutaneous hematoma (<2%)
Petechiae (<2%)
Pruritus (itching) [4]
Rash [3]
Urticaria / hives (<2%)
Wound complications (<2%)
Mucosal
Oral candidiasis (12%) [3]
Cardiovascular
Hypotension [2]
Phlebitis (<2%)
Central Nervous System
Fever (pyrexia) (includes hyperpyrexia) (50%) [9]
Headache (25%) [10]
Vertigo / dizziness (<2%)
Endocrine/Metabolic
Hypoglycemia (<2%)
Gastrointestinal/Hepatic
Abdominal pain (<2%)
Black stools / melena (<2%)
Constipation [6]
Diarrhea (21%) [10]
Hepatotoxicity / liver injury / acute liver injury / drug-induced liver injury (DILI) (<2%)
Loose stools / soft feces [2]
Nausea (6%) [12]
Vomiting [2]
Genitourinary
Vulvovaginal candidiasis (<2%)
Hematologic
Anemia (<2%)
Eosinophilia / eosinophils increased (<2%)
Leukocytopenia (leukopenia) / leukocytes (white blood cells) decreased (<2%)
Neutropenia (neutrophils decreased) (<2%)
Thrombocytopenia / platelets decreased (<2%)
Local
Infusion-related reactions (<2%)
Renal
Nephrotoxicity / kidney injury / acute kidney injury (AKI) / drug-induced kidney injury [2]
Respiratory
Bronchospasm (<2%)
Other
Adverse effects / adverse reactions [4]

DALFAMPRIDINE

Synonyms: Fampridine; 4-aminopyridine; 4-AP
Trade name: Ampyra (Acorda)
Indications: Multiple sclerosis (to improve walking)
Class: Potassium channel blocker
Half-life: 5–6.5 hours
Clinically important, potentially hazardous interactions with: trilaciclib
Important contra-indications noted in the prescribing guidelines for: nursing mothers; pediatric patients
Note: Contra-indicated in patients with a history of seizure, or with moderate or severe renal impairment.

Central Nervous System
Balance disorder (5%)
Gait instability / postural instability [2]
Headache (7%) [6]
Insomnia (9%) [5]
Multiple sclerosis (relapse) (4%)
Paresthesias (4%) [2]
Seizures [5]
Vertigo / dizziness (7%) [10]
Gastrointestinal/Hepatic
Constipation (3%)
Dyspepsia / functional dyspepsia (indigestion) (see also gastroparesis) (2%)
Nausea (7%) [4]
Genitourinary
Urinary tract infection (12%) [2]
Neuromuscular/Skeletal
Asthenia / fatigue (7%) [3]
Back pain (5%)
Respiratory
Nasopharyngitis (4%)
Pharyngolaryngeal pain (2%)
Other
Adverse effects / adverse reactions [6]

DALTEPARIN

Trade name: Fragmin (Pfizer)
Indications: Prophylaxis of deep vein thrombosis
Class: Heparin, low molecular weight
Half-life: 4–8 hours
Clinically important, potentially hazardous interactions with: butabarbital, danaparoid
Important contra-indications noted in the prescribing guidelines for: nursing mothers; pediatric patients
Warning: SPINAL/EPIDURAL HEMATOMA

Skin
Anaphylactoid reactions / anaphylaxis (includes anaphylactic shock) (<10%) [2]
Bullous dermatosis (<10%)
Pruritus (itching) (<10%)
Rash (<10%)

Hair
Alopecia / hair loss [2]
Local
Injection-site hematoma (<10%)
Injection-site pain (<10%)
Other
Allergic reactions (<10%) [3]

DAN-SHEN

Family: Labiatae; Lamiaceae
Scientific name: *Salvia miltiorrhiza*
Indications: Circulation problems, ischemic stroke, angina pectoris, menstrual problems, chronic hepatitis, abdominal masses, insomnia, acne, psoriasis, eczema, bruising, hearing loss
Class: Food supplement, Platelet aggregation inhibitor
Half-life: N/A
Clinically important, potentially hazardous interactions with: none known

---

Hematologic
Anticoagulation [4]
Other
Adverse effects / adverse reactions [3]

DANAPAROID

Trade name: Orgaran (Organon)
Indications: Prevention of postoperative deep thrombosis
Class: Anticoagulant (antithrombotic), Heparinoid
Half-life: ~24 hours
Clinically important, potentially hazardous interactions with: butabarbital, dalteparin, enoxaparin, heparin, nandrolone

---

Skin
Edema / fluid retention (3%)
Peripheral edema (3%)
Pruritus (itching) (4%)
Rash (2–5%)
Hematologic
Thrombocytopenia / platelets decreased [2]
Local
Injection-site hematoma (5%)
Injection-site pain (8–14%)
Injection-site plaques [3]
Other
Infection (2%)

DANAZOL

Indications: Endometriosis, fibrocystic breast disease
Class: Pituitary hormone inhibitor
Half-life: ~4.5 hours
Clinically important, potentially hazardous interactions with: acenocoumarol, acitretin, atorvastatin, cyclosporine, insulin aspart, insulin degludec, insulin detemir, insulin glargine, insulin glulisine, oral contraceptives, paricalcitol, simvastatin, tacrolimus, warfarin
Important contra-indications noted in the prescribing guidelines for: nursing mothers; pediatric patients

---

Skin
Acneiform eruption / acneiform dermatitis / acneiform rash (>10%) [6]
Diaphoresis (3%)
Edema / fluid retention (>10%)
Erythema multiforme [2]
Exanthems [2]
Flushing / rubefaction [3]
Lupus erythematosus (subacute cutaneous lupus erythematosus (SCLE)) [4]
Rash (3%)
Seborrhea [4]
Hair
Alopecia / hair loss [3]
Hirsutism (<10%) [5]
Endocrine/Metabolic
Pseudomenopause [2]
Weight gain [2]
Gastrointestinal/Hepatic
Hepatotoxicity / liver injury / acute liver injury / drug-induced liver injury (DILI) [4]
Neuromuscular/Skeletal
Rhabdomyolysis [5]
Other
Adverse effects / adverse reactions [4]
Death [2]

DAPAGLIFLOZIN

Trade names: Farxiga (AstraZeneca), Qtern (AstraZeneca), Xigduo XR (AstraZeneca)
Indications: Type II diabetes mellitus
Class: Antidiabetic, Sodium-glucose co-transporter 2 (SGLT2) inhibitor ('gliflozin')
Half-life: 13 hours
Clinically important, potentially hazardous interactions with: pioglitazone
Important contra-indications noted in the prescribing guidelines for: the elderly; nursing mothers; pediatric patients
Note: Contra-indicated in patients with severe renal impairment, end-stage renal disease, or undergoing dialysis. Qtern is dapagliflozin and saxagliptin; Xigduo XR is dapagliflozin and metformin.

Skin
Eczema / eczematous reaction / eczematous eruption [2]
Cardiovascular
Hypertension [2]
Hypotension [3]
Central Nervous System
Headache [3]
Vertigo / dizziness [2]
Endocrine/Metabolic
Dehydration [2]
Diabetic ketoacidosis [6]
Dyslipidemia (2–3%)
Euglycemic diabetic ketoacidosis [5]
Hypoglycemia (>10%) [17]
Hypovolemia [2]
Gastrointestinal/Hepatic
Constipation (2%)
Diarrhea [3]
Nausea (3%) [3]
Pancreatitis / acute pancreatitis [4]
Genitourinary
Balanitis (glans penile inflammation) [2]
Dysuria [2]
Genital mycotic infection (particularly in women) (3–8%) [34]
Genitourinary infection / genital infection / reproductive tract infection [3]
Pollakiuria [3]
Urinary frequency (3–4%)
Urinary tract infection (4–6%) [38]
Vulvovaginal candidiasis [2]
Vulvovaginal pruritus [2]
Hematologic
Polycythemia / erythrocytosis [2]
Neuromuscular/Skeletal
Arthralgia [2]
Asthenia / fatigue [2]
Back pain (3–4%) [3]
Pain in extremities (2%)
Renal
Nephrotoxicity / kidney injury / acute kidney injury (AKI) / drug-induced kidney injury [2]
Renal failure [2]
Respiratory
Bronchitis [2]
Cough [2]
Influenza (2–3%) [2]
Nasopharyngitis (6–7%) [7]
Upper respiratory tract infection [5]
Other
Adverse effects / adverse reactions [10]
Dipsia (thirst) / polydipsia [2]
Infection (<10%)

DAPSONE

Trade name: Aczone (Allergan)
Indications: Leprosy, dermatitis herpetiformis, acne
Class: Antibiotic, Antimicrobial, Antimycobacterial (including antitubercular)
Half-life: 10–50 hours
Clinically important, potentially hazardous interactions with: atovaquone/proguanil, chloroquine, didanosine, furazolidone, ganciclovir, hydroxychloroquine, methotrexate, pyrimethamine, rifabutin, rifampin, rifapentine, sulfonamides, trimethoprim, ursodiol
Important contra-indications noted in the prescribing guidelines for: nursing mothers
Note: A hypersensitivity reaction – termed the 'sulfone syndrome' or 'dapsone syndrome' – may infrequently develop during the first six weeks of treatment. This syndrome consists of exfoliative dermatitis, fever, malaise, nausea, anorexia, hepatitis, jaundice, lymphadenopathy and hemolytic anemia.

Skin
AGEP [2]
Bullous dermatosis [2]
Cyanosis / acrocyanosis [2]
Dapsone syndrome [45]
DRESS syndrome (Drug-induced hypersensitivity syndrome) [16]
Erythema multiforme [9]
Erythema nodosum [5]
Exanthems (<5%) [12]
Exfoliative dermatitis [10]
Fixed eruption / fixed drug eruption [5]
Hypersensitivity [21]
Lupus erythematosus (subacute cutaneous lupus erythematosus (SCLE)) [6]
Photosensitivity [9]

Pigmentation (Skin) (includes hyperpigmentation) [6]
Pruritus (itching) [2]
Rash [7]
Stevens-Johnson syndrome and toxic epidermal necrolysis (SJS/TEN) [12]
Urticaria / hives [2]

Nails
Beau's lines (transverse nail bands) [3]

Central Nervous System
Headache (4%) [2]
Insomnia [2]
Peripheral neuropathy [4]

Gastrointestinal/Hepatic
Cholangitis / sclerosing cholangitis [2]
Hepatitis [3]
Hepatotoxicity / liver injury / acute liver injury / drug-induced liver injury (DILI) [3]
Pancreatitis / acute pancreatitis [2]

Hematologic
Agranulocytosis / severe selective neutropenia [8]
Anemia [5]
Hemolysis [9]
Hemolytic anemia [9]
Methemoglobinemia [32]
Pure red cell aplasia [2]

Local
Application-site erythema (13%) [2]
Application-site reactions (18%)

Neuromuscular/Skeletal
Asthenia / fatigue [2]

Respiratory
Cough (2%)
Eosinophilic pneumonia [2]
Nasopharyngitis (5%)
Pharyngitis (sore throat) (2%)
Sinusitis (see also rhinitis / rhinosinusitis) (2%)
Upper respiratory tract infection (3%)

Other
Adverse effects / adverse reactions [4]
Death [6]

DAPTOMYCIN

Trade name: Cubicin (Cubist)
Indications: Complicated skin and skin structure infections, *Staphylococcus aureus* bloodstream infections
Class: Antibiotic, Antibiotic; glycopeptide, Antimicrobial
Half-life: ~8 hours
Clinically important, potentially hazardous interactions with: atorvastatin, cyclosporine, fibrates, HMG-CoA reductase inhibitors, rosuvastatin, statins, tobramycin, typhoid vaccine, warfarin
Important contra-indications noted in the prescribing guidelines for: the elderly; nursing mothers; pediatric patients

---

Skin
AGEP [2]
Anaphylactoid reactions / anaphylaxis (includes anaphylactic shock) [2]
Cellulitis and pseudocellulitis (<2%)
Edema / fluid retention (<7%)
Fungal dermatitis (3%)
Hyperhidrosis (5%)
Pruritus (itching) (3–6%)
Rash (4%)

Cardiovascular
Chest pain (7%)
Hypertension (6%)
Hypotension (2%)

Central Nervous System
Fever (pyrexia) (includes hyperpyrexia) (2%)
Headache (5%)
Insomnia (9%)
Peripheral neuropathy [2]
Vertigo / dizziness (2%)

Endocrine/Metabolic
Creatine phosphokinase (CPK) / creatine kinase increased (hyperCKemia) (7%) [9]
Hyperkalemia [5]

Gastrointestinal/Hepatic
Abdominal pain (<6%)
Constipation (6%)
Diarrhea (5%) [3]
Hepatotoxicity / liver injury / acute liver injury / drug-induced liver injury (DILI) [4]
Nausea (6%) [2]
Vomiting (3%)

Genitourinary
Urinary tract infection (2%)

Hematologic
Eosinophilia / eosinophils increased [2]
Neutropenia (neutrophils decreased) [2]
Thrombocytopenia / platelets decreased [2]

Local
Injection-site reaction (6%)

Neuromuscular/Skeletal
Back pain (<2%)
Myalgia/Myopathy [10]
Rhabdomyolysis [11]

Renal
Nephrotoxicity / kidney injury / acute kidney injury (AKI) / drug-induced kidney injury [3]
Renal failure [4]

Respiratory
Cough (<2%)
Dyspnea / shortness of breath (2%)
Eosinophilic pneumonia [34]
Pharyngolaryngeal pain (8%)
Pneumonia [2]

Other
Adverse effects / adverse reactions [4]

DARATUMUMAB

Trade name: Darzalex (Janssen Biotech)
Indications: Multiple myeloma in patients who have received at least three prior lines of therapy including a proteasome inhibitor (PI) and an immunomodulatory agent or who are double-refractory to a PI and an immunomodulatory agent
Class: Monoclonal antibody
Half-life: 18 days
Clinically important, potentially hazardous interactions with: none known
Pregnancy category: No data available
Important contra-indications noted in the prescribing guidelines for: pediatric patients

---

Skin
Herpes zoster (3%)

Mucosal
Nasal congestion (17%)

Cardiovascular
Atrial fibrillation [2]
Chest pain (12%)
Hypertension (10%)

Central Nervous System
Chills (10%)
Fever (pyrexia) (includes hyperpyrexia) (21%) [3]
Headache (12%)

Endocrine/Metabolic
Appetite decreased (15%)

Gastrointestinal/Hepatic
Constipation (15%)
Diarrhea (16%) [5]
Nausea (27%)
Vomiting (14%)

Hematologic
Anemia (45%) [8]
Hemotoxicity [2]
Lymphopenia (lymphocytopenia) / lymphocytes decreased (72%) [6]
Neutropenia (neutrophils decreased) (60%) [9]
Thrombocytopenia / platelets decreased (48%) [8]

Local
Infusion-related reactions (48%) [13]

Neuromuscular/Skeletal
Arthralgia (17%)
Asthenia / fatigue (39%) [7]
Back pain (23%) [2]
Pain in extremities (15%)

Ocular
Ciliochoroidal effusion / uveal effusion (includes ciliary body effusion) [2]
Glaucoma (includes acute angle-closure glaucoma) [5]

Respiratory
Bronchospasm (<2%) [3]
Cough (21%) [3]
Dyspnea / shortness of breath (15%) [4]
Hypoxia (<2%)
Nasopharyngitis (15%)
Pneumonia (11%) [5]
Respiratory tract infection [2]
Rhinitis / rhinosinusitis (see also sinusitis) (>5%)
Upper respiratory tract infection (20%) [3]

Other
Cytokine release syndrome / cytokine storm [2]
Death [2]

DARBEPOETIN ALFA

Synonym: erythropoiesis stimulating protein
Trade name: Aranesp (Amgen)
Indications: Anemia associated with renal failure and chemotherapy
Class: Colony stimulating factor, Erythropoiesis-stimulating agent (ESA), Erythropoietin
Half-life: 21 hours
Clinically important, potentially hazardous interactions with: none known
Important contra-indications noted in the prescribing guidelines for: nursing mothers; pediatric patients
Note: There is an increased risk of death for patients suffering from chronic renal failure with this drug (6%).
Warning: ERYTHROPOIESIS-STIMULATING AGENTS (ESAs) INCREASE THE RISK OF DEATH, MYOCARDIAL INFARCTION, STROKE, VENOUS THROMBOEMBOLISM, THROMBOSIS OF VASCULAR ACCESS AND

TUMOR PROGRESSION OR RECURRENCE

Skin
Edema / fluid retention (21%)
Peripheral edema (11%)
Pruritus (itching) (8%)
Rash (7%) [2]

Cardiovascular
Hypertension [2]

Central Nervous System
Fever (pyrexia) (includes hyperpyrexia) (9–19%)
Headache [2]
Vertigo / dizziness (8–14%)

Gastrointestinal/Hepatic
Abdominal pain (12%)

Hematologic
Thrombosis [2]

Local
Injection-site pain (7%)

Neuromuscular/Skeletal
Arthralgia (11–13%)
Asthenia / fatigue (9–33%)
Back pain (8%)
Muscle spasm [2]
Myalgia/Myopathy (21%)

Respiratory
Cough (10%)
Influenza- ('flu)-like syndrome (6%)
Upper respiratory tract infection (14%)

Other
Adverse effects / adverse reactions [4]

DARIDOREXANT

Trade name: Quvivo (Idorsia)
Indications: Insomnia
Class: Orexin receptor antagonist
Half-life: approximately 8 hours
Clinically important, potentially hazardous interactions with: CYP3A4 inducers, CYP3A4 inhibitors, diltiazem, efavirenz, itraconazole, ranitidine, ranitidine, rifampin
Pregnancy category: No available data on daridorexant use in pregnant women to evaluate for drug-associated risks of major birth defects, miscarriage, or other adverse maternal or fetal outcomes.
Note: CNS-Depressant Effects and Daytime Impairment: Impairs alertness and motor coordination including morning impairment. Risk increases when used with other central nervous system depressants. Avoid alcohol consumption with daridorexant.

Central Nervous System
Headache (7%) [2]
Somnolence (drowsiness) (5%)
Vertigo / dizziness (3%)

Gastrointestinal/Hepatic
Nausea (3%)

Respiratory
Nasopharyngitis [3]

DARIFENACIN

Trade names: Emselex (Novartis), Enablex (Novartis)
Indications: Overactive bladder
Class: Anticholinergic, Muscarinic antagonist
Half-life: 13–19 hours
Clinically important, potentially hazardous interactions with: anticholinergics, antihistamines, atazanavir, clozapine, cyclosporine, digoxin, disopyramide, domperidone, erythromycin, flecainide, fosamprenavir, haloperidol, imipramine, indinavir, itraconazole, ketoconazole, levodopa, lopinavir, MAO inhibitors, memantine, metoclopramide, nefopam, nelfinavir, nitrates (sublingual), parasympathomimetics, paroxetine hydrochloride, phenothiazines, potent CYP3A4 inhibitors, ritonavir, saquinavir, thioridazine, tipranavir, tricyclic antidepressants, verapamil
Important contra-indications noted in the prescribing guidelines for: nursing mothers; pediatric patients
Note: Contra-indicated in patients with, or at risk for, urinary retention, gastric retention or uncontrolled narrow-angle glaucoma.

Mucosal
Xerostomia (dry mouth) (20%) [12]

Central Nervous System
Headache [2]

Gastrointestinal/Hepatic
Abdominal pain (2%)
Constipation [3]

DAROLUTAMIDE

Synonym: Nubeqa
Trade names: Nubeqa (Bayer), ODM-201 (Bayer)
Indications: Treatment of patients with non-metastatic castration-resistant prostate cancer. Patients should also receive a gonadotropin-releasing hormone (GnRH) analog concurrently or should have had a bilateral orchiectomy
Class: Androgen receptor inhibitor
Half-life: 20 hours
Clinically important, potentially hazardous interactions with: bcrp substrates, CYP3A inducers, CYP3A inhibitors
Pregnancy category: May cause fetal harm and loss of pregnancy when administered to a pregnant female. Males with female partners of reproductive potential are advised to use effective contraception during treatment and for 1 week after the last dose of darolutamide.

Skin
Rash (3%)

Endocrine/Metabolic
AST increased (23%)
Hyperbilirubinemia (16%)

Gastrointestinal/Hepatic
Nausea [2]

Hematologic
Neutropenia (neutrophils decreased) (4% grade 3–4) (20%)

Neuromuscular/Skeletal
Asthenia / fatigue ($<1\% \geq$ grade 3) (16%) [5]
Pain in extremities (6%)

Other
Adverse effects / adverse reactions (serious adverse reactions occurred in 25% of patients) (25%)

DARUNAVIR

Trade names: Prezcobix (Janssen), Prezista (Janssen)
Indications: HIV infection (must be co-administered with ritonavir and with other antiretroviral agents)
Class: Antiretroviral, Covid-19 putative drug, HIV-1 protease inhibitor
Half-life: 15 hours
Clinically important, potentially hazardous interactions with: abacavir, alfuzosin, almotriptan, alosetron, alprazolam, amiodarone, antifungals, apixaban, artemether/lumefantrine, astemizole, atorvastatin, bortezomib, brinzolamide, calcium channel blockers, captopril, carbamazepine, ciclesonide, cisapride, clarithromycin, colchicine, conivaptan, cyclosporine, CYP2D6 substrates, CYP3A4 inhibitors, inducers and substrates, dabigatran, dasatinib, deferasirox, delavirdine, didanosine, dienogest, digoxin, dihydroergotamine, dronedarone, duloxetine, dutasteride, efavirenz, elbasvir & grazoprevir, enfuvirtide, eplerenone, ergotamine, estrogens, etravirine, everolimus, fentanyl, fesoterodine, food, fusidic acid, glecaprevir & pibrentasvir, guanfacine, halofantrine, HMG-CoA reductase inhibitors, indinavir, inhaled corticosteroids, ixabepilone, ketoconazole, lidocaine, lopinavir, lovastatin, maraviroc, meperidine, methadone, methylprednisolone, midazolam, mifepristone, mometasone, nefazodone, nilotinib, nisoldipine, olaparib, P-glycoprotein substrates, paricalcitol, paroxetine hydrochloride, pazopanib, phenobarbital, phenytoin, pimecrolimus, pimozide, prasugrel, pravastatin, protease inhibitors, quetiapine, quinidine, quinine, ranolazine, rifabutin, rifampin, rilpivirine, rivaroxaban, romidepsin, rosuvastatin, salmeterol, saquinavir, saxagliptin, sertraline, sildenafil, silodosin, simeprevir, simvastatin, sirolimus, sorafenib, St John's wort, tacrolimus, tadalafil, tamsulosin, telaprevir, temsirolimus, tenofovir disoproxil, terfenadine, theophylline, tolvaptan, topotecan, trazodone, triazolam, tricyclic antidepressants, vardenafil, viloxazine, voriconazole, warfarin, zidovudine
Important contra-indications noted in the prescribing guidelines for: nursing mothers; pediatric patients
Note: Darunavir is a sulfonamide and can be absorbed systemically. Sulfonamides can produce severe, possibly fatal, reactions such as toxic epidermal necrolysis and Stevens-Johnson syndrome.
Prezcobix is darunavir and cobicistat.

Skin
Angioedema (formerly named angioneurotic edema) (<2%)
Hypersensitivity (<2%) [2]
Pruritus (itching) (<2%)
Rash (6–10%) [9]
Urticaria / hives (<2%)

Central Nervous System
Abnormal dreams (<2%)

Anorexia (2%)
Headache (7%) [6]

Endocrine/Metabolic
Diabetes mellitus (new onset or exacebated) (2%)

Gastrointestinal/Hepatic
Abdominal distension (2%)
Abdominal pain (6%)
Diarrhea (9–14%) [11]
Dyspepsia / functional dyspepsia (indigestion) (see also gastroparesis) (<3%)
Flatulence (<2%)
Gastrointestinal disorder / discomfort [3]
Hepatotoxicity / liver injury / acute liver injury / drug-induced liver injury (DILI) (<2%) [6]
Nausea (4–7%) [6]
Pancreatitis / acute pancreatitis (<2%)
Vomiting (2–5%)

Neuromuscular/Skeletal
Asthenia / fatigue (2–3%)
Osteonecrosis / avascular necrosis (includes steroid-induced osteonecrosis of the femoral head) (<2%)

Other
Adverse effects / adverse reactions [7]

DASATINIB

Trade name: Sprycel (Bristol-Myers Squibb)
Indications: Leukemia (chronic myeloid), acute lymphoblastic leukemia
Class: Antineoplastic / anticancer agent (see also Immune checkpoint inhibitor), Bcr-Abl tyrosine kinase inhibitor / (Breakpoint cluster region Abelson (Bcr-Abl) tyrosine kinase inhibitor, Tyrosine kinase inhibitor, Vascular endothelial growth factor (VEGF) inhibitor / antagonist
Half-life: 3–5 hours
Clinically important, potentially hazardous interactions with: abciximab, alfentanil, alfuzosin, ambrisentan, antacids, anticoagulants, antiplatelet agents, aprepitant, argatroban, artemether/lumefantrine, astemizole, atazanavir, atorvastatin, boceprevir, cabazitaxel, carbamazepine, chloroquine, ciclesonide, cilostazol, cinacalcet, ciprofloxacin, cisapride, clarithromycin, clopidogrel, clozapine, colchicine, conivaptan, cyclosporine, CYP3A4 inhibitors, inducers and substrates, dabigatran, darunavir, deferasirox, dexamethasone, dihydroergotamine, docetaxel, dronedarone, efavirenz, eptifibatide, ergotamine, erythromycin, eszopiclone, famotidine, fentanyl, fesoterodine, gadobutrol, gefitinib, H_2 antagonists, indinavir, itraconazole, ixabepilone, ketoconazole, lopinavir, lurasidone, maraviroc, meloxicam, nefazodone, nelfinavir, nilotinib, omeprazole, pantoprazole, phenobarbital, phenytoin, pimozide, proton pump inhibitors, QT prolonging agents, quinidine, quinine, rifampin, ritonavir, saquinavir, saxagliptin, sildenafil, simvastatin, sirolimus, St John's wort, tacrolimus, tadalafil, temsirolimus, terfenadine, tetrabenazine, thioridazine, tiagabine, tinzaparin, vardenafil, ziprasidone
Important contra-indications noted in the prescribing guidelines for: nursing mothers; pediatric patients

---

Skin
Acneiform eruption / acneiform dermatitis / acneiform rash (<10%) [2]
Cutaneous toxicity / skin toxicity [8]
Dermatitis (<10%)
Eczema / eczematous reaction / eczematous eruption (<10%)
Edema / fluid retention (13–18%) [8]
Erythema [2]
Flushing / rubefaction (<10%)
Herpes (<10%)
Hyperhidrosis (<10%)
Panniculitis [4]
Peripheral edema [3]
Pruritus (itching) (<10%) [5]
Rash (11–21%) [12]
Urticaria / hives (<10%)
Xerosis / xeroderma (<10%)

Hair
Alopecia / hair loss (<10%) [3]
Hair pigmentation [2]

Mucosal
Mucositis (16%)

Cardiovascular
Arrhythmias (<10%)
Cardiac failure (3%)
Cardiotoxicity (left ventricular dysfunction) [2]
Congestive heart failure (2%)
Hypertension (<10%)
Palpitation (<10%)
Pericardial effusion (2–3%) [8]
QT interval prolonged / QT prolongation [4]
Tachycardia (<10%)

Central Nervous System
Anorexia (<10%) [6]
Anxiety [2]
Depression (<10%)
Dysgeusia (taste perversion) (<10%)
Fever (pyrexia) (includes hyperpyrexia) (5–39%)
Headache (12–33%) [11]
Insomnia (<10%)
Neurotoxicity (13%)
Pain (26%) [2]
Peripheral neuropathy (<10%)
Somnolence (drowsiness) (<10%)
Subdural hemorrhage [4]
Vertigo / dizziness (<10%)

Endocrine/Metabolic
ALT increased [2]
Gynecomastia [2]
Hypophosphatemia [2]
Weight gain (<10%)
Weight loss (<10%)

Gastrointestinal/Hepatic
Abdominal distension (<10%)
Abdominal pain (<25%) [2]
Colitis (<10%) [9]
Constipation (<10%)
Diarrhea (18–31%) [22]
Dyspepsia / functional dyspepsia (indigestion) (see also gastroparesis) (<10%)
Enterocolitis (<10%)
Gastritis / pangastritis / gastric irritation (<10%)
Gastrointestinal bleeding (2–8%) [3]
Hemorrhagic colitis [5]
Hepatitis [2]
Hepatotoxicity / liver injury / acute liver injury / drug-induced liver injury (DILI) [2]
Nausea (9–23%) [11]
Vomiting (7–15%) [6]

Hematologic
Anemia [6]
Bleeding (6–26%)
Cytopenia [3]
Febrile neutropenia (<12%)
Hemorrhage [2]
Hemotoxicity [4]
Leukocytopenia (leukopenia) / leukocytes (white blood cells) decreased [2]
Myelosuppression / bone marrow suppression / myelotoxicity [10]
Neutropenia (neutrophils decreased) [9]
Pancytopenia (includes bicytopenia) (<10%)
Thrombocytopenia / platelets decreased [16]

Neuromuscular/Skeletal
Arthralgia (<19%)
Asthenia / fatigue (8%) [18]
Bone pain / joint pain (12–19%) [3]
Myalgia/Myopathy (6–13%) [2]

Ocular
Ocular adverse effect [2]
Reduced visual acuity (<10%)
Vision blurred (<10%)
Visual disturbances (<10%)
Xerophthalmia (dry eyes) (<10%)

Otic
Tinnitus (<10%)

Renal
Nephrotic syndrome [7]
Proteinuria [4]
Renal failure [3]

Respiratory
Chylothorax [14]
Cough (<10%)
Dyspnea / shortness of breath (20%) [5]
Pleural effusion (12–21%) [43]
Pneumonia (<10%) [4]
Pneumonitis (<10%)
Pulmonary hypertension (<10%) [20]
Pulmonary toxicity [4]
Upper respiratory tract infection (<10%)

Other
Adverse effects / adverse reactions [4]
Death [2]
Infection (<14%) [3]
Side effects [2]

DAUNORUBICIN

Synonyms: daunomycin; DNR; rubidomycin
Trade name: DaunoXome (Gilead)
Indications: Acute leukemias
Class: Antibiotic, Antibiotic; anthracycline, Antimicrobial
Half-life: 14–20 hours; 4 hours (intramuscular)
Clinically important, potentially hazardous interactions with: aldesleukin, gadobenate
Important contra-indications noted in the prescribing guidelines for: the elderly; nursing mothers; pediatric patients
Warning: MYOCARDIAL TOXICITY / MYELOSUPPRESSION

Skin
Angioedema (formerly named angioneurotic edema) [4]
Dermatitis [2]
Edema / fluid retention (11%)
Exanthems [2]
Flushing / rubefaction (14%)
Folliculitis (<5%)
Hot flashes / hot flushes (<5%)
Hyperhidrosis (14%)
Lymphadenopathy (<5%)
Neutrophilic eccrine hidradenitis [2]

Pigmentation (Skin) (includes hyperpigmentation) [3]
Pruritus (itching) (7%)
Seborrhea (<5%)
Urticaria / hives [3]
Xerosis / xeroderma (<5%)

Hair
Alopecia / hair loss (8%) [4]

Nails
Leukonychia striata (Mees' lines) [2]
Nail pigmentation [5]

Mucosal
Gingival bleeding (<5%)
Oral lesions [2]
Sialorrhea (ptyalism; hypersalivation) (<5%)
Stomatitis (oral mucositis) (10%)
Xerostomia (dry mouth) (<5%)

Cardiovascular
Chest pain (9–14%)
Hypertension (<5%)
Myocardial toxicity [5]
Palpitation (<5%)
Tachycardia (<5%)

Central Nervous System
Amnesia (<5%)
Anorexia (23%)
Anxiety (<5%)
Cognitive impairment (<5%)
Depression (10%)
Dysgeusia (taste perversion) (<5%)
Fever (pyrexia) (includes hyperpyrexia) [2]
Gait instability / postural instability (<5%)
Hallucinations (<5%)
Headache (25%)
Insomnia (6%)
Meningococcal infection (<5%)
Neurotoxicity (13%)
Rigors (19%)
Seizures (<5%)
Somnolence (drowsiness) (<5%)
Syncope / fainting (<5%)
Tremor (<5%)
Vertigo / dizziness (8%)

Endocrine/Metabolic
Appetite increased (<5%)
Dehydration (<5%)

Gastrointestinal/Hepatic
Abdominal pain (23%)
Black stools / melena (<5%)
Constipation (7%)
Diarrhea (38%)
Dysphagia (<5%)
Gastritis / pangastritis / gastric irritation (<5%)
Gastrointestinal bleeding (<5%)
Hemorrhoids (<5%)
Hepatomegaly (<5%)
Nausea (54%)
Tenesmus (5%)
Vomiting (23%)

Genitourinary
Dysuria (<5%)
Nocturia (<5%)
Polyuria (includes polyuric syndrome) (<5%)

Hematologic
Neutropenia (neutrophils decreased) (15–36%)
Splenomegaly (<5%)

Local
Injection-site inflammation (<5%)
Injection-site necrosis (<10%) [2]
Injection-site ulceration (<10%)

Neuromuscular/Skeletal
Arthralgia (7%)
Asthenia / fatigue (10%)
Ataxia (<5%)
Back pain (16%)
Hyperkinesia (<5%)
Hypertonia (<5%)
Myalgia/Myopathy (7%)

Ocular
Abnormal vision (5%)
Conjunctivitis (conjunctival inflammation) (<5%)
Ocular pain (<5%)

Otic
Ear pain (<5%)
Hearing loss (hypoacusis) (<5%)
Tinnitus (<5%)

Respiratory
Cough (28%)
Dyspnea / shortness of breath (26%)
Hemoptysis (<5%)
Influenza- ('flu)-like syndrome (5%)
PIE syndrome (<5%)
Rhinitis / rhinosinusitis (see also sinusitis) (12%)
Sinusitis (see also rhinitis / rhinosinusitis) (8%)

Other
Dipsia (thirst) / polydipsia (<5%)
Hiccups / singultus (<5%)
Infection (40%)
Tooth decay (<5%)

DECITABINE

Synonym: 5-aza-2'-deoxycytidine
Trade name: Dacogen (MGI Pharma)
Indications: Myelodysplastic syndromes, leukemia
Class: Antineoplastic / anticancer agent (see also Immune checkpoint inhibitor)
Half-life: ~30 minutes
Clinically important, potentially hazardous interactions with: none known
Important contra-indications noted in the prescribing guidelines for: nursing mothers; pediatric patients

---

Skin
Bacterial infection (5%)
Bruise / bruising / contusion / ecchymosis (ecchymoses) (22%)
Candidiasis / candidosis (10%)
Cellulitis and pseudocellulitis (12%)
Edema / fluid retention (18%)
Erythema (14%)
Facial edema (6%)
Hematoma / cutaneous hematoma (5%)
Lymphadenopathy (12%)
Pallor (23%)
Peripheral edema (25%)
Petechiae (39%)
Pruritus (itching) (11%)
Rash (19%) [2]
Sweet's syndrome [2]
Urticaria / hives (6%)

Mucosal
Burning Mouth Syndrome / glossodynia / glossalgia / glossopyrosis (also includes stomatodynia / oral dysesthesia / stomatopyrosis) (5%)
Gingival bleeding (8%)
Lip ulceration (5%)
Mucositis [2]
Oral candidiasis (6%)
Stomatitis (oral mucositis) (12%)
Tongue ulceration (7%)

Cardiovascular
Chest pain (7%)
Hypotension (6%)
QT interval prolonged / QT prolongation [2]

Central Nervous System
Anorexia (16%) [2]
Anxiety (11%)
Confusion (12%)
Fever (pyrexia) (includes hyperpyrexia) (53%) [2]
Headache (28%)
Hypoesthesia / hypesthesia (numbness) (11%)
Insomnia (28%)
Pain (13%)
Rigors (22%)
Vertigo / dizziness (18%)

Endocrine/Metabolic
ALP increased (11%)
Appetite decreased (16%)
AST increased (10%)
Dehydration (6%)
Hyperglycemia (includes glucose increased) (33%)
Hyperkalemia (13%)
Hypoalbuminemia / albumin decreased (24%)
Hypokalemia (22%)
Hypomagnesemia (24%)
Hyponatremia (19%)

Gastrointestinal/Hepatic
Abdominal distension (5%)
Abdominal pain (14%)
Ascites (10%)
Constipation (35%)
Diarrhea (34%) [2]
Dyspepsia / functional dyspepsia (indigestion) (see also gastroparesis) (12%)
Dysphagia (6%)
Gastroesophageal reflux (5%)
Hemorrhoids (8%)
Hepatotoxicity / liver injury / acute liver injury / drug-induced liver injury (DILI) [2]
Loose stools / soft feces (7%)
Nausea (42%) [8]
Vomiting (25%) [5]

Genitourinary
Dysuria (6%)
Urinary frequency (5%)
Urinary tract infection (7%)

Hematologic
Anemia (82%) [5]
Bacteremia (5%)
Febrile neutropenia (29%) [8]
Hemotoxicity [4]
Leukocytopenia (leukopenia) / leukocytes (white blood cells) decreased (28%) [2]
Lymphopenia (lymphocytopenia) / lymphocytes decreased [2]
Myelosuppression / bone marrow suppression / myelotoxicity [11]
Neutropenia (neutrophils decreased) (90%) [13]
Thrombocytopenia / platelets decreased (89%) [9]

Local
Injection-site edema (5%)

Injection-site erythema (5%)

Neuromuscular/Skeletal
Arthralgia (20%)
Asthenia / fatigue (5–12%) [7]
Back pain (17%)
Bone pain / joint pain (6–19%)
Myalgia/Myopathy (5%)

Ocular
Vision blurred (6%)

Respiratory
Cough (40%)
Hypoxia (10%)
Pharyngitis (sore throat) (16%)
Pneumonia (22%) [2]
Pulmonary edema (cardiogenic / non-cardiogenic) (6%)
Sinusitis (see also rhinitis / rhinosinusitis) (5%)

Other
Adverse effects / adverse reactions [2]
Allergic reactions [2]
Death [3]
Infection [5]

DEFERASIROX

Trade names: Exjade (Novartis), Jadenu (Novartis)
Indications: Chronic iron overload due to blood transfusions and in non-transfuson dependent thalassemia syndromes
Class: Chelator, iron
Half-life: 8–16 hours
Clinically important, potentially hazardous interactions with: alfuzosin, aluminum-containing antacids, ambrisentan, aprepitant, cabazitaxel, cholestyramine, cilostazol, colesevelam, colestipol, conivaptan, dabigatran, darunavir, dasatinib, delavirdine, docetaxel, efavirenz, enalapril, estradiol, eszopiclone, fesoterodine, gefitinib, indinavir, ixabepilone, lapatinib, lurasidone, maraviroc, pazopanib, phenobarbital, phenytoin, pioglitazone, repaglinide, rifampin, ritonavir, sildenafil, telithromycin, theophylline, tiagabine, tipranavir, trimethoprim, ulipristal
Important contra-indications noted in the prescribing guidelines for: the elderly; nursing mothers
Warning: RENAL FAILURE, HEPATIC FAILURE, AND GASTROINTESTINAL HEMORRHAGE

Skin
Exanthems [2]
Jaundice (see also cholestasis / cholestatic jaundice) [2]
Rash (2–11%) [24]
Urticaria / hives (4%)

Central Nervous System
Headache (16%) [2]

Endocrine/Metabolic
ALT increased [9]
Appetite decreased [2]
AST increased [4]
Hyperammonemia [4]
Serum creatinine increased [24]

Gastrointestinal/Hepatic
Abdominal pain (21–28%) [13]
Diarrhea (5–20%) [18]
Gastrointestinal bleeding [3]
Gastrointestinal disorder / discomfort [3]
Hepatic failure [4]
Hepatotoxicity / liver injury / acute liver injury / drug-induced liver injury (DILI) [10]
Nausea (2–6%) [20]
Vomiting (10–21%) [7]

Neuromuscular/Skeletal
Arthralgia (7%)
Asthenia / fatigue [3]
Back pain (6%)

Renal
Fanconi syndrome (proximal tubular dysfunction) [17]
Nephrotoxicity / kidney injury / acute kidney injury (AKI) / drug-induced kidney injury [7]
Proteinuria [4]
Renal failure [3]
Renal function abnormal / renal dysfunction [2]

Respiratory
Cough (14%)
Influenza- ('flu)-like syndrome (11%)
Upper respiratory tract infection (9%)

Other
Adverse effects / adverse reactions [16]

DEFERIPRONE

Trade name: Ferriprox (ApoPharma)
Indications: Treatment of patients with transfusional iron overload due to thalassemia syndromes when current chelation therapy is inadequate
Class: Chelator, iron
Half-life: 1.9 hours
Clinically important, potentially hazardous interactions with: antacids containing iron, aluminum, zinc, diclofenac, mineral supplements, probenecid
Important contra-indications noted in the prescribing guidelines for: the elderly; nursing mothers; pediatric patients
Warning: AGRANULOCYTOSIS / NEUTROPENIA

Central Nervous System
Headache (3%)

Endocrine/Metabolic
ALT increased (8%) [5]
Appetite increased (4%)
AST increased [2]
Serum creatinine increased [2]
Weight gain (2%)

Gastrointestinal/Hepatic
Abdominal pain (10%) [2]
Diarrhea (3%) [2]
Dyspepsia / functional dyspepsia (indigestion) (see also gastroparesis) (2%)
Gastrointestinal disorder / discomfort [5]
Hepatotoxicity / liver injury / acute liver injury / drug-induced liver injury (DILI) [3]
Nausea (13%) [4]
Vomiting (10%)

Hematologic
Agranulocytosis / severe selective neutropenia (2%) [16]
Neutropenia (neutrophils decreased) [13]
Thrombocytopenia / platelets decreased [2]

Neuromuscular/Skeletal
Arthralgia (10%) [8]
Arthropathy [5]
Back pain (2%)
Bone pain / joint pain [2]
Pain in extremities (2%)

Renal
Chromaturia (15%)

Other
Adverse effects / adverse reactions [2]
Death [2]

DEFEROXAMINE

Trade name: Desferal (Novartis)
Indications: Hemochromatosis, acute iron overload
Class: Chelator, iron
Half-life: 6.1 hours
Clinically important, potentially hazardous interactions with: ascorbic acid, ferrous sulfate, pericyazine, pericyazine, zinc

---

Skin
Anaphylactoid reactions / anaphylaxis (includes anaphylactic shock) [3]
Hypersensitivity [2]

Central Nervous System
Neurotoxicity [2]

Endocrine/Metabolic
Serum creatinine increased [2]

Local
Injection-site inflammation (<10%)
Injection-site pain (<10%)

Neuromuscular/Skeletal
Arthralgia [6]

Ocular
Night blindness [2]
Retinopathy [12]

Otic
Hearing loss (hypoacusis) [2]
Ototoxicity [7]

Other
Death [3]

DEFIBROTIDE

Trade name: Defitelio (Jazz)
Indications: Hepatic veno-occlusive disease in patients with renal or pulmonary dysfunction following hematopoietic stem-cell transplantation
Class: Oligonucleotide
Half-life: <2 hours
Clinically important, potentially hazardous interactions with: alteplase, heparin
Pregnancy category: No data available
Important contra-indications noted in the prescribing guidelines for: nursing mothers
Note: Contra-indicated for concomitant administration with systemic anticoagulant or fibrinolytic therapy.

Skin
Graft-versus-host reaction (6%)

Mucosal
Epistaxis (nosebleed) (14%)

Cardiovascular
Hypotension (37%) [5]

Central Nervous System
Cerebral hemorrhage (2%)
Intracranial hemorrhage (3%)

Endocrine/Metabolic
Hyperuricemia (2%)

Gastrointestinal/Hepatic
Diarrhea (24%)
Gastrointestinal bleeding (9%) [3]

Nausea (16%)
Vomiting (18%)

Hematologic
Hemorrhage [3]
Sepsis (7%)

Respiratory
Alveolar hemorrhage (pulmonary) (9%)
Pneumonia (5%)
Pulmonary hemorrhage (4%)
Pulmonary toxicity (6%)

Other
Adverse effects / adverse reactions [4]
Infection (3%)

DEFLAZACORT

Trade name: Emflaza (Marathon)
Indications: Duchenne muscular dystrophy
Class: Corticosteroid / Glucocorticoid
Half-life: N/A
Clinically important, potentially hazardous interactions with: carbamazepine, clarithromycin, diltiazem, efavirenz, fluconazole, grapefruit juice, live vaccines, pancuronium, phenytoin, rifampin, verapamil
Pregnancy category: Should be used during pregnancy only if the potential benefit justifies the potential risk to the fetus
Important contra-indications noted in the prescribing guidelines for: the elderly; nursing mothers; pediatric patients

---

Skin
Cushingoid features (33%) [3]
Erythema (8%)
Hypersensitivity [3]
Stevens-Johnson syndrome and toxic epidermal necrolysis (SJS/TEN) [4]

Hair
Hirsutism (10%) [2]

Mucosal
Rhinorrhea (8%)

Central Nervous System
Behavioral disturbances / personality changes [2]
Irritability (8%)

Endocrine/Metabolic
Appetite increased (14%) [2]
Weight gain (20%) [6]

Gastrointestinal/Hepatic
Abdominal pain (6%)

Genitourinary
Pollakiuria (12%)

Ocular
Cataract [3]

Respiratory
Cough (12%)
Nasopharyngitis (10%)
Upper respiratory tract infection (12%)

Other
Adverse effects / adverse reactions [3]
Side effects [2]

DEGARELIX

Trade name: Firmagon (Ferring)
Indications: Advanced hormone-dependent prostate cancer
Class: Gonadotropin-releasing hormone (GnRH) antagonist
Half-life: 43 days
Clinically important, potentially hazardous interactions with: alfuzosin, amiodarone, antipsychotics, artemether/lumefantrine, chloroquine, ciprofloxacin, cisapride, disopyramide, dofetilide, dronedarone, gadobutrol, ibutilide, moxifloxacin, nilotinib, pimozide, QT prolonging agents, quinidine, quinine, sotalol, tetrabenazine, thioridazine, ziprasidone
Important contra-indications noted in the prescribing guidelines for: nursing mothers; pediatric patients

---

Skin
Flushing / rubefaction (<10%) [2]
Hot flashes / hot flushes (26%) [2]
Hyperhidrosis (<5%)

Cardiovascular
Hypertension (6–7%)

Central Nervous System
Chills (4–5%) [2]
Fever (pyrexia) (includes hyperpyrexia) (<5%) [2]
Headache (<5%)
Insomnia (<5%)
Vertigo / dizziness (<5%)

Endocrine/Metabolic
ALT increased (10%)
GGT increased (10%)
Weight gain (9–11%) [3]
Weight loss (<10%)

Gastrointestinal/Hepatic
Constipation (3–5%)
Nausea (<5%)

Genitourinary
Urinary tract infection (2–5%)

Local
Injection-site edema (6%)
Injection-site erythema (17%)
Injection-site nodules (3%)
Injection-site pain (28%) [2]
Injection-site reaction (35–44%) [5]
Injection-site scarring (4%)

Neuromuscular/Skeletal
Arthralgia (4–5%)
Asthenia / fatigue (9–11%)

Respiratory
Influenza- ('flu)-like syndrome (<10%)

DELAVIRDINE

Trade name: Rescriptor (ViiV)
Indications: HIV-1 infection
Class: Antiretroviral, CYP3A4 inhibitor, Non-nucleoside reverse transcriptase inhibitor
Half-life: 2–11 hours
Clinically important, potentially hazardous interactions with: adefovir, alfuzosin, almotriptan, alosetron, alprazolam, amiodarone, amlodipine, amphetamines, amprenavir, anisindione, antacids, anticoagulants, artemether/lumefantrine, astemizole, atomoxetine, atorvastatin, bepridil, bortezomib, brinzolamide, buprenorphine, carbamazepine, carvedilol, cerivastatin, ciclesonide, cimetidine, cisapride, clarithromycin, clopidogrel, codeine, colchicine, conivaptan, cyclosporine, CYP2C19 substrates, CYP2C9 substrates, CYP2D6 substrates, CYP3A4 inducers and substrates, darunavir, deferasirox, dexamethasone, dicumarol, dienogest, dihydroergotamine, diltiazem, dronedarone, dutasteride, eplerenone, ergonovine, ergotamine, estradiol, etravirine, everolimus, famotidine, felodipine, fentanyl, fesoterodine, flecainide, fluticasone propionate, fluvastatin, fosamprenavir, guanfacine, halofantrine, indinavir, isradipine, ixabepilone, lansoprazole, lidocaine, lopinavir, lovastatin, maraviroc, methadone, methylergonovine, methylprednisolone, methysergide, midazolam, mometasone, nebivolol, nelfinavir, nicardipine, nifedipine, nilotinib, nimodipine, nisoldipine, nizatidine, omeprazole, paclitaxel, pantoprazole, paricalcitol, pazopanib, PEG-interferon, phenobarbital, phenytoin, pimecrolimus, pimozide, prasugrel, propafenone, propranolol, protease inhibitors, proton pump inhibitors, quinidine, ranitidine, ranolazine, rifabutin, rifampin, rifapentine, rilpivirine, ritonavir, rivaroxaban, romidepsin, salmeterol, saquinavir, saxagliptin, sildenafil, silodosin, simeprevir, simvastatin, sirolimus, sorafenib, St John's wort, tacrolimus, tadalafil, tamoxifen, tamsulosin, terfenadine, tetrabenazine, thioridazine, tipranavir, tolvaptan, tramadol, trazodone, triazolam, verapamil, warfarin
Important contra-indications noted in the prescribing guidelines for: nursing mothers; pediatric patients

---

Skin
Angioedema (formerly named angioneurotic edema) (<2%)
Bruise / bruising / contusion / ecchymosis (ecchymoses) (<2%)
Cyst / pseudocyst (<2%)
Dermatitis (<2%)
Desquamation (<2%)
Diaphoresis (<2%)
Edema of lip (<2%)
Erythema (<2%)
Erythema multiforme (<2%)
Exanthems (7%)
Folliculitis (<2%)
Fungal dermatitis (<2%)
Nodular eruption (<2%)
Peripheral edema (<2%)
Petechiae (<2%)
Pruritus (itching) (<2%)
Purpura (<2%)
Rash (3–20%) [5]
Seborrhea (<2%)
Stevens-Johnson syndrome and toxic epidermal necrolysis (SJS/TEN) (<2%)
Urticaria / hives (<2%)
Vasculitis (angiitis) / cutaneous vasculitis (angiitis) (<2%)
Vesiculobullous eruption (<2%)
Xerosis / xeroderma (<2%)

Hair
Alopecia / hair loss (<2%)

Nails
Nail changes (<2%)

Mucosal
Aphthous stomatitis / aphthous ulcer / aphtha (aphthae) (<2%)

Gingivitis (<2%)
Oral ulceration (<2%)
Sialorrhea (ptyalism; hypersalivation) (<2%)
Stomatitis (oral mucositis) (<2%)
Tongue edema (<2%)
Xerostomia (dry mouth) (<2%)

Central Nervous System
Anxiety (2–7%)
Depression (4–5%)
Dysgeusia (taste perversion) (<2%)
Fever (pyrexia) (includes hyperpyrexia) (2–7%)
Headache (11–17%)
Insomnia (1–5%)
Pain (2–6%)
Paresthesias (<2%)

Endocrine/Metabolic
Gynecomastia (<2%)

Gastrointestinal/Hepatic
Abdominal pain (2–5%)
Diarrhea (2–9%)
Nausea (9–20%)
Vomiting (3–9%)

Genitourinary
Vulvovaginal candidiasis (<2%)

Neuromuscular/Skeletal
Asthenia / fatigue (5–16%)
Myalgia/Myopathy (<2%)

Respiratory
Bronchitis (4–7%)
Cough (4–10%)
Influenza- ('flu)-like syndrome (2–7%)
Pharyngitis (sore throat) (2–9%)
Sinusitis (see also rhinitis / rhinosinusitis) (1–11%)

Other
Allergic reactions (<2%)

DEMECLOCYCLINE

Trade name: Declomycin (ESP Pharma)
Indications: Various infections caused by susceptible organisms
Class: Antibiotic, Antibiotic; tetracycline, Antimicrobial
Half-life: 10–16 hours
Clinically important, potentially hazardous interactions with: acitretin, amoxicillin, ampicillin, antacids, bacampicillin, BCG vaccine, bismuth, calcium salts, carbenicillin, cloxacillin, coumarins, dairy products, desmopressin, digoxin, dong quai, ergotamine, kaolin, methotrexate, methoxyflurane, methysergide, mezlocillin, nafcillin, oral iron, oral typhoid vaccine, oxacillin, penicillins, phenindione, piperacillin, quinapril, retinoids, St John's wort, strontium ranelate, sucralfate, sulfonylureas, ticarcillin, tripotassium dicitratobismuthate, zinc
Important contra-indications noted in the prescribing guidelines for: nursing mothers; pediatric patients

---

Skin
Fixed eruption / fixed drug eruption [4]
Photosensitivity (<10%) [19]
Phototoxicity [3]

Nails
Photo-onycholysis [6]

DENILEUKIN

Trade name: Ontak (Ligand)
Indications: Cutaneous T-cell lymphoma
Class: Antineoplastic / anticancer agent (see also Immune checkpoint inhibitor)
Half-life: 70–80 minutes
Clinically important, potentially hazardous interactions with: BCG vaccine, belimumab, denosumab, leflunomide, natalizumab, pimecrolimus, roflumilast, sipuleucel-T, tacrolimus, trastuzumab, vaccines
Important contra-indications noted in the prescribing guidelines for: nursing mothers; pediatric patients
Warning: SERIOUS INFUSION REACTIONS, CAPILLARY LEAK SYNDROME AND LOSS OF VISUAL ACUITY

Skin
Diaphoresis (10%)
Edema / fluid retention (47%) [2]
Hypersensitivity (69%) [2]
Peripheral edema (20–26%)
Pruritus (itching) (16–18%)
Rash (20–24%) [2]

Cardiovascular
Hypotension (7–16%) [2]
Vascular leak syndrome [5]

Central Nervous System
Anorexia (9–20%)
Chills (81%) [3]
Dysgeusia (taste perversion) (11%)
Fever (pyrexia) (includes hyperpyrexia) (49–64%) [3]
Headache (26–29%)
Pain (11–13%)
Paresthesias (13%)
Rigors (42–47%)
Vertigo / dizziness (11–13%)

Endocrine/Metabolic
ALT increased (84%) [2]
AST increased (84%)
Hypoalbuminemia / albumin decreased [2]

Gastrointestinal/Hepatic
Diarrhea (22%)
Nausea (47–60%) [4]
Vomiting (13–35%) [3]

Local
Infusion-site reactions [2]

Neuromuscular/Skeletal
Arthralgia (13–16%)
Asthenia / fatigue (17–47%) [4]
Back pain (16–18%) [2]
Myalgia/Myopathy (18–20%) [2]

Ocular
Vision loss [2]

Respiratory
Cough (18–20%)
Dyspnea / shortness of breath (11–13%)
Influenza- ('flu)-like syndrome [2]
Upper respiratory tract infection (13%)

Other
Adverse effects / adverse reactions [3]
Death [2]
Infection (48%)

DENOSUMAB

Trade names: Prolia (Amgen), Xgeva (Amgen)
Indications: Osteoporosis (postmenopausal women), prevention of skeletal-related events in patients with bone metastases from solid tumors
Class: Bone resorption inhibitor, Monoclonal antibody, RANK ligand (RANKL) inhibitor
Half-life: 25–28 days
Clinically important, potentially hazardous interactions with: abatacept, alcohol, azacitidine, betamethasone, cabazitaxel, denileukin, docetaxel, fingolimod, gefitinib, immuosuppressants, leflunomide, lenalidomide, oxaliplatin, pazopanib, pralatrexate, pralatrexate, temsirolimus, triamcinolone
Important contra-indications noted in the prescribing guidelines for: nursing mothers; pediatric patients
Note: Contra-indicated in patients with hypocalcemia. Denosumab-bbdz (Jubbonti and Wyost) biosimilars. Approved 03/05/2024.

Skin
Cellulitis and pseudocellulitis [9]
Dermatitis [2]
Eczema / eczematous reaction / eczematous eruption [10]
Herpes zoster (2%)
Hypersensitivity [3]
Peripheral edema (5%)
Pruritus (itching) (2%)
Rash (3%) [4]

Cardiovascular
Angina (3%)
Atrial fibrillation (2%)
Cardiotoxicity [2]

Central Nervous System
Headache [3]
Insomnia (3%)
Pain [2]
Vertigo / dizziness (5%)

Endocrine/Metabolic
Hypercalcemia [5]
Hypercholesterolemia (7%) [2]
Hypocalcemia (2%) [51]
Hypophosphatemia [6]

Gastrointestinal/Hepatic
Abdominal pain (3%)
Flatulence (2%)
Gastroesophageal reflux (2%)
Hepatotoxicity / liver injury / acute liver injury / drug-induced liver injury (DILI) [2]
Pancreatitis / acute pancreatitis [2]

Genitourinary
Cystitis (includes interstitial cystitis / bladder pain syndrome) (6%)

Hematologic
Anemia (3%) [2]

Neuromuscular/Skeletal
Arthralgia [5]
Asthenia / fatigue (2%) [2]
Back pain (35%) [8]
Bone pain / joint pain (4–8%) [3]
Fractures [10]
Myalgia/Myopathy (3%)
Osteonecrosis / avascular necrosis (includes steroid-induced osteonecrosis of the femoral head) (jaw) [31]
Pain in extremities (12%) [6]

Respiratory
Nasopharyngitis [2]
Pharyngitis (sore throat) (2%)
Pneumonia (4%)
Upper respiratory tract infection (5%)

Other
Adverse effects / adverse reactions [12]
Death [2]
Infection [14]
Malignancies [2]

DESFLURANE

Trade name: Suprane (Baxter)
Indications: Induction or maintenance of anesthesia
Class: Anesthetic; inhalation
Half-life: 5–12 minutes
Clinically important, potentially hazardous interactions with: tramadol
Important contra-indications noted in the prescribing guidelines for: nursing mothers

---

Cardiovascular
QT interval prolonged / QT prolongation [3]

Gastrointestinal/Hepatic
Hepatotoxicity / liver injury / acute liver injury / drug-induced liver injury (DILI) [3]

Respiratory
Cough (34%) [4]

DESIPRAMINE

Trade name: Norpramin (Sanofi-Aventis)
Indications: Depression
Class: Antidepressant; tricyclic, Norepinephrine reuptake inhibitor
Half-life: 7–60 hours
Clinically important, potentially hazardous interactions with: amprenavir, arbutamine, boceprevir, buspirone, cinacalcet, clonidine, cobicistat/elvitegravir/emtricitabine/tenofovir alafenamide, cobicistat/elvitegravir/emtricitabine/tenofovir disoproxil, epinephrine, fentanyl, fluoxetine, formoterol, guanethidine, isocarboxazid, linezolid, lithium, MAO inhibitors, mirabegron, phenelzine, quinolones, sparfloxacin, St John's wort, telaprevir, terbinafine, tramadol, tranylcypromine, tricyclic antidepressants, tryptophan, viloxazine
Important contra-indications noted in the prescribing guidelines for: the elderly; nursing mothers; pediatric patients
Warning: SUICIDALITY AND ANTIDEPRESSANT DRUGS

Skin
Diaphoresis (<10%) [2]
Exanthems [5]
Pigmentation (Skin) (includes hyperpigmentation) (blue-gray) (photosensitive) [3]
Pruritus (itching) [4]
Pseudolymphoma / cutaneous pseudolymphoma [2]
Purpura [2]
Urticaria / hives [3]

Mucosal
Xerostomia (dry mouth) (>10%) [5]

Central Nervous System
Dysgeusia (taste perversion) (>10%)

Other
Allergic reactions [2]
Side effects [2]

DESLORATADINE

Trade name: Clarinex (Schering)
Indications: Allergic rhinitis, urticaria
Class: Histamine H1 receptor antagonist
Half-life: 27 hours
Clinically important, potentially hazardous interactions with: none known
Important contra-indications noted in the prescribing guidelines for: nursing mothers; pediatric patients

---

Skin
Urticaria / hives [2]

Mucosal
Xerostomia (dry mouth) [6]

Central Nervous System
Headache [7]
Seizures [2]
Somnolence (drowsiness) [7]

Gastrointestinal/Hepatic
Diarrhea [2]
Nausea [3]

Neuromuscular/Skeletal
Asthenia / fatigue [8]
Convulsions [2]

Other
Adverse effects / adverse reactions [6]

DESMOPRESSIN

Trade names: DDAVP (Sanofi-Aventis), Minirin (Ferring), Noctiva (Serenity), Stimate (CSL Behring)
Indications: Primary nocturnal enuresis, nocturia due to nocturnal polyuria (Noctiva)
Class: Antidiuretic hormone analog
Half-life: 75 minutes
Clinically important, potentially hazardous interactions with: amitriptyline, citalopram, demeclocycline, hydromorphone, meloxicam, tapentadol
Important contra-indications noted in the prescribing guidelines for: the elderly; nursing mothers; pediatric patients
Warning: Noctiva: HYPONATREMIA

Skin
Flushing / rubefaction (<10%)

Cardiovascular
Myocardial infarction [2]

Central Nervous System
Headache [7]
Seizures [5]

Endocrine/Metabolic
Hyponatremia [16]
SIADH [2]

Local
Injection-site pain (<10%)

DESVENLAFAXINE

Trade name: Pristiq (Wyeth)
Indications: Major depressive disorder
Class: Antidepressant, Serotonin-norepinephrine reuptake inhibitor
Half-life: 11 hours
Clinically important, potentially hazardous interactions with: alcohol, aspirin, CNS-active agents, heparin, ketoconazole, linezolid, lithium, MAO inhibitors, NSAIDs, sibutramine, tramadol, venlafaxine, warfarin
Important contra-indications noted in the prescribing guidelines for: the elderly; nursing mothers; pediatric patients
Warning: SUICIDAL THOUGHTS AND BEHAVIORS

Skin
Hot flashes / hot flushes (<2%)
Hyperhidrosis (10–21%)
Hypersensitivity (2%)
Rash (<2%)

Mucosal
Epistaxis (nosebleed) (<2%)
Xerostomia (dry mouth) (11–25%) [3]

Cardiovascular
Hypertension (<2%)
Hypotension (~2%)
Orthostatic hypotension (<2%)
Palpitation (<3%)
Tachycardia (<2%)

Central Nervous System
Abnormal dreams (2–4%)
Anorexia (5–8%) [2]
Anorgasmia (3–8%)
Anxiety (3–5%)
Chills (<4%)
Dysgeusia (taste perversion) (<2%)
Extrapyramidal symptoms (<2%)
Headache (20–29%) [3]
Impaired concentration (<2%)
Insomnia (9–12%) [3]
Irritability (2%)
Nervousness (<2%) [2]
Paresthesias (<3%)
Seizures (~2%)
Somnolence (drowsiness) (4–12%) [4]
Suicidal ideation [3]
Syncope / fainting (<2%)
Tremor (~3%)
Vertigo / dizziness (10–16%) [5]
Yawning (<4%)

Endocrine/Metabolic
Appetite decreased (5–10%)
Libido decreased (3–6%)
Weight gain (<2%)
Weight loss (<2%)

Gastrointestinal/Hepatic
Constipation (9–14%)
Diarrhea (5–11%)
Nausea (22–41%) [7]
Vomiting (3–9%)

Genitourinary
Ejaculatory dysfunction (<5%)
Erectile dysfunction (3–11%)
Sexual dysfunction (<2%)

Neuromuscular/Skeletal
Asthenia / fatigue (7–11%) [2]

Ocular
Mydriasis (2–6%)
Vision blurred (3–4%)

Otic
Tinnitus (<2%)

DEUTETRABENAZINE

Trade name: Austedo (Teva)
Indications: Chorea associated with Huntington's disease
Class: Vesicular monoamine transporter 2 inhibitor
Half-life: 9–10 hours
Clinically important, potentially hazardous interactions with: alcohol or other sedating drugs, bupropion, dopamine antagonists or antipsychotics, fluoxetine, MAO inhibitors, paroxetine hydrochloride, quinidine, strong CYP2D6 inhibitors, tetrabenazine
Pregnancy category: Based on animal data, may cause fetal harm
Important contra-indications noted in the prescribing guidelines for: the elderly; nursing mothers; pediatric patients
Note: Contra-indicated in suicidal or untreated/ inadequately treated depression, in hepatic impairment. or in patients taking MAO inhibitors, reserpine or tetrabenazine.
Warning: DEPRESSION AND SUICIDALITY

Skin
Hematoma / cutaneous hematoma (4%)
Mucosal
Xerostomia (dry mouth) (9%)
Central Nervous System
Akathisia [3]
Anxiety (4%) [5]
Depression [6]
Headache [2]
Insomnia (7%) [5]
Parkinsonism [2]
Somnolence (drowsiness) (11%) [9]
Suicidal ideation [2]
Vertigo / dizziness (4%)
Gastrointestinal/Hepatic
Constipation (4%)
Diarrhea (9%) [4]
Nausea [2]
Genitourinary
Urinary tract infection (7%)
Neuromuscular/Skeletal
Asthenia / fatigue (9%) [4]
Respiratory
Nasopharyngitis [3]

DEVIL'S CLAW

Family: Pedaliaceae
Scientific names: *Harpagophytum procumbens, Harpagophytum zeyheri*
Indications: Oral: anorexia, arteriosclerosis, rheumatoid arthritis, GI disorders, fibromyalgia, loss of appetite, headache, fever, high cholesterol, menstrual complaints, liver and gallbladder problems. **Topical:** rash, ulcers
Class: Analgesic, Anti-inflammatory
Half-life: 3–6 hours
Clinically important, potentially hazardous interactions with: anesthetics, antacids, antiarrhythmics, anticoagulants, aspirin, beta blockers, histamine H_2-antagonists, hypoglycemics, NSAIDs, sympathomimetics, terfenadine
Note: Devil's claw stimulates stomach acid production, and should be avoided by those with stomach or duodenal ulcers. It should not be taken by people with cardiac arrhythmias or other heart problems.

Other
Adverse effects / adverse reactions [5]

DEXAMETHASONE

Trade names: Decadron (Merck), Dexone (Solvay), Ozurdex (Allergan)
Indications: Antiemetic, arthralgias, dermatoses, diagnostic aid, macular edema following branch retinal vein occlusion (BRVO) or central retinal vein occlusion (CRVO), non-infectious uveitis affecting the posterior segment of the eye
Class: Antiemetic, Corticosteroid / Glucocorticoid, Corticosteroid, systemic, Corticosteroid, topical, Covid-19 putative drug
Half-life: N/A
Clinically important, potentially hazardous interactions with: albendazole, aminoglutethimide, amprenavir, aprepitant, aspirin, bexarotene, boceprevir, carbamazepine, caspofungin, cobicistat/elvitegravir/emtricitabine/ tenofovir alafenamide, cobicistat/elvitegravir/ emtricitabine/tenofovir disoproxil, cyclophosphamide, dasatinib, delavirdine, diuretics, emtricitabine/rilpivirine/tenofovir alafenamide, ephedrine, imatinib, itraconazole, ixabepilone, lapatinib, lenalidomide, live vaccines, lopinavir, methotrexate, midazolam, phenobarbital, phenytoin, praziquantel, primidone, rifampin, rilpivirine, romidepsin, simeprevir, sorafenib, sunitinib, telaprevir, temsirolimus, ticagrelor, vandetanib, warfarin
Important contra-indications noted in the prescribing guidelines for: nursing mothers; pediatric patients

---

Skin
Acneiform eruption / acneiform dermatitis / acneiform rash [6]
AGEP [2]
Anaphylactoid reactions / anaphylaxis (includes anaphylactic shock) [3]
Cutaneous toxicity / skin toxicity [5]
Dermatitis [5]
Edema / fluid retention [4]
Erythema multiforme [3]
Exanthems [4]
Flushing / rubefaction [5]
Herpes zoster [2]
Hyperhidrosis [2]
Hypersensitivity [6]
Peripheral edema [9]
Pigmentation (Skin) (includes hyperpigmentation) [2]
Pruritus (itching) [7]
Pruritus ani et vulvae [2]
Rash [11]
Stevens-Johnson syndrome and toxic epidermal necrolysis (SJS/TEN) [2]
Striae [4]
Xerosis / xeroderma [2]
Mucosal
Oral candidiasis [2]
Cardiovascular
Bradycardia / sinus bradycardia [9]
Cardiac failure [2]
Cardiotoxicity [2]
Hypertension [18]
Myocardial toxicity [11]
Tachycardia [2]
Thromboembolism [3]
Venous thromboembolism [5]
Central Nervous System
Anorexia [2]
Catatonia [2]
Dysgeusia (taste perversion) [3]
Fever (pyrexia) (includes hyperpyrexia) [8]
Headache (<5%) [8]
Hypoesthesia / hypesthesia (numbness) [2]
Insomnia [9]
Leukoencephalopathy / posterior reversible encephalopathy syndrome (PRES) [2]
Neuropsychiatric / neuropsychological adverse effect [6]
Neurotoxicity [10]
Paresthesias [2]
Peripheral neuropathy [28]
Psychosis [6]
Somnolence (drowsiness) [2]
Vertigo / dizziness [3]
Endocrine/Metabolic
ALT increased [2]
AST increased [2]
Cushing's syndrome [3]
Dehydration [3]
Hyperglycemia (includes glucose increased) [9]
Hypokalemia [5]
Hypophosphatemia [4]
Serum creatinine increased [2]
Gastrointestinal/Hepatic
Abdominal distension [2]
Abdominal pain [5]
Constipation [11]
Diarrhea [21]
Dyspepsia / functional dyspepsia (indigestion) (see also gastroparesis) [3]
Gastroesophageal reflux [2]
Gastrointestinal disorder / discomfort [3]
Hepatotoxicity / liver injury / acute liver injury / drug-induced liver injury (DILI) [4]
Nausea [12]
Pancreatitis / acute pancreatitis [2]
Vomiting [7]
Hematologic
Anemia [41]
Febrile neutropenia [8]
Hemoglobin decreased [2]
Hemotoxicity [8]
Leukocytopenia (leukopenia) / leukocytes (white blood cells) decreased [13]
Leukocytosis (elevated white blood cell (WBC) count) [2]
Lymphopenia (lymphocytopenia) / lymphocytes decreased [12]
Myelosuppression / bone marrow suppression / myelotoxicity [5]
Neutropenia (neutrophils decreased) [54]
Sepsis [3]
Thrombocytopenia / platelets decreased [54]
Thrombosis [2]
Local
Infusion-related reactions [2]
Infusion-site reactions [2]
Multi-Organ and/or Multi-Metabolic Adverse Reactions
Pheochromocytoma crisis / paraganglioma crisis [5]

Neuromuscular/Skeletal
Arthralgia [5]
Asthenia / fatigue [45]
Back pain [5]
Bone pain / joint pain [4]
Muscle spasm [5]
Myalgia/Myopathy [6]
Osteonecrosis / avascular necrosis (includes steroid-induced osteonecrosis of the femoral head) [17]
Osteoporosis [4]

Ocular
Cataract (<10%) [10]
Conjunctival hemorrhage (>10%)
Glaucoma (includes acute angle-closure glaucoma) [10]
Intraocular pressure increased (>10%) [15]
Ocular adverse effect [2]
Ocular hypertension (<10%) [8]
Ocular pain (<10%) [6]
Vision blurred [3]

Otic
Ototoxicity [4]

Renal
Nephrotoxicity / kidney injury / acute kidney injury (AKI) / drug-induced kidney injury [2]
Renal failure [2]
Tumor lysis syndrome (TLS) [3]

Respiratory
Cough [4]
Dyspnea / shortness of breath [5]
Pneumonia [14]
Pneumonitis [2]
Upper respiratory tract infection [3]

Other
Adverse effects / adverse reactions [21]
Allergic reactions [2]
Death [11]
Hiccups / singultus [20]
Infection [32]
Side effects [3]

DEXCHLOR-PHENIRAMINE

Trade name: Tanafed (First Horizon)
Indications: Allergic rhinitis, urticaria
Class: Histamine H1 receptor antagonist
Half-life: 20–24 hours
Clinically important, potentially hazardous interactions with: barbiturates, chloral hydrate, ethchlorvynol, glutethimide, phenothiazines, zolpidem

---

Mucosal
Xerostomia (dry mouth) (<10%)

DEXIBUPROFEN

Trade names: Actifen (Gebro), Deltaran (Strathmann), Dexoptifen (Spirig), Seractil (Genus)
Indications: Dental pain, dysmenorrhea, muscular pain and osteoarthritis
Class: Non-steroidal anti-inflammatory (NSAID)
Half-life: 2 hours
Clinically important, potentially hazardous interactions with: aspirin, celecoxib, citalopram, etoricoxib, fluoxetine, NSAIDs, paroxetine hydrochloride, venlafaxine, warfarin
Note: NSAIDs may cause an increased risk of serious cardiovascular and gastrointestinal adverse events, which can be fatal. This risk may increase with duration of use.

DEXKETOPROFEN

Trade names: Enangel (Topical), Keral (Menarini), Ketesse (Pharmaforte)
Indications: Pain
Class: Non-steroidal anti-inflammatory (NSAID)
Half-life: N/A
Clinically important, potentially hazardous interactions with: none known
Note: NSAIDs may cause an increased risk of serious cardiovascular and gastrointestinal adverse events, which can be fatal. This risk may increase with duration of use.

Skin
Photocontact dermatitis [5]

Gastrointestinal/Hepatic
Nausea [3]
Vomiting [2]

Neuromuscular/Skeletal
Asthenia / fatigue [2]

Other
Adverse effects / adverse reactions [2]

DEXLANSOPRAZOLE

Trade name: Dexilant (Takeda)
Indications: Erosive esophagitis, heartburn associated with gastroesophageal reflux disease
Class: Proton pump inhibitor (PPI)
Half-life: <2 hours
Clinically important, potentially hazardous interactions with: atazanavir, clopidogrel, digoxin, emtricitabine/rilpivirine/tenofovir alafenamide, ketoconazole, tacrolimus, warfarin
Important contra-indications noted in the prescribing guidelines for: nursing mothers

---

Skin
Acneiform eruption / acneiform dermatitis / acneiform rash (<2%)
Dermatitis (<2%)
Erythema (<2%)
Hot flashes / hot flushes (<2%)
Lesions (includes skin lesions) (<2%)
Lymphadenopathy (<2%)
Pruritus (itching) (<2%)
Rash (<2%)
Urticaria / hives (<2%)

Mucosal
Mucosal inflammation (<2%)
Oral candidiasis (<2%)
Xerostomia (dry mouth) (<2%)

Cardiovascular
Cardiac disorder / cardiac dysfunction (<2%)

Central Nervous System
Headache [3]

Gastrointestinal/Hepatic
Abdominal pain (4%) [5]
Constipation [2]
Diarrhea (5%) [4]
Flatulence (<3%) [3]
Gastrointestinal disorder / discomfort (<2%)
Nausea (3%) [4]
Vomiting (<2%) [2]

Hematologic
Anemia (<2%)

Ocular
Ocular edema (eye edema) (<2%)
Ocular itching / ocular pruritus (<2%)

Otic
Ear pain (<2%)
Tinnitus (<2%)

Respiratory
Upper respiratory tract infection (2–3%) [4]

Other
Adverse effects / adverse reactions [2]

DEXMEDETOMIDINE

Trade name: Precedex (AbbVie)
Indications: Sedation for intensive care unit intubation
Class: Adrenergic alpha-receptor agonist
Half-life: 2 hours
Clinically important, potentially hazardous interactions with: digoxin, opioids

---

Mucosal
Xerostomia (dry mouth) [2]

Cardiovascular
Asystole [3]
Bradycardia / sinus bradycardia [31]
Cardiac disorder / cardiac dysfunction [2]
Hypotension [23]

Central Nervous System
Delirium [3]
Fever (pyrexia) (includes hyperpyrexia) [10]
Hyperthermia [3]
Pain (3%)
Sedation [2]

Endocrine/Metabolic
Diabetes insipidus [4]

Gastrointestinal/Hepatic
Intestinal pseudo-obstruction (Ogilvie syndrome) [3]
Nausea [3]
Vomiting [2]

Genitourinary
Polyuria (includes polyuric syndrome) [17]

Respiratory
Bradypnea / respiratory rate decreased [2]

Other
Adverse effects / adverse reactions [2]
Infection (2%)

DEXMETHYL-PHENIDATE

Trade name: Focalin (Novartis)
Indications: Attention deficit disorder
Class: Anti-attention deficit hyperactivity disorder (anti-ADHD), CNS stimulant
Half-life: 2–4.5 hours
Clinically important, potentially hazardous interactions with: amitriptyline, clonidine, linezolid, MAO inhibitors, pantoprazole
Important contra-indications noted in the prescribing guidelines for: nursing mothers; pediatric patients
Note: Contra-indicated in patients with marked anxiety, tension and agitation, with glaucoma, or

with motor tics or history/diagnosis of Tourette's syndrome.

Central Nervous System
Fever (pyrexia) (includes hyperpyrexia) (5%)
Headache [4]

Endocrine/Metabolic
Appetite decreased [2]

Gastrointestinal/Hepatic
Abdominal pain (15%) [2]

DEXTRO-AMPHETAMINE

Trade names: Adderall (Shire), Dexedrine (Alliant), Mydayis (Shire)
Indications: Narcolepsy, attention deficit disorder (ADD)
Class: Amphetamine, CNS stimulant
Half-life: 10–12 hours
Clinically important, potentially hazardous interactions with: fluoxetine, fluvoxamine, MAO inhibitors, paroxetine hydrochloride, phenelzine, sertraline, tranylcypromine
Important contra-indications noted in the prescribing guidelines for: nursing mothers; pediatric patients
Warning: ABUSE AND DEPENDENCE

Skin
Diaphoresis (<10%)

Mucosal
Xerostomia (dry mouth) (<10%)

Central Nervous System
Headache [2]
Insomnia [2]

Endocrine/Metabolic
Appetite decreased [2]

Gastrointestinal/Hepatic
Abdominal pain [2]

Neuromuscular/Skeletal
Rhabdomyolysis [10]

DEXTRO-METHORPHAN

Trade names: Robitussin (Wyeth), Vicks Formula 44 (Procter & Gamble)
Indications: Nonproductive cough
Class: Analgesic; narcotic, NMDA receptor antagonist
Half-life: N/A
Clinically important, potentially hazardous interactions with: amiodarone, citalopram, iloperidone, linezolid, lorcaserin, memantine, moclobemide, phenelzine, rasagiline, safinamide, sibutramine, tranylcypromine, valdecoxib, viloxazine
Important contra-indications noted in the prescribing guidelines for: nursing mothers; pediatric patients

Skin
Bullous dermatosis [2]
Fixed eruption / fixed drug eruption [2]

Central Nervous System
Headache [3]
Psychosis [2]
Serotonin syndrome [4]
Vertigo / dizziness [4]

Gastrointestinal/Hepatic
Diarrhea [5]

Genitourinary
Urinary tract infection [2]

Neuromuscular/Skeletal
Dystonia [3]

Other
Adverse effects / adverse reactions [2]

DIATRIZOATE

Trade name: Gastrografin (Schering)
Indications: Imaging (gastrointestinal tract)
Class: Contrast agent, Iodine-containing radiocontrast medium
Half-life: N/A
Clinically important, potentially hazardous interactions with: none known

Skin
Anaphylactoid reactions / anaphylaxis (includes anaphylactic shock) [5]

Hematologic
Thrombocytopenia / platelets decreased [5]

Other
Death [2]

DIAZEPAM

Trade names: Diastat (Xcel), Valium (Roche)
Indications: Anxiety
Class: Benzodiazepine, Skeletal muscle relaxant
Half-life: 20–70 hours
Clinically important, potentially hazardous interactions with: alcohol, amprenavir, barbiturates, buprenorphine, chlorpheniramine, clarithromycin, CNS depressants, cobicistat/elvitegravir/emtricitabine/tenofovir alafenamide, cobicistat/elvitegravir/emtricitabine/tenofovir disoproxil, efavirenz, esomeprazole, eucalyptus, fluoroquinolones, imatinib, indinavir, itraconazole, ivermectin, macrolide antibiotics, MAO inhibitors, methadone, mianserin, nalbuphine, narcotics, nelfinavir, nilutamide, olanzapine, omeprazole, phenothiazines, propranolol, ritonavir, SSRIs, voriconazole
Important contra-indications noted in the prescribing guidelines for: nursing mothers

Skin
Dermatitis (<10%) [3]
Diaphoresis (>10%)
Exanthems [6]
Exfoliative dermatitis [2]
Fixed eruption / fixed drug eruption [2]
Pigmentation (Skin) (includes hyperpigmentation) [2]
Purpura [4]
Rash (>10%) [2]

Mucosal
Nasal discomfort [3]
Xerostomia (dry mouth) (>10%)

Central Nervous System
Amnesia [17]
Dysgeusia (taste perversion) [2]
Hallucinations [2]
Headache [2]
Sedation [3]
Somnolence (drowsiness) [8]
Vertigo / dizziness [2]

Endocrine/Metabolic
Gynecomastia [4]
Porphyria [2]

Local
Injection-site pain [2]
Injection-site phlebitis (>10%) [2]

Neuromuscular/Skeletal
Ataxia [2]

Other
Adverse effects / adverse reactions [4]
Allergic reactions [2]

DIAZOXIDE

Trade name: Hyperstat (Schering)
Indications: Hypoglycemia, hypertension
Class: Vasodilator
Half-life: 20–36 hours
Clinically important, potentially hazardous interactions with: acarbose, acebutolol, alfuzosin, benazepril, captopril, cilazapril, clevidipine, cyclopenthiazide, diclofenac, enalapril, fosinopril, irbesartan, levodopa, levomepromazine, lisinopril, meloxicam, metformin, olmesartan, phenytoin, quinapril, ramipril, saxagliptin, sitagliptin, trandolapril, triamcinolone, trifluoperazine

Skin
Edema / fluid retention [2]
Lichenoid eruption / lichenoid reaction [2]

Hair
Alopecia / hair loss [2]
Hypertrichosis [14]

Endocrine/Metabolic
Diabetic ketoacidosis [2]
Hyperglycemia (includes glucose increased) [4]

DICHLORPHENAMIDE

Trade name: Keveyis (Taro)
Other common trade names: Dichlorophenamide
Indications: Glaucoma (Daranide), primary hyperkalemic or hypokalemic periodic paralysis (Keveyis)
Class: Carbonic anhydrase inhibitor
Half-life: 8 minutes
Clinically important, potentially hazardous interactions with: aspirin, cyclosporine, diflunisal, lithium, metformin, primidone, salicylates, salsalate
Important contra-indications noted in the prescribing guidelines for: the elderly; nursing mothers; pediatric patients

Skin
Rash [2]

Central Nervous System
Cognitive impairment [2]
Depression [2]
Dysgeusia (taste perversion) [3]
Paresthesias [6]

Endocrine/Metabolic
Acidosis (includes lactic acidosis) [3]
Libido decreased [2]
Weight loss [2]

Gastrointestinal/Hepatic
Dyspepsia / functional dyspepsia (indigestion) (see also gastroparesis) [2]

Ocular
Myopia [2]
Renal
Nephrolithiasis (kidney stones / renal calculi) [3]

DICLOFENAC

Trade names: Arthrotec (Pfizer), Cataflam (Novartis), Dicolmax (Galen), Motifene (Daiichi Sankyo), Pennsaid (Mallinckrodt), Solaraze Gel (Nycomed), Voltaren (Novartis), Voltarol (Novartis), Zipsor (Depomed)
Indications: Rheumatoid and osteoarthritis, topical treatment of actinic keratosis, postoperative inflammation in patients who have undergone cataract extraction and for the temporary relief of pain and photophobia in patients undergoing corneal refractive surgery
Class: Non-steroidal anti-inflammatory (NSAID)
Half-life: 1–2 hours
Clinically important, potentially hazardous interactions with: ACE inhibitors, adrenergic neurone blockers, aldosterone antagonists, aliskiren, alpha blockers, angiotensin II receptor antagonists, anticoagulants, aspirin, baclofen, beta blockers, calcium channel blockers, cardiac glycosides, clonidine, clopidogrel, corticosteroids, coumarins, cyclosporine, dabigatran, deferiprone, diazoxide, diuretics, enoxaparin, erlotinib, furosemide, heparins, hydralazine, iloprost, ketorolac, lithium, methotrexate, methyldopa, mifamurtide, minoxidil, moxonidine, nitrates, nitroprusside, penicillamine, pentoxifylline, phenindione, potassium canrenoate, prasugrel, rifampin, ritonavir, rivaroxaban, SSRIs, sulfonylureas, tacrolimus, thiazides, tinzaparin, venlafaxine, voriconazole, warfarin, zidovudine
Pregnancy category: category B for topical use; category C for oral and ophthalmic use; category D in third trimester.
Important contra-indications noted in the prescribing guidelines for: nursing mothers; pediatric patients
Note: NSAIDs may cause an increased risk of serious cardiovascular and gastrointestinal adverse events, which can be fatal. This risk may increase with duration of use.
Contra-indicated in patients who have experienced asthma, urticaria, or allergic-type reactions after taking aspirin or other NSAIDs. Severe, rarely fatal, anaphylactic-like reactions to NSAIDs have been reported in such patients.
Arthrotec is diclofenac and misoprostol.
Warning: RISK OF SERIOUS CARDIOVASCULAR AND GASTROINTESTINAL EVENTS

Skin
Anaphylactoid reactions / anaphylaxis (includes anaphylactic shock) (<3%) [16]
Angioedema (formerly named angioneurotic edema) (<3%) [3]
Bullous dermatosis (<3%) [2]
Dermatitis (<3%) [10]
Dermatitis herpetiformis [2]
DRESS syndrome (Drug-induced hypersensitivity syndrome) [2]
Eczema / eczematous reaction / eczematous eruption (<3%)
Erythema [4]
Erythema multiforme [6]
Exanthems (<5%) [6]
Fixed eruption / fixed drug eruption [4]
Hypersensitivity [5]
Linear IgA bullous dermatosis [7]
Necrosis (skin necrosis) [2]
Nicolau syndrome [18]
Photosensitivity (<3%) [4]
Pruritus (itching) (<10%) [6]
Purpura (<3%) [2]
Purpura fulminans [2]
Rash (>10%) [4]
Stevens-Johnson syndrome and toxic epidermal necrolysis (SJS/TEN) [12]
Urticaria / hives (<3%) [7]
Vasculitis (angiitis) / cutaneous vasculitis (angiitis) [3]
Xerosis / xeroderma [3]
Hair
Alopecia / hair loss (<3%)
Mucosal
Oral erythema multiforme [2]
Tongue edema (<3%)
Xerostomia (dry mouth) (<3%) [2]
Cardiovascular
Atrial fibrillation [2]
Cardiotoxicity [2]
Kounis syndrome / allergic angina syndrome / allergic myocardial infarction [2]
Myocardial infarction [5]
Central Nervous System
Dysgeusia (taste perversion) (<3%)
Headache [2]
Stroke / cerebrovascular accident [3]
Vertigo / dizziness [4]
Gastrointestinal/Hepatic
Abdominal pain [8]
Constipation [3]
Diarrhea [4]
Dyspepsia / functional dyspepsia (indigestion) (see also gastroparesis) [7]
Flatulence [2]
Gastritis / pangastritis / gastric irritation [3]
Gastrointestinal bleeding [7]
Gastrointestinal ulceration [4]
Hepatotoxicity / liver injury / acute liver injury / drug-induced liver injury (DILI) [11]
Nausea [10]
Vomiting [4]
Hematologic
Agranulocytosis / severe selective neutropenia [3]
Anemia [2]
Bleeding [2]
Hemolytic anemia [8]
Local
Application-site reactions [4]
Neuromuscular/Skeletal
Rhabdomyolysis [3]
Renal
Nephrotoxicity / kidney injury / acute kidney injury (AKI) / drug-induced kidney injury [4]
Renal failure [2]
Other
Adverse effects / adverse reactions [12]
Allergic reactions [2]
Death [7]

DICLOXACILLIN

Trade name: Dycill (GSK)
Indications: Infections due to penicillinase-producing staphylococci
Class: Antibiotic, Antibiotic; beta-lactam, Antibiotic; penicillin, Antimicrobial
Half-life: 30–60 minutes
Clinically important, potentially hazardous interactions with: anticoagulants, cyclosporine, imipenem/cilastatin, methotrexate, tetracycline, warfarin

---

Skin
Urticaria / hives [2]
Cardiovascular
Phlebitis [2]

DICUMAROL

Indications: Atrial fibrillation, pulmonary embolism, venous thrombosis
Class: Coumarin
Half-life: 1–4 days
Clinically important, potentially hazardous interactions with: allopurinol, amiodarone, amobarbital, anabolic steroids, anti-thyroid agents, aprobarbital, aspirin, barbiturates, bivalirudin, butabarbital, butalbital, cimetidine, clofibrate, clopidogrel, cyclosporine, delavirdine, disulfiram, fenofibrate, fluconazole, gemfibrozil, glutethimide, imatinib, itraconazole, ketoconazole, levothyroxine, liothyronine, mephobarbital, methimazole, metronidazole, miconazole, penicillins, pentobarbital, phenobarbital, phenylbutazones, piperacillin, prednisone, primidone, propylthiouracil, quinidine, quinine, rifabutin, rifampin, rifapentine, rofecoxib, salicylates, secobarbital, sulfinpyrazone, sulfonamides, testosterone, zileuton
Important contra-indications noted in the prescribing guidelines for: nursing mothers

---

Skin
Dermatitis [2]
Exanthems [5]
Necrosis (skin necrosis) [10]
Purplish erythema (feet and toes) [2]
Purpura [2]
Urticaria / hives [3]
Hair
Alopecia / hair loss (<10%) [5]
Hematologic
Hemorrhage [3]

DICYCLOMINE

Trade name: Bentyl (Aptalis)
Indications: Irritable bowel syndrome
Class: Anticholinergic, Muscarinic antagonist
Half-life: initial: 1.8 hours; terminal: 9–10 hours
Clinically important, potentially hazardous interactions with: antacids, anticholinergics, antiglaucoma agents, arbutamine
Important contra-indications noted in the prescribing guidelines for: nursing mothers; pediatric patients

---

Skin
Exanthems [2]

Rash [2]
Xerosis / xeroderma (>10%)

Mucosal
Xerostomia (dry mouth) (33%) [2]

Central Nervous System
Nervousness (6%)
Somnolence (drowsiness) (9%)
Vertigo / dizziness (40%) [2]

Gastrointestinal/Hepatic
Constipation [2]
Nausea (14%)

Local
Injection-site reaction (>10%)

Neuromuscular/Skeletal
Asthenia / fatigue (7%)

Ocular
Vision blurred (27%)

Other
Death [3]

DIDANOSINE

Trade name: Videx (Bristol-Myers Squibb)
Indications: Advanced HIV infection
Class: Antiretroviral, Nucleoside analog reverse transcriptase inhibitor
Half-life: 1.5 hours
Clinically important, potentially hazardous interactions with: acetaminophen, amprenavir, ciprofloxacin, corticosteroids, dapsone, darunavir, febuxostat, gemifloxacin, indinavir, itraconazole, ketoconazole, levofloxacin, lomefloxacin, lopinavir, moxifloxacin, norfloxacin, ofloxacin, ribavirin, ribavirin, sulfones, tenofovir disoproxil, tetracycline, tipranavir, voriconazole
Important contra-indications noted in the prescribing guidelines for: the elderly; nursing mothers
Warning: PANCREATITIS, LACTIC ACIDOSIS and HEPATOMEGALY with STEATOSIS

Skin
Erythema multiforme [2]
Lipodystrophy / acquired generalized lipodystrophy [2]
Pruritus (itching) (9%)
Rash (9%)
Stevens-Johnson syndrome and toxic epidermal necrolysis (SJS/TEN) [3]

Mucosal
Xerostomia (dry mouth) [4]

Cardiovascular
Myocardial infarction [2]

Central Nervous System
Neurotoxicity [4]

Endocrine/Metabolic
Acidosis (includes lactic acidosis) [6]
Diabetes mellitus [2]
Gynecomastia [3]

Gastrointestinal/Hepatic
Hepatotoxicity / liver injury / acute liver injury / drug-induced liver injury (DILI) [2]
Non-cirrhotic portal hypertension [5]
Pancreatitis / acute pancreatitis [23]

Ocular
Retinopathy [3]

Renal
Fanconi syndrome (proximal tubular dysfunction) [5]
Nephrotoxicity / kidney injury / acute kidney injury (AKI) / drug-induced kidney injury [2]

DIETHYLPROPION

Synonym: amfepramone
Trade name: Tenuate (Sanofi-Aventis)
Indications: Weight reduction
Class: Amphetamine
Half-life: 4–6 hours
Clinically important, potentially hazardous interactions with: fluoxetine, fluvoxamine, linezolid, MAO inhibitors, paroxetine hydrochloride, phenelzine, sertraline, tranylcypromine

---

Skin
Scleroderma [2]

Mucosal
Xerostomia (dry mouth) [2]

Central Nervous System
Insomnia [2]
Vertigo / dizziness [2]

Gastrointestinal/Hepatic
Constipation [2]

DIFLUNISAL

Trade name: Dolobid (Merck)
Indications: Rheumatoid and osteoarthritis
Class: Non-steroidal anti-inflammatory (NSAID)
Half-life: 8–12 hours
Clinically important, potentially hazardous interactions with: acemetacin, dichlorphenamide, indomethacin
Note: NSAIDs may cause an increased risk of serious cardiovascular and gastrointestinal adverse events, which can be fatal. This risk may increase with duration of use.

Skin
Diaphoresis [2]
Erythema multiforme [5]
Erythroderma [2]
Exanthems [4]
Fixed eruption / fixed drug eruption [2]
Pruritus (itching) (<10%) [3]
Rash (3–9%) [3]
Stevens-Johnson syndrome and toxic epidermal necrolysis (SJS/TEN) [10]
Urticaria / hives [6]

Other
Adverse effects / adverse reactions [3]

DIGOXIN

Trade name: Lanoxin (Concordia)
Indications: Congestive heart failure, atrial fibrillation
Class: Antiarrhythmic class IV, Cardiac glycoside, Inotrope
Half-life: 36–48 hours
Clinically important, potentially hazardous interactions with: acarbose, alprazolam, amiodarone, amphotericin B, arbutamine, atorvastatin, azithromycin, bendroflumethiazide, benzthiazide, bisacodyl, boceprevir, bosutinib, bumetanide, canagliflozin, captopril, carbimazole, chlorothiazide, chlorthalidone, cholestyramine, clarithromycin, cobicistat/elvitegravir/emtricitabine/tenofovir alafenamide, cobicistat/elvitegravir/emtricitabine/tenofovir disoproxil, colchicine, conivaptan, cyclopenthiazide, cyclosporine, cyclothiazide, darifenacin, darunavir, demeclocycline, dexlansoprazole, dexmedetomidine, doxycycline, dronedarone, erythromycin, eslicarbazepine, esomeprazole, ethacrynic acid, etravirine, everolimus, ezogabine, fingolimod, flibanserin, flunisolide, furosemide, glycopyrrolate, glycopyrronium, hydrochlorothiazide, hydroflumethiazide, indapamide, indinavir, itraconazole, lapatinib, lenalidomide, liraglutide, lomustine, lopinavir, meloxicam, mepenzolate, metformin, methyclothiazide, metolazone, milnacipran, minocycline, mirabegron, neratinib, nifedipine, nilotinib, omeprazole, oxprenolol, oxytetracycline, pantoprazole, paricalcitol, paroxetine hydrochloride, pemetrexed, phenylbutazone, polythiazide, ponesimod, posaconazole, propafenone, propantheline, quinethazone, quinidine, quinine, rabeprazole, rifampin, roxithromycin, sitagliptin, sodium picosulfate, sorafenib, sotorasib, St John's wort, sunitinib, telaprevir, telithromycin, temozolomide, temsirolimus, teriparatide, tetracycline, thalidomide, thiazide diuretics, ticagrelor, tipranavir, tolvaptan, trichlormethiazide, trimethoprim, troglitazone, tucatinib, ulipristal, valbenazine, venetoclax, verapamil, vibegron, zuclopenthixol
Important contra-indications noted in the prescribing guidelines for: the elderly; nursing mothers; pediatric patients
Note: This is the pure form of Digitalis. Contra-indicated in ventricular fibrillation.

Skin
Cutaneous toxicity / skin toxicity [5]
Exanthems (2%) [2]
Psoriasis [2]

Cardiovascular
Arrhythmias [7]
Atrial fibrillation [4]
Bradycardia / sinus bradycardia [4]
Tachycardia [2]

Central Nervous System
Anorexia [2]
Dementia [2]
Hallucinations, visual [2]

Endocrine/Metabolic
Gynecomastia [2]

Gastrointestinal/Hepatic
Nausea [4]
Vomiting [2]

Neuromuscular/Skeletal
Asthenia / fatigue [2]

Ocular
Dyschromatopsia (green) [6]

Other
Death [5]

DIHYDROERGOTAMINE

Trade names: D.H.E. 45 (Xcel), Migranal (Xcel)
Indications: Prevention of vascular headaches
Class: Ergot alkaloid
Half-life: 1.3–3.9 hours
Clinically important, potentially hazardous interactions with: almotriptan, amprenavir, boceprevir, ceritinib, clarithromycin, crizotinib, darunavir, dasatinib, delavirdine, efavirenz,

eletriptan, eluxadoline, enzalutamide, erythromycin, fosamprenavir, frovatriptan, indinavir, itraconazole, itraconazole, letermovir, methylergonovine, mifepristone, naratriptan, nelfinavir, nilotinib, ombitasvir/paritaprevir/ritonavir, ombitasvir/paritaprevir/ritonavir and dasabuvir, posaconazole, ribociclib, ritonavir, rizatriptan, saquinavir, sibutramine, sumatriptan, telaprevir, telithromycin, tipranavir, troleandomycin, zolmitriptan

---

Skin
- Edema / fluid retention (>10%)
- Necrosis (skin necrosis) [3]

Mucosal
- Xerostomia (dry mouth) (>10%)

Central Nervous System
- Amnesia [2]
- Dysgeusia (taste perversion) [2]
- Headache [5]
- Paresthesias (>10%)
- Vertigo / dizziness [2]

Gastrointestinal/Hepatic
- Nausea [3]

Neuromuscular/Skeletal
- Leg cramps [4]

DIHYDROTACHYSTEROL

Trade names: DHT (Roxane), Hytakerol (Sanofi-Aventis)
Indications: Hypocalcemia associated with hypoparathyroidism
Class: Vitamin D receptor agonist
Half-life: N/A
Clinically important, potentially hazardous interactions with: none known

---

Skin
- Pruritus (itching) (<10%)

DILTIAZEM

Trade names: Cardizem (Biovail), Dilacor XR (Watson), Teczem (Sanofi-Aventis), Tiazac (Forest)
Indications: Angina, essential hypertension
Class: Antiarrhythmic class IV, Calcium channel blocker, CYP3A4 inhibitor
Half-life: 5–8 hours (for extended-release capsules)
Clinically important, potentially hazardous interactions with: acebutolol, alfuzosin, amiodarone, amitriptyline, amprenavir, aprepitant, atazanavir, atenolol, atorvastatin, avanafil, bisoprolol, bosentan, carbamazepine, celiprolol, cilostazol, cobicistat/elvitegravir/emtricitabine/tenofovir alafenamide, cobicistat/elvitegravir/emtricitabine/tenofovir disoproxil, colchicine, copanlisib, corticosteroids, cyclosporine, deflazacort, delavirdine, dronedarone, dutasteride, efavirenz, epirubicin, erythromycin, fingolimod, flibanserin, ivabradine, ivabradine, lumateperone, lurasidone, midostaurin, mifepristone, moricizine, naldemedine, naloxegol, neratinib, nevirapine, nifedipine, olaparib, oxprenolol, ponesimod, posaconazole, ranolazine, silodosin, simvastatin, sonidegib, sulpiride / levosulpiride, telaprevir, venetoclax, voclosporin
Important contra-indications noted in the prescribing guidelines for: the elderly; nursing mothers; pediatric patients
Note: Teczem is diltiazem and enalapril.

Skin
- Acneiform eruption / acneiform dermatitis / acneiform rash [2]
- AGEP [21]
- Angioedema (formerly named angioneurotic edema) [3]
- Cutaneous toxicity / skin toxicity [2]
- Diaphoresis [2]
- Edema / fluid retention (<10%) [4]
- Erythema [2]
- Erythema multiforme (<31%) [11]
- Exanthems [17]
- Exfoliative dermatitis [6]
- Flushing / rubefaction (<10%) [6]
- Hypersensitivity [2]
- Leg ulceration [2]
- Lupus erythematosus (subacute cutaneous lupus erythematosus (SCLE)) [5]
- Palmar–plantar desquamation [2]
- Peripheral edema (5–8%)
- Photosensitivity [12]
- Phototoxicity [2]
- Pigmentation (Skin) (includes hyperpigmentation) [10]
- Pruritus (itching) [6]
- Psoriasis [3]
- Purpura [3]
- Pustules / pustular eruption [2]
- Rash [4]
- Stevens-Johnson syndrome and toxic epidermal necrolysis (SJS/TEN) [6]
- Thickening [2]
- Toxic erythema [2]
- Urticaria / hives [5]
- Vasculitis (angiitis) / cutaneous vasculitis (angiitis) [6]

Hair
- Alopecia / hair loss [2]

Mucosal
- Gingival hyperplasia / gingival hypertrophy / gingival enlargement / gingival overgrowth (21%) [10]
- Xerostomia (dry mouth) [2]

Cardiovascular
- Atrial fibrillation [2]
- Bradycardia / sinus bradycardia [8]
- Cardiogenic shock [2]
- Hypotension [2]
- QT interval prolonged / QT prolongation [2]

Central Nervous System
- Dysgeusia (taste perversion) [2]
- Parkinsonism [3]
- Somnolence (drowsiness) [2]

Neuromuscular/Skeletal
- Rhabdomyolysis [4]

Other
- Side effects [2]

DIMENHYDRINATE

Trade name: Dramamine (Pfizer)
Indications: Motion sickness, dizziness, nausea, vomiting
Class: Antiemetic, Cholinesterase absorption inhibitor
Half-life: N/A
Clinically important, potentially hazardous interactions with: none known
Important contra-indications noted in the prescribing guidelines for: nursing mothers

---

Skin
- Fixed eruption / fixed drug eruption [12]

Mucosal
- Xerostomia (dry mouth) (<10%)

Central Nervous System
- Somnolence (drowsiness) [5]

DIMERCAPROL

Synonym: British anti-Lewisite
Trade name: BAL (Taylor)
Indications: Heavy metal poisoning (arsenic, gold, mercury, lead)
Class: Antidote, Chelator
Half-life: N/A
Clinically important, potentially hazardous interactions with: ferric maltol, ferrous sulfate, insulin, iron, selenium
Note: As an antidote, it is difficult to differentiate side effects due to the drug from those due to the effects of the poison.

DIMETHYL FUMARATE

Synonyms: dimethyl (E) butenedioate; BG-12
Trade names: Fumaderm (Biogen Idec), Tecfidera (Biogen Idec), Zadiva (NanoAlvand)
Indications: Relapsing forms of multiple sclerosis, psoriasis
Class: Fumaric acid ester
Half-life: 1 hour
Clinically important, potentially hazardous interactions with: none known
Important contra-indications noted in the prescribing guidelines for: the elderly; nursing mothers; pediatric patients
Note: Fumaderm is mixed dimethyl fumarate and monoethylfumarate salts.

Skin
- Contact dermatitis (from topical contact) [14]
- Erythema (5%) [2]
- Flushing / rubefaction (40%) [35]
- Pruritus (itching) (8%) [6]
- Rash (8%) [2]

Central Nervous System
- Headache [3]
- Leukoencephalopathy / posterior reversible encephalopathy syndrome (PRES) [6]

Endocrine/Metabolic
- AST increased (4%) [3]

Gastrointestinal/Hepatic
- Abdominal pain (18%) [14]
- Diarrhea (14%) [11]
- Dyspepsia / functional dyspepsia (indigestion) (see also gastroparesis) (5%) [2]
- Gastrointestinal disorder / discomfort [7]

Nausea [7]
Vomiting (9%) [3]

Genitourinary
Albuminuria (6%)
Urinary tract infection [2]

Hematologic
Hemotoxicity [2]
Lymphopenia (lymphocytopenia) / lymphocytes decreased (2%) [17]

Neuromuscular/Skeletal
Asthenia / fatigue [4]

Renal
Proteinuria [2]

Respiratory
Nasopharyngitis [2]

Other
Adverse effects / adverse reactions (gastrointestinal) [20]
Infection [2]

DINOPROSTONE

Trade names: Cervidel (Forest), Prepidil (Pfizer)
Indications: Pregnancy termination, uterine content evacuation, cervical ripening
Class: Prostaglandin
Half-life: 2.5–5 minutes
Clinically important, potentially hazardous interactions with: none known
Note: Dinoprostone is the naturally occurring form of Prostaglandin E2 (PGE2).

DIPHENHYDRAMINE

Trade name: Benadryl (Pfizer)
Indications: Allergic rhinitis, urticaria
Class: Antiemetic, Histamine H1 receptor antagonist, Muscarinic antagonist
Half-life: 2–8 hours
Clinically important, potentially hazardous interactions with: alcohol, anticholinergics, chloral hydrate, CNS depressants, glutethimide, MAO inhibitors
Important contra-indications noted in the prescribing guidelines for: nursing mothers

---

Skin
Anaphylactoid reactions / anaphylaxis (includes anaphylactic shock) [4]
Contact dermatitis [2]
Cutaneous toxicity / skin toxicity [2]
Dermatitis [4]
Eczema / eczematous reaction / eczematous eruption [2]
Fixed eruption / fixed drug eruption [4]
Photosensitivity [3]
Pruritus (itching) [2]
Stevens-Johnson syndrome and toxic epidermal necrolysis (SJS/TEN) [3]

Mucosal
Xerostomia (dry mouth) (<10%)

Cardiovascular
QT interval prolonged / QT prolongation [5]
Torsades de pointes [3]

Central Nervous System
Delirium [3]
Hallucinations, visual [2]
Sedation [2]
Seizures [2]
Somnolence (drowsiness) [7]

Neuromuscular/Skeletal
Dystonia [2]
Rhabdomyolysis [5]

Other
Death [4]

DIPHENOXYLATE

Trade name: Lomotil (Pfizer)
Indications: Diarrhea
Class: Antimotility, Opioid agonist
Half-life: 2.5 hours
Clinically important, potentially hazardous interactions with: oxybutynin
Important contra-indications noted in the prescribing guidelines for: nursing mothers; pediatric patients
Note: Diphenoxylate is almost always prescribed with atropine sulfate.

Mucosal
Xerostomia (dry mouth) (3%)

DIPYRIDAMOLE

Trade names: Aggrenox (Boehringer Ingelheim), Persantine (Boehringer Ingelheim)
Indications: Thromboembolic complications following cardiac valve replacement
Class: Adenosine reuptake inhibitor, Antiplatelet (antithrombotic)
Half-life: 10–12 hours
Clinically important, potentially hazardous interactions with: adenosine, ceftobiprole, clopidogrel, enoxaparin, fondaparinux, regadenoson, reteplase, riociguat, tinzaparin
Important contra-indications noted in the prescribing guidelines for: nursing mothers; pediatric patients
Note: Aggrenox is dipyridamole and aspirin.

Skin
Flushing / rubefaction (3%)
Rash (2%)
Stevens-Johnson syndrome and toxic epidermal necrolysis (SJS/TEN) [3]

Central Nervous System
Headache [4]

Other
Adverse effects / adverse reactions [3]

DIRITHROMYCIN

Trade name: Dynabac (Muro)
Indications: Various infections caused by susceptible organisms
Class: Antibiotic, Antibiotic; macrolide, Antimicrobial
Half-life: 8 hours
Clinically important, potentially hazardous interactions with: pimozide, warfarin

---

Gastrointestinal/Hepatic
Abdominal pain [2]
Diarrhea [2]
Nausea [3]

DISOPYRAMIDE

Trade name: Norpace (Pfizer)
Indications: Ventricular arrhythmias
Class: Antiarrhythmic, Antiarrhythmic class Ia, Muscarinic antagonist
Half-life: 4–10 hours
Clinically important, potentially hazardous interactions with: acebutolol, amiodarone, amisulpride, amitriptyline, arsenic, artemether/lumefantrine, astemizole, atenolol, bisoprolol, celiprolol, ciprofloxacin, clarithromycin, cobicistat/elvitegravir/emtricitabine/tenofovir alafenamide, cobicistat/elvitegravir/emtricitabine/tenofovir disoproxil, darifenacin, degarelix, dronedarone, droperidol, enoxacin, erythromycin, gatifloxacin, gliclazide, glycopyrrolate, glycopyrronium, insulin aspart, insulin degludec, insulin glargine, insulin glulisine, itraconazole, ketoconazole, levomepromazine, lomefloxacin, lurasidone, metformin, moxifloxacin, nevirapine, nilotinib, norfloxacin, ofloxacin, oxprenolol, oxybutynin, pimavanserin, quinine, quinolones, ribociclib, rifapentine, roxithromycin, sildenafil, sotalol, sparfloxacin, sulpiride / levosulpiride, tadalafil, telithromycin, tiotropium, trospium, vandetanib, vardenafil, zuclopenthixol
Important contra-indications noted in the prescribing guidelines for: nursing mothers; pediatric patients

---

Skin
Dermatitis (<3%)
Edema / fluid retention (<3%)
Exanthems (<5%)
Lupus erythematosus (subacute cutaneous lupus erythematosus (SCLE)) [3]
Pruritus (itching) (<3%)
Rash (generalized) (<3%)

Mucosal
Oral lesions (40%)
Xerostomia (dry mouth) (32%) [2]

Cardiovascular
Chest pain (<3%)
Hypotension (<3%)
QT interval prolonged / QT prolongation [8]
Torsades de pointes [13]

Central Nervous System
Anorexia (<3%)
Headache (3–9%)
Nervousness (<3%)
Syncope / fainting (<3%)
Vertigo / dizziness (3–9%)

Endocrine/Metabolic
Hypocalcemia [3]
Hypoglycemia [4]
Hypokalemia (<3%)
Weight gain (<3%)

Gastrointestinal/Hepatic
Abdominal pain (3–9%)
Constipation (11%) [2]
Diarrhea (<3%)
Nausea (3–9%)
Vomiting (<3%)

Genitourinary
Impotence (<3%)
Urinary hesitancy (14%)
Urinary retention (3–9%)

Neuromuscular/Skeletal
Asthenia / fatigue (3–9%)

Ocular
Vision blurred (3–9%)
Xerophthalmia (dry eyes) (3–9%)
Respiratory
Dyspnea / shortness of breath (<3%)

DISTIGMINE

Trade name: Ubretid (Sanofi)
Indications: Post-operative urinary retention, post operative ileus and intestinal atony, adjunct in the treatment of myasthenia gravis
Class: Acetylcholine inhibitor
Half-life: N/A
Clinically important, potentially hazardous interactions with: beta blockers, local anesthetics, muscle relaxants

---

Cardiovascular
Bradycardia / sinus bradycardia [2]

DISULFIRAM

Trade name: Antabuse (Odyssey)
Indications: Alcoholism
Class: Antialcoholism, Antioxidant
Half-life: N/A
Clinically important, potentially hazardous interactions with: acenocoumarol, alcohol, amitriptyline, anisindione, anticoagulants, benznidazole, clobazam, cyclosporine, dicumarol, dronabinol, ethanolamine, ethotoin, fosphenytoin, lopinavir, mephenytoin, metronidazole, omeprazole, oxtriphylline, phenytoin, thalidomide, tipranavir, warfarin
Important contra-indications noted in the prescribing guidelines for: nursing mothers; pediatric patients

---

Skin
Acneiform eruption / acneiform dermatitis / acneiform rash [3]
Bullous dermatosis [2]
Dermatitis [17]
Eczema / eczematous reaction / eczematous eruption [2]
Exanthems [2]
Fixed eruption / fixed drug eruption [2]
Flushing / rubefaction (with alcohol) [5]
Rash (<10%)
Recall reaction (nickel) [4]
Urticaria / hives [3]
Mucosal
Halitosis [2]
Cardiovascular
Hypertension [2]
Hypotension [2]
Polyarteritis nodosa [2]
Tachycardia [2]
Central Nervous System
Dysgeusia (taste perversion) (metallic or garlic aftertaste) (<10%)
Encephalopathy (includes hepatic encephalopathy) [4]
Neurotoxicity [7]
Psychosis [6]
Seizures [3]
Somnolence (drowsiness) [2]
Vertigo / dizziness [2]
Neuromuscular/Skeletal
Asthenia / fatigue [2]
Ocular
Optic neuropathy [2]
Other
Adverse effects / adverse reactions [3]

DOBUTAMINE

Trade name: Dobutrex (Lilly)
Indications: Cardiac surgery, heart failure
Class: Adrenergic beta-receptor agonist, Catecholamine, Inotropic sympathomimetic
Half-life: 2 minutes
Clinically important, potentially hazardous interactions with: furazolidone
Important contra-indications noted in the prescribing guidelines for: the elderly

---

Skin
Pruritus (itching) [2]
Cardiovascular
Arrhythmias [2]
Atrial fibrillation [5]
Cardiomyopathy [2]
Cardiotoxicity [2]
Coronary vasospasm [2]
Hypotension [5]
Myocardial infarction [2]
QT interval prolonged / QT prolongation [2]
Ventricular tachycardia [2]
Central Nervous System
Paresthesias (<10%)
Neuromuscular/Skeletal
Myoclonus (see also hypnic jerk) [7]

DOCETAXEL

Trade name: Taxotere (Sanofi-Aventis)
Indications: Metastatic breast cancer, non-small cell lung cancer, with prednisone in hormone refractory prostate cancer, with cisplatin and fluorouracil for gastric adenocarcinoma and squamous cell carcinoma of the head and neck
Class: Antineoplastic / anticancer agent (see also Immune checkpoint inhibitor), Taxane
Half-life: 11–18 hours
Clinically important, potentially hazardous interactions with: alcohol, aldesleukin, anthracyclines, antifungals, aprepitant, BCG vaccine, conivaptan, cyclosporine, CYP3A4 inhibitors or inducers, dasatinib, deferasirox, denosumab, echinacea, erythromycin, itraconazole, ketoconazole, lapatinib, leflunomide, natalizumab, P-glycoprotein inhibitors or inducers, pimecrolimus, prednisone, ritonavir, sipuleucel-T, sorafenib, St John's wort, tacrolimus, thalidomide, trastuzumab, vaccines, voriconazole
Important contra-indications noted in the prescribing guidelines for: the elderly; nursing mothers; pediatric patients
Note: Contra-indicated in patients with hypersensitivity to docetaxel or polysorbate 80, or with neutrophil counts of <1500 cells/mm^3.
Warning: TOXIC DEATHS, HEPATOTOXICITY, NEUTROPENIA, HYPERSENSITIVITY REACTIONS, and FLUID RETENTION

Skin
AGEP [2]
Anaphylactoid reactions / anaphylaxis (includes anaphylactic shock) [3]
Cutaneous toxicity / skin toxicity (20–48%) [10]
Edema / fluid retention (34%) [26]
Erythema [4]
Exanthems [3]
Facial erythema [2]
Flagellate erythema/pigmentation [3]
Flushing / rubefaction [2]
Hand–foot syndrome (palmar–plantar erythrodysesthesia) [49]
Hypersensitivity (6%) [15]
Peripheral edema [9]
Photosensitivity [6]
Pigmentation (Skin) (includes hyperpigmentation) [2]
Psoriasis [3]
Radiation recall dermatitis [18]
Rash [13]
Recall reaction [3]
Scleroderma [9]
Stevens-Johnson syndrome and toxic epidermal necrolysis (SJS/TEN) [4]
Thrombocytopenic purpura [2]
Toxic erythema of chemotherapy (TEC) [2]
Xerosis / xeroderma [2]
Hair
Alopecia / hair loss (56–76%) [34]
Nails
Beau's lines (transverse nail bands) [3]
Discoloration / nails (dyschromia) [2]
Leukonychia striata (Mees' lines) [2]
Melanonychia [2]
Nail changes [18]
Nail disorder (11–41%) [2]
Nail loss [3]
Nail pigmentation [7]
Onycholysis [15]
Onychopathy [2]
Paronychia [5]
Pyogenic granuloma [2]
Subungual abscess [2]
Subungual hematoma / subungual hemorrhage [2]
Subungual hyperkeratosis [2]
Transverse superficial loss of nail plate [2]
Mucosal
Aphthous stomatitis / aphthous ulcer / aphtha (aphthae) [2]
Mucosal inflammation [2]
Mucositis [15]
Stomatitis (oral mucositis) (19–53%) [26]
Cardiovascular
Capillary leak syndrome [2]
Cardiotoxicity [2]
Hypertension [10]
Hypotension (3%)
Thromboembolism [2]
Central Nervous System
Anorexia [13]
Dysesthesia (4%)
Dysgeusia (taste perversion) (6%) [7]
Fever (pyrexia) (includes hyperpyrexia) (31–35%) [8]
Headache [2]
Mood changes (includes mood disorder) [2]
Neurotoxicity [20]
Pain [5]
Paresthesias (4%) [3]
Peripheral neuropathy [14]
Vertigo / dizziness [2]
Endocrine/Metabolic
ALP increased (4–7%)
ALT increased [5]

Amenorrhea [4]
Appetite decreased [4]
AST increased [4]
Dehydration [2]
Hyperglycemia (includes glucose increased) [3]
Hypomagnesemia [2]
Hyponatremia [4]
Hypophosphatemia [3]

Gastrointestinal/Hepatic
Abdominal pain [4]
Constipation [3]
Diarrhea (23–43%) [51]
Dysphagia [2]
Hepatotoxicity / liver injury / acute liver injury / drug-induced liver injury (DILI) [3]
Nausea (34–42%) [31]
Vomiting (22–23%) [23]

Hematologic
Anemia (65–94%) [26]
Febrile neutropenia (6%) [56]
Granulocytopenia [2]
Hemolytic uremic syndrome [3]
Hemotoxicity [3]
Leukocytopenia (leukopenia) / leukocytes (white blood cells) decreased (84–99%) [36]
Lymphopenia (lymphocytopenia) / lymphocytes decreased [5]
Myelosuppression / bone marrow suppression / myelotoxicity [5]
Neutropenia (neutrophils decreased) (84–99%) [97]
Thrombocytopenia / platelets decreased (8–14%) [14]

Local
Injection-site erythema [2]
Injection-site extravasation [3]
Injection-site pigmentation / injection-site discoloration [3]
Injection-site reaction [2]

Neuromuscular/Skeletal
Arthralgia (3–9%) [3]
Asthenia / fatigue (53–66%) [66]
Bone pain / joint pain [2]
Myalgia/Myopathy (3–23%) [14]

Ocular
Epiphora [8]
Lacrimal duct stenosis / punctal stenosis [2]

Respiratory
Acute respiratory distress syndrome [2]
Cough [2]
Dyspnea / shortness of breath [5]
Interstitial lung disease / interstitial pneumonitis / interstitial pneumonia (cryptogenic organizing pneumonia) / drug-induced interstitial lung disease [18]
Pleural effusion [2]
Pneumonia [3]
Pneumonitis [10]
Pulmonary embolism [2]
Pulmonary toxicity (41%) [4]
Respiratory failure [2]
Upper respiratory tract infection [3]

Other
Adverse effects / adverse reactions [6]
Allergic reactions [2]
Death [22]
Infection (<34%) [9]

DOCOSANOL

Trade name: Abreva (GSK)
Indications: Herpes simplex (labialis)
Class: Antiviral; topical
Half-life: N/A
Clinically important, potentially hazardous interactions with: none known

DOCUSATE

Trade names: Colase (Purdue), Peri-Colase (Purdue), Surfak (Pfizer)
Indications: Constipation
Class: Stimulant laxative
Half-life: N/A
Clinically important, potentially hazardous interactions with: none known

DOFETILIDE

Trade name: Tikosyn (Pfizer)
Indications: Conversion of atrial fibrillation and atrial flutter to normal sinus rhythm
Class: Antiarrhythmic, Antiarrhythmic class III
Half-life: 10 hours
Clinically important, potentially hazardous interactions with: atazanavir, bictegravir/emtricitabine/tenofovir alafenamide, chlorpromazine, cimetidine, co-trimoxazole, degarelix, dolutegravir, fluphenazine, hydrochlorothiazide, itraconazole, ketoconazole, medroxyprogesterone, megestrol, mesoridazine, phenothiazines, prochlorperazine, progestins, promethazine, quinine, ranolazine, thioridazine, trifluoperazine, trilaciclib, trimethoprim, vandetanib, verapamil, voriconazole, zuclopenthixol
Important contra-indications noted in the prescribing guidelines for: nursing mothers; pediatric patients
Note: Contra-indicated in patients with congenital or acquired long QT syndromes.

Skin
Angioedema (formerly named angioneurotic edema) (<2%)
Diaphoresis (>2%)
Edema / fluid retention (<2%)
Peripheral edema (>2%)
Rash (3%)

Cardiovascular
Arrhythmias [2]
Atrioventricular block (<2%)
Chest pain (10%)
QT interval prolonged / QT prolongation [13]
Torsades de pointes (<11%) [30]
Ventricular fibrillation (<5%)
Ventricular tachycardia (3–13%) [2]

Central Nervous System
Headache (11%)
Insomnia (4%)
Paresthesias (<2%)
Vertigo / dizziness (8%)

Gastrointestinal/Hepatic
Abdominal pain (3%)
Diarrhea (3%)
Nausea (5%)

Neuromuscular/Skeletal
Back pain (3%)

Respiratory
Dyspnea / shortness of breath (6%)
Influenza- ('flu)-like syndrome (4%)
Upper respiratory tract infection (7%)

DOLASETRON

Trade name: Anzemet (Sanofi-Aventis)
Indications: Prevention of nausea and vomiting
Class: 5-HT3 antagonist, Serotonin type 3 receptor antagonist (CCR5 co-receptor antagonist)
Half-life: 8 hours
Clinically important, potentially hazardous interactions with: alfuzosin, apomorphine, artemether/lumefantrine, chloroquine, ciprofloxacin, conivaptan, dronedarone, gadobutrol, indacaterol, nilotinib, pimozide, QT prolonging agents, quetiapine, quinine, tetrabenazine, thioridazine, tocilizumab, toremifene, vandetanib, vemurafenib, ziprasidone
Important contra-indications noted in the prescribing guidelines for: the elderly; nursing mothers; pediatric patients

---

Skin
Diaphoresis (<2%)
Edema / fluid retention (<2%)
Peripheral edema (<2%)
Pruritus (itching) (3%)
Rash (<2%)

Cardiovascular
Bradycardia / sinus bradycardia (4–5%)
Hypertension (2%)
Hypotension (5%)
QT interval prolonged / QT prolongation [5]
Tachycardia (2–3%)
Torsades de pointes [2]

Central Nervous System
Chills (<2%)
Fever (pyrexia) (includes hyperpyrexia) (4%)
Headache (7–22%) [13]
Pain (3%)
Shivering (<2%)
Vertigo / dizziness (<4%) [8]

Gastrointestinal/Hepatic
Constipation (<2%)
Diarrhea (2–5%)
Dyspepsia / functional dyspepsia (indigestion) (see also gastroparesis) (2–3%)

Genitourinary
Oliguria (3%)

Neuromuscular/Skeletal
Asthenia / fatigue (3–6%)

DOLUTEGRAVIR

Trade names: Juluca (ViiV), Tivicay (ViiV), Triumeq (ViiV)
Indications: HIV-1 infection
Class: Antiretroviral, Integrase strand transfer inhibitor
Half-life: ~14 hours
Clinically important, potentially hazardous interactions with: dofetilide
Important contra-indications noted in the prescribing guidelines for: nursing mothers; pediatric patients
Note: Triumeq is dolutegravir, abacavir and lamivudine. Juluca is dolutegravir and rilpivirine.

Skin
Hypersensitivity [5]
Pruritus (itching) (<2%)
Rash [3]

Central Nervous System
Abnormal dreams [2]
Headache (<2%) [18]
Insomnia (<3%) [4]
Neuropsychiatric / neuropsychological adverse effect [3]
Neurotoxicity [2]

Endocrine/Metabolic
ALT increased (<2%) [3]
AST increased (<3%)
Creatine phosphokinase (CPK) / creatine kinase increased (hyperCKemia) (<4%)
Hyperglycemia (includes glucose increased) (5–7%)
Serum creatinine increased [3]

Gastrointestinal/Hepatic
Abdominal pain (<2%)
Diarrhea [16]
Flatulence (<2%)
Hepatitis (<2%)
Hepatotoxicity / liver injury / acute liver injury / drug-induced liver injury (DILI) [2]
Nausea [16]
Vomiting (<2%)

Hematologic
Sideroblastic anemia / acquired sideroblastic anemia [2]

Neuromuscular/Skeletal
Asthenia / fatigue (<2%) [3]
Myalgia/Myopathy (<2%)

Renal
Nephrotoxicity / kidney injury / acute kidney injury (AKI) / drug-induced kidney injury (<2%)

Respiratory
Nasopharyngitis [4]
Upper respiratory tract infection [2]

Other
Adverse effects / adverse reactions [7]
Neural tube defects [3]

DOMPERIDONE

Trade name: Motilium (Johnson & Johnson)
Indications: Investigational antiemetic, gastroesophageal reflux disease (GERD), nausea, vomiting
Class: Antiemetic, Dopamine receptor antagonist
Half-life: 7–8 hours
Clinically important, potentially hazardous interactions with: bromocriptine, darifenacin, hydromorphone, ketoconazole, meptazinol, oxybutynin, tiotropium, trospium
Important contra-indications noted in the prescribing guidelines for: nursing mothers; pediatric patients
Note: Use of domperidone has been associated with incidences of cardiac arrhythmias and cardiac arrest. Domperidone-containing products are no longer approved by the FDA, except for an investigational drug application. In response to reports that breastfeeding women may be using domperidone as an unapproved drug to increase milk production, the FDA has advised women not to use domperidone for this purpose.

Mucosal
Xerostomia (dry mouth) [2]

Cardiovascular
Cardiotoxicity [4]
QT interval prolonged / QT prolongation [15]
Ventricular arrhythmia [3]

Central Nervous System
Headache [2]
Neuroleptic malignant syndrome [2]
Tardive syndrome / tardive dyskinesia [2]

Endocrine/Metabolic
Galactorrhea [8]
Gynecomastia [5]

Other
Adverse effects / adverse reactions [2]
Death [6]

DONEPEZIL

Trade names: Aricept (Eisai), Aricept Evess (Eisai)
Indications: Mild, moderate and severe dementia of the Alzheimer's type
Class: Acetylcholinesterase inhibitor, Cholinesterase inhibitor, Parasympathomimetic
Half-life: 50–70 hours
Clinically important, potentially hazardous interactions with: anticholinergics, cholinergic agonists, galantamine, non-depolarising muscle relaxants, ramelteon, succinylcholine
Important contra-indications noted in the prescribing guidelines for: nursing mothers; pediatric patients
Note: Contra-indicated in patients with known hypersensitivity to donepezil hydrochloride or to piperidine derivatives.

Skin
Bruise / bruising / contusion / ecchymosis (ecchymoses) (4–5%)
Diaphoresis [2]
Eczema / eczematous reaction / eczematous eruption (3%)
Purpura (<10%)

Cardiovascular
Atrioventricular block [3]
Bradycardia / sinus bradycardia [9]
Chest pain (2%)
Hypertension [2]
Hypotension (3%)
QT interval prolonged / QT prolongation [5]
Torsades de pointes [2]

Central Nervous System
Abnormal dreams (3%) [3]
Agitation [2]
Anorexia (4–8%) [6]
Confusion (2%) [3]
Delirium [2]
Depression (2–3%) [3]
Emotional lability (2%)
Fever (pyrexia) (includes hyperpyrexia) (3%)
Gait instability / postural instability [2]
Hallucinations (3%)
Headache (4–10%) [7]
Hostility (3%)
Insomnia (5–9%) [5]
Mania [2]
Nervousness (3%)
Neuroleptic malignant syndrome [3]
Pain (3–9%)
Parkinsonism [2]
Somnolence (drowsiness) (2%) [2]
Syncope / fainting (2%) [5]
Tremor [3]
Vertigo / dizziness (2–8%) [7]

Endocrine/Metabolic
Appetite decreased [4]
Creatine phosphokinase (CPK) / creatine kinase increased (hyperCKemia) (3%)
Dehydration (2%)
Hyperlipidemia / lipids elevated (2%)
Weight loss (3%)

Gastrointestinal/Hepatic
Constipation [3]
Diarrhea (10%) [14]
Hepatotoxicity / liver injury / acute liver injury / drug-induced liver injury (DILI) [3]
Nausea (6–11%) [18]
Vomiting (5–8%) [11]

Genitourinary
Enuresis (urinary incontinence) (2%)
Urinary frequency (2%) [2]
Urinary tract infection [3]

Hematologic
Hemorrhage (2%)

Neuromuscular/Skeletal
Arthralgia (2%)
Asthenia / fatigue (5%) [4]
Back pain (3%)
Dystonia [2]
Muscle spasm [2]
Myoclonus (see also hypnic jerk) [2]
Pisa syndrome (pleurothotonus) [2]

Other
Adverse effects / adverse reactions [10]
Infection (11%)

DONG QUAI

Family: Umbelliferae; Apioideae
Scientific name: *Angelica sinensis (Angelica polymorpha sinensis)*
Indications: Menopausal symptoms, PMS, menstrual disorders, anemia, constipation, insomnia, rheumatism, neuralgia, hypertension, hypopigmentation, psoriasis
Class: Immunomodulator, Phytoestrogen
Half-life: N/A
Clinically important, potentially hazardous interactions with: acetaminophen, bexarotene, demeclocycline, gemifloxacin
Note: Some recent research has questioned the efficacy of Dong Quai, and also suggested that it may be a potential carcinogen.

Endocrine/Metabolic
Gynecomastia [2]

DOPAMINE

Trade name: Intropin (Hospira)
Indications: Hemodynamic imbalances present in shock
Class: Adrenergic alpha-receptor agonist, Catecholamine, Inotropic sympathomimetic
Half-life: 2 minutes
Clinically important, potentially hazardous interactions with: ethotoin, fosphenytoin, furazolidone, lurasidone, MAO inhibitors, mephenytoin, phenelzine, phenytoin, quetiapine, tranylcypromine

Important contra-indications noted in the prescribing guidelines for: nursing mothers; pediatric patients

---

Cardiovascular
QT interval prolonged / QT prolongation [2]

Local
Injection-site extravasation [2]
Injection-site necrosis [3]

DORAVIRINE

Trade name: Pifeltro (Merck Sharpe & Dohme)
Indications: indicated in combination with other antiretroviral agents for the treatment of HIV-1 infection in adult patients with no prior antiretroviral treatment history
Class: Non-nucleoside reverse transcriptase inhibitor
Half-life: 15 hours
Clinically important, potentially hazardous interactions with: carbamazepine, efavirenz, enzalutamide, etravirine, mitotane, nevirapine, oxcarbazepine, phenobarbital, phenytoin, rifabutin, rifampin, rifapentine, St John's wort
Pregnancy category: No adequate data to establish risk

Skin
Rash (2%)

Central Nervous System
Headache (6%) [2]
Vertigo / dizziness (3%)

Gastrointestinal/Hepatic
Abdominal pain (5%)
Diarrhea (5%) [2]
Nausea (7%)

Neuromuscular/Skeletal
Asthenia / fatigue (6%)

DORAVIRINE/ LAMIDUVINE/ TENOFOVIR DISOPROXIL

Trade name: Delstrigo (Merck Sharpe & Dohme)
Indications: indicated as a complete regimen for the treatment of HIV-1 infection in adult patients with no antiretroviral treatment history
Half-life: 15 hours (doravirine); 5–7 hours (lamivudine); 17 hours (tenofovir disoproxil)
Clinically important, potentially hazardous interactions with: carbamazepine, enzalutamide, ledipasvir & sofosbuvir, mitotane, oxcarbazepine, phenobarbital, phenytoin, rifabutin, rifampin, rifapentine, sofosbuvir & velpatasvir, St John's wort
Pregnancy category: insufficient data to adequately assess risk
Important contra-indications noted in the prescribing guidelines for: nursing mothers
Note: see also separate profiles for doravirine, lamivudine and tenofovir disoproxil.
Warning: POSTTREATMENT ACUTE EXACERBATION OF HEPATITIS B

Skin
Rash (2%)

Central Nervous System
Abnormal dreams (5%)
Insomnia (4%)
Sensory disturbances (4%)
Sleep disturbances (12%)
Somnolence (drowsiness) (3%)
Vertigo / dizziness (7%)

Gastrointestinal/Hepatic
Diarrhea (3%)
Nausea (5%)

DORIPENEM

Trade name: Doribax (Ortho-McNeil)
Indications: Complicated infections
Class: Antibiotic, Antibiotic; carbapenem, Antimicrobial
Half-life: 1 hour
Clinically important, potentially hazardous interactions with: BCG vaccine, oral typhoid vaccine, probenecid, valproic acid
Important contra-indications noted in the prescribing guidelines for: nursing mothers; pediatric patients

---

Skin
Pruritus (itching) (<3%)
Rash (3%) [3]

Central Nervous System
Headache (16%) [4]
Seizures [3]

Endocrine/Metabolic
ALT increased (2%)
AST increased (2%)

Gastrointestinal/Hepatic
Diarrhea [4]
Nausea [3]

Genitourinary
Vulvovaginalmycotic infection (2%)

Hematologic
Anemia (2–5%)

DORZOLAMIDE

Trade names: Cosopt (Merck), Trusopt (Banyu)
Indications: Glaucoma, ocular hypertension
Class: Carbonic anhydrase inhibitor, Diuretic
Half-life: ~4 months
Clinically important, potentially hazardous interactions with: none known
Important contra-indications noted in the prescribing guidelines for: nursing mothers
Note: Dorzolamide is a sulfonamide and can be absorbed systemically. Sulfonamides can produce severe, possibly fatal, reactions such as toxic epidermal necrolysis and Stevens-Johnson syndrome.
Cosopt is dorzolamide and timolol.

Skin
Contact dermatitis [4]

Central Nervous System
Dysgeusia (taste perversion) (25%) [9]

Ocular
Ocular burning (33%) [5]
Ocular itching / ocular pruritus [5]
Ocular pain [3]
Ocular stinging [10]
Vision blurred [3]

Other
Adverse effects / adverse reactions [2]

DOSTARLIMAB

Trade name: Jemperli (GSK)
Indications: Treatment of advanced endometrial cancer following prior treatment with a platinum-containing drug regimen.

Class: Biologic, Immune checkpoint inhibitor (incl. programmed death receptor-1 (PD-1) inhibitor), Monoclonal antibody, Programmed death receptor-1 (PD-1) inhibitor
Half-life: 25.4 days
Clinically important, potentially hazardous interactions with: none known
Pregnancy category: Based on its mechanism of action, dostarlimab can cause fetal harm when administered in pregnancy. Contraception is advised.
Important contra-indications noted in the prescribing guidelines for: nursing mothers
Note: Dostarlimab may cause immune-mediated adverse reactions.

Skin
Pruritus (itching) (1% grade 3/4) (14%) [2]
Rash [2]

Endocrine/Metabolic
ALP increased (3% grade 3/4) (25%)
ALT increased (3% grade 3/4) (15%)
Appetite decreased (14%) [2]
AST increased (2% grade 3/4) (16%)
Hypercalcemia (2% grade 3/4) (15%)
Hypoalbuminemia / albumin decreased (3% grade 3/4) (30%)
Hypokalemia (2% grade 3/4) (15%)
Hyponatremia (5% grade 3/4) (26%)
Hypothyroidism [2]
Serum creatinine increased (grade 3/4) (27%)

Gastrointestinal/Hepatic
Constipation (1% grade 3/4) (20%)
Diarrhea (2% grade 3/4) (26%) [2]
Nausea (30%) [2]
Vomiting (18%) [2]

Genitourinary
Urinary tract infection (2% grade 3/4) (13%)

Hematologic
Anemia (13% grade 3/4) (24%) [2]
Leukocytopenia (leukopenia) / leukocytes (white blood cells) decreased (3% grade 3/4) (21%)
Lymphopenia (lymphocytopenia) / lymphocytes decreased (9% grade 3/4) (37%)

Neuromuscular/Skeletal
Arthralgia [2]
Asthenia / fatigue (1% grade 3/4) (48%) [2]
Myalgia/Myopathy (12%)

Respiratory
Cough (14%)

DOXACURIUM

Trade name: Nuromax (GSK)
Indications: Neuromuscular blockade
Class: Non-depolarizing neuromuscular blocker
Half-life: 100–200 minutes
Clinically important, potentially hazardous interactions with: amikacin, aminoglycosides, carbamazepine, cyclopropane, enflurane, gentamicin, halothane, isoflurane, kanamycin, methoxyflurane, neomycin, piperacillin, streptomycin, tobramycin
Important contra-indications noted in the prescribing guidelines for: the elderly; nursing mothers; pediatric patients

DOXAZOSIN

Trade name: Cardura (Pfizer)
Indications: Hypertension
Class: Adrenergic alpha-receptor antagonist
Half-life: 19–22 hours
Clinically important, potentially hazardous interactions with: tadalafil, vardenafil, zuclopenthixol
Important contra-indications noted in the prescribing guidelines for: the elderly; nursing mothers; pediatric patients

---

Skin
- Edema / fluid retention (4%)
- Exanthems (2%)

Mucosal
- Xerostomia (dry mouth) (2%) [2]

Cardiovascular
- Hypotension [3]
- Orthostatic hypotension [2]
- Postural hypotension [2]

Central Nervous System
- Headache [2]
- Vertigo / dizziness [9]

Gastrointestinal/Hepatic
- Abdominal pain [2]

Genitourinary
- Erectile dysfunction [3]

Neuromuscular/Skeletal
- Asthenia / fatigue [4]

Ocular
- Floppy iris syndrome [3]

DOXEPIN

Trade names: Adapin (LGM Pharma), Silenor (Somaxon), Sinquan (Pfizer)
Indications: Mental depression, anxiety, insomnia
Class: Antidepressant; tricyclic, Muscarinic antagonist
Half-life: 6–8 hours
Clinically important, potentially hazardous interactions with: alcohol, amprenavir, arbutamine, cholestyramine, clonidine, CNS depressants, epinephrine, formoterol, guanethidine, isocarboxazid, linezolid, MAO inhibitors, phenelzine, QT prolonging agents, quinolones, ramelteon, selegiline, sparfloxacin, sympathomimetics, tranylcypromine
Pregnancy category: pregnancy category is B for topical use
Important contra-indications noted in the prescribing guidelines for: nursing mothers
Warning: SUICIDALITY AND ANTIDEPRESSANT DRUGS

Skin
- Dermatitis (from topical) [9]
- Diaphoresis (<10%)
- Pseudolymphoma / cutaneous pseudolymphoma [2]

Mucosal
- Xerostomia (dry mouth) (>10%) [6]

Cardiovascular
- QT interval prolonged / QT prolongation [2]

Central Nervous System
- Dysgeusia (taste perversion) (>10%)
- Headache [4]
- Somnolence (drowsiness) [7]

DOXERCALCIFEROL

Trade name: Hectorol (Genzyme)
Indications: Secondary hyperparathyroidism in patients with chronic kidney disease on dialysis
Class: Vitamin D receptor agonist
Half-life: 32–37 hours
Clinically important, potentially hazardous interactions with: aminoglutethimide, cholestyramine, erythromycin, ketoconazole, magnesium-containing antacids, mineral oil, phenobarbital
Important contra-indications noted in the prescribing guidelines for: nursing mothers; pediatric patients
Note: Contra-indicated in patients with a tendency towards hypercalcemia or current evidence of vitamin D toxicity.

Skin
- Abscess (3%)
- Edema / fluid retention (34%)
- Pruritus (itching) (8%)

Cardiovascular
- Bradycardia / sinus bradycardia (7%)

Central Nervous System
- Anorexia (5%)
- Headache (28%)
- Sleep-related disorder (3%)
- Vertigo / dizziness (12%)

Endocrine/Metabolic
- Weight gain (5%)

Gastrointestinal/Hepatic
- Constipation (3%)
- Dyspepsia / functional dyspepsia (indigestion) (see also gastroparesis) (5%)
- Nausea (21%)
- Vomiting (21%)

Neuromuscular/Skeletal
- Arthralgia (5%)
- Asthenia / fatigue (28%)

Respiratory
- Dyspnea / shortness of breath (12%)

DOXORUBICIN

Synonym: hydroxydaunomycin
Trade names: Adriamycin (Bedford), Doxil (Tibotec), Rubex (Mead Johnson)
Indications: Carcinomas, leukemias, sarcomas
Class: Antibiotic, Antibiotic; anthracycline, Antimicrobial
Half-life: 20–48 hours
Clinically important, potentially hazardous interactions with: aldesleukin, cabazitaxel, CYP2D6 inhibitors or inducers, CYP3A4 inhibitors or inducers, gadobenate, P-glycoprotein inhibitors or inducers, paclitaxel, sorafenib, stavudine, trastuzumab, zidovudine
Important contra-indications noted in the prescribing guidelines for: nursing mothers
Warning: CARDIOMYOPATHY, SECONDARY MALIGNANCIES, EXTRAVASATION AND TISSUE NECROSIS, and SEVERE MYELOSUPPRESSION

Skin
- Anaphylactoid reactions / anaphylaxis (includes anaphylactic shock) [2]
- Angioedema (formerly named angioneurotic edema) [5]
- Cutaneous toxicity / skin toxicity [12]
- Erythema [2]
- Exanthems [4]
- Exfoliative dermatitis [2]
- Flushing / rubefaction (<10%) [2]
- Hand–foot syndrome (palmar–plantar erythrodysesthesia) [64]
- Hypersensitivity [2]
- Intertrigo [3]
- Lupus erythematosus (subacute cutaneous lupus erythematosus (SCLE)) [3]
- Necrosis (skin necrosis) (local) [5]
- Palmar–plantar erythema (painful) [4]
- Pigmentation (Skin) (includes hyperpigmentation) [15]
- Pruritus (itching) [2]
- Purpura [2]
- Radiation recall dermatitis [8]
- Rash [6]
- Urticaria / hives [10]

Hair
- Alopecia / hair loss (>10%) [41]

Nails
- Beau's lines [3]
- Melanonychia [4]
- Muehrcke's lines [2]
- Nail changes [2]
- Nail pigmentation [17]
- Onycholysis [5]

Mucosal
- Aphthous stomatitis / aphthous ulcer / aphtha (aphthae) [2]
- Mucositis [20]
- Oral lesions [7]
- Stomatitis (oral mucositis) (>10%) [22]
- Tongue pigmentation [3]

Cardiovascular
- Atrial fibrillation [2]
- Cardiomyopathy [7]
- Cardiotoxicity [25]
- Chest pain [2]
- Congestive heart failure [7]
- Myocardial toxicity [4]

Central Nervous System
- Anorexia [3]

Dysgeusia (taste perversion) [2]
Fever (pyrexia) (includes hyperpyrexia) [5]
Headache [3]
Leukoencephalopathy / posterior reversible encephalopathy syndrome (PRES) [4]
Neurotoxicity [4]
Pain [2]
Peripheral neuropathy [9]

Endocrine/Metabolic
ALT increased [3]
Amenorrhea [2]
Hyperglycemia (includes glucose increased) [3]
Hypokalemia [2]
Weight loss [2]

Gastrointestinal/Hepatic
Constipation [4]
Diarrhea [9]
Gastrointestinal perforation / perforated colon / gastric perforation [2]
Hepatotoxicity / liver injury / acute liver injury / drug-induced liver injury (DILI) [6]
Nausea [16]
Pancreatitis / acute pancreatitis [2]
Vomiting [12]

Hematologic
Anemia [19]
Febrile neutropenia [20]
Hemorrhage [2]
Hemotoxicity [2]
Leukocytopenia (leukopenia) / leukocytes (white blood cells) decreased [6]
Myelosuppression / bone marrow suppression / myelotoxicity [2]
Neutropenia (neutrophils decreased) [39]
Thrombocytopenia / platelets decreased [23]

Local
Injection-site erythema [7]
Injection-site extravasation (>10%) [12]
Injection-site necrosis (>10%) [5]
Injection-site reaction [2]
Injection-site ulceration (>10%) [4]

Neuromuscular/Skeletal
Asthenia / fatigue [19]
Bone pain / joint pain [3]
Myalgia/Myopathy [3]

Renal
Nephrotoxicity / kidney injury / acute kidney injury (AKI) / drug-induced kidney injury [2]

Respiratory
Dyspnea / shortness of breath [3]
Pneumonia [4]
Pneumonitis [3]

Other
Adverse effects / adverse reactions [6]
Allergic reactions [4]
Death [11]
Infection [5]

DOXYCYCLINE

Trade names: Adoxa (Bioglan), Doryx (Warner Chilcott), Oracea (Galderma), Vibra-Tabs (Pfizer), Vibramycin-D (Pfizer)
Indications: Various infections caused by susceptible organisms
Class: Antibiotic, Antibiotic; tetracycline, Antimicrobial
Half-life: 12–22 hours
Clinically important, potentially hazardous interactions with: acitretin, amoxicillin, ampicillin, antacids, bacampicillin, barbiturates, BCG vaccine, bismuth, calcium salts, carbamazepine, carbenicillin, cloxacillin, corticosteroids, coumarins, cyclosporine, dairy products, digoxin, ergotamine, kaolin, methotrexate, methoxyflurane, methysergide, mezlocillin, nafcillin, oral contraceptives, oral iron, oral typhoid vaccine, oxacillin, penicillins, phenindione, phenytoin, piperacillin, primidone, quinapril, retinoids, rifampin, St John's wort, strontium ranelate, sucralfate, sulfonylureas, ticarcillin, tripotassium dicitratobismuthate, zinc
Important contra-indications noted in the prescribing guidelines for: nursing mothers; pediatric patients
Note: Drug-induced esophagitis / ulcerative esophagitis, well-documented adverse effects of doxycycline, are often associated with taking the drug while lying down or an inadequate fluid intake.

Skin
AGEP [2]
Angioedema (formerly named angioneurotic edema) [2]
Baboon syndrome / symmetrical drug-related intertriginous and flexural exanthema (SDRIFE) [2]
Candidiasis / candidosis [3]
Erythema multiforme [4]
Exanthems [2]
Fixed eruption / fixed drug eruption [11]
Hypersensitivity [2]
Photosensitivity [21]
Phototoxicity [9]
Pigmentation (Skin) (includes hyperpigmentation) [5]
Pruritus (itching) [3]
Rash [5]
Stevens-Johnson syndrome and toxic epidermal necrolysis (SJS/TEN) [12]
Sweet's syndrome [2]
Urticaria / hives [6]

Nails
Photo-onycholysis [13]

Mucosal
Black tongue / black hairy tongue (lingua villosa nigra) [2]
Mucosal candidiasis [2]

Central Nervous System
Anosmia (smell loss) / smell disorder [2]
Fever (pyrexia) (includes hyperpyrexia) [2]
Headache [4]
Intracranial pressure increased (intracranial hypertension) [3]
Paresthesias [4]
Vertigo / dizziness [3]

Endocrine/Metabolic
Hypoglycemia [2]

Gastrointestinal/Hepatic
Abdominal pain [3]
Diarrhea [4]
Esophagitis [6]
Gastric mucosal injury [2]
Hepatotoxicity / liver injury / acute liver injury / drug-induced liver injury (DILI) [2]
Nausea [5]
Pancreatitis / acute pancreatitis [13]
Peptic ulceration (includes duodenal ulcer, esophageal ulcer) [3]
Ulcerative esophagitis [4]
Vomiting [3]

Genitourinary
Vaginitis (includes vulvitis) [2]

Neuromuscular/Skeletal
Myalgia/Myopathy [2]

Other
Adverse effects / adverse reactions [7]
Allergic reactions [3]
Death [2]
Tooth pigmentation / discoloration (>10%) [6]

DRONABINOL

Synonyms: tetrahydrocannabinol; THC
Trade names: Marinol (AbbVie), Syndros (Insys)
Indications: Chemotherapy-induced nausea, anorexia associated with weight loss in patients with AIDS
Class: Antiemetic, Cannabinoid
Half-life: 19–24 hours
Clinically important, potentially hazardous interactions with: disulfiram, metronidazole
Important contra-indications noted in the prescribing guidelines for: the elderly; nursing mothers; pediatric patients

---

Mucosal
Xerostomia (dry mouth) (<10%)

Central Nervous System
Euphoria / elation (<10%)
Paranoia (<10%)
Somnolence (drowsiness) (<10%) [2]
Vertigo / dizziness (<10%) [6]

Gastrointestinal/Hepatic
Abdominal pain (<10%)
Nausea (<10%) [3]
Vomiting (<10%)

Other
Adverse effects / adverse reactions [4]

DRONEDARONE

Trade name: Multaq (Sanofi-Aventis)
Indications: Atrial fibrillation and atrial flutter
Class: Antiarrhythmic, Antiarrhythmic class III
Half-life: 13–19 hours
Clinically important, potentially hazardous interactions with: amiodarone, amitriptyline, amoxapine, antiarrhythmics, antipsychotics prolonging QT interval, arsenic, atorvastatin, beta blockers, bupivacaine, calcium channel blockers, carbamazepine, citalopram, clarithromycin, conivaptan, coumarins, cyclosporine, CYP3A inducers, dabigatran, darunavir, dasatinib, degarelix, delavirdine, digoxin, diltiazem, disopyramide, dolasetron, efavirenz, erythromycin, fingolimod, grapefruit juice, indinavir, itraconazole, ketoconazole, lapatinib, levobupivacaine, levofloxacin, levomepromazine, metoprolol, moxifloxacin, nefazodone, neratinib, nifedipine, ombitasvir/paritaprevir/ritonavir, ombitasvir/paritaprevir/ritonavir and dasabuvir, oxcarbazepine, pazopanib, phenindione, phenobarbital, phenothiazines, phenytoin, posaconazole, prilocaine, propranolol, rifampin, rifapentine, ritonavir, ropivacaine, rosuvastatin, saquinavir, simvastatin, sirolimus, sotalol, St John's wort, statins, tacrolimus, telavancin, telithromycin, tricyclic antidepressants, venetoclax, verapamil, voriconazole, vorinostat, warfarin, ziprasidone

Important contra-indications noted in the prescribing guidelines for: nursing mothers; pediatric patients
Warning: INCREASED RISK OF DEATH, STROKE AND HEART FAILURE IN PATIENTS WITH DECOMPENSATED HEART FAILURE OR PERMANENT ATRIAL FIBRILLATION

Skin
Anaphylactoid reactions / anaphylaxis (includes anaphylactic shock) [2]
Dermatitis (5%)
Eczema / eczematous reaction / eczematous eruption (5%)
Erythema (5%)
Phototoxicity [2]
Pruritus (itching) (5%)
Rash (5%) [8]

Cardiovascular
Arrhythmias [3]
Bradycardia / sinus bradycardia (3%) [8]
Cardiac failure (new or worsening) [9]
Cardiotoxicity [3]
Congestive heart failure [2]
QT interval prolonged / QT prolongation (28%) [10]
Torsades de pointes [3]

Central Nervous System
Vertigo / dizziness [2]

Endocrine/Metabolic
Serum creatinine increased (51%) [6]

Gastrointestinal/Hepatic
Abdominal pain (4%) [2]
Diarrhea (9%) [14]
Dyspepsia / functional dyspepsia (indigestion) (see also gastroparesis) (2%)
Gastrointestinal disorder / discomfort [4]
Hepatic failure [5]
Hepatotoxicity / liver injury / acute liver injury / drug-induced liver injury (DILI) [9]
Nausea (5%) [12]
Vomiting (2%) [6]

Neuromuscular/Skeletal
Asthenia / fatigue (7%) [3]

Renal
Nephrotoxicity / kidney injury / acute kidney injury (AKI) / drug-induced kidney injury [2]
Renal failure [2]

Respiratory
Pulmonary toxicity [9]

Other
Adverse effects / adverse reactions [3]
Death [2]
Side effects [2]

DROPERIDOL

Trade names: Inapsine (Akorn), Xomolix (ProStrakan)
Indications: Tranquilizer and antiemetic in surgical procedures
Class: Antiemetic, Antipsychotic, Butyrophenone
Half-life: 2.3 hours
Clinically important, potentially hazardous interactions with: amiodarone, amisulpride, amitriptyline, arsenic, atomoxetine, azithromycin, chloroquine, CNS depressants, cyclobenzaprine, disopyramide, duloxetine, eszopiclone, fluoxetine, fluvoxamine, hydromorphone, hydroxychloroquine, levomepromazine, lurasidone, macrolides, metaxalone, milnacipran, moxifloxacin, paliperidone, pentamidine, pimozide, QT prolonging agents, quinine, ramelteon, sertraline, sotalol, sulpiride / levosulpiride, tamoxifen, tapentadol, thiopental, tiagabine, tricyclic antidepressants
Important contra-indications noted in the prescribing guidelines for: nursing mothers; pediatric patients
Note: Contra-indicated in patients with known or suspected QT prolongation.
This product is not available in the European market.
Warning: QT PROLONGATION AND TORSADE DE POINTES

Skin
Anaphylactoid reactions / anaphylaxis (includes anaphylactic shock) [3]
Angioedema (formerly named angioneurotic edema) [2]

Cardiovascular
Arrhythmias [2]
Hypotension [3]
QT interval prolonged / QT prolongation [13]
Torsades de pointes [6]

Central Nervous System
Akathisia [5]
Extrapyramidal symptoms [2]
Neuroleptic malignant syndrome [3]
Restlessness [2]
Sedation [2]

Neuromuscular/Skeletal
Dystonia [7]

Other
Death [3]

DROSPIRENONE/ ESTETROL

Synonyms: DRSP (drospirenone); E4 (estetrol)
Trade name: Nextstellis (Mayne Pharma)
Indications: Indicated for use by females of reproductive potential to prevent pregnancy
Class: Antiandrogen, Estrogen, Hormone, Progestin/estrogen CHC
Half-life: 27 hours (estetrol); 34 hours (drospirenone)
Clinically important, potentially hazardous interactions with: bile acid sequestrants, CYP3A inducers, CYP3A inhibitors
Pregnancy category: Discontinue if pregnancy occurs.
Note: Drospirenone is also marketed (in combination with ethinylestradiol, EE) as the oral contraceptive Yasmin. See under 'Oral Contraceptives' for other combinations of estrogens and progestins.
Warning: FEMALES OVER 35 YEARS OLD WHO SMOKE SHOULD NOT USE DROSPIRENONE/ESTETROL
CIGARETTE SMOKING INCREASES THE RISK OF SERIOUS CARDIOVASCULAR EVENTS FROM COMBINATION ORAL CONTRACEPTIVE USE.

Skin
Acne vulgaris ('acne') (4%)

Central Nervous System
Headache (6%) [2]
Mood changes (includes mood disorder) (9%)

Endocrine/Metabolic
Libido decreased (2%)
Menstrual irregularities (11%)
Weight gain (3%)

Genitourinary
Dysmenorrhea (4%)
Metrorrhagia [2]

Neuromuscular/Skeletal
Breast disorder / breast discomfort (5%)

DROTRECOGIN ALFA

Trade name: Xigris (Lilly)
Indications: Severe sepsis
Class: Recombinant protein C
Half-life: 1.6 hours
Clinically important, potentially hazardous interactions with: abciximab, cilostazol, citalopram, clopidogrel, enoxaparin, eptifibatide, meloxicam, tinzaparin
Important contra-indications noted in the prescribing guidelines for: nursing mothers; pediatric patients
Note: This drug has been withdrawn.

Skin
Purpura (>10%)

Hematologic
Bleeding [8]

DULAGLUTIDE

Trade name: Trulicity (Lilly)
Indications: To improve glycemic control in adults with Type II diabetes mellitus
Class: Antidiabetic, Glucagon-like peptide-1 (GLP-1) receptor agonist
Half-life: 5 days
Clinically important, potentially hazardous interactions with: none known
Important contra-indications noted in the prescribing guidelines for: nursing mothers; pediatric patients
Note: Contra-indicated in patients with a personal or family history of medullary thyroid carcinoma or in patients with multiple endocrine neoplasia syndrome Type 2.
Warning: RISK OF THYROID C-CELL TUMORS

Skin
Bullous pemphigoid / pemphigoid [2]
Hypersensitivity [2]

Cardiovascular
Atrioventricular block (2%)
Tachycardia (3–6%)

Central Nervous System
Headache [3]

Endocrine/Metabolic
Appetite decreased (5–9%) [4]
Hypoglycemia [3]

Gastrointestinal/Hepatic
Abdominal distension [2]
Abdominal pain (7–9%)
Constipation [6]
Diarrhea [26]
Dyspepsia / functional dyspepsia (indigestion) (see also gastroparesis) (4–6%) [3]
Gastrointestinal adverse reaction [2]
Gastrointestinal disorder / discomfort [3]

Nausea (12–21%) [28]
Pancreatitis / acute pancreatitis [5]
Vomiting (6–13%) [19]

Local
Injection-site reaction [5]

Neuromuscular/Skeletal
Asthenia / fatigue (4–6%)

Respiratory
Nasopharyngitis [7]

Other
Adverse effects / adverse reactions (gastrointestinal) [5]

DULOXETINE

Trade names: Cymbalta (Lilly), Yentreve (Lilly)
Indications: Depression
Class: Antidepressant, Noradrenaline reuptake inhibitor, Serotonin reuptake inhibitor
Half-life: 8–17 hours
Clinically important, potentially hazardous interactions with: 5HT1 agonists, alcohol, amitriptyline, artemether/lumefantrine, aspirin, atomoxetine, cimetidine, ciprofloxacin, citalopram, clomipramine, CYP1A2 inducers, CYP2D6 inhibitors and substrates, darunavir, droperidol, enoxacin, fesoterodine, fluoxetine, fluvoxamine, iobenguane, levomepromazine, MAO inhibitors, meperidine, moclobemide, naratriptan, nebivolol, NSAIDs, paroxetine hydrochloride, PEG-interferon, quinidine, sibutramine, SSRIs, St John's wort, tamoxifen, teriflunomide, thioridazine, tramadol, tricyclic antidepressants, tryptophan, venlafaxine, viloxazine, warfarin
Important contra-indications noted in the prescribing guidelines for: nursing mothers; pediatric patients
Warning: SUICIDAL THOUGHTS AND BEHAVIORS

Skin
Diaphoresis (6%) [2]
Flushing / rubefaction (3%)
Hot flashes / hot flushes (>2%)
Hyperhidrosis (7%) [8]
Stevens-Johnson syndrome and toxic epidermal necrolysis (SJS/TEN) [2]

Mucosal
Oropharyngeal pain (>2%)
Xerostomia (dry mouth) (13%) [25]

Cardiovascular
Palpitation (>2%)

Central Nervous System
Agitation (5%)
Anxiety (3%)
Dyskinesia [2]
Headache (14%) [11]
Insomnia (10%) [13]
Paresthesias (>2%)
Restless legs syndrome / Willis-Ekbom disease (includes restless arms syndrome variant) [3]
Serotonin syndrome [5]
Somnolence (drowsiness) (10%) [18]
Suicidal ideation [5]
Tardive syndrome / tardive dyskinesia [4]
Tremor (3%)
Vertigo / dizziness (10%) [17]
Yawning (>2%) [2]

Endocrine/Metabolic
ALT increased [2]
Appetite decreased (8–9%) [3]
Hyponatremia [6]
Libido decreased (4%)
SIADH [6]
Weight loss (>2%)

Gastrointestinal/Hepatic
Abdominal pain (>2%)
Colitis [2]
Constipation (10%) [12]
Diarrhea (9%) [6]
Hepatotoxicity / liver injury / acute liver injury / drug-induced liver injury (DILI) (rare) [4]
Nausea (24%) [27]
Vomiting (>2%) [4]

Genitourinary
Ejaculatory dysfunction (2–5%)
Priapism [2]
Sexual dysfunction [6]

Neuromuscular/Skeletal
Arthralgia (>2%)
Asthenia / fatigue (10%) [15]
Back pain (>2%)
Bone pain / joint pain (4%)
Muscle spasm (3%)

Ocular
Vision blurred (>2%)

Renal
Renal disorder [2]

Respiratory
Cough (>2%)
Influenza (3%)
Nasopharyngitis (5%)
Upper respiratory tract infection (4%)

Other
Adverse effects / adverse reactions [13]
Bruxism (teeth grinding) [3]
Death [2]
Side effects [2]

DUPILUMAB

Trade name: Dupixent (Regeneron)
Indications: Moderate-to-severe atopic dermatitis
Class: Interleukin-4 receptor alpha antagonist, Monoclonal antibody
Half-life: N/A
Clinically important, potentially hazardous interactions with: none known
Pregnancy category: Insufficient evidence to inform drug-associated risk
Important contra-indications noted in the prescribing guidelines for: pediatric patients

Skin
Churg-Strauss syndrome [6]
Dermatitis [2]
Erythroderma [3]
Facial erythema [3]
Granuloma annulare [5]
Herpes simplex (2%) [3]
Psoriasiform dermatitis [2]
Psoriasiform eruption [3]
Psoriasis [8]
Serum sickness [2]
Serum sickness-like reaction [2]
Vitiligo [6]

Hair
Alopecia / hair loss [2]

Mucosal
Oral candidiasis (4%)

Central Nervous System
Headache [7]

Gastrointestinal/Hepatic
Pancreatitis / acute pancreatitis [2]

Hematologic
Eosinophilia / eosinophils increased [9]

Local
Injection-site reaction (10%) [20]

Ocular
Blepharoconjunctivitis [6]
Conjunctivitis (conjunctival inflammation) (10%) [22]
Ectropion / cicatricial ectropion [3]
Ocular adverse effect [4]
Ocular surface disorder / ocular surface disease [10]

Respiratory
Nasopharyngitis [10]
Upper respiratory tract infection [3]

Other
Adverse effects / adverse reactions [4]
Infection [2]

DURVALUMAB

Trade name: Imfinzi (AstraZeneca)
Indications: Locally advanced or metastatic urothelial carcinoma in patients having disease progression following platinum-containing chemotherapy
Class: Antineoplastic / anticancer agent (see also Immune checkpoint inhibitor), Immune checkpoint inhibitor (incl. programmed death receptor-1 (PD-1) inhibitor), Monoclonal antibody, Programmed death-ligand (PD-L1) inhibitor
Half-life: 17 days
Clinically important, potentially hazardous interactions with: none known
Pregnancy category: Can cause fetal harm
Important contra-indications noted in the prescribing guidelines for: the elderly; nursing mothers; pediatric patients

Skin
Lupus erythematosus (subacute cutaneous lupus erythematosus (SCLE)) [2]
Peripheral edema (15%)
Pruritus (itching) [3]
Psoriasis [3]
Rash (11%) [2]

Cardiovascular
Myocarditis, myositis and myasthenia gravis overlap syndrome (Triple-M Syndrome / 3M Syndrome) [3]

Central Nervous System
Encephalitis [4]
Fever (pyrexia) (includes hyperpyrexia) (14%)
Guillain-Barré syndrome / acute inflammatory demyelinating polyradiculoneuropathy / acute motor axonal neuropathy [2]
Paraneoplastic neurological syndromes [4]

Endocrine/Metabolic
ALP increased (4%)
Appetite decreased (19%) [4]
AST increased (2%) [4]
Diabetes mellitus [5]

Diabetic ketoacidosis [2]
Hypercalcemia (3%)
Hyperglycemia (includes glucose increased) (3%)
Hypermagnesemia (4%)
Hyperthyroidism (includes 'thyroid storm') (5–6%)
Hyponatremia (12%)
Hypoparathyroidism [2]
Hypothyroidism (6–10%) [2]
Thyroiditis [3]

Gastrointestinal/Hepatic
Abdominal pain (14%)
Colitis (13%) [3]
Constipation (21%)
Diarrhea (13%) [11]
Hepatitis [2]
Nausea (16%) [3]
Vomiting [3]

Genitourinary
Urinary tract infection (15%)

Hematologic
Agranulocytosis / severe selective neutropenia [2]
Anemia (8%) [2]
Lymphopenia (lymphocytopenia) / lymphocytes decreased (11%)
Thrombocytopenia / platelets decreased [4]

Local
Infusion-related reactions (2%)

Neuromuscular/Skeletal
Arthralgia [2]
Asthenia / fatigue (39%) [11]
Bone pain / joint pain (24%)
Myalgia/Myopathy [4]
Myasthenia gravis [2]

Respiratory
Cough (10%)
Dyspnea / shortness of breath (13%)
Interstitial lung disease / interstitial pneumonitis / interstitial pneumonia (cryptogenic organizing pneumonia) / drug-induced interstitial lung disease [2]
Pneumonitis (2%) [7]

Other
Adverse effects / adverse reactions [4]
Death [7]
Infection (30–38%)

DUTASTERIDE

Trade names: Avodart (GSK), Jalyn (GSK)
Indications: Benign prostatic hyperplasia, male pattern baldness (anecdotal)
Class: 5-alpha reductase inhibitor, Androgen antagonist
Half-life: 3–5 weeks
Clinically important, potentially hazardous interactions with: cimetidine, ciprofloxacin, conivaptan, darunavir, delavirdine, diltiazem, indinavir, ketoconazole, ritonavir, telithromycin, troleandomycin, verapamil, voriconazole
Important contra-indications noted in the prescribing guidelines for: nursing mothers; pediatric patients
Note: Jalyn is dutasteride and tamsulosin.

Endocrine/Metabolic
Gynecomastia [2]
Libido decreased (<3%) [3]

Genitourinary
Ejaculatory dysfunction [3]
Erectile dysfunction [8]
Impotence (<5%)
Sexual dysfunction [7]

Other
Adverse effects / adverse reactions [2]

ECALLANTIDE

Trade name: Kalbitor (Dyax)
Indications: Acute attacks of hereditary angioedema (HAE) in patients 16 years of age and older
Class: Plasma kallikrein inhibitor
Half-life: ~2hours
Clinically important, potentially hazardous interactions with: none known
Important contra-indications noted in the prescribing guidelines for: the elderly; nursing mothers; pediatric patients

---

Skin
Anaphylactoid reactions / anaphylaxis (includes anaphylactic shock) [6]
Pruritus (itching) (5%)

Central Nervous System
Fever (pyrexia) (includes hyperpyrexia) (4%)
Headache (16%) [2]

Gastrointestinal/Hepatic
Abdominal pain (5%)
Diarrhea (13%)
Nausea (5%)
Vomiting (5%)

Local
Injection-site reaction (7%)

Respiratory
Nasopharyngitis (6%)

Other
Adverse effects / adverse reactions [3]

ECHINACEA

Family: Asteraceae; Compositae
Scientific names: *Echinacea angustifola, Echinacea pallida, Echinacea purpurea*
Indications: Colds, upper respiratory infections, peripheral vasodilator, urinary tract infections, yeast infections, ulcers, psoriasis, herpes simplex, septicemia, boils, abscesses, rheumatism, migraine, dyspepsia, eczema, bee stings and hemorrhoids
Class: Immunomodulator
Half-life: N/A
Clinically important, potentially hazardous interactions with: abatacept, alefacept, amiodarone, azacitidine, betamethasone, cabazitaxel, corticosteroids, cyclosporine, docetaxel, gefitinib, ketoconazole, leflunomide, methotrexate, pralatrexate
Note: Individuals with atopy may be more likely to experience an allergic reaction when taking echinacea.

Skin
Anaphylactoid reactions / anaphylaxis (includes anaphylactic shock) [3]
Angioedema (formerly named angioneurotic edema) [2]
Rash [3]
Urticaria / hives [2]

Gastrointestinal/Hepatic
Hepatotoxicity / liver injury / acute liver injury / drug-induced liver injury (DILI) [2]

Ocular
Ocular adverse effect [2]

Other
Adverse effects / adverse reactions [10]
Allergic reactions [2]

ECONAZOLE

Trade name: Gyno-Pervaryl (Janssen)
Indications: Fungal infections caused by Mycotic vulvovaginitis, Mycotic balanitis, *Candida albicans*
Class: Antifungal / antimycotic, Antifungal; imidazole, Antimicrobial
Half-life: N/A
Clinically important, potentially hazardous interactions with: acenocoumarol, condoms, contraceptive diaphragms, imidazole, warfarin

---

Skin
Contact dermatitis [2]

ECULIZUMAB

Trade name: Soliris (Alexion)
Indications: Paroxysmal nocturnal hemoglobinuria, atypical hemolytic uremic syndrome
Class: Complement inhibitor, Covid-19 putative drug, Monoclonal antibody
Half-life: ~12 days
Clinically important, potentially hazardous interactions with: none known
Important contra-indications noted in the prescribing guidelines for: nursing mothers; pediatric patients
Note: Eculizumab-aeeb (Bkemv) is biosimilar to Eculizumab (Soliris). Approved 05/28/2024 Eculizumab-aagh (Epysoli) is biosimilar to Eculizumab (Soliris). Approved 07/19/2024.
Warning: SERIOUS MENINGOCOCCAL INFECTIONS

Skin
Peripheral edema [2]
Pruritus (itching) [2]

Mucosal
Nasal congestion [2]

Cardiovascular
Hypertension [2]

Central Nervous System
Fever (pyrexia) (includes hyperpyrexia) [4]
Headache (44%) [9]
Insomnia [2]
Meningococcal infection [4]
Vertigo / dizziness [3]

Gastrointestinal/Hepatic
Abdominal pain [3]
Diarrhea [4]
Nausea [5]
Vomiting [3]

Genitourinary
Urinary tract infection [3]

Hematologic
Anemia [2]
Leukocytopenia (leukopenia) / leukocytes (white blood cells) decreased [2]

Neuromuscular/Skeletal
Asthenia / fatigue (12%) [5]
Back pain (19%) [3]
Pain in extremities [3]

Respiratory
Cough (12%) [5]
Nasopharyngitis (23%) [6]
Pharyngolaryngeal pain [2]
Upper respiratory tract infection [4]

Other
Adverse effects / adverse reactions [2]
Infection [2]

EDARAVONE

Trade name: Radicava (Mitsubishi Tanabe Pharma)
Indications: Amyotrophic lateral sclerosis
Class: Antioxidant, Neuroprotectant
Half-life: 4–6 hours
Clinically important, potentially hazardous interactions with: none known
Pregnancy category: May cause fetal toxicity based on findings in animal studies
Important contra-indications noted in the prescribing guidelines for: nursing mothers; pediatric patients
Note: Radicava contains sodium bisulfite which may cause allergic type reactions.

Skin
Dermatitis (8%) [2]
Eczema / eczematous reaction / eczematous eruption (7%) [3]
Hematoma / cutaneous hematoma (15%) [3]
Tinea (4%) [2]

Central Nervous System
Gait instability / postural instability (13%) [3]
Headache (10%) [3]
Insomnia [2]

Gastrointestinal/Hepatic
Constipation [2]
Diarrhea [2]
Dysphagia [3]
Hepatotoxicity / liver injury / acute liver injury / drug-induced liver injury (DILI) [2]

Genitourinary
Glycosuria (4%) [3]

Renal
Nephrotoxicity / kidney injury / acute kidney injury (AKI) / drug-induced kidney injury [2]

Respiratory
Hypoxia (6%)
Nasopharyngitis [2]
Respiratory failure (6%) [3]

Other
Adverse effects / adverse reactions [4]

EDOXABAN

Trade name: Savaysa (Daiichi Sankyo)
Indications: Reduce the risk of stroke and systemic embolism in patients with nonvalvular atrial fibrillation, treatment of deep vein thrombosis and pulmonary embolism
Class: Direct factor Xa inhibitor
Half-life: 10–14 hours
Clinically important, potentially hazardous interactions with: anticoagulants, rifampin
Important contra-indications noted in the prescribing guidelines for: nursing mothers; pediatric patients
Note: Contra-indicated in patients with active pathological bleeding.
Warning: REDUCED EFFICACY IN NONVALVULAR ATRIAL FIBRILLATION PATIENTS WITH CRCL>95ml/min, ISCHEMIC EVENTS ON PREMATURE DISCONTINUATION and SPINAL/EPIDURAL HEMATOMA

Skin
Rash (4%)

Mucosal
Epistaxis (nosebleed) (5%)
Gingival bleeding [2]
Oral bleeding (3%)

Gastrointestinal/Hepatic
Diarrhea [2]
Gastrointestinal bleeding (4%)
Hepatotoxicity / liver injury / acute liver injury / drug-induced liver injury (DILI) (5–8%) [2]

Genitourinary
Hematuria (2%) [2]

Hematologic
Anemia (2–10%)
Bleeding (>5%) [13]

Other
Adverse effects / adverse reactions [4]

EDROPHONIUM

Trade names: Enlon (Baxter), Tensilon (Valeant)
Indications: Myasthenia gravis diagnosis
Class: Anesthetic, Cholinesterase inhibitor
Half-life: 1.8 hours
Clinically important, potentially hazardous interactions with: corticosteroids, digitalis, galantamine, pyridostigmine
Note: Anticholinesterase drugs may cause uterine irritability and induce premature labor when given intravenously to pregnant women near term.

Skin
Diaphoresis (>10%)

Mucosal
Sialorrhea (ptyalism; hypersalivation) (>10%)

Cardiovascular
Asystole [2]
Bradycardia / sinus bradycardia [2]
Cardiac failure [3]

Central Nervous System
Syncope / fainting [2]

EFAVIRENZ

Trade names: Atripla (Gilead), Sustiva (Bristol-Myers Squibb)
Indications: HIV infection
Class: Antiretroviral, CYP1A2 inhibitor, CYP3A4 inducer, Non-nucleoside reverse transcriptase inhibitor
Half-life: 52–76 hours
Clinically important, potentially hazardous interactions with: alcohol, alprazolam, amprenavir, aripiprazole, artesunate, atazanavir, atorvastatin, atovaquone, avapritinib, benzodiazepines, bepridil, boceprevir, bortezomib, brentuximab vedotin, budesonide, buprenorphine, bupropion, carbamazepine, carvedilol, caspofungin, chlordiazepoxide, cisapride, citalopram, clarithromycin, clonazepam, clopidogrel, clorazepate, CNS depressants, cobimetinib, colchicine, conivaptan, crizotinib, cyclosporine, CYP2B6 inhibitors and inducers, CYP2C19 substrates, CYP2C9 substrates, CYP3A4 substrates and inducers, darunavir, dasatinib, deferasirox, deflazacort, diazepam, dihydroergotamine, diltiazem, doravirine, dronedarone, elbasvir & grazoprevir, enzalutamide, eplerenone, ergot, etravirine, everolimus, exemestane, fentanyl, finerenone, flurazepam, fosamprenavir, fosphenytoin, gefitinib, glecaprevir & pibrentasvir, grapefruit juice, guanfacine, halofantrine, hydroxyzine, ibrexafungerp, imatinib, indinavir, itraconazole, ixabepilone, lapatinib, lemborexant, levomepromazine, levonorgestrel, linagliptin, lopinavir, lorazepam, lovastatin, lumateperone, lurasidone, maraviroc, methadone, methysergide, midazolam, mifepristone, neratinib, nevirapine, nifedipine, nilotinib, nisoldipine, olaparib, ombitasvir/paritaprevir/ritonavir, ombitasvir/paritaprevir/ritonavir and dasabuvir, oral contraceptives, oxazepam, paclitaxel, palbociclib, pazopanib, phenytoin, pimecrolimus, pimozide, posaconazole, pravastatin, praziquantel, progestogens, propafenone, protease inhibitors, quazepam, raltegravir, ranolazine, rifabutin, rifampin, rilpivirine, ritonavir, rivaroxaban, roflumilast, romidepsin, salmeterol, saquinavir, saxagliptin, sertraline, simeprevir, simvastatin, sirolimus, sofosbuvir & velpatasvir, sofosbuvir/velpatasvir/voxilaprevir, sonidegib, sorafenib, SSRIs, St John's wort, sunitinib, tacrolimus, tadalafil, telaprevir, temazepam, ticagrelor, tipranavir, tocilizumab, tolvaptan, toremifene, triazolam, ulipristal, vandetanib, vemurafenib, venetoclax, vilazodone, vitamin K antagonists, voriconazole, warfarin, zuclopenthixol
Important contra-indications noted in the prescribing guidelines for: the elderly; nursing mothers; pediatric patients
Note: Atripla is efavirenz, emtricitabine and tenofovir disoproxil.

Skin
Cutaneous toxicity / skin toxicity [2]
DRESS syndrome (Drug-induced hypersensitivity syndrome) [2]
Eczema / eczematous reaction / eczematous eruption (<2%)
Erythema (11%)
Exanthems (27%) [3]
Exfoliative dermatitis (<2%)
Flushing / rubefaction (<2%)
Folliculitis (<2%)
Hot flashes / hot flushes (<2%)
Hypersensitivity [5]
Lipodystrophy / acquired generalized lipodystrophy [2]
Peripheral edema (<2%)
Photosensitivity [5]
Pruritus (itching) (11%)
Rash (26%) [16]
Stevens-Johnson syndrome and toxic epidermal necrolysis (SJS/TEN) [5]
Urticaria / hives (<2%)

Hair
Alopecia / hair loss (<2%)

Mucosal
Xerostomia (dry mouth) (<2%)

Cardiovascular
Thrombophlebitis (<2%)

Central Nervous System
Abnormal dreams (<3%) [9]
Aggression (includes anger) [2]
Anorexia (<2%)
Anxiety (13%) [4]
Depression (19%) [9]
Dysgeusia (taste perversion) (<2%)
Hallucinations [2]
Headache (2–8%) [3]
Impaired concentration (3–5%) [5]
Insomnia (7%) [4]
Nervousness (7%)
Neuropsychiatric / neuropsychological adverse effect [2]
Neurotoxicity [14]
Nightmares [3]
Pain (<13%)
Paresthesias (<2%)
Parosmia (<2%)
Psychosis [7]
Sleep-related disorder [2]
Somnolence (drowsiness) (2%) [3]
Suicidal ideation [5]
Tremor (<2%)
Vertigo / dizziness (2–9%) [15]

Endocrine/Metabolic
ALT increased [2]
Dyslipidemia [2]
Gynecomastia [15]

Gastrointestinal/Hepatic
Abdominal pain (2–3%)
Diarrhea (3–14%) [2]
Dyspepsia / functional dyspepsia (indigestion) (see also gastroparesis) (4%)
Hepatic failure [2]
Hepatotoxicity / liver injury / acute liver injury / drug-induced liver injury (DILI) [13]
Nausea (2–10%) [3]
Vomiting (3–6%)

Genitourinary
Urolithiasis / ureteral stones / urinary calculi [3]

Neuromuscular/Skeletal
Asthenia / fatigue (2–8%) [3]
Myalgia/Myopathy (<2%)

Other
Adverse effects / adverse reactions [10]
Teratogenicity [4]

EFINACONAZOLE

Trade name: Jublia (Valeant)
Indications: Onychomycosis
Class: Antifungal / antimycotic, Antifungal; triazole, Antimicrobial
Half-life: 30 hours
Clinically important, potentially hazardous interactions with: none known
Important contra-indications noted in the prescribing guidelines for: nursing mothers; pediatric patients

---

Nails
Onychocryptosis (ingrowing toe nail) (2%)

Local
Application-site dermatitis (2%)
Application-site reactions [5]
Application-site vesicles (2%)

EFLORNITHINE

Trade names: Iwilfin (US WorldMeds, LLC), Vaniqa (Women First)
Indications: Sleeping sickness, hypertrichosis
Class: Ornithine decarboxylase inhibitor
Half-life: 3–3.5 hours (intravenous); 8 hours (topical)
Clinically important, potentially hazardous interactions with: none known
Important contra-indications noted in the prescribing guidelines for: nursing mothers; pediatric patients
Note: Eflornithine hydrochloride.

Skin
Acneiform eruption / acneiform dermatitis / acneiform rash (24%)
Burning / skin burning sensation (4%)
Facial edema (3%)
Pruritus (itching) (4%) [2]
Rash (3%)
Stinging (8%)
Xerosis / xeroderma (2%)

Hair
Alopecia / hair loss (5–10%)
Ingrown (2%)
Pseudofolliculitis barbae (5–15%)

Central Nervous System
Headache (5%)
Paresthesias (4%)
Seizures (7%) [2]
Vertigo / dizziness (<10%)

Gastrointestinal/Hepatic
Diarrhea (<10%)
Vomiting (<10%)

Hematologic
Eosinophilia / eosinophils increased (<10%)

Otic
Hearing impairment (<10%)

ELAGOLIX SODIUM

Trade name: Orilissa (AbbVie)
Indications: indicated for the management of moderate to severe pain associated with endometriosis
Class: Gonadotropin-releasing hormone (GnRH) antagonist
Half-life: 4–6 hours
Clinically important, potentially hazardous interactions with: none known
Pregnancy category: Exposure early in pregnancy may increase the risk of early pregnancy loss.

Skin
Flushing / rubefaction (24–46%)
Rash (6%)

Central Nervous System
Anxiety (3–5%)
Depression (3–6%)
Headache (17–20%)
Insomnia (6–9%)
Irritability (<5%)
Mood changes (includes mood disorder) (5–6%)
Vertigo / dizziness (<5%)

Endocrine/Metabolic
Amenorrhea (4–7%)
Libido decreased (<5%)
Weight gain (<5%)

Gastrointestinal/Hepatic
Abdominal pain (<5%)
Constipation (<5%)
Diarrhea (<5%)
Nausea (11–16%)

Neuromuscular/Skeletal
Arthralgia (3–5%)

ELBASVIR & GRAZOPREVIR

Trade name: Zepatier (Merck)
Indications: Chronic hepatitis C virus genotypes 1 or 4 (with or without ribavirin)
Class: Direct-acting antiviral, Hepatitis C virus NS3/4A protease inhibitor (grazoprevir), Hepatitis C virus NS5A inhibitor (elbasvir)
Half-life: 24 hours (elbasvir); 31 hours (grazoprevir)
Clinically important, potentially hazardous interactions with: atazanavir, atorvastatin, bosentan, carbamazepine, cobicistat/elvitegravir/emtricitabine/tenofovir disoproxil, cyclosporine, darunavir, efavirenz, fluvastatin, ketoconazole, lopinavir, lovastatin, modafinil, moderate CYP3A inducers, nafcillin, OATP1B1/3 inhibitors, phenytoin, rifampin, rosuvastatin, saquinavir, simvastatin, strong CYP3A inducers, tacrolimus, tipranavir
Pregnancy category: No available data; contra-indicated in pregnant women and in men with pregnant partners when administered with ribavirin
Important contra-indications noted in the prescribing guidelines for: pediatric patients
Note: Contra-indicated in patients with moderate or severe hepatic impairment (Child-Pugh B or C).

Central Nervous System
Headache (10–11%) [10]

Gastrointestinal/Hepatic
Abdominal pain (2%)
Diarrhea (2%) [3]
Hepatotoxicity / liver injury / acute liver injury / drug-induced liver injury (DILI) [2]
Nausea (11%) [9]

Hematologic
Anemia [2]

Neuromuscular/Skeletal
Asthenia / fatigue (5–11%) [10]

Other
Adverse effects / adverse reactions [3]

ELETRIPTAN

Trade name: Relpax (Pfizer)
Indications: Migraine headaches
Class: 5-HT1 agonist, Serotonin receptor agonist, Triptan
Half-life: 4–5 hours
Clinically important, potentially hazardous interactions with: clarithromycin, dihydroergotamine, itraconazole, ketoconazole, methysergide, nefazodone, nelfinavir, paclitaxel, ritonavir, SNRIs, SSRIs, telithromycin, triptans, troleandomycin, voriconazole

Important contra-indications noted in the prescribing guidelines for: nursing mothers; pediatric patients
Note: Contra-indicated in patients with history, symptoms, or signs of ischemic cardiac, cerebrovascular, or peripheral vascular syndromes, or in patients with uncontrolled hypertension.

Skin
Flushing / rubefaction (2%)
Mucosal
Xerostomia (dry mouth) (2–4%)
Cardiovascular
Chest pain (<4%) [3]
Central Nervous System
Headache (3–4%)
Neurotoxicity [2]
Paresthesias (3–4%)
Somnolence (drowsiness) (3–7%) [2]
Vertigo / dizziness (3–7%)
Warm feeling (includes feeling hot) (2%)
Gastrointestinal/Hepatic
Abdominal pain (<2%)
Dyspepsia / functional dyspepsia (indigestion) (see also gastroparesis) (<2%)
Dysphagia (<2%)
Nausea (3–7%) [5]
Vomiting [2]
Neuromuscular/Skeletal
Asthenia / fatigue (4–10%) [4]
Other
Adverse effects / adverse reactions [2]

ELIGLUSTAT

Trade name: Cerdelga (Genzyme)
Indications: Gaucher disease
Class: Glucosylceramide synthase inhibitor
Half-life: 7–9 hours
Clinically important, potentially hazardous interactions with: carbamazepine, grapefruit juice, phenobarbital, phenytoin, rifampin, St John's wort, strong or moderate CYP2D6 inhibitors
Important contra-indications noted in the prescribing guidelines for: nursing mothers; pediatric patients

---

Skin
Rash (5%)
Mucosal
Oropharyngeal pain (10%)
Cardiovascular
Palpitation (5%) [3]
Central Nervous System
Headache (13–40%) [2]
Migraine (10%)
Vertigo / dizziness (8%)
Gastrointestinal/Hepatic
Abdominal pain (10%) [2]
Constipation (5%)
Diarrhea (12%) [2]
Dyspepsia / functional dyspepsia (indigestion) (see also gastroparesis) (7%)
Flatulence (10%)
Gastroesophageal reflux (7%)
Nausea (10–12%)
Neuromuscular/Skeletal
Asthenia / fatigue (8–14%)
Back pain (12%)
Pain in extremities (11%)
Respiratory
Cough (7%)
Other
Adverse effects / adverse reactions [2]

ELTROMBOPAG

Trade names: Promacta (Novartis), Revolade (Novartis)
Indications: Thrombocytopenic purpura, severe aplastic anemia in patients with insufficient response to immunosuppressive therapy
Class: Thrombopoietin receptor (TPO) agonist
Half-life: 21–32 hours
Clinically important, potentially hazardous interactions with: antacids, atorvastatin, dairy products, eluxadoline, lopinavir, mineral supplements, olmesartan, rosuvastatin, selenium, zinc
Important contra-indications noted in the prescribing guidelines for: nursing mothers; pediatric patients
Warning: RISK FOR HEPATIC DECOMPENSATION IN PATIENTS WITH CHRONIC HEPATITIS C

Skin
Peripheral edema (3–4%)
Pigmentation (Skin) (includes hyperpigmentation) [2]
Rash (3–7%)
Hair
Alopecia / hair loss (2%)
Mucosal
Oropharyngeal pain (4%)
Xerostomia (dry mouth) (2%)
Cardiovascular
Myocardial infarction [2]
Thromboembolism [5]
Venous thromboembolism [4]
Central Nervous System
Dysgeusia (taste perversion) (4%)
Fever (pyrexia) (includes hyperpyrexia) [2]
Headache (10–21%) [12]
Ischemic stroke / cerebral infarction (includes transient ischemic attack) [2]
Paresthesias (3%)
Endocrine/Metabolic
ALP increased (2%)
ALT increased (5–6%) [6]
AST increased (4%)
Hyperbilirubinemia [2]
Gastrointestinal/Hepatic
Abdominal pain [2]
Constipation [2]
Diarrhea (9%) [2]
Hepatic (liver) disorder / hepatobiliary disorder / hepatic (liver) dysfunction [3]
Hepatotoxicity / liver injury / acute liver injury / drug-induced liver injury (DILI) [5]
Nausea (4–9%) [5]
Vomiting (6%)
Genitourinary
Urinary tract infection (5%)
Hematologic
Bleeding [3]
Myelosuppression / bone marrow suppression / myelotoxicity [2]
Neutropenia (neutrophils decreased) [2]
Thrombocytopenia / platelets decreased [3]
Thrombosis [6]
Neuromuscular/Skeletal
Arthralgia (3%) [2]
Asthenia / fatigue (3–4%) [5]
Back pain (3%)
Myalgia/Myopathy (5%)
Pain in extremities (7%)
Ocular
Cataract (5%) [3]
Renal
Renal failure [3]
Respiratory
Cough (5%)
Nasopharyngitis [4]
Pharyngitis (sore throat) (4%)
Upper respiratory tract infection (7%) [3]
Other
Adverse effects / adverse reactions [8]

ELUXADOLINE

Trade name: Viberzi (Forest)
Indications: Irritable bowel syndrome with diarrhea
Class: Opioid mu receptor agonist
Half-life: 4–6 hours
Clinically important, potentially hazardous interactions with: alfentanil, alosetron, anticholinergics, atazanavir, bupropion, ciprofloxacin, clarithromycin, cyclosporine, dihydroergotamine, eltrombopag, ergotamine, fentanyl, fluconazole, gemfibrozil, lopinavir, opioids, paroxetine hydrochloride, paroxetine mesylate, pimozide, quinidine, rifampin, ritonavir, rosuvastatin, saquinavir, sirolimus, tacrolimus, tipranavir
Pregnancy category: Insufficient evidence to inform drug-associated risk
Important contra-indications noted in the prescribing guidelines for: pediatric patients
Note: Contra-indicated in patients with known or suspected biliary duct obstruction, or sphincter of Oddi disease or dysfunction; alcoholism, alcohol abuse, alcohol addiction, or drink more than 3 alcoholic beverages/day; a history of pancreatitis; structural diseases of the pancreas, including known or suspected pancreatic duct obstruction; severe hepatic impairment (Child-Pugh Class C); severe constipation or sequelae from constipation, or known or suspected mechanical gastrointestinal obstruction.

Skin
Rash (3%)
Central Nervous System
Euphoria / elation (<2%)
Sedation (<2%)
Somnolence (drowsiness) (<2%)
Vertigo / dizziness (3%) [2]
Endocrine/Metabolic
ALT increased (2–3%)
AST increased (<2%)
Gastrointestinal/Hepatic
Abdominal distension (3%) [2]
Abdominal pain (6–7%) [4]
Constipation (7–8%) [7]
Flatulence (3%)
Gastroenteritis (<3%) [2]
Gastroesophageal reflux (<2%)
Nausea (7–8%) [5]
Pancreatitis / acute pancreatitis [7]
Vomiting (4%) [3]

Respiratory
Asthma (<2%)
Bronchitis (3%)
Bronchospasm (<2%)
Nasopharyngitis (3–4%) [2]
Respiratory failure (<2%)
Wheezing (<2%)

Other
Adverse effects / adverse reactions [2]

EMAPALUMAB

Trade name: Gamifant (Novimmune)
Indications: Adult and pediatric (newborn and older) patients with primary hemophagocytic lymphohistiocytosis (HLH) with refractory, recurrent or progressive disease or intolerance with conventional HLH therapy
Class: Anti-interferon-gamma (IFNγ) monoclonal antibody, Covid-19 putative drug, Monoclonal antibody
Half-life: ~22 days
Clinically important, potentially hazardous interactions with: none known
Pregnancy category: There are no available data in pregnant women to inform a drug-associated risk of adverse developmental outcomes.
Important contra-indications noted in the prescribing guidelines for: nursing mothers
Note: Until more data become available, emapalumab should be used with caution during breastfeeding, especially while nursing a newborn or preterm infant.
Emapalumab-Lzsg is a biosimilar to Emapalumab.

Skin
Peripheral edema (<10%)
Rash (12%)

Mucosal
Epistaxis (nosebleed) (<10%)

Cardiovascular
Bradycardia / sinus bradycardia (<10%)
Hypertension (41%)
Tachycardia (12%)

Central Nervous System
Fever (pyrexia) (includes hyperpyrexia) (24%)
Irritability (12%)

Endocrine/Metabolic
Hypokalemia (15%)

Gastrointestinal/Hepatic
Abdominal pain (12%)
Constipation (15%)
Diarrhea (12%)
Gastrointestinal hemorrhage (fatal / 1 case) (<10%)
Vomiting (<10%)

Hematologic
Lymphocytosis / lymphocytes increased (12%)

Local
Infusion-related reactions (27%)

Neuromuscular/Skeletal
Asthenia / fatigue (<10%)

Renal
Nephrotoxicity / kidney injury / acute kidney injury (AKI) / drug-induced kidney injury (<10%)

Respiratory
Cough (12%)
Dyspnea / shortness of breath (<10%)
Tachypnea / respiratory rate increased (12%)

Other
Cytomegalovirus infection (12%)
Death (2 cases) (6%)
Infection (≥3% serious) (56%)

EMPAGLIFLOZIN

Trade names: Glyxambi (Boehringer Ingelheim), Jardiance (Boehringer Ingelheim), Synjardy (Boehringer Ingelheim)
Indications: Type II diabetes mellitus. Repurposed for the treatment of glycogen storage disease type Ib (GSD Ib)
Class: Antidiabetic, Sodium-glucose co-transporter 2 (SGLT2) inhibitor ('gliflozin')
Half-life: 12 hours
Clinically important, potentially hazardous interactions with: none known
Important contra-indications noted in the prescribing guidelines for: nursing mothers; pediatric patients
Note: Contra-indicated in patients with severe renal impairment, end stage renal disease, or on dialysis. Glyxambi is empagliflozin and linagliptin; Synjardy is empagliflozin and metformin.

Central Nervous System
Headache [2]
Vertigo / dizziness [2]

Endocrine/Metabolic
Diabetic ketoacidosis [5]
Euglycemic diabetic ketoacidosis [2]
Hypoglycemia [7]

Gastrointestinal/Hepatic
Constipation [2]
Pancreatitis / acute pancreatitis [6]

Genitourinary
Genital mycotic infection (2–6%) [13]
Genitourinary infection / genital infection / reproductive tract infection [2]
Pollakiuria [4]
Urinary frequency (3%)
Urinary tract infection (8–9%) [11]

Neuromuscular/Skeletal
Myalgia/Myopathy [2]

Respiratory
Nasopharyngitis [4]

Other
Adverse effects / adverse reactions [8]
Death [2]
Dipsia (thirst) / polydipsia (2%)

EMTRICITABINE

Trade names: Atripla (Gilead), Complera (Gilead), Descovy (Gilead), Emtriva (Gilead), Truvada (Gilead)
Indications: HIV-1 infection
Class: Antiretroviral, Nucleoside analog reverse transcriptase inhibitor
Half-life: ~10 hours
Clinically important, potentially hazardous interactions with: cobicistat/elvitegravir/emtricitabine/tenofovir disoproxil, ganciclovir, lamivudine, ribavirin, valganciclovir
Important contra-indications noted in the prescribing guidelines for: nursing mothers
Note: Emtricitabine is a fluorinated derivative of lamivudine. Atripla is emtricitabine, efavirenz and tenofovir disoproxil; Complera is emtricitabine, rilpivirine and tenofovir disoproxil; Descovy is emtricitabine and tenofovir alafenamide; Truvada is emtricitabine and tenofovir disoproxil. See also separate profiles for emtricitabine in combination with cobicistat, elvitegravir and tenofovir disoproxil or tenofovir alafenamide.
Warning: LACTIC ACIDOSIS / SEVERE HEPATOMEGALY WITH STEATOSIS and POST TREATMENT EXACERBATION OF HEPATITIS B

Skin
Exanthems (17%)
Pigmentation (Skin) (includes hyperpigmentation) (palms and soles) (32%)
Pruritus (itching) (17–30%)
Pustules / pustular eruption (17–30%)
Rash (17–30%) [6]
Urticaria / hives (17–30%)
Vesiculobullous eruption (17–30%)

Central Nervous System
Abnormal dreams (2–11%) [3]
Anxiety [2]
Depression (6–9%)
Fever (pyrexia) (includes hyperpyrexia) (18%)
Headache (13–22%) [6]
Insomnia (7–16%)
Neurotoxicity [5]
Paresthesias (6%)
Peripheral neuropathy (4%)
Somnolence (drowsiness) [2]
Vertigo / dizziness (4–25%) [4]

Gastrointestinal/Hepatic
Abdominal pain (8–14%) [2]
Diarrhea (20–23%) [6]
Dyspepsia / functional dyspepsia (indigestion) (see also gastroparesis) (4–8%)
Gastroenteritis (11%)
Hepatic failure [2]
Hepatotoxicity / liver injury / acute liver injury / drug-induced liver injury (DILI) [2]
Nausea (13–18%) [7]
Vomiting (9–23%) [4]

Hematologic
Anemia (7%)
Pure red cell aplasia [2]

Neuromuscular/Skeletal
Arthralgia (3–5%)
Asthenia / fatigue (12–16%) [4]
Myalgia/Myopathy (4–6%) [2]

Otic
Otitis (otitis externa, otitis media, otitis interna) (23%)

Respiratory
Cough (14–28%)
Pneumonia (15%)
Rhinitis / rhinosinusitis (see also sinusitis) (12–20%)

Other
Adverse effects / adverse reactions [5]
Allergic reactions (17–30%)
Infection (44%)

EMTRICITABINE/ RILPIVIRINE/ TENOFOVIR ALAFENAMIDE

Trade name: Odefsey (Gilead)
Indications: HIV-1 infection
Class: Hepatitis B virus necleoside analog reverse transcriptase inhibitor (tenofovir alafenamide), Non-nucleoside reverse transcriptase inhibitor (rilpivirine), Nucleoside analog reverse transcriptase inhibitor (emtricitabine)
Half-life: 10 hours (emtricitabine); 50 hours (rilpivirine); <1 hour (tenofovir alafenamide)
Clinically important, potentially hazardous interactions with: carbamazepine, dexamethasone, dexlansoprazole, esomeprazole, lansoprazole, omeprazole, oxcarbazepine, pantoprazole, phenobarbital, phenytoin, rabeprazole, rifampin, rifapentine, St John's wort
Pregnancy category: Insufficient evidence to inform drug-associated risk
Important contra-indications noted in the prescribing guidelines for: nursing mothers; pediatric patients
Warning: LACTIC ACIDOSIS/SEVERE HEPATOMEGALY WITH STEATOSIS and POST TREATMENT ACUTE EXACERBATION OF HEPATITIS B

Central Nervous System
Depression (<2%)
Headache (<2%)
Insomnia (<2%)

ENALAPRIL

Trade names: Innovace (Merck Sharpe & Dohme), Lexxel (AstraZeneca), Teczem (Sanofi-Aventis), Vaseretic (Valeant), Vasotec (Valeant)
Indications: Hypertension, symptomatic congestive heart failure, asymptomatic left ventricular dysfunction
Class: Angiotensin-converting enzyme (ACE) inhibitor, Antihypertensive, Vasodilator
Half-life: 11 hours
Clinically important, potentially hazardous interactions with: alcohol, aldesleukin, allopurinol, alpha blockers, alprostadil, amifostine, amiloride, angiotensin II receptor antagonists, antacids, antidiabetics, antihypertensives, antipsychotics, anxiolytics and hypnotics, aprotinin, azathioprine, baclofen, beta blockers, calcium channel blockers, clonidine, conivaptan, corticosteroids, cyclosporine, CYP3A4 inducers, deferasirox, diazoxide, diuretics, eplerenone, estrogens, everolimus, general anesthetics, gold & gold compounds, grapefruit juice, heparins, hydralazine, hypotensives, insulin, levodopa, lithium, MAO inhibitors, metformin, methyldopa, methylphenidate, minoxidil, moxisylyte, moxonidine, nitrates, nitroprusside, NSAIDs, pentoxifylline, phosphodiesterase 5 inhibitors, potassium salts, prostacyclin analogues, quinine, rituximab, salicylates, sirolimus, spironolactone, sulfonylureas, tadalafil, temsirolimus, tizanidine, tolvaptan, triamterene, trimethoprim
Pregnancy category: category C in first trimester; category D in second and third trimesters
Important contra-indications noted in the prescribing guidelines for: nursing mothers
Note: Lexxel is enalapril and felodipine; Teczem is enalapril and diltiazem; Vaseretic is enalapril and hydrochlorothiazide. Hydrochlorothiazide is a sulfonamide and can be absorbed systemically. Sulfonamides can produce severe, possibly fatal, reactions such as toxic epidermal necrolysis and Stevens-Johnson syndrome.
Contra-indicated in patients with a history of angioedema with or without previous ACE inhibitor treatment.
Warning: FETAL TOXICITY

Skin
Angioedema (formerly named angioneurotic edema) [76]
Bullous pemphigoid / pemphigoid [2]
Exanthems [9]
Flushing / rubefaction [4]
Lichenoid eruption / lichenoid reaction [2]
Lupus erythematosus (subacute cutaneous lupus erythematosus (SCLE)) [2]
Pemphigus [11]
Pemphigus foliaceus [2]
Peripheral edema [2]
Photosensitivity [2]
Pruritus (itching) [3]
Psoriasis [3]
Rash [5]
Urticaria / hives [5]
Vasculitis (angiitis) / cutaneous vasculitis (angiitis) [2]

Mucosal
Burning Mouth Syndrome / glossodynia / glossalgia / glossopyrosis (also includes stomatodynia / oral dysesthesia / stomatopyrosis) [2]
Oral lesions [4]
Oral ulceration [2]
Tongue edema [4]

Cardiovascular
Hypotension [2]

Central Nervous System
Ageusia (taste loss) / taste disorder [4]
Dysgeusia (taste perversion) (<10%) [7]
Headache (5%)
Vertigo / dizziness (4–8%) [2]

Endocrine/Metabolic
Hyperkalemia [4]
SIADH [3]

Gastrointestinal/Hepatic
Hepatotoxicity / liver injury / acute liver injury / drug-induced liver injury (DILI) [3]
Intestinal angioedema [3]
Pancreatitis / acute pancreatitis [2]

Neuromuscular/Skeletal
Asthenia / fatigue (<3%)
Pseudopolymyalgia [2]

Renal
Nephrotoxicity / kidney injury / acute kidney injury (AKI) / drug-induced kidney injury [2]

Respiratory
Cough (8–23%) [41]

Other
Adverse effects / adverse reactions [9]
Death [4]

ENCORAFENIB

Trade name: Braftovi (Array Biopharma Inc)
Indications: in combination with binimetinib, for the treatment of patients with unresectable or metastatic melanoma with a BRAF V600E or V600K mutation
Class: BRAF inhibitor, Kinase inhibitor
Half-life: 3.5 hours
Clinically important, potentially hazardous interactions with: none known
Pregnancy category: can cause fetal harm
Important contra-indications noted in the prescribing guidelines for: nursing mothers

---

Skin
Acneiform eruption / acneiform dermatitis / acneiform rash (3–8%)
Erythema (7–16%)
Hand–foot syndrome (palmar–plantar erythrodysesthesia) (7–51%) [3]
Hyperkeratosis (23–57%)
Nevi (naevi) [3]
Panniculitis (<10%)
Pruritus (itching) (13–31%)
Rash (22–41%)
Xerosis / xeroderma (16–38%)

Hair
Alopecia / hair loss (14–56%)

Central Nervous System
Dysgeusia (taste perversion) (6–13%)
Fever (pyrexia) (includes hyperpyrexia) (18%)
Headache (22%)
Paresis (<10%)
Peripheral neuropathy (12%)
Vertigo / dizziness (15%)

Endocrine/Metabolic
ALP increased (21%)
ALT increased (29%)
AST increased (27%)
Creatine phosphokinase (CPK) / creatine kinase increased (hyperCKemia) [2]
GGT increased (45%)
Hyperglycemia (includes glucose increased) (28%)
Hypermagnesemia (10%)
Hyponatremia (18%)
Serum creatinine increased (93%)

Gastrointestinal/Hepatic
Abdominal pain (28%)
Constipation (22%)
Nausea (41%)
Pancreatitis / acute pancreatitis (<10%)
Vomiting (30%)

Hematologic
Anemia (36%)
Hemorrhage (19%)
Leukocytopenia (leukopenia) / leukocytes (white blood cells) decreased (13%)
Lymphopenia (lymphocytopenia) / lymphocytes decreased (13%)
Neutropenia (neutrophils decreased) (13%)

Neuromuscular/Skeletal
Arthralgia (26–44%)
Asthenia / fatigue (43%)
Back pain (9–15%)
Myalgia/Myopathy (23–33%) [2]
Pain in extremities (11%)

ENFLURANE

Trade name: Ethrane (Baxter)
Indications: Maintenance of general anesthesia
Class: Anesthetic; inhalation
Half-life: N/A
Clinically important, potentially hazardous interactions with: cisatracurium, doxacurium, mivacurium, pancuronium, rapacuronium

---

Cardiovascular
Arrhythmias [3]
Myocardial ischemia [2]

Central Nervous System
Headache [2]
Seizures [15]

Neuromuscular/Skeletal
Rhabdomyolysis [2]

Other
Death [3]

ENFUVIRTIDE

Trade name: Fuzeon (Roche)
Indications: HIV-1 infection (in combination with other antiretroviral agents)
Class: Antiretroviral, HIV cell fusion inhibitor
Half-life: 3.8 hours
Clinically important, potentially hazardous interactions with: darunavir, indinavir, tipranavir
Important contra-indications noted in the prescribing guidelines for: the elderly; nursing mothers

---

Skin
Folliculitis (2%)
Herpes simplex (4%)
Hypersensitivity [3]
Papillomas (4%)
Pruritus (itching) (62%)

Mucosal
Xerostomia (dry mouth) (2%)

Central Nervous System
Anorexia (2%)
Depression (9%)

Endocrine/Metabolic
ALT increased (<4%)
Appetite decreased (3%)
Creatine phosphokinase (CPK) / creatine kinase increased (hyperCKemia) (3–7%)
Weight loss (7%)

Gastrointestinal/Hepatic
Abdominal pain (4%)
Pancreatitis / acute pancreatitis (3%)

Hematologic
Eosinophilia / eosinophils increased (2–9%)

Local
Injection-site bruising (52%)
Injection-site erythema (91%)
Injection-site induration (90%)
Injection-site nodules (80%) [4]
Injection-site pain (96%)
Injection-site pruritus (65%)
Injection-site reaction (98%) [27]
Injection-site scleroderma [2]

Neuromuscular/Skeletal
Asthenia / fatigue (16%) [2]
Myalgia/Myopathy (3%)
Pain in extremities (3%)

Ocular
Conjunctivitis (conjunctival inflammation) (2%)

Respiratory
Cough (4%)
Influenza- ('flu)-like syndrome (2%)
Pneumonia (3%)
Sinusitis (see also rhinitis / rhinosinusitis) (6%)

Other
Infection [3]

ENOXACIN

Trade name: Penetrex (Sanofi-Aventis)
Indications: Urinary tract infections
Class: Antibiotic, Antibiotic; fluoroquinolone, Antimicrobial
Half-life: 3–6 hours
Clinically important, potentially hazardous interactions with: amiodarone, arsenic, bepridil, bretylium, disopyramide, duloxetine, erythromycin, fenbufen, oxtriphylline, phenothiazines, procainamide, quinidine, roflumilast, sotalol, tricyclic antidepressants
Important contra-indications noted in the prescribing guidelines for: nursing mothers; pediatric patients
Note: Fluoroquinolones are associated with an increased risk of tendinitis and tendon rupture in all ages. This risk is further increased in older patients usually over 60 years of age, in patients taking corticosteroid drugs, and in patients with kidney, heart or lung transplants.
Fluoroquinolones may exacerbate muscle weakness in persons with myasthenia gravis.

Skin
Photosensitivity [5]
Phototoxicity [5]

Other
Adverse effects / adverse reactions [2]

ENOXAPARIN

Trade names: Clexane (Sanofi-Aventis), Lovenox (Sanofi-Aventis)
Indications: Prevention of deep vein thrombosis, ischemic complications of unstable angina and non-Q wave myocardial infarction, treatment of acute ST-segment elevation myocardial infarction
Class: Heparin, low molecular weight
Half-life: 4.5 hours
Clinically important, potentially hazardous interactions with: ACE inhibitors, angiotensin II receptor antagonists, anticoagulants, aspirin, butabarbital, clopidogrel, danaparoid, diclofenac, dipyridamole, drotrecogin alfa, iloprost, infused nitrates, ketorolac, NSAIDs, platelet inhibitors, rivaroxaban, salicylates, sulfinpyrazone
Important contra-indications noted in the prescribing guidelines for: nursing mothers; pediatric patients
Note: Epidural or spinal hematomas may occur in patients who are anticoagulated with low molecular weight heparins or heparinoids and are receiving neuraxial anesthesia or undergoing spinal puncture.
Contra-indicated in patients with active major bleeding; thrombocytopenia with a positive *in vitro* test for anti-platelet antibody in the presence of enoxaparin; hypersensitivity to heparin or pork products; hypersensitivity to benzyl alcohol (multi-dose formulation only).
Warning: SPINAL/EPIDURAL HEMATOMA

Skin
Anaphylactoid reactions / anaphylaxis (includes anaphylactic shock) [3]
Angioedema (formerly named angioneurotic edema) [2]
Bruise / bruising / contusion / ecchymosis (ecchymoses) (2%)
Bullous hemorrhagic dermatosis / hemorrhagic bullae [10]
DRESS syndrome (Drug-induced hypersensitivity syndrome) [2]
Edema / fluid retention (3%)
Erythema (<10%) [2]
Exanthems [2]
Hematoma / cutaneous hematoma [11]
Hypersensitivity [7]
Necrosis (skin necrosis) [6]
Peripheral edema (3%)
Pruritus (itching) [2]
Purpura (<10%)

Cardiovascular
Venous thromboembolism [2]

Endocrine/Metabolic
ALT increased [4]
AST increased [3]

Gastrointestinal/Hepatic
Hepatotoxicity / liver injury / acute liver injury / drug-induced liver injury (DILI) [6]

Genitourinary
Hematuria [3]

Hematologic
Bleeding [9]
Hemorrhage [4]
Thrombocythemia (thrombocytosis) / platelets increased [7]
Thrombocytopenia / platelets decreased [7]

Local
Injection-site necrosis [4]
Injection-site plaques [2]

Other
Adverse effects / adverse reactions [5]
Death [2]

ENTACAPONE

Trade names: Comtan (Orion), Comtess (Orion), Stalevo (Orion)
Indications: Parkinsonism
Class: Catechol-O-methyl transferase inhibitor
Half-life: 2.4 hours
Clinically important, potentially hazardous interactions with: amitriptyline, MAO inhibitors, paroxetine hydrochloride, phenelzine, rasagiline, tranylcypromine, venlafaxine
Important contra-indications noted in the prescribing guidelines for: nursing mothers; pediatric patients

---

Skin
Diaphoresis (2%)
Purpura (2%)

Mucosal
Xerostomia (dry mouth) (3%)

Central Nervous System
Anxiety (2%)
Dyskinesia (25%) [3]
Hyperactivity (10%)

Hypokinesia (9%)
Parkinsonism (17%)
Somnolence (drowsiness) (2%)
Vertigo / dizziness (8%) [2]

Gastrointestinal/Hepatic
Abdominal pain (8%)
Constipation (6%)
Diarrhea (10%) [3]
Dyspepsia / functional dyspepsia (indigestion) (see also gastroparesis) (2%)
Flatulence (2%)
Nausea (14%) [3]
Vomiting (4%)

Genitourinary
Melanuria (10%) [2]

Neuromuscular/Skeletal
Asthenia / fatigue (8%)
Back pain (4%)

Respiratory
Dyspnea / shortness of breath (3%)

ENTECAVIR

Trade name: Baraclude (Bristol-Myers Squibb)
Indications: Chronic hepatitis B virus infection
Class: Antiviral, Guanosine nucleoside analog
Half-life: ~24 hours
Clinically important, potentially hazardous interactions with: none known
Important contra-indications noted in the prescribing guidelines for: nursing mothers; pediatric patients
Warning: SEVERE ACUTE EXACERBATIONS OF HEPATITIS B, PATIENTS CO-INFECTED WITH HIV AND HBV, and LACTIC ACIDOSIS AND HEPATOMEGALY

Skin
Rash [2]

Hair
Alopecia / hair loss [2]

Central Nervous System
Headache (2–4%) [4]
Neurotoxicity [3]
Peripheral neuropathy [2]
Vertigo / dizziness [2]

Endocrine/Metabolic
Acidosis (includes lactic acidosis) [6]
ALT increased (2–12%) [2]
Creatine phosphokinase (CPK) / creatine kinase increased (hyperCKemia) (<2%)
Hypophosphatemia [2]

Gastrointestinal/Hepatic
Abdominal pain [3]
Diarrhea [2]
Nausea [2]
Pancreatitis / acute pancreatitis [3]

Genitourinary
Hematuria (9%)

Neuromuscular/Skeletal
Asthenia / fatigue (<3%) [7]
Myalgia/Myopathy [3]

Respiratory
Cough [2]
Upper respiratory tract infection [2]

Other
Adverse effects / adverse reactions [4]

ENTRECTINIB

Trade name: Rozlytrek (Genentech)
Indications: Treatment of adult patients with metastatic non-small cell lung cancer whose tumors are ROS1-positive.
Treatment of adult and pediatric patients 12 years of age and older with solid tumors that have a neurotrophic tyrosine receptor kinase gene fusion without a known acquired resistance mutation.
Treatment of solid tumors that are metastatic or have progressed following treatment or have no satisfactory alternative therapy.

Class: Anaplastic lymphoma kinase (ALK) inhibitor, Kinase inhibitor, Tropomyosin receptor kinase inhibitor
Half-life: 20 hours; 40 hours (major metabolite)
Clinically important, potentially hazardous interactions with: moderate and strong CYP3A inducers, moderate and strong CYP3A inhibitors
Pregnancy category: Can cause fetal harm. Advise females of reproductive potential of the potential risk to a fetus and use of effective contraception. Advise not to breastfeed.
Important contra-indications noted in the prescribing guidelines for: nursing mothers

---

Skin
Edema / fluid retention (1% ≥ grade 3) (40%)
Rash (<1% ≥ grade 3) (18%)

Cardiovascular
Congestive heart failure (3%)
Hypotension (3% ≥ grade 3) (18%)
QT interval prolonged / QT prolongation (3%)

Central Nervous System
Cognitive impairment (5% ≥ grade 3) (27%)
Dysesthesia (<1% ≥ grade 3) (34%)
Dysgeusia (taste perversion) (<1% ≥ grade 3) (44%)
Fall (8%)
Fever (pyrexia) (includes hyperpyrexia) (1% ≥ grade 3) (21%)
Headache (<1% ≥ grade 3) (18%)
Mood changes (includes mood disorder) (<1% ≥ grade 3) (10%)
Peripheral neuropathy (1% ≥ grade 3) (18%)
Sleep-related disorder (<1% ≥ grade 3) (14%)
Syncope / fainting (4%)
Vertigo / dizziness (<1% ≥ grade 3) (38%)

Endocrine/Metabolic
ALP increased (1% grade 3 or 4) (25%)
ALT increased (3& grade 3 or 4) (38%)
Appetite decreased (<1% ≥ grade 3) (13%)
AST increased (3% grade 3 or 4) (44%)
Dehydration (1% ≥ grade 3) (10%)
Hyperamylasemia (5% grade 3 or 4) (26%)
Hyperkalemia (2% grade 3 or 4) (25%)
Hyperlipasemia (10% grade 3 or 4) (28%)
Hypernatremia (1% grade 3 or 4) (35%)
Hyperuricemia (10% grade 3 or 4) (52%)
Hypoalbuminemia / albumin decreased (3% grade 3 or 4) (28%)
Hypocalcemia (2% grade 3 or 4) (34%)
Hypophosphatemia (7% grade 3 or 4) (30%)
Serum creatinine increased (2% grade 3 or 4) (73%)
Weight gain (7% ≥ grade 3) (25%)

Gastrointestinal/Hepatic
Abdominal pain (1% ≥ grade 3) (16%)
Constipation (1% ≥ grade 3) (46%)
Diarrhea (2% ≥ grade 3) (35%)
Dysphagia (10%)
Nausea (<1% ≥ grade 3) (34%)
Vomiting (1% ≥ grade 3) (24%)

Genitourinary
Urinary tract infection (2% ≥ grade 3) (13%)

Hematologic
Anemia (9% grade 3 or 4) (67%)
Lymphopenia (lymphocytopenia) / lymphocytes decreased (12% grade 3 or 4) (40%)
Neutropenia (neutrophils decreased) (7% grade 3 or 4) (28%)

Neuromuscular/Skeletal
Arthralgia (<1% ≥ grade 3) (21%)
Asthenia / fatigue (48%)
Ataxia (<1% ≥ grade 3) (17%)
Back pain (1% ≥ grade 3) (12%)
Fractures (6%)
Muscle weakness (<1% ≥ grade 3) (12%)
Myalgia/Myopathy (1% ≥ grade 3) (28%)
Pain in extremities (<1% ≥ grade 3) (11%)

Ocular
Vision disorders (<1% ≥ grade 3) (21%)

Respiratory
Cough (<1% ≥ grade 3) (24%)
Dyspnea / shortness of breath (6% ≥ grade 3) (30%)
Hypoxia (4%)
Pleural effusion (8%)
Pneumonia (serious) (4%)
Pulmonary embolism (4%)
Respiratory tract infection (6% ≥ grade 3) (10%)

ENZALUTAMIDE

Trade name: Xtandi (Medivation)
Indications: Metastatic castration-resistant prostate cancer in patients who have previously received docetaxel
Class: Androgen antagonist
Half-life: 8–9 days
Clinically important, potentially hazardous interactions with: alfentanil, bosentan, carbamazepine, copanlisib, cyclosporine, dihydroergotamine, doravirine, doravirine/lamiduvine/tenofovir disoproxil, efavirenz, ergotamine, fentanyl, fostemsavir, gemfibrozil, itraconazole, midazolam, midostaurin, modafinil, nafcillin, neratinib, omeprazole, phenobarbital, phenytoin, pimozide, quinidine, rifabutin, rifampin, rifapentine, sirolimus, St John's wort, tacrolimus, warfarin
Pregnancy category: not indicated for use in women
Important contra-indications noted in the prescribing guidelines for: nursing mothers; pediatric patients

---

Skin
Hot flashes / hot flushes (20%) [11]
Peripheral edema (15%) [3]
Pruritus (itching) (4%)
Xerosis / xeroderma (4%)

Mucosal
Epistaxis (nosebleed) (3%)
Cardiovascular
Cardiotoxicity [2]
Congestive heart failure [3]
Hypertension (6%) [5]
Central Nervous System
Amnesia (>2%)
Anxiety (7%)
Cognitive impairment (4%)
Gait instability / postural instability [3]
Hallucinations (2%)
Headache (12%) [4]
Hypoesthesia / hypesthesia (numbness) (4%)
Insomnia (9%)
Paresthesias (7%) [2]
Seizures [13]
Spinal cord compression (7%)
Vertigo / dizziness (10%) [2]
Endocrine/Metabolic
ALT increased (10%)
Appetite decreased [8]
Gynecomastia [2]
Weight loss [3]
Gastrointestinal/Hepatic
Constipation [5]
Diarrhea (22%) [10]
Hepatotoxicity / liver injury / acute liver injury / drug-induced liver injury (DILI) [2]
Nausea [6]
Vomiting [2]
Genitourinary
Hematuria (7%) [2]
Pollakiuria (5%)
Urinary tract infection [2]
Hematologic
Anemia [3]
Neutropenia (neutrophils decreased) (15%)
Thrombocytopenia / platelets decreased [2]
Neuromuscular/Skeletal
Arthralgia (21%) [5]
Asthenia / fatigue (51%) [29]
Back pain (26%) [6]
Bone pain / joint pain (15%) [8]
Fractures (4%) [2]
Respiratory
Bronchitis (>2%)
Dyspnea / shortness of breath [2]
Laryngitis (>2%)
Nasopharyngitis (>2%)
Pharyngitis (sore throat) (>2%)
Pneumonia (>2%)
Sinusitis (see also rhinitis / rhinosinusitis) (>2%)
Upper respiratory tract infection (11%) [3]
Other
Adverse effects / adverse reactions [8]
Death [3]

EPHEDRA

Family: Gnetaceae
Scientific names: *Ephedra equisetina, Ephedra intermedia, Ephedra sinica, Ephedra vulgaris*
Indications: Bronchospasm, asthma, bronchitis, allergy, appetite suppressant, colds, flu, fever, chills, edema, headache, anhidrosis, diuretic, joint and bone pain
Class: Ephedrine alkaloid, Stimulant
Half-life: N/A
Clinically important, potentially hazardous interactions with: acetazolamide, amitriptyline, caffeine, clevidipine, cocoa, corticosteroids, guanethidine, guarana, MAO inhibitors, phenelzine, selegiline, sibutramine, sodium bicarbonate
Note: Banned in the USA.

Cardiovascular
Cardiotoxicity [2]
Hypertension [4]
Palpitation [2]
Tachycardia [3]
Central Nervous System
Seizures [7]
Other
Adverse effects / adverse reactions [4]
Death [5]
Side effects [2]

EPHEDRINE

Trade names: Rynatuss (MedPointe), Vicks Vatronol (Procter & Gamble)
Indications: Nasal congestion, acute hypotensive states, asthma
Class: Adrenergic alpha-receptor agonist, Sympathomimetic
Half-life: 3–6 hours
Clinically important, potentially hazardous interactions with: antihypertensives, dexamethasone, furazolidone, guanethidine, iobenguane, levomepromazine, MAO inhibitors, methyldopa, oxprenolol, phenelzine, phenylpropanolamine, selegiline, tranylcypromine, tricyclic antidepressants
Important contra-indications noted in the prescribing guidelines for: nursing mothers

Skin
Dermatitis [5]
Diaphoresis (<10%)
Fixed eruption / fixed drug eruption [6]
Pallor (<10%)
Urticaria / hives [2]
Mucosal
Xerostomia (dry mouth) (<10%)
Central Nervous System
Trembling (<10%)
Tremor (<10%)

EPINASTINE

Synonym: relastat
Trade name: Elestat (Allergan)
Indications: Allergic conjunctivitis
Class: Histamine H1 receptor antagonist
Half-life: 12 hours
Clinically important, potentially hazardous interactions with: none known

Central Nervous System
Headache (~10%)
Ocular
Ocular burning (<10%)
Ocular hemorrhage (<10%)
Respiratory
Cough (<3%)
Rhinitis / rhinosinusitis (see also sinusitis) (~10%)
Sinusitis (see also rhinitis / rhinosinusitis) (~10%)
Upper respiratory tract infection (~10%)

EPINEPHRINE

Synonym: adrenaline
Trade names: Adrenaclick (Amedra), Adrenalin (JHP Pharmaceuticals), Auvi-Q (Sanofi-Aventis), Epipen (Mylan)
Indications: Cardiac arrest, hay fever, asthma, anaphylaxis
Class: Catecholamine, Sympathomimetic
Half-life: N/A
Clinically important, potentially hazardous interactions with: albuterol, alpha blockers, amitriptyline, amoxapine, atenolol, beta blockers, carteolol, chlorpromazine, clomipramine, clozapine, cocaine, desipramine, doxepin, ergotamine, furazolidone, halothane, imipramine, insulin aspart, insulin degludec, insulin detemir, insulin glargine, insulin glulisine, levalbuterol, lisdexamfetamine, lurasidone, MAO inhibitors, metoprolol, milnacipran, nadolol, nortriptyline, oxprenolol, penbutolol, phenelzine, phenoxybenzamine, phenylephrine, pindolol, prazosin, propranolol, protriptyline, sympathomimetics, terbutaline, thioridazine, timolol, tranylcypromine, tricyclic antidepressants, trimipramine, vasopressors
Important contra-indications noted in the prescribing guidelines for: the elderly

Skin
Dermatitis [4]
Diaphoresis (<10%) [2]
Flushing / rubefaction (<10%)
Necrosis (skin necrosis) [3]
Pemphigus (cicatricial) [2]
Cardiovascular
Arrhythmias [3]
Chest pain [2]
Hypertension [3]
Hypotension [4]
Myocardial infarction [5]
Palpitation [3]
QT interval prolonged / QT prolongation [2]
Ventricular tachycardia [2]
Central Nervous System
Anxiety [2]
Trembling (<10%)
Tremor [3]
Gastrointestinal/Hepatic
Nausea [2]

EPIRUBICIN

Trade name: Ellence (Pfizer)
Indications: Adjuvant therapy in primary breast cancer
Class: Antibiotic, Antibiotic; anthracycline, Antimicrobial
Half-life: 33 hours
Clinically important, potentially hazardous interactions with: amlodipine, bepridil, cimetidine, diltiazem, felodipine, isradipine, nicardipine, nifedipine, nimodipine, nisoldipine, verapamil
Important contra-indications noted in the prescribing guidelines for: nursing mothers
Warning: SEVERE OR LIFE-THREATENING HEMATOLOGICAL AND OTHER ADVERSE REACTIONS

Skin
Erythroderma (5%)
Hand–foot syndrome (palmar–plantar erythrodysesthesia) [5]
Hot flashes / hot flushes (5–39%)
Pruritus (itching) (9%)
Rash (<9%) [2]
Vasculitis (angiitis) / cutaneous vasculitis (angiitis) [2]

Hair
Alopecia / hair loss (69–95%) [19]

Mucosal
Mucositis [5]
Stomatitis (oral mucositis) [9]

Cardiovascular
Cardiotoxicity [3]
QT interval prolonged / QT prolongation [3]

Central Nervous System
Anorexia [5]
Dysgeusia (taste perversion) [2]
Fever (pyrexia) (includes hyperpyrexia) [2]
Headache [2]
Neurotoxicity [2]
Peripheral neuropathy [4]

Endocrine/Metabolic
ALT increased [2]
Amenorrhea [2]
AST increased [2]

Gastrointestinal/Hepatic
Abdominal pain [2]
Constipation [3]
Diarrhea [7]
Hepatotoxicity / liver injury / acute liver injury / drug-induced liver injury (DILI) [2]
Nausea [13]
Vomiting [11]

Hematologic
Anemia [9]
Febrile neutropenia [5]
Leukocytopenia (leukopenia) / leukocytes (white blood cells) decreased [4]
Neutropenia (neutrophils decreased) [13]
Thrombocytopenia / platelets decreased [5]

Local
Injection-site reaction (3–20%)

Neuromuscular/Skeletal
Arthralgia [2]
Asthenia / fatigue (6%) [9]
Myalgia/Myopathy (55%) [5]

Other
Allergic reactions [2]

EPLERENONE

Trade name: Inspra (Pfizer)
Indications: Hypertension
Class: Aldosterone antagonist / mineralocorticoid receptor antagonist (MRA), Diuretic
Half-life: 4–6 hours
Clinically important, potentially hazardous interactions with: ACE inhibitors, angiotensin II receptor antagonist, aprepitant, benazepril, captopril, conivaptan, darunavir, delavirdine, efavirenz, enalapril, erythromycin, fluconazole, grapefruit juice, indinavir, irbesartan, itraconazole, ketoconazole, lapatinib, lisinopril, meloxicam, nelfinavir, olmesartan, quinapril, ramipril, saquinavir, St John's wort, telithromycin, tipranavir, trimethoprim, verapamil, voriconazole

---

Central Nervous System
Vertigo / dizziness (3%)

Endocrine/Metabolic
Hyperkalemia [4]

Neuromuscular/Skeletal
Asthenia / fatigue (2%)

Respiratory
Cough (2%)
Influenza- ('flu)-like syndrome (2%)

EPOETIN ALFA

Synonyms: erythropoietin; EPO
Trade names: Epogen (Amgen), Eprex (Janssen-Cilag), Procrit (Ortho)
Indications: Anemia
Class: Erythropoiesis-stimulating agent (ESA), Erythropoietin
Half-life: 4–13 hours (in patients with chronic renal failure)
Clinically important, potentially hazardous interactions with: none known
Important contra-indications noted in the prescribing guidelines for: nursing mothers
Note: Epoetin alfa-epbx (Retacrit) is biosimilar to Epoetin alfa (Epogen/Procrit). Approved 05/15/2018.
Warning: ERYTHROPOIESIS-STIMULATING AGENTS (ESAs) INCREASE THE RISK OF DEATH, MYOCARDIAL INFARCTION, STROKE, VENOUS THROMBOEMBOLISM, THROMBOSIS OF VASCULAR ACCESS AND TUMOR PROGRESSION OR RECURRENCE

Skin
Angioedema (formerly named angioneurotic edema) (<5%)
Edema / fluid retention (17%)
Pruritus (itching) (12–21%) [2]
Rash (2–19%)

Cardiovascular
Hypertension (3–28%)

Central Nervous System
Fever (pyrexia) (includes hyperpyrexia) (10–42%) [2]
Hallucinations, visual [2]
Headache (5–18%)
Paresthesias (11%)

Gastrointestinal/Hepatic
Constipation [2]
Nausea (35–56%)

Hematologic
Thrombocytopenia / platelets decreased [2]

Local
Injection-site reaction (7%)

Neuromuscular/Skeletal
Arthralgia (10–16%)

Respiratory
Cough (4–26%)
Dyspnea / shortness of breath [2]

EPOPROSTENOL

Trade names: Flolan (GSK), Veletri (Actelion)
Indications: Pulmonary arterial hypertension
Class: Vasodilator, peripheral
Half-life: 6 minutes
Clinically important, potentially hazardous interactions with: anticoagulants, antihypertensives, diuretics, vasodilators
Important contra-indications noted in the prescribing guidelines for: the elderly; nursing mothers; pediatric patients
Note: Contra-indicated in patients with heart failure induced by reduced left ventricular ejection fraction.

Skin
Diaphoresis (41%)
Flushing / rubefaction [6]
Pruritus (itching) (4%)
Rash (10%) [3]

Cardiovascular
Bradycardia / sinus bradycardia (5%) [2]
Cardiac failure (31%)
Chest pain (11%) [2]
Hypotension (16%) [5]
Tachycardia (35%) [2]

Central Nervous System
Agitation (11%)
Anxiety (21%) [2]
Chills (25%)
Fever (pyrexia) (includes hyperpyrexia) (25%)
Headache (83%) [13]
Insomnia (9%)
Paresthesias (12%)
Seizures (4%)
Somnolence (drowsiness) (4%)
Syncope / fainting (13%)
Tremor (21%)

Endocrine/Metabolic
Weight loss (27%)

Gastrointestinal/Hepatic
Abdominal pain (14%)
Diarrhea [2]
Nausea [5]

Hematologic
Sepsis (25%)

Local
Injection-site infection (21%)
Injection-site pain (13%)

Neuromuscular/Skeletal
Back pain (13%)
Jaw pain (54%) [6]
Myalgia/Myopathy (44%)

Respiratory
Alveolar hemorrhage (pulmonary) [2]
Dyspnea / shortness of breath (2%)
Influenza- ('flu)-like syndrome (25%)
Pneumonia [2]

Other
Adverse effects / adverse reactions [3]

EPROSARTAN

Trade name: Teveten (AbbVie)
Indications: Hypertension
Class: Angiotensin receptor antagonist (blocker), Antihypertensive
Half-life: 5–9 hours
Clinically important, potentially hazardous interactions with: none known
Pregnancy category: category C in first trimester; category D in second and third trimesters
Important contra-indications noted in the prescribing guidelines for: nursing mothers; pediatric patients
Warning: FETAL TOXICITY

Central Nervous System
Dysgeusia (taste perversion) [2]
Vertigo / dizziness [2]
Gastrointestinal/Hepatic
Abdominal pain (2%)
Neuromuscular/Skeletal
Arthralgia (2%)
Asthenia / fatigue (2%)
Respiratory
Cough (4%) [3]
Pharyngitis (sore throat) (4%)
Rhinitis / rhinosinusitis (see also sinusitis) (4%)
Upper respiratory tract infection (8%) [2]
Other
Adverse effects / adverse reactions [3]

EPTIFIBATIDE

Trade name: Integrilin (Merck)
Indications: Acute coronary syndrome, unstable angina
Class: Antiplatelet (antithrombotic), Glycoprotein IIb/IIIa inhibitor
Half-life: 2.5 hours
Clinically important, potentially hazardous interactions with: anticoagulants, antiplatelet agents, collagenase, dasatinib, drotrecogin alfa, fondaparinux, glucosamine, ibritumomab, iloprost, lepirudin, NSAIDs, pentoxifylline, salicylates, thrombolytic agents, tositumomab & iodine[131]
Important contra-indications noted in the prescribing guidelines for: nursing mothers; pediatric patients
Note: Contra-indicated in patients with a history of bleeding diathesis, or evidence of active abnormal bleeding within the previous 30 days; severe hypertension not adequately controlled on antihypertensive therapy; major surgery within the preceding 6 weeks; history of stroke within 30 days or any history of hemorrhagic stroke; current or planned administration of another parenteral GP IIb/IIIa inhibitor; or dependency on renal dialysis.

Cardiovascular
Hypotension (7%)
Hematologic
Bleeding [3]
Hemorrhage (<10%)
Thrombocytopenia / platelets decreased [25]
Thrombosis [4]
Other
Death [2]

ERDAFITINIB

Synonym: Balversa
Trade name: Balversa (Janssen Biotech)
Class: Fibroblast growth factor receptor inhibitor, Tyrosine kinase inhibitor
Half-life: 59 hours
Clinically important, potentially hazardous interactions with: CYP2C9 or CYP3A4 inhibitors, CYP2C9 or CYP3A4 inducers, serum phosphate level-altering agents, CYP3A4 substrates, oct2 substrates, P-gp substrates
Pregnancy category: Based on the mechanism of action and findings in animal reproduction studies, BALVERSA can cause fetal harm when administered to a pregnant woman. There are no available data on BALVERSA use in pregnant women to inform a drug-associated risk.

Skin
Dry skin (≥20%)
Hand–foot syndrome (palmar–plantar erythrodysesthesia) (6% grade 3–4) (26%)
Hair
Alopecia / hair loss (26%)
Nails
Discoloration / nails (dyschromia) (11%)
Onycholysis (10% grade 3–4) (41%)
Paronychia (3% grade 3–4) (17%)
Mucosal
Oropharyngeal pain (1% grade 3–4) (11%)
Stomatitis (oral mucositis) (9% grade 3–4) (56%) [3]
Xerostomia (dry mouth) (45%) [3]
Central Nervous System
Dysgeusia (taste perversion) (1% grade 3–4) (37%) [3]
Fever (pyrexia) (includes hyperpyrexia) (1% grade 3–4) (14%)
Endocrine/Metabolic
ALP increased (1% grade 3–4) (41%)
ALT increased (1% grade 3–4) (41%)
Appetite decreased (38%) [2]
AST increased (30%)
Glucose dysregulation (10%)
Hypercalcemia (3% grade 3–4) (22%)
Hyperkalemia (16%)
Hyperphosphatemia (1% grade 3–4) (76%) [4]
Hypoalbuminemia / albumin decreased (37%)
Hypomagnesemia (1% grade 3–4) (30%)
Hyponatremia (16% grade 3–4) (40%)
Hypophosphatemia (9% grade 3–4) (24%)
Serum creatinine increased (52% (5% grade 3–4))
Weight loss (16%)
Gastrointestinal/Hepatic
Abdominal pain (2% grade 3–4) (23%)
Constipation (1% grade 3–4) (28%)
Diarrhea (2% grade 3–4) (47%)
Nausea (1% grade 3–4) (21%) [2]
Vomiting (2% grade 3–4) (13%)
Genitourinary
Hematuria (2% grade 3–4) (11%)
Urinary tract infection (6% grade 3–4) (17%)
Hematologic
Hemoglobin decreased (3% grade 3–4) (35%)
Leukocytopenia (leukopenia) / leukocytes (white blood cells) decreased (17%)
Neutropenia (neutrophils decreased) (2% grade 3–4) (10%)
Thrombocytopenia / platelets decreased (1% grade 3–4) (19%)
Neuromuscular/Skeletal
Arthralgia (11%)
Asthenia / fatigue (10% grade 3–4) (54%) [2]
Musculoskeletal pain (20%)
Ocular
Conjunctivitis (conjunctival inflammation) (11%)
Dry eye (keratoconjunctivitis sicca) (6% grade 3–4) (28%)
Lacrimation (10%)
Vision blurred (17%)
Respiratory
Dyspnea / shortness of breath (2% grade 3–4) (10%)
Other
Adverse effects / adverse reactions (67% grade 3–4) (100%)

ERDOSTEINE

Trade name: Erdotin (Galen)
Indications: Chronic obstructive pulmonary disease (COPD)
Class: Mucolytic
Half-life: N/A
Clinically important, potentially hazardous interactions with: none known

ERGOCALCIFEROL

Synonyms: viosterol; vitamin D_2
Trade name: Drisdol (Sanofi-Aventis)
Indications: Rickets, hypoparathyroidism
Class: Vitamin
Half-life: 19–48 hours
Clinically important, potentially hazardous interactions with: cholestyramine, cyclopenthiazide, orlistat, paricalcitol

---

Skin
Pruritus (itching) (<10%)
Central Nervous System
Dysgeusia (taste perversion) (<10%)
Endocrine/Metabolic
Hypercalcemia [3]
Other
Adverse effects / adverse reactions [2]

ERGOTAMINE

Trade name: Wigrettes (Organon)
Indications: Migraine, migraine variants
Class: Ergot alkaloid
Half-life: 2 hours
Clinically important, potentially hazardous interactions with: acebutolol, almotriptan, amprenavir, azithromycin, boceprevir, ceritinib, chlortetracycline, crizotinib, darunavir, dasatinib, delavirdine, demeclocycline, doxycycline, eluxadoline, enzalutamide, epinephrine, erythromycin, indinavir, itraconazole, letermovir,

lopinavir, lymecycline, methylergonovine, mifepristone, minocycline, naratriptan, nelfinavir, nilotinib, ombitasvir/paritaprevir/ritonavir, ombitasvir/paritaprevir/ritonavir and dasabuvir, oxytetracycline, posaconazole, propyphenazone, ribociclib, ritonavir, telaprevir, telithromycin, tetracycline, tigecycline, tipranavir, troleandomycin, voriconazole, warfarin
Important contra-indications noted in the prescribing guidelines for: nursing mothers
Note: Ergotamine is excreted in breast milk and may cause symptoms of vomiting, diarrhea, weak pulse and unstable blood pressure in nursing infants.

Skin
Cutaneous toxicity / skin toxicity [4]
Cardiovascular
Valvulopathy [3]
Respiratory
Pleural effusion [2]

ERIBULIN

Trade name: Halaven (Eisai)
Indications: Metastatic breast cancer in patients who have previously received at least two chemotherapeutic regimens (prior therapy should have included an anthracycline and a taxane in either the adjuvant or metastatic setting), unresectable or metastatic liposarcoma in patients who have received a prior anthracycline-containing regimen
Class: Antineoplastic / anticancer agent (see also Immune checkpoint inhibitor), Microtubule inhibitor
Half-life: 40 hours
Clinically important, potentially hazardous interactions with: none known
Pregnancy category: No available data but caused embryo-fetal toxicity in animal studies
Important contra-indications noted in the prescribing guidelines for: nursing mothers; pediatric patients

---

Skin
Peripheral edema (5–10%)
Rash (5–10%)
Hair
Alopecia / hair loss (45%) [12]
Mucosal
Mucosal inflammation (9%)
Mucositis [2]
Stomatitis (oral mucositis) (5–10%) [2]
Xerostomia (dry mouth) (5–10%)
Central Nervous System
Anorexia (20%) [3]
Depression (5–10%)
Dysgeusia (taste perversion) (5–10%)
Fever (pyrexia) (includes hyperpyrexia) (21%) [2]
Headache (19%)
Insomnia (5–10%)
Neurotoxicity [7]
Peripheral neuropathy (35%) [30]
Vertigo / dizziness (5–10%)
Endocrine/Metabolic
ALT increased [3]
Appetite decreased [2]
Hypokalemia (5–10%)
Weight loss (21%)
Gastrointestinal/Hepatic
Abdominal pain (5–10%)
Constipation (25%) [2]
Diarrhea (18%) [3]
Dyspepsia / functional dyspepsia (indigestion) (see also gastroparesis) (5–10%)
Gastrointestinal disorder / discomfort [2]
Hepatotoxicity / liver injury / acute liver injury / drug-induced liver injury (DILI) [2]
Nausea (35%) [10]
Vomiting (18%)
Genitourinary
Urinary tract infection (10%)
Hematologic
Anemia (58%) [17]
Febrile neutropenia (5%) [18]
Leukocytopenia (leukopenia) / leukocytes (white blood cells) decreased [22]
Lymphopenia (lymphocytopenia) / lymphocytes decreased [5]
Neutropenia (neutrophils decreased) (82%) [66]
Thrombocytopenia / platelets decreased [4]
Thrombosis [2]
Neuromuscular/Skeletal
Arthralgia (22%)
Asthenia / fatigue (54%) [33]
Back pain (16%)
Muscle spasm (5–10%)
Myalgia/Myopathy (22%)
Pain in extremities (11%)
Ocular
Lacrimation (increased) (5–10%)
Respiratory
Cough (14%)
Dyspnea / shortness of breath (16%) [2]
Upper respiratory tract infection (5–10%)
Other
Adverse effects / adverse reactions [7]
Death [3]

ERLOTINIB

Trade name: Tarceva (OSI)
Indications: Non-small cell lung cancer, pancreatic cancer (with gemcitabine)
Class: Antineoplastic / anticancer agent (see also Immune checkpoint inhibitor), Biologic, Epidermal growth factor receptor (EGFR) inhibitor / antagonist, Tyrosine kinase inhibitor
Half-life: ~36 hours
Clinically important, potentially hazardous interactions with: atazanavir, capecitabine, carbamazepine, ciprofloxacin, clarithromycin, diclofenac, itraconazole, ketoconazole, meloxicam, nefazodone, nelfinavir, omeprazole, pantoprazole, phenobarbital, phenytoin, rifabutin, rifampin, rifapentine, ritonavir, saquinavir, St John's wort, troleandomycin, voriconazole, warfarin
Important contra-indications noted in the prescribing guidelines for: nursing mothers; pediatric patients

---

Skin
Acne keloid [2]
Acneiform eruption / acneiform dermatitis / acneiform rash [30]
AGEP [3]
Cutaneous toxicity / skin toxicity [10]
Dermatitis [5]
DRESS syndrome (Drug-induced hypersensitivity syndrome) [2]
Erosive pustular dermatosis [2]
Erythema (18%)
Exanthems [3]
Folliculitis [9]
Hand–foot syndrome (palmar–plantar erythrodysesthesia) [3]
Papulopustular eruption [9]
Pruritus (itching) (13%) [10]
Purpura [3]
Rash (75%) [119]
Rosacea [2]
Xerosis / xeroderma (12%) [13]
Hair
Alopecia / hair loss [10]
Folliculitis decalvans [3]
Hair changes [4]
Hypertrichosis [4]
Nails
Nail changes [3]
Paronychia [14]
Mucosal
Mucositis [10]
Stomatitis (oral mucositis) (17%) [12]
Cardiovascular
Hypertension [5]
Central Nervous System
Anorexia [9]
Fever (pyrexia) (includes hyperpyrexia) [2]
Neurotoxicity [2]
Endocrine/Metabolic
ALT increased [3]
Appetite decreased [4]
AST increased [3]
Dehydration [3]
Hyperglycemia (includes glucose increased) [3]
Gastrointestinal/Hepatic
Abdominal pain (11%)
Cholangitis / sclerosing cholangitis [2]
Diarrhea [73]
Gastrointestinal bleeding [3]
Hepatotoxicity / liver injury / acute liver injury / drug-induced liver injury (DILI) [13]
Nausea [18]
Pneumatosis intestinalis / pneumatosis cystoides intestinalis [2]
Vomiting [10]
Hematologic
Anemia [12]
Febrile neutropenia [2]
Hemotoxicity [2]
Leukocytopenia (leukopenia) / leukocytes (white blood cells) decreased [5]
Neutropenia (neutrophils decreased) [14]
Thrombocytopenia / platelets decreased [10]
Neuromuscular/Skeletal
Asthenia / fatigue (52%) [33]
Rhabdomyolysis [2]
Ocular
Conjunctivitis (conjunctival inflammation) (12%) [3]
Corneal perforation [2]
Ectropion / cicatricial ectropion [4]
Ocular adverse effect [3]
Periorbital rash [2]
Trichomegaly [13]
Respiratory
Cough (33%)
Dyspnea / shortness of breath [4]
Pneumonia [2]

Pneumonitis [7]
Pneumothorax [2]
Pulmonary toxicity [15]

Other
Adverse effects / adverse reactions [12]
Death [10]
Infection (24%) [7]

ERTAPENEM

Trade name: Invanz (Merck)
Indications: Severe resistant bacterial infections caused by susceptible organisms
Class: Antibiotic, Antibiotic; carbapenem, Antimicrobial
Half-life: 4 hours
Clinically important, potentially hazardous interactions with: probenecid
Important contra-indications noted in the prescribing guidelines for: the elderly; nursing mothers

---

Skin
Edema / fluid retention (3%)
Erythema (<2%)
Pruritus (itching) (<2%)
Rash (2–3%)
Wound complications [2]

Cardiovascular
Phlebitis (2%)
Thrombophlebitis (2%)

Central Nervous System
Delirium [2]
Encephalopathy (includes hepatic encephalopathy) [7]
Hallucinations [2]
Neurotoxicity [9]
Peripheral neuropathy [2]
Seizures [7]

Gastrointestinal/Hepatic
Nausea [2]

Genitourinary
Vaginitis (includes vulvitis) (<3%)

Local
Injection-site extravasation (2%)

Respiratory
Cough (<2%)

Other
Death (2%)

ERYTHROMYCIN

Trade names: Eryc (Warner Chilcott), PCE (AbbVie)
Indications: Various infections caused by susceptible organisms
Class: Antibiotic, Antibiotic; macrolide, Antimicrobial, CYP3A4 inhibitor
Half-life: 1.4–2 hours
Clinically important, potentially hazardous interactions with: afatinib, alfentanil, aminophylline, amisulpride, amoxicillin, ampicillin, anticonvulsants, arsenic, astemizole, atorvastatin, avanafil, benzodiazepines, bosentan, bromocriptine, buprenorphine, bupropion, carbamazepine, cilostazol, ciprofloxacin, cisapride, clindamycin, clindamycin/tretinoin, clopidogrel, clozapine, colchicine, cyclosporine, CYP3A inhibitors, darifenacin, dasatinib, digoxin, dihydroergotamine, diltiazem, disopyramide, docetaxel, doxercalciferol, dronedarone, enoxacin, eplerenone, ergotamine, estradiol, eszopiclone, everolimus, finerenone, flibanserin, fluconazole, fluoxetine, fluvastatin, gatifloxacin, HMG-CoA reductase inhibitors, imatinib, indacaterol, itraconazole, ketoconazole, levodopa, lomefloxacin, lorazepam, lovastatin, lumateperone, methadone, methylergonovine, methylprednisolone, methysergide, midazolam, mifepristone, mizolastine, moxifloxacin, naldemedine, naloxegol, neratinib, nintedanib, nitrazepam, norfloxacin, ofloxacin, olaparib, oliceridine, oxtriphylline, paroxetine hydrochloride, pentamidine, pimecrolimus, pimozide, pitavastatin, pravastatin, quetiapine, quinolones, ranolazine, relugolix, repaglinide, rilpivirine, rivaroxaban, roflumilast, rosuvastatin, rupatadine, sertraline, sildenafil, silodosin, simeprevir, simvastatin, sparfloxacin, sulpiride / levosulpiride, tacrolimus, tadalafil, tamsulosin, terfenadine, tezacaftor/ivacaftor, tramadol, triamcinolone, triazolam, troleandomycin, vardenafil, venetoclax, verapamil, vilazodone, vinblastine, warfarin, zafirlukast, zaleplon, zolpidem, zuclopenthixol
Important contra-indications noted in the prescribing guidelines for: the elderly; nursing mothers

---

Skin
AGEP [3]
Anaphylactoid reactions / anaphylaxis (includes anaphylactic shock) [2]
Baboon syndrome / symmetrical drug-related intertriginous and flexural exanthema (SDRIFE) [2]
Dermatitis (systemic) [4]
Exanthems (<5%) [4]
Fixed eruption / fixed drug eruption [6]
Hypersensitivity (<10%) [3]
Rash [3]
Stevens-Johnson syndrome and toxic epidermal necrolysis (SJS/TEN) [13]
Urticaria / hives [4]

Mucosal
Oral candidiasis (<10%)

Cardiovascular
QT interval prolonged / QT prolongation [5]
Torsades de pointes [8]

Gastrointestinal/Hepatic
Abdominal pain [3]
Diarrhea [4]
Nausea [4]

Local
Injection-site phlebitis (<10%) [2]

Neuromuscular/Skeletal
Rhabdomyolysis [4]

Otic
Tinnitus [3]

Other
Allergic reactions (<2%) [3]

ESCITALOPRAM

Trade name: Lexapro (Forest)
Indications: Major depressive disorders, anxiety
Class: Antidepressant, Selective serotonin reuptake inhibitor (SSRI)
Half-life: 27–32 hours
Clinically important, potentially hazardous interactions with: alcohol, bupropion, gilteritinib, MAO inhibitors, methylphenidate, omeprazole, selegiline, St John's wort, sumatriptan, telaprevir, valerian
Important contra-indications noted in the prescribing guidelines for: the elderly; nursing mothers; pediatric patients
Note: Escitalopram is the (S)-form of citalopram (q.v.).
Warning: SUICIDALITY AND ANTIDEPRESSANT DRUGS

Skin
Diaphoresis (5%)
Hot flashes / hot flushes (<10%)
Rash (<10%) [3]

Mucosal
Epistaxis (nosebleed) [3]
Oral vesiculation (<19%)
Xerostomia (dry mouth) (6%) [6]

Cardiovascular
Bradycardia / sinus bradycardia [3]
QT interval prolonged / QT prolongation [9]
Torsades de pointes [2]

Central Nervous System
Anxiety [3]
Headache (24%) [5]
Insomnia (9–12%) [5]
Paresthesias (<10%)
Parkinsonism [2]
Rabbit syndrome (oral vertical dyskinesia) [2]
Restless legs syndrome / Willis-Ekbom disease (includes restless arms syndrome variant) [5]
Serotonin syndrome [5]
Somnolence (drowsiness) (6–13%) [7]
Tremor (<10%)
Vertigo / dizziness (5%) [7]

Endocrine/Metabolic
Galactorrhea [4]
Hyponatremia [4]
SIADH [7]
Weight gain [3]

Gastrointestinal/Hepatic
Abdominal pain [3]
Constipation [2]
Diarrhea [4]
Dyspepsia / functional dyspepsia (indigestion) (see also gastroparesis) [2]
Hepatotoxicity / liver injury / acute liver injury / drug-induced liver injury (DILI) [3]
Nausea [12]
Vomiting [3]

Genitourinary
Ejaculatory dysfunction (9–14%)
Sexual dysfunction [5]

Neuromuscular/Skeletal
Asthenia / fatigue [4]
Hypnic jerks / hypnagogic jerk / sleep start (twitch) / myoclonic jerk [4]
Myalgia/Myopathy (<10%)

Ocular
Glaucoma (includes acute angle-closure glaucoma) [4]

Otic
Tinnitus (<10%)

Respiratory
Cough (<10%)
Influenza- ('flu)-like syndrome (5%)

Other
Adverse effects / adverse reactions [3]
Allergic reactions (<10%)
Toothache (odontalgia) (<10%)

ESLICARBAZEPINE

Trade names: Aptiom (Sunovion), Zebinix (Eisai)
Indications: Partial-onset seizures
Class: Anticonvulsant (see also antiepileptic (anti-seizure)), Antiepileptic (anti-seizure)
Half-life: 13–20 hours
Clinically important, potentially hazardous interactions with: carbamazepine, digoxin, lamotrigine, levetiracetam, MAO inhibitors, oral contraceptives, oxcarbazepine, phenytoin, topiramate, valproic acid, warfarin
Important contra-indications noted in the prescribing guidelines for: nursing mothers; pediatric patients

---

Skin
Peripheral edema (<2%)
Rash (<3%) [4]
Cardiovascular
Hypertension (<2%)
Central Nervous System
Balance disorder (3%)
Depression (<3%)
Dysarthria (<2%)
Gait instability / postural instability (2%)
Headache (13–15%) [16]
Incoordination [3]
Insomnia (2%)
Seizures [2]
Somnolence (drowsiness) (11–18%) [24]
Tremor (2–4%)
Vertigo / dizziness (20–28%) [28]
Endocrine/Metabolic
Hyponatremia (2%) [7]
Gastrointestinal/Hepatic
Constipation (2%)
Diarrhea (2–4%)
Nausea (10–16%) [14]
Vomiting (6–10%) [7]
Genitourinary
Urinary tract infection (2%)
Neuromuscular/Skeletal
Asthenia / fatigue (4–7%) [12]
Ataxia (4–6%)
Ocular
Diplopia (double vision) (9–11%) [10]
Nystagmus (<2%)
Vision blurred (5–6%) [4]
Vision impaired (<2%)
Respiratory
Cough (<2%)
Nasopharyngitis [3]
Other
Adverse effects / adverse reactions [4]

ESMOLOL

Trade name: Brevibloc (Baxter)
Indications: Tachyarrhythmias, tachycardia
Class: Adrenergic beta-receptor antagonist, Antiarrhythmic class II
Half-life: 9 minutes
Clinically important, potentially hazardous interactions with: clonidine, verapamil
Important contra-indications noted in the prescribing guidelines for: nursing mothers; pediatric patients

---

Skin
Diaphoresis (>10%)
Cardiovascular
Bradycardia / sinus bradycardia [5]
Hypotension [12]
Local
Injection-site pain (8%)
Injection-site reaction (<10%)
Other
Death [2]

ESOMEPRAZOLE

Trade name: Nexium (AstraZeneca)
Indications: Gastroesophageal reflux disease
Class: Proton pump inhibitor (PPI)
Half-life: 1.5 hours
Clinically important, potentially hazardous interactions with: benzodiazepines, chlordiazepoxide, cilostazol, clonazepam, clopidogrel, clorazepate, diazepam, digoxin, emtricitabine/rilpivirine/tenofovir alafenamide, flurazepam, lorazepam, midazolam, oxazepam, posaconazole, quazepam, rifampin, rilpivirine, St John's wort, temazepam, tipranavir, voriconazole
Important contra-indications noted in the prescribing guidelines for: nursing mothers; pediatric patients

---

Skin
DRESS syndrome (Drug-induced hypersensitivity syndrome) [2]
Fixed eruption / fixed drug eruption [2]
Lupus erythematosus (subacute cutaneous lupus erythematosus (SCLE)) [3]
Cardiovascular
Chest pain [2]
Central Nervous System
Dysgeusia (taste perversion) [3]
Fever (pyrexia) (includes hyperpyrexia) [2]
Headache (8–11%) [6]
Somnolence (drowsiness) [2]
Vertigo / dizziness [3]
Endocrine/Metabolic
Hypomagnesemia [3]
Gastrointestinal/Hepatic
Abdominal pain [3]
Constipation [3]
Diarrhea [7]
Nausea [5]
Vomiting [4]
Neuromuscular/Skeletal
Rhabdomyolysis [2]
Respiratory
Bronchitis (4%)
Other
Adverse effects / adverse reactions [6]

ESTAZOLAM

Indications: Insomnia
Class: Benzodiazepine
Half-life: 10–24 hours
Clinically important, potentially hazardous interactions with: cobicistat/elvitegravir/emtricitabine/tenofovir alafenamide, cobicistat/elvitegravir/emtricitabine/tenofovir disoproxil, indinavir, ritonavir

---

Skin
Diaphoresis (<10%)
Flushing / rubefaction (<10%)
Pruritus (itching) (<10%)
Rash (>10%)
Urticaria / hives (<10%)
Mucosal
Sialopenia (>10%)
Xerostomia (dry mouth) (>10%)
Central Nervous System
Dysgeusia (taste perversion) (<10%)
Paresthesias (<10%)
Genitourinary
Vaginal pruritus (<10%)
Neuromuscular/Skeletal
Myalgia/Myopathy (<10%)
Other
Adverse effects / adverse reactions [2]

ESTRADIOL

Trade names: Alora (Watson), Climara (Bayer), Divigel (Upsher-Smith), Elestrin (Azur Pharma), Esclim (Women First), Estrace (Bristol-Myers Squibb) (Warner Chilcott), Estraderm (Novartis), Estring (Pharmacia & Upjohn), Estrogel (Ascend), Evamist (KV Pharm), Fempatch (Pfizer), Gynodiol (Barr), Innofem (Novo Nordisk), Menostar (Bayer), Vagifem (Novo Nordisk), Vivelle (Novartis), Vivelle-Dot (Novartis)
Indications: Menopausal symptoms, hypoestrogenism due to hypogonadism, castration or primary ovarian failure, postmenopausal osteoporosis
Class: Estrogen, Hormone
Half-life: 1.75±2.87 hours
Clinically important, potentially hazardous interactions with: alcohol, amprenavir, anastrozole, ascorbic acid, atorvastatin, boceprevir, carbamazepine, chenodiol, clarithromycin, colesevelam, conivaptan, corticosteroids, CYP1A2 inducers, CYP3A4 inducers, deferasirox, delavirdine, erythromycin, folic acid, grapefruit juice, itraconazole, ketoconazole, lopinavir, minocycline, oxtriphylline, P-glycoprotein inhibitors or inducers, PEG-interferon, phenobarbital, rifampin, ritonavir, ropinirole, saxagliptin, somatropin, St John's wort, telaprevir, thyroid products, tipranavir, ursodiol
Important contra-indications noted in the prescribing guidelines for: the elderly; nursing mothers; pediatric patients
Note: See also separate entry for estrogens.
Warning: ENDOMETRIAL CANCER, CARDIOVASCULAR DISORDERS, BREAST CANCER and PROBABLE DEMENTIA

Central Nervous System
Headache [2]
Endocrine/Metabolic
Mastodynia (7%)
Gastrointestinal/Hepatic
Nausea [3]
Genitourinary
Metrorrhagia (4%)
Respiratory
Nasopharyngitis (10%)
Upper respiratory tract infection (6%)
Other
Adverse effects / adverse reactions [3]

ESTRAMUSTINE

Trade name: Emcyt (Pfizer)
Indications: Prostate carcinoma
Class: Alkylating agent, Nitrosourea
Half-life: 20 hours
Clinically important, potentially hazardous interactions with: aldesleukin
Pregnancy category: not indicated for use in women

Skin
Angioedema (formerly named angioneurotic edema) [2]
Edema / fluid retention (>10%) [4]
Peripheral edema [2]
Pruritus (itching) (2%) [2]
Purpura (3%)
Xerosis / xeroderma (2%)

Cardiovascular
Thrombophlebitis (3%)

Endocrine/Metabolic
Gynecomastia (>10%) [5]
Mastodynia (66%)

Gastrointestinal/Hepatic
Diarrhea [3]
Nausea [3]

Hematologic
Anemia [3]
Febrile neutropenia [2]
Leukocytopenia (leukopenia) / leukocytes (white blood cells) decreased [2]
Neutropenia (neutrophils decreased) [5]

Local
Injection-site thrombophlebitis (<10%) [3]

Neuromuscular/Skeletal
Asthenia / fatigue [3]

Other
Allergic reactions [2]
Death [2]

ESTROGENS

Trade names: Estrace (Warner Chilcott), Estraderm (Novartis), Estratab (Solvay), Menest (Monarch), Ogen (Pfizer), Premarin (Wyeth)
Indications: Menopausal symptoms, hypoestrogenism due to hypogonadism, castration or primary ovarian failure, postmenopausal osteoporosis
Class: Estrogen
Half-life: N/A
Clinically important, potentially hazardous interactions with: acarbose, acebutolol, alfuzosin, amitriptyline, anastrozole, aprepitant, atazanavir, beclomethasone, betamethasone, captopril, cilazapril, darunavir, enalapril, flunisolide, fosinopril, hydrocortisone, indinavir, insulin aspart, insulin degludec, insulin detemir, insulin glargine, lisinopril, metformin, minocycline, nelfinavir, olmesartan, oxtriphylline, penicillin G, penicillin V, prednisone, quinapril, ramipril, saxagliptin, sitagliptin, somatropin, terbinafine, tipranavir, trandolapril, triamcinolone, ursodiol, voriconazole
Important contra-indications noted in the prescribing guidelines for: nursing mothers
Note: Estrogen administration to women who are breastfeeding has been shown to decrease the quantity and quality of the milk. Estrogens are not indicated for the prevention of postpartum breast engorgement. A Women's Health Initiative (WHI) estrogen alone study reported increased risks of stroke and deep vein thrombosis (DVT) in postmenopausal women (50–79 years of age) and an increased risk of developing probable dementia in postmenopausal women over 65 years of age. Large and repeated doses of estrogen over an extended time period have been shown to accelerate epiphyseal closure, which could result in short adult stature if treatment is initiated before the completion of physiologic puberty in normally developing children. Estrogen treatment of prepubertal girls also induces premature breast development and vaginal cornification, and may induce gynecomastia.

Skin
Acneiform eruption / acneiform dermatitis / acneiform rash (5%)
Angioedema (formerly named angioneurotic edema) [4]
Dermatitis [2]
Erythema nodosum [2]
Exanthems [4]
Flushing / rubefaction (5%) [2]
Lupus erythematosus (subacute cutaneous lupus erythematosus (SCLE)) [11]
Melasma [2]
Papulovesicular eruption [2]
Photosensitivity [3]
Pigmentation (Skin) (includes hyperpigmentation) [2]
Pruritus (itching) [7]
Tumors [3]
Urticaria / hives [4]

Hair
Alopecia / hair loss [2]
Hirsutism [2]

Endocrine/Metabolic
Gynecomastia (>10%) [9]
Mastodynia (>10%) [3]
Porphyria [2]
Porphyria cutanea tarda [21]

Gastrointestinal/Hepatic
Pancreatitis / acute pancreatitis [4]

Local
Injection-site pain (<10%)

ESZOPICLONE

Trade names: Imovane (Sanofi-Aventis), Lunesta (Sunovion), Zimovane (Sanofi-Aventis)
Indications: Insomnia
Class: Hypnotic, non-benzodiazepine
Half-life: 6 hours
Clinically important, potentially hazardous interactions with: alcohol, antifungals, cimetidine, CNS depressants, conivaptan, CYP3A4 inhibitors and inducers, dasatinib, deferasirox, droperidol, erythromycin, ethanol, flumazenil, ketoconazole, levomepromazine, lorazepam, nefazodone, nelfinavir, olanzapine, rifampin, ritonavir, St John's wort, telithromycin, tricyclic antidepressants, valerian, voriconazole
Important contra-indications noted in the prescribing guidelines for: the elderly; nursing mothers; pediatric patients

---

Skin
Pruritus (itching) (<4%)
Rash (<5%)

Mucosal
Xerostomia (dry mouth) (3–7%) [5]

Central Nervous System
Abnormal dreams (<3%)
Amnesia [3]
Anxiety (<3%)
Confusion (<3%)
Depression (<4%)
Dysgeusia (taste perversion) (8–34%) [22]
Hallucinations (<3%)
Headache (13–21%) [9]
Nervousness (<5%)
Neurotoxicity (<3%)
Pain (4–5%)
Somnolence (drowsiness) (8–10%) [2]
Vertigo / dizziness [3]

Endocrine/Metabolic
Gynecomastia (<3%)
Libido decreased (<3%)

Gastrointestinal/Hepatic
Diarrhea (2–4%)
Dyspepsia / functional dyspepsia (indigestion) (see also gastroparesis) (2–6%)
Nausea (4–5%) [2]
Vomiting (<3%)

Genitourinary
Dysmenorrhea (<3%)
Urinary tract infection (<3%)

Other
Adverse effects / adverse reactions [4]
Infection (3–10%)

ETAMSYLATE

Trade name: Dicynene (Sanofi-Aventis)
Indications: Primary and IUD-induced menorrhagia
Class: Hemostatic, Vitamin K
Half-life: 4–8 hours
Clinically important, potentially hazardous interactions with: none known
Important contra-indications noted in the prescribing guidelines for: nursing mothers

ETANERCEPT

Trade names: Enbrel (Amgen), Erelzi (Sandoz)
Indications: Rheumatoid arthritis, polyarticular juvenile idiopathic arthritis in patients aged 2 years or older, psoriatic arthritis, ankylosing spondylitis, plaque psoriasis
Class: Anti-Tumor Necrosis Factor-alpha (TNF-α antagonist), Antipsoriatic agent, Biologic, Biologic disease-modifying antirheumatic drug (bDMARD), Cytokine inhibitor, Disease-modifying antirheumatic drug (DMARD)
Half-life: 4–13 days
Clinically important, potentially hazardous interactions with: abatacept, anakinra, cyclophosphamide, live vaccines
Important contra-indications noted in the prescribing guidelines for: the elderly; nursing mothers; pediatric patients
Note: TNF inhibitors should be used in patients with heart failure only after consideration of other treatment options. Contra-indicated in patients with sepsis. TNF inhibitors are contra-indicated in patients with a personal or family history of multiple sclerosis or demyelinating disease. TNF inhibitors should not be administered to patients with moderate to severe heart failure (New York Heart Association Functional Class III/IV).

Etanercept-szzs (Erelzi) is biosimilar to Etanercept (Enbrel). Approved 08/30/2016
Etanercept-ykro (Eticovo)) is biosimilar to Etanercept (Enbrel). Approved 04/25/2019.
Warning: SERIOUS INFECTIONS AND MALIGNANCIES

Skin
Abscess [2]
Anaphylactoid reactions / anaphylaxis (includes anaphylactic shock) [2]
Carcinoma [2]
Cellulitis and pseudocellulitis [2]
Dermatitis [3]
Dermatomyositis [4]
Exanthems [2]
Granulomas [2]
Granulomatous reaction [5]
Henoch-Schönlein purpura / IgA vasculitis / immunoglobulin A vasculitis [3]
Herpes zoster [6]
Hidradenitis suppurativa (acne inversa) [2]
Leprosy (Hansen disease) [2]
Lichen planus (includes hypertrophic lichen planus) [2]
Lichenoid eruption / lichenoid reaction [3]
Lupus erythematosus (subacute cutaneous lupus erythematosus (SCLE)) [25]
Lupus syndrome / drug-induced lupus (DIL) [4]
Lymphoma [3]
Melanoma [2]
Nodular eruption [3]
Pruritus (itching) (2–5%) [2]
Psoriasis [21]
Pustules / pustular eruption [2]
Rash (3–13%) [8]
Sarcoidosis / sarcoid-like reaction (cutaneous sarcoidosis) [10]
Squamous cell carcinoma [4]
Urticaria / hives (2%) [3]
Vasculitis (angiitis) / cutaneous vasculitis (angiitis) [23]

Hair
Alopecia / hair loss [5]

Mucosal
Gingivitis [2]

Cardiovascular
Atrial fibrillation [2]
Cardiotoxicity [2]
Congestive heart failure [2]
Hypertension [2]

Central Nervous System
Demyelinating neuropathy / demyelination [3]
Fever (pyrexia) (includes hyperpyrexia) (2–3%) [3]
Headache [20]
Leukoencephalopathy / posterior reversible encephalopathy syndrome (PRES) [3]
Multiple sclerosis [2]
Neurotoxicity [4]
Paresthesias [2]
Peripheral neuropathy [2]
Vertigo / dizziness [3]

Endocrine/Metabolic
ALT increased [3]
Hypertriglyceridemia (includes triglycerides increased) [2]
Thyroiditis [3]
Weight gain [2]

Gastrointestinal/Hepatic
Abdominal pain [4]
Colitis [2]
Crohn's disease [5]
Diarrhea (8–16%) [5]
Gastroenteritis [3]
Hepatotoxicity / liver injury / acute liver injury / drug-induced liver injury (DILI) [5]
Inflammatory bowel disease [2]
Nausea [5]

Genitourinary
Cystitis (includes interstitial cystitis / bladder pain syndrome) [2]
Urinary tract infection [2]

Hematologic
Leukocytopenia (leukopenia) / leukocytes (white blood cells) decreased [2]
Macrophage activation syndrome [2]
Neutropenia (neutrophils decreased) [3]
Pancytopenia (includes bicytopenia) [3]
Thrombocytopenia / platelets decreased [2]

Local
Injection-site reaction (37–43%) [65]

Neuromuscular/Skeletal
Arthralgia [3]
Asthenia / fatigue [7]
Back pain [2]
Myalgia/Myopathy [2]
Myasthenia gravis [3]

Ocular
Uveitis / anterior uveitis / posterior uveitis / panuveitis [13]

Otic
Otitis (otitis externa, otitis media, otitis interna) [2]

Renal
Nephrotoxicity / kidney injury / acute kidney injury (AKI) / drug-induced kidney injury [2]

Respiratory
Asthma [2]
Bronchitis [5]
Cough [4]
Influenza- ('flu)-like syndrome [3]
Laryngitis [2]
Nasopharyngitis [6]
Pharyngitis (sore throat) [5]
Pneumonia [7]
Pneumonitis [2]
Pulmonary toxicity [4]
Rhinitis / rhinosinusitis (see also sinusitis) [4]
Sinusitis (see also rhinitis / rhinosinusitis) [5]
Tuberculosis [2]
Upper respiratory tract infection (38–65%) [14]

Other
Adverse effects / adverse reactions [38]
Allergic reactions (<3%)
Cancer [2]
Death [7]
Infection (50–81%) [47]
Malignancies (<3%) [4]
Neoplasms [2]

ETHACRYNIC ACID

Trade name: Edecrin (Merck)
Indications: Edema
Class: Diuretic, loop
Half-life: 2-4 hours
Clinically important, potentially hazardous interactions with: amikacin, aminoglycosides, digoxin, gentamicin, kanamycin, neomycin, streptomycin, tobramycin

Skin
Vasculitis (angiitis) / cutaneous vasculitis (angiitis) [2]

Otic
Ototoxicity [4]

ETHAMBUTOL

Trade name: Myambutol (Stat Trade)
Indications: Tuberculosis
Class: Antimycobacterial (including antitubercular)
Half-life: 3–4 hours
Clinically important, potentially hazardous interactions with: cortisone, zinc
Important contra-indications noted in the prescribing guidelines for: nursing mothers; pediatric patients

Skin
Bullous dermatosis [2]
Dermatitis [2]
DRESS syndrome (Drug-induced hypersensitivity syndrome) [5]
Erythema multiforme [2]
Exanthems (<5%) [4]
Hypersensitivity [3]
Lichenoid eruption / lichenoid reaction [3]
Lupus erythematosus (subacute cutaneous lupus erythematosus (SCLE)) [2]
Photosensitivity [2]
Pruritus (itching) [4]
Rash [2]
Stevens-Johnson syndrome and toxic epidermal necrolysis (SJS/TEN) [4]
Urticaria / hives [2]

Central Nervous System
Peripheral neuropathy [2]

Ocular
Amblyopia [2]
Ocular toxicity [9]
Optic neuritis / papillitis [5]
Optic neuropathy [14]
Vision impaired [2]

Renal
Nephrotoxicity / kidney injury / acute kidney injury (AKI) / drug-induced kidney injury [2]

Other
Adverse effects / adverse reactions [4]

ETHANOLAMINE

Trade name: Ethamolin (GSK)
Indications: Bleeding esophageal varices
Class: Sclerosant, local
Half-life: N/A
Clinically important, potentially hazardous interactions with: acitretin, amobarbital, aprobarbital, butabarbital, disulfiram, insulin, mephobarbital, pentobarbital, phenobarbital, primidone, secobarbital, thiopental

Skin
Dermatitis [5]

Genitourinary
Hemoglobinuria [2]

ETHCHLORVYNOL

Indications: Insomnia
Class: Sedative
Half-life: 10–20 hours
Clinically important, potentially hazardous interactions with: antihistamines, brompheniramine, buclizine, chlorpheniramine, clemastine, dexchlorpheniramine, meclizine, tripelennamine

---

Skin
Bullous dermatosis (from overdose) [2]
Rash (<10%)

Central Nervous System
Dysgeusia (taste perversion) (>10%)

ETHIONAMIDE

Trade name: Trecator-SC (Wyeth)
Indications: Tuberculosis
Class: Antibiotic, Antimicrobial, Antimycobacterial (including antitubercular)
Half-life: 2–3 hours
Clinically important, potentially hazardous interactions with: none known

---

Skin
Acneiform eruption / acneiform dermatitis / acneiform rash [3]
Exanthems [2]
Pellagra [2]
Photosensitivity [2]
Urticaria / hives (<5%)

Hair
Alopecia / hair loss [3]

Central Nervous System
Dysgeusia (taste perversion) (<10%)
Peripheral neuropathy [3]

Endocrine/Metabolic
Gynecomastia [3]
Hypothyroidism [3]

Other
Adverse effects / adverse reactions [5]

ETHOSUXIMIDE

Trade name: Zarontin (Pfizer)
Indications: Absence (petit mal) seizures
Class: Antiepileptic; succinimide
Half-life: 50–60 hours
Clinically important, potentially hazardous interactions with: antipsychotics, carbamazepine, chloroquine, cobicistat/elvitegravir/emtricitabine/tenofovir alafenamide, cobicistat/elvitegravir/emtricitabine/tenofovir disoproxil, hydroxychloroquine, isoniazid, levomepromazine, lisdexamfetamine, MAO inhibitors, mefloquine, nevirapine, orlistat, phenobarbital, phenytoin, primidone, risperidone, SSRIs, St John's wort, tricyclic antidepressants, valproic acid, zuclopenthixol
Important contra-indications noted in the prescribing guidelines for: nursing mothers
Note: Cases of birth defects have been reported with ethosuximide.

Skin
Exanthems (<5%) [2]
Lupus erythematosus (subacute cutaneous lupus erythematosus (SCLE)) (>10%) [22]
Raynaud's phenomenon [3]
Stevens-Johnson syndrome and toxic epidermal necrolysis (SJS/TEN) (>10%)
Urticaria / hives (<5%)

Hematologic
Agranulocytosis / severe selective neutropenia [2]

Other
Side effects (3%)

ETHOTOIN

Trade name: Peganone (Ovation)
Indications: Tonic-clonic (grand mal) seizures
Class: Antiepileptic; hydantoin
Half-life: 3–9 hours
Clinically important, potentially hazardous interactions with: chloramphenicol, cyclosporine, disulfiram, dopamine, imatinib, itraconazole, phenacemide

ETHOXZOLAMIDE

Trade names: Cardase (Pharmacia & Upjohn), Ethamide (Allergan)
Other common trade names: Ethoxazolamide, Ethoxyzolamide, Etoxzolamide
Indications: Glaucoma, duodenal ulcers, may be used as a diuretic in the treatment of epileptic seizures
Class: Carbonic anhydrase inhibitor, Sulfonamide
Half-life: 2.5–5.5 hours
Clinically important, potentially hazardous interactions with: amphotericin B, corticosteroids, lithium, procainamide, quinidine
Note: Ethoxzolamide is a sulfonamide and can be absorbed systemically. Sulfonamides can produce severe, possibly fatal, reactions such as toxic epidermal necrolysis and Stevens-Johnson syndrome.

Central Nervous System
Depression [2]
Dysgeusia (taste perversion) [2]
Paresthesias [2]

Endocrine/Metabolic
Acidosis (includes lactic acidosis) [2]
Libido decreased [2]
Weight loss [2]

Gastrointestinal/Hepatic
Dyspepsia / functional dyspepsia (indigestion) (see also gastroparesis) [2]

Neuromuscular/Skeletal
Asthenia / fatigue [2]

Ocular
Myopia [3]

Renal
Nephrolithiasis (kidney stones / renal calculi) [2]

ETIDRONATE

Trade name: Didronel (Procter & Gamble)
Indications: Paget's disease, osteoporosis
Class: Bisphosphonate
Half-life: 6 hours
Clinically important, potentially hazardous interactions with: ferrous sulfate
Important contra-indications noted in the prescribing guidelines for: nursing mothers; pediatric patients

---

Gastrointestinal/Hepatic
Esophagitis [2]

Neuromuscular/Skeletal
Fractures [6]
Osteomalacia [3]
Pseudogout [2]
Skeletal toxicity [2]

ETODOLAC

Trade name: Lodine (Wyeth)
Indications: Pain
Class: COX-2 inhibitor, Non-steroidal anti-inflammatory (NSAID)
Half-life: 7 hours
Clinically important, potentially hazardous interactions with: aspirin, methotrexate
Important contra-indications noted in the prescribing guidelines for: the elderly; nursing mothers; pediatric patients
Note: NSAIDs may cause an increased risk of serious cardiovascular and gastrointestinal adverse events, which can be fatal. This risk may increase with duration of use.

Skin
Exanthems [2]
Facial edema [2]
Fixed eruption / fixed drug eruption [2]
Pruritus (itching) (<10%) [7]
Rash (>10%) [5]
Vasculitis (angiitis) / cutaneous vasculitis (angiitis) [2]

Gastrointestinal/Hepatic
Abdominal pain [3]
Constipation [2]
Dyspepsia / functional dyspepsia (indigestion) (see also gastroparesis) [4]
Nausea [3]

Other
Adverse effects / adverse reactions [2]

ETOMIDATE

Trade name: Hypnomidate (Janssen)
Indications: Intravenous induction agent of anesthesia
Class: Hypnotic
Half-life: 3–5 hours
Clinically important, potentially hazardous interactions with: sedatives

---

Skin
Anaphylactoid reactions / anaphylaxis (includes anaphylactic shock) [4]

Cardiovascular
Hypotension [2]
Tachycardia [3]

Central Nervous System
Seizures [10]

Endocrine/Metabolic
Adrenal insufficiency (hypoadrenalism) / Addisonian crisis (includes Addison's disease) [4]

Gastrointestinal/Hepatic
Nausea [2]
Vomiting [2]

Neuromuscular/Skeletal
Myoclonus (see also hypnic jerk) [26]

Respiratory
Pneumonia [2]

ETOPOSIDE

Trade name: VePesid (Bristol-Myers Squibb)
Indications: Lymphomas, carcinomas
Class: Topoisomerase 2 inhibitor
Half-life: 4–11 hours
Clinically important, potentially hazardous interactions with: aldesleukin, atovaquone, atovaquone/proguanil, cyclosporine, gadobenate, prednisolone, St John's wort
Important contra-indications noted in the prescribing guidelines for: the elderly; nursing mothers; pediatric patients

---

Skin
Anaphylactoid reactions / anaphylaxis (includes anaphylactic shock) (<2%) [3]
Cutaneous toxicity / skin toxicity [2]
Erythema [3]
Exanthems [4]
Flushing / rubefaction [3]
Hand–foot syndrome (palmar–plantar erythrodysesthesia) [4]
Hypersensitivity [9]
Pigmentation (Skin) (includes hyperpigmentation) [2]
Radiation recall dermatitis [3]
Rash [2]
Stevens-Johnson syndrome and toxic epidermal necrolysis (SJS/TEN) [3]

Hair
Alopecia / hair loss (8–66%) [10]

Mucosal
Mucositis (>10%)
Oral lesions (<5%) [2]
Stomatitis (oral mucositis) (<10%) [2]

Central Nervous System
Anorexia [4]
Leukoencephalopathy / posterior reversible encephalopathy syndrome (PRES) [2]
Neurotoxicity [3]

Endocrine/Metabolic
Hyponatremia [2]

Gastrointestinal/Hepatic
Diarrhea [3]
Hepatotoxicity / liver injury / acute liver injury / drug-induced liver injury (DILI) [3]
Nausea [8]
Vomiting [8]

Hematologic
Anemia [9]
Febrile neutropenia [7]
Leukocytopenia (leukopenia) / leukocytes (white blood cells) decreased [5]
Myeloid leukemia [2]
Myelosuppression / bone marrow suppression / myelotoxicity [2]
Neutropenia (neutrophils decreased) [14]
Thrombocytopenia / platelets decreased [11]
Thrombotic microangiopathy [2]

Neuromuscular/Skeletal
Asthenia / fatigue [3]
Rhabdomyolysis [3]

Renal
Nephrotoxicity / kidney injury / acute kidney injury (AKI) / drug-induced kidney injury [4]

Respiratory
Pneumonitis [3]
Pulmonary toxicity [2]

Other
Adverse effects / adverse reactions [3]
Allergic reactions (<2%)
Death [3]
Infection [5]

ETORICOXIB

Trade name: Arcoxia (MSD)
Indications: Rheumatoid arthritis, osteoarthritis, ankylosing spondylitis, chronic low back pain, dysmenorrhea, acute gouty arthritis
Class: COX-2 inhibitor, Non-steroidal anti-inflammatory (NSAID)
Half-life: 22 hours
Clinically important, potentially hazardous interactions with: ACE inhibitors, cyclosporine, dexibuprofen, lithium, methotrexate, rifampin, tacrolimus, warfarin
Pregnancy category: Contra-indicated in pregnancy
Important contra-indications noted in the prescribing guidelines for: nursing mothers; pediatric patients
Note: NSAIDs may cause an increased risk of serious cardiovascular and gastrointestinal adverse events, which can be fatal. This risk may increase with duration of use.

Skin
Angioedema (formerly named angioneurotic edema) [3]
Fixed eruption / fixed drug eruption [11]
Stevens-Johnson syndrome and toxic epidermal necrolysis (SJS/TEN) [8]
Urticaria / hives [4]

Mucosal
Oral mucosal fixed drug eruption [2]

Cardiovascular
Cardiotoxicity [6]
Hypertension [3]
Myocardial infarction [2]

Central Nervous System
Stroke / cerebrovascular accident [2]

Other
Adverse effects / adverse reactions [4]

ETRAVIRINE

Trade name: Intelence (Tibotec)
Indications: HIV infection
Class: Non-nucleoside reverse transcriptase inhibitor
Half-life: 41 hours
Clinically important, potentially hazardous interactions with: atazanavir, atorvastatin, carbamazepine, clarithromycin, clopidogrel, darunavir, delavirdine, digoxin, doravirine, efavirenz, fosamprenavir, ibrexafungerp, indinavir, lemborexant, lumateperone, maraviroc, nelfinavir, neratinib, nevirapine, non-nucleoside reverse transcriptase inhibitors, olaparib, palbociclib, phenobarbital, phenytoin, rifabutin, rifampin, rifapentine, rilpivirine, ritonavir, sildenafil, simeprevir, St John's wort, tadalafil, telithromycin, tipranavir, vardenafil, venetoclax, voriconazole
Important contra-indications noted in the prescribing guidelines for: nursing mothers; pediatric patients

---

Skin
Facial edema (<2%)
Hyperhidrosis (<2%)
Lipohypertrophy (<2%)
Prurigo (<2%)
Rash (9%) [17]
Xerosis / xeroderma (<2%)

Mucosal
Stomatitis (oral mucositis) (<2%)
Xerostomia (dry mouth) (<2%)

Cardiovascular
Angina (<2%)
Atrial fibrillation (<2%)
Hypertension (3%)
Myocardial infarction (<2%)

Central Nervous System
Abnormal dreams (<2%)
Amnesia (<2%)
Anorexia (<2%)
Anxiety (<2%)
Confusion (<2%)
Disorientation (<2%)
Headache (3%) [3]
Hypersomnia (<2%)
Hypoesthesia / hypesthesia (numbness) (<2%)
Insomnia (<2%)
Nervousness (<2%)
Neurotoxicity [3]
Nightmares (<2%)
Paresthesias (<2%)
Peripheral neuropathy (3%)
Seizures (<2%)
Sleep-related disorder (<2%)
Somnolence (drowsiness) (<2%)
Syncope / fainting (<2%)
Tremor (<2%)
Vertigo / dizziness (<2%)

Endocrine/Metabolic
Diabetes mellitus (<2%)
Dyslipidemia (<2%)
Gynecomastia (<2%)

Gastrointestinal/Hepatic
Abdominal distension (<2%)
Abdominal pain (3%)
Constipation (<2%)
Diarrhea [3]
Flatulence (<2%)
Gastritis / pangastritis / gastric irritation (<2%)
Gastroesophageal reflux (<2%)
Hematemesis (<2%)
Hepatic failure (<2%)
Hepatomegaly (<2%)
Hepatotoxicity / liver injury / acute liver injury / drug-induced liver injury (DILI) [2]
Nausea [4]
Pancreatitis / acute pancreatitis (<2%)
Retching (<2%)

Hematologic
Hemolytic anemia (<2%)

Neuromuscular/Skeletal
Asthenia / fatigue (3%)

Ocular
Vision blurred (<2%)

Renal
Renal failure (<2%)

Respiratory
Bronchospasm (<2%)
Dyspnea / shortness of breath (<2%)

Other
Adverse effects / adverse reactions [6]

EUCALYPTUS

Family: Myrtaceae
Scientific names: *Eucalyptus bicostata, Eucalyptus fruticetorum, Eucalyptus globulus, Eucalyptus odorata, Eucalyptus pauciflora, Eucalyptus polybractea, Eucalyptus smithii*
Indications: Asthma, bronchitis, cough, croup, fever, joint and muscle pains, nasal congestion, sore throats, rheumatism. Flavoring, fragrance, toothpaste, substances used in root canal fillings
Class: Anti-inflammatory, Diuretic
Half-life: N/A
Clinically important, potentially hazardous interactions with: aminophylline, amitriptyline, borage, carisoprodol, coltsfoot, comfrey, diazepam, insulin, lansoprazole, nelfinavir, pantoprazole
Note: [O] = Oral.

EVENING PRIMROSE

Family: Onagraceae
Scientific names: *Oenothera biennis, Oenothera muricata, Oenothera purpurata, Oenothera rubricaulis, Oenothera suaveolens*
Indications: Mastalgia, osteoporosis, atopic dermatitis, rheumatoid arthritis, hypercholesterolemia, chronic fatigue syndrome, neurodermatitis, ulcerative colitis, irritable bowel syndrome. Used in soaps and cosmetics
Class: Anti-inflammatory, Gamma linoleic acid
Half-life: N/A
Clinically important, potentially hazardous interactions with: aspirin, chlorpromazine, fluphenazine, phenothiazine
Note: The Medicines Control Agency (MCA) has withdrawn licenses for prescription evening primrose drug products under the brand names of Epogam and Efamast. This was because there is not enough evidence that they are effective.

Other
Adverse effects / adverse reactions [3]

EVEROLIMUS

Trade names: Afinitor (Novartis), Certican (Novartis), Zortress (Novartis)
Indications: Prophylaxis of organ rejection in adults following kidney or liver transplant, advanced renal cell carcinoma, neuroendocrine tumors of pancreatic, gastrointestinal or lung origin, breast cancer in post-menopausal women with advanced hormone-receptor positive, HER2-negative type cancer, renal angiomyolipoma and tuberous sclerosis complex, subependymal giant cell astrocytoma associated with tuberous sclerosis
Class: Antineoplastic / anticancer agent (see also Immune checkpoint inhibitor), Immunosuppressant, mTOR inhibitor
Half-life: ~30 hours
Clinically important, potentially hazardous interactions with: aprepitant, atazanavir, atorvastatin, benazepril, captopril, clarithromycin, clozapine, conivaptan, cyclosporine, darunavir, delavirdine, digoxin, efavirenz, enalapril, erythromycin, grapefruit juice, indinavir, itraconazole, ketoconazole, lapatinib, lisinopril, live vaccines, nelfinavir, oxcarbazepine, phenytoin, posaconazole, quinapril, ramipril, ribociclib, rifampin, rifapentine, ritonavir, saquinavir, St John's wort, telithromycin, venetoclax, verapamil, viloxazine, voriconazole
Important contra-indications noted in the prescribing guidelines for: nursing mothers; pediatric patients
Warning: In immunosuppression therapy: MALIGNANCIES AND SERIOUS INFECTIONS, KIDNEY GRAFT THROMBOSIS; NEPHROTOXICITY
In heart transplantation: MORTALITY

Skin
Acneiform eruption / acneiform dermatitis / acneiform rash (3–25%) [5]
Angioedema (formerly named angioneurotic edema) [4]
Baboon syndrome / symmetrical drug-related intertriginous and flexural exanthema (SDRIFE) [2]
Cellulitis and pseudocellulitis (21%)
Contact dermatitis (14%)
Cutaneous toxicity / skin toxicity [9]
Dermatitis [2]
Edema / fluid retention (39%) [6]
Erythema (4%) [2]
Exanthems [4]
Excoriations (14%)
Hand–foot syndrome (palmar–plantar erythrodysesthesia) (5%) [9]
Hypersensitivity [2]
Lymphedema [2]
Peripheral edema (4–39%) [8]
Pityriasis rosea (4%)
Pruritus (itching) (14–21%) [5]
Rash (18–59%) [51]
Tinea (18%)
Xerosis / xeroderma (13–18%)

Nails
Nail disorder (4–22%) [2]

Mucosal
Aphthous stomatitis / aphthous ulcer / aphtha (aphthae) [5]
Epistaxis (nosebleed) (18–22%) [3]
Mucosal inflammation (19%) [3]
Mucositis [18]
Nasal congestion (14%)
Oral ulceration [4]
Oropharyngeal pain (11%)
Rhinorrhea (3%)
Stomatitis (oral mucositis) (44–86%) [88]
Xerostomia (dry mouth) (8–11%)

Cardiovascular
Chest pain (5%)
Hypertension (4–13%) [14]
Tachycardia (3%)

Central Nervous System
Anorexia (25%) [12]
Anxiety (7%)
Chills (4%)
Dysgeusia (taste perversion) (10–19%) [2]
Fever (pyrexia) (includes hyperpyrexia) (20–32%) [7]
Headache (18–30%) [4]
Insomnia (9%)
Migraine (30%)
Pain [2]
Peripheral neuropathy [2]
Seizures (29%)
Somnolence (drowsiness) (7%)
Tremor [2]
Vertigo / dizziness (7–14%)

Endocrine/Metabolic
ALT increased (21–48%) [4]
Amenorrhea [2]
Appetite decreased (30%) [5]
AST increased (25–56%) [3]
Diabetes mellitus (2–10%) [2]
Dyslipidemia [2]
GGT increased [2]
Hypercholesterolemia [9]
Hyperglycemia (includes glucose increased) [40]
Hyperlipidemia / lipids elevated [9]
Hypertriglyceridemia (includes triglycerides increased) [3]
Hypokalemia [5]
Hypomagnesemia [2]
Hyponatremia [3]
Hypophosphatemia [5]
Hypothyroidism [2]
Serum creatinine increased (19–50%) [4]
Weight loss (9–28%) [3]

Gastrointestinal/Hepatic
Abdominal pain (9–36%) [4]
Constipation (11–14%)
Diarrhea (25–50%) [36]
Dysphagia (4%)
Gastritis / pangastritis / gastric irritation (7%)
Gastroenteritis (18%)
Gastrointestinal bleeding [3]
Hemorrhoids (5%)
Hepatotoxicity / liver injury / acute liver injury / drug-induced liver injury (DILI) [8]
Nausea (26–32%) [12]
Pancreatitis / acute pancreatitis [2]
Vomiting (20–29%) [3]

Genitourinary
Urinary tract infection (15%)

Hematologic
Anemia [40]
Cytopenia [2]
Febrile neutropenia [5]
Hemoglobin decreased (86–92%) [2]
Hemolytic uremic syndrome [2]
Hemorrhage (3%) [3]
Hemotoxicity [5]
Immunosupression [2]
Leukocytopenia (leukopenia) / leukocytes (white blood cells) decreased [5]
Lymphopenia (lymphocytopenia) / lymphocytes decreased [8]
Neutropenia (neutrophils decreased) [19]
Sepsis [2]
Thrombocytopenia / platelets decreased [24]

Neuromuscular/Skeletal
Arthralgia (15%)
Asthenia / fatigue (7–45%) [64]
Back pain (15%)
Jaw pain (3%)
Muscle spasm (10%)
Pain in extremities (10–14%)

Ocular
Conjunctivitis (conjunctival inflammation) (2%)
Eyelid edema / palpebral edema / blepharedema (4%) [2]
Ocular hyperemia (4%)

Otic
Otitis (otitis externa, otitis media, otitis interna) (36%)

Renal
Nephrotoxicity / kidney injury / acute kidney injury (AKI) / drug-induced kidney injury [7]
Proteinuria (7%) [17]
Renal failure (3%) [3]

Respiratory
Cough (21–30%) [6]
Dyspnea / shortness of breath (20–24%) [8]
Interstitial lung disease / interstitial pneumonitis / interstitial pneumonia (cryptogenic organizing pneumonia) / drug-induced interstitial lung disease [2]
Nasopharyngitis (25%)
Pharyngitis (sore throat) (11%)
Pharyngolaryngeal pain (4%)
Pleural effusion (7%)
Pneumocystis jirovecii pneumonia [5]
Pneumonia [11]
Pneumonitis (14–17%) [46]
Pulmonary toxicity [11]
Rhinitis / rhinosinusitis (see also sinusitis) (25%)
Sinusitis (see also rhinitis / rhinosinusitis) (39%)
Upper respiratory tract infection (25–82%) [3]

Other
Adverse effects / adverse reactions [32]
Death [10]
Infection (18%) [32]
Side effects [2]

EVOLOCUMAB

Trade name: Repatha (Amgen)
Indications: Heterozygous or homozygous familial hypercholesterolemia where additional lowering of low density lipoprotein cholesterol is required, hyperlipidemia
Class: Monoclonal antibody, Proprotein convertase subtilisin kexin type 9 (PCSK9) inhibitor
Half-life: 11–17 days
Clinically important, potentially hazardous interactions with: none known
Pregnancy category: No data available but likely to cross the placenta in second and third trimester
Important contra-indications noted in the prescribing guidelines for: pediatric patients

---

Mucosal
Nasal congestion [3]
Oropharyngeal pain [3]

Cardiovascular
Hypertension (2%)

Central Nervous System
Headache (4%) [11]
Neurotoxicity [2]
Vertigo / dizziness (3%)

Endocrine/Metabolic
Creatine phosphokinase (CPK) / creatine kinase increased (hyperCKemia) [9]

Gastrointestinal/Hepatic
Diarrhea (3%) [6]
Gastroenteritis (2%) [2]
Hepatotoxicity / liver injury / acute liver injury / drug-induced liver injury (DILI) [5]
Nausea [4]

Genitourinary
Urinary tract infection (<4%)

Local
Injection-site bruising [4]
Injection-site edema [2]
Injection-site erythema [3]
Injection-site pain [7]
Injection-site reaction (3–5%) [10]

Neuromuscular/Skeletal
Arthralgia (2%) [9]
Asthenia / fatigue [3]
Back pain (2–6%) [10]
Bone pain / joint pain (3%) [4]
Muscle spasm [7]
Myalgia/Myopathy (3%) [11]
Pain in extremities [5]

Respiratory
Cough (<4%) [4]
Influenza (<6%) [10]
Nasopharyngitis (4–10%) [14]
Pharyngitis (sore throat) [2]
Sinusitis (see also rhinitis / rhinosinusitis) (3%) [2]
Upper respiratory tract infection (2–6%) [12]

Other
Adverse effects / adverse reactions [8]
Allergic reactions (5%)

EXEMESTANE

Trade name: Aromasin (Pfizer)
Indications: Advanced breast cancer
Class: Aromatase inhibitor
Half-life: 24 hours
Clinically important, potentially hazardous interactions with: efavirenz, oxcarbazepine, rifapentine
Important contra-indications noted in the prescribing guidelines for: nursing mothers; pediatric patients

---

Skin
Cellulitis and pseudocellulitis [2]
Diaphoresis (6–12%) [2]
Edema / fluid retention (7%)
Hot flashes / hot flushes (30%) [7]
Lymphedema (2–5%)
Peripheral edema (9%) [2]
Pruritus (itching) (2–5%)
Radiation recall dermatitis [2]
Rash (2–5%) [6]

Hair
Alopecia / hair loss (2–5%)

Mucosal
Stomatitis (oral mucositis) [11]

Central Nervous System
Dysgeusia (taste perversion) [2]
Headache [3]
Insomnia [2]
Paresthesias (2–5%)
Tumor pain (30%)

Endocrine/Metabolic
Hyperglycemia (includes glucose increased) [5]

Gastrointestinal/Hepatic
Cholestatic liver injury / cholestatic hepatitis [2]
Diarrhea [4]
Nausea [2]

Hematologic
Anemia [3]

Neuromuscular/Skeletal
Arthralgia [4]
Asthenia / fatigue [7]
Back pain [2]
Bone pain / joint pain [2]
Myalgia/Myopathy [2]

Respiratory
Dyspnea / shortness of breath [2]
Pneumonitis [6]
Pulmonary toxicity [2]

Other
Adverse effects / adverse reactions [2]

EXENATIDE

Trade names: Bydureon (Amylin), Byetta (Amylin)
Indications: Type II diabetes mellitus
Class: Antidiabetic, Glucagon-like peptide-1 (GLP-1) receptor agonist, Incretin mimetic, Insulin secretagogue
Half-life: 2.4 hours
Clinically important, potentially hazardous interactions with: acetaminophen, alcohol, antibiotics, corticosteroids, lovastatin, oral contraceptives, pegvisomant, prandial insulin, somatropin, sulfonylureas, thiazide diuretics, vitamin K antagonists, warfarin
Important contra-indications noted in the prescribing guidelines for: nursing mothers; pediatric patients
Note: Risk of thyroid C-cell tumors with exenatide extended release formulations. Bydureon is contra-indicated in patients with a personal or family history of medullary thyroid carcinoma or in patients with multiple endocrine neoplasia syndrome Type 2.

Skin
Anaphylactoid reactions / anaphylaxis (includes anaphylactic shock) [3]
Hyperhidrosis (<10%)
Urticaria / hives [2]

Cardiovascular
Cardiotoxicity [2]

Central Nervous System
Chills (<2%)
Headache (<10%) [9]
Vertigo / dizziness (<10%) [4]

Endocrine/Metabolic
Appetite decreased (<10%) [3]
Hypoglycemia (>5%) [7]

Gastrointestinal/Hepatic
Abdominal distension (<10%)
Abdominal pain (<10%) [2]
Constipation (>5%) [3]
Diarrhea (<11%) [19]
Dyspepsia / functional dyspepsia (indigestion) (see also gastroparesis) (<10%)
Flatulence (2%)
Gastroenteritis (<10%)
Gastroesophageal reflux (3%)
Gastrointestinal disorder / discomfort [3]
Nausea (<11%) [46]
Pancreatitis / acute pancreatitis [12]
Vomiting (~10%) [27]

Genitourinary
Urinary tract infection [2]

Local
- Injection-site erythema (5–7%)
- Injection-site nodules (~10%) [4]
- Injection-site pruritus (5–6%) [2]
- Injection-site reaction [8]

Neuromuscular/Skeletal
- Asthenia / fatigue (<10%)

Renal
- Nephrotoxicity / kidney injury / acute kidney injury (AKI) / drug-induced kidney injury [2]
- Renal failure [3]

Respiratory
- Nasopharyngitis [2]

Other
- Adverse effects / adverse reactions [10]
- Cancer [2]
- Death [2]

EZETIMIBE

Trade names: Ezetrol (Merck), Liptruzet (Merck Sharpe & Dohme), Vytorin (MSD), Zetia (Merck)
Indications: Hypercholesterolemia
Class: Cholesterol inhibitor
Half-life: 22 hours
Clinically important, potentially hazardous interactions with: cholestyramine, cyclosporine, fenofibrate, gemfibrozil, HMG-CoA reductase inhibitors, ritonavir
Pregnancy category: Pregnancy category is X when combined with a statin.
Important contra-indications noted in the prescribing guidelines for: nursing mothers
Note: Liptruzet is ezetimibe and atorvastatin; vytorin is ezetimibe and simvastatin.

Skin
- Rash [3]

Central Nervous System
- Headache [5]
- Vertigo / dizziness [4]

Endocrine/Metabolic
- Creatine phosphokinase (CPK) / creatine kinase increased (hyperCKemia) [8]

Gastrointestinal/Hepatic
- Abdominal pain (2%)
- Diarrhea [4]
- Hepatotoxicity / liver injury / acute liver injury / drug-induced liver injury (DILI) [6]
- Nausea [4]
- Pancreatitis / acute pancreatitis [3]

Genitourinary
- Urinary tract infection [2]

Hematologic
- Thrombocytopenia / platelets decreased [2]

Local
- Injection-site erythema [2]
- Injection-site reaction [6]

Neuromuscular/Skeletal
- Arthralgia (4%) [3]
- Asthenia / fatigue [2]
- Back pain (4%) [4]
- Bone pain / joint pain [4]
- Muscle spasm [3]
- Myalgia/Myopathy (5%) [16]
- Pain in extremities [2]

Respiratory
- Cough (2%)
- Influenza [3]
- Nasopharyngitis [5]
- Upper respiratory tract infection [3]

Other
- Adverse effects / adverse reactions [8]

EZOGABINE

Synonym: retigabine
Trade names: Potiga (GSK), Trobalt (GSK)
Indications: Epilepsy
Class: Anticonvulsant (see also antiepileptic (anti-seizure)), Potassium channel opener
Half-life: 7–11 hours
Clinically important, potentially hazardous interactions with: alcohol, carbamazepine, digoxin, phenytoin
Important contra-indications noted in the prescribing guidelines for: the elderly; nursing mothers; pediatric patients
Note: In 2013, the FDA placed a black boxed warning on the retigabine (ezogabine) drug label, related to risks of retinal abnormalities, potential vision loss, and blue discoloration of the skin, nail, mucous membrane, and eyes. Retigabine was withdrawn in the UK from the beginning of 2017.
Warning: RETINAL ABNORMALITIES AND POTENTIAL VISION LOSS

Skin
- Hyperhidrosis (<2%)
- Peripheral edema (<2%)
- Pigmentation (Skin) (includes hyperpigmentation) [2]

Mucosal
- Mucosal membrane pigmentation [4]
- Xerostomia (dry mouth) (<2%)

Central Nervous System
- Amnesia (2%)
- Anxiety (3%)
- Aphasia (4%)
- Balance disorder (4%)
- Confusion (9%) [6]
- Disorientation (2%)
- Dysarthria (4%) [3]
- Dysphasia (2%)
- Gait instability / postural instability (4%)
- Hallucinations (<2%)
- Headache [6]
- Hypokinesia (<2%)
- Impaired concentration (6%)
- Incoordination (7%)
- Memory loss/memory impaired (6%)
- Neurotoxicity [3]
- Paresthesias (3%)
- Somnolence (drowsiness) (22%) [14]
- Speech disorder [3]
- Tremor (8%) [3]
- Vertigo / dizziness (31%) [14]

Endocrine/Metabolic
- Appetite increased (<2%)
- Weight gain (dose related) (3%)

Gastrointestinal/Hepatic
- Constipation (3%)
- Dyspepsia / functional dyspepsia (indigestion) (see also gastroparesis) (2%)
- Dysphagia (<2%)
- Nausea (7%) [5]

Genitourinary
- Dysuria (2%)
- Hematuria (2%)
- Urinary hesitancy (2%)
- Urinary retention (<2%) [6]
- Urinary tract infection [3]

Neuromuscular/Skeletal
- Asthenia / fatigue (20%) [11]
- Ataxia [3]
- Myoclonus (see also hypnic jerk) (<2%)

Ocular
- Diplopia (double vision) (7%) [2]
- Ocular pigmentation [5]
- Vision blurred (5%) [2]

Renal
- Chromaturia (2%)

Respiratory
- Influenza (3%)

Other
- Adverse effects / adverse reactions [2]

FACTOR VIII - VON WILLEBRAND FACTOR

Trade names: Alphanate (Grifols), Haemate (CSL Behring), Opivate (BPL)
Indications: Control and prevention of bleeding in patients with hemophilia A, surgical procedures in patients with von Willebrand disease in whom desmopressin is either ineffective or contraindicated
Class: Antihemorrhagic, Coagulation factor VIII
Half-life: 12.4 hours
Clinically important, potentially hazardous interactions with: none known

---

Skin
- Peripheral edema (<10%)
- Pruritus (itching) (<10%)
- Rash (<10%)

Central Nervous System
- Fever (pyrexia) (includes hyperpyrexia) (<10%)
- Headache (<10%)
- Rigors (<10%)
- Somnolence (drowsiness) (<10%)
- Vertigo / dizziness (<10%)

Local
- Infusion-site erythema (<10%)
- Infusion-site pain (<10%)
- Infusion-site rash (<10%)

FAMOTIDINE

Trade names: Duexis (Horizon), Pepcid (Valeant)
Indications: Duodenal ulcer, gastric ulcer, gastroesophageal reflux disease
Class: Histamine H2 receptor antagonist
Half-life: 2.5–3.5 hours
Clinically important, potentially hazardous interactions with: acalabrutinib, atazanavir, cefditoren, dasatinib, delavirdine, rilpivirine, sotorasib, thalidomide
Important contra-indications noted in the prescribing guidelines for: nursing mothers
Note: Duexis is famotidine and ibuprofen.

Skin
- Dermatitis [3]
- Peripheral edema [2]
- Pruritus (itching) [2]
- Rash [3]
- Urticaria / hives [3]
- Vasculitis (angiitis) / cutaneous vasculitis (angiitis) [2]

Cardiovascular
Hypertension [3]
Central Nervous System
Confusion [2]
Delirium [3]
Fever (pyrexia) (includes hyperpyrexia) [2]
Headache (5%) [4]
Neurotoxicity [2]
Somnolence (drowsiness) [2]
Endocrine/Metabolic
Hypomagnesemia [2]
Hypophosphatemia [2]
Gastrointestinal/Hepatic
Abdominal pain [2]
Diarrhea (2%) [3]
Dyspepsia / functional dyspepsia (indigestion) (see also gastroparesis) [3]
Gastroesophageal reflux [2]
Nausea [4]
Vomiting [4]
Genitourinary
Urinary tract infection [2]
Hematologic
Eosinophilia / eosinophils increased [2]
Thrombocytopenia / platelets decreased [2]
Neuromuscular/Skeletal
Arthralgia [2]
Back pain [2]
Respiratory
Influenza [2]
Sinusitis (see also rhinitis / rhinosinusitis) [2]
Upper respiratory tract infection [2]

FARICIMAB

Trade name: Vabysmo (Genentech)
Indications: 1. Neovascular (wet) age-related macular degeneration. 2. Diabetic macular edema.

Class: Angiopoietin-2 inhibitor, Vascular endothelial growth factor (VEGF) inhibitor / antagonist
Half-life: 7.5 days (estimated)
Clinically important, potentially hazardous interactions with: none known
Pregnancy category: No adequate and well-controlled studies of faricimab administration in pregnant women..
Note: Faricimab is contraindicated in patients with: ocular or periocular infections; active intraocular inflammation; a known hypersensitivity to faricimab or any of its excipients. Hypersensitivity reactions may manifest as rash, pruritus, urticaria, erythema, or severe intraocular inflammation.

Ocular
Conjunctival hemorrhage (7%)
Intraocular inflammation (1–2%)
Intraocular pressure increased (3%)
Ocular pain (2–3%)
Vitreous floaters / floaters / myodesopsia / myiodesopsia / muscae volitantes (3%)
Other
Adverse effects / adverse reactions [2]

FEBUXOSTAT

Trade name: Uloric (Takeda)
Indications: Hyperuricemia in gout
Class: Xanthine oxidase inhibitor
Half-life: 5–8 hours
Clinically important, potentially hazardous interactions with: aminophylline, azathioprine, didanosine, mercaptopurine, oxtriphylline, theophylline

---

Skin
Rash (2%) [7]
Stevens-Johnson syndrome and toxic epidermal necrolysis (SJS/TEN) [2]
Cardiovascular
Cardiac disorder / cardiac dysfunction [2]
Cardiotoxicity [2]
Cardiovascular adverse effect (includes major adverse cardiovascular events (MACE)) [3]
Central Nervous System
Headache [5]
Vertigo / dizziness [5]
Gastrointestinal/Hepatic
Diarrhea [9]
Hepatotoxicity / liver injury / acute liver injury / drug-induced liver injury (DILI) (5%) [14]
Nausea [7]
Vomiting [2]
Hematologic
Agranulocytosis / severe selective neutropenia [2]
Neuromuscular/Skeletal
Arthralgia [5]
Bone pain / joint pain [2]
Gouty tophi (flare) [3]
Joint disorder [2]
Respiratory
Upper respiratory tract infection [2]
Other
Adverse effects / adverse reactions [7]

FEDRATINIB HYDROCHLORIDE

Trade name: Inrebic (Impact Biomedicines)
Indications: Treatment of adult patients with intermediate-2 or high-risk primary or secondary (post-polycythemia vera or post-essential thrombocythemia) myelofibrosis
Class: Janus kinase-2 inhibitor, Kinase inhibitor
Half-life: ~114 hours
Clinically important, potentially hazardous interactions with: CYP3A4 and CYP2C19 inhibitors, strong and moderate CYP3A4 inducers, strong CYP3A4 inhibitors
Pregnancy category: There are no available data on the use of fedratinib in pregnant women to evaluate for a drug-associated risk of major birth defects, miscarriage or adverse maternal or fetal outcomes.
Important contra-indications noted in the prescribing guidelines for: nursing mothers
Note: Avoid use in patients with severe hepatic impairment. Advise patients not to breastfeed.
Warning:
SERIOUS AND FATAL ENCEPHALOPATHY, INCLUDING WERNICKE'S, HAS OCCURRED IN PATIENTS TREATED WITH FEDRATINIB. WERNICKE'S ENCEPHALOPATHY IS A NEUROLOGIC EMERGENCY. ASSESS THIAMINE LEVELS IN ALL PATIENTS PRIOR TO STARTING FEDRATINIB, PERIODICALLY DURING TREATMENT, AND AS CLINICALLY INDICATED. DO NOT START FEDRATINIB IN PATIENTS WITH THIAMINE DEFICIENCY; REPLETE THIAMINE PRIOR TO TREATMENT INITIATION. IF ENCEPHALOPATHY IS SUSPECTED, IMMEDIATELY DISCONTINUE FEDRATINIB AND INITIATE PARENTERAL THIAMINE. MONITOR UNTIL SYMPTOMS RESOLVE OR IMPROVE AND THIAMINE LEVELS NORMALIZE.

Cardiovascular
Cardiac failure (5%)
Hypertension (3%)
Central Nervous System
Encephalopathy (includes hepatic encephalopathy) (including Wernicke's encephalopathy) (fatal / 1 case) [3]
Headache (9%)
Vertigo / dizziness (8%)
Endocrine/Metabolic
ALT increased (9%)
AST increased (5%)
Hyperamylasemia (2%)
Hyperlipasemia (10%)
Serum creatinine increased (1% ≥ grade 3) (10%)
Weight gain (9%)
Gastrointestinal/Hepatic
Diarrhea (5% ≥ grade 3) (66%) [2]
Nausea (62%) [2]
Vomiting (3% ≥ grade 3) (39%) [2]
Genitourinary
Dysuria (6%)
Urinary tract infection (6%)
Hematologic
Anemia (30% ≥ grade 3) (40%) [4]
Thrombocytopenia / platelets decreased (12%) [2]
Neuromuscular/Skeletal
Asthenia / fatigue (5% ≥ grade 3) (19%)
Bone pain / joint pain (8%)
Muscle spasm (12%)
Pain in extremities (10%)
Other
Adverse effects / adverse reactions (serious ≥ 2%) (21%)

FELBAMATE

Trade name: Felbatol (MedPointe)
Indications: Partial seizures
Class: Anticonvulsant (see also antiepileptic (anti-seizure))
Half-life: 13–23 hours
Clinically important, potentially hazardous interactions with: levonorgestrel, ulipristal
Important contra-indications noted in the prescribing guidelines for: nursing mothers
Note: Contraindicated in patients with a history of any blood dyscrasia or hepatic dysfunction.
Warning: APLASTIC ANEMIA and HEPATIC FAILURE

Skin
Acneiform eruption / acneiform dermatitis / acneiform rash (3%)
Facial edema (3%)
Rash (4%) [2]
Stevens-Johnson syndrome and toxic epidermal necrolysis (SJS/TEN) [2]

Mucosal
Xerostomia (dry mouth) (3%)

Central Nervous System
Dysgeusia (taste perversion) (6%)
Paresthesias (4%)

Endocrine/Metabolic
Hypophosphatemia (3%)
Weight loss [2]

Gastrointestinal/Hepatic
Constipation (7%)
Diarrhea (5%)
Dyspepsia / functional dyspepsia (indigestion) (see also gastroparesis) (9%)
Hepatotoxicity / liver injury / acute liver injury / drug-induced liver injury (DILI) [4]
Vomiting (9%)

Genitourinary
Urinary tract infection (3%)
Vaginal bleeding (intramenstual) (3%)

Hematologic
Anemia [4]

Neuromuscular/Skeletal
Myalgia/Myopathy (3%)

Ocular
Diplopia (double vision) (3%)

Otic
Otitis (otitis externa, otitis media, otitis interna) (3%)

Respiratory
Rhinitis / rhinosinusitis (see also sinusitis) (7%)
Upper respiratory tract infection (9%)

Other
Side effects [2]

FELODIPINE

Trade names: Lexxel (AstraZeneca), Plendil (AstraZeneca)
Indications: Hypertension
Class: Calcium channel blocker
Half-life: 11–16 hours
Clinically important, potentially hazardous interactions with: amprenavir, atazanavir, boceprevir, carbamazepine, cobicistat/elvitegravir/emtricitabine/tenofovir alafenamide, cobicistat/elvitegravir/emtricitabine/tenofovir disoproxil, delavirdine, epirubicin, grapefruit juice, imatinib, indinavir, itraconazole, lopinavir, paclitaxel, posaconazole, telaprevir, venetoclax
Important contra-indications noted in the prescribing guidelines for: the elderly; nursing mothers; pediatric patients
Note: Lexxel is felodipine and enalapril.

Skin
Erythema (2%)
Exanthems [2]
Facial edema (2%)
Flushing / rubefaction (>25%) [10]
Peripheral edema (22%) [6]
Rash (2%)
Telangiectasia [2]
Urticaria / hives (2%)

Mucosal
Gingival hyperplasia / gingival hypertrophy / gingival enlargement / gingival overgrowth (2–10%) [6]

Central Nervous System
Paresthesias (2%)

Neuromuscular/Skeletal
Myalgia/Myopathy (2%)

FENOFIBRATE

Trade name: Tricor (AbbVie)
Indications: Hyperlipidemia
Class: Fibrate, Lipid regulator
Half-life: 20 hours
Clinically important, potentially hazardous interactions with: atorvastatin, colchicine, dicumarol, ezetimibe, lovastatin, nicotinic acid, rosuvastatin, statins, warfarin
Important contra-indications noted in the prescribing guidelines for: the elderly; nursing mothers; pediatric patients

---

Skin
Photosensitivity [11]
Phototoxicity [2]
Pruritus (itching) (4%)
Rash (2–8%) [3]

Endocrine/Metabolic
Gynecomastia [2]

Gastrointestinal/Hepatic
Hepatotoxicity / liver injury / acute liver injury / drug-induced liver injury (DILI) [15]
Pancreatitis / acute pancreatitis [3]

Hematologic
Thrombocytopenia / platelets decreased [2]

Neuromuscular/Skeletal
Myalgia/Myopathy [11]
Rhabdomyolysis [19]

Renal
Nephrotoxicity / kidney injury / acute kidney injury (AKI) / drug-induced kidney injury [3]
Renal failure [3]

Other
Adverse effects / adverse reactions (<10%)

FENOLDOPAM

Trade name: Corlopam (AbbVie) (Neurex)
Indications: Hypertension (severe), hypertensive emergency
Class: Dopamine receptor agonist
Half-life: ~5 minutes
Clinically important, potentially hazardous interactions with: none known

FENTANYL

Trade names: Actiq (Cephalon), Duragesic (Janssen)
Indications: Chronic pain
Class: Analgesic; opioid, Anesthetic
Half-life: ~7 hours
Clinically important, potentially hazardous interactions with: amiodarone, amprenavir, aprepitant, atazanavir, ceritinib, cimetidine, conivaptan, crizotinib, darunavir, dasatinib, delavirdine, desipramine, efavirenz, eluxadoline, enzalutamide, indinavir, itraconazole, ketoconazole, lapatinib, letermovir, lopinavir, mifepristone, nelfinavir, nevirapine, nifedipine, osimertinib, ranitidine, ribociclib, rifapentine, ritonavir, saquinavir, telithromycin, voriconazole
Important contra-indications noted in the prescribing guidelines for: nursing mothers; pediatric patients
Note: Contra-indicated in opioid non-tolerant patients, and for the management of acute or postoperative pain including headache/migraines and dental pain.
Warning: ADDICTION, ABUSE, and MISUSE; LIFE-THREATENING RESPIRATORY DEPRESSION; ACCIDENTAL EXPOSURE; NEONATAL OPIOID WITHDRAWAL SYNDROME; CYTOCHROME P450 3A4 INTERACTION.
EXPOSURE TO HEAT (for topical patches)

Skin
Anaphylactoid reactions / anaphylaxis (includes anaphylactic shock) [6]
Diaphoresis (>10%) [2]
Edema / fluid retention (>10%)
Erythema (at application site) [3]
Flushing / rubefaction (3–10%)
Pruritus (itching) (3–44%) [30]
Rash [3]

Mucosal
Xerostomia (dry mouth) (>10%) [3]

Cardiovascular
Bradycardia / sinus bradycardia (>10%) [3]
Hypotension [9]
Tachycardia [2]

Central Nervous System
Agitation [2]
Anorexia [2]
Coma [2]
Confusion (>10%)
Delirium [2]
Depression (>10%)
Hallucinations [2]
Headache (>10%)
Hyperalgesia [2]
Leukoencephalopathy / posterior reversible encephalopathy syndrome (PRES) [6]
Neuroleptic malignant syndrome [2]
Sedation [3]
Serotonin syndrome [4]
Somnolence (drowsiness) [15]
Vertigo / dizziness [13]

Endocrine/Metabolic
Adrenal insufficiency (hypoadrenalism) / Addisonian crisis (includes Addison's disease) [3]

Gastrointestinal/Hepatic
Constipation (>10%) [11]
Nausea (>10%) [33]
Vomiting (>10%) [23]

Local
Application-site erythema [2]

Neuromuscular/Skeletal
Asthenia / fatigue (>10%) [2]
Chest wall rigidity [6]
Myoclonus (see also hypnic jerk) [3]

Ocular
Miosis (>10%)

Respiratory
Cough [18]
Respiratory depression [8]

Other
Adverse effects / adverse reactions [8]
Death [7]

FERRIC CARBOXYMALTOSE (INJECTION)

Trade names: Ferinject (Vifor Pharma), Injectafer (American Reagent)
Indications: Iron deficiency anemia in adult patients
Class: Iron supplement
Half-life: 7–12 hours
Clinically important, potentially hazardous interactions with: none known
Note: Serious hypersensitivity reactions, including anaphylactic-type reactions, some of which have been life-threatening and fatal, have been reported in patients receiving ferric carboxymaltose injection. Patients may present with shock, clinically significant hypotension, loss of consciousness, and/or collapse. Monitor patients for signs and symptoms of hypersensitivity during and after Injectafer administration for at least 30 minutes and until clinically stable following completion of the infusion. Only administer when personnel and therapies are immediately available for the treatment of serious hypersensitivity reactions.

Skin
Hot flashes / hot flushes (4%)

Cardiovascular
Hypertension (4%)

Central Nervous System
Vertigo / dizziness (2%)

Endocrine/Metabolic
Hypophosphatemia (2%) [5]

Gastrointestinal/Hepatic
Nausea (7%)
Vomiting (2%)

Other
Adverse effects / adverse reactions [4]

FERRIC MALTOL

Synonym: Accrufer
Trade name: Accrufer (Shield Therapeutics)
Indications: Treatment of iron deficiency in adults
Class: Iron supplement
Half-life: n/a
Clinically important, potentially hazardous interactions with: dimercaprol
Pregnancy category: An overdose of iron in pregnant women may carry a risk for spontaneous abortion, gestational diabetes and fetal malformation.

Gastrointestinal/Hepatic
Abdominal pain (3%)
Constipation (4%)
Diarrhea (4%)
Feces discolored (4%)
Flatulence (5%)
Nausea (2%)
Vomiting (2%)

FERROUS SULFATE

Trade names: Feosol (Meda), Fer-In-Sol (Mead Johnson), Feratab (Upsher-Smith)
Indications: Iron deficiency anemia
Class: Iron supplement
Half-life: 6 hours
Clinically important, potentially hazardous interactions with: antacids, caffeine, calcium supplements, cimetidine, deferoxamine, dimercaprol, etidronate, fluoroquinolones, pancreatin, pancrelipase, penicillamine, tetracylines, trientine, zinc

Gastrointestinal/Hepatic
Gastritis / pangastritis / gastric irritation [5]

Other
Adverse effects / adverse reactions [2]

FERUMOXYTOL

Trade name: Feraheme (AMG Pharma)
Indications: Iron deficiency anemia in adults with chronic kidney disease
Class: Iron supplement
Half-life: 15 hours
Clinically important, potentially hazardous interactions with: none known
Important contra-indications noted in the prescribing guidelines for: the elderly; nursing mothers; pediatric patients
Note: May cause hypersensitivity reactions, hypotension and iron overload. Feraheme may transiently affect magnetic resonance (MRI) imaging for up to 3 months following dosage. Contra-indicated in patients with evidence of iron overload or anemia not caused by iron deficiency.

Skin
Anaphylactoid reactions / anaphylaxis (includes anaphylactic shock) [4]
Hypersensitivity [3]
Pruritus (itching) [5]
Rash [2]
Urticaria / hives [2]

Cardiovascular
Hypotension (3%) [3]

Central Nervous System
Headache [6]
Vertigo / dizziness (3%) [3]

Gastrointestinal/Hepatic
Abdominal pain [2]
Nausea (3%) [6]
Vomiting [2]

Local
Injection-site pain [3]

Neuromuscular/Skeletal
Asthenia / fatigue [2]
Back pain [2]

Respiratory
Dyspnea / shortness of breath [3]

Other
Adverse effects / adverse reactions [2]

FESOTERODINE

Trade name: Toviaz (Pfizer)
Indications: Overactive bladder syndrome, urinary incontinence, urgency and frequency
Class: Muscarinic antagonist
Half-life: 7 hours; 4 hours (oral)
Clinically important, potentially hazardous interactions with: alcohol, amantadine, anticholinergics, antidepressants, antimuscarinics, atazanavir, botulinum toxin (A & B), carbamazepine, cinacalcet, clarithromycin, conivaptan, CYP2D6 inhibitors, CYP3A4 inhibitors, CYP3AF inhibitors, darunavir, dasatinib, deferasirox, delavirdine, duloxetine, indinavir, itraconazole, ketoconazole, nefazodone, nelfinavir, PEG-interferon, phenobarbital, phenytoin, pramlintide, rifampin, ritonavir, saquinavir, secretin, St John's wort, telithromycin, terbinafine, tipranavir, tocilizumab, voriconazole
Important contra-indications noted in the prescribing guidelines for: nursing mothers; pediatric patients
Note: Contra-indicated in patients with urinary retention, gastric retention, or uncontrolled narrow-angle glaucoma.

Mucosal
Xerostomia (dry mouth) (19–35%) [29]

Central Nervous System
Headache [3]

Gastrointestinal/Hepatic
Constipation (4–6%) [17]
Diarrhea (<10%)
Dyspepsia / functional dyspepsia (indigestion) (see also gastroparesis) (<2%) [2]
Nausea (<2%) [2]

Genitourinary
Dysuria (<2%)
Urinary retention [2]
Urinary tract infection (3–4%) [3]

Neuromuscular/Skeletal
Back pain (2%)

Ocular
Vision blurred [2]
Xerophthalmia (dry eyes) (<4%) [2]

Respiratory
Upper respiratory tract infection (2–3%)

Other
Adverse effects / adverse reactions [3]

FEVERFEW

Family: Asteraceae; Compositae
Scientific names: *Chrysanthemum parthenium, Pyrethrum parthenium, Tanacetum parthenium*
Indications: Fever, headache, migraine, menstrual irregularities, arthritis, psoriasis, allergy, asthma, tinnitus, vertigo, nausea, cold, earache, orthopedic disorders, swollen feet, diarrhea, dyspepsia
Class: Antipyretic
Half-life: N/A
Clinically important, potentially hazardous interactions with: anticoagulants, NSAIDs

Skin
Angioedema (formerly named angioneurotic edema) (lips) [3]
Dermatitis [4]

Mucosal
Oral ulceration [3]
Central Nervous System
Ageusia (taste loss) / taste disorder [2]
Other
Adverse effects / adverse reactions [4]

FEXINIDAZOLE

Synonym: Fexinidazole Winthrop
Trade name: Fexinidazole (Sanofi)
Indications: Treatment of both first-stage (hemolymphatic) and second-stage (meningoencephalitic) human African trypanosomiasis due to *Trypanosoma brucei gambiense*
Class: Antimicrobial, Antiprotozoal
Clinically important, potentially hazardous interactions with: adefovir, bupropion, carbamazepine, cefaclor, clarithromycin, diazepam, dofetilide, duloxetine, efavirenz, erythromycin, fluconazole, furosemide, itraconazole, lansoprazole, lovastatin, mephenytoin, metformin, midazolam, nisoldipine, phenytoin, rifampin, saquinavir, simvastatin, St John's wort, tacrine, theophylline, tizanidine, voriconazole
Pregnancy category: Insufficient to evaluate for a drug-associated risk of major birth defects or miscarriage.
Note: Avoid concomitant use of herbal medicines and supplements during treatment with fexinidazole.

Skin
Hot flashes / hot flushes (5%)
Hyperhidrosis (3%)
Pruritus (itching) (4%)
Mucosal
Sialorrhea (ptyalism; hypersalivation) (6%)
Cardiovascular
Chest pain (9%)
Hypertension (5%)
Palpitation (5%)
Central Nervous System
Agitation (4%)
Anxiety (4%)
Behavioral disturbances / personality changes (3%)
Extrapyramidal symptoms (3%)
Gait instability / postural instability (5%)
Headache (35%) [2]
Insomnia (28%)
Paresthesias (2%)
Tremor (22%)
Vertigo / dizziness (19%)
Warm feeling (includes feeling hot) (10%)
Endocrine/Metabolic
Appetite decreased (21%)
Hypoalbuminemia / albumin decreased (9%)
Hypocalcemia (14%)
Gastrointestinal/Hepatic
Abdominal distension (3%)
Abdominal pain (10%)
Constipation (5%)
Dyspepsia / functional dyspepsia (indigestion) (see also gastroparesis) (13%)
Gastritis / pangastritis / gastric irritation (3%)
Nausea (26%)
Vomiting (28%) [2]
Hematologic
Neutropenia (neutrophils decreased) (6%)
Neuromuscular/Skeletal
Asthenia / fatigue (23%)
Back pain (11%)
Muscle spasm (3%)
Neck pain (9%)
Ocular
Photophobia (2%)
Respiratory
Cough (6%)
Dyspnea / shortness of breath (2%)

FEXOFENADINE

Trade name: Allegra (Sanofi-Aventis)
Indications: Allergic rhinitis, pruritus, urticaria
Class: Histamine H1 receptor antagonist
Half-life: 14.4 hours
Clinically important, potentially hazardous interactions with: neratinib, St John's wort
Important contra-indications noted in the prescribing guidelines for: the elderly; nursing mothers; pediatric patients

---

Skin
Stevens-Johnson syndrome and toxic epidermal necrolysis (SJS/TEN) [2]
Urticaria / hives [3]
Central Nervous System
Headache (5–11%) [2]

FINASTERIDE

Trade names: Propecia (Merck), Proscar (Merck)
Indications: Benign prostatic hypertrophy, male-pattern baldness
Class: 5-alpha reductase inhibitor, Androgen antagonist, Enzyme inhibitor
Half-life: 5–8 hours
Clinically important, potentially hazardous interactions with: none known
Pregnancy category: Contra-indicated in women
Important contra-indications noted in the prescribing guidelines for: nursing mothers; pediatric patients
Note: UK reports of persistent sexual dysfunction after discontinuation of finasteride Since the first report was received in November 1992, the UK's MHRA has received 426 Yellow Card reports up until 5 April 2024 of finasteride (both 1mg and 5mg formulations) and sexual dysfunction, including reports of erectile dysfunction and decreased sex drive. In almost half of these reports, the outcome was recorded as 'not recovered' or 'not resolved'. UK reports of psychiatric dysfunction with finasteride Since the first report was received in February 1993, the UK's MHRA has received 281 reports of finasteride and depressed mood disorders and suicidal and self-injurious behaviours, up until 5 April 2024.

Skin
Folliculitis [2]
Rash [3]
Urticaria / hives [2]
Xerosis / xeroderma [2]
Hair
Hirsutism [3]
Cardiovascular
Postural hypotension [2]
Central Nervous System
Depression [7]
Headache [2]
Vertigo / dizziness (7%) [3]
Endocrine/Metabolic
Gynecomastia (<2%) [17]
Libido decreased (2–10%) [10]
Mastodynia (<2%)
Menstrual irregularities [2]
Genitourinary
Ejaculatory dysfunction [11]
Erectile dysfunction [9]
Impotence (5–19%)
Sexual dysfunction [8]
Neuromuscular/Skeletal
Asthenia / fatigue (5%) [3]
Myalgia/Myopathy (severe) [2]
Other
Adverse effects / adverse reactions [8]

FINERENONE

Trade name: Kerendia (Bayer)
Indications: Reduction of the risk of hospitalization and mortality in patients with, for example, heart failure, chronic kidney disease.
Class: Aldosterone antagonist / mineralocorticoid receptor antagonist (MRA)
Half-life: 2–3 hours
Clinically important, potentially hazardous interactions with: amiodarone, CYP3A4 inducers, CYP3A4 inhibitors, efavirenz, erythromycin, grapefruit juice, itraconazole
Pregnancy category: No available data in pregnancy to evaluate for a drug-associated risk of major birth defects, miscarriage or adverse maternal or fetal outcomes.
Important contra-indications noted in the prescribing guidelines for: nursing mothers
Note: More frequent serum potassium monitoring is advised in patients receiving concomitant therapy with drugs or supplements that increase serum potassium.

Cardiovascular
Hypotension (5%)
Endocrine/Metabolic
Hyperkalemia (18%) [6]

FINGOLIMOD

Trade name: Gilenya (Novartis)
Indications: Multiple sclerosis
Class: Covid-19 putative drug, Immunosuppressant
Half-life: 6–9 days
Clinically important, potentially hazardous interactions with: BCG vaccine, beta blockers, class Ia antiarrhythmics, class III antiarrhythmics, conivaptan, cyproterone, denosumab, digoxin, diltiazem, dronedarone, ketoconazole, leflunomide, live vaccines, natalizumab, PEG-interferon, pimecrolimus, QT prolonging drugs, roflumilast, sipuleucel-T, tacrolimus, tocilizumab, trastuzumab, typhoid vaccine, verapamil, yellow fever vaccine

Important contra-indications noted in the prescribing guidelines for: nursing mothers; pediatric patients
Note: Contra-indicated in patients with recent (within the last 6 months) occurrence of: myocardial infarction, unstable angina, stroke, transient ischemic attack, decompensated heart failure requiring hospitalization, or Class III/IV heart failure; history or presence of Mobitz Type II 2nd degree or 3rd degree AV block or sick sinus syndrome, unless patient has a pacemaker; baseline QT interval ≥500 ms; or is receiving treatment with Class Ia or Class III anti-arrhythmic drugs.

Skin
Basal cell carcinoma [4]
Eczema / eczematous reaction / eczematous eruption (3%)
Herpes (9%) [6]
Herpes simplex [3]
Herpes zoster [3]
Kaposi's sarcoma [2]
Lymphoma [2]
Melanoma [2]
Pruritus (itching) (3%)
Skin cancer [3]
Tinea (4%)
Varicella zoster [5]

Hair
Alopecia / hair loss (4%)

Cardiovascular
Asystole [2]
Atrial fibrillation [2]
Atrioventricular block [20]
Bradycardia / sinus bradycardia (4%) [25]
Cardiac failure [2]
Cardiotoxicity [3]
Hypertension (6%) [10]

Central Nervous System
Depression (8%)
Encephalopathy (includes hepatic encephalopathy) [2]
Headache (25%) [11]
Leukoencephalopathy / posterior reversible encephalopathy syndrome (PRES) [6]
Migraine (5%)
Paresthesias (5%)
Vertigo / dizziness (7%) [2]

Endocrine/Metabolic
ALT increased (14%) [3]
AST increased (14%)
GGT increased (5%)
Weight loss (5%)

Gastrointestinal/Hepatic
Diarrhea (12%) [4]
Gastroenteritis (5%)
Hepatotoxicity / liver injury / acute liver injury / drug-induced liver injury (DILI) [11]

Genitourinary
Urinary tract infection [2]

Hematologic
Leukocytopenia (leukopenia) / leukocytes (white blood cells) decreased (3%) [2]
Lymphopenia (lymphocytopenia) / lymphocytes decreased (4%) [15]

Neuromuscular/Skeletal
Asthenia / fatigue (3%) [5]
Back pain (12%) [6]

Ocular
Macular edema [23]
Ocular pain (3%)
Vision blurred (4%)

Respiratory
Bronchitis (8%)
Cough (10%) [4]
Dyspnea / shortness of breath (8%) [2]
Influenza (13%) [4]
Nasopharyngitis [5]
Pulmonary toxicity [4]
Respiratory tract infection [2]
Sinusitis (see also rhinitis / rhinosinusitis) (7%)
Upper respiratory tract infection [2]

Other
Adverse effects / adverse reactions [13]
Death [7]
Infection [18]
Neoplasms [2]

FISH OILS

Scientific names: *docosahexaenoic acid (DHA), eicosapentaenoic acid (EPA), Omega-3 fatty acids*
Indications: Albuminuria, anorexia nervosa, cardiovascular disease, hypertension, lupus erythematosus, macular degeneration, osteoarthritis, otitis media, psoriasis
Class: Anti-inflammatory, Lipid regulator
Half-life: N/A
Clinically important, potentially hazardous interactions with: none known
Note: More than 25 mL or 3 g per day can decrease blood coagulation and increase the risk of bleeding. Fish oils contain a significant amount of vitamins A and D and high doses may be toxic.

Central Nervous System
Dysgeusia (taste perversion) [2]

FLAVOXATE

Trade name: Urispas (Ortho-McNeil)
Indications: Dysuria, urgency, nocturia
Class: Anticholinergic, Muscarinic antagonist
Half-life: Onset of action: 55–60 minutes
Clinically important, potentially hazardous interactions with: anticholinergics, arbutamine
Important contra-indications noted in the prescribing guidelines for: nursing mothers; pediatric patients

---

Mucosal
Xerostomia (dry mouth) (>10%)

Ocular
Glaucoma (includes acute angle-closure glaucoma) [2]

FLECAINIDE

Trade name: Tambocor (3M)
Indications: Atrial fibrillation
Class: Antiarrhythmic, Antiarrhythmic class Ic
Half-life: 12–16 hours
Clinically important, potentially hazardous interactions with: acebutolol, amiodarone, amisulpride, amitriptyline, artemether/lumefantrine, boceprevir, cinacalcet, clozapine, cobicistat/elvitegravir/emtricitabine/tenofovir alafenamide, cobicistat/elvitegravir/emtricitabine/tenofovir disoproxil, darifenacin, delavirdine, fosamprenavir, lopinavir, mirabegron, quinine, ritonavir, telaprevir, tipranavir
Important contra-indications noted in the prescribing guidelines for: nursing mothers; pediatric patients

---

Skin
Diaphoresis (<3%)
Edema / fluid retention (4%)
Flushing / rubefaction (<3%)
Psoriasis [2]
Rash (<3%)

Cardiovascular
Arrhythmias [7]
Atrial fibrillation [3]
Atrial flutter [3]
Atrioventricular block [2]
Bradycardia / sinus bradycardia [4]
Brugada syndrome [5]
Bundle branch block [5]
Cardiomyopathy [2]
Cardiotoxicity [4]
Chest pain (5%)
Congestive heart failure [2]
Extrasystoles [2]
Hypotension [2]
Palpitation (6%)
QT interval prolonged / QT prolongation [7]
Supraventricular tachycardia [2]
Tachycardia [3]
Torsades de pointes [4]
Ventricular dysfunction (left ventricular dysfunction / right ventricular dysfunction) [2]

Central Nervous System
Headache (10%) [4]
Hyperesthesia (<10%)
Neurotoxicity [3]
Seizures [2]
Syncope / fainting [2]
Tremor (5%)
Vertigo / dizziness (19%) [5]

Gastrointestinal/Hepatic
Abdominal pain (3%)
Constipation (4%)
Diarrhea (<3%) [2]
Nausea (9%) [3]

Neuromuscular/Skeletal
Asthenia / fatigue (5–8%)

Ocular
Vision blurred [2]
Visual disturbances (16%) [3]

Respiratory
Dyspnea / shortness of breath (10%)

Other
Adverse effects / adverse reactions [2]

FLIBANSERIN

Trade name: Addyi (Sprout)
Indications: Hypoactive sexual desire disorder in premenopausal women
Class: Serotonin type 1A receptor agonist, Serotonin type 2A receptor antagonist
Half-life: 11 hours
Clinically important, potentially hazardous interactions with: alcohol, amprenavir, atazanavir, boceprevir, carbamazepine, ciprofloxacin, clarithromycin, conivaptan, digoxin, diltiazem, erythromycin, fluconazole, fosamprenavir, grapefruit juice, indinavir, itraconazole, ketoconazole, nefazodone, nelfinavir, phenobarbital, phenytoin, posaconazole, rifabutin, rifampin, rifapentine,

ritonavir, saquinavir, St John's wort, telaprevir, telithromycin, verapamil
Pregnancy category: No data available
Important contra-indications noted in the prescribing guidelines for: the elderly; nursing mothers; pediatric patients
Warning: HYPOTENSION AND SYNCOPE IN CERTAIN SETTINGS

Mucosal
Xerostomia (dry mouth) (2%) [2]
Central Nervous System
Anxiety (2%)
Insomnia (5%) [4]
Sedation [2]
Somnolence (drowsiness) (11%) [10]
Vertigo / dizziness (2%) [11]
Gastrointestinal/Hepatic
Abdominal pain (2%)
Constipation (2%)
Nausea (10%) [7]
Neuromuscular/Skeletal
Asthenia / fatigue (9%) [5]

FLORBETAPIR F18

Trade name: Amyvid (Avid Pharmaceuticals)
Indications: Postiron Emission Tomography (PET) imaging
Class: Radiopharmaceutical, diagnostic agent
Half-life: 110 minutes
Clinically important, potentially hazardous interactions with: none known
Important contra-indications noted in the prescribing guidelines for: nursing mothers; pediatric patients
Note: Florbetapir F18 injection emits radiation. Use procedures to minimize radiation exposure.

Central Nervous System
Headache (2%)

FLUCLOXACILLIN

Trade name: Floxapen (Actavis)
Indications: Infections due to sensitive Gram-positive organisms
Class: Antibiotic, Antibiotic; beta-lactam, Antibiotic; penicillin, Antimicrobial
Half-life: 53 minutes
Clinically important, potentially hazardous interactions with: oral contraceptives, probenecid
Important contra-indications noted in the prescribing guidelines for: nursing mothers

Skin
AGEP [2]
Endocrine/Metabolic
Acidosis (includes lactic acidosis) [2]
Hypokalemia [2]
Gastrointestinal/Hepatic
Hepatotoxicity / liver injury / acute liver injury / drug-induced liver injury (DILI) [22]
Hematologic
Anemia [2]
Renal
Nephrotoxicity / kidney injury / acute kidney injury (AKI) / drug-induced kidney injury [4]

FLUCONAZOLE

Trade name: Diflucan (Pfizer)
Indications: Candidiasis
Class: Antifungal / antimycotic, Antifungal; triazole, Antimicrobial, CYP3A4 inhibitor
Half-life: 25–30 hours
Clinically important, potentially hazardous interactions with: alprazolam, amphotericin B, anisindione, anticoagulants, atorvastatin, avanafil, avapritinib, betamethasone, bosentan, celecoxib, citalopram, clobazam, clopidogrel, deflazacort, dicumarol, eluxadoline, eplerenone, erythromycin, flibanserin, irbesartan, ivacaftor, lemborexant, lesinurad, lumateperone, methadone, midazolam, mifepristone, naldemedine, neratinib, nevirapine, olaparib, ospemifene, pantoprazole, phenobarbital, phenytoin, pimecrolimus, propranolol, quetiapine, ramelteon, rifapentine, rilpivirine, rimegepant, ruxolitinib, selumetinib, simeprevir, sonidegib, sulfonylureas, temsirolimus, terbinafine, tezacaftor/ivacaftor, tipranavir, tofacitinib, trabectedin, triamcinolone, ubrogepant, venetoclax, vinblastine, vincristine, voclosporin, voxelotor, warfarin, zidovudine
Pregnancy category: fluconazole is pregnancy category C for vaginal candidiasis
Important contra-indications noted in the prescribing guidelines for: the elderly; nursing mothers

Skin
AGEP [5]
Erythema multiforme [5]
Exfoliative dermatitis [2]
Fixed eruption / fixed drug eruption [10]
Hypersensitivity (<4%)
Rash (2%) [4]
Stevens-Johnson syndrome and toxic epidermal necrolysis (SJS/TEN) [11]
Hair
Alopecia / hair loss [5]
Nails
Nail changes [2]
Mucosal
Oral ulceration [2]
Cardiovascular
Hypotension [2]
QT interval prolonged / QT prolongation [7]
Torsades de pointes [11]
Central Nervous System
Dysgeusia (taste perversion) [2]
Headache (2–13%) [3]
Neurotoxicity [2]
Endocrine/Metabolic
Adrenal insufficiency (hypoadrenalism) / Addisonian crisis (includes Addison's disease) [5]
Gastrointestinal/Hepatic
Abdominal pain [2]
Diarrhea [2]
Hepatotoxicity / liver injury / acute liver injury / drug-induced liver injury (DILI) [4]
Nausea (2–7%)
Neuromuscular/Skeletal
Rhabdomyolysis [4]
Renal
Renal failure [2]
Other
Adverse effects / adverse reactions [5]

FLUCYTOSINE

Trade name: Ancobon (Valeant)
Indications: Candidal and cryptococcal infections
Class: Antimycobacterial (including antitubercular)
Half-life: 3–8 hours
Clinically important, potentially hazardous interactions with: amphotericin B, tegafur/gimeracil/oteracil
Important contra-indications noted in the prescribing guidelines for: nursing mothers; pediatric patients

Skin
Exanthems [2]
Photosensitivity [2]
Rash (<10%)

FLUDARABINE

Trade names: Fludara (Genzyme), Oforta (Sanofi-Aventis)
Indications: Chronic lymphocytic leukemia (B-cell)
Class: Antimetabolite, Antineoplastic / anticancer agent (see also Immune checkpoint inhibitor)
Half-life: 9 hours
Clinically important, potentially hazardous interactions with: aldesleukin, clofazimine, live vaccines, pentostatin
Important contra-indications noted in the prescribing guidelines for: nursing mothers; pediatric patients
Note: Severe neurologic effects, including blindness, coma, and death were observed in dose-ranging studies in patients with acute leukemia when fludarabine phosphate was administered at high doses. Instances of life-threatening and sometimes fatal autoimmune hemolytic anemia have been reported after one or more cycles of treatment with fludarabine phosphate.
Warning: CNS TOXICITY, HEMOLYTIC ANEMIA, AND PULMONARY TOXICITY

Skin
Anaphylactoid reactions / anaphylaxis (includes anaphylactic shock) (<3%)
Diaphoresis (14%)
Edema / fluid retention (8–19%)
Herpes simplex (7–8%)
Herpes zoster [2]
Paraneoplastic pemphigus [4]
Peripheral edema (7%)
Pruritus (itching) (<3%)
Rash (4–15%)
Hair
Alopecia / hair loss (<10%)
Mucosal
Mucositis (2%)
Stomatitis (oral mucositis) (9%)
Cardiovascular
Aneurysm (<2%)
Angina (6%)
Arrhythmias (<4%)
Chest pain (5%)
Congestive heart failure (<4%)
Myocardial infarction (<4%)
Phlebitis (<3%)
Supraventricular tachycardia (<4%)

Central Nervous System
Anorexia (7–34%)
Chills (11–19%)
Fever (pyrexia) (includes hyperpyrexia) (11–69%) [2]
Headache (3–9%)
Leukoencephalopathy / posterior reversible encephalopathy syndrome (PRES) [9]
Neurotoxicity [3]
Pain (5–22%)
Paresthesias (4–12%)
Sleep-related disorder (<3%)
Stroke / cerebrovascular accident (<4%)

Endocrine/Metabolic
Hyperglycemia (includes glucose increased) (<6%)
Weight loss (<6%)

Gastrointestinal/Hepatic
Abdominal pain (8–10%)
Cholelithiasis (gallstones in the gall bladder or the bile duct) (3%)
Constipation (<3%)
Diarrhea (5–15%)
Esophagitis (3%)
Gastrointestinal bleeding (3–13%) [2]
Hepatotoxicity / liver injury / acute liver injury / drug-induced liver injury (DILI) [2]
Nausea (<36%)

Genitourinary
Dysuria (3–4%)
Hematuria (<3%)
Urinary hesitancy (3%)
Urinary tract infection (4–15%)

Hematologic
Anemia [3]
Cytopenia [2]
Febrile neutropenia [2]
Hemolytic anemia [3]
Hemotoxicity [3]
Leukocytopenia (leukopenia) / leukocytes (white blood cells) decreased [2]
Myelosuppression / bone marrow suppression / myelotoxicity [5]
Neutropenia (neutrophils decreased) [6]
Sepsis [2]
Thrombocytopenia / platelets decreased [4]
Thrombosis (<3%)

Neuromuscular/Skeletal
Asthenia / fatigue (6–65%)
Back pain (4–9%)
Myalgia/Myopathy (>10%)

Ocular
Visual disturbances (3–15%)

Otic
Hearing loss (hypoacusis) (2–6%)

Respiratory
Bronchitis (<9%)
Cough (6–44%)
Dyspnea / shortness of breath (<22%)
Hemoptysis (<6%)
Influenza- ('flu)-like syndrome (5–8%)
Pharyngitis (sore throat) (9%)
Pneumonia (3–22%) [3]
Pneumonitis (6%)
Pulmonary toxicity [4]
Rhinitis / rhinosinusitis (see also sinusitis) (3–11%)
Sinusitis (see also rhinitis / rhinosinusitis) (<5%)
Upper respiratory tract infection (2–14%)

Other
Adverse effects / adverse reactions [2]
Death [4]
Infection (12–44%) [6]

FLUDEOXYGLUCOSE F18

Indications: Positron emission tomography (PET) imaging
Class: Radiopharmaceutical, diagnostic agent
Half-life: 110 minutes
Clinically important, potentially hazardous interactions with: none known
Important contra-indications noted in the prescribing guidelines for: nursing mothers
Note: Fludeoxyglucose F18 injection emits radiation. Use procedures to minimize radiation exposure. Use alternatives to breast feeding (e.g., stored breast milk or infant formula) for at least 10 half-lives of radioactive decay, if Fludeoxyglucose F18 injection is administered to a woman who is breast-feeding.

FLUMAZENIL

Trade name: Romazicon (Roche)
Indications: Benzodiazepine overdose
Class: Benzodiazepine antagonist
Half-life: terminal: 41–79 minutes
Clinically important, potentially hazardous interactions with: alcohol, eszopiclone, nalmefene, neuromuscular blockers
Important contra-indications noted in the prescribing guidelines for: nursing mothers

---

Skin
Diaphoresis (3–9%)
Flushing / rubefaction (<3%)
Hot flashes / hot flushes (<10%)

Mucosal
Xerostomia (dry mouth) (<10%)

Central Nervous System
Paresthesias (<10%)
Seizures [17]
Tremor (<10%)

FLUNISOLIDE

Trade names: Aerobid (Roche), Nasalide (Ivax), Nasarel (Ivax)
Indications: Asthma, rhinitis
Class: Corticosteroid / Glucocorticoid, Corticosteroid, inhaled
Half-life: N/A
Clinically important, potentially hazardous interactions with: aspirin, cyclosporine, digoxin, diuretics, estrogens, ketoconazole, live vaccines, oral contraceptives, phenobarbital, phenytoin, rifampin, warfarin

---

Central Nervous System
Dysgeusia (taste perversion) [3]
Headache [4]

FLUOCINOLONE

Trade names: Capex (Galderma), Derma-Smoothe (Hill Dermac), Retisert (Bausch & Lomb), Synalar (Medicis)
Indications: Dermatoses, asthma, inflammatory ocular conditions
Class: Corticosteroid / Glucocorticoid, Corticosteroid, topical
Half-life: N/A
Clinically important, potentially hazardous interactions with: live vaccines
Important contra-indications noted in the prescribing guidelines for: nursing mothers; pediatric patients
Note: Derma-Smoothe is formulated with refined peanut oil and should be used with caution in peanut-sensitive individuals.

Ocular
Cataract [11]
Glaucoma (includes acute angle-closure glaucoma) [2]
Intraocular pressure increased [11]
Ocular pressure [3]

Other
Adverse effects / adverse reactions [2]

FLUORIDES

Indications: Caries prevention (topical), osteoporosis prevention (oral)
Class: Chemical
Half-life: N/A
Clinically important, potentially hazardous interactions with: caffeine

---

Skin
Acneiform eruption / acneiform dermatitis / acneiform rash [2]
Burning / skin burning sensation [12]
Cutaneous toxicity / skin toxicity [27]
Dermatitis [4]
Edema / fluid retention [2]
Erythema [2]
Hypersensitivity [6]
Necrosis (skin necrosis) [2]
Pruritus (itching) [5]
Urticaria / hives [7]

Mucosal
Oral ulceration [2]
Stomatitis (oral mucositis) [3]

Central Nervous System
Headache [2]

Gastrointestinal/Hepatic
Abdominal pain [2]

Neuromuscular/Skeletal
Arthralgia [5]
Bone pain / joint pain [12]
Skeletal fluorosis [35]

Ocular
Cataract [2]

Other
Adverse effects / adverse reactions [9]
Death [7]
Tooth fluorosis / dental fluorosis [39]

FLUOROURACIL

Trade names: 5-fluorouracil (Taj), Carac (Valeant), Efudex (Valeant), Fluoroplex (Allergan), Fluorouracil Injection, USP (Bioniche), Tolak (Hill Dermac)
Indications: Palliative management of malignant neoplasms especially of the gastrointestinal tract, breast, liver and pancreas, topical therapy for actinic keratoses. Advanced pancreatic cancer (in combination with oxaliplatin/irinotecan/ leucovorin (FOLFIRINOX or FOLFOXIRI)). Used in combination with leucovorin and irinotecan (FOLFIRI) for treatment of advanced-stage and metastatic colorectal cancer. Used in combination with leucovorin and oxaliplatin (FOLFOX, mFOLFOX6) for treatment of colorectal cancer
Class: Antimetabolite, Antineoplastic / anticancer agent (see also Immune checkpoint inhibitor), Fluoropyrimidine
Half-life: 8–20 minutes
Clinically important, potentially hazardous interactions with: aldesleukin, bromelain, cimetidine, granulocyte colony-stimulating factor (G-CSF), metronidazole, tegafur/gimeracil/ oteracil, tegafur/gimeracil/oteracil, tinidazole
Important contra-indications noted in the prescribing guidelines for: nursing mothers; pediatric patients
Note: Contra-indicated in patients with dihydropyrimidine dehydrogenase deficiency. Tolak cream contains peanut oil and should be used with caution in peanut-sensitive individuals.

Skin
- Acneiform eruption / acneiform dermatitis / acneiform rash [3]
- Acral erythema [4]
- Actinic keratoses [4]
- Anaphylactoid reactions / anaphylaxis (includes anaphylactic shock) [2]
- Cutaneous toxicity / skin toxicity [5]
- Dermatitis (>10%) [4]
- Eczema / eczematous reaction / eczematous eruption [2]
- Edema / fluid retention [2]
- Erythema [4]
- Erythema multiforme [3]
- Exanthems (<10%) [3]
- Folliculitis [2]
- Hand–foot syndrome (palmar–plantar erythrodysesthesia) (<38%) [54]
- Lupus erythematosus (subacute cutaneous lupus erythematosus (SCLE)) [6]
- Palmar–plantar pigmentation [2]
- Peripheral edema [2]
- Photosensitivity [3]
- Pigmentation (Skin) (includes hyperpigmentation) [11]
- Pruritus (itching) [5]
- Radiation recall dermatitis [3]
- Rash [8]
- Recall reaction [3]
- Seborrheic dermatitis [3]
- Ulcerations [2]
- Xerosis / xeroderma (<10%) [3]

Hair
- Alopecia / hair loss (>10%) [19]

Nails
- Nail pigmentation [3]
- Paronychia [3]

Mucosal
- Epistaxis (nosebleed) [2]
- Mucosal inflammation [2]
- Mucositis (<79%) [18]
- Oral ulceration [2]
- Stomatitis (oral mucositis) (>10%) [31]
- Tongue pigmentation [2]

Cardiovascular
- Acute coronary syndrome [3]
- Angina [9]
- Bradycardia / sinus bradycardia [2]
- Cardiac failure [5]
- Cardiomyopathy [4]
- Cardiotoxicity [20]
- Coronary vasospasm [2]
- Hypertension [12]
- Myocardial infarction [4]
- QT interval prolonged / QT prolongation [4]
- Takotsubo syndrome [3]
- Thromboembolism [2]
- Venous thromboembolism [2]
- Ventricular tachycardia [2]

Central Nervous System
- Anorexia [13]
- Dysgeusia (taste perversion) [2]
- Encephalopathy (includes hepatic encephalopathy) [5]
- Fever (pyrexia) (includes hyperpyrexia) [6]
- Headache [2]
- Insomnia [2]
- Leukoencephalopathy / posterior reversible encephalopathy syndrome (PRES) [32]
- Neurotoxicity [12]
- Peripheral neuropathy [7]
- Syncope / fainting [2]
- Vertigo / dizziness [2]

Endocrine/Metabolic
- Acidosis (includes lactic acidosis) [2]
- ALP increased [2]
- ALT increased [2]
- AST increased [2]
- Hyperammonemia [6]
- Hyperglycemia (includes glucose increased) [3]
- Hypocalcemia [2]
- Hypokalemia [3]
- Hypomagnesemia [3]
- Hyponatremia [3]
- Serum creatinine increased [2]
- SIADH [4]
- Weight loss [2]

Gastrointestinal/Hepatic
- Abdominal pain [4]
- Constipation [4]
- Diarrhea [40]
- Gastrointestinal perforation / perforated colon / gastric perforation [2]
- Hepatotoxicity / liver injury / acute liver injury / drug-induced liver injury (DILI) [8]
- Nausea [31]
- Vomiting [23]

Hematologic
- Anemia [21]
- Febrile neutropenia [23]
- Hemolytic uremic syndrome [3]
- Leukocytopenia (leukopenia) / leukocytes (white blood cells) decreased [18]
- Lymphopenia (lymphocytopenia) / lymphocytes decreased [2]
- Myelosuppression / bone marrow suppression / myelotoxicity [4]
- Neutropenia (neutrophils decreased) [60]
- Thrombocytopenia / platelets decreased [21]

Local
- Application-site edema [2]
- Application-site pruritus [3]
- Injection-site burning [2]
- Injection-site desquamation [4]
- Injection-site edema [3]
- Injection-site erythema [4]
- Injection-site necrosis [2]
- Injection-site pain [2]
- Injection-site ulceration [2]

Neuromuscular/Skeletal
- Asthenia / fatigue [26]

Ocular
- Ectropion / cicatricial ectropion [2]
- Epiphora [2]
- Lacrimal duct stenosis / punctal stenosis [3]
- Ocular inflammation [2]

Renal
- Proteinuria [5]

Respiratory
- Dysphonia (includes voice disorders / voice changes) [2]
- Pneumonia [2]
- Pulmonary embolism [2]

Other
- Adverse effects / adverse reactions [9]
- Death [7]
- Infection [7]
- Side effects [2]

FLUOXETINE

Trade names: Prozac (Lilly), Sarafem (Warner Chilcott), Symbyax (Lilly)
Indications: Depression, obsessive-compulsive disorder
Class: Antidepressant, Selective serotonin reuptake inhibitor (SSRI)
Half-life: 2–3 days
Clinically important, potentially hazardous interactions with: alprazolam, amoxapine, amphetamines, astemizole, clarithromycin, clopidogrel, clozapine, desipramine, deutetrabenazine, dexibuprofen, dextroamphetamine, diethylpropion, droperidol, duloxetine, erythromycin, gilteritinib, haloperidol, iloperidone, imipramine, insulin aspart, insulin degludec, insulin glargine, insulin glulisine, isocarboxazid, linezolid, lithium, MAO inhibitors, mazindol, meperidine, methamphetamine, midazolam, moclobemide, nifedipine, nortriptyline, olanzapine, oliceridine, PEG-interferon, phendimetrazine, phenelzine, phentermine, phenylpropanolamine, phenytoin, pimozide, propranolol, pseudoephedrine, rasagiline, risperidone, selegiline, serotonin agonists, sibutramine, St John's wort, sumatriptan, sympathomimetics, tramadol, tranylcypromine, trazodone, tricyclic antidepressants, troleandomycin, tryptophan, valbenazine, vortioxetine, zolmitriptan
Important contra-indications noted in the prescribing guidelines for: the elderly; nursing mothers; pediatric patients
Note: Increased risk of suicidal thinking and behavior in children, adolescents, and young adults taking antidepressants for Major Depressive Disorder (MDD) and other psychiatric disorders. Sarafem is not approved for use in pediatric patients with MDD and obsessive compulsive disorder. Symbyax is not approved for use in children and adolescents.

Symbyax is fluoxetine and olanzapine.
Warning: SUICIDAL THOUGHTS AND BEHAVIORS

Skin
Bruise / bruising / contusion / ecchymosis (ecchymoses) [2]
Cutaneous toxicity / skin toxicity [2]
Diaphoresis (8%) [3]
Exanthems (4%) [7]
Flushing / rubefaction (<2%)
Mycosis fungoides [2]
Phototoxicity [2]
Pruritus (itching) (2%) [4]
Pseudolymphoma / cutaneous pseudolymphoma [4]
Rash (6%) [4]
Raynaud's phenomenon [2]
Serum sickness-like reaction [2]
Stevens-Johnson syndrome and toxic epidermal necrolysis (SJS/TEN) [3]
Urticaria / hives (4%) [5]
Vasculitis (angiitis) / cutaneous vasculitis (angiitis) [2]

Hair
Alopecia / hair loss [9]

Mucosal
Black tongue / black hairy tongue (lingua villosa nigra) [3]
Oral ulceration [2]
Xerostomia (dry mouth) (12%) [7]

Cardiovascular
Hypertension [2]
Orthostatic hypotension [2]
QT interval prolonged / QT prolongation [7]
Torsades de pointes [2]

Central Nervous System
Akathisia [6]
Amnesia [2]
Anxiety [2]
Delirium [3]
Depression [2]
Dysgeusia (taste perversion) (2%)
Extrapyramidal symptoms [3]
Hallucinations [3]
Hallucinations, visual [4]
Headache (<27%) [3]
Insomnia [3]
Neuroleptic malignant syndrome [2]
Paresthesias [2]
Parkinsonism [2]
Restless legs syndrome / Willis-Ekbom disease (includes restless arms syndrome variant) [4]
Seizures [6]
Serotonin syndrome [15]
Somnolence (drowsiness) [4]
Stuttering (dysphemia) / stammering [2]
Suicidal ideation [11]
Tremor (2–10%) [2]
Vertigo / dizziness [4]

Endocrine/Metabolic
Gynecomastia [2]
Libido decreased [2]
SIADH [20]
Weight gain [4]

Gastrointestinal/Hepatic
Nausea [4]
Pancreatitis / acute pancreatitis [2]

Genitourinary
Priapism [2]
Sexual dysfunction [6]

Neuromuscular/Skeletal
Asthenia / fatigue [3]
Rhabdomyolysis [2]

Other
Adverse effects / adverse reactions [4]
Bruxism (teeth grinding) [4]
Death [3]

FLUOXYMESTERONE

Trade name: Halotestin (Pfizer)
Indications: Breast carcinoma, hypogonadism, anemia
Class: Anabolic steroid
Half-life: 9.2 hours
Clinically important, potentially hazardous interactions with: anticoagulants, cyclosporine, warfarin

Skin
Acneiform eruption / acneiform dermatitis / acneiform rash (>10%) [12]
Edema / fluid retention (>10%)
Flushing / rubefaction (<5%)

Hair
Alopecia / hair loss [2]
Hirsutism (<10%) [9]

Endocrine/Metabolic
Mastodynia (>10%)

Genitourinary
Priapism (>10%)

FLUPHENAZINE

Trade name: Prolixin (Bristol-Myers Squibb)
Indications: Psychoses
Class: Antipsychotic, Phenothiazine
Half-life: 84–96 hours
Clinically important, potentially hazardous interactions with: antihistamines, arsenic, chlorpheniramine, clozapine, dofetilide, evening primrose, quinolones, sparfloxacin
Important contra-indications noted in the prescribing guidelines for: nursing mothers

Skin
Rash (<10%)
Vitiligo [2]

Central Nervous System
Neuroleptic malignant syndrome [14]
Parkinsonism [3]
Somnolence (drowsiness) [4]

Endocrine/Metabolic
Galactorrhea (<10%)
Gynecomastia (<10%)
Mastodynia (<10%)

Genitourinary
Priapism [2]

Neuromuscular/Skeletal
Dystonia [3]

Ocular
Maculopathy [3]

FLUPREDNISOLONE

Trade names: Alphadrol (Pharmacia & Upjohn), Isopredon (Sanofi-Aventis), Selectren (Sanofi-Aventis)
Indications: Inflammation
Class: Anti-inflammatory, Corticosteroid / Glucocorticoid
Half-life: N/A
Clinically important, potentially hazardous interactions with: none known

Skin
Edema / fluid retention [2]

Cardiovascular
Hypertension [5]

Endocrine/Metabolic
Hypokalemia [5]

Neuromuscular/Skeletal
Rhabdomyolysis [4]

FLURAZEPAM

Trade names: Dalmane (Valeant), Flurazepam (Watson)
Indications: Insomnia
Class: Benzodiazepine
Half-life: 40–114 hours
Clinically important, potentially hazardous interactions with: amprenavir, chlorpheniramine, clarithromycin, cobicistat/elvitegravir/emtricitabine/tenofovir alafenamide, cobicistat/elvitegravir/emtricitabine/tenofovir disoproxil, efavirenz, esomeprazole, imatinib, indinavir, nelfinavir, ritonavir

Skin
Dermatitis (<10%)
Diaphoresis (>10%)
Rash (>10%)

Mucosal
Sialopenia (>10%)
Sialorrhea (ptyalism; hypersalivation) (<10%)
Xerostomia (dry mouth) (>10%)

Central Nervous System
Dysgeusia (taste perversion) (metallic taste) (3%)

Other
Adverse effects / adverse reactions [2]

FLURBIPROFEN

Trade name: Ansaid (Pfizer)
Indications: Rheumatoid arthritis, osteoarthritis
Class: Non-steroidal anti-inflammatory (NSAID)
Half-life: 3–4 hours
Clinically important, potentially hazardous interactions with: ACE inhibitors, aspirin, furosemide, lithium, methotrexate
Important contra-indications noted in the prescribing guidelines for: the elderly; nursing mothers
Note: NSAIDs may cause an increased risk of serious cardiovascular and gastrointestinal adverse events, which can be fatal. This risk may increase with duration of use.
Elderly patients are at greater risk for serious gastrointestinal events.

Warning: CARDIOVASCULAR AND GASTROINTESTINAL RISKS

Skin
Eczema / eczematous reaction / eczematous eruption (3–9%)
Edema / fluid retention (3–9%)
Exanthems [3]
Fixed eruption / fixed drug eruption [2]
Hypersensitivity [4]
Pruritus (itching) (<5%)
Rash (<3%)
Stevens-Johnson syndrome and toxic epidermal necrolysis (SJS/TEN) [2]

Mucosal
Oral lichenoid eruption [2]

Central Nervous System
Headache [4]

Renal
Nephrotoxicity / kidney injury / acute kidney injury (AKI) / drug-induced kidney injury [2]

Other
Side effects (6%) [2]

FLUTICASONE FUROATE

Synonym: FF
Trade names: Arnuity (GSK), Breo (GSK)
Indications: Asthma
Class: Corticosteroid / Glucocorticoid, Corticosteroid, inhaled
Half-life: 24 hours
Clinically important, potentially hazardous interactions with: cobicistat/elvitegravir/emtricitabine/tenofovir alafenamide
Important contra-indications noted in the prescribing guidelines for: nursing mothers; pediatric patients
Note: Breo is fluticasone furoate and vilanterol.

Mucosal
Epistaxis (nosebleed) [2]
Nasal congestion (3%)
Oral candidiasis (<3%) [9]
Oropharyngeal pain (3–4%) [9]

Cardiovascular
Extrasystoles [2]
Hypertension [2]

Central Nervous System
Fever (pyrexia) (includes hyperpyrexia) [4]
Headache (6–13%) [18]
Vertigo / dizziness [2]

Gastrointestinal/Hepatic
Abdominal pain (3%)
Gastroenteritis (3%)
Nausea [2]

Neuromuscular/Skeletal
Arthralgia (3%) [3]
Back pain (3%) [6]
Fractures [3]

Respiratory
Asthma [2]
Bronchitis (7–12%) [6]
Cough (<3%) [10]
Dysphonia (includes voice disorders / voice changes) (2–3%) [6]
Influenza (7%) [5]
Nasopharyngitis (8–13%) [15]
Pharyngitis (sore throat) (3–6%) [7]
Pneumonia [3]
Rhinitis / rhinosinusitis (see also sinusitis) (3%) [4]
Sinusitis (see also rhinitis / rhinosinusitis) (4–7%) [8]
Upper respiratory tract infection (6%) [13]

Other
Adverse effects / adverse reactions [11]
Toothache (odontalgia) (3%) [2]

FLUTICASONE PROPIONATE

Synonym: FP
Trade names: Advair (GSK), Cutivate (GSK) (Nycomed), Flonase (GSK), Flovent (GSK), Flutiform (Napp)
Indications: Dermatoses, rhinitis, maintenance treatment of asthma (as inhalation)
Class: Corticosteroid / Glucocorticoid, Corticosteroid, inhaled, Corticosteroid, topical
Half-life: 8 hours
Clinically important, potentially hazardous interactions with: amprenavir, atazanavir, boceprevir, clarithromycin, cobicistat/elvitegravir/emtricitabine/tenofovir alafenamide, cobicistat/elvitegravir/emtricitabine/tenofovir disoproxil, delavirdine, indinavir, itraconazole, ketoconazole, live vaccines, lopinavir, nefazodone, nelfinavir, oral contraceptives, ritonavir, saquinavir, telaprevir, telithromycin
Important contra-indications noted in the prescribing guidelines for: nursing mothers; pediatric patients
Note: Advair is fluticasone propionate and salmeterol; Flutiform is fluticasone propionate and formoterol. [INH] = Inhalation.

Skin
Burning / skin burning sensation [2]
Perioral dermatitis [2]
Pruritus (itching) (6%) [3]
Rash (8%)
Vasculitis (angiitis) / cutaneous vasculitis (angiitis) [3]

Mucosal
Nasal congestion (16%)
Oral candidiasis (<31%) [12]
Oropharyngeal pain (3–22%) [4]

Cardiovascular
Hypertension [2]

Central Nervous System
Fever (pyrexia) (includes hyperpyrexia) (<7%) [2]
Headache (2–14%) [15]
Pain (10%)
Vertigo / dizziness [2]

Endocrine/Metabolic
Cushing's syndrome [5]

Gastrointestinal/Hepatic
Abdominal pain (2–4%)
Nausea (<9%)
Vomiting (<9%)

Genitourinary
Urinary tract infection [2]

Neuromuscular/Skeletal
Arthralgia (17%)
Asthenia / fatigue (16%)
Back pain [6]
Bone pain / joint pain (2–5%)
Myalgia/Myopathy (12%) [2]

Ocular
Cataract [INH] [2]

Respiratory
Asthma (exacerbation) [6]
Bronchitis (2–8%) [3]
COPD (exacerbation) [3]
Cough (<9%) [8]
Dysphonia (includes voice disorders / voice changes) (9%) [9]
Nasopharyngitis [10]
Pharyngitis (sore throat) [3]
Pneumonia [6]
Rhinitis / rhinosinusitis (see also sinusitis) (<13%) [2]
Sinusitis (see also rhinitis / rhinosinusitis) (>3%) [4]
Upper respiratory tract infection (14–31%) [8]

Other
Adverse effects / adverse reactions [10]
Infection (2–5%) [6]

FLUVASTATIN

Trade name: Lescol (Novartis)
Indications: Hypercholesterolemia
Class: HMG-CoA reductase inhibitor / statin
Half-life: 1.2 hours
Clinically important, potentially hazardous interactions with: azithromycin, bosentan, ciprofibrate, clarithromycin, colchicine, cyclosporine, delavirdine, elbasvir & grazoprevir, erythromycin, gemfibrozil, imatinib, letermovir, mifepristone, red rice yeast
Important contra-indications noted in the prescribing guidelines for: nursing mothers

---

Skin
Lupus erythematosus (subacute cutaneous lupus erythematosus (SCLE)) [2]
Rash (3%)

Central Nervous System
Headache (9%)

Endocrine/Metabolic
Creatine phosphokinase (CPK) / creatine kinase increased (hyperCKemia) [2]

Gastrointestinal/Hepatic
Diarrhea (5%)
Dyspepsia / functional dyspepsia (indigestion) (see also gastroparesis) (8%)
Hepatotoxicity / liver injury / acute liver injury / drug-induced liver injury (DILI) [5]

Neuromuscular/Skeletal
Asthenia / fatigue (3%)
Myalgia/Myopathy (5%) [4]
Rhabdomyolysis [13]

Respiratory
Sinusitis (see also rhinitis / rhinosinusitis) (3%)
Upper respiratory tract infection (16%)

Other
Allergic reactions (3%)

FLUVOXAMINE

Trade name: Luvox (Solvay)
Indications: Obsessive-compulsive disorder, depression
Class: Antidepressant, CYP1A2 inhibitor, CYP3A4 inhibitor, Selective serotonin reuptake inhibitor (SSRI)
Half-life: 15 hours
Clinically important, potentially hazardous interactions with: alosetron, alprazolam, aminophylline, amphetamines, anagrelide, asenapine, astemizole, bendamustine, clobazam, clopidogrel, clozapine, dextroamphetamine, diethylpropion, droperidol, duloxetine, isocarboxazid, linezolid, lumateperone, MAO inhibitors, mazindol, methadone, methamphetamine, neratinib, olanzapine, oxtriphylline, phendimetrazine, phenelzine, phentermine, phenylpropanolamine, pirfenidone, propranolol, pseudoephedrine, ramelteon, rasagiline, roflumilast, ropivacaine, selegiline, sibutramine, St John's wort, sumatriptan, sympathomimetics, tacrine, tasimelteon, tizanidine, tramadol, tranylcypromine, trazodone, troleandomycin, tryptophan, ubrogepant, zolmitriptan
Important contra-indications noted in the prescribing guidelines for: the elderly; nursing mothers; pediatric patients
Warning: SUICIDALITY AND ANTIDEPRESSANT DRUGS

Skin
Diaphoresis (<7%)
Photosensitivity [3]

Mucosal
Oral lesions (10%)
Xerostomia (dry mouth) (<14%) [2]

Cardiovascular
Chest pain (3%)
Palpitation (3%)
QT interval prolonged / QT prolongation [3]

Central Nervous System
Akathisia [2]
Anorexia (6–14%)
Anxiety (5–8%)
Dysgeusia (taste perversion) (3%)
Headache (22–35%)
Insomnia (21–35%)
Neuroleptic malignant syndrome [2]
Pain (10%)
Seizures [2]
Serotonin syndrome [6]
Somnolence (drowsiness) (22–27%)
Tremor (5–8%)
Vertigo / dizziness (11–15%)
Yawning (2–5%)

Endocrine/Metabolic
Galactorrhea [2]
Libido decreased (2–10%)
SIADH [2]

Gastrointestinal/Hepatic
Diarrhea (16–18%)
Dyspepsia / functional dyspepsia (indigestion) (see also gastroparesis) (8–10%)
Nausea (34–40%)

Genitourinary
Ejaculatory dysfunction (8–11%)
Sexual dysfunction [2]

Neuromuscular/Skeletal
Asthenia / fatigue (14–26%) [3]
Dystonia [3]
Myalgia/Myopathy (5%)

Respiratory
Pharyngitis (sore throat) (6%)
Upper respiratory tract infection (9%)

FOLFIRI

Indications: A combination of folinic acid (leucovorin), fluorouracil and irinotecan for the treatment of advanced-stage and metastatic colorectal cancer
Clinically important, potentially hazardous interactions with: see individual drugs of this combination for drug interactions
Note: FOLFOX and related chemotherapeutic combinations FOLFOX: A combination of leucovorin (folinic acid), fluorouracil, and oxaliplatin. FOLFOX-4, FOLFOX-6, FOLFOX-7 are different regimens for the administration of FOLFOX. FOLFIRI: A combination of leucovorin (folinic acid), fluorouracil, and irinotecan. FOLFIRINOX (also known as FOLFOXIRI): A combination of leucovorin (folinic acid), fluorouracil, irinotecan, and oxaliplatin. For the individual drugs in these combinations, refer to leucovorin, fluorouracil, oxaliplatin and irinotecan, respectively. .

FOLFIRINOX

Synonym: FOLFOXIRI
Indications: A combination of folinic acid (leucovorin) fluorouracil, irinotecan and oxaliplatin for the treatment of advanced pancreatic cancer
Clinically important, potentially hazardous interactions with: see individual drugs of this combination for drug interactions
Note: FOLFOX and related chemotherapeutic combinations FOLFOX: A combination of leucovorin (folinic acid), fluorouracil, and oxaliplatin. FOLFOX-4, FOLFOX-6, FOLFOX-7 are different regimens for the administration of FOLFOX. FOLFIRI: A combination of leucovorin (folinic acid), fluorouracil, and irinotecan. FOLFIRINOX (also known as FOLFOXIRI): A combination of leucovorin (folinic acid), fluorouracil, irinotecan, and oxaliplatin. For the individual drugs in these combinations, refer to leucovorin, fluorouracil, oxaliplatin and irinotecan, respectively. .

FOLFOX

Synonym: mFOLFOX6
Indications: A combination of fluorouracil, leucovorin and oxaliplatin for the treatment of colorectal cancer.
Other names for this combination: mFOLFOX6

Clinically important, potentially hazardous interactions with: none known
Note: FOLFOX and related chemotherapeutic combinations FOLFOX: A combination of leucovorin (folinic acid), fluorouracil, and oxaliplatin. FOLFOX-4, FOLFOX-6, FOLFOX-7 are different regimens for the administration of FOLFOX. FOLFIRI: A combination of leucovorin (folinic acid), fluorouracil, and irinotecan. FOLFIRINOX (also known as FOLFOXIRI): A combination of leucovorin (folinic acid), fluorouracil, irinotecan, and oxaliplatin. For the individual drugs in these combinations, refer to leucovorin, fluorouracil, oxaliplatin and irinotecan, respectively.

FOLIC ACID

Synonyms: folacin; folate; vitamin B_9
Indications: Anemias
Class: Vitamin
Half-life: N/A
Clinically important, potentially hazardous interactions with: balsalazide, estradiol, raltitrexed

---

Skin
Anaphylactoid reactions / anaphylaxis (includes anaphylactic shock) [3]
Exanthems [2]
Pruritus (itching) [2]
Urticaria / hives [2]

FOMEPIZOLE

Trade name: Antizol (Orphan Medical)
Indications: Toxicity to methanol and ethylene glycol
Class: Antidote
Half-life: not calculated; varies with dose
Clinically important, potentially hazardous interactions with: alcohol
Note: As an antidote, it is difficult to differentiate side effects due to the drug from those due to the effects of the poison.

Skin
Facial flushing (~3%)
Rash (~3%) [2]

Mucosal
Oral vesiculation (~3%)

Cardiovascular
Phlebitis (<10%)

Central Nervous System
Dysgeusia (taste perversion) (6%)
Parosmia (<10%)
Seizures (~3%)
Vertigo / dizziness (6%) [2]

Local
Application-site reactions (<10%)
Injection-site inflammation (<10%)
Injection-site pain (<10%)

Neuromuscular/Skeletal
Back pain (<10%)

Other
Hiccups / singultus (<10%)

FONDAPARINUX

Trade name: Arixtra (Mylan)
Indications: Prophylaxis of deep vein thrombosis
Class: Anticoagulant (antithrombotic), Heparinoid
Half-life: 17–21 hours
Clinically important, potentially hazardous interactions with: abciximab, anagrelide, anticoagulants, cilostazol, clopidogrel, dabigatran, dipyridamole, eptifibatide, nandrolone, salicylates, ticlopidine, tirofiban

Important contra-indications noted in the prescribing guidelines for: the elderly; nursing mothers; pediatric patients
Warning: SPINAL/EPIDURAL HEMATOMAS

Skin
- Bullous dermatosis (3%)
- Edema / fluid retention (9%)
- Hematoma / cutaneous hematoma [2]
- Hypersensitivity [4]
- Purpura (4%)
- Rash (8%)

Central Nervous System
- Pain (2%)

Gastrointestinal/Hepatic
- Hepatotoxicity / liver injury / acute liver injury / drug-induced liver injury (DILI) [2]

Local
- Injection-site bleeding (<10%)
- Injection-site pruritus (<10%)

FORMOTEROL

Trade names: Dulera (Merck Sharpe & Dohme), Foradil (Novartis), Perforomist (Mylan), Symbicort (AstraZeneca)
Indications: Asthma, bronchospasm
Class: Beta-2 adrenergic agonist, Bronchodilator
Half-life: 10–14 hours
Clinically important, potentially hazardous interactions with: beta blockers, clomipramine, desipramine, doxepin, imipramine, iobenguane, nortriptyline, protriptyline, trimipramine
Important contra-indications noted in the prescribing guidelines for: nursing mothers; pediatric patients
Note: Dulera is formoterol and mometasone; Symbicort is formoterol and budesonide.
Warning: ASTHMA-RELATED DEATH

Skin
- Pruritus (itching) (2%)

Mucosal
- Xerostomia (dry mouth) (<3%) [4]

Cardiovascular
- Atrial fibrillation [2]
- Chest pain (2%)
- Hypertension [2]
- Myocardial infarction [2]
- Palpitation [2]

Central Nervous System
- Anxiety (2%)
- Fever (pyrexia) (includes hyperpyrexia) (2%)
- Headache [9]
- Insomnia (2%)
- Tremor (2%) [7]
- Vertigo / dizziness (2–3%) [3]

Gastrointestinal/Hepatic
- Diarrhea (5%) [2]
- Nausea (5%)
- Vomiting (2%)

Genitourinary
- Urinary tract infection [2]

Neuromuscular/Skeletal
- Back pain (4%)
- Cramps (2%)
- Leg cramps (2%)
- Muscle spasm [2]

Respiratory
- Asthma (exacerbation) [4]
- Bronchitis (5%) [2]
- Cough [7]
- Dysphonia (includes voice disorders / voice changes) [3]
- Dyspnea / shortness of breath (2%) [2]
- Nasopharyngitis [9]
- Pharyngitis (sore throat) (4%) [2]
- Pneumonia [2]
- Rhinitis / rhinosinusitis (see also sinusitis) [2]
- Upper respiratory tract infection (7%) [3]

Other
- Adverse effects / adverse reactions [3]
- Death [2]
- Infection (17%)

FOSAMPRENAVIR

Trade name: Lexiva (ViiV)
Indications: HIV infections (in combination with other antiretrovirals)
Class: Antiretroviral, HIV-1 protease inhibitor
Half-life: 7.7 hours
Clinically important, potentially hazardous interactions with: amiodarone, atorvastatin, avanafil, bepridil, carbamazepine, darifenacin, delavirdine, dihydroergotamine, efavirenz, etravirine, flecainide, flibanserin, itraconazole, ketoconazole, lidocaine, lopinavir, lovastatin, midazolam, mifepristone, nevirapine, olaparib, phenobarbital, phenytoin, pimozide, posaconazole, propafenone, quinidine, quinine, rifabutin, rifampin, rilpivirine, ritonavir, rivaroxaban, rosuvastatin, sildenafil, simeprevir, simvastatin, St John's wort, tadalafil, telaprevir, telithromycin, tipranavir, triazolam, vardenafil, warfarin
Important contra-indications noted in the prescribing guidelines for: the elderly; nursing mothers; pediatric patients
Note: Fosamprenavir is a sulfonamide and can be absorbed systemically. Sulfonamides can produce severe, possibly fatal, reactions such as toxic epidermal necrolysis and Stevens-Johnson syndrome.
Fosamprenavir is a prodrug of amprenavir (see separate entry).

Skin
- Hypersensitivity [2]
- Pruritus (itching) (7%)
- Rash (~19%) [5]

Central Nervous System
- Depression (8%)
- Headache (19%)
- Paresthesias (oral) (2%)

Gastrointestinal/Hepatic
- Abdominal pain (5%)
- Diarrhea [3]
- Hepatotoxicity / liver injury / acute liver injury / drug-induced liver injury (DILI) [2]
- Vomiting [2]

Neuromuscular/Skeletal
- Asthenia / fatigue (10%)

Respiratory
- Bronchitis [2]
- Cough [2]
- Nasopharyngitis [3]
- Rhinitis / rhinosinusitis (see also sinusitis) [2]
- Upper respiratory tract infection [2]

Other
- Adverse effects / adverse reactions [4]

FOSCARNET

Trade name: Foscavir (AstraZeneca)
Indications: Cytomegalovirus retinitis in patients with AIDS
Class: Antiviral, DNA and RNA polymerase inhibitor
Half-life: ~3 hours
Clinically important, potentially hazardous interactions with: adefovir, cyclosporine, pentamidine
Important contra-indications noted in the prescribing guidelines for: the elderly; nursing mothers; pediatric patients
Warning: RENAL IMPAIRMENT; SEIZURES

Skin
- Diaphoresis (>5%)
- Exanthems (>5%) [2]
- Facial edema (>5%)
- Flushing / rubefaction (<5%)
- Pigmentation (Skin) (includes hyperpigmentation) (>5%)
- Pruritus (itching) (>5%)
- Rash (generalized) (>5%) [2]
- Seborrhea (>5%)
- Ulcerations (>5%)

Mucosal
- Oral ulceration [5]
- Ulcerative stomatitis (>5%)

Central Nervous System
- Dysgeusia (taste perversion) (>5%)
- Paresthesias (<10%)

Genitourinary
- Penile ulceration (4–30%) [17]
- Vulvar ulceration [2]

Local
- Injection-site pain (<10%)

Neuromuscular/Skeletal
- Myalgia/Myopathy (>5%)

Renal
- Nephrotoxicity / kidney injury / acute kidney injury (AKI) / drug-induced kidney injury [2]

Other
- Crystal precipitation [2]

FOSFOMYCIN

Trade name: Monurol (Forest)
Indications: Urinary tract infections
Class: Antibiotic, Antimicrobial
Half-life: 3–9 hours
Clinically important, potentially hazardous interactions with: none known
Important contra-indications noted in the prescribing guidelines for: the elderly; nursing mothers; pediatric patients

---

Skin
- Anaphylactoid reactions / anaphylaxis (includes anaphylactic shock) [3]
- Rash [3]

Central Nervous System
- Headache (4%)

Endocrine/Metabolic
- Hypokalemia [2]

Gastrointestinal/Hepatic
- Abdominal pain [3]
- Diarrhea (9%) [6]

Hepatotoxicity / liver injury / acute liver injury / drug-induced liver injury (DILI) [2]
Loose stools / soft feces [2]
Nausea (4%) [4]

Genitourinary
Vaginitis (includes vulvitis) (6%)

Local
Injection-site pain [2]

Other
Adverse effects / adverse reactions [3]

FOSINOPRIL

Trade name: Monopril (Bristol-Myers Squibb)
Indications: Hypertension, heart failure
Class: Angiotensin-converting enzyme (ACE) inhibitor, Antihypertensive, Vasodilator
Half-life: 12 hours
Clinically important, potentially hazardous interactions with: alcohol, aldesleukin, allopurinol, alpha blockers, alprostadil, amifostine, amiloride, angiotensin II receptor blocking agents, antacids, antidiabetics, antihypertensives, antipsychotics, anxiolytics and hypnotics, azathioprine, baclofen, beta blockers, calcium channel blockers, clonidine, corticosteroids, cyclosporine, diazoxide, diuretics, estrogens, general anesthetics, gold & gold compounds, heparins, hydralazine, hypotensives, insulin, levodopa, lithium, MAO inhibitors, metformin, methyldopa, minoxidil, moxisylyte, moxonidine, nitrates, nitroprusside, NSAIDs, pentoxifylline, phosphodiesterase 5 inhibitors, potassium salts, prostacyclin analogues, rituximab, sirolimus, spironolactone, sulfonylureas, temsirolimus, tizanidine, tolvaptan, triamterene, trimethoprim
Pregnancy category: category C in first trimester; category D in second and third trimesters
Important contra-indications noted in the prescribing guidelines for: nursing mothers
Warning: USE IN PREGNANCY

Skin
Angioedema (formerly named angioneurotic edema) [3]

Respiratory
Cough [3]

FOSPHENYTOIN

Trade name: Cerebyx (Eisai)
Indications: Seizure prophylaxis, status epilepticus
Class: Antiepileptic; hydantoin
Half-life: 15 minutes
Clinically important, potentially hazardous interactions with: chloramphenicol, cyclosporine, disulfiram, dopamine, efavirenz, imatinib, itraconazole, lacosamide, tinidazole
Note: Fosphenytoin is a prodrug of phenytoin (see separate entry).

Skin
Pruritus (itching) (49%) [5]
Purple glove syndrome [2]

Mucosal
Xerostomia (dry mouth) (4%)

Cardiovascular
Hypotension [2]

Central Nervous System
Dysgeusia (taste perversion) (3%)
Hyperesthesia (2%)
Paresthesias (4%) [3]

FOSTEMSAVIR

Synonym: Fostemsavir tromethamine
Trade name: Rukobia (ViiV)
Indications: HIV-1 infection
Class: Antiretroviral, Antiviral
Half-life: 11 hours
Clinically important, potentially hazardous interactions with: carbamazepine, CYP3A4 inducers, enzalutamide, mitotane, phenytoin, rifampin, St John's wort
Pregnancy category: Insufficient human data to adequately assess a drug-associated risk of birth defects and miscarriage.
Important contra-indications noted in the prescribing guidelines for: nursing mothers
Note: HIV-1–infected mothers are recommended not to breastfeed their infants. Fostemsavir is a prodrug of temsavir.

Skin
Pruritus (itching) (with concomitant therapy) (<2%)
Rash (with concomitant therapy) (3%)

Cardiovascular
QT interval prolonged / QT prolongation (with concomitant therapy) (<2%)

Central Nervous System
Dysgeusia (taste perversion) (with concomitant therapy) (<2%)
Headache (with concomitant therapy) (4%)
Peripheral neuropathy (with concomitant therapy) (<2%)
Sleep disturbances (with concomitant therapy) (3%)
Somnolence (drowsiness) (with concomitant therapy) (2%)
Vertigo / dizziness (with concomitant therapy) (<2%)

Endocrine/Metabolic
ALT increased (with concomitant therapy) (5%)
AST increased (with concomitant therapy) (4%)
Creatine phosphokinase (CPK) / creatine kinase increased (hyperCKemia) (with concomitant therapy) (2%)
Hyperbilirubinemia (with concomitant therapy) (3%)
Hypercholesterolemia (with concomitant therapy) (5%)
Hyperglycemia (includes glucose increased) (with concomitant therapy) (4%)
Hyperlipasemia (with concomitant therapy) (5%)
Hypertriglyceridemia (includes triglycerides increased) (with concomitant therapy) (5%)
Hyperuricemia (with concomitant therapy) (3%)
Immune Reconstitution Inflammatory Syndrome (with concomitant therapy) (2%)
Serum creatinine increased (with concomitant therapy) (19%)

Gastrointestinal/Hepatic
Abdominal pain (with concomitant therapy) (3%)
Diarrhea (with concomitant therapy) (4%)
Dyspepsia / functional dyspepsia (indigestion) (see also gastroparesis) (with concomitant therapy) (3%)
Nausea (with concomitant therapy) (10%)
Vomiting (with concomitant therapy) (2%)

Hematologic
Hemoglobin decreased (with concomitant therapy) (6%)
Neutropenia (neutrophils decreased) (with concomitant therapy) (4%)

Neuromuscular/Skeletal
Asthenia / fatigue (with concomitant therapy) (3%)
Myalgia/Myopathy (with concomitant therapy) (<2%)

FREMANEZUMAB

Trade names: Ajovy (Teva), TEV-48125 (Teva)
Indications: Migraine in adults
Class: Calcitonin gene-related peptide (CGRP) receptor antagonist, Monoclonal antibody
Half-life: ~31 days
Clinically important, potentially hazardous interactions with: none known
Pregnancy category: There are no adequate data on the developmental risk associated with the use of fremanexumab in pregnant women. The long half life of fremanezumab should be a consideration for women who are pregnant or plan to become pregnant while using fremanezumab.
Note: Contraindicated in patients with serious hypersensitivity to fremanezumab or to any of the excipients.
Fremanezumab-Vfrm is biosimilar to Fremanezumab.

Local
Injection-site erythema [2]
Injection-site induration [2]
Injection-site pain [2]
Injection-site reaction (45%) [2]

Respiratory
Nasopharyngitis [2]

FROVATRIPTAN

Trade names: Frova (Vernalis), Migard (Menarini)
Indications: Migraine headaches
Class: 5-HT1 agonist, Serotonin receptor agonist, Triptan
Half-life: 26 hours
Clinically important, potentially hazardous interactions with: dihydroergotamine, methysergide, SNRIs, SSRIs, triptans
Important contra-indications noted in the prescribing guidelines for: nursing mothers; pediatric patients

Skin
Flushing / rubefaction (4%) [3]

Mucosal
Sialopenia (3%)
Xerostomia (dry mouth) (3%) [3]

Cardiovascular
Chest pain (2%) [3]

Central Nervous System
Headache (4%) [4]

Paresthesias (4%) [4]
Somnolence (drowsiness) (>2%)
Vertigo / dizziness (4%) [6]

Gastrointestinal/Hepatic
Dyspepsia / functional dyspepsia (indigestion) (see also gastroparesis) (2%) [2]
Nausea (>2%) [4]

Neuromuscular/Skeletal
Asthenia / fatigue (5%) [6]
Bone pain / joint pain (3%) [2]

Other
Adverse effects / adverse reactions [6]

FULVESTRANT

Trade name: Faslodex (AstraZeneca)
Indications: Metastatic breast cancer
Class: Estrogen receptor antagonist
Half-life: ~40 days
Clinically important, potentially hazardous interactions with: none known
Important contra-indications noted in the prescribing guidelines for: nursing mothers; pediatric patients

---

Skin
Diaphoresis (5%)
Edema / fluid retention (9%)
Hot flashes / hot flushes (6–7%) [11]
Peripheral edema (9%)
Rash (7%) [2]

Mucosal
Stomatitis (oral mucositis) [3]

Cardiovascular
Chest pain (7%)
Vasodilation (18%) [3]

Central Nervous System
Anorexia (4–9%) [2]
Anxiety (5%)
Depression (6%)
Fever (pyrexia) (includes hyperpyrexia) (6%) [2]
Headache (7–8%) [8]
Insomnia (7%)
Pain (19%) [2]
Paresthesias (6%)
Vertigo / dizziness (7%)

Endocrine/Metabolic
ALP increased (>15%)
ALT increased (>15%) [2]
AST increased (>15%)
Hyperglycemia (includes glucose increased) [2]

Gastrointestinal/Hepatic
Abdominal pain (12%)
Constipation (4–13%) [2]
Diarrhea (12%) [5]
Gastrointestinal disorder / discomfort [4]
Nausea (10–26%) [11]
Vomiting (6–13%) [3]

Genitourinary
Urinary tract infection (6%) [2]
Vaginitis (includes vulvitis) [2]

Hematologic
Anemia (5%) [5]
Febrile neutropenia [3]
Leukocytopenia (leukopenia) / leukocytes (white blood cells) decreased [4]
Neutropenia (neutrophils decreased) [7]
Thrombocytopenia / platelets decreased [2]

Local
Injection-site pain (9–12%) [5]
Injection-site reaction (11%) [5]

Neuromuscular/Skeletal
Arthralgia (3–8%) [5]
Asthenia / fatigue (6–22%) [8]
Back pain (8–14%)
Bone pain / joint pain (3–16%) [4]
Joint disorder [6]
Myalgia/Myopathy [2]
Pain in extremities (7%)

Respiratory
Cough (5–10%)
Dyspnea / shortness of breath (4–15%) [2]
Influenza- ('flu)-like syndrome (7%)
Nasopharyngitis [2]
Pharyngitis (sore throat) (16%)

Other
Adverse effects / adverse reactions [7]

FURAZOLIDONE

Indications: Various infections caused by susceptible organisms
Class: Antibiotic, Antibiotic; nitrofuran, Antimicrobial
Half-life: N/A
Clinically important, potentially hazardous interactions with: amphetamines, benzphetamine, chloroquine, dapsone, dobutamine, dopamine, ephedrine, epinephrine, meperidine, morphine, phenylephrine, phenylpropanolamine, pseudoephedrine, sympathomimetics

---

Skin
Dermatitis [4]
Erythema multiforme [2]
Rash [2]

Central Nervous System
Anorexia [2]
Vertigo / dizziness [3]

Gastrointestinal/Hepatic
Diarrhea [2]
Nausea [3]

Neuromuscular/Skeletal
Asthenia / fatigue [2]

FUROSEMIDE

Trade name: Lasix (Sanofi-Aventis)
Indications: Edema
Class: Diuretic, loop
Half-life: ~2 hours
Clinically important, potentially hazardous interactions with: acemetacin, aliskiren, amikacin, amyl nitrite, celecoxib, diclofenac, digoxin, flurbiprofen, gentamicin, hyaluronic acid, hydrocortisone, kanamycin, mivacurium, neomycin, piroxicam, probenecid, streptomycin, tobramycin, tolmetin
Important contra-indications noted in the prescribing guidelines for: the elderly; nursing mothers; pediatric patients
Note: Furosemide is a sulfonamide and can be absorbed systemically. Sulfonamides can produce severe, possibly fatal, reactions such as toxic epidermal necrolysis and Stevens-Johnson syndrome.

Skin
AGEP [2]
Anaphylactoid reactions / anaphylaxis (includes anaphylactic shock) [2]
Bullous dermatosis [16]
Bullous pemphigoid / pemphigoid [11]
Erythema multiforme [3]
Exanthems (12%) [7]
Exfoliative dermatitis [3]
Lichenoid eruption / lichenoid reaction [2]
Linear IgA bullous dermatosis [2]
Photosensitivity (<10%) [2]
Phototoxicity [4]
Pruritus (itching) [2]
Purpura [3]
Pustules / pustular eruption [3]
Stevens-Johnson syndrome and toxic epidermal necrolysis (SJS/TEN) [6]
Sweet's syndrome [2]
Urticaria / hives [3]
Vasculitis (angiitis) / cutaneous vasculitis (angiitis) [7]

Mucosal
Xerostomia (dry mouth) [3]

Cardiovascular
Hypotension [2]

Endocrine/Metabolic
Electrolyte imbalance / electrolyte disorder / electrolyte abnormalities / dyselectrolytemia [2]
Porphyria cutanea tarda [3]

Gastrointestinal/Hepatic
Pancreatitis / acute pancreatitis [3]

Hematologic
Hemolytic anemia [3]

Otic
Hearing loss (hypoacusis) [2]
Ototoxicity [4]

Renal
Nephrotoxicity / kidney injury / acute kidney injury (AKI) / drug-induced kidney injury [2]

Other
Adverse effects / adverse reactions [3]
Side effects [2]

FUSIDIC ACID

Trade names: Fucidin (Leo), Fucithalmic (Leo)
Indications: Angular cheilitis, bacterial infections, ocular infections
Class: Antibiotic, Antimicrobial
Half-life: N/A
Clinically important, potentially hazardous interactions with: atorvastatin, darunavir, indinavir, rosuvastatin, simvastatin, tipranavir

---

Skin
Dermatitis [7]
Jaundice (see also cholestasis / cholestatic jaundice) [3]
Rash [2]

Gastrointestinal/Hepatic
Hepatotoxicity / liver injury / acute liver injury / drug-induced liver injury (DILI) [2]

Neuromuscular/Skeletal
Rhabdomyolysis [9]

Renal
Nephrotoxicity / kidney injury / acute kidney injury (AKI) / drug-induced kidney injury [2]

GABAPENTIN

Trade names: Horizant (GSK), Neurontin (Pfizer)
Indications: Postherpetic neuralgia in adults, seizures
Class: Anticonvulsant (see also antiepileptic (anti-seizure)), GABA analog, Gabapentinoid
Half-life: 5–7 hours
Clinically important, potentially hazardous interactions with: none known
Important contra-indications noted in the prescribing guidelines for: the elderly; nursing mothers; pediatric patients
Note: Gabapentin (Neurontin) and risk of abuse and dependence: new scheduling requirements from 1 April 2019 (UK) As of 1 April 2019 in the UK, gabapentin is controlled under the Misuse of Drugs Act 1971 as a Class C substance and scheduled under the Misuse of Drugs Regulations 2001 as Schedule 3. Patients should be evaluated carefully for a history of drug abuse before prescribing gabapentin and patients should be observed for development of signs of abuse and dependence.
Gabapentin enacarbil is a prodrug of gabapentin.

Skin
Bullous pemphigoid / pemphigoid [2]
DRESS syndrome (Drug-induced hypersensitivity syndrome) [2]
Edema / fluid retention [5]
Exanthems [2]
Peripheral edema (8%) [14]
Rash [2]
Stevens-Johnson syndrome and toxic epidermal necrolysis (SJS/TEN) [2]

Hair
Alopecia / hair loss [2]

Mucosal
Xerostomia (dry mouth) (5%)

Cardiovascular
Atrial fibrillation [2]

Central Nervous System
Aggression (includes anger) [2]
Coma [3]
Confusion [4]
Delirium [2]
Fever (pyrexia) (includes hyperpyrexia) (10%)
Gait instability / postural instability (2%) [4]
Hallucinations, visual [2]
Headache (3%) [9]
Incoordination (2%)
Myokymia / twitching / fasciculation [2]
Neurotoxicity [4]
Psychosis [2]
Sedation [5]
Seizures [4]
Somnolence (drowsiness) (21%) [41]
Tremor [3]
Vertigo / dizziness (17–28%) [52]

Endocrine/Metabolic
Hypoglycemia [3]
Weight gain (2%) [8]

Gastrointestinal/Hepatic
Abdominal pain (3%)
Constipation (4%) [2]
Diarrhea (6%)
Fecal incontinence [2]
Flatulence (2%) [2]
Nausea (4%) [5]
Vomiting (3%) [3]

Genitourinary
Enuresis (urinary incontinence) [5]
Priapism [2]
Sexual dysfunction [5]
Urinary retention [2]

Neuromuscular/Skeletal
Asthenia / fatigue (6%) [13]
Ataxia (3%) [10]
Dystonia [2]
Myalgia/Myopathy [5]
Myasthenia gravis [3]
Myoclonus (see also hypnic jerk) [7]
Rhabdomyolysis [5]

Ocular
Diplopia (double vision) [2]
Nystagmus [2]
Vision blurred (3%)

Otic
Hearing loss (hypoacusis) [2]

Respiratory
Respiratory depression [3]

Other
Adverse effects / adverse reactions [7]
Infection (5%)

GADOBENATE

Synonym: gadobenate dimeglumine
Trade name: Multihance (Bracco)
Indications: Magnetic resonance imaging and magnetic resonance angiography
Class: Contrast agent, Gadolinium-based contrast agent (GBCA)
Half-life: 1–2 hours
Clinically important, potentially hazardous interactions with: cisplatin, daunorubicin, doxorubicin, etoposide, methotrexate, paclitaxel, tamoxifen, vincristine
Important contra-indications noted in the prescribing guidelines for: nursing mothers; pediatric patients
Warning: NEPHROGENIC SYSTEMIC FIBROSIS (NSF)

Skin
Anaphylactoid reactions / anaphylaxis (includes anaphylactic shock) [4]
Urticaria / hives [2]

Cardiovascular
Cardiac arrest [4]

Gastrointestinal/Hepatic
Nausea [6]
Vomiting [4]

Respiratory
Dyspnea / shortness of breath [2]

Other
Adverse effects / adverse reactions [10]
Death [2]

GADOBUTROL

Trade name: Gadovist (Bayer)
Indications: Magnetic resonance imaging
Class: Gadolinium-based contrast agent (GBCA)
Half-life: 90 minutes
Clinically important, potentially hazardous interactions with: amitriptyline, arsenic, citalopram, dasatinib, degarelix, dolasetron, lapatinib, levofloxacin, moxifloxacin, pazopanib, telavancin, telithromycin, voriconazole, vorinostat, ziprasidone
Important contra-indications noted in the prescribing guidelines for: nursing mothers; pediatric patients
Warning: NEPHROGENIC SYSTEMIC FIBROSIS (NSF)

Skin
Anaphylactoid reactions / anaphylaxis (includes anaphylactic shock) [5]

Central Nervous System
Headache (2%) [2]

Gastrointestinal/Hepatic
Nausea [6]
Vomiting [3]

Renal
Nephrogenic systemic fibrosis [2]

Other
Adverse effects / adverse reactions [4]

GADOXETATE

Trade names: Eovist (Bayer), Primovist (Bayer)
Indications: Magnetic resonance imaging (MRI) of the liver
Class: Gadolinium-based contrast agent (GBCA)
Half-life: ~1.0 hour
Clinically important, potentially hazardous interactions with: anionic drugs, rifampin
Important contra-indications noted in the prescribing guidelines for: nursing mothers; pediatric patients
Warning: NEPHROGENIC SYSTEMIC FIBROSIS

Central Nervous System
Headache [4]
Paresthesias [2]
Parosmia [2]

Gastrointestinal/Hepatic
Nausea [5]

Local
Injection-site pain [2]

Neuromuscular/Skeletal
Back pain [2]

Respiratory
Dyspnea / shortness of breath [3]

GALANTAMINE

Trade names: Razadyne (Janssen), Reminyl (Janssen)
Indications: Alzheimer's disease
Class: Acetylcholinesterase inhibitor, Cholinesterase inhibitor
Half-life: ~7 hours
Clinically important, potentially hazardous interactions with: bethanechol, cimetidine, donepezil, edrophonium, paroxetine hydrochloride, physostigmine, pilocarpine, rivastigmine, succinylcholine, tacrine
Important contra-indications noted in the prescribing guidelines for: nursing mothers; pediatric patients
Note: Originally derived from snowdrop (*Galanthus* sp) bulbs.

Skin
Peripheral edema (>2%)

Purpura (>2%)

Cardiovascular

Bradycardia / sinus bradycardia (2%) [5]
QT interval prolonged / QT prolongation [5]

Central Nervous System

Anorexia (7–9%) [2]
Depression (7%)
Headache (8%) [2]
Insomnia (5%)
Somnolence (drowsiness) (4%)
Syncope / fainting (2%) [3]
Tremor (3%)
Vertigo / dizziness (9%) [4]

Endocrine/Metabolic

Weight loss (5–7%)

Gastrointestinal/Hepatic

Abdominal pain (5%)
Diarrhea (6–12%) [5]
Dyspepsia / functional dyspepsia (indigestion) (see also gastroparesis) (5%)
Nausea (6–24%) [7]
Vomiting (4–13%) [7]

Genitourinary

Hematuria (3%)
Urinary tract infection (8%)

Hematologic

Anemia (3%)

Neuromuscular/Skeletal

Asthenia / fatigue (5%)
Pisa syndrome (pleurothotonus) [4]

Respiratory

Rhinitis / rhinosinusitis (see also sinusitis) (4%)
Upper respiratory tract infection (>2%)

Other

Adverse effects / adverse reactions [3]

GANCICLOVIR

Trade name: Cytovene (Roche)
Indications: Cytomegalovirus retinitis in immunocompromised patients
Class: Antiviral, Guanine nucleoside analog
Half-life: 2.5–3.6 hours
Clinically important, potentially hazardous interactions with: abacavir, amphotericin B, cobicistat/elvitegravir/emtricitabine/tenofovir alafenamide, cobicistat/elvitegravir/emtricitabine/tenofovir disoproxil, dapsone, emtricitabine, imipenem/cilastatin, imipenem/cilastatin/relebactam, tenofovir disoproxil, zidovudine
Important contra-indications noted in the prescribing guidelines for: the elderly; nursing mothers; pediatric patients
Warning: GRANULOCYTOPENIA, ANEMIA AND THROMBOCYTOPENIA

Skin

Exanthems (2–5%) [2]
Pruritus (itching) (5%)
Rash (>10%)

Cardiovascular

Phlebitis (2%)

Central Nervous System

Agitation [2]
Paresthesias (6–10%)

Local

Injection-site inflammation (2%)
Injection-site pain (4%)

GARLIC

Family: Liliaceae
Scientific name: *Allium sativum*
Indications: Hypertension, hypercholesterolemia, atherosclerosis, earache, menstrual disorders, allergy, flu, arthritis, diarrhea, bacterial and fungal infections, tinea corporis, tinea pedis, onychomycosis, vaginitis
Class: Immunomodulator
Half-life: N/A
Clinically important, potentially hazardous interactions with: arsenic, atazanavir, chlorpropamide, HIV medications, tipranavir

---

Skin

Anaphylactoid reactions / anaphylaxis (includes anaphylactic shock) [2]
Burning / skin burning sensation [9]
Dermatitis [20]
Hypersensitivity [2]

Gastrointestinal/Hepatic

Esophagitis [2]

Hematologic

Bleeding [2]

Other

Adverse effects / adverse reactions [4]
Allergic reactions [4]

GATIFLOXACIN

Trade names: Tequin (Bristol-Myers Squibb), Zymar (Allergan), Zymaxid (Allergan)
Indications: Various infections caused by susceptible organisms
Class: Antibiotic, Antibiotic; fluoroquinolone, Antimicrobial, Drug-resistant antituberculosis agent
Half-life: 7–14 hours
Clinically important, potentially hazardous interactions with: amiodarone, arsenic, asenapine, bepridil, bretylium, disopyramide, erythromycin, phenothiazines, pimavanserin, procainamide, quinidine, sotalol, tricyclic antidepressants, zinc
Important contra-indications noted in the prescribing guidelines for: nursing mothers; pediatric patients
Note: Fluoroquinolones are associated with an increased risk of tendinitis and tendon rupture in all ages. This risk is further increased in older patients usually over 60 years of age, in patients taking corticosteroid drugs, and in patients with kidney, heart or lung transplants. Fluoroquinolones may exacerbate muscle weakness in persons with myasthenia gravis.

Skin

Diaphoresis (<3%)
Peripheral edema (3%)
Photosensitivity [2]
Rash (3%)

Mucosal

Glossitis (inflammation of the tongue) (3%)
Oral candidiasis (3%)
Oral ulceration (3%)
Stomatitis (oral mucositis) (3%)

Cardiovascular

Torsades de pointes [3]

Central Nervous System

Chills (<3%)
Delirium [2]
Dysgeusia (taste perversion) (<4%) [2]
Headache (<4%)
Paresthesias (3%)
Psychosis [2]
Seizures [3]
Tremor (3%)
Vertigo / dizziness (<2%) [2]

Endocrine/Metabolic

Hyperglycemia (includes glucose increased) [3]
Hypoglycemia [2]

Gastrointestinal/Hepatic

Hepatotoxicity / liver injury / acute liver injury / drug-induced liver injury (DILI) [5]

Genitourinary

Vaginitis (includes vulvitis) (6%)

Local

Injection-site reaction (5%) [2]

Ocular

Conjunctival edema (<4%)
Conjunctival hemorrhage (<4%)
Conjunctivitis (conjunctival inflammation) (5–10%)
Eyelid edema / palpebral edema / blepharedema (<4%)
Keratitis (ocular keratitis) / corneal inflammation) (5–10%)
Lacrimation (increased) (5–10%)
Ocular discharge (<4%)
Ocular itching / ocular pruritus (<4%)
Ocular pain (<4%)
Reduced visual acuity (<4%)
Xerophthalmia (dry eyes) (<4%)

GEFITINIB

Trade name: Iressa (AstraZeneca)
Indications: Advanced non-small cell lung cancer
Class: Antineoplastic / anticancer agent (see also Immune checkpoint inhibitor), Biologic, Epidermal growth factor receptor (EGFR) inhibitor / antagonist, Tyrosine kinase inhibitor
Half-life: 48 hours
Clinically important, potentially hazardous interactions with: antifungals, BCG vaccine, boceprevir, carbamazepine, cardiac glycosides, clozapine, conivaptan, CYP3A4 inhibitors and inducers, dasatinib, deferasirox, denosumab, echinacea, efavirenz, grapefruit juice, itraconazole, leflunomide, natalizumab, phenobarbital, phenytoin, pimecrolimus, ranitidine, rifampin, rifapentine, sipuleucel-T, St John's wort, tacrolimus, topotecan, trastuzumab, vaccines, vitamin K antagonists, voriconazole, warfarin
Important contra-indications noted in the prescribing guidelines for: nursing mothers; pediatric patients

---

Skin

Acneiform eruption / acneiform dermatitis / acneiform rash (25–33%) [34]
Cutaneous adverse reaction (includes severe cutaneous adverse drug reaction (SCAR)) [2]
Cutaneous toxicity / skin toxicity [12]
Desquamation (39%) [2]
Exanthems [3]
Folliculitis [4]
Hand–foot syndrome (palmar–plantar erythrodysesthesia) [3]

Papulopustular eruption [3]
Peripheral edema (2%)
Pruritus (itching) (8–9%) [6]
Rash (43–54%) [69]
Seborrhea [2]
Stevens-Johnson syndrome and toxic epidermal necrolysis (SJS/TEN) [2]
Ulcerations [2]
Xerosis / xeroderma (13–26%) [13]

Hair
Alopecia / hair loss [6]
Hypertrichosis [2]

Nails
Nail changes (17%)
Paronychia (6%) [16]
Pyogenic granuloma [2]

Mucosal
Mucositis [4]
Stomatitis (oral mucositis) [10]

Cardiovascular
Hypertension [3]

Central Nervous System
Anorexia (7–10%) [2]

Endocrine/Metabolic
ALT increased [10]
Appetite decreased [3]
AST increased [8]
Dehydration [2]
Hyponatremia [2]
Weight loss (3–5%)

Gastrointestinal/Hepatic
Abdominal pain [3]
Constipation [2]
Diarrhea (48–67%) [44]
Gastrointestinal perforation / perforated colon / gastric perforation [2]
Hepatic (liver) disorder / hepatobiliary disorder / hepatic (liver) dysfunction [2]
Hepatotoxicity / liver injury / acute liver injury / drug-induced liver injury (DILI) [28]
Nausea (13–18%) [12]
Pneumatosis intestinalis / pneumatosis cystoides intestinalis [3]
Vomiting (9–12%) [6]

Genitourinary
Bladder disorder [2]
Cystitis (includes interstitial cystitis / bladder pain syndrome) [3]

Hematologic
Anemia [5]
Neutropenia (neutrophils decreased) [7]
Thrombocytopenia / platelets decreased [3]

Neuromuscular/Skeletal
Asthenia / fatigue [13]
Myalgia/Myopathy [2]

Ocular
Amblyopia (2%)
Blepharitis [3]
Conjunctivitis (conjunctival inflammation) [2]
Corneal erosion [2]

Renal
Immunoglobulin A (IgA) nephropathy (Berger's disease) [2]
Nephritis / interstitial nephritis / tubulointerstitial nephritis [2]
Nephrotoxicity / kidney injury / acute kidney injury (AKI) / drug-induced kidney injury [2]
Proteinuria [2]

Respiratory
Alveolar hemorrhage (pulmonary) [2]
Dyspnea / shortness of breath (2%)
Pneumonia [2]
Pneumonitis [4]
Pulmonary toxicity [16]

Other
Adverse effects / adverse reactions [12]
Death [8]

GEMCITABINE

Trade name: Gemzar (Lilly)
Indications: Pancreatic carcinoma as a single agent, ovarian cancer (with carboplatin), breast cancer (with paclitaxel), non-small cell lung cancer (with cisplatin)
Class: Antimetabolite, Antineoplastic / anticancer agent (see also Immune checkpoint inhibitor)
Half-life: 42–94 minutes for short infusions; 4–11 hours for longer infusions
Clinically important, potentially hazardous interactions with: aldesleukin
Important contra-indications noted in the prescribing guidelines for: nursing mothers; pediatric patients

---

Skin
Acneiform eruption / acneiform dermatitis / acneiform rash [3]
AGEP [4]
Bullous dermatosis [2]
Cellulitis and pseudocellulitis [13]
Cutaneous toxicity / skin toxicity [7]
Dermatitis [6]
Dermatomyositis [2]
Eczema / eczematous reaction / eczematous eruption (13%)
Edema / fluid retention (13%) [4]
Erysipelas [2]
Exanthems [2]
Hand–foot syndrome (palmar–plantar erythrodysesthesia) [22]
Hypersensitivity [3]
Lipodermatosclerosis [3]
Livedo reticularis / livedo racemosa [2]
Necrosis (skin necrosis) [3]
Peripheral edema (20%) [4]
Petechiae (16%)
Pruritus (itching) (13%) [2]
Radiation recall dermatitis (<74%) [17]
Rash (30%) [35]
Raynaud's phenomenon [3]
Scleroderma [2]
Seborrheic keratoses [2]
Stevens-Johnson syndrome and toxic epidermal necrolysis (SJS/TEN) [3]
Sweet's syndrome [2]
Thrombocytopenic purpura [7]
Toxic erythema of chemotherapy (TEC) [2]
Vasculitis (angiitis) / cutaneous vasculitis (angiitis) [3]

Hair
Alopecia / hair loss (15%) [15]

Mucosal
Mucositis [7]
Stomatitis (oral mucositis) (11%) [14]

Cardiovascular
Arrhythmias [3]
Atrial fibrillation [4]
Capillary leak syndrome [11]
Cardiotoxicity [3]
Hypertension [3]
Hypotension [2]
Large-vessel vasculitis (includes giant cell arteritis) [2]
Myocardial infarction [3]
Thromboembolism [2]
Venous thromboembolism [4]

Central Nervous System
Anorexia [13]
Fever (pyrexia) (includes hyperpyrexia) (41%) [13]
Leukoencephalopathy / posterior reversible encephalopathy syndrome (PRES) [4]
Neurotoxicity [11]
Pain [2]
Paresthesias (10%) [2]
Peripheral neuropathy [8]
Somnolence (drowsiness) (11%)

Endocrine/Metabolic
ALT increased [6]
Appetite decreased [2]
AST increased [6]
Dehydration [2]
Hyperglycemia (includes glucose increased) [2]
Hypomagnesemia [7]
Hyponatremia [3]

Gastrointestinal/Hepatic
Abdominal pain [2]
Cholangitis / sclerosing cholangitis [2]
Constipation [3]
Diarrhea (19%) [26]
Gastrointestinal bleeding [2]
Hepatic (liver) disorder / hepatobiliary disorder / hepatic (liver) dysfunction [2]
Hepatotoxicity / liver injury / acute liver injury / drug-induced liver injury (DILI) [11]
Nausea (69%) [29]
Vomiting (69%) [22]

Genitourinary
Hematuria (30%)

Hematologic
Anemia (70%) [42]
Febrile neutropenia [20]
Hemolytic uremic syndrome [34]
Hemotoxicity [7]
Leukocytopenia (leukopenia) / leukocytes (white blood cells) decreased (62%) [30]
Myelosuppression / bone marrow suppression / myelotoxicity [10]
Neutropenia (neutrophils decreased) (61%) [96]
Thrombocytopenia / platelets decreased (30%) [68]
Thrombosis [3]
Thrombotic microangiopathy [8]

Local
Injection-site reaction (4%)

Neuromuscular/Skeletal
Asthenia / fatigue (18%) [50]
Myalgia/Myopathy (>10%) [7]

Renal
Nephrotoxicity / kidney injury / acute kidney injury (AKI) / drug-induced kidney injury [5]
Renal failure [2]

Respiratory
Dyspnea / shortness of breath (10–23%) [2]
Influenza- ('flu)-like syndrome (19%) [2]
Interstitial lung disease / interstitial pneumonitis / interstitial pneumonia (cryptogenic organizing pneumonia) / drug-induced interstitial lung disease [8]
Pneumonitis [4]
Pulmonary toxicity [11]

Other
Adverse effects / adverse reactions [9]

Allergic reactions (4%)
Death [13]
Infection (16%) [11]

GEMFIBROZIL

Trade name: Lopid (Pfizer)
Indications: Hyperlipidemia
Class: Fibrate, Lipid regulator
Half-life: 2 hours
Clinically important, potentially hazardous interactions with: atorvastatin, bexarotene, colchicine, cyclosporine, dicumarol, eluxadoline, enzalutamide, ezetimibe, fluvastatin, interferon alfa, lovastatin, nicotinic acid, ombitasvir/paritaprevir/ritonavir and dasabuvir, ozanimod, paclitaxel, pioglitazone, pitavastatin, pravastatin, repaglinide, rosiglitazone, rosuvastatin, roxithromycin, selexipag, simvastatin, treprostinil, tucatinib, warfarin
Important contra-indications noted in the prescribing guidelines for: nursing mothers; pediatric patients
Note: Contra-indicated in patients with preexisting gallbladder disease.

Skin
Eczema / eczematous reaction / eczematous eruption (2%)
Exanthems (3%) [2]
Psoriasis [3]
Rash (2%)

Central Nervous System
Headache [3]

Gastrointestinal/Hepatic
Abdominal pain (10%)
Dyspepsia / functional dyspepsia (indigestion) (see also gastroparesis) (20%)
Hepatotoxicity / liver injury / acute liver injury / drug-induced liver injury (DILI) [2]
Pancreatitis / acute pancreatitis [2]

Neuromuscular/Skeletal
Asthenia / fatigue (2%)
Compartment syndrome [2]
Myalgia/Myopathy [5]
Rhabdomyolysis [35]

Other
Death [2]

GEMIFLOXACIN

Trade name: Factive (LG Life Sciences)
Indications: Infections due to various microorganisms
Class: Antibiotic, Antibiotic; fluoroquinolone, Antimicrobial
Half-life: 4–12 hours
Clinically important, potentially hazardous interactions with: antacids, BCG vaccine, calcium salts, corticosteroids, didanosine, dong quai, insulin, iron salts, magnesium salts, mycophenolate, NSAIDs, probenecid, quinapril, sevelamer, St John's wort, sucralfate, sulfonylureas, typhoid vaccine, vitamin K antagonists, zinc
Important contra-indications noted in the prescribing guidelines for: the elderly; nursing mothers; pediatric patients
Note: Fluoroquinolones are associated with an increased risk of tendinitis and tendon rupture in all ages. This risk is further increased in older patients usually over 60 years of age, in patients taking corticosteroid drugs, and in patients with kidney, heart or lung transplants.
Fluoroquinolones may exacerbate muscle weakness in persons with myasthenia gravis.
The incidence of rash increases significantly when duration of therapy exceeds seven days, reaching 7.4% at 14 days.
Warning: SERIOUS ADVERSE REACTIONS INCLUDING TENDINITIS, TENDON RUPTURE, PERIPHERAL NEUROPATHY, CENTRIAL NERVOUS SYSTEM EFFECTS and EXACERBATION OF MYASTHENIA GRAVIS

Skin
Photosensitivity [2]
Rash (2–7%) [7]

Cardiovascular
QT interval prolonged / QT prolongation [2]

Central Nervous System
Vertigo / dizziness (2%)

Gastrointestinal/Hepatic
Abdominal pain (2%)
Diarrhea (5%)
Nausea (4%)
Vomiting (2%)

Genitourinary
Vaginitis (includes vulvitis) [4]

Other
Adverse effects / adverse reactions [2]

GEMTUZUMAB

Trade name: Mylotarg (Wyeth)
Indications: Acute myeloid leukemia
Class: Antineoplastic / anticancer agent (see also Immune checkpoint inhibitor), Monoclonal antibody
Half-life: 45 hours (initial dose)
Clinically important, potentially hazardous interactions with: none known
Important contra-indications noted in the prescribing guidelines for: nursing mothers; pediatric patients
Warning: HEPATOTOXICITY

Skin
Bruise / bruising / contusion / ecchymosis (ecchymoses) (10%)
Herpes simplex (21%)
Peripheral edema (14%)
Petechiae (19%)
Pruritus (itching) (6%)
Rash (18%)

Mucosal
Gingival bleeding (9%)
Mucositis [4]
Stomatitis (oral mucositis) (25%)

Cardiovascular
Veno-occlusive disease [2]

Central Nervous System
Chills (66%)
Headache (37%)
Pain (18%)

Gastrointestinal/Hepatic
Hepatotoxicity / liver injury / acute liver injury / drug-induced liver injury (DILI) [5]
Nausea [2]
Vomiting [2]

Hematologic
Febrile neutropenia [3]
Hemorrhage [2]
Leukocytopenia (leukopenia) / leukocytes (white blood cells) decreased [2]
Neutropenia (neutrophils decreased) [7]
Thrombocytopenia / platelets decreased (50%) [5]

Local
Infusion-related reactions [2]
Injection-site reaction (22%)

Neuromuscular/Skeletal
Arthralgia (10%)

Other
Infection (9%) [5]

GENTAMICIN

Trade names: Garamycin (Schering), Genoptic (Allergan)
Indications: Various infections caused by susceptible organisms
Class: Antibiotic, Antibiotic; aminoglycoside, Antimicrobial
Half-life: 2–4 hours
Clinically important, potentially hazardous interactions with: adefovir, aldesleukin, aminoglycosides, atracurium, bumetanide, carbenicillin, cephalexin, cephalothin, cobicistat/elvitegravir/emtricitabine/tenofovir alafenamide, doxacurium, ethacrynic acid, furosemide, methoxyflurane, non-polarizing muscle relaxants, pancuronium, pipecuronium, polypeptide antibiotics, rocuronium, succinylcholine, teicoplanin, torsemide, tubocurarine, vecuronium
Important contra-indications noted in the prescribing guidelines for: the elderly; nursing mothers
Note: Aminoglycosides may cause neurotoxicity and/or nephrotoxicity.

Skin
Anaphylactoid reactions / anaphylaxis (includes anaphylactic shock) [2]
Dermatitis [8]
Edema / fluid retention (<10%)
Erythema (<10%)
Exanthems [5]
Photosensitivity [2]
Pruritus (itching) (<10%)

Hair
Alopecia / hair loss [2]

Local
Injection-site necrosis [5]

Otic
Ototoxicity [12]
Tinnitus [4]

Renal
Bartter-like syndrome [3]
Fanconi syndrome (proximal tubular dysfunction) [2]
Nephrotoxicity / kidney injury / acute kidney injury (AKI) / drug-induced kidney injury [14]

GILTERITINIB

Trade name: Xospata (Astellas)
Indications: indicated for the treatment of adult patients who have relapsed or refractory acute myeloid leukemia (AML) with a FLT3 mutation as detected by an FDA-approved test
Class: Kinase inhibitor
Half-life: 113 hours
Clinically important, potentially hazardous interactions with: escitalopram, fluoxetine, sertraline
Pregnancy category: can cause fetal harm
Important contra-indications noted in the prescribing guidelines for: nursing mothers

---

Skin
Edema / fluid retention (34%)
Rash (30%)

Mucosal
Stomatitis (oral mucositis) (26%)

Cardiovascular
Cardiac failure (4%)
Hypertension (10%)
Hypotension (21%)
Pericardial effusion (3%)
Pericarditis (2%)
QT interval prolonged / QT prolongation (7%)

Central Nervous System
Dysgeusia (taste perversion) (11%)
Fever (pyrexia) (includes hyperpyrexia) (35%)
Headache (21%)
Insomnia (14%)
Vertigo / dizziness (20%)

Endocrine/Metabolic
ALP increased (65%)
ALT increased (78%)
Appetite decreased (15%)
AST increased (78%)
Creatine phosphokinase (CPK) / creatine kinase increased (hyperCKemia) (54%)
Hyperbilirubinemia (11%)
Hyperglycemia (includes glucose increased) (86%)
Hypertriglyceridemia (includes triglycerides increased) (81%)
Hypoalbuminemia / albumin decreased (58%)
Hypocalcemia (61%)
Hypokalemia (35%)
Hyponatremia (32%)
Hypophosphatemia (48%)
Serum creatinine increased (94%)

Gastrointestinal/Hepatic
Abdominal pain (17%)
Constipation (27%)
Diarrhea (34%)
Nausea (27%)
Vomiting (20%)

Hematologic
Sepsis (15%)
Thrombocytopenia / platelets decreased [2]

Neuromuscular/Skeletal
Arthralgia (42%)
Asthenia / fatigue (40%)
Myalgia/Myopathy (42%)

Renal
Renal function abnormal / renal dysfunction (19%)

Respiratory
Cough (25%)
Dyspnea / shortness of breath (34%)
Pneumonia (30%)

GINGER

Family: Zingiberaceae
Scientific name: *Zingiber officinale*
Indications: Colic, dyspepsia, flatulence, rheumatoid arthritis, loss of appetite, nausea, vomiting, upper respiratory infections, cough, bronchitis, burns, tinnitus, flavoring agent, fragrance component
Class: Carminative, Oleoresin
Half-life: N/A
Clinically important, potentially hazardous interactions with: arsenic, clevidipine, squill

---

Gastrointestinal/Hepatic
Diarrhea [2]
Nausea [2]

GINKGO BILOBA

Family: Ginkgoaceae
Scientific name: *Ginkgo biloba (Mericon)*
Indications: Dementia, memory loss, headache, tinnitus, dizziness, mood disturbances, hearing disorders, intermittent claudication, attention deficit hyperactivity disorder, premenstrual syndrome, heart disease
Class: Food supplement, Vascular stimulant
Half-life: N/A
Clinically important, potentially hazardous interactions with: anticoagulants, aspirin, diuretics, NSAIDs, platelet inhibitors, SSRIs, St John's wort, thiazide diuretics, trazodone
Note: *Ginkgo biloba* is the oldest living tree species in the world. Ginkgo is the most frequently prescribed herbal medicine in Germany.

Skin
Dermatitis [3]
Exanthems [2]
Fixed eruption / fixed drug eruption [2]

Cardiovascular
Hypertension [2]

Central Nervous System
Cerebral hemorrhage [2]
Seizures [5]

Hematologic
Bleeding [2]

Ocular
Ocular adverse effect [2]

Other
Adverse effects / adverse reactions [9]

GINSENG

Family: Araliaceae; oriental ginseng
Scientific name: *Panax ginseng*
Indications: General tonic, improving stamina, cognitive function, concentration, diuretic, antidepressant, gastritis, neurasthenia, impotence, fever, hangover, cancer, cardiovascular diseases
Class: Immunomodulator
Half-life: N/A
Clinically important, potentially hazardous interactions with: alcohol, arsenic, aspirin, caffeine, clevidipine, phenelzine, squill, tamoxifen
Note: Ginseng has been used for medicinal purposes for more than 2000 years. Approximately 6,000,000 Americans use it regularly.

Skin
Stevens-Johnson syndrome and toxic epidermal necrolysis (SJS/TEN) [2]

Cardiovascular
Hypertension [2]

Central Nervous System
Insomnia [2]
Mania [4]

Endocrine/Metabolic
Mastodynia [3]

Gastrointestinal/Hepatic
Hepatotoxicity / liver injury / acute liver injury / drug-induced liver injury (DILI) [2]

Other
Adverse effects / adverse reactions [8]
Side effects [2]

GLATIRAMER

Synonym: copolymer-1
Trade names: Copaxone (Teva), Glatopa (Novartis)
Indications: Multiple sclerosis
Class: Immunomodulator
Half-life: N/A
Clinically important, potentially hazardous interactions with: Hemophilus B vaccine
Important contra-indications noted in the prescribing guidelines for: the elderly; nursing mothers; pediatric patients

---

Skin
Acneiform eruption / acneiform dermatitis / acneiform rash (>2%)
Anaphylactoid reactions / anaphylaxis (includes anaphylactic shock) [3]
Bruise / bruising / contusion / ecchymosis (ecchymoses) (8%)
Cyst / pseudocyst (2%)
Diaphoresis (15%)
Eczema / eczematous reaction / eczematous eruption (8%)
Edema / fluid retention (8%)
Erythema (4%)
Facial edema (6%)
Flushing / rubefaction [6]
Herpes simplex (4%)
Hyperhidrosis (15%)
Hypersensitivity (3%)
Lipoatrophy [3]
Nicolau syndrome [5]
Nodular eruption (2%)
Panniculitis [2]

Peripheral edema (7%)
Pruritus (itching) (4%)
Purpura (8%)
Rash (18%)
Urticaria / hives [2]

Hair
Alopecia / hair loss (>2%)

Nails
Nail changes (>2%)

Mucosal
Oral vesiculation (6%)
Xerostomia (dry mouth) (>2%)

Cardiovascular
Chest pain (13%) [3]
Palpitation (7%) [7]
Vasodilation (20%) [2]

Central Nervous System
Anxiety (13%) [4]
Chills (4%)
Depression (>2%)
Dysgeusia (taste perversion) (>2%)
Fever (pyrexia) (includes hyperpyrexia) (6%)
Hyperesthesia (>2%)
Migraine (4%)
Pain (28%) [3]
Paresthesias (>2%) [2]
Tremor (7%)
Vertigo / dizziness (>2%)

Endocrine/Metabolic
Mastodynia (>2%)

Gastrointestinal/Hepatic
Hepatotoxicity / liver injury / acute liver injury / drug-induced liver injury (DILI) [3]
Nausea (15%) [2]
Vomiting (7%)

Genitourinary
Urinary tract infection [2]
Vaginitis (includes vulvitis) (4%)

Local
Injection-site bleeding (5%)
Injection-site ecchymoses (>2%)
Injection-site edema [2]
Injection-site erythema (66%) [4]
Injection-site induration (13%) [3]
Injection-site inflammation (49%)
Injection-site lipoatrophy/lipohypertrophy [2]
Injection-site pain (73%) [3]
Injection-site pruritus (40%) [3]
Injection-site reaction (6–67%) [15]
Injection-site urticaria (5%)

Neuromuscular/Skeletal
Arthralgia (24%)
Asthenia / fatigue (19%)
Myalgia/Myopathy (>2%)

Otic
Tinnitus (>2%)

Respiratory
Cough (>2%)
Dyspnea / shortness of breath [4]
Influenza- ('flu)-like syndrome (26%)
Sinusitis (see also rhinitis / rhinosinusitis) (>2%)

Other
Adverse effects / adverse reactions [5]
Infection (50%) [2]

GLECAPREVIR & PIBRENTASVIR

Trade name: Mavyret (AbbVie)
Indications: Chronic HCV genotype 1–6 infection
Class: Direct-acting antiviral, Hepatitis C virus NS3/4A protease inhibitor (glecaprevir), Hepatitis C virus NS5A inhibitor (pibrentasvir)
Half-life: 6 hours (glecaprevir); 13 hours (pibrentasvir)
Clinically important, potentially hazardous interactions with: atazanavir, atorvastatin, carbamazepine, cyclosporine, darunavir, efavirenz, lopinavir, lovastatin, oral contraceptives, rifampin, ritonavir, simvastatin, St John's wort
Pregnancy category: Insufficient evidence to inform drug-associated risk
Important contra-indications noted in the prescribing guidelines for: nursing mothers; pediatric patients
Note: Contra-indicated in patients with severe hepatic impairment (Child-Pugh C).
Warning: RISK OF HEPATITIS B VIRUS REACTIVATION IN PATIENTS COINFECTED WITH HCV AND HBV

Skin
Pruritus (itching) [12]

Central Nervous System
Headache (13%) [12]

Endocrine/Metabolic
Hyperbilirubinemia (<4%) [4]

Gastrointestinal/Hepatic
Diarrhea [2]
Nausea (8%) [6]

Neuromuscular/Skeletal
Asthenia / fatigue (11%) [14]

Other
Adverse effects / adverse reactions [9]

GLICLAZIDE

Trade names: Diamicron (Servier), Diamicron MR (Servier)
Indications: Non-insulin dependent diabetes mellitus
Class: Sulfonylurea
Half-life: 10–12 hours
Clinically important, potentially hazardous interactions with: beta andrenergic blocking agents, chloramphenicol, cimetidine, clofibrate, coumarin derivatives, disopyramide, MAO inhibitors, miconazole, phenylbutazone, salicylates, sulfonamides, tetracycline
Important contra-indications noted in the prescribing guidelines for: pediatric patients
Note: Gliclazide is a sulfonamide and can be absorbed systemically. Sulfonamides can produce severe, possibly fatal, reactions such as toxic epidermal necrolysis and Stevens-Johnson syndrome.

Endocrine/Metabolic
Hypoglycemia [2]

Gastrointestinal/Hepatic
Hepatotoxicity / liver injury / acute liver injury / drug-induced liver injury (DILI) [2]
Pancreatitis / acute pancreatitis [2]

Neuromuscular/Skeletal
Arthralgia (<5%)
Back pain (<5%)

Respiratory
Bronchitis (<5%)

GLIMEPIRIDE

Trade names: Amaryl (Sanofi-Aventis), Avandaryl (GSK)
Indications: Non-insulin dependent diabetes Type II
Class: Antidiabetic, Hypoglycemic (antihyperglycemic) agent, Sulfonylurea
Half-life: 5–9 hours
Clinically important, potentially hazardous interactions with: none known
Important contra-indications noted in the prescribing guidelines for: the elderly; nursing mothers; pediatric patients
Note: Glimepiride is a sulfonamide and can be absorbed systemically. Sulfonamides can produce severe, possibly fatal, reactions such as toxic epidermal necrolysis and Stevens-Johnson syndrome
Avandaryl is glimepiride and rosiglitazone.

Central Nervous System
Headache [4]
Vertigo / dizziness [2]

Endocrine/Metabolic
Hypoglycemia [12]
Weight gain [3]

Gastrointestinal/Hepatic
Diarrhea [5]
Dyspepsia / functional dyspepsia (indigestion) (see also gastroparesis) [2]
Nausea [4]
Pancreatitis / acute pancreatitis [2]

Genitourinary
Genital mycotic infection [4]
Urinary tract infection [3]

Neuromuscular/Skeletal
Arthralgia [2]

Other
Adverse effects / adverse reactions [5]

GLIPIZIDE

Trade names: Glucotrol (Pfizer), Metaglip (Bristol-Myers Squibb)
Indications: Non-insulin dependent diabetes Type II
Class: Antidiabetic, Hypoglycemic (antihyperglycemic) agent, Sulfonylurea
Half-life: 2–4 hours
Clinically important, potentially hazardous interactions with: none known
Important contra-indications noted in the prescribing guidelines for: the elderly; nursing mothers; pediatric patients
Note: Glipizide is a sulfonamide and can be absorbed systemically. Sulfonamides can produce severe, possibly fatal, reactions such as toxic epidermal necrolysis and Stevens-Johnson syndrome.

Skin
Photosensitivity (<10%)
Pruritus (itching) (<3%)
Rash (<10%)

Stevens-Johnson syndrome and toxic epidermal necrolysis (SJS/TEN) [2]
Urticaria / hives (<10%)

Central Nervous System
Hyperesthesia (<3%)
Paresthesias (<3%)

Endocrine/Metabolic
Hypoglycemia [3]

Neuromuscular/Skeletal
Myalgia/Myopathy (<3%)

Other
Adverse effects / adverse reactions [2]

GLUCAGON

Trade name: Glucagon Emergency Kit (Lilly)
Indications: Hypoglycemic reactions
Class: Hormone, polypeptide
Half-life: 3–10 minutes
Clinically important, potentially hazardous interactions with: insulin degludec, insulin glargine, insulin glulisine, warfarin

---

Skin
Erythema necrolyticum migrans [2]
Exanthems [7]
Folliculitis [2]
Pyoderma gangrenosum [3]
Rash [2]
Sweet's syndrome [7]
Urticaria / hives (<10%) [2]
Vasculitis (angiitis) / cutaneous vasculitis (angiitis) [9]

Local
Injection-site reaction [3]

GLUCOSAMINE

Trade names: Arthro-Aid (NutraSense), Glucosamine sulfate (Rottapharm)
Indications: Arthritis, osteoarthritis, cartilage repair and maintenance, strained joints, improving joint function and range of motion, alleviating joint pain
Class: Amino sugar, Food supplement
Half-life: N/A
Clinically important, potentially hazardous interactions with: abciximab, cilostazol, citalopram, clopidogrel, eptifibatide, meloxicam

---

Mucosal
Oral vesiculation (7%)

Central Nervous System
Depression (6%)

Gastrointestinal/Hepatic
Dyspepsia / functional dyspepsia (indigestion) (see also gastroparesis) [2]
Hepatotoxicity / liver injury / acute liver injury / drug-induced liver injury (DILI) [3]
Nausea [2]

Neuromuscular/Skeletal
Asthenia / fatigue (9%) [2]

Other
Adverse effects / adverse reactions (6%) [5]
Allergic reactions (4%) [2]

GLYBURIDE

Synonyms: glibenclamide; glybenclamide
Trade names: Diabeta (Sanofi-Aventis), Glucovance (Bristol-Myers Squibb), Glynase (Pfizer), Micronase (Pfizer)
Indications: Non-insulin dependent diabetes Type II
Class: Antidiabetic, Hypoglycemic (antihyperglycemic) agent, Sulfonylurea
Half-life: 5–16 hours
Clinically important, potentially hazardous interactions with: bosentan, colesevelam, letermovir, norfloxacin
Note: Glyburide is a sulfonamide and can be absorbed systemically. Sulfonamides can produce severe, possibly fatal, reactions such as toxic epidermal necrolysis and Stevens-Johnson syndrome.
Glucovance is glyburide and metformin.

Skin
Erythema (<5%)
Exanthems (<5%) [3]
Flushing / rubefaction [2]
Linear IgA bullous dermatosis [2]
Pemphigus [2]
Photosensitivity (<10%) [5]
Pruritus (itching) (<10%) [3]
Psoriasis [2]
Purpura [2]
Rash (<10%)
Urticaria / hives (<5%) [4]
Vasculitis (angiitis) / cutaneous vasculitis (angiitis) [5]

Endocrine/Metabolic
Hypoglycemia [2]
Weight gain [2]

Other
Adverse effects / adverse reactions [3]

GLYCOPYRROLATE

Synonyms: glycopyrronium bromide, glycopyrronium tosylate
Trade names: Cuvposa (Shionogi), Robinul (Forte), Seebri Neohaler (Novartis), Utibron Neohaler (Novartis)
Indications: Duodenal ulcer, irritable bowel syndrome, hyperhidrosis
Class: Anticholinergic, Muscarinic antagonist, Non-depolarizing muscle relaxant
Half-life: N/A
Clinically important, potentially hazardous interactions with: anticholinergics, arbutamine, belladonna alkaloids, digoxin, disopyramide, meperidine, phenothiazines, procainamide, quinidine, ritodrine, tricyclic antidepressants
Important contra-indications noted in the prescribing guidelines for: the elderly; nursing mothers; pediatric patients
Note: Utibron Neohaler is glycopyrrolate and indacaterol.

Skin
Flushing / rubefaction (30%)
Photosensitivity (<10%)
Rash [2]
Xerosis / xeroderma (>10%)

Mucosal
Nasal congestion (30%)
Xerostomia (dry mouth) (40%) [12]

Cardiovascular
Bradycardia / sinus bradycardia [2]

Central Nervous System
Headache (15%) [2]

Gastrointestinal/Hepatic
Constipation (35%) [2]
Vomiting (40%)

Genitourinary
Urinary retention (15%)

Local
Application-site pruritus [2]
Injection-site irritation (>10%)

Ocular
Mydriasis [4]
Vision blurred [2]

Respiratory
Nasopharyngitis [2]
Sinusitis (see also rhinitis / rhinosinusitis) (15%)
Upper respiratory tract infection (15%)

GOLD & GOLD COMPOUNDS

Synonyms: auranofin; aurothioglucose
Trade names: Myochrysine (Merck), Myocrisin (Sanofi-Aventis), Ridaura (Prometheus), Solganal (Schering)
Indications: Rheumatoid arthritis
Class: Disease-modifying antirheumatic drug (DMARD)
Half-life: 5 days
Clinically important, potentially hazardous interactions with: ACE inhibitors, benazepril, captopril, cilazapril, enalapril, fosinopril, lisinopril, penicillamine, phenytoin, quinapril, ramipril, trandolapril
Important contra-indications noted in the prescribing guidelines for: nursing mothers; pediatric patients
Note: Contra-indicated in patients with a history of any of the following gold-induced disorders: anaphylactic reactions, necrotizing enterocolitis, pulmonary fibrosis, exfoliative dermatitis, bone marrow aplasia or other severe hematologic disorders. Adverse reactions can occur months after therapy has been discontinued.

Skin
Acneiform eruption / acneiform dermatitis / acneiform rash [2]
Bullous dermatosis [3]
Chrysiasis (blue-green pigmentation) [3]
Cutaneous toxicity / skin toxicity [5]
Dermatitis [64]
Eczema / eczematous reaction / eczematous eruption [3]
Erythema multiforme [2]
Erythema nodosum [4]
Exanthems (>5%) [10]
Exfoliative dermatitis [9]
Granuloma annulare [2]
Herpes zoster [2]
Lichen planus (includes hypertrophic lichen planus) (<32%) [11]
Lichenoid eruption / lichenoid reaction [8]
Lupus erythematosus (subacute cutaneous lupus erythematosus (SCLE)) [3]
Pemphigus [3]
Photosensitivity [2]

Pigmentation (Skin) (includes hyperpigmentation) [20]
Pityriasis rosea [10]
Pruritus (itching) (17%) [10]
Pseudolymphoma / cutaneous pseudolymphoma [3]
Purpura [3]
Rash (24%) [12]
Seborrheic dermatitis [3]
Squamous cell carcinoma [2]
Stevens-Johnson syndrome and toxic epidermal necrolysis (SJS/TEN) [4]
Urticaria / hives (<10%) [7]
Vasculitis (angiitis) / cutaneous vasculitis (angiitis) [4]

Hair
Alopecia / hair loss (<10%) [7]

Nails
Nail dystrophy [2]
Nail pigmentation [3]

Mucosal
Aphthous stomatitis / aphthous ulcer / aphtha (aphthae) [4]
Cheilitis (inflammation of the lips) [2]
Gingivitis (>10%) [2]
Glossitis (inflammation of the tongue) (>10%) [2]
Mucocutaneous reactions [4]
Oral lichen planus [3]
Oral pigmentation [2]
Oral ulceration [6]
Stomatitis (oral mucositis) (13%) [22]

Cardiovascular
Myocardial infarction [2]

Central Nervous System
Dysgeusia (taste perversion) [4]
Neurotoxicity [5]
Syncope / fainting [3]

Gastrointestinal/Hepatic
Abdominal pain (14%)
Diarrhea (47%) [5]
Hepatotoxicity / liver injury / acute liver injury / drug-induced liver injury (DILI) [2]
Loose stools / soft feces (47%)
Nausea (10%) [3]
Vomiting [2]

Hematologic
Leukocytopenia (leukopenia) / leukocytes (white blood cells) decreased [2]
Thrombocytopenia / platelets decreased [4]

Renal
Nephrotoxicity / kidney injury / acute kidney injury (AKI) / drug-induced kidney injury [2]
Proteinuria [5]

Respiratory
Pneumonitis [2]

Other
Death [4]

GOLDENSEAL

Family: Ranunculaceae
Scientific name: *Hydrastis canadensis*
Indications: Oral: Anorexia, fever, hemorrhoids, hemorrhage, liver disorders, menstrual disorders, rhinitis, upper respiratory tract infections, urinary tract infections. **Topical:** Acne, conjunctivitis, dandruff, earache, eczema, eye inflammation, herpes, itching, mouthwash, rash, ringworm, tinnitus, wounds
Class: Immunomodulator, Isoquinolone alkaloid
Half-life: N/A
Clinically important, potentially hazardous interactions with: clevidipine

GOLIMUMAB

Trade name: Simponi (Centocor)
Indications: Rheumatoid arthritis, psoriatic arthritis, ankylosing spondylitis, ulcerative colitis
Class: Anti-Tumor Necrosis Factor-alpha (TNF-α antagonist), Biologic, Biologic disease-modifying antirheumatic drug (bDMARD), Disease-modifying antirheumatic drug (DMARD), Monoclonal antibody
Half-life: 2 weeks
Clinically important, potentially hazardous interactions with: abatacept, anakinra, live vaccines
Important contra-indications noted in the prescribing guidelines for: nursing mothers; pediatric patients
Note: TNF inhibitors should be used in patients with heart failure only after consideration of other treatment options. TNF inhibitors are contra-indicated in patients with a personal or family history of multiple sclerosis or demyelinating disease. TNF inhibitors should not be administered to patients with moderate to severe heart failure (New York Heart Association Functional Class III/IV).
Warning: SERIOUS INFECTIONS AND MALIGNANCY

Skin
Lupus erythematosus (subacute cutaneous lupus erythematosus (SCLE)) [3]
Psoriasis [2]
Rash [4]

Cardiovascular
Hypertension [2]

Central Nervous System
Headache [7]

Endocrine/Metabolic
ALT increased [4]
AST increased [3]

Gastrointestinal/Hepatic
Colitis [2]
Diarrhea [4]
Nausea [6]

Genitourinary
Urinary tract infection [2]

Hematologic
Sepsis [4]

Local
Injection-site erythema [7]
Injection-site reaction (6%) [7]

Neuromuscular/Skeletal
Arthralgia [3]
Asthenia / fatigue [3]

Respiratory
Cough [2]
Nasopharyngitis (6%) [7]
Pneumonia [4]
Pulmonary toxicity [2]
Tuberculosis [2]
Upper respiratory tract infection (7%) [8]

Other
Adverse effects / adverse reactions [15]
Death [3]
Infection (28%) [19]
Malignancies [6]

GOSERELIN

Trade name: Zoladex (AstraZeneca)
Indications: Breast and prostate carcinoma, endometriosis
Class: Gonadotropin-releasing hormone (GnRH) agonist
Half-life: 5 hours
Clinically important, potentially hazardous interactions with: none known
Pregnancy category: category D in patients with advanced breast cancer
Important contra-indications noted in the prescribing guidelines for: nursing mothers; pediatric patients

---

Skin
Acneiform eruption / acneiform dermatitis / acneiform rash (>20%)
Anaphylactoid reactions / anaphylaxis (includes anaphylactic shock) [3]
Diaphoresis (>20%)
Edema / fluid retention (<10%)
Hot flashes / hot flushes (>10%) [5]
Peripheral edema (>20%)
Pruritus (itching) (<5%)
Rash (<10%)
Seborrhea (>20%)

Hair
Hirsutism (>5%)

Cardiovascular
Arrhythmias (<5%)
Chest pain (<5%)
Congestive heart failure (>5%)
Hypertension (<5%)
Myocardial infarction (<5%)
Vasodilation (>5%)

Central Nervous System
Anorexia (>5%)
Anxiety (<5%)
Chills (<5%)
Depression (>20%) [2]
Emotional lability (>20%)
Fever (pyrexia) (includes hyperpyrexia) (<5%)
Headache (>20%)
Insomnia (>5%)
Nervousness (<5%)
Pain (>10%)
Stroke / cerebrovascular accident (<5%)
Vertigo / dizziness (>5%)

Endocrine/Metabolic
Appetite increased (<5%)
Breast atrophy (>20%)
Gynecomastia (>10%)
Hyperglycemia (includes glucose increased) (in men) (<5%)
Libido decreased (>20%)
Libido increased (in women) (>10%)

Mastodynia (<10%)
Weight gain (<5%)

Gastrointestinal/Hepatic
Abdominal pain (>5%)
Constipation (<5%)
Diarrhea (<5%)
Gastrointestinal ulceration (<5%)
Nausea (>5%)
Vomiting (<5%)

Genitourinary
Dyspareunia (>10%)
Urinary obstruction (<5%)
Urinary tract infection (<5%)
Vaginitis (includes vulvitis) (>20%)

Hematologic
Anemia (<5%)

Local
Infusion-site reactions (>5%)
Injection-site pain (<10%)

Neuromuscular/Skeletal
Arthralgia [4]
Asthenia / fatigue (>10%)
Back pain (>5%)
Gouty tophi (<5%)
Hypertonia (<5%)
Leg cramps (<5%)
Myalgia/Myopathy (<5%)

Respiratory
COPD (>5%)
Dysphonia (includes voice disorders / voice changes) (<5%)
Influenza- ('flu)-like syndrome (<5%)
Pharyngitis (sore throat) (<5%)

Other
Infection (>10%)

GRANISETRON

Trade names: Kytril (Roche), Sancuso (ProStrakan), Sustol (Heron)
Indications: Chemotherapy-related emesis
Class: 5-HT3 antagonist, Antiemetic, Serotonin type 3 receptor antagonist
Half-life: 3–4 hours; cancer patients: 10–12 hours
Clinically important, potentially hazardous interactions with: apomorphine, apomorphine, vandetanib
Important contra-indications noted in the prescribing guidelines for: nursing mothers; pediatric patients

---

Hair
Alopecia / hair loss (3%)

Central Nervous System
Dysgeusia (taste perversion) (2%)
Headache [12]
Vertigo / dizziness [3]

Gastrointestinal/Hepatic
Constipation [9]

Neuromuscular/Skeletal
Asthenia / fatigue [2]

GRANULOCYTE COLONY-STIMULATING FACTOR (G-CSF)

Synonyms: filgrastim; sargramostim; pegfilgrastim; mecapegfilgrastim (pegfilgrastim biosimilar)
Trade names: Granix (Sicor), Leukine (Bayer) (Berlex), Neulasta (Amgen), Neupogen (Amgen), Zarxio (Novartis)
Indications: Bone marrow allograft and autograft
Class: Biologic, Colony stimulating factor, Covid-19 putative drug, Hematopoietic
Half-life: filgrastim: 3.5 hours; sargramostim: 2–3 hours; pegfilgrastim: 15–80 hours; tbo-filgrastim: 3–4 hours
Clinically important, potentially hazardous interactions with: fluorouracil
Important contra-indications noted in the prescribing guidelines for: nursing mothers; pediatric patients
Note: rGM-CSF is granulocyte-macrophage colony-stimulating factor; rG-CSF is granulocyte colony-stimulating factor.

Skin
Anaphylactoid reactions / anaphylaxis (includes anaphylactic shock) [4]
Erythema [5]
Erythema nodosum [2]
Exanthems (5–63%) [11]
Exfoliative dermatitis (10%)
Flushing / rubefaction (>10%)
Graft-versus-host reaction [4]
Leukocytoclastic vasculitis (angiitis) [4]
Lymphoproliferative disease / lymphoproliferative disorder [2]
Peripheral edema (<10%)
Pruritus (itching) (<5%) [5]
Psoriasis [5]
Pyoderma gangrenosum [4]
Rash (<40%) [8]
Sweet's syndrome [45]
Urticaria / hives [4]
Vasculitis (angiitis) / cutaneous vasculitis (angiitis) [9]

Hair
Alopecia / hair loss (>10%)

Mucosal
Mucositis (40%) [2]
Stomatitis (oral mucositis) (>10%) [2]

Cardiovascular
Aortitis / periaortitis [5]
Capillary leak syndrome [6]
Large-vessel vasculitis (includes giant cell arteritis) [9]

Central Nervous System
Anorexia [2]
Carotidynia / Fay syndrome / Transient Perivascular Inflammation of the Carotid artery (TIPIC) syndrome [3]
Fever (pyrexia) (includes hyperpyrexia) (5–50%) [21]
Headache (39–80%) [13]
Neurotoxicity [2]
Pain [2]
Vertigo / dizziness (>5%)

Gastrointestinal/Hepatic
Colitis [2]
Hepatotoxicity / liver injury / acute liver injury / drug-induced liver injury (DILI) [3]
Nausea [5]

Hematologic
Anemia [3]
Febrile neutropenia [6]
Leukocytosis (elevated white blood cell (WBC) count) [5]
Neutropenia (neutrophils decreased) [4]
Thrombocytopenia / platelets decreased [3]

Local
Injection-site pain (1–10%)
Injection-site pruritus [2]
Injection-site reaction (>5%) [6]

Neuromuscular/Skeletal
Arthralgia [5]
Asthenia / fatigue [11]
Back pain [2]
Bone pain / joint pain (13–84%) [46]
Musculoskeletal pain [2]
Myalgia/Myopathy (>10%) [4]
Rhabdomyolysis [2]

Renal
Nephrotoxicity / kidney injury / acute kidney injury (AKI) / drug-induced kidney injury [4]

Respiratory
Influenza- ('flu)-like syndrome [2]
Pneumonitis [2]
Respiratory distress [2]

Other
Adverse effects / adverse reactions (19%) [14]
Allergic reactions (19%)
Death [6]
Infection [3]

GRAPEFRUIT JUICE

Family: Rutaceae
Scientific names: *Citrus decumana, Citrus maxima, Citrus paradisi*
Indications: Atherosclerosis, anti-cancer agent, cholesterol reduction, psoriasis, weight reduction, source of potassium, vitamin C, and fiber
Class: CYP3A4 inhibitor, Food supplement
Half-life: N/A
Clinically important, potentially hazardous interactions with: abemaciclib, alprazolam, ambrisentan, amiodarone, amitriptyline, aprepitant, astemizole, atorvastatin, bexarotene, brigatinib, buspirone, cabazitaxel, cabozantinib, ceritinib, cilostazol, colchicine, copanlisib, corticosteroids, crizotinib, cyclosporine, deflazacort, dronedarone, efavirenz, eliglustat, enalapril, eplerenone, estradiol, everolimus, felodipine, finerenone, flibanserin, gefitinib, ibrutinib, indinavir, itraconazole, ivabradine, ivacaftor, ixabepilone, lapatinib, lercanidipine, lomitapide, lonafarnib, lovastatin, lumateperone, midazolam, midostaurin, mifepristone, naloxegol, neratinib, nifedipine, nilotinib, nisoldipine, olaparib, palbociclib, pazopanib, pimozide, ponatinib, prednisolone, prednisone, propafenone, ranolazine, red rice yeast, regorafenib, repaglinide, ribociclib, rosiglitazone, rupatadine, ruxolitinib, sildenafil, simvastatin, sunitinib, tacrolimus, tadalafil, temsirolimus, terfenadine, tezacaftor/ivacaftor, tolvaptan, ubrogepant, vardenafil, venetoclax, voriconazole, warfarin

---

Skin
Cutaneous toxicity / skin toxicity [2]

Central Nervous System
Headache [3]
Neuromuscular/Skeletal
Rhabdomyolysis [3]
Other
Adverse effects / adverse reactions [2]

GREEN TEA

Family: Theaceae
Scientific names: *Camellia sinensis, Camellia thea, Camellia theifera, Thea bohea, Thea sinensis, Thea viridis*
Indications: Improving cognitive performance, stomach disorders, nausea, vomiting, diarrhea, anticancer, headaches, Crohn's disease. **Topical**: soothe sunburn, bleeding gums, reduce sweating
Class: Anti-Tumor Necrosis Factor-alpha (TNF-α antagonist), Food supplement, Xanthine alkaloid
Half-life: N/A
Clinically important, potentially hazardous interactions with: none known
Note: Tea is consumed as a beverage.

Gastrointestinal/Hepatic
Hepatotoxicity / liver injury / acute liver injury / drug-induced liver injury (DILI) [11]
Other
Adverse effects / adverse reactions [6]

GRISEOFULVIN

Trade names: Fulvicin (Schering), Grifulvin V (Ortho), Gris-PEG (Pedinol)
Indications: Fungal infections of the skin, hair and nails
Class: Antifungal / antimycotic, Antimicrobial
Half-life: 9–24 hours
Clinically important, potentially hazardous interactions with: alcohol, amphotericin B, levonorgestrel, liraglutide, midazolam, thalidomide, ulipristal
Important contra-indications noted in the prescribing guidelines for: nursing mothers; pediatric patients

---

Skin
Angioedema (formerly named angioneurotic edema) [3]
Bullous dermatosis [2]
Cold urticaria [2]
Erythema multiforme [6]
Exanthems [6]
Exfoliative dermatitis [2]
Fixed eruption / fixed drug eruption [7]
Lichenoid eruption / lichenoid reaction [2]
Lupus erythematosus (subacute cutaneous lupus erythematosus (SCLE)) [14]
Petechiae [2]
Photosensitivity (<10%) [18]
Pigmentation (Skin) (includes hyperpigmentation) [2]
Pruritus (itching) [4]
Rash (>10%)
Serum sickness-like reaction [3]
Stevens-Johnson syndrome and toxic epidermal necrolysis (SJS/TEN) [7]
Urticaria / hives (>10%) [5]
Vasculitis (angiitis) / cutaneous vasculitis (angiitis) [2]
Mucosal
Oral candidiasis (<10%)

Central Nervous System
Dysgeusia (taste perversion) [3]
Endocrine/Metabolic
Gynecomastia [2]
Porphyria [12]
Other
Adverse effects / adverse reactions [2]
Allergic reactions (<5%)

GUANABENZ

Indications: Hypertension
Class: Adrenergic alpha-receptor agonist
Half-life: 7–10 hours
Clinically important, potentially hazardous interactions with: none known

---

Skin
Edema / fluid retention (<3%)
Pruritus (itching) (<3%)
Rash (<3%)
Mucosal
Xerostomia (dry mouth) (28%) [5]
Central Nervous System
Dysgeusia (taste perversion) (<3%)
Endocrine/Metabolic
Gynecomastia (<3%)

GUANADREL

Indications: Hypertension
Class: Adrenergic alpha-receptor agonist
Half-life: 5–45 hours (terminal)
Clinically important, potentially hazardous interactions with: none known

---

Skin
Peripheral edema (29%)
Mucosal
Glossitis (inflammation of the tongue) (8%)
Xerostomia (dry mouth) (2%)
Central Nervous System
Paresthesias (25%)

GUANETHIDINE

Trade name: Ismelin (Novartis)
Indications: Hypertension
Class: Adrenergic alpha-receptor agonist
Half-life: 5–10 days
Clinically important, potentially hazardous interactions with: amitriptyline, amoxapine, benzphetamine, bisoprolol, chlorpromazine, clomipramine, cyclopenthiazide, desipramine, doxepin, ephedra, ephedrine, imipramine, insulin, insulin degludec, insulin detemir, insulin glargine, insulin glulisine, minoxidil, nortriptyline, oxprenolol, pericyazine, protriptyline, sotalol, tricyclic antidepressants, trimipramine, zuclopenthixol, zuclopenthixol acetate, zuclopenthixol decanoate, zuclopenthixol dihydrochloride

---

Skin
Peripheral edema (>10%)
Mucosal
Glossitis (inflammation of the tongue) (5%)
Xerostomia (dry mouth) (<10%)
Central Nervous System
Paresthesias (16%)

GUANFACINE

Trade name: Tenex (ESP)
Indications: Hypertension, attention deficit hyperactivity disorder (ADHD)
Class: Adrenergic alpha-receptor agonist, Anti-attention deficit hyperactivity disorder (anti-ADHD), Imidazoline receptor agonist
Half-life: 10–30 hours
Clinically important, potentially hazardous interactions with: conivaptan, darunavir, delavirdine, efavirenz, indinavir, oxcarbazepine, rifapentine, telithromycin, voriconazole

---

Skin
Dermatitis (<3%)
Diaphoresis (<3%) [3]
Pruritus (itching) (<3%)
Purpura (<3%)
Mucosal
Xerostomia (dry mouth) (47%) [9]
Cardiovascular
Bradycardia / sinus bradycardia [4]
Hypotension [3]
Central Nervous System
Dysgeusia (taste perversion) (<3%)
Headache [6]
Insomnia [2]
Irritability [3]
Paresthesias (<3%)
Sedation [2]
Somnolence (drowsiness) [8]
Vertigo / dizziness [4]
Gastrointestinal/Hepatic
Abdominal pain [3]
Constipation [2]
Neuromuscular/Skeletal
Asthenia / fatigue [6]
Respiratory
Nasopharyngitis [4]
Other
Dipsia (thirst) / polydipsia [2]

GUARANA

Family: Sapindaceae
Scientific names: *Paullinia cupana, Paullinia sorbilis*
Indications: Aphrodisiac, diarrhea, fatigue, fever, heart problems, headache, mental alertness, neuralgia, weight loss. Cosmetic products, anti-cellulite creams, shampoo for hair loss. Flavoring
Class: Stimulant, mild
Half-life: N/A
Clinically important, potentially hazardous interactions with: caffeine, clozapine, ephedra, MAO inhibitors
Note: The main constituent of guarana is caffeine. It contains more than twice as much caffeine as coffee or tea. Excessive consumption of caffeine is contraindicated for persons with high blood pressure, cardiac disorders, diabetes, ulcers, and epilepsy. See also separate profile for caffeine.

Central Nervous System
Seizures [2]
Other
Adverse effects / adverse reactions [7]

GUSELKUMAB

Trade name: Tremfya (Janssen Biotech)
Indications: Moderate-to-severe plaque psoriasis
Class: Interleukin-17 (IL-17) antagonist / interleukin-17 inhibitor, Interleukin-23 inhibitor, Monoclonal antibody
Half-life: 15–18 days
Clinically important, potentially hazardous interactions with: live vaccines
Pregnancy category: Insufficient evidence to inform drug-associated risk
Important contra-indications noted in the prescribing guidelines for: nursing mothers; pediatric patients

---

Skin
Pruritus (itching) [2]
Central Nervous System
Headache (5%) [8]
Gastrointestinal/Hepatic
Diarrhea (2%)
Hepatotoxicity / liver injury / acute liver injury / drug-induced liver injury (DILI) (3%)
Local
Injection-site erythema [2]
Injection-site reaction (5%) [2]
Neuromuscular/Skeletal
Arthralgia (3%) [2]
Back pain [3]
Respiratory
Nasopharyngitis [15]
Upper respiratory tract infection (14%) [10]
Other
Adverse effects / adverse reactions [2]
Infection [6]

HALOFANTRINE

Trade name: Halfan (GSK)
Indications: Malaria
Class: Antimalarial
Half-life: 6–10 days
Clinically important, potentially hazardous interactions with: aprepitant, artemether/ lumefantrine, chloroquine, conivaptan, darunavir, delavirdine, efavirenz, indinavir, itraconazole, ketoconazole, mefloquine, nilotinib, quinine, ribociclib, sulpiride / levosulpiride, telithromycin, voriconazole

---

Skin
Pruritus (itching) (3%) [3]
Rash [2]
Cardiovascular
Palpitation [2]
QT interval prolonged / QT prolongation [14]
Ventricular tachycardia [2]
Central Nervous System
Anorexia (5%)
Headache (5%)
Rigors (2%)
Vertigo / dizziness (5%)
Gastrointestinal/Hepatic
Abdominal pain (10%) [4]
Diarrhea (5%) [2]
Nausea (10%) [2]
Vomiting (10%) [2]
Respiratory
Cough (3%)
Other
Death [6]

HALOPERIDOL

Trade name: Haldol (Ortho-McNeil)
Indications: Schizophrenia, Tourette's disorder
Class: Antiemetic, Antipsychotic
Half-life: 20 hours
Clinically important, potentially hazardous interactions with: acemetacin, arsenic, benztropine, citalopram, clozapine, darifenacin, fluoxetine, itraconazole, lisdexamfetamine, lithium, meloxicam, methotrexate, moxifloxacin, nilotinib, oxybutynin, propranolol, quinine, ribociclib, sotalol, sulpiride / levosulpiride, tetrabenazine, tiotropium, trospium, vandetanib, venlafaxine
Important contra-indications noted in the prescribing guidelines for: the elderly; pediatric patients
Warning: INCREASED MORTALITY IN ELDERLY PATIENTS WITH DEMENTIA-RELATED PSYCHOSIS

Skin
Cellulitis and pseudocellulitis [2]
Diaphoresis [2]
Photosensitivity [3]
Seborrheic dermatitis [2]
Hair
Alopecia areata [2]
Mucosal
Xerostomia (dry mouth) [4]
Cardiovascular
Arrhythmias [2]
QT interval prolonged / QT prolongation [23]
Torsades de pointes [12]
Ventricular arrhythmia [2]
Central Nervous System
Agitation [4]
Akathisia [9]
Catatonia [2]
Delirium [3]
Extrapyramidal symptoms [9]
Fever (pyrexia) (includes hyperpyrexia) [2]
Headache [2]
Insomnia [4]
Neuroleptic malignant syndrome [37]
Parkinsonism [10]
Rabbit syndrome (oral vertical dyskinesia) [2]
Sedation [3]
Somnolence (drowsiness) [6]
Tardive syndrome / tardive dyskinesia (<37%) [5]
Tremor [7]
Vertigo / dizziness [3]
Endocrine/Metabolic
Galactorrhea [4]
Hyperprolactinemia [2]
Hypoglycemia [2]
SIADH [3]
Weight gain [2]
Gastrointestinal/Hepatic
Constipation [2]
Pancreatitis / acute pancreatitis [2]
Genitourinary
Priapism [3]
Urinary retention [3]
Hematologic
Pancytopenia (includes bicytopenia) [2]
Local
Injection-site reaction [4]
Neuromuscular/Skeletal
Dystonia [5]
Myoclonus (see also hypnic jerk) [3]
Rhabdomyolysis [7]
Respiratory
Pneumonia [2]
Other
Adverse effects / adverse reactions [5]
Death [7]

HALOTHANE

Indications: Induction and maintenance of general anesthesia
Class: Anesthetic; inhalation
Half-life: N/A
Clinically important, potentially hazardous interactions with: aminophylline, atracurium, carbetocin, cisatracurium, doxacurium, epinephrine, ergometrine, labetalol, mivacurium, non-depolarizing muscle relaxants, oxprenolol, oxytocin, pancuronium, rapacuronium, rifampin, vecuronium, xanthines

---

Skin
Acneiform eruption / acneiform dermatitis / acneiform rash [3]
Gastrointestinal/Hepatic
Hepatotoxicity / liver injury / acute liver injury / drug-induced liver injury (DILI) [2]
Neuromuscular/Skeletal
Rhabdomyolysis [5]

HAWTHORN (FRUIT, LEAF, FLOWER EXTRACT)

Family: Rosaceae
Scientific names: *Crataegus laevigata, Crataegus monogyna, Crataegus oxyacantha, Crataegus pentagyna*
Indications: Amenorrhea, arrhythmias, atherosclerosis, diuretic, hyperlipidemia, hypertension, hypotension, sedative, appetite stimulant, arthritis, enteritis, indigestion, sore throats. **Topical**: boils, sores and ulcers
Class: Cardio-stimulant
Half-life: N/A
Clinically important, potentially hazardous interactions with: clevidipine, squill, vasodilators
Note: The American Herbal Products Association (AHPA) gives hawthorn a class I safety rating, indicating that it is very safe. However, hawthorn should be used with caution in patients with heart disease.

Skin
Hypersensitivity [2]
Rash (hands) [4]
Cardiovascular
Circulatory collapse [2]
Palpitation [2]

Central Nervous System
- Headache [2]
- Migraine [2]
- Vertigo / dizziness [4]

Gastrointestinal/Hepatic
- Hepatotoxicity / liver injury / acute liver injury / drug-induced liver injury (DILI) [2]

Other
- Adverse effects / adverse reactions [2]

HEMOPHILUS B VACCINE

Trade names: ActHIB (Sanofi-Aventis), Comvax (Merck), HibTITER (Lederle), OmniHIB (GSK), PedivaxHIB (Merck), ProHIBIT (Connaught)
Indications: Hemophilus B immunization
Class: Vaccine
Half-life: N/A
Clinically important, potentially hazardous interactions with: azathioprine, basiliximab, corticosteroids, cyclosporine, daclizumab, glatiramer, mycophenolate, sirolimus, tacrolimus

---

Skin
- Erythema [2]

HENNA

Family: Lythraceae
Scientific names: *Lawsonia alba, Lawsonia inermis*
Indications: Analgesic, antipyretic, seborrheic dermatitis, fungal infections, gastrointestinal ulcers, sunscreen, dandruff, scabies, headache, jaundice, decorative tattoos, Used in cosmetics, body paint, hair dyes, hair care products
Class: Anti-inflammatory
Half-life: N/A
Clinically important, potentially hazardous interactions with: none known
Note: Black Henna is henna plus paraphenylenediamine (PPD). PPD is added to henna to make it stain black. PPD is a transdermal toxin and may be used alone as hair dye or to stain skin black. Other products called 'black henna' may have indigo or food dyes added, and are generally not harmful to the skin.
Adverse side effects to pure henna are rare; those reported above may be due to additives. Henna tattoos were popularized by the singer, Madonna. Her black patterns, however, were created with body paint, not henna.

Skin
- Angioedema (formerly named angioneurotic edema) [3]
- Dermatitis [34]
- Edema / fluid retention [3]
- Erythema [3]
- Hypersensitivity [10]
- Lichenoid eruption / lichenoid reaction [4]
- Pigmentation (Skin) (includes hyperpigmentation) [3]
- Pruritus (itching) [3]
- Urticaria / hives [3]

Other
- Adverse effects / adverse reactions [2]
- Allergic reactions [3]
- Death [3]

HEPARIN

Trade names: Hep-Flush (Wyeth), Viaflex (Baxter)
Indications: Venous thrombosis, pulmonary embolism, intravascular coagulation, peripheral arterial embolism
Class: Anticoagulant (antithrombotic), Heparinoid
Half-life: 2 hours
Clinically important, potentially hazardous interactions with: acenocoumarol, aliskiren, antihistamines, aspirin, balsalazide, bivalirudin, butabarbital, ceftobiprole, dabigatran, danaparoid, defibrotide, desvenlafaxine, iloprost, inotersen, nandrolone, nicotine, nitroglycerin, palifermin, piperacillin/tazobactam, salicylates, tirofiban, warfarin
Important contra-indications noted in the prescribing guidelines for: the elderly
Note: A higher incidence of bleeding has been reported in patients over 60 years of age, especially women. Contra-indicated in patients with severe thrombocyopenia.

Skin
- Anaphylactoid reactions / anaphylaxis (includes anaphylactic shock) [4]
- Bruise / bruising / contusion / ecchymosis (ecchymoses) [4]
- Bullous hemorrhagic dermatosis / hemorrhagic bullae [8]
- Dermatitis [6]
- Erythema [2]
- Exanthems [2]
- Hypersensitivity [17]
- Lesions (includes skin lesions) [2]
- Livedo reticularis / livedo racemosa [2]
- Necrosis (skin necrosis) [57]
- Petechiae [2]
- Purpura (>10%)
- Stevens-Johnson syndrome and toxic epidermal necrolysis (SJS/TEN) [3]
- Urticaria / hives [6]
- Vasculitis (angiitis) / cutaneous vasculitis (angiitis) [6]

Hair
- Alopecia / hair loss [2]

Mucosal
- Gingivitis (>10%)

Central Nervous System
- Cerebral venous sinus thrombosis (includes cavernous sinus thrombosis) [2]

Endocrine/Metabolic
- Hyperkalemia [2]

Genitourinary
- Priapism [6]

Hematologic
- Bleeding [2]
- Hemorrhage [7]
- Thrombocythemia (thrombocytosis) / platelets increased [2]
- Thrombocytopenia / platelets decreased [139]
- Thrombosis [10]

Local
- Injection-site eczematous eruption [5]
- Injection-site induration [4]
- Injection-site necrosis [4]
- Injection-site plaques [2]

Other
- Allergic reactions (<10%) [3]
- Death [7]

HOPS

Family: Cannabaceae
Scientific name: *Humulus lupulus*
Indications: Insomnia, anxiety, diuretic, appetite stimulant. Flavoring in foods and beverages
Class: Cannabinoid, Phytoestrogen, Sedative
Half-life: N/A
Clinically important, potentially hazardous interactions with: none known

---

Skin
- Urticaria / hives [2]

HORSE CHESTNUT (BARK, FLOWER, LEAF, SEED)

Family: Hippocastanaceae
Scientific name: *Aesculus hippocastanum*
Indications: Oral: malaria, dysentery, tinnitus, pancreatitis, cough, arthritis, rheumatism, chronic venous insufficiency. **Topical**: lupus, skin ulcers eczema, phlebitis, varicose veins, hemorrhoids, rectal problems
Class: Diuretic
Half-life: N/A
Clinically important, potentially hazardous interactions with: NSAIDs
Note: The active ingredient is a toxic glycoside, escin.

Other
- Adverse effects / adverse reactions (mild) [2]

HORSETAIL

Family: Equisetaceae
Scientific names: *Equisetum arvense, Equisetum myriochaetum, Equisetum ramosissimum, Equisetum telmateia*
Indications: Oral: Alopecia, diabetes, hepatitis, bacterial infections, osteoarthritis, pressure ulcers, urinary tract infections. **Topical:** burns
Class: Anti-inflammatory, Antioxidant, Diuretic
Half-life: N/A
Clinically important, potentially hazardous interactions with: diuretics, nicotine

---

Gastrointestinal/Hepatic
- Hepatotoxicity / liver injury / acute liver injury / drug-induced liver injury (DILI) [2]

HYALURONIC ACID

Synonym: Hyaluronan
Trade names: Euflexxa (Ferring), Hyalgan (Sanofi-Aventis), Hylan G-F 20 (Synvisc), Juvederm (Allergan), Perlane (Q-Med AB), Restylane Fine Lines (Medicis), Vitrase (ISTA Pharma)
Indications: **Oral**: joint disorders **Injection**: adjunct in eye surgery, viscosupplementation in orthopedics, cosmetic surgery **Topical**: wounds, burns, skin ulcers, stomatitis
Class: Dermal filler, Food supplement, Glycoaminoglycan
Half-life: 2.5–5.5 minutes
Clinically important, potentially hazardous interactions with: furosemide, local anesthetics, NSAIDs, oral anticoagulants
Important contra-indications noted in the prescribing guidelines for: nursing mothers; pediatric patients
Note: Most reported reactions relate to orthopedic use.

Skin
- Acneiform eruption / acneiform dermatitis / acneiform rash (<29%)
- Anaphylactoid reactions / anaphylaxis (includes anaphylactic shock) [2]
- Angioedema (formerly named angioneurotic edema) [6]
- Bruise / bruising / contusion / ecchymosis (ecchymoses) [3]
- Churg-Strauss syndrome [12]
- Dermatitis (24%) [2]
- Edema / fluid retention [9]
- Erythema [6]
- Erythema multiforme [2]
- Facial edema [3]
- Granulomatous reaction [2]
- Hematoma / cutaneous hematoma [2]
- Herpes simplex [2]
- Hypersensitivity [6]
- Induration [2]
- Inflammation [7]
- Livedo reticularis / livedo racemosa [2]
- Necrosis (skin necrosis) [5]
- Nodular eruption [2]
- Pigmentation (Skin) (includes hyperpigmentation) [2]
- Pruritus (itching) [4]

Hair
- Alopecia / hair loss [3]

Cardiovascular
- Arterial occlusion [3]
- Hypertension (4%)
- Vascular occlusion [7]

Central Nervous System
- Pain [4]

Gastrointestinal/Hepatic
- Nausea (2%)

Local
- Injection-site bruising [4]
- Injection-site ecchymoses [2]
- Injection-site edema (20%) [13]
- Injection-site erythema (47%) [9]
- Injection-site granuloma [2]
- Injection-site nodules [3]
- Injection-site pain (8–47%) [16]
- Injection-site pruritus [2]
- Injection-site reaction (<11%) [12]

Neuromuscular/Skeletal
- Arthralgia [9]
- Back pain (5%)
- Chondritis (<11%) [2]
- Gouty tophi [3]
- Tendinitis (2%)

Ocular
- Blindness [2]
- Ophthalmoplegia [3]
- Orbital inflammation [2]
- Vision loss [3]

Other
- Adverse effects / adverse reactions [15]
- Infection [2]

HYDRALAZINE

Trade names: Apresazide (Novartis), Apresoline (Novartis), Ser-Ap-Es (Novartis)
Indications: Hypertension
Class: Vasodilator
Half-life: 3–7 hours
Clinically important, potentially hazardous interactions with: acebutolol, alfuzosin, captopril, cilazapril, diclofenac, enalapril, fosinopril, levodopa, levomepromazine, lisinopril, meloxicam, olmesartan, quinapril, ramipril, trandolapril, triamcinolone, trifluoperazine, zuclopenthixol
Note: Apresazide is hydralazine and hydrochlorothiazide; Ser-Ap-Es is hydralazine, reserpine and hydrochlorothiazide. Hydrochlorothiazide is a sulfonamide and can be absorbed systemically. Sulfonamides can produce severe, possibly fatal, reactions such as toxic epidermal necrolysis and Stevens-Johnson syndrome.

Skin
- Anti-neutrophil cytoplasmic antibody (ANCA) vasculitis (angiitis) [14]
- Edema / fluid retention [2]
- Exanthems [4]
- Flushing / rubefaction (>10%)
- Lupus erythematosus (subacute cutaneous lupus erythematosus (SCLE)) (7%) [114]
- Lupus syndrome / drug-induced lupus (DIL) [6]
- Photosensitivity [2]
- Purpura [3]
- Stevens-Johnson syndrome and toxic epidermal necrolysis (SJS/TEN) [2]
- Sweet's syndrome [7]
- Ulcerations [2]
- Vasculitis (angiitis) / cutaneous vasculitis (angiitis) [17]

Mucosal
- Oral ulceration [2]
- Orogenital ulceration [2]

Gastrointestinal/Hepatic
- Cholestatic liver injury / cholestatic hepatitis [2]
- Hepatitis [2]
- Hepatotoxicity / liver injury / acute liver injury / drug-induced liver injury (DILI) [4]

Renal
- Glomerulonephritis (includes membranous nephropathy) [8]
- Nephritis / interstitial nephritis / tubulointerstitial nephritis [4]

Respiratory
- Alveolar hemorrhage (pulmonary) [2]
- Pulmonary-renal syndrome [2]

HYDROCHLOROTHIAZIDE

Trade names: Accuretic (Pfizer), Aldactazide (Pfizer), Aldoril (Merck), Atacand HCT (AstraZeneca), Avalide (Bristol-Myers Squibb), Capozide (Par), Diovan HCT (Novartis), Dyazide (GSK), Hyzaar (Merck), Inderide (Wyeth), Lopressor (Novartis), Lotensin (Novartis), Lotensin HCT (Novartis), Micardis (Boehringer Ingelheim), Microzide (Watson), Moduretic (Merck), Prinzide (Merck), Tekturna HCT (Novartis), Teveten HCT (Biovail), Uniretic (Schwarz), Vaseretic (Biovail), Zestoretic (AstraZeneca), Ziac (Barr)
Indications: Edema
Class: Diuretic, thiazide
Half-life: 5.6–14.8 hours
Clinically important, potentially hazardous interactions with: digoxin, dofetilide, lithium, zinc
Important contra-indications noted in the prescribing guidelines for: nursing mothers; pediatric patients
Note: Hydrochlorothiazide is a sulfonamide and can be absorbed systemically. Sulfonamides can produce severe, possibly fatal, reactions such as toxic epidermal necrolysis and Stevens-Johnson syndrome.
Hydrochlorothiazide is often used in combination, e.g. with aliskiren (Tekturna HCT); amiloride (Moduretic); benazepril (Lotensin HCT); bisoprolol (Ziac); captopril (Capozide); enalapril (Vaseretic); irbesartan (Avalide); lisinopril (Prinzide and Zestoretic); losartan (Hyzaar); methyldopa (Aldoril); moexipril (Uniretic); spironolactone (Aldactazide); triamterene (Dyazide and Maxzide).

Skin
- AGEP [2]
- Baboon syndrome / symmetrical drug-related intertriginous and flexural exanthema (SDRIFE) [2]
- Dermatitis [2]
- Diaphoresis [2]
- Edema / fluid retention [3]
- Erythema annulare centrifugum [2]
- Lichenoid eruption / lichenoid reaction [5]
- Lupus erythematosus (subacute cutaneous lupus erythematosus (SCLE)) [16]
- Peripheral edema [5]
- Photosensitivity [21]
- Phototoxicity [5]
- Purpura [7]
- Rash [2]
- Stevens-Johnson syndrome and toxic epidermal necrolysis (SJS/TEN) [2]
- Vasculitis (angiitis) / cutaneous vasculitis (angiitis) [3]

Cardiovascular
- Capillary leak syndrome [2]
- Hypotension [6]
- Orthostatic hypotension [2]

Central Nervous System
- Headache [7]
- Vertigo / dizziness [10]

Endocrine/Metabolic
Hypokalemia [5]
Hyponatremia [5]
Serum creatinine increased [2]
SIADH [4]

Gastrointestinal/Hepatic
Diarrhea [2]
Nausea [2]
Pancreatitis / acute pancreatitis [6]

Hematologic
Hemolytic anemia [4]

Neuromuscular/Skeletal
Asthenia / fatigue [3]

Ocular
Glaucoma (includes acute angle-closure glaucoma) [2]

Renal
Nephrotoxicity / kidney injury / acute kidney injury (AKI) / drug-induced kidney injury [2]

Respiratory
Upper respiratory tract infection [3]

Other
Adverse effects / adverse reactions [5]
Death [3]

HYDROCODONE

Trade names: Duratuss (UCB), Entex HC (Andrx), Hycotuss (Endo), Hydromet (Actavis), Hysingla ER (Purdue), Lortab (UCB), Maxidone (Watson), Norco (Watson), Tussionex (Celltech), Vicodin (AbbVie), Vicoprofen (AbbVie), Zohydro ER (Pernix), Zydone (Endo)
Indications: Acute pain, coughing
Class: Opiate agonist
Half-life: 3.8 hours
Clinically important, potentially hazardous interactions with: alcohol, buprenorphine, butorphanol, CYP3A4 inhibitors or inducers, MAO inhibitors, nalbuphine, pentazocine
Important contra-indications noted in the prescribing guidelines for: nursing mothers; pediatric patients
Note: Hydrocodone is included in many combination drugs. Other medications that can be included in these preparations include: phenylpropanolamine, phenylephrine, pyrilamine, pseudoephedrine, acetaminophen, ibuprofen, and others. Zohydro ER is the first extended-release, single-entity hydrocodone-containing drug product approved by the FDA and reflects the newly updated labeling requirements recently announced by the FDA.
Warning: ADDICTION, ABUSE, AND MISUSE; LIFE-THREATENING RESPIRATORY DEPRESSION; ACCIDENTAL INGESTION; NEONATAL OPIOID WITHDRAWAL SYNDROME; INTERACTION WITH ALCOHOL; and CYTOCHROME P450 3A4 INTERACTION

Skin
Hot flashes / hot flushes (<10%)
Hyperhidrosis (<10%)
Peripheral edema (<3%)
Pruritus (itching) (3%) [2]
Rash (<10%)

Mucosal
Xerostomia (dry mouth) (3%)

Cardiovascular
Chest pain (<10%)

Central Nervous System
Fever (pyrexia) (includes hyperpyrexia) (<10%)
Headache [2]
Migraine (<10%)
Paresthesias (<10%)
Somnolence (drowsiness) (<5%) [4]
Tremor (3%)
Vertigo / dizziness (2–3%) [4]

Endocrine/Metabolic
Dehydration (<10%)
GGT increased (<10%)
Hypokalemia (<10%)

Gastrointestinal/Hepatic
Abdominal pain (2–3%)
Constipation (8–11%) [7]
Gastroesophageal reflux (<10%)
Nausea (7–10%) [9]
Vomiting [8]

Genitourinary
Urinary tract infection (<5%)

Neuromuscular/Skeletal
Arthralgia (<10%)
Asthenia / fatigue (<4%)
Back pain (<4%) [2]
Bone pain / joint pain (<10%)
Muscle spasm (<3%)
Myalgia/Myopathy (<10%)
Neck pain (<10%)
Pain in extremities (<10%)

Respiratory
Cough (<10%)
Dyspnea / shortness of breath (<10%)
Respiratory depression [2]
Upper respiratory tract infection (<3%)

HYDROCORTISONE

Trade names: Ala-Cort (Del-Ray), Cortef (Pharmacia), Cortenema (Solvay), Hydrocortone (Merck), Hytone (Dermik), Solu-Cortef (Pharmacia)
Indications: Arthralgias, asthma, inflammatory ocular conditions, rhinitis
Class: Corticosteroid / Glucocorticoid, Corticosteroid, topical
Half-life: N/A
Clinically important, potentially hazardous interactions with: amphotericin B, chlorotrianisene, colestyramine, diuretics, estrogens, furosemide, insulin, live vaccines, methotrexate, oral contraceptives, pancuronium, phenobarbital, phenytoin, rifampin

---

Skin
Anaphylactoid reactions / anaphylaxis (includes anaphylactic shock) [18]
Dermatitis [11]
Eczema / eczematous reaction / eczematous eruption [4]
Hypersensitivity [6]
Pruritus (itching) [2]
Rash [2]
Urticaria / hives [5]

Cardiovascular
Bradycardia / sinus bradycardia [3]
Hypertension [2]

Neuromuscular/Skeletal
Myalgia/Myopathy [5]
Osteonecrosis / avascular necrosis (includes steroid-induced osteonecrosis of the femoral head) [2]

Other
Allergic reactions [10]
Infection [2]

HYDROMORPHONE

Trade names: Dilaudid (AbbVie), Exalgo (Mallinckrodt), Jurnista (Janssen-Cilag), Palladone (Napp)
Indications: Pain
Class: Opiate agonist
Half-life: 1–3 hours; 2 hours (IV)
Clinically important, potentially hazardous interactions with: alcohol, alvimopan, ammonium chloride, amphetamines, anticholinergics, anxiolytics and hypnotics, buprenorphine, butorphanol, cimetidine, CNS depressants, desmopressin, domperidone, droperidol, linezolid, MAO inhibitors, metoclopramide, moclobemide, nalbuphine, pegvisomant, pentazocine, phenothiazines, sodium oxybate, SSRIs, St John's wort, succinylcholine, thiazide diuretics
Important contra-indications noted in the prescribing guidelines for: nursing mothers; pediatric patients
Note: OROS hydromorphone prolonged release (Jurnista) is a once-daily formulation of hydromorphone that utilizes OROS (osmotic-controlled release oral delivery system) technology to deliver the drug at a near constant rate.
Warning: ADDICTION, ABUSE, AND MISUSE; LIFE-THREATENING RESPIRATORY DEPRESSION; ACCIDENTAL INGESTION; NEONATAL OPIOID WITHDRAWAL SYNDROME; and INTERACTION WITH ALCOHOL

Skin
Flushing / rubefaction (<10%)
Pruritus (itching) (<11%) [12]

Mucosal
Xerostomia (dry mouth) (<10%)

Cardiovascular
Bradycardia / sinus bradycardia [2]
Hypotension [2]

Central Nervous System
Agitation [3]
Dysgeusia (taste perversion) [3]
Hallucinations [2]
Headache [5]
Hyperalgesia [3]
Somnolence (drowsiness) [6]
Tremor [2]
Vertigo / dizziness [10]

Endocrine/Metabolic
Appetite decreased [2]

Gastrointestinal/Hepatic
Constipation [11]
Nausea [18]
Vomiting [11]

Neuromuscular/Skeletal
Asthenia / fatigue [5]
Myoclonus (see also hypnic jerk) [3]

Other
Adverse effects / adverse reactions [7]

HYDROQUINONE

Trade names: Ambi (Johnson & Johnson), Lustra (Taro)
Indications: Ultraviolet induced dyschromia and discoloration resulting from the use of oral contraceptives, pregnancy, hormone replacement therapy, or skin trauma
Class: Depigmentation agent
Half-life: N/A
Clinically important, potentially hazardous interactions with: none known
Important contra-indications noted in the prescribing guidelines for: nursing mothers; pediatric patients

Skin
- Acneiform eruption / acneiform dermatitis / acneiform rash [2]
- Burning / skin burning sensation [2]
- Contact dermatitis (localized) [2]
- Depigmentation [2]
- Erythema [4]
- Ochronosis [15]
- Peeling [2]
- Pigmentation (Skin) (includes hyperpigmentation) [3]
- Pruritus (itching) [2]
- Scaling [2]
- Striae [2]
- Xerosis / xeroderma [2]

Other
- Adverse effects / adverse reactions [4]

HYDROXY-CHLOROQUINE

Trade name: Plaquenil (Sanofi-Aventis)
Indications: Malaria, lupus erythematosus, rheumatoid arthritis
Class: Antimalarial, Antimicrobial, Antiprotozoal, Covid-19 putative drug, Disease-modifying antirheumatic drug (DMARD)
Half-life: 32–50 days
Clinically important, potentially hazardous interactions with: chloroquine, cholestyramine, dapsone, droperidol, ethosuximide, lacosamide, lanthanum, moxifloxacin, neostigmine, oxcarbazepine, penicillamine, tiagabine, typhoid vaccine, vigabatrin, yellow fever vaccine
Important contra-indications noted in the prescribing guidelines for: nursing mothers; pediatric patients

Skin
- AGEP [28]
- Bullous dermatosis [2]
- Cutaneous adverse reaction (includes severe cutaneous adverse drug reaction (SCAR)) [2]
- DRESS syndrome (Drug-induced hypersensitivity syndrome) [5]
- Erythema annulare centrifugum [3]
- Erythema multiforme [3]
- Erythroderma [5]
- Exanthems (<5%) [4]
- Exfoliative dermatitis [3]
- Lichenoid eruption / lichenoid reaction [4]
- Photosensitivity [6]
- Phototoxicity [3]
- Pigmentation (Skin) (includes hyperpigmentation) (<10%) [23]
- Pruritus (itching) (>10%) [13]
- Psoriasis (exacerbation) [17]
- Rash (<10%) [5]
- Stevens-Johnson syndrome and toxic epidermal necrolysis (SJS/TEN) [4]
- Sweet's syndrome [2]
- Thrombocytopenic purpura [2]
- Urticaria / hives [2]

Hair
- Alopecia / hair loss [2]
- Hair pigmentation (bleaching) (<10%) [8]

Nails
- Nail pigmentation [3]

Mucosal
- Oral pigmentation [7]
- Stomatitis (oral mucositis) [2]

Cardiovascular
- Cardiomyopathy [12]
- Cardiotoxicity [4]
- Cardiovascular adverse effect (includes major adverse cardiovascular events (MACE)) [4]
- QT interval prolonged / QT prolongation [7]
- Torsades de pointes [2]
- Ventricular arrhythmia [3]

Central Nervous System
- Anorexia [2]
- Dysgeusia (taste perversion) [2]
- Headache [2]
- Neurotoxicity [3]

Endocrine/Metabolic
- Hypoglycemia [6]
- Porphyria [7]
- Weight loss [2]

Gastrointestinal/Hepatic
- Diarrhea [6]
- Dysphagia [2]
- Gastrointestinal adverse reaction [5]
- Hepatotoxicity / liver injury / acute liver injury / drug-induced liver injury (DILI) [2]
- Nausea [6]
- Vomiting [4]

Hematologic
- Anemia [3]
- Neutropenia (neutrophils decreased) [2]
- Thrombocytopenia / platelets decreased [4]

Neuromuscular/Skeletal
- Asthenia / fatigue [3]
- Myalgia/Myopathy [9]

Ocular
- Maculopathy [6]
- Ocular adverse effect [2]
- Ocular toxicity [9]
- Reduced visual acuity [2]
- Retinal adverse effect [2]
- Retinopathy [31]
- Vision blurred [3]

Otic
- Hearing loss (hypoacusis) [2]

Renal
- Renal phospholipidosis [4]

Other
- Adverse effects / adverse reactions [15]
- Death [4]

HYDROXYUREA

Synonym: hydroxycarbamide
Trade names: Droxia (Bristol-Myers Squibb), Hydrea (Bristol-Myers Squibb)
Indications: Leukemia, malignant tumors
Class: Antineoplastic / anticancer agent (see also Immune checkpoint inhibitor), Antiretroviral
Half-life: 3–4 hours
Clinically important, potentially hazardous interactions with: adefovir, aldesleukin

Skin
- Acral erythema [8]
- Atrophy / Skin atrophy [4]
- Dermatitis [3]
- Dermatomyositis [30]
- Exanthems (<10%)
- Fixed eruption / fixed drug eruption [4]
- Ichthyosis [3]
- Keratoses [2]
- Leg ulceration (29%) [20]
- Lichen planus (includes hypertrophic lichen planus) [3]
- Lichenoid eruption / lichenoid reaction [3]
- Lupus erythematosus (subacute cutaneous lupus erythematosus (SCLE)) [3]
- Palmar–plantar desquamation [6]
- Pigmentation (Skin) (includes hyperpigmentation) (<58%) [19]
- Poikiloderma [3]
- Pruritus (itching) [3]
- Purpura [2]
- Radiation recall dermatitis [2]
- Squamous cell carcinoma [2]
- Telangiectasia [2]
- Tumors [5]
- Ulcerations [29]
- Vasculitis (angiitis) / cutaneous vasculitis (angiitis) [6]
- Xerosis / xeroderma (<10%) [7]

Hair
- Alopecia / hair loss (<10%) [8]

Nails
- Atrophic nails (onychatrophy) [3]
- Melanonychia [9]
- Nail changes [4]
- Nail dystrophy [2]
- Nail pigmentation [19]
- Onycholysis [2]

Mucosal
- Oral lesions [2]
- Oral pigmentation [2]
- Oral squamous cell carcinoma [2]
- Oral ulceration [8]
- Stomatitis (oral mucositis) (>10%) [4]
- Tongue pigmentation (<29%) [3]

Gastrointestinal/Hepatic
- Pancreatitis / acute pancreatitis [3]

Genitourinary
- Genital ulceration [3]

Other
- Adverse effects / adverse reactions [2]
- Death [2]
- Side effects (7–35%) [3]

HYDROXYZINE

Trade names: Atarax (Pfizer), Vistaril (Pfizer)
Indications: Anxiety and tension, pruritus
Class: Histamine H1 receptor antagonist, Muscarinic antagonist
Half-life: 3–7 hours
Clinically important, potentially hazardous interactions with: alcohol, barbiturates, CNS depressants, efavirenz, lurasidone, narcotics, non-narcotic analgesics
Important contra-indications noted in the prescribing guidelines for: nursing mothers

Skin
AGEP [3]
Anaphylactoid reactions / anaphylaxis (includes anaphylactic shock) [2]
Angioedema (formerly named angioneurotic edema) [3]
Erythema multiforme [2]
Exanthems [3]
Fixed eruption / fixed drug eruption [3]
Urticaria / hives [4]

Mucosal
Xerostomia (dry mouth) (12%) [6]

Cardiovascular
Torsades de pointes [3]

Central Nervous System
Somnolence (drowsiness) [6]

Gastrointestinal/Hepatic
Vomiting [2]

Genitourinary
Priapism [2]

HYOSCYAMINE

Trade names: IB-Stat (InKline), Levbid (Schwarz), Levsin (Schwarz), Levsin/SL (Schwarz), Levsinex (Schwarz), Nulev (Schwarz)
Indications: Treatment of gastrointestinal tract disorders caused by spasm, adjunctive therapy for peptic ulcers, cystitis, Parkinsonism, biliary and renal colic
Class: Anticholinergic, Muscarinic antagonist
Half-life: N/A
Clinically important, potentially hazardous interactions with: anticholinergics, arbutamine
Important contra-indications noted in the prescribing guidelines for: the elderly; nursing mothers; pediatric patients

Skin
Photosensitivity (<10%)
Xerosis / xeroderma (>10%)

Mucosal
Xerostomia (dry mouth) (>10%)

Cardiovascular
Tachycardia [2]

Local
Injection-site inflammation (>10%)

IBANDRONATE

Synonym: ibandronic acid
Trade names: Bondronat (Roche), Boniva (Roche)
Indications: Postmenopausal osteoporosis
Class: Bisphosphonate
Half-life: 37–157 hours
Clinically important, potentially hazardous interactions with: alcohol, aminoglycosides, antacids, calcium salts, food, magnesium salts, NSAIDs, oral iron
Important contra-indications noted in the prescribing guidelines for: nursing mothers; pediatric patients

Skin
Rash (<2%)

Cardiovascular
Hypertension (6–7%)

Central Nervous System
Fever (pyrexia) (includes hyperpyrexia) (~9%) [4]
Headache (3–7%)
Vertigo / dizziness (<4%)

Endocrine/Metabolic
Hypercholesterolemia (5%)
Hypocalcemia [3]
Hypophosphatemia [2]

Gastrointestinal/Hepatic
Abdominal pain (5–8%)
Constipation (3–4%)
Diarrhea (4–7%) [2]
Dyspepsia / functional dyspepsia (indigestion) (see also gastroparesis) (6–12%) [4]
Gastritis / pangastritis / gastric irritation (2%)
Gastrointestinal disorder / discomfort [3]
Nausea (5%) [4]
Vomiting (3%) [4]

Genitourinary
Urinary tract infection (2–6%)

Neuromuscular/Skeletal
Arthralgia (3–6%) [2]
Asthenia / fatigue (4%) [3]
Back pain (4–14%)
Bone pain / joint pain [3]
Cramps (2%)
Joint disorder (4%)
Myalgia/Myopathy (<6%)
Osteonecrosis / avascular necrosis (includes steroid-induced osteonecrosis of the femoral head) [16]
Pain in extremities (<8%)

Ocular
Ocular adverse effect [2]

Respiratory
Bronchitis (3–10%)
Influenza- ('flu)-like syndrome (<4%) [7]
Nasopharyngitis (4%)
Pharyngitis (sore throat) (3%)
Pneumonia (6%)
Upper respiratory tract infection (2–34%)

Other
Adverse effects / adverse reactions [5]
Allergic reactions (3%)
Infection (4%)
Tooth disorder (4%)

IBREXAFUNGERP

Trade name: Brexafemme (Scynexis)
Indications: Vulvovaginal candidiasis
Class: Antifungal / antimycotic, Antimicrobial
Half-life: approximately 20 hours
Clinically important, potentially hazardous interactions with: bosentan, carbamazepine, CYP3A inducers, CYP3A inhibitors, efavirenz, etravirine, itraconazole, ketoconazole, long acting barbiturates, phenytoin, rifampin, St John's wort
Pregnancy category: May cause fetal harm based on animal studies. Advise females of reproductive potential to use effective contraception during treatment.
Note: Prior to initiating treatment, verify pregnancy status in females of reproductive potential.

Skin
Rash (<2%)

Central Nervous System
Vertigo / dizziness (3%)

Endocrine/Metabolic
Hypertransaminasemia (hepatic transaminitis) / elevated transaminases (<2%)

Gastrointestinal/Hepatic
Abdominal pain (11%)
Diarrhea (17%) [2]
Flatulence (<2%)
Nausea (12%) [2]
Vomiting (2%)

Genitourinary
Dysmenorrhea (<2%)
Vaginal bleeding (<2%)

Neuromuscular/Skeletal
Back pain (<2%)

IBRITUMOMAB

Trade name: Zevalin (Biogen)
Indications: Non-Hodgkin's lymphoma
Class: Antineoplastic / anticancer agent (see also Immune checkpoint inhibitor), Biologic, CD20-directed cytolytic monoclonal antibody, Monoclonal antibody
Half-life: 30 hours
Clinically important, potentially hazardous interactions with: argatroban, cilostazol, citalopram, clopidogrel, dabigatran, eptifibatide, meloxicam, tinzaparin
Important contra-indications noted in the prescribing guidelines for: nursing mothers; pediatric patients
Warning: SERIOUS INFUSION REACTIONS, PROLONGED AND SEVERE CYTOPENIAS, and SEVERE CUTANEOUS AND MUCOCUTANEOUS REACTIONS

Skin
Angioedema (formerly named angioneurotic edema) (5%)
Bruise / bruising / contusion / ecchymosis (ecchymoses) (7%)
Diaphoresis (4%)
Flushing / rubefaction (6%)
Hyperhidrosis (8%)
Peripheral edema (8%)
Petechiae (8%)
Pruritus (itching) (7%)

Purpura (7%)
Rash (7%)
Urticaria / hives (4%)

Mucosal
Epistaxis (nosebleed) (5%)

Cardiovascular
Hypertension (7%)

Central Nervous System
Anorexia (8%)
Chills (24%)
Fever (pyrexia) (includes hyperpyrexia) (10%)
Leukoencephalopathy / posterior reversible encephalopathy syndrome (PRES) [2]
Pain (13%)
Vertigo / dizziness (7%)

Gastrointestinal/Hepatic
Abdominal pain (17%)
Diarrhea (11%)
Nausea (18%)

Genitourinary
Urinary tract infection (7%)

Hematologic
Anemia (22%)
Hemotoxicity [7]
Leukocytopenia (leukopenia) / leukocytes (white blood cells) decreased [2]
Lymphopenia (lymphocytopenia) / lymphocytes decreased (26%)
Myelosuppression / bone marrow suppression / myelotoxicity [2]
Neutropenia (neutrophils decreased) [4]
Thrombocytopenia / platelets decreased (62%) [8]

Neuromuscular/Skeletal
Arthralgia (7%)
Asthenia / fatigue (15–33%)
Back pain (8%)
Myalgia/Myopathy (9%)

Respiratory
Bronchitis (8%)
Cough (11%)
Influenza- ('flu)-like syndrome (8%)
Nasopharyngitis (19%)
Pharyngolaryngeal pain (7%)
Rhinitis / rhinosinusitis (see also sinusitis) (8%)
Sinusitis (see also rhinitis / rhinosinusitis) (7%)

Other
Adverse effects / adverse reactions [2]
Allergic reactions (2%)
Infection (29%) [3]

IBRUTINIB

Trade name: Imbruvica (Pharmacyclics)
Indications: Mantle cell lymphoma
Class: Bruton's tyrosine kinase (BTK) inhibitor
Half-life: 4–6 hours
Clinically important, potentially hazardous interactions with: carbamazepine, clarithromycin, grapefruit juice, itraconazole, ketoconazole, phenytoin, posaconazole, rifampin, St John's wort, strong or moderate CYP3A inhibitors or inducers, telithromycin, viloxazine, voriconazole
Important contra-indications noted in the prescribing guidelines for: nursing mothers; pediatric patients

Skin
Bruise / bruising / contusion / ecchymosis (ecchymoses) (30%) [4]
Cellulitis and pseudocellulitis [3]
Cutaneous toxicity / skin toxicity (14%) [3]
Neutrophilic dermatosis [3]
Panniculitis [2]
Peripheral edema (35%) [4]
Petechiae (11%)
Pyoderma gangrenosum [2]
Rash (25%) [5]

Mucosal
Epistaxis (nosebleed) (11%)
Stomatitis (oral mucositis) (17%)

Cardiovascular
Atrial fibrillation [22]
Hypertension [8]
Hypotension [2]
Pericardial effusion [7]
Ventricular dysfunction (left ventricular dysfunction / right ventricular dysfunction) [2]

Central Nervous System
Fever (pyrexia) (includes hyperpyrexia) (18%) [5]
Headache (13%) [2]
Peripheral neuropathy [2]
Vertigo / dizziness (14%)

Endocrine/Metabolic
Appetite decreased (21%) [2]
Dehydration (12%) [2]
Hyperuricemia (15%) [2]
Hypokalemia [2]
Hyponatremia [2]

Gastrointestinal/Hepatic
Abdominal pain (24%)
Constipation (25%)
Diarrhea (51%) [34]
Dyspepsia / functional dyspepsia (indigestion) (see also gastroparesis) (11%)
Hepatotoxicity / liver injury / acute liver injury / drug-induced liver injury (DILI) [2]
Nausea (31%) [19]
Vomiting (24%) [5]

Genitourinary
Urinary tract infection (14%) [2]

Hematologic
Anemia [15]
Bleeding [17]
Cytopenia [4]
Febrile neutropenia [4]
Hemorrhage [4]
Lymphocytosis / lymphocytes increased [2]
Neutropenia (neutrophils decreased) [21]
Sepsis [2]
Thrombocytopenia / platelets decreased [18]

Neuromuscular/Skeletal
Arthralgia (11%) [4]
Asthenia / fatigue (14–41%) [24]
Bone pain / joint pain (37%)
Muscle spasm (14%) [2]

Ocular
Uveitis / anterior uveitis / posterior uveitis / panuveitis [4]

Renal
Tumor lysis syndrome (TLS) [3]

Respiratory
Cough (19%) [3]
Dyspnea / shortness of breath (27%)
Pneumonia (14%) [11]
Sinusitis (see also rhinitis / rhinosinusitis) (13%) [2]
Upper respiratory tract infection (34%) [6]

Other
Adverse effects / adverse reactions [7]
Death [2]
Infection [15]

IBUPROFEN

Trade names: Advil (Wyeth), Motrin (McNeil), Vicoprofen (AbbVie)
Indications: Arthritis, pain
Class: Non-steroidal anti-inflammatory (NSAID)
Half-life: 2–4 hours
Clinically important, potentially hazardous interactions with: aspirin, ciprofibrate, diuretics, methotrexate, methyl salicylate, NSAIDs, oxycodone hydrochloride, salicylates, tacrine, tacrolimus, urokinase, voriconazole
Pregnancy category: category C prior to 30 weeks gestation; category D starting at 30 weeks gestation
Note: NSAIDs may cause an increased risk of serious cardiovascular and gastrointestinal adverse events, which can be fatal. This risk may increase with duration of use. September 2022: Codeine with ibuprofen – EMA warning for serious renal and gastrointestinal harms The European Medicine Agency Pharmacovigilance Risk Assessment Committee has recommended a change to the product information for codeine with ibuprofen combination medicines to include a warning of serious harms, including death, particularly when taken for prolonged periods at higher than recommended doses. The recommendation is based on several cases of renal, gastrointestinal and metabolic toxicities that have been reported in association with cases of abuse of and dependence from codeine with ibuprofen combinations, some of which have been fatal. .

Skin
AGEP [5]
Anaphylactoid reactions / anaphylaxis (includes anaphylactic shock) [5]
Angioedema (formerly named angioneurotic edema) [8]
Bullous dermatosis [3]
Bullous pemphigoid / pemphigoid [2]
Dermatitis [5]
DRESS syndrome (Drug-induced hypersensitivity syndrome) [4]
Erythema multiforme [12]
Erythema nodosum (<5%)
Exanthems [9]
Fixed eruption / fixed drug eruption [17]
Hypersensitivity [5]
Lupus erythematosus (subacute cutaneous lupus erythematosus (SCLE)) [5]
Nicolau syndrome [2]
Peripheral edema [2]
Photosensitivity [6]
Pruritus (itching) (<5%) [7]
Pseudoporphyria [2]
Psoriasis (palms) [2]
Rash (>10%) [4]
Stevens-Johnson syndrome and toxic epidermal necrolysis (SJS/TEN) [22]
Urticaria / hives (>10%) [10]
Vasculitis (angiitis) / cutaneous vasculitis (angiitis) [8]
Vesiculobullous eruption [2]

Hair
Alopecia / hair loss [2]
Cardiovascular
Cardiotoxicity [2]
Hypertension [4]
Kounis syndrome / allergic angina syndrome / allergic myocardial infarction [4]
Central Nervous System
Aseptic meningitis [21]
Headache [4]
Somnolence (drowsiness) [2]
Gastrointestinal/Hepatic
Abdominal pain [6]
Constipation [4]
Diarrhea [4]
Dyspepsia / functional dyspepsia (indigestion) (see also gastroparesis) [5]
Gastroesophageal reflux [2]
Gastrointestinal bleeding [2]
Gastrointestinal disorder / discomfort [4]
Hepatotoxicity / liver injury / acute liver injury / drug-induced liver injury (DILI) [5]
Nausea [8]
Pancreatitis / acute pancreatitis [2]
Vanishing bile duct syndrome / ductopenia [3]
Vomiting [6]
Genitourinary
Urinary tract infection [2]
Hematologic
Leukocytopenia (leukopenia) / leukocytes (white blood cells) decreased [2]
Pancytopenia (includes bicytopenia) [2]
Thrombocytopenia / platelets decreased [5]
Neuromuscular/Skeletal
Arthralgia [2]
Back pain [2]
Rhabdomyolysis [3]
Ocular
Amblyopia [2]
Optic neuritis / papillitis [2]
Periorbital edema [3]
Visual disturbances [2]
Otic
Hearing loss (hypoacusis) [2]
Tinnitus [2]
Renal
Nephritis / interstitial nephritis / tubulointerstitial nephritis [6]
Nephrotoxicity / kidney injury / acute kidney injury (AKI) / drug-induced kidney injury [4]
Respiratory
Influenza [2]
Sinusitis (see also rhinitis / rhinosinusitis) [2]
Upper respiratory tract infection [2]
Other
Adverse effects / adverse reactions [15]

IBUTILIDE

Trade name: Corvert (Pfizer)
Indications: Atrial fibrillation and flutter
Class: Antiarrhythmic, Antiarrhythmic class III
Half-life: 2–12 hours
Clinically important, potentially hazardous interactions with: degarelix
Important contra-indications noted in the prescribing guidelines for: nursing mothers; pediatric patients

Cardiovascular
Bradycardia / sinus bradycardia [4]
Hypotension [2]
QT interval prolonged / QT prolongation [5]
Tachycardia (3%)
Torsades de pointes [14]
Ventricular arrhythmia [4]
Ventricular tachycardia [6]
Central Nervous System
Headache (4%)
Gastrointestinal/Hepatic
Nausea (2%) [3]

ICATIBANT

Trade name: Firazyr (Sanofi)
Indications: Hereditary angioedema (HAE) in adults
Class: Bradykinin B2 receptor antagonist
Half-life: 1–2 hours
Clinically important, potentially hazardous interactions with: ACE inhibitors

Skin
Angioedema (formerly named angioneurotic edema) (<10%) [2]
Burning / skin burning sensation (10%)
Erythema (10%)
Pruritus (itching) (10%)
Rash (<10%)
Mucosal
Nasal congestion (<10%)
Central Nervous System
Headache (<10%) [2]
Vertigo / dizziness (<10%)
Gastrointestinal/Hepatic
Abdominal pain (<10%)
Nausea (<10%)
Local
Injection-site edema [2]
Injection-site erythema [2]
Injection-site pain [2]
Injection-site reaction [12]
Neuromuscular/Skeletal
Asthenia / fatigue (<10%)

IDARUBICIN

Synonyms: 4-demethoxydaunorubicin; 4-DMDR
Trade name: Idamycin (Pfizer)
Indications: Acute myeloid leukemia
Class: Antibiotic, Antibiotic; anthracycline, Antimicrobial
Half-life: 14–35 hours (oral)
Clinically important, potentially hazardous interactions with: aldesleukin
Important contra-indications noted in the prescribing guidelines for: nursing mothers; pediatric patients

Skin
Rash (>10%) [4]
Urticaria / hives (>10%)
Hair
Alopecia / hair loss (77%) [8]
Mucosal
Mucositis (50%) [5]
Stomatitis (oral mucositis) (>10%)
Gastrointestinal/Hepatic
Diarrhea [3]
Hepatotoxicity / liver injury / acute liver injury / drug-induced liver injury (DILI) [2]
Nausea [2]
Vomiting [2]
Hematologic
Febrile neutropenia [2]
Neutropenia (neutrophils decreased) [2]
Other
Infection [2]

IDEBENONE

Trade names: Catena (Santhera), Mnesis (Takeda)
Indications: Alzheimer's dementia, cardiovascular disease, cerebrovascular disease, demyelination, depression, Friedreich's ataxia, improving memory, Leber's hereditary optic neuropathy
Class: Coenzyme Q10 analog
Half-life: N/A
Clinically important, potentially hazardous interactions with: none known

Skin
Contact dermatitis [2]
Central Nervous System
Headache [2]
Gastrointestinal/Hepatic
Loose stools / soft feces [2]
Other
Adverse effects / adverse reactions [2]

IDELALISIB

Trade name: Zydelig (Gilead)
Indications: Relapsed chronic lymphocytic leukemia (with rituximab), follicular B-cell non-Hodgkin lymphoma, small lymphocytic lymphoma
Class: Phosphoinositide 3-kinase (Phosphatidylinositol 3-kinase) (PI3K) inhibitor
Half-life: 8 hours
Clinically important, potentially hazardous interactions with: carbamazepine, copanlisib, midostaurin, neratinib, phenytoin, rifampin, St John's wort, strong CYP3A inducers and substrates
Important contra-indications noted in the prescribing guidelines for: nursing mothers; pediatric patients
Warning: FATAL AND SERIOUS TOXICITIES: HEPATIC, SEVERE DIARRHEA, COLITIS, PNEUMONITIS, and INTESTINAL PERFORATION

Skin
Cutaneous toxicity / skin toxicity [2]
Diaphoresis (12%)
Peripheral edema (10%)
Rash (21%) [8]
Central Nervous System
Chills [5]
Fever (pyrexia) (includes hyperpyrexia) [11]
Headache (11%)
Insomnia (12%)
Endocrine/Metabolic
ALT increased (50%) [8]
Appetite decreased (16%) [3]
AST increased (41%) [8]
Gastrointestinal/Hepatic
Abdominal pain (26%)

Colitis [6]
Constipation [2]
Diarrhea (47%) [18]
Gastrointestinal perforation / perforated colon / gastric perforation [2]
Hepatotoxicity / liver injury / acute liver injury / drug-induced liver injury (DILI) [10]
Nausea (29%) [8]
Vomiting (15%) [3]

Hematologic
Anemia [6]
Febrile neutropenia [6]
Neutropenia (neutrophils decreased) [8]
Thrombocytopenia / platelets decreased [6]

Neuromuscular/Skeletal
Asthenia / fatigue (30%) [8]

Respiratory
Cough (29%) [5]
Dyspnea / shortness of breath (17%)
Pneumonia (25%) [10]
Pneumonitis [5]
Upper respiratory tract infection (12%) [3]

Other
Adverse effects / adverse reactions [3]
Infection [2]
Side effects [2]

IFOSFAMIDE

Trade name: Ifex (Bristol-Myers Squibb)
Indications: Cancers, sarcomas, leukemias, lymphomas
Class: Alkylating agent
Half-life: 4–15 hours
Clinically important, potentially hazardous interactions with: aldesleukin, aprepitant

---

Skin
Cutaneous toxicity / skin toxicity [2]
Dermatitis (<10%)
Pigmentation (Skin) (includes hyperpigmentation) (<10%) [2]

Hair
Alopecia / hair loss (50–100%) [6]

Nails
Ridging (<10%)

Cardiovascular
Phlebitis (2%)

Central Nervous System
Anorexia [2]
Confusion [2]
Delirium [2]
Encephalopathy (includes hepatic encephalopathy) [15]
Neurotoxicity [12]
Seizures [2]

Endocrine/Metabolic
SIADH [2]

Gastrointestinal/Hepatic
Hepatotoxicity / liver injury / acute liver injury / drug-induced liver injury (DILI) [2]
Nausea [7]
Pancreatitis / acute pancreatitis [2]
Vomiting [7]

Hematologic
Anemia [3]
Febrile neutropenia [2]
Leukocytopenia (leukopenia) / leukocytes (white blood cells) decreased [3]
Myelosuppression / bone marrow suppression / myelotoxicity [2]
Neutropenia (neutrophils decreased) [4]
Thrombocytopenia / platelets decreased [4]

Neuromuscular/Skeletal
Asthenia / fatigue [2]
Osteomalacia [2]

Renal
Fanconi syndrome (proximal tubular dysfunction) [4]
Nephrotoxicity / kidney injury / acute kidney injury (AKI) / drug-induced kidney injury [35]

Other
Allergic reactions (<10%)
Death [2]
Infection [2]

ILOPERIDONE

Trade name: Fanapt (Vanda)
Indications: Schizophrenia
Class: Antipsychotic, Antipsychotic, atypical
Half-life: 18–33 hours
Clinically important, potentially hazardous interactions with: alcohol, dextromethorphan, fluoxetine, itraconazole, ketoconazole, paroxetine hydrochloride, QT prolonging agents
Important contra-indications noted in the prescribing guidelines for: the elderly; nursing mothers; pediatric patients
Warning: INCREASED MORTALITY IN ELDERLY PATIENTS WITH DEMENTIA-RELATED PSYCHOSIS

Skin
Rash (2%)

Mucosal
Nasal congestion (8%) [3]
Xerostomia (dry mouth) (10%) [10]

Cardiovascular
Hypotension (3%)
Orthostatic hypotension (3%) [4]
QT interval prolonged / QT prolongation [8]
Tachycardia (12%) [5]

Central Nervous System
Akathisia (2%) [3]
Anxiety [2]
Headache [3]
Insomnia (18%) [3]
Sedation [4]
Somnolence (drowsiness) (15%) [9]
Tremor (3%)
Vertigo / dizziness (20%) [12]

Endocrine/Metabolic
Weight gain (9%) [11]

Gastrointestinal/Hepatic
Diarrhea (7%)
Dyspepsia / functional dyspepsia (indigestion) (see also gastroparesis) [3]
Nausea (10%) [2]

Genitourinary
Ejaculatory dysfunction (2%) [2]
Priapism [2]

Neuromuscular/Skeletal
Arthralgia (3%)
Asthenia / fatigue (6%) [2]

Respiratory
Dyspnea / shortness of breath (2%)
Nasopharyngitis (3%)
Upper respiratory tract infection (3%)

ILOPROST

Trade name: Ventavis (Schering) (Cotherix)
Indications: Pulmonary arterial hypertension, peripheral neuropathy
Class: Antihypertensive, Prostaglandin, Vasodilator
Half-life: 20–30 minutes
Clinically important, potentially hazardous interactions with: anticoagulants, aspirin, clopidogrel, coumarins, diclofenac, enoxaparin, eptifibatide, heparin, meloxicam, NSAIDs, phenindione, tinzaparin, tirofiban
Important contra-indications noted in the prescribing guidelines for: the elderly; nursing mothers; pediatric patients
Note: Ventavis is for oral inhalation only.

Skin
Flushing / rubefaction (27%) [12]

Cardiovascular
Angina [3]
Hypotension (11%) [4]
Palpitation (7%)

Central Nervous System
Headache (30%) [17]
Vertigo / dizziness (8%)

Neuromuscular/Skeletal
Back pain (7%)
Jaw pain [2]
Myalgia/Myopathy (6%)

Respiratory
Cough (39%) [7]

IMATINIB

Trade name: Gleevec (Novartis)
Indications: Chronic myeloid leukemia
Class: Antineoplastic / anticancer agent (see also Immune checkpoint inhibitor), Bcr-Abl tyrosine kinase inhibitor / (Breakpoint cluster region Abelson (Bcr-Abl) tyrosine kinase inhibitor, Biologic, Tyrosine kinase inhibitor
Half-life: 18 hours
Clinically important, potentially hazardous interactions with: acetaminophen, amlodipine, anisindione, anticoagulants, aprepitant, atorvastatin, barbiturates, benzodiazepines, butabarbital, carbamazepine, chlordiazepoxide, clarithromycin, clonazepam, clorazepate, corticosteroids, cyclosporine, dexamethasone, diazepam, dicumarol, efavirenz, erythromycin, ethotoin, felodipine, flurazepam, fluvastatin, fosphenytoin, isradipine, itraconazole, ketoconazole, lorazepam, lovastatin, mephenytoin, mephobarbital, midazolam, mifepristone, neratinib, nicardipine, nifedipine, nimodipine, nisoldipine, olaparib, oxazepam, oxcarbazepine, pentobarbital, phenobarbital, phenytoin, pimozide, pravastatin, primidone, quazepam, rifampin, rifapentine, safinamide, secobarbital, simvastatin, St John's wort, tafamidis meglumine, temazepam, voriconazole, warfarin
Important contra-indications noted in the prescribing guidelines for: nursing mothers

---

Skin
Acneiform eruption / acneiform dermatitis / acneiform rash [3]
AGEP [7]
Cutaneous toxicity / skin toxicity [9]

Diaphoresis (13%)
DRESS syndrome (Drug-induced hypersensitivity syndrome) [5]
Edema / fluid retention (<5%) [40]
Erythema (<10%) [5]
Erythema multiforme [2]
Erythroderma [4]
Exanthems [9]
Exfoliative dermatitis [4]
Facial edema (<10%) [3]
Hand–foot syndrome (palmar–plantar erythrodysesthesia) [3]
Hypomelanosis [5]
Lichen planus (includes hypertrophic lichen planus) [7]
Lichenoid eruption / lichenoid reaction [15]
Mycosis fungoides [2]
Neutrophilic eccrine hidradenitis [3]
Panniculitis [3]
Pemphigus [2]
Peripheral edema (<10%) [5]
Petechiae (<10%)
Photosensitivity (<10%) [3]
Pigmentation (Skin) (includes hyperpigmentation) [14]
Pityriasis rosea [6]
Pruritus (itching) (6–10%) [3]
Pseudolymphoma / cutaneous pseudolymphoma [3]
Pseudoporphyria [6]
Psoriasis [3]
Pyoderma gangrenosum [2]
Rash (32–39%) [27]
Squamous cell carcinoma [2]
Stevens-Johnson syndrome and toxic epidermal necrolysis (SJS/TEN) [15]
Sweet's syndrome [4]
Urticaria / hives [3]
Vasculitis (angiitis) / cutaneous vasculitis (angiitis) [2]
Xerosis / xeroderma (<10%) [2]

Hair
Alopecia / hair loss (10–15%) [2]
Follicular mucinosis [2]

Nails
Nail dystrophy [2]
Nail pigmentation [2]

Mucosal
Mucositis [2]
Oral lichenoid eruption [3]
Oral pigmentation [4]
Oral ulceration [3]

Cardiovascular
Cardiac failure [2]
Cardiotoxicity [2]
Congestive heart failure [2]
Pericardial effusion [3]
QT interval prolonged / QT prolongation [2]

Central Nervous System
Anorexia [4]
Chills (11%)
Depression (15%) [2]
Fever (pyrexia) (includes hyperpyrexia) (13–41%) [3]
Headache (19–37%) [5]
Hypoesthesia / hypesthesia (numbness) (<10%)
Insomnia (10–19%)
Pain [2]
Subdural hemorrhage [2]
Tremor [3]
Vertigo / dizziness [2]

Endocrine/Metabolic
Creatine phosphokinase (CPK) / creatine kinase increased (hyperCKemia) [2]
Gynecomastia [7]
Hypophosphatemia [6]
Hypothyroidism [2]
Porphyria cutanea tarda [3]
Weight gain (5–32%) [3]

Gastrointestinal/Hepatic
Abdominal pain [5]
Ascites [2]
Constipation (9–16%) [2]
Diarrhea (25–59%) [21]
Dyspepsia / functional dyspepsia (indigestion) (see also gastroparesis) [2]
Gastric antral vascular ectasia (GAVE) [5]
Gastrointestinal bleeding [3]
Hepatotoxicity / liver injury / acute liver injury / drug-induced liver injury (DILI) (6–12%) [20]
Nausea (42–73%) [21]
Ulcerative colitis [2]
Vomiting (23–58%) [14]

Hematologic
Anemia [12]
Febrile neutropenia [2]
Hemotoxicity [5]
Hypofibrinogenemia [2]
Hypogammaglobulinemia [3]
Leukocytopenia (leukopenia) / leukocytes (white blood cells) decreased [3]
Myelosuppression / bone marrow suppression / myelotoxicity [2]
Neutropenia (neutrophils decreased) [14]
Pure red cell aplasia [2]
Thrombocytopenia / platelets decreased [12]

Neuromuscular/Skeletal
Arthralgia (21–26%) [4]
Asthenia / fatigue (29–75%) [23]
Bone pain / joint pain (11–31%) [13]
Muscle spasm [10]
Myalgia/Myopathy (16–62%) [12]
Osteonecrosis / avascular necrosis (includes steroid-induced osteonecrosis of the femoral head) [3]

Ocular
Epiphora (25%)
Eyelid edema / palpebral edema / blepharedema [2]
Optic edema [3]
Periorbital edema (33%) [15]

Otic
Hearing loss (hypoacusis) [4]

Renal
Fanconi syndrome (proximal tubular dysfunction) [2]
Nephrotoxicity / kidney injury / acute kidney injury (AKI) / drug-induced kidney injury [3]
Renal failure [2]

Respiratory
Cough (11–27%)
Dyspnea / shortness of breath (21%)
Nasopharyngitis (10–31%)
Pharyngitis (sore throat) (10–15%)
Pleural effusion [5]
Pneumonitis (4–13%) [2]
Pulmonary toxicity [2]
Rhinitis / rhinosinusitis (see also sinusitis) (17%)
Upper respiratory tract infection (3–21%)

Other
Adverse effects / adverse reactions [16]
Death [3]
Side effects [2]

IMIDAPRIL

Indications: Hypertension
Class: Angiotensin-converting enzyme (ACE) inhibitor, Antihypertensive
Half-life: 2 hours
Clinically important, potentially hazardous interactions with: allopurinol, azathioprine, procainamide
Important contra-indications noted in the prescribing guidelines for: nursing mothers; pediatric patients

---

Respiratory
Cough [7]

IMIPENEM/CILASTATIN

Synonym: imipemide
Trade name: Primaxin (Merck)
Indications: Various infections caused by susceptible organisms
Class: Antibiotic, Antibiotic; carbapenem, Antimicrobial, Thienamycin
Half-life: 1 hour
Clinically important, potentially hazardous interactions with: amoxicillin, ampicillin, azlocillin, bacampicillin, carbenicillin, cloxacillin, cyclosporine, dicloxacillin, ganciclovir, methicillin, mezlocillin, nafcillin, oxacillin, penicillin G, penicillin V, piperacillin, ticarcillin

---

Skin
Exanthems (<5%) [3]
Pruritus (itching) [3]
Rash (4%)
Urticaria / hives [3]

Cardiovascular
Phlebitis (3%)
Thrombophlebitis (3%)

Central Nervous System
Seizures [2]

Gastrointestinal/Hepatic
Diarrhea [2]
Nausea [4]
Vomiting [4]

Local
Injection-site pain [2]
Injection-site phlebitis (<4%) [4]

Other
Allergic reactions (<3%) [2]

IMIPRAMINE

Trade name: Tofranil (Mallinckrodt)
Indications: Depression
Class: Antidepressant; tricyclic, Muscarinic antagonist
Half-life: 6–18 hours
Clinically important, potentially hazardous interactions with: amprenavir, arbutamine, artemether/lumefantrine, clonidine, cobicistat/elvitegravir/emtricitabine/tenofovir alafenamide, cobicistat/elvitegravir/emtricitabine/tenofovir disoproxil, darifenacin, epinephrine, fluoxetine, formoterol, guanethidine, iobenguane, isocarboxazid, labetalol, linezolid, MAO inhibitors, phenelzine, propranolol, quinolones,

ropivacaine, sparfloxacin, tranylcypromine, zaleplon, zolpidem
Warning: SUICIDALITY AND ANTIDEPRESSANT DRUGS

Skin
- Diaphoresis (<25%) [8]
- Exanthems (<6%) [6]
- Exfoliative dermatitis [4]
- Photosensitivity [3]
- Pigmentation (Skin) (includes hyperpigmentation) [13]
- Pruritus (itching) (3%) [6]
- Purpura [3]
- Urticaria / hives [6]

Hair
- Alopecia / hair loss [2]

Mucosal
- Glossitis (inflammation of the tongue) [2]
- Oral lesions [3]
- Stomatitis (oral mucositis) [2]
- Xerostomia (dry mouth) (>10%) [16]

Cardiovascular
- QT interval prolonged / QT prolongation [3]
- Tachycardia [2]

Central Nervous System
- Dysgeusia (taste perversion) (metallic taste) (>10%) [2]
- Parkinsonism (<10%)

Endocrine/Metabolic
- Galactorrhea [2]
- SIADH [4]

Neuromuscular/Skeletal
- Asthenia / fatigue [2]

Otic
- Tinnitus [4]

IMIQUIMOD

Trade names: Aldara (3M), Zyclara (Graceway)
Indications: External genital and perianal warts, actinic keratoses
Class: Antiviral, Immunomodulator
Half-life: N/A
Clinically important, potentially hazardous interactions with: none known
Important contra-indications noted in the prescribing guidelines for: nursing mothers; pediatric patients

Skin
- Angioedema (formerly named angioneurotic edema) [2]
- Burning / skin burning sensation (9–31%) [7]
- Crusting [3]
- Depigmentation [3]
- Eczema / eczematous reaction / eczematous eruption (<10%)
- Edema / fluid retention (12–17%) [2]
- Erosions (10–32%) [5]
- Erythema (33–85%) [14]
- Erythema multiforme [9]
- Excoriations (18–25%) [2]
- Flaking (18–67%) [3]
- Fungal dermatitis (<10%)
- Herpes simplex (<10%)
- Hypomelanosis [2]
- Induration (5%)
- Lichen planus (includes hypertrophic lichen planus) [3]
- Lupus erythematosus (subacute cutaneous lupus erythematosus (SCLE)) [3]
- Lymphadenopathy (2%)
- Pemphigus [4]
- Pemphigus foliaceus [3]
- Pigmentation (Skin) (includes hyperpigmentation) [3]
- Pityriasis rubra pilaris [4]
- Pruritus (itching) (22–75%) [10]
- Psoriasis [6]
- Scabbing (4%)
- Scar [3]
- Seborrheic keratoses (<10%)
- Stevens-Johnson syndrome and toxic epidermal necrolysis (SJS/TEN) [4]
- Tenderness (local) (12%) [2]
- Ulcerations (5–10%) [6]
- Vesiculation (2–3%)
- Vitiligo [7]

Hair
- Alopecia / hair loss (<10%)
- Poliosis [2]

Cardiovascular
- Chest pain (<10%)

Central Nervous System
- Anorexia (<10%)
- Anxiety (<10%)
- Fever (pyrexia) (includes hyperpyrexia) (<10%) [2]
- Headache (<10%) [4]
- Neurotoxicity [2]
- Pain (2–11%) [6]
- Rigors (<10%)
- Vertigo / dizziness (<10%)

Gastrointestinal/Hepatic
- Nausea (<10%) [2]
- Vomiting (<10%)

Genitourinary
- Urinary tract infection (<10%)

Hematologic
- Lymphopenia (lymphocytopenia) / lymphocytes decreased [2]

Local
- Application-site burning (<10%)
- Application-site edema (<10%) [4]
- Application-site erythema (<10%) [3]
- Application-site pruritus (<10%) [5]
- Application-site reactions [9]

Neuromuscular/Skeletal
- Asthenia / fatigue (<10%) [3]
- Back pain (<10%)
- Myalgia/Myopathy (<10%) [2]

Respiratory
- Cough (<10%)
- Influenza- ('flu)-like syndrome (<3%) [3]
- Pharyngitis (sore throat) (<10%)
- Rhinitis / rhinosinusitis (see also sinusitis) (<10%)
- Sinusitis (see also rhinitis / rhinosinusitis) (<10%)
- Upper respiratory tract infection (<10%)

Other
- Adverse effects / adverse reactions [7]

IMMUNE GLOBULIN IV

Synonyms: IGIV; IVIG; Octagam; intravenous immunoglobulin (IVIg)
Trade names: Gamimune (Bayer), Gammagard (Baxter), Gammar PIV (ZLB Behring), Gamunex (Bayer), Iveegam (Baxter), Panzyga (Octapharma), Venoglobulin (Alpha Therapeutics)
Indications: Immunodeficiency in patients unable to produce sufficient amounts of IgG antibodies
Class: Covid-19 putative drug, Immunomodulator
Half-life: N/A
Clinically important, potentially hazardous interactions with: live vaccines
Important contra-indications noted in the prescribing guidelines for: nursing mothers
Warning: THROMBOSIS, RENAL DYSFUNCTION and ACUTE RENAL FAILURE

Skin
- Anaphylactoid reactions / anaphylaxis (includes anaphylactic shock) [5]
- Eczema / eczematous reaction / eczematous eruption [4]
- Flushing / rubefaction [2]
- Lichenoid eruption / lichenoid reaction [2]
- Pompholyx / dyshidrotic eczema [3]
- Rash [2]
- Stevens-Johnson syndrome and toxic epidermal necrolysis (SJS/TEN) [2]
- Vasculitis (angiitis) / cutaneous vasculitis (angiitis) [4]

Cardiovascular
- Hypertension [5]
- Myocardial infarction [2]
- Palpitation [2]
- Thromboembolism [4]

Central Nervous System
- Aseptic meningitis [13]
- Chills [5]
- Fever (pyrexia) (includes hyperpyrexia) [13]
- Headache [23]

Endocrine/Metabolic
- Hypertransaminasemia (hepatic transaminitis) / elevated transaminases [2]

Gastrointestinal/Hepatic
- Abdominal pain [2]
- Diarrhea [2]
- Hepatitis [3]
- Hepatotoxicity / liver injury / acute liver injury / drug-induced liver injury (DILI) [2]
- Nausea [11]
- Vomiting [3]

Hematologic
- Anemia [2]
- Hemolysis [2]
- Hemolytic anemia [5]
- Neutropenia (neutrophils decreased) [6]
- Thrombocytopenia / platelets decreased [4]
- Thrombosis [3]

Local
- Application-site pain (16%)
- Infusion-related reactions [6]
- Injection-site edema [2]
- Injection-site erythema [2]

Neuromuscular/Skeletal
- Arthralgia [3]
- Asthenia / fatigue [5]
- Back pain [3]
- Bone pain / joint pain [2]
- Myalgia/Myopathy [4]

Renal
Nephrotoxicity / kidney injury / acute kidney injury (AKI) / drug-induced kidney injury [6]
Renal failure [3]

Respiratory
Cough [2]
Dyspnea / shortness of breath [2]
Pulmonary embolism [2]

Other
Adverse effects / adverse reactions [10]

INACTIVATED POLIO VACCINE

Trade names: IMOVAX Polio (Sanofi-Aventis), IPV (Sanofi-Aventis)
Indications: Polio immunization
Class: Vaccine
Half-life: 4 years
Clinically important, potentially hazardous interactions with: immunosuppressants
Important contra-indications noted in the prescribing guidelines for: nursing mothers

---

Central Nervous System
Fever (pyrexia) (includes hyperpyrexia) [2]

INAMRINONE

Synonym: amrinone
Indications: Congestive heart failure
Class: Phosphodiesterase inhibitor
Half-life: 4.6 hours
Clinically important, potentially hazardous interactions with: anagrelide
Important contra-indications noted in the prescribing guidelines for: nursing mothers; pediatric patients

INDACATEROL

Trade names: Arcapta Neohaler (Novartis), Onbrez Breezhaler (Novartis), Utibron Neohaler (Novartis)
Indications: Long term, once-daily maintenance bronchodilator treatment of airflow obstruction in chronic obstructive pulmonary disease (COPD), including chronic bronchitis and/or emphysema
Class: Beta-2 adrenergic agonist, Bronchodilator
Half-life: 40–56 hours
Clinically important, potentially hazardous interactions with: acetazolamide, adrenergics, aminophylline, arsenic, corticosteroids, diuretics, dolasetron, erythromycin, ketoconazole, MAO inhibitors, pazopanib, QT prolonging agents, ritonavir, steroids, telavancin, theophylline, tricyclic antidepressants, verapamil, xanthine derivatives
Important contra-indications noted in the prescribing guidelines for: nursing mothers; pediatric patients
Note: Studies in asthma patients showed that long-acting beta$_2$-adrenergic agonists may increase the risk of asthma-related death. Contra-indicated in patients with asthma without use of a long-term asthma control medication. Utibron Neohaler is indacaterol and glycopyrrolate.
Warning: ASTHMA-RELATED DEATH

Mucosal
Oropharyngeal pain [2]

Cardiovascular
QT interval prolonged / QT prolongation [2]

Central Nervous System
Headache (5%) [4]
Pain (oropharyngeal) (2%)

Endocrine/Metabolic
Hyperglycemia (includes glucose increased) [2]

Gastrointestinal/Hepatic
Nausea (2%)

Respiratory
Asthma [2]
COPD (exacerbation) [8]
Cough (7%) [11]
Dyspnea / shortness of breath [2]
Influenza [2]
Nasopharyngitis (5%) [7]
Upper respiratory tract infection [4]

Other
Adverse effects / adverse reactions [7]
Death [2]

INDAPAMIDE

Trade name: Lozol (Sanofi-Aventis)
Indications: Edema
Class: Diuretic, thiazide
Half-life: 14–18 hours
Clinically important, potentially hazardous interactions with: digoxin, lithium, zinc
Important contra-indications noted in the prescribing guidelines for: the elderly; nursing mothers; pediatric patients
Note: Indapamide is a sulfonamide and can be absorbed systemically. Sulfonamides can produce severe, possibly fatal, reactions such as toxic epidermal necrolysis and Stevens-Johnson syndrome.

Skin
Angioedema (formerly named angioneurotic edema) [3]
Erythema multiforme [2]
Flushing / rubefaction (<5%)
Pemphigus foliaceus [2]
Peripheral edema (<5%) [2]
Pruritus (itching) (<5%) [2]
Rash (<5%) [4]
Stevens-Johnson syndrome and toxic epidermal necrolysis (SJS/TEN) [4]
Urticaria / hives (<5%)
Vasculitis (angiitis) / cutaneous vasculitis (angiitis) (<5%)

Mucosal
Xerostomia (dry mouth) (<5%) [2]

Cardiovascular
QT interval prolonged / QT prolongation [5]

Central Nervous System
Paresthesias (<5%)
Vertigo / dizziness [2]

Endocrine/Metabolic
Hypokalemia [4]
Hyponatremia [4]

Ocular
Myopia [5]

INDINAVIR

Trade name: Crixivan (Merck)
Indications: HIV infection
Class: Antiretroviral, CYP3A4 inhibitor, HIV-1 protease inhibitor
Half-life: ~1.8 hours
Clinically important, potentially hazardous interactions with: abiraterone, alfuzosin, almotriptan, alosetron, alprazolam, amiodarone, amprenavir, antacids, antiarrhythmics, antifungal agents, artemether/lumefantrine, astemizole, atazanavir, atorvastatin, atovaquone, atovaquone/proguanil, avanafil, bepridil, bortezomib, bosentan, brigatinib, brinzolamide, cabazitaxel, cabozantinib, calcifediol, calcium channel blockers, carbamazepine, chlordiazepoxide, ciclesonide, cisapride, clarithromycin, clonazepam, clorazepate, colchicine, conivaptan, copanlisib, corticosteroids, crizotinib, cyclosporine, CYP3A4 inducers and substrates, darifenacin, darunavir, dasatinib, deferasirox, delavirdine, diazepam, didanosine, dienogest, digoxin, dihydroergotamine, dronedarone, dutasteride, efavirenz, enfuvirtide, eplerenone, ergot derivatives, ergotamine, estazolam, estrogens, etravirine, everolimus, felodipine, fentanyl, fesoterodine, flibanserin, flurazepam, fluticasone propionate, food, fusidic acid, grapefruit juice, guanfacine, H_2-antagonists, halazepam, halofantrine, HMG-CoA reductase inhibitors, itraconazole, ixabepilone, ketoconazole, lapatinib, lidocaine, lomitapide, lopinavir, lovastatin, maraviroc, meperidine, methylergonovine, methylprednisolone, methysergide, midazolam, midostaurin, mifepristone, mometasone, nefazodone, nelfinavir, neratinib, nevirapine, nicardipine, nifedipine, nilotinib, nisoldipine, olaparib, P-glycoprotein inhibitors and inducers, paclitaxel, palbociclib, pantoprazole, paricalcitol, pazopanib, PEG-interferon, phenobarbital, phenytoin, pimavanserin, pimecrolimus, pimozide, ponatinib, prasugrel, protease inhibitors, proton pump inhibitors, quazepam, quinidine, quinine, ranolazine, ribociclib, rifabutin, rifampin, rifapentine, rilpivirine, rivaroxaban, romidepsin, rosuvastatin, ruxolitinib, salmeterol, saxagliptin, sildenafil, silodosin, simeprevir, simvastatin, sirolimus, solifenacin, sorafenib, St John's wort, sunitinib, tacrolimus, tadalafil, tamsulosin, telithromycin, temsirolimus, tenofovir disoproxil, theophylline, ticagrelor, tolvaptan, trazodone, triazolam, tricyclic antidepressants, valproic acid, vardenafil, vemurafenib, venetoclax, venlafaxine, vorapaxar, zidovudine
Important contra-indications noted in the prescribing guidelines for: nursing mothers; pediatric patients
Note: Protease inhibitors cause dyslipidemia which includes elevated triglycerides and cholesterol and redistribution of body fat centrally to produce the so-called 'protease paunch', breast enlargement, facial atrophy, and 'buffalo hump'.

Skin
Bromhidrosis (<2%)
Dermatitis (<2%)
Diaphoresis (<2%)
Flushing / rubefaction (<2%)
Folliculitis (<2%)

Herpes simplex (<2%)
Herpes zoster (<2%)
Jaundice (see also cholestasis / cholestatic jaundice) (2%)
Lipodystrophy / acquired generalized lipodystrophy [8]
Lipomatosis [2]
Pruritus (itching) [2]
Rash [2]
Seborrhea (<2%)
Stevens-Johnson syndrome and toxic epidermal necrolysis (SJS/TEN) [2]
Xerosis / xeroderma [2]

Hair
Alopecia / hair loss [5]

Nails
Onychocryptosis (ingrowing toe nail) [2]
Paronychia [5]
Pyogenic granuloma [3]

Mucosal
Aphthous stomatitis / aphthous ulcer / aphtha (aphthae) (<2%)
Cheilitis (inflammation of the lips) [4]
Gingivitis (<2%)

Central Nervous System
Anorexia (3%)
Dysesthesia (<2%)
Dysgeusia (taste perversion) (3%)
Fever (pyrexia) (includes hyperpyrexia) (2%)
Headache (5%)
Hyperesthesia (<2%)
Paresthesias (<2%)
Somnolence (drowsiness) (2%)
Vertigo / dizziness (3%)

Endocrine/Metabolic
ALT increased (5%)
Appetite increased (2%)
AST increased (4%)
Creatine phosphokinase (CPK) / creatine kinase increased (hyperCKemia) [2]
Diabetes mellitus [2]
Gynecomastia [4]
Porphyria (acute) [2]

Gastrointestinal/Hepatic
Abdominal pain (17%) [2]
Diarrhea (3%)
Dyspepsia / functional dyspepsia (indigestion) (see also gastroparesis) (2%)
Nausea (12%)
Vomiting (8%)

Genitourinary
Crystalluria [2]
Dysuria (2%)

Neuromuscular/Skeletal
Asthenia / fatigue (2%)
Back pain (8%)
Myalgia/Myopathy with lovastatin or simvastatin (<2%)

Ocular
Eyelid edema / palpebral edema / blepharedema (<2%)

Renal
Nephrolithiasis (kidney stones / renal calculi) (9%) [5]
Nephrotoxicity / kidney injury / acute kidney injury (AKI) / drug-induced kidney injury [14]

Respiratory
Cough (2%)

Other
Bruxism (teeth grinding) (<2%)

INDOMETHACIN

Synonym: indometacin
Indications: Arthritis
Class: Non-steroidal anti-inflammatory (NSAID)
Half-life: 4.5 hours
Clinically important, potentially hazardous interactions with: aldesleukin, aspirin, atenolol, cyclopenthiazide, dasiglucagon, diflunisal, diuretics, methotrexate, NSAIDs, prednisolone, prednisone, sermorelin, tiludronate, torsemide, triamterene, urokinase
Important contra-indications noted in the prescribing guidelines for: nursing mothers; pediatric patients
Note: NSAIDs may cause an increased risk of serious cardiovascular and gastrointestinal adverse events, which can be fatal. This risk may increase with duration of use.
Warning: RISK OF SERIOUS CARDIOVASCULAR AND GASTROINTESTINAL EVENTS

Skin
Angioedema (formerly named angioneurotic edema) [2]
Bullous dermatosis [2]
Dermatitis [5]
Dermatitis herpetiformis (exacerbation) [2]
Edema / fluid retention (3–9%)
Exanthems (<5%) [7]
Fixed eruption / fixed drug eruption [3]
Pruritus (itching) (<10%) [3]
Psoriasis [7]
Purpura [5]
Rash (>10%)
Stevens-Johnson syndrome and toxic epidermal necrolysis (SJS/TEN) [6]
Urticaria / hives [7]
Vasculitis (angiitis) / cutaneous vasculitis (angiitis) [5]

Mucosal
Oral lesions (<7%) [2]
Oral ulceration [4]

Central Nervous System
Headache [2]
Psychosis [3]

Gastrointestinal/Hepatic
Gastrointestinal bleeding [2]
Gastrointestinal perforation / perforated colon / gastric perforation [3]
Gastrointestinal ulceration [3]
Pancreatitis / acute pancreatitis [2]

Ocular
Periorbital edema [2]

Otic
Tinnitus [2]

Other
Adverse effects / adverse reactions [8]

INDORAMIN

Trade names: Baratol (Amdipharm), Doralese Tiltab (GSK)
Indications: Hypertension, alpha blockade, benign prostatic hyperplasia
Class: Alpha 1 adrenoreceptor antagonist
Half-life: 5 hours
Clinically important, potentially hazardous interactions with: anesthetics, antidepressants, antihypertensives, anxiolytics, beta-blockers, calcium channel blockers, diuretics, MAO inhibitors, moxisylyte

---

Central Nervous System
Sedation (>10%)
Somnolence (drowsiness) (>10%)

INFIGRATINIB

Trade name: Truseltiq (Helsinn)
Indications: Cholangiocarcinoma (in adults with previously treated, unresectable locally advanced or metastatic cholangiocarcinoma with a fibroblast growth factor receptor 2 (FGFR2) fusion or other rearrangement)
Class: Fibroblast growth factor receptor inhibitor, Kinase inhibitor
Half-life: 33.5 hours
Clinically important, potentially hazardous interactions with: antacids, CYP3A inducers, CYP3A inhibitors, histamine-2 (H2) receptor antagonists, itraconazole, lansoprazole, proton pump inhibitors, rifampin
Pregnancy category: Insufficient data on use in pregnant women. Advise against breastfeeding during treatment and for 1 month after the last dose.
Note: Infigratinib can cause retinal pigment epithelial detachment (RPED), which may result in symptoms such as blurred vision. Perform a comprehensive ophthalmic examination including optical coherence tomography prior to initiation of infigratinib, at 1 month, at 3 months, and then every 3 months thereafter during treatment.

Skin
Dry skin (23%)
Edema / fluid retention (17%)
Hand–foot syndrome (palmar–plantar erythrodysesthesia) (33%)

Hair
Alopecia / hair loss (38%)

Nails
Nail toxicity (57%)

Mucosal
Epistaxis (nosebleed) (18%)
Stomatitis (oral mucositis) (56%)
Xerostomia (dry mouth) (25%)

Central Nervous System
Dysgeusia (taste perversion) (32%)
Fever (pyrexia) (includes hyperpyrexia) (15%)
Headache (17%)

Endocrine/Metabolic
ALP increased (54%)
ALT increased (51%)
Appetite decreased (22%)
AST increased (38%)
Hyperbilirubinemia (24%)
Hypercalcemia (43%)
Hypercholesterolemia (18%)
Hyperkalemia (17%)
Hyperlipasemia (44%)
Hyperphosphatemia (13% grade 3/4) (90%) [2]
Hypertriglyceridemia (includes triglycerides increased) (38%)
Hyperuricemia (37%)
Hypoalbuminemia / albumin decreased (24%)
Hypocalcemia (10%)
Hypokalemia (21%)

Hyponatremia (20% grade 3/4) (41%)
Hypophosphatemia (31% grade 3/4) (64%)
Serum creatinine increased (93%)
Weight loss (15%)

Gastrointestinal/Hepatic
Abdominal pain (26%)
Constipation (30%)
Diarrhea (24%)
Dyspepsia / functional dyspepsia (indigestion) (see also gastroparesis) (17%)
Nausea (19%)
Vomiting (21%)

Hematologic
Hemoglobin decreased (53%)
Leukocytopenia (leukopenia) / leukocytes (white blood cells) decreased (26%)
Lymphopenia (lymphocytopenia) / lymphocytes decreased (43%)
Neutropenia (neutrophils decreased) (14%)
Thrombocytopenia / platelets decreased (37%)

Neuromuscular/Skeletal
Arthralgia (32%)
Asthenia / fatigue (44%)
Pain in extremities (17%)

Ocular
Dry eye (keratoconjunctivitis sicca) (44%)
Eyelash changes (25%)
Retinal pigment epithelial detachment (RPED) (asymptomatic RPED) (11%)
Vision blurred (21%)

INFLIXIMAB

Synonym: CT-P13 is biosimilar infliximab
Trade names: Inflectra (Celltrion), Remicade (Centocor), Remsima (Celltrion), Renflexis (Samsung Bioepsis)
Indications: Crohn's disease, ulcerative colitis, rheumatoid arthritis, ankylosing spondylitis, psoriatic arthritis, plaque psoriasis
Class: Anti-Tumor Necrosis Factor-alpha (TNF-α antagonist), Antipsoriatic agent, Biologic, Biologic disease-modifying antirheumatic drug (bDMARD), Cytokine inhibitor, Disease-modifying antirheumatic drug (DMARD), Monoclonal antibody
Half-life: 8–10 days
Clinically important, potentially hazardous interactions with: abatacept, anakinra, live vaccines, methotrexate, tocilizumab
Important contra-indications noted in the prescribing guidelines for: the elderly; nursing mothers
Note: TNF inhibitors should be used in patients with heart failure only after consideration of other treatment options.
Contra-indicated in patients with a personal or family history of multiple sclerosis or demyelinating disease. TNF inhibitors should not be administered to patients with moderate to severe heart failure (New York Heart Association Functional Class III/IV). Infliximab-dyyb (Inflectra) is biosimilar to Infliximab (Remicade). Approved 04/05/2016 Infliximab-abda (Renflexis) is biosimilar to Infliximab (Remicade). Approved 04/21/2017 Infliximab-qbtx (Ixifi) is biosimilar to Infliximab (Remicade). Approved 12/13/2017 Infliximab-axxq (Avsola) is biosimilar to Infliximab (Remicade). Approved 12/06/2019 Infliximab-dyyb (Zymfentra) is biosimilar to Infliximab. Approved 10/20/2023.

Warning: SERIOUS INFECTIONS and MALIGNANCY

Skin
Abscess [4]
Acneiform eruption / acneiform dermatitis / acneiform rash [6]
AGEP [2]
Anaphylactoid reactions / anaphylaxis (includes anaphylactic shock) [11]
Angioedema (formerly named angioneurotic edema) [2]
Baboon syndrome / symmetrical drug-related intertriginous and flexural exanthema (SDRIFE) [2]
Candidiasis / candidosis (5%) [4]
Cellulitis and pseudocellulitis [5]
Cutaneous toxicity / skin toxicity [2]
Dermatitis [4]
Eczema / eczematous reaction / eczematous eruption [5]
Edema / fluid retention [3]
Erythema multiforme [4]
Exanthems [4]
Flushing / rubefaction [2]
Folliculitis [2]
Hand–foot syndrome (palmar–plantar erythrodysesthesia) [2]
Henoch-Schönlein purpura / IgA vasculitis / immunoglobulin A vasculitis [5]
Herpes [2]
Herpes simplex [4]
Herpes zoster [11]
Hidradenitis suppurativa (acne inversa) [2]
Hypersensitivity [11]
Lesions (includes skin lesions) [2]
Leukocytoclastic vasculitis (angiitis) [6]
Lichen planus (includes hypertrophic lichen planus) [4]
Lichenoid eruption / lichenoid reaction [4]
Lupus erythematosus (subacute cutaneous lupus erythematosus (SCLE)) [35]
Lupus syndrome / drug-induced lupus (DIL) [14]
Lymphoma [9]
Molluscum contagiosum [2]
Nevi (naevi) [2]
Palmoplantar pustulosis [3]
Pityriasis lichenoides / pityriasis lichenoides chronica / pityriasis lichenoides et varioliformis acuta [3]
Pruritus (itching) (7%) [8]
Pseudolymphoma / cutaneous pseudolymphoma [2]
Psoriasiform eruption [4]
Psoriasis [57]
Pustules / pustular eruption [5]
Pyoderma gangrenosum [2]
Rash (10%) [13]
Sarcoidosis / sarcoid-like reaction (cutaneous sarcoidosis) [5]
Serum sickness [2]
Serum sickness-like reaction (<3%) [5]
Stevens-Johnson syndrome and toxic epidermal necrolysis (SJS/TEN) [3]
Urticaria / hives [7]
Vasculitis (angiitis) / cutaneous vasculitis (angiitis) [18]
Vitiligo [8]

Hair
Alopecia / hair loss [8]
Alopecia areata [4]
Lichen planopilaris [2]

Cardiovascular
Cardiotoxicity [2]
Chest pain [4]
Hypertension (7%) [3]
Palpitation [2]
Pericarditis [3]
Tachycardia [2]

Central Nervous System
Aseptic meningitis [2]
Chills (5–9%) [2]
Demyelinating neuropathy / demyelination [4]
Depression [3]
Fever (pyrexia) (includes hyperpyrexia) (7%) [10]
Headache (18%) [12]
Leukoencephalopathy / posterior reversible encephalopathy syndrome (PRES) [2]
Neurotoxicity [8]
Pain (8%) [3]
Paresthesias (<4%) [2]
Peripheral neuropathy [8]
Seizures [2]
Suicidal ideation [2]
Vertigo / dizziness [3]

Endocrine/Metabolic
ALT increased [2]

Gastrointestinal/Hepatic
Abdominal pain (12%) [4]
Colitis [2]
Crohn's disease (26%)
Diarrhea (12%)
Dyspepsia / functional dyspepsia (indigestion) (see also gastroparesis) (10%)
Hepatitis [13]
Hepatotoxicity / liver injury / acute liver injury / drug-induced liver injury (DILI) [18]
Nausea (21%) [3]
Pancreatitis / acute pancreatitis [2]

Genitourinary
Cystitis (includes interstitial cystitis / bladder pain syndrome) [2]
Urinary tract infection (8%) [3]

Hematologic
Hemolytic anemia [2]
Neutropenia (neutrophils decreased) [5]
Sepsis [2]
Thrombocytopenia / platelets decreased [5]

Local
Application-site reactions (mild) (<4%) [6]
Infusion-related reactions [26]
Infusion-site reactions (20%) [13]
Injection-site reaction (6%) [9]

Neuromuscular/Skeletal
Arthralgia (<8%) [16]
Asthenia / fatigue (9%) [5]
Back pain (8%)
Myalgia/Myopathy (5%) [8]
Polymyositis [2]

Ocular
Optic neuritis / papillitis [3]
Uveitis / anterior uveitis / posterior uveitis / panuveitis [3]

Renal
Nephrotoxicity / kidney injury / acute kidney injury (AKI) / drug-induced kidney injury [2]

Respiratory
Bronchitis (10%)
Cough (12%) [3]
Dyspnea / shortness of breath (6%) [4]
Influenza [2]

Interstitial lung disease / interstitial pneumonitis / interstitial pneumonia (cryptogenic organizing pneumonia) / drug-induced interstitial lung disease [9]
Pharyngitis (sore throat) (12%)
Pleural effusion [2]
Pneumonia [12]
Pulmonary toxicity [6]
Respiratory tract infection [2]
Rhinitis / rhinosinusitis (see also sinusitis) (8%)
Sinusitis (see also rhinitis / rhinosinusitis) (14%) [5]
Tuberculosis [17]
Upper respiratory tract infection (32%) [8]

Other
Adverse effects / adverse reactions [48]
Allergic reactions [8]
Death [15]
Infection (36%) [67]
Malignancies [2]
Neoplasms [2]
Nocardiosis [3]
Side effects [2]
Systemic reactions [2]

INFLUENZA VACCINE

Trade names: Afluria (Seqirus), Agrippal (Chiron), Comvax (Merck), Fluad (Novartis), Fluarix (GSK), FluMist (Medimmune) (Wyeth), Flurix (GSK), Fluviral (Shire), Inflexal V (Berna Biotech), Invivac (Solvay), Vaxigrip (Sanofi-Aventis)
Indications: Influenza prevention
Class: Vaccine
Half-life: N/A
Clinically important, potentially hazardous interactions with: aminophylline, carbamazepine, cyclosporine, mercaptopurine, phenobarbital, phenytoin, prednisone, vincristine, warfarin
Important contra-indications noted in the prescribing guidelines for: pediatric patients
Note: Inactivated influenza vaccine should not be given to persons with anaphylactic hypersensitivity to eggs or other components of the vaccine. For current data on influenza in the USA consult the Centers for Disease Control and Protection website (www.cdc.gov/flu).

Skin
Anaphylactoid reactions / anaphylaxis (includes anaphylactic shock) (rare) [4]
Henoch-Schönlein purpura / IgA vasculitis / immunoglobulin A vasculitis [2]
Hypersensitivity [2]
Linear IgA bullous dermatosis [2]
Purpura [2]
Rash [3]
Serum sickness-like reaction [2]
Vasculitis (angiitis) / cutaneous vasculitis (angiitis) [10]

Central Nervous System
Fever (pyrexia) (includes hyperpyrexia) [15]
Guillain-Barré syndrome / acute inflammatory demyelinating polyradiculoneuropathy / acute motor axonal neuropathy [11]
Headache [11]
Seizures [3]
Syncope / fainting [2]

Gastrointestinal/Hepatic
Abdominal pain [2]

Hematologic
Thrombocytopenia / platelets decreased [2]

Local
Injection-site edema [4]
Injection-site erythema [7]
Injection-site induration [5]
Injection-site inflammation [3]
Injection-site pain (20–28%) [16]
Injection-site reaction [4]

Neuromuscular/Skeletal
Arthralgia [2]
Asthenia / fatigue [8]
Myalgia/Myopathy [11]
Polymyositis [4]

Ocular
Oculorespiratory syndrome [15]
Optic neuritis / papillitis [2]

Respiratory
Asthma [2]
Cough [2]

Other
Adverse effects / adverse reactions [9]
Side effects [4]
Systemic reactions (injection site) [5]

INOTERSEN

Trade name: Tegsedi (Ionis Pharms Inc)
Indications: indicated for treatment of the polyneuropathy of hereditary transthyretin-mediated amyloidosis in adults
Class: Transthyretin-directed antisense oligonucleotide
Half-life: 32.3 days
Clinically important, potentially hazardous interactions with: adenosine, aspirin, clopidogrel, heparin, prasugrel, ticagrelor, ticlopidine, warfarin
Pregnancy category: no data on the associated developmental risk
Warning: THROMBOCYTOPENIA AND GLOMERULONEPHRITIS

Skin
Bacterial infection (7%)
Peripheral edema (19%)

Mucosal
Xerostomia (dry mouth) (5%)

Cardiovascular
Arrhythmias (13%)
Orthostatic hypotension (8%)

Central Nervous System
Chills (18%)
Fever (pyrexia) (includes hyperpyrexia) (20%)
Headache (26%)
Paresthesias (10%)
Presyncope (13%)
Syncope / fainting (13%)

Endocrine/Metabolic
Appetite decreased (10%)

Gastrointestinal/Hepatic
Nausea (31%)
Vomiting (15%)

Hematologic
Anemia (17%)
Eosinophilia / eosinophils increased (5%)
Thrombocytopenia / platelets decreased (24%) [2]

Local
Injection-site reaction (Includes bruising, erythema, hematoma, hemorrhage, induration, inflammation, mass, edema, pain, pruritus, rash, swelling, and urticaria) (49%)

Neuromuscular/Skeletal
Arthralgia (13%)
Asthenia / fatigue (25%)
Myalgia/Myopathy (15%)

Renal
Renal function abnormal / renal dysfunction (14%)

Respiratory
Dyspnea / shortness of breath (9%)
Influenza (8%)

INOTUZUMAB OZOGAMICIN

Trade name: Besponsa (Wyeth)
Indications: Relapsed or refractory B-cell precursor acute lymphoblastic leukemia
Class: Antibody-drug conjugate (ADC), CD22-directed antibody-drug conjugate
Half-life: 12 days
Clinically important, potentially hazardous interactions with: none known
Pregnancy category: Can cause fetal harm
Important contra-indications noted in the prescribing guidelines for: nursing mothers; pediatric patients
Warning: HEPATOTOXICITY, INCLUDING HEPATIC VENOOCCLUSIVE DISEASE (ALSO KNOWN AS SINUSOIDAL OBSTRUCTION SYNDROME) and INCREASED RISK OF POSTHEMATOPOIETIC STEM CELL TRANSPLANT NONRELAPSE MORTALITY

Skin
Hypersensitivity (2%)

Mucosal
Stomatitis (oral mucositis) (13%)

Cardiovascular
Hypotension [2]
Veno-occlusive disease (23%) [6]

Central Nervous System
Chills (11%)
Fever (pyrexia) (includes hyperpyrexia) (32%) [4]
Headache (28%) [2]

Endocrine/Metabolic
ALP increased (13%)
ALT increased (>10%) [2]
Appetite decreased (12%)
AST increased (>10%) [3]
GGT increased (21%)
Hyperbilirubinemia (21%) [6]
Hyperlipasemia (9%)
Hyperuricemia (4%)

Gastrointestinal/Hepatic
Abdominal distension (6%)
Abdominal pain (23%)
Ascites (4%)
Constipation (16%)
Diarrhea (17%)
Hepatotoxicity / liver injury / acute liver injury / drug-induced liver injury (DILI) (14%) [4]
Nausea (31%) [4]
Vomiting (15%)

Hematologic
Anemia (36%)
Febrile neutropenia (26%) [2]
Hemorrhage (33%)
Leukocytopenia (leukopenia) / leukocytes (white blood cells) decreased (35%) [3]
Lymphopenia (lymphocytopenia) / lymphocytes decreased (18%) [4]
Myelosuppression / bone marrow suppression / myelotoxicity (>10%)
Neutropenia (neutrophils decreased) (49%) [10]
Pancytopenia (includes bicytopenia) (2%)
Sepsis [2]
Thrombocytopenia / platelets decreased (51%) [11]

Local
Infusion-related reactions (2%)

Neuromuscular/Skeletal
Asthenia / fatigue (35%) [2]

Respiratory
Pneumonia [2]

Other
Death [2]
Infection (48%) [3]

INSULIN

Trade names: Humulin (Lilly), Iletin Lente (Lilly), Novolin R (Novo Nordisk), Velosulin (Novo Nordisk)
Indications: Diabetes
Class: Antidiabetic, CYP1A2 inducer, Hormone, polypeptide
Half-life: N/A
Clinically important, potentially hazardous interactions with: acebutolol, alcohol, captopril, cilazapril, ciprofloxacin, dimercaprol, enalapril, ethanolamine, eucalyptus, fosinopril, gemifloxacin, guanethidine, hydrocortisone, lanreotide, levofloxacin, lisinopril, moxifloxacin, nifedipine, ofloxacin, pegvisomant, pioglitazone, propranolol, quinapril, ramipril, semaglutide, sermorelin, sotalol, trandolapril, vidarabine, zofenopril
Important contra-indications noted in the prescribing guidelines for: nursing mothers; pediatric patients
Note: About 25% of patients with insulin allergy have a concomitant history of penicillin allergy. Various forms of insulin are available - see other insulin profiles for reaction details.

Skin
Acanthosis nigricans [3]
Anaphylactoid reactions / anaphylaxis (includes anaphylactic shock) (<10%) [10]
Angioedema (formerly named angioneurotic edema) [6]
Dermatitis [2]
Diaphoresis (<10%)
Edema / fluid retention (<10%) [4]
Hyperkeratosis [3]
Hypersensitivity [5]
Lipoatrophy (<10%) [29]
Lipodystrophy / acquired generalized lipodystrophy [26]
Lipohypertrophy (<10%) [11]
Pallor (<10%)
Peripheral edema [4]
Pruritus (itching) (<10%) [4]
Purpura [2]
Urticaria / hives (<10%) [17]
Vasculitis (angiitis) / cutaneous vasculitis (angiitis) [2]

Central Nervous System
Headache [2]
Paresthesias (<10%)
Tremor (<10%)

Endocrine/Metabolic
Amyloidosis (localized) [2]
Hypoglycemia [8]
Weight gain [6]

Gastrointestinal/Hepatic
Nausea [2]
Vomiting [2]

Local
Injection-site induration [4]
Injection-site pruritus [2]
Injection-site reaction [3]

Respiratory
Cough [2]
Nasopharyngitis [2]

Other
Adverse effects / adverse reactions [2]
Allergic reactions (local) [14]

INSULIN ASPART

Trade names: NovoLog (Novo Nordisk), NovoRapid (Novo Nordisk), Ryzodeg (Novo Nordisk)
Indications: Diabetes mellitus
Class: Hormone, polypeptide
Half-life: 81 minutes
Clinically important, potentially hazardous interactions with: ACE inhibitors, alcohol, atypical antipsychotics, beta blockers, clonidine, corticosteroids, danazol, disopyramide, diuretics, epinephrine, estrogens, fibrates, fluoxetine, isoniazid, isoniazid, lithium salts, MAO inhibitors, niacin, octreotide, oral contraceptives, pentamidine, phenothiazine derivatives, pramlintide, propoxyphene, salbutamol, salicylates, somatropin, sulfonamide antibiotics, terbutaline, thyroid hormones
Important contra-indications noted in the prescribing guidelines for: the elderly; pediatric patients
Note: Ryzodeg is insulin aspart and insulin degludec; various forms of insulin are available - see other insulin profiles for reaction details.

Skin
Lipodystrophy / acquired generalized lipodystrophy (>5%)
Peripheral edema (>5%)

Nails
Onychomycosis (10%)

Cardiovascular
Chest pain (5%)

Central Nervous System
Headache (12%) [3]
Hyporeflexia (11%)

Endocrine/Metabolic
Diabetic ketoacidosis [2]
Hypoglycemia (75%) [6]
Weight gain (>5%)

Gastrointestinal/Hepatic
Abdominal pain (5%)
Diarrhea (5%)
Nausea (7%)

Genitourinary
Urinary tract infection (8%)

Respiratory
Nasopharyngitis [3]
Sinusitis (see also rhinitis / rhinosinusitis) (5%)

INSULIN DEGLUDEC

Trade names: Ryzodeg (Novo Nordisk), Tresiba (Novo Nordisk), Xultophy (Novo Nordisk)
Indications: Diabetes mellitus
Class: Human insulin analog, long-acting
Half-life: 25 hours
Clinically important, potentially hazardous interactions with: ACE inhibitors, albuterol, alcohol, angiotensin II receptor blocking agents, beta blockers, clonidine, clozapine, corticosteroids, danazol, DDP-4-inhibitors, disopyramide, diuretics, epinephrine, estrogens, fibrates, fluoxetine, GLP-1 receptor agonists, glucagon, guanethidine, isoniazid, lithium, MAO inhibitors, niacin, octreotide, olanzapine, oral contraceptives, pentamidine, pentoxifylline, phenothiazines, pramlintide, propoxyphene, protease inhibitors, reserpine, salicylates, SGLT-2 inhibitors, somatropin, sulfonamide antibiotics, terbutaline, thyroid hormones
Important contra-indications noted in the prescribing guidelines for: the elderly; nursing mothers; pediatric patients
Note: Contra-indicated during episodes of hypoglycemia. Ryzodeg is insulin degludec and insulin aspart; Xultophy is insulin degludec and liraglutide; various forms of insulin are available - see other insulin profiles for reaction details.

Skin
Hypersensitivity [2]
Peripheral edema (<3%)

Central Nervous System
Headache (9–12%) [11]

Endocrine/Metabolic
Diabetic ketoacidosis [2]
Hypoglycemia [10]

Gastrointestinal/Hepatic
Diarrhea (6%) [6]
Gastroenteritis (5%)
Nausea [7]
Vomiting [2]

Local
Injection-site reaction (4%) [6]

Ocular
Retinopathy [2]

Respiratory
Nasopharyngitis (13–24%) [12]
Sinusitis (see also rhinitis / rhinosinusitis) (5%)
Upper respiratory tract infection (8–12%) [3]

Other
Adverse effects / adverse reactions [4]

INSULIN DETEMIR

Trade name: Levemir (Novo Nordisk)
Indications: Diabetes (Type I or II)
Class: Human insulin analog, long-acting
Half-life: 5–7 hours
Clinically important, potentially hazardous interactions with: albuterol, alcohol, antipsychotics, beta blockers, clonidine, clozapine, corticosteroids, danazol, diuretics, epinephrine, estrogens, guanethidine, isoniazid, lithium, niacin, olanzapine, oral antidiabetics, oral contraceptives, pentamidine, phenothiazines, propranolol, protease inhibitors, reserpine, somatropin, terbutaline, thiazolidinediones, thyroid hormones
Important contra-indications noted in the prescribing guidelines for: the elderly; nursing mothers; pediatric patients
Note: Various forms of insulin are available - see other insulin profiles for reaction details.

Central Nervous System
Fever (pyrexia) (includes hyperpyrexia) (10%)
Headache (7–31%) [3]

Endocrine/Metabolic
Hyperglycemia (includes glucose increased) [2]
Hypoglycemia [4]

Gastrointestinal/Hepatic
Abdominal pain (6–13%)
Gastroenteritis (6–17%)
Nausea (7%)
Vomiting (7%)

Local
Injection-site reaction (3–4%) [4]

Neuromuscular/Skeletal
Back pain (8%)

Respiratory
Bronchitis (5%)
Cough (8%)
Influenza- ('flu)-like syndrome (6–14%)
Pharyngitis (sore throat) (10–17%)
Rhinitis / rhinosinusitis (see also sinusitis) (7%)
Upper respiratory tract infection (13–36%)

Other
Allergic reactions [3]
Infection (viral) (7%)

INSULIN GLARGINE

Trade names: Basaglar (Lilly), Lantus (Sanofi-Aventis), Soliqua (Sanofi-Aventis)
Indications: Diabetes (Type I or II)
Class: Hormone analog, polypeptide
Half-life: N/A
Clinically important, potentially hazardous interactions with: ACE inhibitors, albuterol, alcohol, beta blockers, clonidine, clozapine, corticosteroids, danazol, disopyramide, diuretics, epinephrine, estrogens, fibrates, fluoxetine, glucagon, guanethidine, isoniazid, lithium, MAO inhibitors, niacin, olanzapine, oral antidiabetic products, oral contraceptives, pentamidine, pentoxifylline, phenothiazine derivatives, pramlintide, propoxyphene, propranolol, protease inhibitors, reserpine, salicylates, somatostain analogs, somatropin, sulfonamide antibiotics, terbutaline, thyroid hormones
Important contra-indications noted in the prescribing guidelines for: nursing mothers; pediatric patients
Note: Soliqua is insulin glargine and lixisenatide; various forms of insulin are available - see other insulin profiles for reaction details. insulin glargine-yfgn (Semglee) is biosimilar. Approved 07/28/2021 Insulin glargine-aglr (Rezvoglar) is biosimilar. Approved 12/17/2021.

Skin
Lipoatrophy [2]
Peripheral edema (20%)

Central Nervous System
Depression (11%)
Headache (6–10%) [4]

Endocrine/Metabolic
Diabetic ketoacidosis [2]
Hypoglycemia [7]

Gastrointestinal/Hepatic
Diarrhea (11%) [6]
Nausea [5]
Vomiting [4]

Genitourinary
Urinary tract infection (11%)

Local
Injection-site pain (3%)
Injection-site reaction [4]

Neuromuscular/Skeletal
Arthralgia (14%)
Back pain (13%)
Pain in extremities (13%)

Ocular
Cataract (18%)
Retinopathy [2]

Respiratory
Bronchitis (15%)
Cough (12%)
Influenza (19%)
Nasopharyngitis [6]
Pharyngitis (sore throat) (8%)
Rhinitis / rhinosinusitis (see also sinusitis) (5%)
Sinusitis (see also rhinitis / rhinosinusitis) (19%)
Upper respiratory tract infection (11–29%) [3]

Other
Adverse effects / adverse reactions [6]
Infection (9–14%)

INSULIN GLULISINE

Trade name: Apidra (Sanofi-Aventis)
Indications: Diabetes
Class: Insulin analog
Half-life: 13–42 minutes
Clinically important, potentially hazardous interactions with: ACE inhibitors, albuterol, alcohol, anitpsychotics, beta blockers, clonidine, clozapine, corticosteroids, danazol, disopyramide, diuretics, epinephrine, fibrates, fluoxetine, glucagon, guanethidine, isoniazid, lithium, MAO inhibitors, niacin, oral antidiabetic agents, oral contraceptives, pentamidine, pentoxifylline, phenothiazine derivatives, pramlintide, propoxyphene, propranolol, protease inhibitors, reserpine, salicylates, somatostatin analogs, somatropin, sulfonamide antibiotics, terbutaline, thyroid hormones
Important contra-indications noted in the prescribing guidelines for: nursing mothers; pediatric patients
Note: Various forms of insulin are available - see other insulin profiles for reaction details.

Skin
Peripheral edema (8%)

Cardiovascular
Hypertension (4%)

Central Nervous System
Headache (7%)

Endocrine/Metabolic
Hypoglycemia (6–7%) [3]

Local
Injection-site reaction (10%) [2]

Neuromuscular/Skeletal
Arthralgia (6%)

Respiratory
Influenza (4–6%)
Nasopharyngitis (8–11%)
Upper respiratory tract infection (7–11%)

INTERFERON ALFA

Synonyms: IFN; INF
Trade names: Infergen (Intermune), Intron A (Schering), Rebetron (Schering), Roferon-A (Roche)
Indications: Chronic hepatitis C virus infection, hairy cell leukemia
Class: Biologic, Immunomodulator, Interferon
Half-life: 2 hours
Clinically important, potentially hazardous interactions with: aldesleukin, amitriptyline, captopril, gemfibrozil, metaxalone, methadone, ribavirin, telbivudine, theophylline, theophylline derivatives, zafirlukast, zidovudine
Pregnancy category: pregnancy category will be X when used in combination with ribavirin
Important contra-indications noted in the prescribing guidelines for: nursing mothers; pediatric patients
Note: Many of the adverse reactions depend on the nature of the disease being treated. Either hairy cell leukemia [L] or AIDS-related Kaposi's sarcoma [K].

Skin
Angioedema (formerly named angioneurotic edema) [3]
Bullous dermatosis [4]
Cutaneous toxicity / skin toxicity [4]
Dermatitis (6%)
Eczema / eczematous reaction / eczematous eruption [6]
Edema / fluid retention [L] (11%) [2]
Erythema [2]
Exanthems [3]
Herpes simplex [2]
Kaposi's sarcoma [2]
Lichen planus (includes hypertrophic lichen planus) [9]
Linear IgA bullous dermatosis [3]
Livedo reticularis / livedo racemosa [2]
Lupus erythematosus (subacute cutaneous lupus erythematosus (SCLE)) [18]
Lupus syndrome / drug-induced lupus (DIL) [2]
Necrosis (skin necrosis) [6]
Pemphigus [2]
Photosensitivity [2]

Pigmentation (Skin) (includes hyperpigmentation) [3]
Pruritus (itching) 13% [L] 5–7% [K] (13%) [4]
Psoriasis [24]
Purpura [2]
Rash 44% [L] 11% [K] [5]
Raynaud's phenomenon [11]
Sarcoidosis / sarcoid-like reaction (cutaneous sarcoidosis) [47]
Seborrheic dermatitis [2]
Thrombocytopenic purpura [2]
Urticaria / hives [K] (<3%) [3]
Vasculitis (angiitis) / cutaneous vasculitis (angiitis) [7]
Vitiligo [9]

Hair
Alopecia / hair loss (23%) [16]
Hair pigmentation [3]
Hypertrichosis [3]
Straight hair [2]

Mucosal
Aphthous stomatitis / aphthous ulcer / aphtha (aphthae) [2]
Oral lichen planus [7]
Sjögren's syndrome (see also sicca syndrome) [4]
Stomatitis (oral mucositis) (<10%)
Xerostomia (dry mouth) (>10%) [4]

Cardiovascular
Cardiotoxicity [2]
Hypertension [3]
Hypotension [2]

Central Nervous System
Ageusia (taste loss) / taste disorder [2]
Anorexia [5]
Anosmia (smell loss) / smell disorder [4]
Anxiety [3]
Chills [4]
Depression (5–15%) [25]
Dysgeusia (taste perversion) [K] (25%) [2]
Fever (pyrexia) (includes hyperpyrexia) (37%) [7]
Headache (54%) [6]
Impaired concentration [2]
Insomnia (19%)
Irritability [3]
Neurotoxicity [4]
Paresthesias 8% [L] (12%)
Parkinsonism [3]
Restless legs syndrome / Willis-Ekbom disease (includes restless arms syndrome variant) [2]
Rigors (35%)
Seizures [2]
Suicidal ideation [6]
Tremor [2]
Vertigo / dizziness (16%) [2]

Endocrine/Metabolic
ALT increased [2]
AST increased [2]
Hyperglycemia (includes glucose increased) [2]
Hyperthyroidism (includes 'thyroid storm') [3]
Thyroid dysfunction [5]
Thyroiditis [3]
Weight loss (16%) [5]

Gastrointestinal/Hepatic
Abdominal pain (15%)
Constipation [2]
Crohn's disease [2]
Diarrhea (24%) [6]
Hepatotoxicity / liver injury / acute liver injury / drug-induced liver injury (DILI) [2]
Nausea (24%) [8]
Pancreatitis / acute pancreatitis [7]
Vomiting [5]

Genitourinary
Impotence [2]

Hematologic
Anemia (11%) [8]
Febrile neutropenia [2]
Hemolytic uremic syndrome [6]
Leukocytopenia (leukopenia) / leukocytes (white blood cells) decreased [6]
Lymphopenia (lymphocytopenia) / lymphocytes decreased (14%)
Neutropenia (neutrophils decreased) (21%) [5]
Thrombocytopenia / platelets decreased [8]

Local
Injection-site alopecia [2]
Injection-site erythema [2]
Injection-site induration [3]
Injection-site necrosis [16]

Neuromuscular/Skeletal
Arthralgia (28%) [4]
Asthenia / fatigue (56%) [11]
Back pain (9%)
Myalgia/Myopathy 69% [L] 71% [K] [11]
Myasthenia gravis [11]
Rhabdomyolysis [3]

Ocular
Eyelashes – hypertrichosis (eyelash megalotrichosis) [3]
Optic neuropathy [4]
Retinopathy [6]
Vision blurred (4%)

Otic
Tinnitus [4]

Renal
Nephrotoxicity / kidney injury / acute kidney injury (AKI) / drug-induced kidney injury [3]
Proteinuria [2]

Respiratory
Cough [2]
Dyspnea / shortness of breath (13%) [2]
Influenza- ('flu)-like syndrome (>10%) [11]
Pulmonary hypertension [3]

Other
Adverse effects / adverse reactions [6]
Infection [4]
Vogt-Koyanagi-Harada syndrome [6]

INTERFERON BETA

Trade names: Avonex (Biogen), Betaferon (Bayer), Betaseron (Bayer), Plegridy (Biogen), Rebif (Merck)
Indications: Relapsing multiple sclerosis, cancers
Class: Covid-19 putative drug, Immunomodulator, Interferon
Half-life: 10 hours
Clinically important, potentially hazardous interactions with: theophylline, theophylline derivatives, zidovudine
Important contra-indications noted in the prescribing guidelines for: nursing mothers; pediatric patients

---

Skin
Cyst / pseudocyst (4%)
Diaphoresis (23%)
Edema / fluid retention (generalized) (8%)
Herpes simplex (2–3%)
Herpes zoster (3)
Hypersensitivity (3%)
Lipoatrophy [2]
Lupus erythematosus (subacute cutaneous lupus erythematosus (SCLE)) [8]
Nevi (naevi) (3%)
Nicolau syndrome [2]
Psoriasis [2]
Rash [2]
Raynaud's phenomenon [2]
Sarcoidosis / sarcoid-like reaction (cutaneous sarcoidosis) [2]
Thrombocytopenic purpura [4]
Urticaria / hives (5%)
Vasculitis (angiitis) / cutaneous vasculitis (angiitis) [4]

Hair
Alopecia / hair loss (4%)

Mucosal
Mucosal bleeding (12–38%)

Cardiovascular
Capillary leak syndrome [3]

Central Nervous System
Chills (21%)
Depression [8]
Fever (pyrexia) (includes hyperpyrexia) [4]
Headache [5]
Multiple sclerosis [2]
Pain (52%)
Paresthesias [2]
Psychosis [2]
Seizures (2%) [2]
Vertigo / dizziness (35%)

Endocrine/Metabolic
Mastodynia (7%)
Thyroid dysfunction [4]

Gastrointestinal/Hepatic
Hepatotoxicity / liver injury / acute liver injury / drug-induced liver injury (DILI) [6]

Genitourinary
Vaginitis (includes vulvitis) (4%)

Hematologic
Hemolytic uremic syndrome [3]
Thrombocytopenia / platelets decreased [2]
Thrombotic microangiopathy [4]

Local
Injection-site ecchymoses (2%)
Injection-site erythema [2]
Injection-site inflammation (3%)
Injection-site necrosis [3]
Injection-site purpura (2%)
Injection-site reaction (4%) [10]

Neuromuscular/Skeletal
Arthralgia [2]
Asthenia / fatigue [3]
Myalgia/Myopathy (44%)
Rhabdomyolysis [2]

Ocular
Retinopathy [3]

Renal
Nephrotoxicity / kidney injury / acute kidney injury (AKI) / drug-induced kidney injury [2]

Respiratory
Influenza- ('flu)-like syndrome (61%) [15]
Upper respiratory tract infection (31%)

Other
Adverse effects / adverse reactions [4]
Death [4]
Infection (11%) [3]

INTERFERON GAMMA

Trade name: Actimmune (Horizon)
Indications: Chronic granulomatous disease, severe malignant osteopetrosis
Class: Immunomodulator, Interferon
Half-life: 6 hours
Clinically important, potentially hazardous interactions with: tasonermin, typhoid vaccine
Pregnancy category: May cause fetal toxicity based on findings in animal studies
Important contra-indications noted in the prescribing guidelines for: nursing mothers; pediatric patients

---

Skin
Rash (17%)

Central Nervous System
Chills (14%) [3]
Fever (pyrexia) (includes hyperpyrexia) (52%) [8]
Headache (33%) [3]

Gastrointestinal/Hepatic
Diarrhea (14%)
Nausea (10%)
Vomiting (13%)

Hematologic
Lymphopenia (lymphocytopenia) / lymphocytes decreased [2]

Local
Injection-site erythema (14%) [2]

Neuromuscular/Skeletal
Arthralgia (2%)
Asthenia / fatigue (14%) [3]
Myalgia/Myopathy (6%)

Respiratory
Influenza- ('flu)-like syndrome [4]

IOBENGUANE

Synonyms: metaiodobenzylguanidine; MIBG
Trade name: AdreView (GE Healthcare)
Indications: Detection of primary or metastatic pheochromocytoma or neuroblastoma as an adjunct to other diagnostic tests
Class: Radiopharmaceutical, diagnostic agent
Half-life: 13 hours
Clinically important, potentially hazardous interactions with: amitriptyline, amoxapine, citalopram, cocaine, duloxetine, ephedrine, formoterol, formoterol, imipramine, labetalol, levalbuterol, lisdexamfetamine, phenylephrine, phenylpropanolamine, pseudoephedrine, reserpine, salmeterol, SSRIs, terbutaline
Important contra-indications noted in the prescribing guidelines for: nursing mothers; pediatric patients

---

Skin
Flushing / rubefaction (<2%)
Pruritus (itching) (<2%)
Rash (<2%)

Cardiovascular
Hypertension [3]

Central Nervous System
Vertigo / dizziness (<2%)

Local
Injection-site hemorrhage (<2%)

IODIXANOL

Trade name: Visipaque (Amersham Health)
Indications: Angiocardiography
Class: Contrast agent, Iodine-containing radiocontrast medium
Half-life: 2 hours
Clinically important, potentially hazardous interactions with: none known

---

Skin
AGEP [2]
Anaphylactoid reactions / anaphylaxis (includes anaphylactic shock) [2]
Erythema (2%)
Pruritus (itching) (<2%)
Rash (2%)

Central Nervous System
Dysgeusia (taste perversion) (4%)
Encephalopathy (includes hepatic encephalopathy) [2]
Headache [2]
Vertigo / dizziness (2%)

Renal
Nephrotoxicity / kidney injury / acute kidney injury (AKI) / drug-induced kidney injury [3]

IODOQUINOL

Synonym: diiodohydroxyquin
Indications: Acute and chronic intestinal amebiasis, blastocystis hominis infections
Class: Amebicide
Half-life: N/A
Clinically important, potentially hazardous interactions with: none known
Note: Ineffective for amebic hepatitis or hepatic abscess.

Central Nervous System
Peripheral neuropathy [2]

Ocular
Blindness [4]
Optic atrophy [3]

IOHEXOL

Trade name: Omnipaque (GE Healthcare)
Indications: Diagnostic aid in myelography, angiography and computerized tomography procedures
Class: Contrast agent, Iodine-containing radiocontrast medium
Half-life: variable
Clinically important, potentially hazardous interactions with: corticosteroids

---

Skin
Pruritus (itching) [2]

Mucosal
Sialadenitis [2]

Central Nervous System
Dysgeusia (taste perversion) [2]
Encephalopathy (includes hepatic encephalopathy) [5]
Headache (18%) [7]

Neuromuscular/Skeletal
Myalgia/Myopathy (8%)

Ocular
Photophobia (2%)
Vision blurred (2%)

Renal
Nephrotoxicity / kidney injury / acute kidney injury (AKI) / drug-induced kidney injury [3]

Other
Death [2]

IOMEPROL

Trade name: Iomeron (Bracco)
Indications: X-ray contrast medium
Class: Contrast agent
Half-life: 0.5–1.9 hours
Clinically important, potentially hazardous interactions with: corticosteroids, vasopressors
Important contra-indications noted in the prescribing guidelines for: nursing mothers

---

Skin
AGEP [2]

Central Nervous System
Headache (<10%)

Gastrointestinal/Hepatic
Nausea (<10%) [4]
Vomiting [2]

Hematologic
Hemolytic anemia [4]

Local
Injection-site pain (<10%)

IPILIMUMAB

Trade name: Yervoy (Bristol-Myers Squibb)
Indications: Melanoma
Class: Antineoplastic / anticancer agent (see also Immune checkpoint inhibitor), Biologic, CTLA-4-blocking monoclonal antibody, Immune checkpoint inhibitor (incl. programmed death receptor-1 (PD-1) inhibitor), Monoclonal antibody
Half-life: 15 days
Clinically important, potentially hazardous interactions with: none known
Important contra-indications noted in the prescribing guidelines for: nursing mothers; pediatric patients
Warning: IMMUNE-MEDIATED ADVERSE REACTIONS

Skin
Cutaneous toxicity / skin toxicity [4]
Dermatitis (12%) [14]
Dermatomyositis [4]
DRESS syndrome (Drug-induced hypersensitivity syndrome) [3]
Erythema [6]
Erythema multiforme [2]
Exanthems [6]
Granulomas [5]
Lupus erythematosus (subacute cutaneous lupus erythematosus (SCLE)) [2]
Lymphadenopathy [3]
Pruritus (itching) (21–31%) [24]
Psoriasis [2]
Rash (19–29%) [34]
Sarcoidosis / sarcoid-like reaction (cutaneous sarcoidosis) [7]
Stevens-Johnson syndrome and toxic epidermal necrolysis (SJS/TEN) [5]
Sweet's syndrome [3]
Thrombotic thrombocytopenic purpura [3]

Transient acantholytic dermatosis (Grover's disease) [3]
Urticaria / hives (2%) [3]
Vasculitis (angiitis) / cutaneous vasculitis (angiitis) [4]
Vitiligo [4]

Hair
Alopecia / hair loss [3]

Cardiovascular
Atrial fibrillation [2]
Cardiomyopathy [2]
Cardiotoxicity [3]
Large-vessel vasculitis (includes giant cell arteritis) [3]
Myocarditis [10]
Myocarditis, myositis and myasthenia gravis overlap syndrome (Triple-M Syndrome / 3M Syndrome) [5]
Pericarditis [4]

Central Nervous System
Anorexia [3]
Aseptic meningitis [2]
Chills [2]
Encephalitis [9]
Encephalopathy (includes hepatic encephalopathy) [5]
Fever (pyrexia) (includes hyperpyrexia) [4]
Guillain-Barré syndrome / acute inflammatory demyelinating polyradiculoneuropathy / acute motor axonal neuropathy [10]
Headache (14%) [4]
Leukoencephalopathy / posterior reversible encephalopathy syndrome (PRES) [2]
Meningoencephalitis [4]
Neurotoxicity [6]

Endocrine/Metabolic
Adrenal insufficiency (hypoadrenalism) / Addisonian crisis (includes Addison's disease) [7]
ALT increased [14]
AST increased [12]
Autosplenectomy [2]
Diabetes mellitus [8]
Diabetic ketoacidosis [5]
Hyperamylasemia [4]
Hyperlipasemia [5]
Hyperthyroidism (includes 'thyroid storm') [5]
Hyponatremia [3]
Hypophysitis [54]
Hypopituitarism (<4%)
Hypothyroidism [16]
Thyroid dysfunction [5]
Thyroiditis [17]
Thyrotoxicosis [3]
Weight loss [2]

Gastrointestinal/Hepatic
Abdominal pain [3]
Colitis (5–8%) [69]
Constipation [2]
Diarrhea (32–37%) [56]
Enterocolitis (7%) [9]
Gastritis / pangastritis / gastric irritation [3]
Gastrointestinal perforation / perforated colon / gastric perforation [5]
Hepatitis [22]
Hepatotoxicity / liver injury / acute liver injury / drug-induced liver injury (DILI) (<2%) [22]
Ileus / adynamic ileus / paralytic ileus [2]
Nausea [6]
Pancreatitis / acute pancreatitis [6]
Vomiting [2]

Genitourinary
Cystitis (includes interstitial cystitis / bladder pain syndrome) [2]

Hematologic
Anemia [4]
Aplastic anemia [2]
Coagulopathy / coagulation dysfunction / clotting factor deficiency (includes disseminated intravascular coagulation / DIC) [2]
Eosinophilia / eosinophils increased [4]
Hemolytic anemia [2]
Hemophagocytic lymphohistiocytosis / hemophagocytic syndrome [3]
Neutropenia (neutrophils decreased) [7]
Pure red cell aplasia [2]
Thrombocytopenia / platelets decreased [6]

Local
Infusion-related reactions [4]
Injection-site reaction [2]

Neuromuscular/Skeletal
Arthralgia [5]
Asthenia / fatigue (34–41%) [14]
Myalgia/Myopathy [8]
Myasthenia gravis [8]
Polymyalgia rheumatica [4]
Rhabdomyolysis [2]

Ocular
Iridocyclitis [3]
Ocular adverse effect [3]
Optic neuropathy [2]
Orbital (ocular) myositis [2]
Orbital inflammation [6]
Retinitis [2]
Uveitis / anterior uveitis / posterior uveitis / panuveitis [10]
Xerophthalmia (dry eyes) [2]

Renal
Nephritis / interstitial nephritis / tubulointerstitial nephritis [3]
Nephrotoxicity / kidney injury / acute kidney injury (AKI) / drug-induced kidney injury [9]
Renal failure [4]
Tumor lysis syndrome (TLS) [2]

Respiratory
Cough [2]
Dyspnea / shortness of breath [3]
Pneumonia [5]
Pneumonitis [11]

Other
Adverse effects / adverse reactions [32]
Cytokine release syndrome / cytokine storm [3]
Death [20]
Vogt-Koyanagi-Harada syndrome [5]

IPRATROPIUM

Trade names: Atrovent (Boehringer Ingelheim), Combivent (Boehringer Ingelheim), Duoneb (Mylan Specialty), Ipratropium Steri-Neb (Ivax), Rinatec (Boehringer Ingelheim)
Indications: Bronchospasm
Class: Anticholinergic, Muscarinic antagonist
Half-life: 2 hours
Clinically important, potentially hazardous interactions with: anticholinergics
Important contra-indications noted in the prescribing guidelines for: nursing mothers
Note: Combivent is ipratropium and albuterol.

Mucosal
Oral lesions (<5%)
Oral ulceration [2]
Xerostomia (dry mouth) (3%) [3]

Central Nervous System
Dysgeusia (taste perversion) [2]
Trembling (<10%)

Ocular
Mydriasis [2]

Other
Adverse effects / adverse reactions [2]

IRBESARTAN

Trade names: Aprovel (Bristol-Myers Squibb), Avalide (Bristol-Myers Squibb), Avapro (Sanofi-Aventis)
Indications: Hypertension, diabetic nephropathy
Class: Angiotensin receptor antagonist (blocker), Antihypertensive
Half-life: 11–15 hours
Clinically important, potentially hazardous interactions with: ACE inhibitors, adrenergic neurone blockers, alcohol, aldesleukin, aldosterone antagonists, aliskiren, alpha blockers, alprostadil, amifostine, antihypertensives, antipsychotics, anxiolytics and hypnotics, baclofen, beta blockers, calcium channel blockers, carvedilol, clonidine, corticosteroids, cyclosporine, CYP2C8 and CYP2C9 substrates, diazoxide, diuretics, eplerenone, fluconazole, general anesthetics, heparins, hypotensives, levodopa, lithium, MAO inhibitors, methyldopa, methylphenidate, moxisylyte, moxonidine, nitrates, NSAIDs, pentoxifylline, phosphodiesterase 5 inhibitors, potassium salts, prostacyclin analogues, rifamycin derivatives, rituximab, tacrolimus, tizanidine, tolvaptan, trimethoprim
Pregnancy category: category C in first trimester; category D in second and third trimesters
Important contra-indications noted in the prescribing guidelines for: nursing mothers; pediatric patients
Note: Avalide is irbesartan and hydrochlorothiazide. Hydrochlorothiazide is a sulfonamide which can be absorbed systemically. Sulfonamides can produce severe, possibly fatal, reactions such as toxic epidermal necrolysis and Stevens-Johnson syndrome.
Warning: FETAL TOXICITY

Skin
Angioedema (formerly named angioneurotic edema) [3]
Edema / fluid retention (<10%)
Peripheral edema [2]
Rash (<10%)

Gastrointestinal/Hepatic
Pancreatitis / acute pancreatitis [2]

Respiratory
Cough [2]

IRINOTECAN

Trade names: Camptosar (Pfizer), Onivyde (Merrimack)
Indications: Metastatic colorectal carcinoma (Camptosar), metastatic adenocarcinoma of the pancreas (Onivyde - in combination with fluorouracil and leucovorin). Advanced pancreatic cancer in combination with oxaliplatin/ fluorouracil/leucovorin (FOLFIRINOX or FOLFOXIRI). Used in combination with fluorouracil and leucovorin (FOLFIRI) for treatment of advanced-stage and metastatic colorectal cancer
Class: Antineoplastic / anticancer agent (see also Immune checkpoint inhibitor), Topoisomerase I inhibitor
Half-life: 6–10 hours
Clinically important, potentially hazardous interactions with: aprepitant, atazanavir, bevacizumab, itraconazole, ketoconazole, lapatinib, safinamide, sorafenib, St John's wort, strong CYP3A4 inhibitors, voriconazole
Important contra-indications noted in the prescribing guidelines for: the elderly; nursing mothers; pediatric patients
Warning: DIARRHEA and MYELOSUPPRESSION (Camptosar). SEVERE NEUTROPENIA and SEVERE DIARRHEA (Onivyde)

Skin
- Acneiform eruption / acneiform dermatitis / acneiform rash [4]
- Cutaneous toxicity / skin toxicity [4]
- Exfoliative dermatitis (14%)
- Flushing / rubefaction (11%)
- Hand–foot syndrome (palmar–plantar erythrodysesthesia) [6]
- Pruritus (itching) [4]
- Rash (46%) [7]

Hair
- Alopecia / hair loss (13–61%) [25]

Mucosal
- Mucositis (30%) [4]
- Stomatitis (oral mucositis) (<14%) [6]

Cardiovascular
- Bradycardia / sinus bradycardia [2]
- Hypertension [11]
- Hypotension (5%) [2]
- Thrombophlebitis (<10%)
- Vasodilation (6%)

Central Nervous System
- Anorexia (44%) [19]
- Chills (14%)
- Confusion (3%)
- Dysarthria [12]
- Fever (pyrexia) (includes hyperpyrexia) (44%) [3]
- Insomnia [2]
- Myokymia / twitching / fasciculation [2]
- Neurotoxicity [5]
- Pain (23%)
- Somnolence (drowsiness) (9%)
- Vertigo / dizziness (21%)

Endocrine/Metabolic
- Dehydration [4]

Gastrointestinal/Hepatic
- Abdominal pain (68%) [4]
- Constipation (32%) [3]
- Diarrhea (83%) [55]
- Gastrointestinal perforation / perforated colon / gastric perforation [2]
- Hepatotoxicity / liver injury / acute liver injury / drug-induced liver injury (DILI) [4]
- Nausea (82%) [25]
- Vomiting (63%) [22]

Hematologic
- Anemia (97%) [22]
- Febrile neutropenia [17]
- Leukocytopenia (leukopenia) / leukocytes (white blood cells) decreased (96%) [15]
- Lymphopenia (lymphocytopenia) / lymphocytes decreased [2]
- Neutropenia (neutrophils decreased) (96%) [57]
- Thrombocytopenia / platelets decreased (96%) [12]

Neuromuscular/Skeletal
- Asthenia / fatigue (69%) [25]

Renal
- Proteinuria [5]

Respiratory
- Cough (20%)
- Dyspnea / shortness of breath (22%)
- Pneumonia (4%) [5]

Other
- Adverse effects / adverse reactions [4]
- Allergic reactions (9%)
- Death [7]
- Infection (14%) [4]

ISAVUCONAZONIUM SULFATE

Synonym: Isavuconazole
Trade name: Cresemba (Astellas)
Indications: Invasive aspergillosis, mucormycosis
Class: Antifungal / antimycotic, Antifungal; triazole, Antimicrobial
Half-life: 130 hours
Clinically important, potentially hazardous interactions with: carbamazepine, ketoconazole, rifampin, ritonavir, St John's wort, strong CYP3A4 inducers or inhibitors
Important contra-indications noted in the prescribing guidelines for: nursing mothers; pediatric patients
Note: Isavuconazonium sulfate is the water-soluble prodrug of isavuconazole. Contra-indicated in patients with familial short QT syndrome.

Skin
- Dermatitis (<5%)
- Erythema (<5%)
- Exfoliative dermatitis (<5%)
- Hypersensitivity (<5%)
- Peripheral edema (15%)
- Petechiae (<5%)
- Pruritus (itching) (8%)
- Rash (9%)
- Urticaria / hives (<5%)

Hair
- Alopecia / hair loss (<5%)

Mucosal
- Gingivitis (<5%)
- Stomatitis (oral mucositis) (<5%)

Cardiovascular
- Atrial fibrillation (<5%)
- Atrial flutter (<5%)
- Bradycardia / sinus bradycardia (<5%)
- Cardiac arrest (<5%)
- Chest pain (9%)
- Extrasystoles (<5%)
- Hypotension (8%) [2]
- Palpitation (<5%)
- QT interval shortening (<5%)
- Thrombophlebitis (<5%)

Central Nervous System
- Anxiety (8%)
- Chills (<5%)
- Confusion (<5%)
- Delirium (9%)
- Depression (<5%)
- Dysgeusia (taste perversion) (<5%)
- Encephalopathy (includes hepatic encephalopathy) (<5%)
- Gait instability / postural instability (<5%)
- Hallucinations (<5%)
- Headache (17%)
- Hypoesthesia / hypesthesia (numbness) (<5%)
- Insomnia (11%)
- Migraine (<5%)
- Paresthesias (<5%)
- Peripheral neuropathy (<5%)
- Seizures (<5%)
- Somnolence (drowsiness) (<5%)
- Stupor (<5%)
- Syncope / fainting (<5%)
- Tremor (<5%)
- Vertigo / dizziness (<5%)

Endocrine/Metabolic
- Appetite decreased (9%)
- Hypoalbuminemia / albumin decreased (<5%)
- Hypoglycemia (<5%)
- Hypokalemia (19%)
- Hypomagnesemia (5%)
- Hyponatremia (<5%)

Gastrointestinal/Hepatic
- Abdominal distension (<5%)
- Abdominal pain (17%)
- Cholecystitis (calculous / acalculous) (<5%)
- Cholelithiasis (gallstones in the gall bladder or the bile duct) (<5%)
- Constipation (14%)
- Diarrhea (24%) [3]
- Dyspepsia / functional dyspepsia (indigestion) (see also gastroparesis) (6%)
- Gastritis / pangastritis / gastric irritation (<5%)
- Hepatic failure (<5%)
- Hepatomegaly (<5%)
- Hepatotoxicity / liver injury / acute liver injury / drug-induced liver injury (DILI) (17%) [2]
- Nausea (28%) [4]
- Vomiting (25%)

Genitourinary
- Hematuria (<5%)

Hematologic
- Agranulocytosis / severe selective neutropenia (<5%)
- Leukocytopenia (leukopenia) / leukocytes (white blood cells) decreased (<5%)
- Pancytopenia (includes bicytopenia) (<5%)

Local
- Injection-site reaction (6%)

Neuromuscular/Skeletal
- Asthenia / fatigue (11%)
- Back pain (10%)
- Bone pain / joint pain (<5%)
- Myalgia/Myopathy (<5%)

Neck pain (<5%)

Ocular
Optic neuropathy (<5%)

Otic
Tinnitus (<5%)

Renal
Proteinuria (<5%)
Renal failure (10%)

Respiratory
Bronchospasm (<5%)
Dyspnea / shortness of breath (17%)
Respiratory failure (7%)
Tachypnea / respiratory rate increased (<5%)

Other
Adverse effects / adverse reactions [3]

ISOCARBOXAZID

Trade name: Marplan (Validus)
Indications: Depression
Class: Antidepressant, Monoamine oxidase (MAO) inhibitor
Half-life: N/A
Clinically important, potentially hazardous interactions with: amitriptyline, amoxapine, bupropion, citalopram, clomipramine, desipramine, doxepin, fluoxetine, fluvoxamine, imipramine, meperidine, nefazodone, nortriptyline, opicapone, paroxetine hydrochloride, pizotifen, protriptyline, rizatriptan, sertraline, sibutramine, sumatriptan, trimipramine, tryptophan, valbenazine, venlafaxine, viloxazine, zolmitriptan
Important contra-indications noted in the prescribing guidelines for: nursing mothers; pediatric patients
Warning: SUICIDALITY AND ANTIDEPRESSANT DRUGS

Skin
Exanthems (7%)
Peripheral edema (<10%)
Photosensitivity (4%)
Pruritus (itching) (4%)

Mucosal
Xerostomia (dry mouth) (<10%) [2]

Central Nervous System
Vertigo / dizziness [2]

ISOETHARINE

Indications: Bronchial asthma
Class: Adrenergic beta-receptor agonist
Half-life: N/A
Clinically important, potentially hazardous interactions with: phenelzine
Important contra-indications noted in the prescribing guidelines for: pediatric patients

---

Mucosal
Xerostomia (dry mouth) (<10%)

Central Nervous System
Trembling (<10%)

ISOFLURANE

Trade name: Forane (Baxter)
Indications: Maintenance of general anesthesia
Class: Anesthetic; inhalation
Half-life: N/A
Clinically important, potentially hazardous interactions with: cisatracurium, doxacurium, mivacurium, muscle relaxants, pancuronium, rapacuronium

---

Central Nervous System
Hallucinations [2]
Malignant hyperthermia [2]

Gastrointestinal/Hepatic
Hepatotoxicity / liver injury / acute liver injury / drug-induced liver injury (DILI) [2]

Other
Death [3]

ISONIAZID

Synonyms: INH; isonicotinic acid hydrazide
Trade names: Rifamate (Sanofi-Aventis), Rifater (Sanofi-Aventis)
Indications: Tuberculosis
Class: Antibiotic, Antimicrobial, Antimycobacterial (including antitubercular)
Half-life: <4 hours
Clinically important, potentially hazardous interactions with: acetaminophen, betamethasone, ethosuximide, insulin aspart, insulin degludec, insulin detemir, insulin glargine, insulin glulisine, itraconazole, levodopa, metformin, phenytoin, prednisolone, propranolol, rifampin, rifapentine, safinamide, triamcinolone

---

Skin
Acneiform eruption / acneiform dermatitis / acneiform rash [7]
AGEP [2]
Angioedema (formerly named angioneurotic edema) [2]
Bullous dermatosis [2]
Cutaneous toxicity / skin toxicity [2]
Dermatitis [3]
DRESS syndrome (Drug-induced hypersensitivity syndrome) [7]
Erythema multiforme [2]
Erythroderma [2]
Exanthems [4]
Exfoliative dermatitis [5]
Hypersensitivity [7]
Lichenoid eruption / lichenoid reaction [3]
Lupus erythematosus (subacute cutaneous lupus erythematosus (SCLE)) [59]
Peripheral edema [22]
Photosensitivity [6]
Pruritus (itching) [3]
Purpura [7]
Pustules / pustular eruption [3]
Rash [2]
Stevens-Johnson syndrome and toxic epidermal necrolysis (SJS/TEN) [12]
Urticaria / hives (<5%) [4]
Vasculitis (angiitis) / cutaneous vasculitis (angiitis) [2]

Hair
Alopecia / hair loss [3]

Mucosal
Oral lesions [2]

Central Nervous System
Cerebellitis [6]
Fever (pyrexia) (includes hyperpyrexia) [3]
Hallucinations [3]
Hallucinations, visual [2]
Mania [2]
Neurotoxicity [2]
Peripheral neuropathy [3]
Psychosis [4]
Seizures [9]

Endocrine/Metabolic
Gynecomastia [4]

Gastrointestinal/Hepatic
Hepatotoxicity / liver injury / acute liver injury / drug-induced liver injury (DILI) [41]
Pancreatitis / acute pancreatitis [5]

Hematologic
Pure red cell aplasia [4]
Sideroblastic anemia / acquired sideroblastic anemia [4]

Neuromuscular/Skeletal
Arthralgia [2]
Rhabdomyolysis (3%) [4]

Ocular
Optic neuritis / papillitis [3]
Optic neuropathy [2]

Renal
Nephrotoxicity / kidney injury / acute kidney injury (AKI) / drug-induced kidney injury [2]

Respiratory
Influenza- ('flu)-like syndrome [2]
Interstitial lung disease / interstitial pneumonitis / interstitial pneumonia (cryptogenic organizing pneumonia) / drug-induced interstitial lung disease [2]
Pleural effusion [2]
Pneumonitis [4]

Other
Adverse effects / adverse reactions [8]
Death [4]
Side effects (2%) [2]

ISOPROTERENOL

Trade name: Isuprel (Hospira)
Indications: Bronchospasm, ventricular arrhythmias
Class: Adrenergic beta-receptor agonist, Catecholamine, Sympathomimetic
Half-life: 2.5–5 minutes
Clinically important, potentially hazardous interactions with: amitriptyline, oxtriphylline
Important contra-indications noted in the prescribing guidelines for: nursing mothers; pediatric patients

---

Skin
Diaphoresis (<10%)
Flushing / rubefaction (<10%)

Mucosal
Xerostomia (dry mouth) (>10%)

Cardiovascular
Bradycardia / sinus bradycardia [2]
Myocardial toxicity [2]
Palpitation [3]
Tachycardia [2]

ISOSORBIDE

Indications: Acute angle-closure glaucoma
Class: Diuretic
Half-life: 5–9.5 hours
Clinically important, potentially hazardous interactions with: sildenafil
Note: Various forms of isosorbide are available – see other isosorbide profiles for reaction details.

Central Nervous System
Headache [10]

ISOSORBIDE DINITRATE

Trade names: Dilatrate-SR (Schwarz), Isordil (Wyeth), Sorbitrate (AstraZeneca)
Indications: Angina pectoris
Class: Nitrate, Vasodilator
Half-life: 4 hours (oral)
Clinically important, potentially hazardous interactions with: sildenafil
Important contra-indications noted in the prescribing guidelines for: the elderly; nursing mothers; pediatric patients
Note: Various forms of isosorbide are available – see other isosorbide profiles for reaction details.

Skin
Flushing / rubefaction (>10%)

Central Nervous System
Headache [3]

ISOSORBIDE MONO-NITRATE

Trade names: Imdur (Schering), Monoket (Schwarz)
Indications: Angina pectoris
Class: Nitrate, Vasodilator
Half-life: ~4 hours
Clinically important, potentially hazardous interactions with: sildenafil
Important contra-indications noted in the prescribing guidelines for: the elderly; nursing mothers; pediatric patients
Note: Various forms of isosorbide are available – see other isosorbide profiles for reaction details.

Skin
Flushing / rubefaction (>10%) [2]
Peripheral edema [2]

Cardiovascular
Palpitation [2]

Central Nervous System
Headache [7]
Vertigo / dizziness [2]

Other
Adverse effects / adverse reactions [2]

ISOTRETINOIN

Synonym: 13-*cis*-retinoic acid
Trade names: Accutane (Roche), Amnesteem (Genpharm), Claravis (Barr), Roaccutane (Roche)
Indications: Cystic acne
Class: Retinoid
Half-life: 21–24 hours
Clinically important, potentially hazardous interactions with: acitretin, alcohol (ethyl), antacids, bexarotene, carbamazepine, cholestyramine, co-trimoxazole, corticosteroids, dairy products, minocycline, oral contraceptives, phenytoin, retinoids, sarecycline, St John's wort, tetracycline, tetracyclines, vitamin A
Important contra-indications noted in the prescribing guidelines for: nursing mothers; pediatric patients
Note: Oral retinoids can cause birth defects, and women should avoid isotretinoin when pregnant or trying to conceive.
April 2023. In the UK, 'The Isotretinoin Expert Working Group of the Commission on Human Medicines' has made recommendations to strengthen the safety of isotretinoin treatment. Recommendations include new warnings, the need for consistent monitoring requirements for psychiatric side effects, the introduction of new monitoring requirements for sexual side effects, and additional oversight of the initiation of treatment for patients younger than 18 years.

Skin
Abscess [3]
Acne fulminans (acne maligna) [3]
Acneiform eruption / acneiform dermatitis / acneiform rash [20]
AGEP [2]
Angioedema (formerly named angioneurotic edema) [3]
Desquamation (palms and soles) (5%)
Diaphoresis [2]
Edema / fluid retention (subcutaneous, recurrent) [3]
Erythema nodosum [4]
Exfoliative dermatitis (<10%)
Facial edema (<10%)
Facial erythema [3]
Granulation tissue [4]
Keloid [5]
Pallor (<10%)
Photosensitivity (>10%) [7]
Pigmentation (Skin) (includes hyperpigmentation) [2]
Pityriasis rosea [2]
Pruritus (itching) (<5%) [5]
Pyoderma gangrenosum [3]
Rash [3]
Seborrheic dermatitis [2]
Skin fragility [3]
Sweet's syndrome [2]
Urticaria / hives [2]
Vasculitis (angiitis) / cutaneous vasculitis (angiitis) [4]
Xanthomas [2]
Xerosis / xeroderma (>10%) [12]

Hair
Alopecia / hair loss (16%) [3]
Curly hair [3]

Nails
Brittle nails [2]
Elkonyxis [2]
Median canaliform dystrophy [3]
Onycholysis [3]
Paronychia [4]
Pyogenic granuloma [8]

Mucosal
Cheilitis (inflammation of the lips) (>90%) [19]
Epistaxis (nosebleed) [3]
Mucositis [2]
Xerostomia (dry mouth) (>10%) [5]

Central Nervous System
Depression [7]
Headache [7]
Hypersomnia [3]
Pseudotumor cerebri [4]
Psychosis [6]

Endocrine/Metabolic
ALT increased [2]
Amenorrhea [2]
AST increased [2]
Gynecomastia [2]
Hypercholesterolemia [3]
Hyperlipidemia / lipids elevated [2]
Hypertriglyceridemia (includes triglycerides increased) [6]
Menstrual irregularities [3]

Gastrointestinal/Hepatic
Abdominal pain [3]
Hepatotoxicity / liver injury / acute liver injury / drug-induced liver injury (DILI) [3]
Pancreatitis / acute pancreatitis [12]

Genitourinary
Hematuria [3]
Urethritis [3]

Hematologic
Neutropenia (neutrophils decreased) [2]

Neuromuscular/Skeletal
Arthralgia [4]
Asthenia / fatigue [2]
Myalgia/Myopathy [8]
Rhabdomyolysis [3]
Sacroiliitis [5]
Stiff person syndrome [2]

Ocular
Myopia [2]
Ocular adverse effect [2]
Photophobia [2]
Xerophthalmia (dry eyes) [2]

Other
Adverse effects / adverse reactions [11]
Side effects [2]
Teratogenicity [9]

ISOXSUPRINE

Indications: Peripheral vascular disease, Raynaud's phenomenon
Class: Adrenergic beta-receptor agonist
Half-life: N/A
Clinically important, potentially hazardous interactions with: none known
Important contra-indications noted in the prescribing guidelines for: pediatric patients

---

Cardiovascular
Tachycardia [3]

ISRADIPINE

Trade name: DynaCirc (Reliant)
Indications: Hypertension
Class: Calcium channel blocker
Half-life: 8 hours
Clinically important, potentially hazardous interactions with: amprenavir, delavirdine, epirubicin, imatinib, phenytoin

Skin
Edema / fluid retention (7%) [6]
Exanthems (2%)
Flushing / rubefaction (2–9%) [9]
Pruritus (itching) (<6%)
Rash (2%)

Mucosal
Oral lesions (6%)

Cardiovascular
QT interval prolonged / QT prolongation [2]

Central Nervous System
Headache (9%)
Vertigo / dizziness (9%)

ISTRADEFYLLINE

Trade name: Nourianz (Kyowa Kirin)
Indications: Indicated as adjunctive treatment to levodopa/carbidopa in adult patients with Parkinson's disease (PD) experiencing "off" episodes
Class: Adenosine A2A receptor agonist
Half-life: approximately 83 hours
Clinically important, potentially hazardous interactions with: strong CYP3A4 inducers, strong CYP3A4 inhibitors
Pregnancy category: There are no adequate data on the developmental risk associated with the use of istradefylline in pregnant women.
Note: Use during pregnancy is not recommended. Women of childbearing potential should be advised to use contraception during treatment with istradefylline. Because of the potential risk of exacerbating psychosis, patients with a major psychotic disorder should not be treated with istradefylline.

Skin
Rash (2%)

Central Nervous System
Dyskinesia (17%) [4]
Hallucinations (6%) [2]
Hallucinations, visual [2]
Insomnia (6%)
Vertigo / dizziness (6%)

Endocrine/Metabolic
ALP increased (2%)
Appetite decreased (3%)
Glucose dysregulation (2%)
Uremia (2%)

Gastrointestinal/Hepatic
Constipation (6%)
Diarrhea (2%)
Nausea (6%)

Respiratory
Upper respiratory tract inflammation (2%)

ITRACONAZOLE

Trade names: Onmel (Merz), Sporanox (Janssen)
Indications: Onychomycosis, deep mycoses, oropharyngeal candidiasis (oral solution only)
Class: Antifungal / antimycotic, Antifungal; triazole, Antimicrobial, CYP3A4 inhibitor
Half-life: 21 hours
Clinically important, potentially hazardous interactions with: abiraterone, acalabrutinib, afatinib, alfentanil, alfuzosin, aliskiren, alprazolam, amphotericin B, amprenavir, anisindione, antacids, aprepitant, aripiprazole, artemether/lumefantrine, astemizole, atazanavir, atorvastatin, avanafil, avapritinib, boceprevir, bosentan, brigatinib, budesonide, buspirone, busulfan, cabazitaxel, cabozantinib, calcifediol, calcium channel blockers, capmatinib, carbamazepine, cerivastatin, ciclesonide, cilostazol, cimetidine, cinacalcet, cisapride, clarithromycin, clopidogrel, clorazepate, cobicistat/elvitegravir/emtricitabine/tenofovir alafenamide, cobicistat/elvitegravir/emtricitabine/tenofovir disoproxil, cobimetinib, colchicine, conivaptan, copanlisib, corticosteroids, coumarins, crizotinib, cyclophosphamide, cyclosporine, cyproterone, dabigatran, darifenacin, dasatinib, dexamethasone, diazepam, dicumarol, didanosine, digoxin, dihydroergotamine, dihydropyridines, disopyramide, docetaxel, dofetilide, dronedarone, efavirenz, eletriptan, enzalutamide, eplerenone, ergotamine, erlotinib, erythromycin, estradiol, ethotoin, everolimus, felodipine, fentanyl, fesoterodine, flibanserin, fluticasone propionate, fosamprenavir, fosphenytoin, gefitinib, grapefruit juice, halofantrine, haloperidol, histamine H_2-antagonists, HMG-CoA reductase inhibitors, ibrexafungerp, ibrutinib, iloperidone, imatinib, indinavir, infigratinib, irinotecan, isoniazid, ivabradine, ixabepilone, lapatinib, lemborexant, lercanidipine, levomethadyl, lomitapide, lopinavir, lovastatin, lumateperone, lurasidone, mephenytoin, methadone, methylergonovine, methylprednisolone, methysergide, micafungin, midazolam(oral), midostaurin, mifepristone, mizolastine, naldemedine, neratinib, nevirapine, nilotinib, nisoldipine, olaparib, omeprazole, oral hypoglycemics, osimertinib, paclitaxel, palbociclib, paliperidone, pantoprazole, pazopanib, pemigatinib, phenobarbital, phenytoin, pimavanserin, pimecrolimus, pimozide, ponatinib, pralsetinib, prednisolone, prednisone, proton pump inhibitors, quetiapine, quinidine, ranolazine, reboxetine, regorafenib, repaglinide, ribociclib, rifabutin, rifampin, rilpivirine, rimegepant, rimonabant, ripretinib, ritonavir, rivaroxaban, romidepsin, ruxolitinib, saquinavir, selpercatinib, sildenafil, silodosin, simeprevir, simvastatin, sirolimus, solifenacin, sonidegib, sotorasib, sunitinib, tacrolimus, tadalafil, talazoparib, telaprevir, telithromycin, temsirolimus, terfenadine, tezacaftor/ivacaftor, ticagrelor, tolterodine, tolvaptan, triamcinolone, triazolam, trimetrexate, tucatinib, ubrogepant, ulipristal, valbenazine, vardenafil, vemurafenib, venetoclax, vinblastine, vincristine, vinflunine, vinorelbine, voclosporin, vorapaxar, warfarin
Important contra-indications noted in the prescribing guidelines for: nursing mothers
Note: Contra-indicated in patients with evidence of ventricular dysfunction such as congestive heart failure (CHF) or a history of CHF except for the treatment of life-threatening or other serious infections.
Warning: CONGESTIVE HEART FAILURE, CARDIAC EFFECTS AND DRUG INTERACTIONS

Skin
AGEP [3]
Angioedema (formerly named angioneurotic edema) [2]
Baboon syndrome / symmetrical drug-related intertriginous and flexural exanthema (SDRIFE) [2]
Diaphoresis (3%)
Edema / fluid retention (<4%) [11]
Exanthems (<3%) [7]
Peripheral edema (4%)
Phototoxicity [2]
Pruritus (itching) (<3%) [8]
Rash (8%) [10]
Urticaria / hives [3]
Vasculitis (angiitis) / cutaneous vasculitis (angiitis) [2]

Hair
Alopecia / hair loss [3]

Mucosal
Xerostomia (dry mouth) [3]

Cardiovascular
Cardiac arrest [2]
Cardiac failure [4]
Congestive heart failure [4]
Hypertension (3%) [3]
QT interval prolonged / QT prolongation [5]
Torsades de pointes [2]

Central Nervous System
Fever (pyrexia) (includes hyperpyrexia) [2]
Headache (4%) [3]
Neurotoxicity [5]
Peripheral neuropathy [4]
Seizures [2]
Tremor [2]
Vertigo / dizziness [2]

Endocrine/Metabolic
ALT increased [2]
AST increased [2]
Hyperbilirubinemia [2]
Hypertriglyceridemia (includes triglycerides increased) [2]
Hypokalemia [6]

Gastrointestinal/Hepatic
Abdominal pain (2–6%) [5]
Constipation [2]
Diarrhea [4]
Hepatitis [2]
Hepatotoxicity / liver injury / acute liver injury / drug-induced liver injury (DILI) [8]
Nausea (5–7%) [8]
Pancreatitis / acute pancreatitis [2]
Vomiting [3]

Hematologic
Leukocytopenia (leukopenia) / leukocytes (white blood cells) decreased [2]
Thrombocytopenia / platelets decreased [2]

Neuromuscular/Skeletal
Asthenia / fatigue [3]
Back pain [2]
Rhabdomyolysis [7]

Renal
Renal failure [2]

Respiratory
Cough (4%)

Dyspnea / shortness of breath (2%)
Influenza- ('flu)-like syndrome [2]
Pneumonia (2%)

Other
Adverse effects / adverse reactions [8]
Death [4]
Side effects [2]

IVABRADINE

Trade names: Corlanor (Amgen), Procoralan (Servier)
Indications: Chronic stable angina pectoris
Class: Cardiotonic agent, HCN channel blocker
Half-life: 2 hours
Clinically important, potentially hazardous interactions with: azole antifungals, clarithromycin, CYP3A4 inducers, diltiazem, grapefruit juice, itraconazole, ketoconazole, macrolide antibiotics, nefazodone, nelfinavir, pentamidine, phenytoin, rifampin, ritonavir, sotalol, St John's wort, strong or moderate CYP3A4 inhibitors, telithromycin, verapamil
Important contra-indications noted in the prescribing guidelines for: nursing mothers; pediatric patients

---

Cardiovascular
Atrial fibrillation (8%) [4]
Atrioventricular block (<10%)
Bradycardia / sinus bradycardia (10%) [7]
Hypertension (9%)

Central Nervous System
Headache (2–5%) [2]
Vertigo / dizziness (<10%) [3]

Gastrointestinal/Hepatic
Nausea [2]

Neuromuscular/Skeletal
Myalgia/Myopathy (<10%)

Ocular
Luminous phenomena (14%) [5]
Photopsia [3]
Vision blurred (<10%) [3]
Visual disturbances [3]

IVACAFTOR

Trade name: Kalydeco (Vertex)
Indications: Cystic fibrosis in patients aged 6 years and older who have a *G551D* mutation in the *CFTR* gene
Class: CFTR potentiator
Half-life: 12 hours
Clinically important, potentially hazardous interactions with: CYP3A inducers or inhibitors, fluconazole, grapefruit juice, ketoconazole, rifampin, St John's wort
Important contra-indications noted in the prescribing guidelines for: nursing mothers; pediatric patients
Note: See also separate profiles for lumacaftor/ivacaftor and tezacaftor/ivacaftor.

Skin
Acneiform eruption / acneiform dermatitis / acneiform rash (4–7%)
Rash (13%) [6]

Mucosal
Nasal congestion (20%) [7]
Oropharyngeal pain (22%) [7]

Cardiovascular
Chest pain (4–7%)

Central Nervous System
Fever (pyrexia) (includes hyperpyrexia) [2]
Headache (24%) [8]
Vertigo / dizziness (9%) [4]

Endocrine/Metabolic
AST increased (4–7%)

Gastrointestinal/Hepatic
Abdominal pain (16%) [4]
Diarrhea (13%) [6]
Hepatotoxicity / liver injury / acute liver injury / drug-induced liver injury (DILI) [3]
Nausea (12%) [3]
Vomiting [2]

Neuromuscular/Skeletal
Arthralgia (4–7%)
Myalgia/Myopathy (4–7%)

Otic
Otitis (otitis externa, otitis media, otitis interna) [2]

Respiratory
Cough [5]
Hemoptysis [2]
Nasopharyngitis (15%) [4]
Rhinitis / rhinosinusitis (see also sinusitis) (4–7%)
Upper respiratory tract infection (22%) [7]
Wheezing (4–7%)

Other
Adverse effects / adverse reactions [4]

IVERMECTIN

Trade names: Sklice (Sanofi Pasteur), Soolantra (Galderma), Stromectol (Merck)
Indications: Various infections caused by susceptible helmintic organisms
Class: Anthelmintic, Covid-19 putative drug
Half-life: 16–35 hours
Clinically important, potentially hazardous interactions with: alprazolam, barbiturates, benzodiazepines, diazepam, midazolam, valproic acid
Important contra-indications noted in the prescribing guidelines for: nursing mothers; pediatric patients

---

Skin
Edema / fluid retention (10–53%) [7]
Exanthems (<34%) [3]
Facial edema [3]
Pruritus (itching) (38–71%) [14]
Rash (<93%) [6]
Stevens-Johnson syndrome and toxic epidermal necrolysis (SJS/TEN) [2]
Urticaria / hives (23%)

Cardiovascular
Tachycardia (4%)

Central Nervous System
Fever (pyrexia) (includes hyperpyrexia) (23%) [3]
Headache [6]
Psychosis [2]
Vertigo / dizziness (3%) [6]

Gastrointestinal/Hepatic
Abdominal pain [5]
Nausea [2]

Neuromuscular/Skeletal
Arthralgia (9%)
Asthenia / fatigue [3]
Myalgia/Myopathy (20%) [3]

Other
Adverse effects / adverse reactions [6]
Side effects (mild) [3]

IXABEPILONE

Trade name: Ixempra (Bristol-Myers Squibb)
Indications: Breast cancer (advanced or metastatic)
Class: Antineoplastic / anticancer agent (see also Immune checkpoint inhibitor), Epithilone
Half-life: 52 hours
Clinically important, potentially hazardous interactions with: amprenavir, atazanavir, carbamazepine, clarithromycin, conivaptan, darunavir, dasatinib, deferasirox, delavirdine, dexamethasone, efavirenz, grapefruit juice, indinavir, itraconazole, ketoconazole, nefazodone, nelfinavir, oxcarbazepine, phenobarbital, phenytoin, rifabutin, rifampin, rifapentine, ritonavir, saquinavir, St John's wort, telithromycin, voriconazole
Important contra-indications noted in the prescribing guidelines for: nursing mothers; pediatric patients
Note: Often prescribed along with capecitabine. Patients with diabetes may be at increased risk of severe neuropathy.

Skin
Cutaneous toxicity / skin toxicity [2]
Edema / fluid retention (9%)
Exfoliative dermatitis (2%)
Hand–foot syndrome (palmar–plantar erythrodysesthesia) (8%)
Hot flashes / hot flushes (6%)
Hypersensitivity (5%)
Pigmentation (Skin) (includes hyperpigmentation) (2%)
Pruritus (itching) (6%)
Rash (9%)

Hair
Alopecia / hair loss (48%) [2]

Nails
Nail disorder (9%)

Mucosal
Mucositis (29%) [2]
Stomatitis (oral mucositis) (29%)

Cardiovascular
Chest pain (5%)

Central Nervous System
Anorexia (19%) [2]
Dysgeusia (taste perversion) (6%)
Fever (pyrexia) (includes hyperpyrexia) (8%)
Headache (11%)
Insomnia (5%)
Neurotoxicity [5]
Pain (8%)
Peripheral neuropathy (63%) [3]
Vertigo / dizziness (7%)

Endocrine/Metabolic
Dehydration (2%)
Weight loss (6%)

Gastrointestinal/Hepatic
Abdominal pain (13%)
Constipation (16%) [2]
Diarrhea (22%) [2]
Gastroesophageal reflux (6%)
Nausea (42%) [2]
Vomiting (29%)

Hematologic
Anemia (6%) [3]
Febrile neutropenia (3%)
Leukocytopenia (leukopenia) / leukocytes (white blood cells) decreased (36%) [2]
Neutropenia (neutrophils decreased) (31%) [5]
Thrombocytopenia / platelets decreased (5%)

Neuromuscular/Skeletal
Arthralgia [3]
Asthenia / fatigue (56%) [6]
Bone pain / joint pain (23%)
Myalgia/Myopathy (49%) [2]

Ocular
Lacrimation (4%)

Respiratory
Cough (2%)
Dyspnea / shortness of breath (9%)
Upper respiratory tract infection (6%)

IXAZOMIB

Trade name: Ninlaro (Millennium)
Indications: Multiple myeloma (in combination with lenalidomide and dexamethasone) in patients who have received at least one prior therapy
Class: Proteasome inhibitor
Half-life: 10 days
Clinically important, potentially hazardous interactions with: carbamazepine, phenytoin, rifampin, St John's wort, strong CYP3A inducers
Pregnancy category: Can cause fetal harm
Important contra-indications noted in the prescribing guidelines for: nursing mothers; pediatric patients
Note: See separate profiles for dexamethasone and lenalidomide.

Skin
Acneiform eruption / acneiform dermatitis / acneiform rash [3]
Erythema [4]
Erythema multiforme [2]
Exanthems [8]
Exfoliative dermatitis [4]
Facial edema [2]
Hyperhidrosis [4]
Peripheral edema (25%) [4]
Petechiae [3]
Pigmentation (Skin) (includes hyperpigmentation) [3]
Pruritus (itching) [4]
Rash (19%) [10]
Sweet's syndrome [5]
Urticaria / hives [2]
Xerosis / xeroderma [3]

Hair
Alopecia / hair loss [2]

Central Nervous System
Chills [2]
Fever (pyrexia) (includes hyperpyrexia) [4]
Insomnia [2]
Peripheral neuropathy (28%) [14]

Endocrine/Metabolic
Appetite decreased [4]
Dehydration [3]
Hypokalemia [2]

Gastrointestinal/Hepatic
Abdominal pain [2]
Constipation (34%) [4]
Diarrhea (42%) [14]
Nausea (26%) [12]
Vomiting (22%) [11]

Hematologic
Anemia [11]
Leukocytopenia (leukopenia) / leukocytes (white blood cells) decreased [4]
Lymphopenia (lymphocytopenia) / lymphocytes decreased [6]
Neutropenia (neutrophils decreased) (67%) [15]
Thrombocytopenia / platelets decreased (78%) [21]

Neuromuscular/Skeletal
Asthenia / fatigue [12]
Back pain (21%)

Ocular
Conjunctivitis (conjunctival inflammation) (6%)
Vision blurred (6%)
Xerophthalmia (dry eyes) (5%)

Renal
Renal failure [2]

Respiratory
Dyspnea / shortness of breath [2]
Pneumonia [3]
Upper respiratory tract infection (19%)

Other
Adverse effects / adverse reactions [6]
Infection [3]

IXEKIZUMAB

Trade name: Taltz (Lilly)
Indications: Moderate-to-severe plaque psoriasis, active psoriatic arthritis
Class: Biologic, Interleukin-17 (IL-17) antagonist / interleukin-17 inhibitor, Monoclonal antibody
Half-life: 13 days
Clinically important, potentially hazardous interactions with: live vaccines
Pregnancy category: Insufficient evidence to inform drug-associated risk
Important contra-indications noted in the prescribing guidelines for: pediatric patients

---

Skin
Candidiasis / candidosis [3]
Eczema / eczematous reaction / eczematous eruption [3]
Hypersensitivity [6]
Peripheral edema [2]
Pruritus (itching) [2]
Tinea [2]
Urticaria / hives [3]
Vitiligo [4]

Central Nervous System
Headache [8]

Endocrine/Metabolic
ALT increased [2]
AST increased [2]

Gastrointestinal/Hepatic
Colitis [5]
Crohn's disease [4]
Nausea (2%)

Hematologic
Neutropenia (neutrophils decreased) (11%) [4]
Thrombocytopenia / platelets decreased (3%)

Local
Injection-site erythema [4]
Injection-site pain [3]
Injection-site reaction (17%) [22]

Neuromuscular/Skeletal
Arthralgia [2]

Otic
Ear infection (2%)

Respiratory
Bronchitis [3]
Interstitial lung disease / interstitial pneumonitis / interstitial pneumonia (cryptogenic organizing pneumonia) / drug-induced interstitial lung disease [3]
Nasopharyngitis [14]
Sinusitis (see also rhinitis / rhinosinusitis) [2]
Upper respiratory tract infection (14%) [14]

Other
Adverse effects / adverse reactions [9]
Death [5]
Infection [8]

JOJOBA OIL

Family: Simmondsiaceae
Scientific names: *Buxus chinensis, Simmondsia chinensis*
Indications: Moisturizer in cosmetics and hair care products, edible oil
Half-life: N/A
Clinically important, potentially hazardous interactions with: none known

---

Skin
Dermatitis [2]

JUNIPER

Family: Cupressaceae
Scientific names: *Juniperus communis, Juniperus oxycedrus, Juniperus phoenicea, Juniperus virginiana*
Indications: Cystitis, urethritis, urinary tract infections, flatulent colic, rheumatism, arthritis, gout, leucorrhea, blenorrhea, scrofula. **Topical:** joint pain, muscle pain, neuralgia, chronic eczema. **Inhalant:** bronchitis, lung infections. Condiment, flavor component (gin, Chartreuse, bitters), perfume
Class: Anti-inflammatory
Half-life: N/A
Clinically important, potentially hazardous interactions with: loop diuretics, thiazide diuretics

KANAMYCIN

Indications: Various infections caused by susceptible organisms
Class: Antibiotic, Antibiotic; aminoglycoside, Antimicrobial, Drug-resistant antituberculosis agent
Half-life: 2–4 hours
Clinically important, potentially hazardous interactions with: aldesleukin, atracurium, bacitracin, bumetanide, doxacurium, ethacrynic acid, furosemide, methoxyflurane, neostigmine, non-depolarizing muscle relaxants, pancuronium, polypeptide antibiotics, rocuronium, succinylcholine, teicoplanin, torsemide, vecuronium

Important contra-indications noted in the prescribing guidelines for: nursing mothers
Note: Aminoglycosides may cause neurotoxicity and/or nephrotoxicity.

Skin
Edema / fluid retention (>10%)
Pruritus (itching) (<10%)
Rash (<10%)
Otic
Hearing loss (hypoacusis) [2]
Ototoxicity [8]
Renal
Nephrotoxicity / kidney injury / acute kidney injury (AKI) / drug-induced kidney injury [2]

KAVA

Family: Piperaceae
Scientific name: *Piper methysticum*
Indications: Psychosis, depression, headache, migraines, colds, rheumatism, cystitis, vaginal prolapse, otitis, abscesses, antistress, analgesic, local anesthetic, anticonvulsant
Class: Anxiolytic
Half-life: N/A
Clinically important, potentially hazardous interactions with: alcohol, alprazolam, amitriptyline, benzodiazepines
Note: Products containing kava have been implicated in cases of severe liver toxicity. Serious adverse effects include hepatitis, cirrhosis and liver failure. At least one patient required a liver transplant. Kava has now been banned in many countries
Kava was discovered by Captain Cook, who named the plant "intoxicating pepper." In the South Pacific, kava is a popular social drink, similar to alcohol in Western societies.

Central Nervous System
Coma [2]
Gastrointestinal/Hepatic
Hepatotoxicity / liver injury / acute liver injury / drug-induced liver injury (DILI) [13]
Other
Adverse effects / adverse reactions [8]
Side effects [3]

KETAMINE

Synonym: Esketamine (S-isomer)
Trade names: Ketalar (Monarch), Spravato (S-isomer) (Janssen) (S-ketamine)
Indications: Induction of anesthesia, treatment-resistant depression (S-isomer)
Class: Anesthetic, NMDA receptor antagonist (S-isomer)
Half-life: 2–3 hours
Clinically important, potentially hazardous interactions with: memantine, mivacurium
Note: The S-form, S-ketamine (esketamine; Spravato) is indicated, in conjunction with an oral antidepressant, for the treatment of treatment-resistant depression in adults. Ketamine has become a popular recreational drug of abuse. Acute adverse effects following recreational use are diverse and can include impaired consciousness, dizziness, irrational behaviour, hallucinations, abdominal pain and vomiting. Chronic use can result in impaired verbal information processing, cystitis and cholangiopathy. (2022) The FDA became aware of safety reports involving compounded intranasal ketamine to treat psychiatric disorders which may be putting patients at risk. Compounded drugs are not FDA-approved, which means FDA has not evaluated their safety, effectiveness, or quality prior to marketing. Ketamine hydrochloride (tradename: Ketalar) is a Schedule III controlled substance that is FDA-approved as an intravenous or intramuscular injection solution for induction and maintenance of general anesthesia. Ketamine is a racemic mixture consisting of two mirror image molecules, R- and S-ketamine. FDA-approved labeling for ketamine contains warnings and precautions on hemodynamic instability, emergence reactions (vivid dreams, hallucinations, or delirium), respiratory depression, and drug-induced liver injury, among others. Ketamine is not FDA-approved for the treatment of any psychiatric disorder. However, the "S" form of ketamine, which is derived from ketamine and known as Spravato (esketamine), is a Schedule III controlled substance that was approved by FDA in 2019 as a nasal spray for treatment-resistant depression in adults and depressive symptoms in adults with major depressive disorder with acute suicidal ideation or behavior, in conjunction with an oral antidepressant. Because of the potential risks associated with Spravato (esketamine), including sedation, dissociation, and abuse or misuse, its label contains Boxed Warnings, and Spravato is subject to strict safety controls on dispensing and administration under a safety program called a Risk Evaluation and Mitigation Strategy (REMS). The Spravato REMS program requires Spravato (esketamine) to be dispensed and administered in health care settings that are certified in the REMS. Spravato (esketamine) cannot be dispensed for use outside the certified healthcare setting. Patients must be monitored inside the healthcare setting after administration for a minimum of two hours until patients are safe to leave. Though esketamine is derived from racemic ketamine, they are not the same drug. Animal studies have shown that racemic ketamine can cause lesions in the brains of rodents; the relevance of this finding to humans is unknown. Animal studies with esketamine do not show these brain lesions. .

Skin
Pruritus (itching) [3]
Rash (<10%)
Mucosal
Sialorrhea (ptyalism; hypersalivation) [2]
Cardiovascular
Bradycardia / sinus bradycardia [4]
Hypertension [7]
Hypotension [5]
Tachycardia [2]
Central Nervous System
Agitation [6]
Amnesia [2]
Cognitive impairment [3]
Dissociation (psychology) [11]
Dysgeusia (taste perversion) [3]
Hallucinations [18]
Headache [11]
Mania [4]
Nightmares [2]
Sedation [4]
Seizures [4]
Somnolence (drowsiness) [4]
Suicidal ideation [3]
Tremor (>10%)
Vertigo / dizziness [17]
Endocrine/Metabolic
SIADH [2]
Gastrointestinal/Hepatic
Cholangiopathy [7]
Hepatotoxicity / liver injury / acute liver injury / drug-induced liver injury (DILI) [2]
Nausea [19]
Vomiting [14]
Genitourinary
Bladder disorder [3]
Cystitis (includes interstitial cystitis / bladder pain syndrome) [12]
Uropathy [9]
Local
Injection-site pain (<10%)
Neuromuscular/Skeletal
Asthenia / fatigue [2]
Ocular
Vision blurred [3]
Renal
Nephropathy [3]
Respiratory
Apnea [4]
Hypoxia [3]
Laryngospasm (laryngeal dystonia / spasmodic dysphonia) [4]
Other
Adverse effects / adverse reactions [20]

KETOCONAZOLE

Trade name: Nizoral (Janssen)
Indications: Fungal infections
Class: Antifungal / antimycotic, Antifungal; imidazole, Antimicrobial, CYP3A4 inhibitor
Half-life: initial: 2 hours; terminal: 8 hours
Clinically important, potentially hazardous interactions with: abemaciclib, abiraterone, afatinib, alcohol, alfuzosin, aliskiren, alitretinoin, almotriptan, alprazolam, amphotericin B, amprenavir, anisindione, anticoagulants, aprepitant, aripiprazole, astemizole, atazanavir, avanafil, axitinib, beclomethasone, bedaquiline, benzodiazepines, betrixaban, boceprevir, bosentan, bosutinib, brentuximab vedotin, brigatinib, budesonide, buprenorphine, cabazitaxel, cabozantinib, caffeine, calcifediol, ceritinib, chlordiazepoxide, ciclesonide, cilostazol, cimetidine, cinacalcet, cisapride, clopidogrel, clorazepate, cobicistat/elvitegravir/emtricitabine/tenofovir alafenamide, cobicistat/elvitegravir/emtricitabine/tenofovir disoproxil, colchicine, conivaptan, copanlisib, crizotinib, cyclosporine, cyproterone, dabigatran, darifenacin, darunavir, dasatinib, desvenlafaxine, dexlansoprazole, dicumarol, didanosine, disopyramide, docetaxel, dofetilide, domperidone, doxercalciferol, dronedarone, dutasteride, echinacea, elbasvir & grazoprevir, eletriptan, eplerenone, erlotinib, erythromycin, estradiol, eszopiclone, everolimus, fentanyl, fesoterodine, fingolimod, flibanserin, flunisolide, fluticasone propionate, fosamprenavir, gastric alkanizers, halofantrine, HMG-CoA reductase inhibitors, ibrexafungerp, ibrutinib, iloperidone, imatinib, indacaterol, indinavir, irinotecan, isavuconazonium sulfate, ivabradine,

ivacaftor, ixabepilone, lanthanum, lapatinib, levomilnacipran, lomitapide, lopinavir, lurasidone, macitentan, maraviroc, mefloquine, methadone, methylergonovine, methylprednisolone, midazolam, midostaurin, mizolastine, mometasone, naldemedine, neratinib, nevirapine, nilotinib, nisoldipine, non-sedating antihistamines, olaparib, oliceridine, omeprazole, ospemifene, oxybutynin, paclitaxel, palbociclib, pantoprazole, paricalcitol, pazopanib, pimavanserin, pimecrolimus, pimozide, pomalidomide, ponatinib, prednisolone, prednisone, proton-pump inhibitors, quetiapine, quinidine, rabeprazole, ramelteon, ranolazine, reboxetine, regorafenib, ribociclib, rifampin, rilpivirine, rimonabant, ritonavir, rivaroxaban, roflumilast, romidepsin, ropivacaine, rupatadine, ruxolitinib, saquinavir, saxagliptin, sildenafil, silodosin, simeprevir, simvastatin, solifenacin, sonidegib, sucralfate, sunitinib, tacrolimus, tadalafil, tamsulosin, tasimelteon, telaprevir, telithromycin, temsirolimus, tezacaftor/ivacaftor, ticagrelor, tiotropium, tofacitinib, tolterodine, tolvaptan, trabectedin, tramadol, triamcinolone, triazolam, trospium, ubrogepant, ulipristal, valbenazine, vardenafil, vemurafenib, venetoclax, venlafaxine, vilazodone, vinblastine, vincristine, voclosporin, vorapaxar, warfarin, zaleplon, ziprasidone, zolpidem, zotarolimus
Warning: HEPATOTOXICITY, QT PROLONGATION AND DRUG INTERACTIONS LEADING TO QT PROLONGATION

Skin
Anaphylactoid reactions / anaphylaxis (includes anaphylactic shock) [3]
Angioedema (formerly named angioneurotic edema) [3]
Dermatitis [3]
Exanthems (<9%) [7]
Exfoliative dermatitis [2]
Fixed eruption / fixed drug eruption [2]
Hypersensitivity [3]
Pigmentation (Skin) (includes hyperpigmentation) [3]
Pruritus (itching) (<9%) [5]
Purpura [2]
Rash (<3%) [3]
Urticaria / hives (<3%) [2]
Xerosis / xeroderma [3]

Hair
Alopecia / hair loss (<4%) [4]

Mucosal
Gingivitis [2]
Oral lesions (<5%) [3]
Oral lichenoid eruption [2]
Oral pigmentation [3]

Cardiovascular
QT interval prolonged / QT prolongation [5]

Central Nervous System
Chills (<3%)
Fever (pyrexia) (includes hyperpyrexia) [2]
Headache [2]
Neurotoxicity [3]

Endocrine/Metabolic
Gynecomastia (<3%) [8]

Gastrointestinal/Hepatic
Hepatotoxicity / liver injury / acute liver injury / drug-induced liver injury (DILI) [18]
Nausea (3–10%) [5]
Vomiting (3–10%)

Hematologic
Eosinophilia / eosinophils increased [2]

Neuromuscular/Skeletal
Asthenia / fatigue [3]
Rhabdomyolysis [3]

Other
Adverse effects / adverse reactions [6]
Death [5]

KETOPROFEN

Trade names: Orudis (Sanofi-Aventis), Oruvail (Wyeth)
Indications: Arthritis
Class: Non-steroidal anti-inflammatory (NSAID)
Half-life: 1.5–4 hours
Clinically important, potentially hazardous interactions with: aspirin, caffeine, methotrexate, probenecid
Important contra-indications noted in the prescribing guidelines for: nursing mothers; pediatric patients
Note: NSAIDs may cause an increased risk of serious cardiovascular and gastrointestinal adverse events, which can be fatal. This risk may increase with duration of use.

Skin
Anaphylactoid reactions / anaphylaxis (includes anaphylactic shock) [4]
Contact dermatitis [5]
Dermatitis [29]
Eczema / eczematous reaction / eczematous eruption [3]
Erythema [4]
Exanthems [3]
Peripheral edema (<3%)
Photoallergic reaction [2]
Photocontact dermatitis [6]
Photosensitivity [36]
Pruritus (itching) (<10%) [4]
Pseudoporphyria [2]
Rash (>10%)
Urticaria / hives [6]

Gastrointestinal/Hepatic
Abdominal pain (3–9%) [2]
Constipation [2]
Diarrhea (3–9%)
Dyspepsia / functional dyspepsia (indigestion) (see also gastroparesis) (11%) [2]
Gastrointestinal bleeding [2]
Nausea (3–9%) [2]
Pancreatitis / acute pancreatitis [3]

Local
Application-site reactions [2]

Renal
Renal function abnormal / renal dysfunction (3–9%)

Other
Adverse effects / adverse reactions [11]
Allergic reactions [2]

KETOROLAC

Trade names: Acular (Allergan), Toradol (Roche)
Indications: Pain, relief of inflammation following cataract surgery (ophthalmic solution)
Class: Analgesic; non-opioid, Non-steroidal anti-inflammatory (NSAID)
Half-life: 2–8 hours
Clinically important, potentially hazardous interactions with: aspirin, buprenorphine, dabigatran, diclofenac, enoxaparin, meloxicam, methotrexate, probenecid, rivaroxaban, salicylates, tiagabine, tinzaparin
Important contra-indications noted in the prescribing guidelines for: nursing mothers; pediatric patients
Note: Ketorolac trometamol is an injectable formulation (trometamol = TRIS buffer).
Warning: GASTROINTESTINAL, CARDIOVASCULAR, RENAL, AND BLEEDING RISK

Skin
Anaphylactoid reactions / anaphylaxis (includes anaphylactic shock) [8]
Dermatitis (3–9%)
Diaphoresis (<10%) [2]
Edema / fluid retention (<10%)
Exanthems (3–9%)
Hematoma / cutaneous hematoma [2]
Hypersensitivity [2]
Pruritus (itching) (<10%)
Purpura (<10%)
Rash (<10%)

Mucosal
Stomatitis (oral mucositis) (<10%)
Xerostomia (dry mouth) [2]

Cardiovascular
Hypertension (<10%)

Central Nervous System
Aseptic meningitis [2]
Headache (>10%) [4]
Somnolence (drowsiness) [3]
Vertigo / dizziness [4]

Gastrointestinal/Hepatic
Abdominal pain (>10%)
Constipation (<10%)
Diarrhea (7%) [2]
Dyspepsia / functional dyspepsia (indigestion) (see also gastroparesis) (>10%)
Flatulence (<10%)
Gastrointestinal bleeding [6]
Gastrointestinal ulceration (<10%) [2]
Nausea (>10%) [12]
Vomiting (<10%) [8]

Hematologic
Anemia (<10%)
Prothrombin time (INR) increased (<10%)

Local
Injection-site pain (<10%)

Ocular
Corneal melting (see also corneal ulceration) [5]
Ocular burning [2]

Otic
Tinnitus (<10%)

Renal
Renal function abnormal / renal dysfunction (<10%)

Other
Adverse effects / adverse reactions [10]
Death [3]
Side effects [2]

KETOTIFEN

Trade name: Zaditor (Novartis)
Indications: Allergic conjunctivitis
Class: Histamine H1 receptor antagonist
Half-life: 22 hours
Clinically important, potentially hazardous interactions with: metformin
Important contra-indications noted in the prescribing guidelines for: pediatric patients

---

Skin
Pruritus (itching) (<10%)
Rash (<10%)

Central Nervous System
Headache (10–25%)

Ocular
Conjunctivitis (conjunctival inflammation) (<5%)
Keratitis (ocular keratitis) / corneal inflammation) (<5%)
Lacrimation (<5%)
Mydriasis (<5%)
Ocular burning (<5%)
Ocular discharge (<5%)
Ocular pain (<5%)
Ocular stinging (<5%)
Photophobia (<5%)
Xerophthalmia (dry eyes) (<5%)

Respiratory
Influenza- ('flu)-like syndrome (<5%)
Pharyngitis (sore throat) (<5%)
Rhinitis / rhinosinusitis (see also sinusitis) (10–25%)

Other
Allergic reactions (<10%)

L-CARNITINE

Indications: Improves lipid metabolism, red blood cell count, and antioxidant status, chronic fatigue syndrome, dementia, angina, post-MI cardioprotection, congestive heart failure, valproate toxicity, anorexia
Class: Food supplement
Half-life: N/A
Clinically important, potentially hazardous interactions with: none known
Note: Mixed D-, L-carnitine has been associated with myasthenic syndrome.

LABETALOL

Trade name: Trandate (Prometheus)
Indications: Hypertension
Class: Adrenergic beta-receptor antagonist, Antiarrhythmic class II
Half-life: 3–8 hours
Clinically important, potentially hazardous interactions with: cimetidine, halothane, imipramine, iobenguane, tricyclic antidepressants
Important contra-indications noted in the prescribing guidelines for: nursing mothers; pediatric patients
Note: Cutaneous side effects of beta-receptor blockers are clinically polymorphous. They apparently appear after several months of continuous therapy.

Skin
Anaphylactoid reactions / anaphylaxis (includes anaphylactic shock) [2]
Edema / fluid retention (<2%)
Exanthems (<5%) [4]
Flushing / rubefaction (19%)
Lichenoid eruption / lichenoid reaction [4]
Lupus erythematosus (subacute cutaneous lupus erythematosus (SCLE)) [4]
Pityriasis rubra pilaris [2]
Pruritus (itching) (<10%) [3]
Psoriasis (exacerbation) [3]
Raynaud's phenomenon [2]
Scalp tingling [3]

Cardiovascular
Bradycardia / sinus bradycardia [3]
Hypotension [6]

Central Nervous System
Dysgeusia (taste perversion) (<10%)
Paresthesias (7%) [2]

Neuromuscular/Skeletal
Myalgia/Myopathy [4]

Other
Side effects (6%) [2]

LACOSAMIDE

Trade name: Vimpat (UCB Pharma)
Indications: Partial-onset seizures
Class: Anticonvulsant (see also antiepileptic (anti-seizure)), Antiepileptic (anti-seizure)
Half-life: 13 hours
Clinically important, potentially hazardous interactions with: alcohol, antipsychotics, carbamazepine, chloroquine, fosphenytoin, hydroxychloroquine, lamotrigine, MAO inhibitors, mefloquine, orlistat, phenobarbital, phenytoin, pregabalin, SSRIs, St John's wort, tricyclic antidepressants
Important contra-indications noted in the prescribing guidelines for: the elderly; nursing mothers; pediatric patients

---

Skin
Angioedema (formerly named angioneurotic edema) [2]
Pruritus (itching) (2%)
Rash [6]
Stevens-Johnson syndrome and toxic epidermal necrolysis (SJS/TEN) [3]

Cardiovascular
Atrioventricular block [4]
Bradycardia / sinus bradycardia [4]
Hypotension [3]
Sinus node dysfunction (sick sinus syndrome) [2]

Central Nervous System
Balance disorder (4%)
Depression (2%) [2]
Gait instability / postural instability (2%) [4]
Headache (13%) [18]
Incoordination [2]
Irritability [3]
Memory loss/memory impaired (2%)
Sedation [5]
Seizures [6]
Somnolence (drowsiness) (7%) [20]
Status epilepticus [2]
Tic disorder [2]
Tremor (7%) [4]
Vertigo / dizziness (31%) [44]

Endocrine/Metabolic
Weight gain [2]

Gastrointestinal/Hepatic
Diarrhea (4%)
Nausea (11%) [20]
Pancreatitis / acute pancreatitis [3]
Vomiting (9%) [12]

Hematologic
Agranulocytosis / severe selective neutropenia [2]

Local
Injection-site pain (2%)

Neuromuscular/Skeletal
Asthenia / fatigue (2–9%) [10]
Ataxia (8%) [10]
Back pain [2]

Ocular
Abnormal vision [3]
Diplopia (double vision) (11%) [15]
Nystagmus (5%) [3]
Vision blurred (8%) [4]

Respiratory
Nasopharyngitis [3]
Upper respiratory tract infection [2]

Other
Adverse effects / adverse reactions [10]

LACTOBACILLUS

Family: Lactobacillaceae
Scientific names: *Lactobacillus acidophilus, Lactobacillus amylovorus, Lactobacillus brevis, Lactobacillus bulgaricus, Lactobacillus casei, Lactobacillus crispatus, Lactobacillus delbrueckii, Lactobacillus fermentum, Lactobacillus gallinarum, Lactobacillus johnsonii, Lactobacillus paracasei, Lactobacillus plantarum, Lactobacillus reuteri, Lactobacillus rhamnosus, Lactobacillus salivarius, Lactobacillus sporogenes*
Indications: Oral: Acne, allergic rhinitis, atopic allergy, diarrhea, *Helicobacter pylori* infection, irritable bowel syndrome, rotavirus, ulcerative colitis, urinary tract infections. **Suppository**: vaginitis, urinary tract infections
Class: Immunomodulator, Probiotic
Half-life: N/A
Clinically important, potentially hazardous interactions with: none known
Note: Immune-deficient subjects or those with mucosal disease may experience serious adverse effects.

LAMIVUDINE

Synonym: 3TC
Trade names: Combivir (ViiV), Epivir (ViiV), Epzicom (ViiV), Triumeq (ViiV), Trizivir (ViiV)
Indications: HIV progression
Class: Antiretroviral, Nucleoside analog reverse transcriptase inhibitor
Half-life: 5–7 hours
Clinically important, potentially hazardous interactions with: cobicistat/elvitegravir/emtricitabine/tenofovir disoproxil, emtricitabine, trimethoprim
Note: Combivir is lamivudine and zidovudine; Epzicom is lamivudine and abacavir; Triumeq is abacavir, dolutegravir and lamivudine; Trizivir is lamivudine, abacavir and zidovudine.

Skin
Angioedema (formerly named angioneurotic edema) [2]
Exanthems [2]
Hypersensitivity [4]
Jaundice (see also cholestasis / cholestatic jaundice) [2]
Pigmentation (Skin) (includes hyperpigmentation) [2]
Pruritus (itching) [3]
Rash (9%) [10]
Stevens-Johnson syndrome and toxic epidermal necrolysis (SJS/TEN) [5]

Hair
Alopecia / hair loss [3]

Central Nervous System
Abnormal dreams [2]
Chills (<10%)
Headache [6]
Insomnia [3]
Neurotoxicity [2]
Paresthesias (>10%)
Peripheral neuropathy [3]
Vertigo / dizziness [4]

Endocrine/Metabolic
Acidosis (includes lactic acidosis) [3]

Gastrointestinal/Hepatic
Abdominal pain [4]
Diarrhea [5]
Hepatotoxicity / liver injury / acute liver injury / drug-induced liver injury (DILI) [3]
Nausea [7]
Pancreatitis / acute pancreatitis [4]
Vomiting [2]

Hematologic
Anemia [2]
Pure red cell aplasia [3]

Neuromuscular/Skeletal
Asthenia / fatigue [5]
Myalgia/Myopathy (8%)
Rhabdomyolysis [3]

Renal
Nephrotoxicity / kidney injury / acute kidney injury (AKI) / drug-induced kidney injury [2]

Respiratory
Upper respiratory tract infection [3]

Other
Adverse effects / adverse reactions [10]

LAMOTRIGINE

Trade name: Lamictal (GSK)
Indications: Epilepsy
Class: Anticonvulsant (see also antiepileptic (anti-seizure)), Antiepileptic (anti-seizure), Mood stabilizer
Half-life: 24 hours
Clinically important, potentially hazardous interactions with: cenobamate, eslicarbazepine, lacosamide, oral contraceptives, rufinamide
Important contra-indications noted in the prescribing guidelines for: the elderly; nursing mothers
Warning: SERIOUS SKIN RASHES

Skin
Angioedema (formerly named angioneurotic edema) (<10%)
DRESS syndrome (Drug-induced hypersensitivity syndrome) [38]
Erythema (<10%) [2]
Erythema multiforme [4]
Exanthems (<10%) [19]
Hot flashes / hot flushes (<10%)
Hypersensitivity (<10%) [30]
Lupus erythematosus (subacute cutaneous lupus erythematosus (SCLE)) [5]
Lupus syndrome / drug-induced lupus (DIL) [2]
Photosensitivity [2]
Pruritus (itching) (3%) [3]
Rash (10–20%) [57]
Stevens-Johnson syndrome and toxic epidermal necrolysis (SJS/TEN) (<10%) [89]

Hair
Alopecia / hair loss [2]

Mucosal
Xerostomia (dry mouth) (6%)

Cardiovascular
Brugada syndrome [4]

Central Nervous System
Agitation [2]
Aseptic meningitis [4]
Fever (pyrexia) (includes hyperpyrexia) [2]
Hallucinations [3]
Hallucinations, visual [2]
Headache [7]
Insomnia (5–10%)
Mania [4]
Nervousness [2]
Neuroleptic malignant syndrome [2]
Pain (5%)
Seizures [9]
Somnolence (drowsiness) (9%) [8]
Suicidal ideation [2]
Tic disorder [3]
Tremor [5]
Vertigo / dizziness [9]

Endocrine/Metabolic
SIADH [2]

Gastrointestinal/Hepatic
Abdominal pain (6%)
Hepatotoxicity / liver injury / acute liver injury / drug-induced liver injury (DILI) [4]
Nausea [4]

Genitourinary
Urinary frequency (<5%)
Vaginitis (includes vulvitis) (4%)

Hematologic
Agranulocytosis / severe selective neutropenia [3]
Hemophagocytic lymphohistiocytosis / hemophagocytic syndrome [3]

Neuromuscular/Skeletal
Asthenia / fatigue (8%) [4]
Ataxia (2–5%) [3]
Rhabdomyolysis [3]

Ocular
Abnormal vision (2–5%)
Diplopia (double vision) [5]
Downbeat nystagmus [2]
Nystagmus (2–5%) [3]
Ocular adverse effect [2]
Tubulointerstitial nephritis and uveitis syndrome [2]

Renal
Nephrotoxicity / kidney injury / acute kidney injury (AKI) / drug-induced kidney injury [3]

Respiratory
Cough (5%)
Influenza- ('flu)-like syndrome (7%)
Pharyngitis (sore throat) (5%)
Rhinitis / rhinosinusitis (see also sinusitis) (7%)

Other
Adverse effects / adverse reactions [8]
Allergic reactions [2]
Death [8]
Multiorgan failure [2]
Side effects [2]
Teratogenicity [6]

LANREOTIDE

Trade names: Somatuline Autogel (Ipsen), Somatuline Depot (Ipsen), Somatuline LA (Ipsen)
Indications: Acromegaly, carcinoid syndrome, thyrotrophic adenoma
Class: Somatostatin analog
Half-life: 2 hours (immediate release) 5 days (sustained release).
Clinically important, potentially hazardous interactions with: antidiabetics, bromocriptine, cyclosporine, insulin, metformin, repaglinide, sulfonylureas
Important contra-indications noted in the prescribing guidelines for: nursing mothers; pediatric patients

---

Hair
Alopecia / hair loss [2]

Cardiovascular
Bradycardia / sinus bradycardia (5–18%)
Hypertension (5%)

Central Nervous System
Headache (7%)
Pain (7%)

Endocrine/Metabolic
Diabetes mellitus (7%)
Hyperglycemia (includes glucose increased) (7%)
Hypoglycemia (7%)
Weight loss (5–11%)

Gastrointestinal/Hepatic
Abdominal pain (7–19%) [9]
Cholelithiasis (gallstones in the gall bladder or the bile duct) (2–17%) [2]
Constipation (8%)
Diarrhea (31–65%) [7]
Flatulence (6–14%) [4]
Loose stools / soft feces (6%)
Nausea (11%) [3]
Steatorrhea (fatty stool) [2]
Vomiting (7%)

Hematologic
Anemia (5–14%)

Local
Injection-site induration [3]
Injection-site pain (4%) [4]
Injection-site reaction (6–22%) [3]

Neuromuscular/Skeletal
Arthralgia (7%) [2]
Asthenia / fatigue [2]

Other
Adverse effects / adverse reactions [2]

LANSOPRAZOLE

Trade name: Prevacid (TAP)
Indications: Active duodenal ulcer
Class: Proton pump inhibitor (PPI)
Half-life: 2 hours
Clinically important, potentially hazardous interactions with: bosutinib, clopidogrel, delavirdine, emtricitabine/rilpivirine/tenofovir alafenamide, emtricitabine/rilpivirine/tenofovir alafenamide, eucalyptus, infigratinib, neratinib, prednisone, rilpivirine, sucralfate
Important contra-indications noted in the prescribing guidelines for: nursing mothers

Skin
Anaphylactoid reactions / anaphylaxis (includes anaphylactic shock) [7]
Erythema multiforme [2]
Facial edema [2]
Hypersensitivity [3]
Lupus erythematosus (subacute cutaneous lupus erythematosus (SCLE)) [3]
Peripheral edema [2]
Pruritus (itching) (3–10%)
Rash (3–10%)
Stevens-Johnson syndrome and toxic epidermal necrolysis (SJS/TEN) [5]
Urticaria / hives [3]

Mucosal
Stomatitis (oral mucositis) [2]

Central Nervous System
Dysgeusia (taste perversion) [3]
Headache (3%) [4]
Vertigo / dizziness [2]

Endocrine/Metabolic
Gynecomastia [2]
Hypomagnesemia [2]

Gastrointestinal/Hepatic
Abdominal pain [2]
Colitis [2]
Constipation [2]
Diarrhea (<5%) [6]
Hepatitis [2]
Nausea [2]

Hematologic
Thrombocytopenia / platelets decreased [2]

Renal
Nephrotoxicity / kidney injury / acute kidney injury (AKI) / drug-induced kidney injury [2]

Other
Death [2]

LANTHANUM

Trade name: Fosrenol (Shire)
Indications: Hyperphosphatemia in end-stage renal disease
Class: Chelator
Half-life: 53 hours
Clinically important, potentially hazardous interactions with: chloroquine, ciprofloxacin, hydroxychloroquine, ketoconazole, levofloxacin, levothyroxine, moxifloxacin, norfloxacin, ofloxacin, quinolones
Important contra-indications noted in the prescribing guidelines for: nursing mothers; pediatric patients
Note: Contra-indicated in patients with bowel obstruction, ileus, and/or fecal impaction.

Central Nervous System
Headache (21%)

Gastrointestinal/Hepatic
Abdominal pain (5%) [2]
Constipation [2]
Gastrointestinal disorder / discomfort [2]
Nausea (11%) [3]
Vomiting (9%)

Other
Adverse effects / adverse reactions [2]

LAPATINIB

Trade name: Tykerb (Novartis)
Indications: Breast cancer
Class: Antineoplastic / anticancer agent (see also Immune checkpoint inhibitor), Epidermal growth factor receptor (EGFR) inhibitor / antagonist, HER2/neu receptor antagonist (HER2 receptor antagonist), Tyrosine kinase inhibitor
Half-life: 24 hours
Clinically important, potentially hazardous interactions with: alfuzosin, artemether/lumefantrine, atazanavir, carbamazepine, chloroquine, ciprofloxacin, clarithromycin, clozapine, colchicine, conivaptan, CYP2C8 substrates, CYP3A4 inhibitors or inducers, dabigatran, deferasirox, dexamethasone, digoxin, docetaxel, dronedarone, efavirenz, eplerenone, everolimus, fentanyl, food, gadobutrol, grapefruit juice, histamine H_2-antagonists, indinavir, irinotecan, itraconazole, ketoconazole, nefazodone, nelfinavir, nilotinib, omeprazole, P-glycoprotein inducers, paclitaxel, pantoprazole, pazopanib, phenobarbital, phenytoin, pimecrolimus, pimozide, posaconazole, proton pump inhibitors, QT prolonging agents, quinine, repaglinide, rifabutin, rifampin, rifapentin, ritonavir, rivaroxaban, safinamide, salmeterol, saquinavir, saxagliptin, silodosin, St John's wort, telithromycin, tetrabenazine, thioridazine, tolvaptan, topotecan, voriconazole, ziprasidone
Important contra-indications noted in the prescribing guidelines for: nursing mothers; pediatric patients
Note: Lapitinib is used in conjunction with capecitabine.
Warning: HEPATOXICITY

Skin
Acneiform eruption / acneiform dermatitis / acneiform rash (90%) [4]
Cutaneous toxicity / skin toxicity [7]
Depigmentation (21%)
Hand–foot syndrome (palmar–plantar erythrodysesthesia) (53%) [10]
Inflammation (15%)
Pruritus (itching) [3]
Rash (28%) [26]
Xerosis / xeroderma (10%)

Hair
Alopecia / hair loss [2]

Nails
Paronychia [4]

Mucosal
Mucosal inflammation (15%)
Mucositis [2]
Stomatitis (oral mucositis) (14%)

Central Nervous System
Anorexia (24%) [2]
Insomnia (10%)

Endocrine/Metabolic
ALT increased (37%) [5]
AST increased (49%) [4]
Hyperbilirubinemia [3]

Gastrointestinal/Hepatic
Abdominal pain (15%)
Diarrhea (65%) [45]
Dyspepsia / functional dyspepsia (indigestion) (see also gastroparesis) (11%)
Hepatotoxicity / liver injury / acute liver injury / drug-induced liver injury (DILI) [11]
Nausea (44%) [10]
Vomiting (26%) [7]

Hematologic
Anemia [5]
Febrile neutropenia [2]
Leukocytopenia (leukopenia) / leukocytes (white blood cells) decreased [4]
Lymphopenia (lymphocytopenia) / lymphocytes decreased [2]
Neutropenia (neutrophils decreased) [8]

Neuromuscular/Skeletal
Asthenia / fatigue (12%) [19]
Back pain (11%)
Bone pain / joint pain [2]
Pain in extremities (12%)

Otic
Tinnitus (14%)

Respiratory
Dyspnea / shortness of breath (12%) [2]

Other
Adverse effects / adverse reactions [11]
Death [2]

LARONIDASE

Trade name: Aldurazyme (Genzyme)
Indications: Mucopolysaccharidosis I
Class: Enzyme
Half-life: 1.5–3.6 hours
Clinically important, potentially hazardous interactions with: none known

Skin
Facial edema (9%)
Flushing / rubefaction (23%)
Peripheral edema (9%)
Rash (36%)

Cardiovascular
Chest pain (9%)

Central Nervous System
Paresthesias (14%)

Local
Application-site pain (9%)
Application-site reactions (18%)

LASMIDITAN

Trade name: Reyvow (Eli Lilly and Co)
Indications: Indicated for the acute treatment of migraine with or without aura in adults
Class: Serotonin type 1F receptor agonist
Half-life: ~5.7 hours
Clinically important, potentially hazardous interactions with: CNS depressants, heart rate lowering drugs, P-gp or bcrp substrates, serotonergic drugs
Pregnancy category: There are no adequate data on the developmental risk associated with use in pregnant women.

Note: Not indicated for the preventive treatment of migraine.

Central Nervous System
Anxiety (<2%)
Cognitive impairment (<2%)
Euphoria / elation (<2%)
Hallucinations (<2%)
Incoordination (<2%)
Paresthesias (9%) [7]
Sedation (7%)
Sleep-related disorder (<2%)
Somnolence (drowsiness) [8]
Vertigo / dizziness (17%) [10]

Gastrointestinal/Hepatic
Nausea (4%) [5]
Vomiting (4%)

Neuromuscular/Skeletal
Asthenia / fatigue (6%) [7]
Muscle weakness (2%) [2]

Ocular
Vision impaired (<2%)

Respiratory
Dyspnea / shortness of breath (<2%)

LATANOPROST

Trade name: Xalatan (Pfizer)
Indications: Reduction of elevated intraocular pressure in open angle glaucoma or ocular hypertension
Class: Prostaglandin analog, Prostaglandin receptor agonist
Half-life: 17 minutes
Clinically important, potentially hazardous interactions with: thimerosal
Important contra-indications noted in the prescribing guidelines for: nursing mothers; pediatric patients

---

Skin
Pigmentation (Skin) (includes hyperpigmentation) [2]
Pruritus (itching) [2]
Rash (<10%)

Cardiovascular
Angina (<10%)
Chest pain (<10%)

Central Nervous System
Headache [4]
Vertigo / dizziness [2]

Neuromuscular/Skeletal
Arthralgia (<10%)
Back pain (<10%)
Myalgia/Myopathy (<10%)

Ocular
Blepharitis [3]
Conjunctival hyperemia / conjunctival injection [20]
Deepening of upper lid sulcus [5]
Eyelashes – hypertrichosis (eyelash megalotrichosis) [15]
Eyelashes – pigmentation [9]
Eyelid edema / palpebral edema / blepharedema (<4%) [2]
Eyelid erythema (<4%)
Eyelid pain (<10%)
Eyelid pigmentation [4]
Eyelid pruritus (2%)
Foreign body sensation [6]
Intraocular pressure increased [2]
Iris pigmentation [7]
Keratitis (ocular keratitis) / corneal inflammation) [3]
Macular edema [7]
Ocular adverse effect [7]
Ocular hyperemia [5]
Ocular itching / ocular pruritus [8]
Ocular pigmentation (5%) [13]
Periorbitopathy / periorbital syndrome [2]
Uveitis / anterior uveitis / posterior uveitis / panuveitis [5]
Vision blurred [4]
Xerophthalmia (dry eyes) (<10%)

Respiratory
Influenza- ('flu)-like syndrome (<10%)
Upper respiratory tract infection (<10%)

Other
Allergic reactions (<10%)

LAVENDER

Family: Lamiaceae
Scientific names: *Lavandula angustifolia, Lavandula dentata, Lavandula spica, Lavandula vera*
Indications: Restlessness, insomnia, loss of appetite, flatulence, colic, giddiness, nervous headache, migraine, toothache, sprains, neuralgia, rheumatism, acne, pimples, nausea, vomiting. Flavoring, fragrance, insect repellent
Class: Anxiolytic
Half-life: N/A
Clinically important, potentially hazardous interactions with: none known

---

Skin
Dermatitis [4]

Endocrine/Metabolic
Gynecomastia [2]

LEDIPASVIR & SOFOSBUVIR

Trade name: Harvoni (Gilead)
Indications: Hepatitis C
Class: Covid-19 putative drug, Hepatitis C virus NS5A inhibitor (ledipasvir), Hepatitis C virus nucleotide analog NS5B polymerase inhibitor (sofosbuvir)
Half-life: 47 hours (ledipasvir); <27 hours (sofosbuvir)
Clinically important, potentially hazardous interactions with: amiodarone, carbamazepine, cobicistat/elvitegravir/emtricitabine/tenofovir disoproxil, doravirine/lamiduvine/tenofovir disoproxil, oxcarbazepine, phenobarbital, phenytoin, rifabutin, rifampin, rifapentine, ritonavir, rosuvastatin, simeprevir, St John's wort, tenofovir disoproxil
Pregnancy category: Insufficient evidence to inform drug-associated risk; contra-indicated in pregnancy when given with ribavirin
Important contra-indications noted in the prescribing guidelines for: nursing mothers; pediatric patients
Note: See also separate entry for sofosbuvir.

Skin
Pruritus (itching) [7]
Rash [6]

Cardiovascular
Bradycardia / sinus bradycardia [3]

Central Nervous System
Headache (11–17%) [41]
Insomnia (3–6%) [14]
Irritability [5]
Vertigo / dizziness [3]

Endocrine/Metabolic
Hypophosphatemia [2]

Gastrointestinal/Hepatic
Constipation [2]
Diarrhea (3–7%) [14]
Hepatotoxicity / liver injury / acute liver injury / drug-induced liver injury (DILI) [3]
Nausea (6–9%) [22]

Hematologic
Anemia [8]

Neuromuscular/Skeletal
Arthralgia [3]
Asthenia / fatigue (7–18%) [39]
Muscle spasm [2]
Myalgia/Myopathy [3]

Renal
Nephrotoxicity / kidney injury / acute kidney injury (AKI) / drug-induced kidney injury [3]

Respiratory
Cough [4]
Dyspnea / shortness of breath [3]
Nasopharyngitis [3]
Upper respiratory tract infection [7]

Other
Adverse effects / adverse reactions [8]
Infection [2]

LEFLUNOMIDE

Trade name: Arava (Sanofi-Aventis)
Indications: Rheumatoid arthritis
Class: Disease-modifying antirheumatic drug (DMARD), Tyrosine kinase inhibitor
Half-life: 14–15 days
Clinically important, potentially hazardous interactions with: alefacept, azacitidine, BCG vaccine, betamethasone, cabazitaxel, carvedilol, cholestyramine(unless drug elimination required), CYP2C9 substrates, denileukin, denosumab, docetaxel, echinacea, fingolimod, gefitinib, immunosuppressants, lenalidomide, live vaccines, methotrexate, natalizumab, oxaliplatin, pazopanib, pemetrexed, phenytoin, pimecrolimus, pralatrexate, pralatrexate, rifampin, tacrolimus, temsirolimus, teriflunomide, tolbutamide, trastuzumab, triamcinolone, typhoid vaccine, vitamin K antagonists, warfarin, yellow fever vaccine
Important contra-indications noted in the prescribing guidelines for: nursing mothers; pediatric patients

---

Skin
Acneiform eruption / acneiform dermatitis / acneiform rash (<10%)
Bullous dermatosis [3]
Dermatitis (<10%)
Diaphoresis (<10%)
DRESS syndrome (Drug-induced hypersensitivity syndrome) [6]
Eczema / eczematous reaction / eczematous eruption (2%)
Lichenoid eruption / lichenoid reaction [2]
Lupus erythematosus (subacute cutaneous lupus erythematosus (SCLE)) [9]
Nodular eruption (<10%)
Peripheral edema (<10%)

Pigmentation (Skin) (includes hyperpigmentation) (<10%)
Pruritus (itching) (4%) [3]
Purpura (<10%)
Rash (10%) [17]
Stevens-Johnson syndrome and toxic epidermal necrolysis (SJS/TEN) [5]
Ulcerations (<10%) [3]
Vasculitis (angiitis) / cutaneous vasculitis (angiitis) (<10%) [4]
Xerosis / xeroderma (2%)

Hair

Alopecia / hair loss (10%) [21]
Alopecia areata [3]
Hair pigmentation (<10%)

Nails

Nail changes (<10%)

Mucosal

Gingivitis (<10%)
Oral candidiasis (3%)
Oral ulceration (3%)
Stomatitis (oral mucositis) (3%)
Xerostomia (dry mouth) (<10%)

Cardiovascular

Hypertension (10%) [7]

Central Nervous System

Anorexia (3%)
Dysgeusia (taste perversion) (<10%)
Fever (pyrexia) (includes hyperpyrexia) [2]
Headache (7%) [2]
Leukoencephalopathy / posterior reversible encephalopathy syndrome (PRES) [2]
Neurotoxicity [2]
Pain (2%)
Paresthesias (2%)
Peripheral neuropathy [3]
Vertigo / dizziness (4%)

Endocrine/Metabolic

ALT increased [3]
Weight loss [3]

Gastrointestinal/Hepatic

Abdominal pain (6%)
Diarrhea (17%) [10]
Dyspepsia / functional dyspepsia (indigestion) (see also gastroparesis) (5%) [4]
Gastroenteritis (3%)
Hepatotoxicity / liver injury / acute liver injury / drug-induced liver injury (DILI) [20]
Nausea (9%) [6]
Vomiting (3%)

Genitourinary

Urinary tract infection (5%)

Hematologic

Leukocytopenia (leukopenia) / leukocytes (white blood cells) decreased [2]
Neutropenia (neutrophils decreased) [2]
Pancytopenia (includes bicytopenia) [2]

Neuromuscular/Skeletal

Asthenia / fatigue (3%)
Back pain (5%)
Myalgia/Myopathy (<10%)
Rhabdomyolysis [2]
Synovial effusions (2%)
Tendinopathy/Tendon rupture (<10%)

Renal

Nephrotoxicity / kidney injury / acute kidney injury (AKI) / drug-induced kidney injury [2]

Respiratory

Bronchitis (7%)
Cough (increased) (3%)
Influenza- ('flu)-like syndrome (2%)
Interstitial lung disease / interstitial pneumonitis / interstitial pneumonia (cryptogenic organizing pneumonia) / drug-induced interstitial lung disease [2]
Pharyngitis (sore throat) (3%)
Pneumonia (2%)
Pneumonitis [3]
Pulmonary hypertension [2]
Pulmonary toxicity [4]
Sinusitis (see also rhinitis / rhinosinusitis) (2%)
Upper respiratory tract infection (4–15%)

Other

Adverse effects / adverse reactions [7]
Allergic reactions (2%) [6]
Death [2]
Infection (4%) [5]
Tooth disorder (<10%)

LEMBOREXANT

Trade name: Dayvigo (Eisai)
Indications: Adult patients with insomnia
Class: Orexin receptor antagonist
Half-life: 17–19 hours
Clinically important, potentially hazardous interactions with: bosentan, carbamazepine, chlorzoxazone, clarithromycin, CYP3A inhibitors and inducers, efavirenz, etravirine, fluconazole, itraconazole, modafinil, ranitidine, rifampin, St John's wort, verapamil
Pregnancy category: No available data in pregnant women to evaluate for drug-associated risks of major birth defects, miscarriage or adverse maternal or fetal outcomes.
Note: Impairs alertness and motor coordination including morning impairment. Risk increases with dose and if used with other central nervous system depressants. .

Central Nervous System

Abnormal dreams (1–2%)
Headache (5–6%) [2]
Sleep-related disorder (1–2%)
Somnolence (drowsiness) (7–10%) [5]

LEMON BALM

Family: Labiatae
Scientific name: *Melissa officinalis*
Indications: Oral: Alzheimer's disease, anxiety, attention deficit disorder, colic, dementia, depression, hyperactivity, hyperthyroidism, insomnia, menstrual cramps, fevers, headache. **Topical:** genital herpes, herpes simplex, insect bites, insect repellent, muscle tension, skin irritation
Class: Carminative, Immunomodulator
Half-life: N/A
Clinically important, potentially hazardous interactions with: none known

---

Other

Adverse effects / adverse reactions [2]

LENALIDOMIDE

Trade name: Revlimid (Celgene)
Indications: Transfusion-dependent anemia due to myeloplastic syndromes, multiple myeloma (in combination with dexamethasone)
Class: Biologic, Immunomodulator, Thalidomide analog
Half-life: 3–5 hours
Clinically important, potentially hazardous interactions with: abatacept, anakinra, canakinumab, certolizumab, denosumab, dexamethasone, digoxin, erythropoietin stimulating agents, estrogen containing therapies, leflunomide, natalizumab, pimecrolimus, rilonacept, sipuleucel-T, tacrolimus, trastuzumab, vaccines
Important contra-indications noted in the prescribing guidelines for: nursing mothers; pediatric patients
Warning: FETAL RISK, HEMATOLOGIC TOXICITY, and DEEP VEIN THOMBOSIS AND PULMONARY EMBOLISM

Skin

Bruise / bruising / contusion / ecchymosis (ecchymoses) (5–8%)
Cellulitis and pseudocellulitis (5%)
Cutaneous toxicity / skin toxicity [7]
DRESS syndrome (Drug-induced hypersensitivity syndrome) [4]
Edema / fluid retention (10%)
Erythema (5%)
Exanthems [3]
Folliculitis [2]
Graft-versus-host reaction [2]
Hyperhidrosis (7%) [2]
Peripheral edema (26%) [5]
Pigmentation (Skin) (includes hyperpigmentation) [2]
Pruritus (itching) (42%) [3]
Psoriasis [2]
Pyoderma gangrenosum [2]
Rash (36%) [22]
Stevens-Johnson syndrome and toxic epidermal necrolysis (SJS/TEN) [10]
Sweet's syndrome [3]
Tumors [5]
Xerosis / xeroderma (14%) [2]

Mucosal

Epistaxis (nosebleed) (15%)
Xerostomia (dry mouth) (7%)

Cardiovascular

Cardiac failure [2]
Cardiotoxicity [2]
Chest pain (5%)
Hypertension (6%) [2]
Palpitation (5%)
Thromboembolism [6]
Venous thromboembolism [13]

Central Nervous System

Anorexia (10%)
Depression (5%)
Dysgeusia (taste perversion) (6%)
Fever (pyrexia) (includes hyperpyrexia) (21%) [5]
Headache (20%)
Hypoesthesia / hypesthesia (numbness) (7%)
Insomnia (10%) [4]
Neurotoxicity (7%) [8]
Pain (7%)
Peripheral neuropathy (5%) [17]
Rigors (6%)

Somnolence (drowsiness) [2]
Tremor (21%)
Vertigo / dizziness (20%)

Endocrine/Metabolic
ALT increased (8%) [3]
Appetite decreased (7%)
AST increased [2]
Hyperglycemia (includes glucose increased) [3]
Hypocalcemia (9%)
Hypokalemia (11%) [5]
Hypomagnesemia (6%)
Hyponatremia [2]
Hypophosphatemia [3]
Hypothyroidism (7%)
Weight loss (20%)

Gastrointestinal/Hepatic
Abdominal pain (8–12%)
Constipation (24%) [11]
Diarrhea (49%) [20]
Gastrointestinal disorder / discomfort [4]
Hepatotoxicity / liver injury / acute liver injury / drug-induced liver injury (DILI) [3]
Loose stools / soft feces (6%)
Nausea (24%) [10]
Vomiting (10%) [6]

Genitourinary
Urinary tract infection (11%)

Hematologic
Anemia (31%) [32]
Cytopenia [3]
Febrile neutropenia (5%) [9]
Hemotoxicity [13]
Leukocytopenia (leukopenia) / leukocytes (white blood cells) decreased (8%) [14]
Lymphopenia (lymphocytopenia) / lymphocytes decreased (5%) [9]
Myelosuppression / bone marrow suppression / myelotoxicity [6]
Neutropenia (neutrophils decreased) (59%) [68]
Thrombocytopenia / platelets decreased (62%) [60]
Thrombosis [4]

Local
Infusion-related reactions [2]
Infusion-site reactions [2]
Injection-site reaction [2]

Neuromuscular/Skeletal
Arthralgia (21%) [4]
Asthenia / fatigue (15–31%) [38]
Back pain (21%) [4]
Bone pain / joint pain (14%)
Cramps (33%)
Muscle spasm [5]
Myalgia/Myopathy (18%) [3]
Osteonecrosis / avascular necrosis (includes steroid-induced osteonecrosis of the femoral head) [2]
Pain in extremities (12%)

Ocular
Vision blurred (17%)

Renal
Nephrotoxicity / kidney injury / acute kidney injury (AKI) / drug-induced kidney injury [3]
Tumor lysis syndrome (TLS) [3]

Respiratory
Acute respiratory distress syndrome [2]
Alveolar hemorrhage (pulmonary) [2]
Bronchitis (11%)
Cough (20%) [6]
Dyspnea / shortness of breath (7–17%) [4]
Interstitial lung disease / interstitial pneumonitis / interstitial pneumonia (cryptogenic organizing pneumonia) / drug-induced interstitial lung disease [3]
Nasopharyngitis (23%)
Pharyngitis (sore throat) (16%)
Pneumonia (12%) [10]
Pneumonitis [6]
Pulmonary toxicity [3]
Rhinitis / rhinosinusitis (see also sinusitis) (7%)
Sinusitis (see also rhinitis / rhinosinusitis) (8%)
Upper respiratory tract infection (15%) [4]

Other
Adverse effects / adverse reactions [14]
Cancer [3]
Death [4]
Infection [22]
Malignancies (secondary) [6]
Teratogenicity [2]

LENVATINIB

Trade name: Lenvima (Eisai)
Indications: Differentiated thyroid cancer, renal cell cancer (in combination with everolimus)
Class: Angiogenesis inhibitor / antiangiogenic agent, RET (Rearranged during Transfection) kinase inhibitor, Tyrosine kinase inhibitor, Vascular endothelial growth factor (VEGF) inhibitor / antagonist
Half-life: 28 hours
Clinically important, potentially hazardous interactions with: none known
Pregnancy category: Can cause fetal harm
Important contra-indications noted in the prescribing guidelines for: nursing mothers; pediatric patients

---

Skin
Cutaneous toxicity / skin toxicity [3]
Exanthems (21%)
Hand–foot syndrome (palmar–plantar erythrodysesthesia) (32%) [16]
Hyperkeratosis (7%)
Peripheral edema (21%) [3]
Rash (21%)

Hair
Alopecia / hair loss (12%)

Mucosal
Aphthous stomatitis / aphthous ulcer / aphtha (aphthae) (41%)
Burning Mouth Syndrome / glossodynia / glossalgia / glossopyrosis (also includes stomatodynia / oral dysesthesia / stomatopyrosis) (25%)
Epistaxis (nosebleed) (12%)
Gingivitis (10%)
Glossitis (inflammation of the tongue) (41%)
Mucosal inflammation (41%)
Oral ulceration (41%)
Oropharyngeal pain (25%)
Parotitis (10%)
Stomatitis (oral mucositis) (41%) [5]
Xerostomia (dry mouth) (17%)

Cardiovascular
Cardiotoxicity [2]
Hypertension (73%) [41]
Hypotension (9%)
QT interval prolonged / QT prolongation (9%)
Takotsubo syndrome [2]

Central Nervous System
Anorexia [7]
Dysgeusia (taste perversion) (18%)
Encephalopathy (includes hepatic encephalopathy) [4]
Headache (38%) [4]
Insomnia (12%)
Leukoencephalopathy / posterior reversible encephalopathy syndrome (PRES) [7]
Vertigo / dizziness (15%)

Endocrine/Metabolic
ALP increased (>5%)
ALT increased (4%) [2]
Appetite decreased (54%) [13]
AST increased (5%) [2]
Creatine phosphokinase (CPK) / creatine kinase increased (hyperCKemia) (3%)
Dehydration (9%)
Hyperbilirubinemia (>5%) [2]
Hypercalcemia (>5%)
Hypercholesterolemia (>5%)
Hyperkalemia (>5%)
Hypoalbuminemia / albumin decreased (>5%)
Hypocalcemia (9%)
Hypoglycemia (>5%)
Hypokalemia (6%)
Hypomagnesemia (>5%)
Hypothyroidism [6]
Weight loss (51%) [9]

Gastrointestinal/Hepatic
Abdominal pain (31%) [3]
Constipation (29%) [3]
Diarrhea (67%) [21]
Dyspepsia / functional dyspepsia (indigestion) (see also gastroparesis) (13%)
Nausea (47%) [7]
Vomiting (36%) [5]

Genitourinary
Hematuria [2]
Urinary tract infection (11%)

Hematologic
Anemia [2]
Hemorrhage [2]
Leukocytopenia (leukopenia) / leukocytes (white blood cells) decreased [2]
Neutropenia (neutrophils decreased) [2]
Thrombocytopenia / platelets decreased [6]

Neuromuscular/Skeletal
Arthralgia (62%)
Asthenia / fatigue (67%) [23]
Back pain (62%)
Bone pain / joint pain (62%)
Myalgia/Myopathy (62%)
Pain in extremities (62%)

Renal
Nephrotic syndrome [3]
Proteinuria (34%) [24]
Renal failure [3]

Respiratory
Cough (24%)
Dysphonia (includes voice disorders / voice changes) (31%) [2]
Interstitial lung disease / interstitial pneumonitis / interstitial pneumonia (cryptogenic organizing pneumonia) / drug-induced interstitial lung disease [4]
Nasopharyngitis [2]
Pneumothorax [4]

Other
Adverse effects / adverse reactions [7]
Death [3]
Tooth disorder (10%)

LEPIRUDIN

Trade name: Refludan (ZLB Behring)
Indications: Anticoagulation in heparin-induced thrombocytopenia (HIT) and associated thromboembolic disease
Class: Anticoagulant (antithrombotic), Thrombin inhibitor
Half-life: 1.3 hours
Clinically important, potentially hazardous interactions with: abciximab, acenocoumarol, clopidogrel, eptifibatide, streptokinase, thrombolytics, ticlopidine, tirofiban, vitamin K antagonists, warfarin
Important contra-indications noted in the prescribing guidelines for: the elderly; nursing mothers; pediatric patients
Note: Contra-indicated in patients with a generalized hemostatic abnormality such as hemophilia, Christmas disease, idiopathic thrombocytopenic purpura and in patients with active bleeding from a local lesion such as acute ulcer or ulcerating carcinoma; in patients who have had recent cranial, spinal, eye or ear surgery or trauma; hypersensitivity to hirudins; shock.

Skin
Anaphylactoid reactions / anaphylaxis (includes anaphylactic shock) [3]

Hematologic
Bleeding [4]

Respiratory
Bronchospasm (>10%)
Cough (>10%)
Dyspnea / shortness of breath (>10%)
Stridor (>10%)

Other
Death [3]

LESINURAD

Trade names: Duzallo (AstraZeneca), Zurampic (AstraZeneca)
Indications: Gout-associated hyperuricemia (in combination with a xanthine oxidase inhibitor)
Class: URAT1 inhibitor, Uricosuric
Half-life: 5 hours
Clinically important, potentially hazardous interactions with: amiodarone, carbamazepine, CYP2C9 inducers or inhibitors, CYP3A substrates, fluconazole, rifampin, valproic acid
Pregnancy category: No available data
Important contra-indications noted in the prescribing guidelines for: nursing mothers; pediatric patients
Note: Contra-indicated in patients with severe renal impairment (including end stage renal disease, kidney transplant recipients or patients on dialysis), tumor lysis syndrome or Lesch-Nylan syndrome. Duzallo is lesinurad and allopurinol (see separate entry).
Warning: RISK OF ACUTE RENAL FAILURE, MORE COMMON WHEN USED WITHOUT A XANTHINE OXIDASE INHIBITOR

Cardiovascular
Cardiotoxicity (<2%)

Central Nervous System
Headache (5%) [2]
Vertigo / dizziness [2]

Endocrine/Metabolic
Serum creatinine increased (4–8%) [3]

Gastrointestinal/Hepatic
Diarrhea [2]
Gastroesophageal reflux (3%)

Neuromuscular/Skeletal
Back pain [2]

Renal
Nephrolithiasis (kidney stones / renal calculi) (<3%)
Renal failure (<4%)

Respiratory
Influenza (5%)
Nasopharyngitis [2]

LETERMOVIR

Trade name: Prevymis (Merck Sharpe & Dohme)
Indications: Prophylaxis of cytomegalovirus (CMV) infection and disease in adult CMV-seropositive recipients of an allogeneic hematopoietic stem cell transplant
Class: Antiviral, Viral terminase complex inhibitor
Half-life: 12 hours
Clinically important, potentially hazardous interactions with: alfentanil, amiodarone, atorvastatin, cyclosporine, dihydroergotamine, ergotamine, fentanyl, fluvastatin, glyburide, lovastatin, midazolam, omeprazole, pantoprazole, phenytoin, pimozide, pitavastatin, pravastatin, quinidine, repaglinide, rifampin, rosiglitazone, rosuvastatin, simvastatin, sirolimus, tacrolimus, voriconazole, warfarin
Pregnancy category: No adequate human data available
Important contra-indications noted in the prescribing guidelines for: nursing mothers; pediatric patients

---

Skin
Peripheral edema (14%)

Cardiovascular
Atrial fibrillation (3%)
Tachycardia (4%)

Central Nervous System
Headache (14%)

Endocrine/Metabolic
Serum creatinine increased (2–17%) [3]

Gastrointestinal/Hepatic
Abdominal pain (12%)
Diarrhea (26%)
Gastroenteritis [3]
Nausea (27%) [2]
Vomiting (19%) [2]

Hematologic
Anemia (2–41%)
Neutropenia (neutrophils decreased) (4–19%)
Thrombocytopenia / platelets decreased (17–27%)

Neuromuscular/Skeletal
Asthenia / fatigue (13%)

Respiratory
Cough (14%)
Dyspnea / shortness of breath [3]
Nasopharyngitis [3]

LETROZOLE

Trade name: Femara (Novartis)
Indications: Breast cancer
Class: Aromatase inhibitor
Half-life: ~2 days
Clinically important, potentially hazardous interactions with: none known
Important contra-indications noted in the prescribing guidelines for: nursing mothers; pediatric patients

---

Skin
Exanthems (5%)
Hot flashes / hot flushes (6%) [10]
Hyperhidrosis (<5%)
Leukocytoclastic vasculitis (angiitis) [2]
Pruritus (itching) (2%) [2]
Psoriasis (5%)
Rash (<10%) [8]
Vesiculation (5%)

Hair
Alopecia / hair loss (<5%) [7]

Mucosal
Stomatitis (oral mucositis) [4]
Xerostomia (dry mouth) [2]

Cardiovascular
Cardiac failure [2]
Hypertension [5]
Myocardial toxicity [2]

Central Nervous System
Anorexia [3]
Depression [3]
Fever (pyrexia) (includes hyperpyrexia) [3]
Headache [5]
Insomnia [3]
Mood changes (includes mood disorder) [3]
Pain [2]
Peripheral neuropathy [2]
Vertigo / dizziness [2]

Endocrine/Metabolic
ALT increased [3]
AST increased [4]
Hypercholesterolemia [3]
Hyperglycemia (includes glucose increased) [5]
Libido decreased [2]

Gastrointestinal/Hepatic
Constipation [3]
Diarrhea [10]
Nausea [12]
Vomiting [6]

Genitourinary
Vaginal dryness [4]

Hematologic
Anemia [5]
Febrile neutropenia [3]
Leukocytopenia (leukopenia) / leukocytes (white blood cells) decreased [6]
Neutropenia (neutrophils decreased) [12]
Thrombocytopenia / platelets decreased [3]

Neuromuscular/Skeletal
Arthralgia [13]
Asthenia / fatigue [16]
Back pain [5]
Bone pain / joint pain [4]
Myalgia/Myopathy [7]
Osteoporosis [7]

Respiratory
Cough [2]
Dyspnea / shortness of breath [3]

Other
Adverse effects / adverse reactions [2]
Infection [4]

LEUCOVORIN

Synonyms: citrovorum factor; folinic acid
Indications: Overdose of methotrexate, in combination with fluorouracil in the palliative treatment of patients with colorectal cancer. Advanced pancreatic cancer (in combination with oxaliplatin/irinotecan/fluorouracil (FOLFIRINOX or FOLFOXIRI)). Used in combination with fluorouracil and irinotecan (FOLFIRI) for treatment of advanced-stage and metastatic colorectal cancer. Used in combination with fluorouracil and oxaliplatin (FOLFOX, mFOLFOX6) for treatment of colorectal cancer
Class: Antidote, Chemotherapy modulating agent, Folate analogue
Half-life: 15 minutes
Clinically important, potentially hazardous interactions with: capecitabine, glucarpidase, trimethoprim

---

Skin
Cutaneous toxicity / skin toxicity [3]
Hand–foot syndrome (palmar–plantar erythrodysesthesia) [3]
Rash [6]
Hair
Alopecia / hair loss [2]
Mucosal
Mucositis [8]
Stomatitis (oral mucositis) [7]
Cardiovascular
Hypertension [8]
Central Nervous System
Anorexia [8]
Neurotoxicity [5]
Peripheral neuropathy [5]
Endocrine/Metabolic
ALP increased [2]
Hyperammonemia [2]
Gastrointestinal/Hepatic
Abdominal pain [2]
Constipation [2]
Diarrhea [31]
Hepatic failure [2]
Nausea [18]
Vomiting [14]
Hematologic
Anemia [10]
Febrile neutropenia [9]
Leukocytopenia (leukopenia) / leukocytes (white blood cells) decreased [7]
Neutropenia (neutrophils decreased) [36]
Thrombocytopenia / platelets decreased [6]
Neuromuscular/Skeletal
Asthenia / fatigue [13]
Renal
Proteinuria [4]
Respiratory
Pneumonia [2]
Other
Adverse effects / adverse reactions [3]
Death [3]
Infection [3]

LEUPROLIDE

Synonym: leuprorelin
Trade names: Eligard (Sanofi-Aventis), Lupron (TAP), Lupron Depot-Ped (AbbVie), Viadur (Bayer)
Indications: Prostate carcinoma, endometriosis
Class: Gonadotropin-releasing hormone (GnRH) agonist
Half-life: 3–4 hours
Clinically important, potentially hazardous interactions with: none known
Important contra-indications noted in the prescribing guidelines for: nursing mothers

---

Skin
Anaphylactoid reactions / anaphylaxis (includes anaphylactic shock) [3]
Bruise / bruising / contusion / ecchymosis (ecchymoses) (<5%)
Dermatitis (5%)
Dermatitis herpetiformis [2]
Edema / fluid retention (<10%)
Flushing / rubefaction (61%) [3]
Granulomas [4]
Hot flashes / hot flushes (12%) [7]
Peripheral edema (4–12%)
Pigmentation (Skin) (includes hyperpigmentation) (<5%)
Pruritus (itching) (<5%)
Rash (<10%)
Vasculitis (angiitis) / cutaneous vasculitis (angiitis) [2]
Xerosis / xeroderma (<5%)
Hair
Alopecia / hair loss (<5%)
Cardiovascular
Thrombophlebitis (2%)
Central Nervous System
Dysgeusia (taste perversion) (<5%)
Paresthesias (<5%)
Endocrine/Metabolic
Gynecomastia (7%)
Mastodynia (7%)
Local
Injection-site granuloma [6]
Injection-site induration [2]
Injection-site inflammation (2%)
Injection-site pain [2]
Injection-site reaction (24%)
Neuromuscular/Skeletal
Myalgia/Myopathy [2]
Osteoporosis [2]
Ocular
Diplopia (double vision) [2]

LEVALBUTEROL

Trade name: Xopenex (Sepracor)
Indications: Bronchospasm
Class: Beta-2 adrenergic agonist, Bronchodilator
Half-life: 3.3–4.0 hours
Clinically important, potentially hazardous interactions with: alpha blockers, atomoxetine, beta blockers, betahistine, cannabinoids, epinephrine, iobenguane, loop diuretics, MAO inhibitors, sympathomimetics, tricyclic antidepressants

---

Skin
Diaphoresis (<2%)
Central Nervous System
Chills (<2%)
Hyperesthesia (<2%)
Pain (<3%)
Paresthesias (<2%)
Tremor (~7%)
Neuromuscular/Skeletal
Leg cramps (~3%)
Myalgia/Myopathy (<2%)
Ocular
Ocular itching / ocular pruritus (<2%)
Respiratory
Cough (<4%)
Influenza- ('flu)-like syndrome (<4%)

LEVAMISOLE

Trade name: Ergamisol (Janssen)
Indications: Susceptible helmintic organism infections, colorectal carcinoma
Class: Antineoplastic / anticancer agent (see also Immune checkpoint inhibitor), Immunomodulator
Half-life: 2–6 hours
Clinically important, potentially hazardous interactions with: alcohol, aldesleukin
Note: Levamisole is a known contaminant of street cocaine.
Levamisole has been withdrawn in Canada and the USA.

Skin
Cutaneous toxicity / skin toxicity [3]
Dermatitis (<10%)
Edema / fluid retention (<10%)
Exanthems (2–10%) [7]
Fixed eruption / fixed drug eruption [2]
Lichenoid eruption / lichenoid reaction [3]
Necrosis (skin necrosis) [5]
Pruritus (itching) [5]
Purpura [7]
Pyoderma gangrenosum [3]
Rash [9]
Urticaria / hives [4]
Vasculitis (angiitis) / cutaneous vasculitis (angiitis) [20]
Hair
Alopecia / hair loss (<10%)
Mucosal
Oral lesions (<10%) [5]
Oral ulceration [2]
Stomatitis (oral mucositis) (<10%) [2]
Central Nervous System
Dysgeusia (taste perversion) (<10%) [2]
Leukoencephalopathy / posterior reversible encephalopathy syndrome (PRES) [19]
Paresthesias (<10%)
Hematologic
Agranulocytosis / severe selective neutropenia [5]
Leukocytopenia (leukopenia) / leukocytes (white blood cells) decreased [2]
Neutropenia (neutrophils decreased) [7]
Neuromuscular/Skeletal
Arthralgia [2]
Myalgia/Myopathy (<10%)
Renal
Glomerulonephritis (includes membranous nephropathy) [2]

Other
- Cocaine/Levamisole-Associated Autoimmune Syndrome (see also oronasal midline defect) [2]
- Infection (<10%)
- Side effects (<20%)

LEVETIRACETAM

Trade names: Elepsia XR (Sun Pharma), Keppra (UCB)
Indications: Partial onset seizures
Class: Anticonvulsant (see also antiepileptic (anti-seizure))
Half-life: 7 hours
Clinically important, potentially hazardous interactions with: carbamazepine, eslicarbazepine
Important contra-indications noted in the prescribing guidelines for: nursing mothers

---

Skin
- Anaphylactoid reactions / anaphylaxis (includes anaphylactic shock) [2]
- DRESS syndrome (Drug-induced hypersensitivity syndrome) [11]
- Erythema [2]
- Erythema multiforme [2]
- Hypersensitivity [2]
- Rash [6]
- Stevens-Johnson syndrome and toxic epidermal necrolysis (SJS/TEN) [5]
- Urticaria / hives [2]

Central Nervous System
- Aggression (includes anger) [10]
- Agitation [6]
- Anorexia [3]
- Behavioral disturbances / personality changes [8]
- Compulsions / obsessive-compulsive symptoms / obsessive-compulsive disorder [2]
- Confusion [2]
- Delirium [2]
- Depression [9]
- Encephalopathy (includes hepatic encephalopathy) [4]
- Fever (pyrexia) (includes hyperpyrexia) [3]
- Headache (25%) [13]
- Irritability [13]
- Nervousness [3]
- Neurotoxicity [3]
- Paresthesias (2%)
- Psychosis [6]
- Seizures [4]
- Sleep-related disorder [2]
- Somnolence (drowsiness) [20]
- Suicidal ideation [4]
- Vertigo / dizziness (9–18%) [23]

Endocrine/Metabolic
- Creatine phosphokinase (CPK) / creatine kinase increased (hyperCKemia) [3]
- Libido decreased [2]
- Weight gain [4]

Gastrointestinal/Hepatic
- Abdominal pain [2]
- Diarrhea [2]
- Hepatotoxicity / liver injury / acute liver injury / drug-induced liver injury (DILI) [4]
- Nausea [4]
- Vomiting [4]

Genitourinary
- Sexual dysfunction [2]

Hematologic
- Hemotoxicity [2]
- Pancytopenia (includes bicytopenia) [4]
- Thrombocytopenia / platelets decreased [4]

Neuromuscular/Skeletal
- Asthenia / fatigue (<22%) [21]
- Osteoporosis [2]
- Rhabdomyolysis [9]

Renal
- Nephrotoxicity / kidney injury / acute kidney injury (AKI) / drug-induced kidney injury [4]

Respiratory
- Influenza [2]
- Nasopharyngitis [5]
- Upper respiratory tract infection [2]

Other
- Adverse effects / adverse reactions [15]
- Death [2]
- Infection (13–26%) [7]

LEVOBETAXOLOL

Trade name: Betaxon (Alcon)
Indications: Chronic open-angle glaucoma, ocular hypertension
Class: Adrenergic beta-receptor antagonist
Half-life: 20 hours
Clinically important, potentially hazardous interactions with: none known

---

Skin
- Breast abscess (<2%)
- Dermatitis (<2%)
- Psoriasis (<2%)

Hair
- Alopecia / hair loss (<2%)

Central Nervous System
- Dysgeusia (taste perversion) (<2%)

Neuromuscular/Skeletal
- Tendinopathy/Tendon rupture (<2%)

Ocular
- Ocular transient discomfort (11%)

Otic
- Tinnitus (<2%)

Other
- Infection (<2%)

LEVOBUNOLOL

Trade name: Betagan (Allergan)
Indications: Glaucoma, ocular hypertension
Class: Adrenergic beta-receptor antagonist
Half-life: N/A
Clinically important, potentially hazardous interactions with: none known
Note: Peak effect: 1–7 days.

Skin
- Dermatitis [8]

Hair
- Alopecia / hair loss (1–10%)

LEVOBUPIVACAINE

Trade name: Chirocaine (Purdue)
Indications: Regional anesthesia for surgery, postoperative pain management
Class: Anesthetic; local
Half-life: 1.3 hours
Clinically important, potentially hazardous interactions with: adenosine, dronedarone

---

Skin
- Pruritus (itching) (4%)

Central Nervous System
- Hyperesthesia (3%)
- Pain (7–18%)
- Paresthesias (2%)
- Seizures [6]
- Shivering [2]

Gastrointestinal/Hepatic
- Nausea [2]
- Vomiting [2]

Neuromuscular/Skeletal
- Back pain (6%)

LEVOCETIRIZINE

Trade name: Xyzal (UCB Pharma)
Indications: Allergic rhinitis, chronic idiopathic urticaria
Class: Histamine H1 receptor antagonist
Half-life: 6–10 hours
Clinically important, potentially hazardous interactions with: none known
Important contra-indications noted in the prescribing guidelines for: the elderly; nursing mothers; pediatric patients

---

Skin
- Fixed eruption / fixed drug eruption [3]

Mucosal
- Xerostomia (dry mouth) (2–3%)

Central Nervous System
- Headache [2]
- Sedation [2]
- Somnolence (drowsiness) (5–6%)

Gastrointestinal/Hepatic
- Hepatotoxicity / liver injury / acute liver injury / drug-induced liver injury (DILI) [2]

Neuromuscular/Skeletal
- Asthenia / fatigue (<4%)

Respiratory
- Nasopharyngitis (4–6%)
- Pharyngitis (sore throat) (<2%)

LEVODOPA

Synonyms: L-dopa; carbidopa
Trade names: Duopa, Rytary (Impax), Sinemet (Bristol-Myers Squibb), Stalevo (Orion)
Indications: Parkinsonism
Class: Dopamine precursor
Half-life: 1–3 hours
Clinically important, potentially hazardous interactions with: ACE inhibitors, acebutolol, alfuzosin, alpha blockers, amisulpride, ampicillin, angiotensin II receptor antagonists, anti-hypertensives, antimuscarinics, antipsychotics, baclofen, benzodiazepines, beta blockers, bupropion, calcium channel blockers, captopril, chloramphenicol, cholestyramine, cilazapril,

clobazam, clonidine, darifenacin, diazoxide, diuretics, dopamine D_2 receptor antagonists, enalapril, erythromycin, fosinopril, hydralazine, irbesartan, iron salts, isoniazid, levomepromazine, linezolid, lisinopril, MAO inhibitors, memantine, methyldopa, metoclopramide, minoxidil, moclobemide, moxonidine, nitrates, olanzapine, olmesartan, oral iron, oxybutynin, paliperidone, papaverine, pericyazine, phenelzine, phenytoin, probenecid, pyridoxine, quetiapine, quinapril, ramipril, rifampin, risperidone, sapropterin, selegiline, sodium nitroprusside, sulpiride / levosulpiride, tetrabenazine, tiotropium, trandolapril, tranylcypromine, tricyclic antidepressants, trospium, volatile liquid general anesthetics, ziprasidone, zuclopenthixol, zuclopenthixol acetate, zuclopenthixol decanoate, zuclopenthixol dihydrochloride

Important contra-indications noted in the prescribing guidelines for: nursing mothers; pediatric patients

Note: Levodopa is always used in conjuntion with carbidopa. Stalevo is levodopa, carbidopa and entacapone. Contra-indicated in patients with narrow-angle glaucoma or those with a history of melanoma.

Skin
- Chromhidrosis (<10%)
- Edema / fluid retention [2]
- Exanthems [2]
- Lupus erythematosus (subacute cutaneous lupus erythematosus (SCLE)) [2]
- Melanoma [28]
- Rash [3]

Hair
- Hair pigmentation [2]

Nails
- Nail growth [2]

Mucosal
- Xerostomia (dry mouth) (<10%) [2]

Cardiovascular
- Hypotension [2]
- Orthostatic hypotension [4]

Central Nervous System
- Agitation [2]
- Anosmia (smell loss) / smell disorder [2]
- Anxiety [2]
- Confusion [3]
- Delusions [2]
- Depression [3]
- Dyskinesia [54]
- Gait instability / postural instability [4]
- Hallucinations [12]
- Hallucinations, visual [2]
- Insomnia [6]
- Narcolepsy [2]
- Neuroleptic malignant syndrome [7]
- Neurotoxicity [3]
- Psychosis [6]
- Restless legs syndrome / Willis-Ekbom disease (includes restless arms syndrome variant) [5]
- Somnolence (drowsiness) [5]
- Suicidal ideation [2]
- Tardive syndrome / tardive dyskinesia [2]
- Vertigo / dizziness [5]

Endocrine/Metabolic
- Hyponatremia [3]
- Weight loss [3]

Gastrointestinal/Hepatic
- Abdominal pain [2]
- Constipation [5]
- Diarrhea [3]
- Hepatotoxicity / liver injury / acute liver injury / drug-induced liver injury (DILI) [2]
- Nausea [11]
- Vomiting [5]

Neuromuscular/Skeletal
- Arthralgia [2]
- Asthenia / fatigue [2]
- Back pain [2]

Ocular
- Ocular adverse effect [2]
- Ocular dyskinesia [5]

Other
- Adverse effects / adverse reactions [4]
- Hiccups / singultus [3]

LEVOFLOXACIN

Trade names: Iquix (Santen), Levaquin (Ortho-McNeil), Quixin (Johnson & Johnson), Tavanic (Sanofi-Aventis)

Indications: Various infections caused by susceptible organisms, inhalational anthrax (post exposure)

Class: Antibiotic, Antibiotic; fluoroquinolone, Antibiotic; quinolone, Antimicrobial, Drug-resistant antituberculosis agent

Half-life: 6–8 hours

Clinically important, potentially hazardous interactions with: alfuzosin, aminophylline, amiodarone, antacids, antidiabetics, arsenic, artemether/lumefantrine, BCG vaccine, chloroquine, ciprofloxacin, corticosteroids, cyclosporine, didanosine, dronedarone, gadobutrol, insulin, lanthanum, mycophenolate, nilotinib, NSAIDs, oral iron, oral typhoid vaccine, phenindione, pimozide, probenecid, QT prolonging agents, quinine, strontium ranelate, sucralfate, sulfonylureas, tetrabenazine, thioridazine, vitamin K antagonists, warfarin, zinc, ziprasidone, zolmitriptan

Important contra-indications noted in the prescribing guidelines for: the elderly; nursing mothers

Note: Fluoroquinolones are associated with an increased risk of tendinitis and tendon rupture in all ages. This risk is further increased in older patients usually over 60 years of age, in patients taking corticosteroid drugs, and in patients with kidney, heart or lung transplants.
Fluoroquinolones may exacerbate muscle weakness in persons with myasthenia gravis.
Levofloxacin is the levo- or (S)-isomer of the racemic form, Ofloxacin. See Ofloxacin for the adverse reactions of the racemic form.

Warning: SERIOUS ADVERSE REACTIONS INCLUDING TENDINITIS, TENDON RUPTURE, PERIPHERAL NEUROPATHY, CENTRIAL NERVOUS SYSTEM EFFECTS and EXACERBATION OF MYASTHENIA GRAVIS

Skin
- AGEP [2]
- Anaphylactoid reactions / anaphylaxis (includes anaphylactic shock) [6]
- DRESS syndrome (Drug-induced hypersensitivity syndrome) [4]
- Erythema [2]
- Erythema nodosum (<3%)
- Exanthems [2]
- Fixed eruption / fixed drug eruption [2]
- Hypersensitivity [5]
- Photosensitivity [3]
- Phototoxicity [5]
- Pruritus (itching) (2%) [3]
- Purpura [3]
- Radiation recall dermatitis [2]
- Rash (2%) [2]
- Stevens-Johnson syndrome and toxic epidermal necrolysis (SJS/TEN) [6]
- Vasculitis (angiitis) / cutaneous vasculitis (angiitis) [3]

Cardiovascular
- Kounis syndrome / allergic angina syndrome / allergic myocardial infarction [2]
- Myocardial infarction [2]
- Palpitation [2]
- QT interval prolonged / QT prolongation [5]
- Torsades de pointes [6]

Central Nervous System
- Anorexia [2]
- Anxiety [2]
- Delirium [6]
- Depression [2]
- Dysgeusia (taste perversion) [2]
- Hallucinations [2]
- Headache (6%) [6]
- Insomnia (4%) [3]
- Peripheral neuropathy [3]
- Psychosis [4]
- Seizures [9]
- Vertigo / dizziness [6]

Endocrine/Metabolic
- ALT increased [3]
- AST increased [3]
- Hypoglycemia [4]

Gastrointestinal/Hepatic
- Abdominal pain [3]
- Constipation (3%)
- Diarrhea (5%) [4]
- Hepatotoxicity / liver injury / acute liver injury / drug-induced liver injury (DILI) [5]
- Nausea (7%) [6]
- Pancreatitis / acute pancreatitis [4]
- Vomiting [3]

Genitourinary
- Vaginitis (includes vulvitis) (2%)

Hematologic
- Thrombocytopenia / platelets decreased [5]

Neuromuscular/Skeletal
- Arthralgia [5]
- Myalgia/Myopathy [4]
- Myasthenia gravis (exacerbation) [3]
- Rhabdomyolysis [4]
- Tendinitis [2]
- Tendinopathy/Tendon rupture [38]

Renal
- Nephrotoxicity / kidney injury / acute kidney injury (AKI) / drug-induced kidney injury [8]

Other
- Adverse effects / adverse reactions [14]
- Death [5]
- Side effects [2]

LEVOLEUCOVORIN

Trade names: Fusilev (Spectrum), Isovorin (Pfizer)
Indications: Antidote for folic acid antagonists, various cancers in combination with other medications
Class: Antidote, Chemotherapy modulating agent, Folate analogue
Half-life: 4–8 hours
Clinically important, potentially hazardous interactions with: trimethoprim
Important contra-indications noted in the prescribing guidelines for: nursing mothers
Note: As an antidote, it is difficult to differentiate side effects due to the drug from those due to the effects of the poison.

Hematologic
Neutropenia (neutrophils decreased) [2]

LEVOMEPROMAZINE

Synonym: methotrimeprazine
Trade name: Nozinan (Sanofi-Aventis)
Indications: Pain, anxiety and distress in people with terminal illness, psychosis, schizophrenia
Class: Antipsychotic, Neuroleptic, Phenothiazine
Half-life: ~20 hours
Clinically important, potentially hazardous interactions with: ACE inhibitors, adrenergic neurone blockers, alcohol, alpha blockers, amantadine, amiodarone, angiotensin II receptor antagonists, antacids, antiarrhythmics prolonging QT interval, antimuscarinics, antiolytics and hypnotics, apomorphine, arsenic, artemether/lumefantrine, atomoxetine, barbiturates, beta blockers, bromocriptine, cabergoline, caffeine, calcium channel blockers, carbamazepine, cimetidine, clonidine, cyclobenzaprine, diazoxide, disopyramide, diuretics, dronedarone, droperidol, duloxetine, efavirenz, ephedrine, eszopiclone, ethosuximide, general anesthetics, histamine, hydralazine, kaolin, levodopa, lithium, lurasidone, memantine, metaxalone, methyldopa, metoclopramide, milnacipran, minoxidil, moxifloxacin, moxonidine, myelosuppressives, nitrates, nitroprusside, opioid analgesics, oxcarbazepine, paliperidone, pentamidine, pergolide, phenytoin, pimozide, pramipexole, primidone, ramelteon, ritonavir, ropinirole, rotigotine, saquinavir, sodium oxybate, sodium phenylbutyrate, sotalol, succinylcholine, sulfonylureas, sympathomimetics, tetrabenazine, tiagabine, tramadol, tricyclic antidepressants, valproic acid
Important contra-indications noted in the prescribing guidelines for: the elderly
Note: Elderly patients with dementia-related psychosis treated with antipsychotic drugs are at an increased risk of death. Nozinan is not indicated for the treatment of patients with dementia-related psychosis.
Contraindicated in cases of coma or CNS depression due to alcohol, hypnotics, analgesics or narcotics; also in patients with blood dyscrasia, hepatic problems or a sensitivity to phenothiazines.
Not available in the USA.

Endocrine/Metabolic
Hyponatremia [2]

LEVOMILNACIPRAN

Trade name: Fetzima (Forest)
Indications: Major depressive disorder
Class: Antidepressant, Serotonin-norepinephrine reuptake inhibitor
Half-life: 12 hours
Clinically important, potentially hazardous interactions with: ketoconazole, MAO inhibitors, NSAIDs
Important contra-indications noted in the prescribing guidelines for: nursing mothers; pediatric patients
Warning: SUICIDAL THOUGHTS AND BEHAVIORS

Skin
Hyperhidrosis (9%) [9]
Pruritus (itching) (<2%)
Rash (2%)
Urticaria / hives (<2%)
Xerosis / xeroderma (<2%)

Mucosal
Xerostomia (dry mouth) [4]

Cardiovascular
Angina (<2%)
Extrasystoles (<2%)
Hypertension (3%) [2]
Hypotension (3%)
Palpitation (5%) [5]
Tachycardia (6%) [9]

Central Nervous System
Aggression (includes anger) (<2%)
Agitation (<2%)
Extrapyramidal symptoms (<2%)
Headache [5]
Insomnia [3]
Migraine (<2%)
Panic attack (<2%)
Paresthesias (<2%)
Syncope / fainting (<2%)
Vertigo / dizziness [4]
Yawning (<2%)

Endocrine/Metabolic
Appetite decreased (3%)

Gastrointestinal/Hepatic
Abdominal pain (<2%)
Constipation (9%) [9]
Flatulence (<2%)
Nausea (17%) [10]
Vomiting (5%) [5]

Genitourinary
Ejaculatory dysfunction (5%) [4]
Erectile dysfunction (6%) [7]
Hematuria (<2%)
Pollakiuria (<2%)
Testicular pain / orchialgia / orchidalgia (4%)
Urinary hesitancy (4%) [3]

Ocular
Conjunctival hemorrhage (<2%)
Vision blurred (<2%)
Xerophthalmia (dry eyes) (<2%)

Renal
Proteinuria (<2%)

Respiratory
Upper respiratory tract infection [2]

Other
Adverse effects / adverse reactions [2]
Bruxism (teeth grinding) (<2%)

LEVONORGESTREL

Trade names: Kyleena (Bayer), Mirena (Bayer), Plan B (Duramed)
Indications: Intrauterine contraception, treatment of heavy menstrual bleeding, emergency contraception
Class: Hormone, Progestogen
Half-life: 17 hours
Clinically important, potentially hazardous interactions with: barbiturates, bosentan, carbamazepine, CYP3A4 inducers and inhibitors, efavirenz, felbamate, griseofulvin, nevirapine, oxcarbazepine, phenytoin, rifabutin, rifampin, St John's wort, topiramate, ulipristal
Important contra-indications noted in the prescribing guidelines for: the elderly; nursing mothers; pediatric patients

Skin
Acneiform eruption / acneiform dermatitis / acneiform rash [2]

Central Nervous System
Headache (17%) [8]
Vertigo / dizziness (11%)

Endocrine/Metabolic
Amenorrhea [3]
Mastodynia (11%) [2]
Menstrual irregularities (26%) [7]
Weight gain [2]

Gastrointestinal/Hepatic
Abdominal pain (18%)
Diarrhea (5%)
Nausea (23%) [8]
Vomiting (6%) [3]

Genitourinary
Dysmenorrhea [2]
Metrorrhagia [2]
Vaginal bleeding [4]

Neuromuscular/Skeletal
Asthenia / fatigue (17%)

Other
Adverse effects / adverse reactions [3]

LEVOTHYROXINE

Synonyms: L-thyroxine sodium; T_4
Trade names: Levothyroid (Forest), Levoxyl (Monarch), Synthroid (AbbVie), Unithroid (Watson)
Indications: Hypothyroidism
Class: Thyroid hormone, synthetic
Half-life: 6–7 days
Clinically important, potentially hazardous interactions with: colesevelam, dicumarol, lanthanum, oral anticoagulants, orlistat, propranolol, raloxifene, red rice yeast, ritonavir, warfarin

Skin
Angioedema (formerly named angioneurotic edema) [2]
Urticaria / hives [3]

Cardiovascular
Circulatory collapse [2]

Central Nervous System
Restless legs syndrome / Willis-Ekbom disease (includes restless arms syndrome variant) [2]

Endocrine/Metabolic
Thyrotoxicosis [3]
Gastrointestinal/Hepatic
Hepatic (liver) disorder / hepatobiliary disorder / hepatic (liver) dysfunction [2]
Neuromuscular/Skeletal
Bone loss / bone disorder [2]
Fractures [2]
Other
Adverse effects / adverse reactions [2]
Side effects [2]

LICORICE

Family: Fabaceae; Leguminosae
Scientific names: *Glycyrrhiza glabra, Glycyrrhiza uralensis*
Indications: Upper respiratory tract infection, gastric and duodenal ulcers, bronchitis, colic, dry cough, arthritis, lupus, sore throat, malaria, sores, abscesses, contact dermatitis. Flavoring in foods, beverages and tobacco
Class: Anti-inflammatory
Half-life: N/A
Clinically important, potentially hazardous interactions with: alclometasone, cascara, clevidipine, squill

---

Skin
Edema / fluid retention [2]
Cardiovascular
Hypertension [10]
Torsades de pointes [3]
Endocrine/Metabolic
Hypokalemia [5]
Mineralocorticoid excess / apparent mineralocorticoid excess [3]
Neuromuscular/Skeletal
Rhabdomyolysis [22]
Ocular
Ocular adverse effect [2]
Other
Adverse effects / adverse reactions [2]

LIDOCAINE

Synonyms: lignocaine; xylocaine
Trade names: Anamantle HC (Doak), ELA-Max (Ferndale), EMLA (AstraZeneca), Lidoderm (Endo), Xylocaine (AstraZeneca)
Indications: Ventricular arrhythmias, topical anesthesia
Class: Anesthetic; local, Antiarrhythmic, Antiarrhythmic class Ib
Half-life: terminal: 1.5–2 hours
Clinically important, potentially hazardous interactions with: amiodarone, amprenavir, antiarrhythmics, atazanavir, cimetidine, cobicistat/elvitegravir/emtricitabine/tenofovir alafenamide, cobicistat/elvitegravir/emtricitabine/tenofovir disoproxil, darunavir, delavirdine, fosamprenavir, indinavir, lopinavir, mivacurium, nevirapine, nilutamide, oxprenolol, propranolol, telaprevir
Important contra-indications noted in the prescribing guidelines for: nursing mothers; pediatric patients

---

Skin
Anaphylactoid reactions / anaphylaxis (includes anaphylactic shock) [7]
Angioedema (formerly named angioneurotic edema) [3]
Cutaneous toxicity / skin toxicity [3]
Dermatitis [27]
Eczema / eczematous reaction / eczematous eruption [3]
Edema / fluid retention [2]
Erythema [3]
Erythema multiforme [2]
Exanthems [2]
Exfoliative dermatitis [2]
Fixed eruption / fixed drug eruption [2]
Hypersensitivity [9]
Pruritus (itching) [3]
Urticaria / hives [5]
Cardiovascular
Bradycardia / sinus bradycardia [2]
Central Nervous System
Paresthesias [2]
Seizures [14]
Shivering (<10%)
Hematologic
Methemoglobinemia [4]
Local
Application-site erythema [2]
Application-site reactions [3]
Injection-site pain [2]
Otic
Tinnitus [3]
Other
Adverse effects / adverse reactions [3]
Death [3]
Hoigne's syndrome [2]

LINACLOTIDE

Trade name: Linzess (Forest)
Indications: Irritable bowel syndrome with constipation and chronic idiopathic constipation
Class: Amino acid, Guanylate cyclase-C agonist
Half-life: N/A
Clinically important, potentially hazardous interactions with: none known
Important contra-indications noted in the prescribing guidelines for: nursing mothers; pediatric patients
Note: Contra-indicated in patients with known or suspected mechanical gastrointestinal obstruction.
Warning: PEDIATRIC RISK

Central Nervous System
Headache (4%)
Gastrointestinal/Hepatic
Abdominal distension (2–3%)
Abdominal pain (7%) [4]
Diarrhea (16–20%) [26]
Dyspepsia / functional dyspepsia (indigestion) (see also gastroparesis) (<2%)
Flatulence (4–6%) [4]
Gastroenteritis (3%)
Gastroesophageal reflux (<2%)
Vomiting (<2%)
Neuromuscular/Skeletal
Asthenia / fatigue (<2%)
Respiratory
Sinusitis (see also rhinitis / rhinosinusitis) (3%)
Upper respiratory tract infection (5%)

LINAGLIPTIN

Trade names: Glyxambi (Boehringer Ingelheim), Tradjenta (Boehringer Ingelheim)
Indications: Type II diabetes mellitus
Class: Antidiabetic, Dipeptidyl peptidase-4 (DPP-4) (gliptin) inhibitor
Half-life: 12 hours
Clinically important, potentially hazardous interactions with: efavirenz, rifampin
Important contra-indications noted in the prescribing guidelines for: nursing mothers; pediatric patients
Note: Linagliptin should not be used in patients with Type I diabetes or for the treatment of diabetic ketoacidosis, and has not been studied in combination with insulin. Glyxambi is linagliptin and empagliflozin.

Cardiovascular
Cardiotoxicity [3]
Hypertension [4]
Central Nervous System
Headache [5]
Endocrine/Metabolic
Diabetes mellitus [2]
Hyperglycemia (includes glucose increased) [2]
Hyperlipidemia / lipids elevated [2]
Hypertriglyceridemia (includes triglycerides increased) [2]
Hypoglycemia [18]
Gastrointestinal/Hepatic
Constipation [2]
Diarrhea [2]
Nausea [3]
Pancreatitis / acute pancreatitis [4]
Genitourinary
Genital mycotic infection [2]
Urinary tract infection [4]
Neuromuscular/Skeletal
Arthralgia [2]
Back pain [3]
Pain in extremities [2]
Respiratory
Cough [4]
Nasopharyngitis [9]
Upper respiratory tract infection [6]
Other
Adverse effects / adverse reactions [19]
Infection [3]

LINCOMYCIN

Trade name: Lincocin (Pfizer)
Indications: Various infections caused by susceptible organisms
Class: Antibiotic, Antibiotic; lincosamide, Antimicrobial
Half-life: 2–11.5 hours
Clinically important, potentially hazardous interactions with: mivacurium
Important contra-indications noted in the prescribing guidelines for: nursing mothers; pediatric patients

---

Skin
AGEP [3]
Dermatitis [2]
Stevens-Johnson syndrome and toxic epidermal necrolysis (SJS/TEN) [2]

Other
Allergic reactions (<5%)

LINEZOLID

Trade name: Zyvox (Pfizer)
Indications: Various infections caused by susceptible organisms
Class: Antibiotic, Antibiotic; oxazolidinone, Antimicrobial
Half-life: 4–5 hours
Clinically important, potentially hazardous interactions with: alcohol, alpha blockers, altretamine, amitriptyline, amoxapine, amphetamines, anilidopiperidine opioids, antihypertensives, atomoxetine, beta blockers, buprenorphine, bupropion, buspirone, caffeine, carbamazepine, clomipramine, cyclobenzaprine, desipramine, desvenlafaxine, dexmethylphenidate, dextromethorphan, diethylpropion, doxapram, doxepin, fluoxetine, fluvoxamine, hydromorphone, imipramine, levodopa, lithium, MAO inhibitors, maprotiline, meperidine, methadone, methyldopa, methylphenidate, mirtazapine, nortriptyline, oral typhoid vaccine, ozanimod, paroxetine hydrochloride, paroxetine mesylate, paroxetine mesylate, propoxyphene, protriptyline, reserpine, rifampin, safinamide, serotonin 5-HT1D receptor agonists, serotonin/norepinephrine reuptake inhibitors, sertraline, sibutramine, SSRIs, tapentadol, tetrabenazine, tetrahydrozoline, tramadol, trazodone, tricyclic antidepressants, trimipramine, tryptophan, venlafaxine
Important contra-indications noted in the prescribing guidelines for: nursing mothers

---

Skin
Cellulitis and pseudocellulitis [2]
Cutaneous adverse reaction (includes severe cutaneous adverse drug reaction (SCAR)) [2]
Edema / fluid retention (2%)
Fungal dermatitis (2%)
Pruritus (itching) [2]
Rash (<7%) [4]
Stevens-Johnson syndrome and toxic epidermal necrolysis (SJS/TEN) [2]

Mucosal
Black tongue / black hairy tongue (lingua villosa nigra) [13]

Central Nervous System
Dysgeusia (taste perversion) (<2%) [2]
Encephalopathy (includes hepatic encephalopathy) [2]
Fever (pyrexia) (includes hyperpyrexia) (2–14%)
Headache (<11%) [6]
Insomnia (3%)
Leukoencephalopathy / posterior reversible encephalopathy syndrome (PRES) [2]
Neurotoxicity [5]
Peripheral neuropathy [19]
Seizures (3%)
Serotonin syndrome [27]
Vertigo / dizziness (2%)

Endocrine/Metabolic
Acidosis (includes lactic acidosis) [39]
ALP increased (<4%)
ALT increased (2–10%)
AST increased (2–5%)
Hyperlactatemia [3]
Hypoglycemia [6]
Hypokalemia (3%)
Hyponatremia [6]
SIADH [3]

Gastrointestinal/Hepatic
Abdominal pain (<2%)
Constipation (2%) [2]
Diarrhea (3–11%) [12]
Gastrointestinal bleeding (2%)
Gastrointestinal disorder / discomfort [3]
Hepatotoxicity / liver injury / acute liver injury / drug-induced liver injury (DILI) [2]
Loose stools / soft feces (<2%)
Nausea (3–10%) [11]
Pancreatitis / acute pancreatitis [4]
Vomiting (<10%) [5]

Genitourinary
Candidal vaginitis (<2%)

Hematologic
Anemia (<6%) [14]
Hemoglobin decreased [2]
Hemotoxicity [2]
Leukocytopenia (leukopenia) / leukocytes (white blood cells) decreased [4]
Myelosuppression / bone marrow suppression / myelotoxicity [13]
Pancytopenia (includes bicytopenia) [9]
Pure red cell aplasia [6]
Sepsis (8%)
Sideroblastic anemia / acquired sideroblastic anemia [2]
Thrombocytopenia / platelets decreased (<5%) [38]

Local
Injection-site reaction (3%)

Ocular
Optic neuropathy [19]

Renal
Nephrotoxicity / kidney injury / acute kidney injury (AKI) / drug-induced kidney injury [2]
Renal function abnormal / renal dysfunction [2]

Respiratory
Apnea (2%)
Cough (<2%)
Dyspnea / shortness of breath (3%)
Pneumonia (3%)
Upper respiratory tract infection (4%)

Other
Adverse effects / adverse reactions (4%) [18]
Allergic reactions (4%)
Death [6]
Tooth pigmentation / discoloration [7]

LINSEED

Family: Linaceae
Scientific name: *Linum usitatissimum*
Indications: Dry mouth, menopause, osteoporosis, heart disease, catarrh, bronchitis, furunculosis, pleuritic pains, constipation, high cholesterol, benign prostatic hyperplasia, bladder inflammation, gastritis, enteritis, irritable bowel syndrome. **Topical:** poultice for skin inflammation. **Ophthalmologic:** oil used for removal of foreign bodies from the eye
Class: Anti-inflammatory
Half-life: N/A
Clinically important, potentially hazardous interactions with: none known
Note: Linum is cultivated for both its stem fibers (the source of linen and some paper) and its seeds (oil used in cooking and in margarine). The oil is used in paints and varnishes and the seed residues are used in cattle cake.

Skin
Anaphylactoid reactions / anaphylaxis (includes anaphylactic shock) [3]

LIOTHYRONINE

Synonym: T_3 sodium
Trade names: Cytomel (Pfizer), Triostat (Par)
Indications: Hypothyroidism
Class: Thyroid hormone, synthetic
Half-life: 16–49 hours
Clinically important, potentially hazardous interactions with: anticoagulants, dicumarol, warfarin

---

Skin
Urticaria / hives [3]

LIRAGLUTIDE

Trade names: Saxenda (Novo Nordisk), Victoza (Novo Nordisk), Xultophy (Novo Nordisk)
Indications: To improve glycemic control in adults with Type II diabetes mellitus (Victoza). Adjunct for the treatment of obesity and for weight loss management in defined populations and health conditions (Saxenda).

Class: Anti-obesity / weight loss pharmacotherapy, Antidiabetic, Glucagon-like peptide-1 (GLP-1) receptor agonist
Half-life: 13 hours
Clinically important, potentially hazardous interactions with: acetaminophen, atorvastatin, digoxin, griseofulvin, lisinopril, warfarin
Important contra-indications noted in the prescribing guidelines for: nursing mothers; pediatric patients
Note: Contra-indicated in patients with a personal or family history of medullary thyroid carcinoma or in patients with multiple endocrine neoplasia syndrome Type 2. Xultophy is liraglutide and insulin degludec.
Warning: RISK OF THYROID C-CELL TUMORS

Skin
Hypersensitivity [4]

Cardiovascular
Cardiotoxicity [2]
Hypertension (3%)

Central Nervous System
Headache (~5%) [8]
Vertigo / dizziness (6%) [3]

Endocrine/Metabolic
Appetite decreased [7]
Hypoglycemia [12]
Weight loss [6]

Gastrointestinal/Hepatic
Abdominal distension [2]
Abdominal pain [4]
Cholelithiasis (gallstones in the gall bladder or the bile duct) [3]
Constipation (10%) [13]
Diarrhea (17%) [33]

Dyspepsia / functional dyspepsia (indigestion) (see also gastroparesis) [5]
Gastrointestinal disorder / discomfort [8]
Nausea (28%) [65]
Pancreatitis / acute pancreatitis [14]
Vomiting (11%) [32]

Genitourinary
Urinary tract infection (6%)

Local
Injection-site reaction (2%) [4]

Neuromuscular/Skeletal
Arthralgia [2]
Asthenia / fatigue [4]
Back pain (5%) [4]

Renal
Nephrotoxicity / kidney injury / acute kidney injury (AKI) / drug-induced kidney injury [2]

Respiratory
Influenza (7%) [2]
Nasopharyngitis (5%) [6]
Sinusitis (see also rhinitis / rhinosinusitis) (6%)
Upper respiratory tract infection (10%) [4]

Other
Adverse effects / adverse reactions [16]
Malignant neoplasms (11%)

LISDEXAMFETAMINE

Trade name: Vyvanse (Shire)
Indications: Attention-deficit hyperactivity disorder (ADHD)
Class: Anti-attention deficit hyperactivity disorder (anti-ADHD), CNS stimulant, Dextroamphetamine prodrug
Half-life: 1 hour
Clinically important, potentially hazardous interactions with: acetazolamide, ammonium chloride, analgesics, antacids, antihistamines, antihypertensives, antipsychotics, atomoxetine, cannabinoids, carbonic anhydrase inhibitors, chlorpromazine, epinephrine, ethosuximide, haloperidol, iobenguane, lithium, MAO inhibitors, meperidine, methenamine, phenobarbital, phenytoin, propoxyphene, sympathomimetics, tricyclic antidepressants, urinary alkalinizing agents
Important contra-indications noted in the prescribing guidelines for: nursing mothers; pediatric patients
Warning: ABUSE AND DEPENDENCE

Skin
Hyperhidrosis (3%)
Rash (3%)

Mucosal
Xerostomia (dry mouth) (4–26%) [23]

Cardiovascular
Hypertension (3%) [2]
Tachycardia [3]

Central Nervous System
Agitation (3%)
Anorexia (5%) [3]
Anxiety [9]
Fever (pyrexia) (includes hyperpyrexia) (2%)
Headache [32]
Insomnia (13–23%) [31]
Irritability (10%) [21]
Restlessness (3%)
Sleep-related disorder [2]
Somnolence (drowsiness) (2%) [2]
Tic disorder (2%) [2]
Vertigo / dizziness (5%) [6]

Endocrine/Metabolic
Appetite decreased (27–39%) [31]
Libido decreased (<2%)
Weight loss (9%) [9]

Gastrointestinal/Hepatic
Abdominal pain (12%) [12]
Constipation [2]
Diarrhea (7%)
Nausea (6–7%) [10]
Vomiting (9%) [3]

Genitourinary
Erectile dysfunction (<2%)

Neuromuscular/Skeletal
Asthenia / fatigue [3]
Back pain [2]
Muscle spasm [2]

Respiratory
Dyspnea / shortness of breath (2%)
Influenza [2]
Nasopharyngitis [6]
Sinusitis (see also rhinitis / rhinosinusitis) [2]
Upper respiratory tract infection [12]

Other
Adverse effects / adverse reactions [6]

LISINOPRIL

Trade names: Prinivil (Merck), Prinzide (Merck), Zestoretic (AstraZeneca), Zestril (AstraZeneca)
Indications: Hypertension, as adjunctive therapy in the management of heart failure, short-term treatment following myocardial infarction in hemodynamically stable patients
Class: Angiotensin-converting enzyme (ACE) inhibitor
Half-life: 12 hours
Clinically important, potentially hazardous interactions with: alcohol, aldesleukin, allopurinol, alpha blockers, alprostadil, amifostine, amiloride, angiotensin II receptor antagonists, antacids, antidiabetics, antihypertensives, antipsychotics, anxiolytics and hypnotics, aprotinin, azathioprine, baclofen, beta blockers, calcium channel blockers, clonidine, corticosteroids, cyclosporine, diazoxide, diuretics, eplerenone, estrogens, everolimus, general anesthetics, gold & gold compounds, heparins, hydralazine, hypotensives, insulin, levodopa, liraglutide, lithium, MAO inhibitors, metformin, methyldopa, methylphenidate, minoxidil, moxisylyte, moxonidine, nitrates, nitroprusside, NSAIDs, pentoxifylline, phosphodiesterase 5 inhibitors, potassium salts, prostacyclin analogues, rituximab, salicylates, sirolimus, spironolactone, sulfonylureas, temsirolimus, tizanidine, tolvaptan, triamterene, trimethoprim, yohimbine
Pregnancy category: category C in first trimester; category D in second and third trimesters
Important contra-indications noted in the prescribing guidelines for: nursing mothers; pediatric patients
Note: Prinzide and Zestoretic are lisinopril and hydrochlorothiazide. Hydrochlorothiazide is a sulfonamide and can be absorbed systemically. Sulfonamides can produce severe, possibly fatal, reactions such as toxic epidermal necrolysis and Stevens-Johnson syndrome.
Contra-indicated in patients with a history of angioedema related to previous treatment with an ACE inhibitor and in patients with hereditary or idiopathic angioedema.
Warning: FETAL TOXICITY

Skin
Angioedema (formerly named angioneurotic edema) [44]
Edema of lip [2]
Exanthems (3%) [4]
Exfoliative dermatitis [2]
Flushing / rubefaction [2]
Kaposi's sarcoma [2]
Lichenoid eruption / lichenoid reaction [2]
Pemphigus foliaceus [2]
Pityriasis rosea [2]
Purpura [2]
Rash (2%) [5]
Urticaria / hives [2]

Mucosal
Tongue edema [3]

Cardiovascular
Hypotension (<4%) [3]

Central Nervous System
Headache (4–6%)
Vertigo / dizziness (5–12%)

Endocrine/Metabolic
Hyperkalemia [3]

Gastrointestinal/Hepatic
Hepatotoxicity / liver injury / acute liver injury / drug-induced liver injury (DILI) [2]
Intestinal angioedema [14]
Pancreatitis / acute pancreatitis [16]

Neuromuscular/Skeletal
Asthenia / fatigue (3%)

Respiratory
Cough (4–9%) [15]
Upper respiratory tract infection (<2%)

Other
Death [4]

LITHIUM

Trade names: Eskalith (GSK), Lithobid (Solvay)
Indications: Manic-depressive states
Class: Antipsychotic, Mood stabilizer
Half-life: 18–24 hours
Clinically important, potentially hazardous interactions with: aceclofenac, acemetacin, acetazolamide, acitretin, amitriptyline, arsenic, benazepril, bendroflumethiazide, benzthiazide, captopril, celecoxib, chlorothiazide, chlorthalidone, cilazapril, citalopram, clozapine, cyclopenthiazide, desipramine, desvenlafaxine, dichlorphenamide, diclofenac, enalapril, ethoxzolamide, etoricoxib, fluoxetine, flurbiprofen, fosinopril, haloperidol, hydrochlorothiazide, hydroflumethiazide, indapamide, insulin degludec, insulin detemir, insulin glargine, insulin glulisine, irbesartan, levomepromazine, linezolid, lisdexamfetamine, lisinopril, lorcaserin, lurasidone, mazindol, mazindol, meloxicam, meperidine, mesoridazine, methyclothiazide, metolazone, metronidazole, milnacipran, neostigmine, olanzapine, olmesartan, paliperidone, paroxetine hydrochloride, pericyazine, phenylbutazone, piroxicam, polythiazide, quinapril, quinethazone, ramipril, rocuronium, rofecoxib, sacubitril/valsartan, sacubitril/valsartan, sibutramine, sulpiride / levosulpiride, tenoxicam, tetrabenazine,

thalidomide, thiazides, tinidazole, tolmetin, trandolapril, trichlormethiazide, trifluoperazine, valdecoxib, venlafaxine, xipamide, ziprasidone, zofenopril, zuclopenthixol

---

Skin
Acneiform eruption / acneiform dermatitis / acneiform rash [21]
Angioedema (formerly named angioneurotic edema) [2]
Atopic dermatitis (3%)
Cutaneous toxicity / skin toxicity [2]
Darier's disease / keratosis follicularis [3]
Dermatitis [4]
Dermatitis herpetiformis [3]
DRESS syndrome (Drug-induced hypersensitivity syndrome) [2]
Edema / fluid retention [3]
Erythema [2]
Exanthems [11]
Exfoliative dermatitis [3]
Follicular keratosis [3]
Folliculitis [5]
Hidradenitis suppurativa (acne inversa) [5]
Ichthyosis [2]
Keratosis pilaris [2]
Linear IgA bullous dermatosis [4]
Lupus erythematosus (subacute cutaneous lupus erythematosus (SCLE)) [5]
Myxedema [10]
Papulo-nodular lesions (elbows) [2]
Pruritus (itching) [9]
Psoriasis (2%) [59]
Purpura [2]
Pustules / pustular eruption [2]
Rash (<10%)
Seborrheic dermatitis [3]
Ulcerations (lower extremities) [5]
Urticaria / hives [3]
Vasculitis (angiitis) / cutaneous vasculitis (angiitis) [4]

Hair
Alopecia / hair loss (10–19%) [18]
Alopecia areata (2%) [3]

Nails
Nail dystrophy [2]

Mucosal
Lichenoid stomatitis [3]
Oral ulceration [4]
Sialorrhea (ptyalism; hypersalivation) [4]
Stomatitis (oral mucositis) [2]
Xerostomia (dry mouth) [6]

Cardiovascular
Atrioventricular block [3]
Bradycardia / sinus bradycardia [11]
Brugada syndrome [5]
QT interval prolonged / QT prolongation [4]
Sinus node dysfunction (sick sinus syndrome) [4]
Takotsubo syndrome [3]

Central Nervous System
Amnesia [2]
Delirium [3]
Dysgeusia (taste perversion) (>10%) [2]
Dyskinesia [2]
Hallucinations [2]
Neuroleptic malignant syndrome [9]
Neurotoxicity [5]
Parkinsonism [8]
Pseudohallucinations [2]
Restless legs syndrome / Willis-Ekbom disease (includes restless arms syndrome variant) [4]
Serotonin syndrome [5]
Somnambulism (sleepwalking; noctambulism) [4]
Tardive syndrome / tardive dyskinesia [5]
Tremor [5]

Endocrine/Metabolic
Diabetes insipidus [6]
Hypercalcemia [4]
Hyperparathyroidism [6]
Hyperthyroidism (includes 'thyroid storm') [2]
Hypothyroidism [5]
Myxedema coma / myxedema crisis [5]
Thyroid dysfunction [2]
Thyrotoxicosis [2]
Weight gain [4]

Genitourinary
Polyuria (includes polyuric syndrome) [3]
Priapism [5]

Neuromuscular/Skeletal
Myasthenia gravis [2]
Rhabdomyolysis [3]

Renal
Minimal change disease (minimal change glomerulopathy) [2]
Nephrogenic diabetes insipidus / arginine vasopressin resistance [9]
Nephropathy [3]
Nephrotic syndrome [2]
Nephrotoxicity / kidney injury / acute kidney injury (AKI) / drug-induced kidney injury [15]

Other
Adverse effects / adverse reactions [6]
Death [2]
Dipsia (thirst) / polydipsia [2]
Side effects (23–33%) [4]
Teratogenicity [3]

LIXISENATIDE

Trade names: Adlyxin (Sanofi-Aventis), Lyxumia (Sanofi-Aventis), Soliqua (Sanofi-Aventis)
Indications: To improve glycemic control in adults with Type II diabetes mellitus
Class: Antidiabetic, Glucagon-like peptide-1 (GLP-1) receptor agonist
Half-life: 3 hours
Clinically important, potentially hazardous interactions with: none known
Pregnancy category: Use during pregnancy only if the potential benefit justifies the potential risk to the fetus
Important contra-indications noted in the prescribing guidelines for: nursing mothers; pediatric patients
Note: Soliqua is lixisenatide and insulin glargine. Repurposed for investigation into the treatment of Parkinson's disease.

Central Nervous System
Headache (9%) [3]
Vertigo / dizziness (7%) [2]

Endocrine/Metabolic
Hypoglycemia (3%) [8]

Gastrointestinal/Hepatic
Abdominal distension (2%)
Abdominal pain (2%)
Constipation (3%)
Diarrhea (8%) [10]
Dyspepsia / functional dyspepsia (indigestion) (see also gastroparesis) (3%)
Nausea (25%) [26]
Vomiting (10%) [25]

Local
Injection-site reaction (4%) [2]

Other
Adverse effects / adverse reactions [3]
Allergic reactions [2]

LOFEXIDINE

Trade names: BritLofex (Britannia), Lucemyra (US WorldMeds, LLC)
Indications: mitigation of opioid withdrawal symptoms to facilitate abrupt opioid discontinuation in adults
Class: Adrenergic alpha2-receptor agonist
Half-life: ~12 hours
Clinically important, potentially hazardous interactions with: methadone, naltrexone
Pregnancy category: The safety of lofexidine in pregnant women has not been established.

Mucosal
Xerostomia (dry mouth) (10–11%) [4]

Cardiovascular
Bradycardia / sinus bradycardia (24–32%) [4]
Hypotension (30%) [9]
Orthostatic hypotension (29–42%) [3]
QT interval prolonged / QT prolongation [2]

Central Nervous System
Insomnia (51–55%) [2]
Sedation (12–13%) [5]
Somnolence (drowsiness) (11–13%) [4]
Syncope / fainting (<5%)
Vertigo / dizziness (19–23%) [3]

Otic
Tinnitus (<5%)

Other
Adverse effects / adverse reactions [2]

LOMITAPIDE

Trade name: Juxtapid (Aegerion)
Indications: Homozygous familial hypercholesterolemia
Class: Lipid regulator
Half-life: 39.7 hours
Clinically important, potentially hazardous interactions with: bile acid sequestrants, boceprevir, clarithromycin, conivaptan, grapefruit juice, indinavir, itraconazole, ketoconazole, lopinavir, lovastatin, mibefradil, nefazodone, nelfinavir, oral contraceptives, P-glycoprotein substrates, posaconazole, ritonavir, saquinavir, simvastatin, strong or moderate CYP3A4 inhibitors, telaprevir, telithromycin, viloxazine, voriconazole, warfarin
Important contra-indications noted in the prescribing guidelines for: nursing mothers; pediatric patients
Warning: RISK OF HEPATOTOXICITY

Mucosal
Nasal congestion (10%)

Cardiovascular
Angina (10%)
Chest pain (24%)
Palpitation (10%)

Central Nervous System
Fever (pyrexia) (includes hyperpyrexia) (10%)

Headache (10%)
Vertigo / dizziness (10%)

Endocrine/Metabolic
ALT increased (17%) [3]
Weight loss (24%)

Gastrointestinal/Hepatic
Abdominal pain (21–34%)
Constipation (21%)
Defecation (urgency) (10%)
Diarrhea (79%) [3]
Dyspepsia / functional dyspepsia (indigestion) (see also gastroparesis) (38%) [3]
Flatulence (21%)
Gastroenteritis (14%)
Gastroesophageal reflux (10%)
Gastrointestinal adverse reaction [2]
Hepatotoxicity / liver injury / acute liver injury / drug-induced liver injury (DILI) [6]
Nausea (65%) [2]
Tenesmus (10%)
Vomiting (34%) [3]

Neuromuscular/Skeletal
Asthenia / fatigue (17%)
Back pain (14%)

Respiratory
Influenza (21%)
Nasopharyngitis (17%)
Pharyngolaryngeal pain (14%)

Other
Adverse effects / adverse reactions [6]

LOMUSTINE

Trade name: CeeNU (Bristol-Myers Squibb)
Indications: Brain tumors, lymphomas, melanoma, Hodgkin's disease
Class: Alkylating agent, Nitrosourea
Half-life: 16–48 hours
Clinically important, potentially hazardous interactions with: aldesleukin, cimetidine, clozapine, digoxin, phenytoin
Important contra-indications noted in the prescribing guidelines for: the elderly; nursing mothers

---

Skin
Rash (<10%)

Mucosal
Stomatitis (oral mucositis) (<10%)

Cardiovascular
Hypertension [2]

Gastrointestinal/Hepatic
Hepatotoxicity / liver injury / acute liver injury / drug-induced liver injury (DILI) [2]
Vomiting [2]

Hematologic
Hemotoxicity [2]
Neutropenia (neutrophils decreased) [3]
Thrombocytopenia / platelets decreased [3]

Neuromuscular/Skeletal
Asthenia / fatigue [2]

LONAFARNIB

Trade name: Zokinvy (Eiger Biopharmaceuticals)
Indications: Reduction of the risk of mortality in Hutchinson-Gilford Progeria Syndrome. For treatment of processing-deficient Progeroid Laminopathies with *either* heterozygous LMNA mutation with progerin-like protein accumulation *or* homozygous or compound heterozygous *ZMPSTE24* mutations.

Class: Farnesyltransferase inhibitor
Half-life: approximately 4–6 hours
Clinically important, potentially hazardous interactions with: atorvastatin, CYP2C9 inhibitors, CYP3A inducers, CYP3A inhibitors, grapefruit juice, loperamide, lovastatin, midazolam, simvastatin
Pregnancy category: Can cause fetal harm. Advise females of reproductive potential of the risk to a fetus and to use effective contraception.
Note: Based on animal studies, may impair fertility. Advise females and males of the adverse reproductive potential of lonafarnib.

Skin
Pruritus (itching) (8%)
Rash (11%)

Mucosal
Epistaxis (nosebleed) (21%)
Mucositis (8%)

Cardiovascular
Hypertension (29%)

Central Nervous System
Cerebral ischemia (11%)
Depression (5%)
Fever (pyrexia) (includes hyperpyrexia) (14%)
Headache (37%)

Endocrine/Metabolic
ALT increased (27%)
Appetite decreased (53%)
AST increased (35%)
Bicarbonate decreased (33%)
Dehydration (5%)
Electrolyte imbalance / electrolyte disorder / electrolyte abnormalities / dyselectrolytemia (43%)
Weight loss (37%)

Gastrointestinal/Hepatic
Abdominal pain (48%)
Constipation (22%)
Diarrhea (81%)
Flatulence (6%)
Nausea (56%)
Vomiting (90%)

Hematologic
Myelosuppression / bone marrow suppression / myelotoxicity (35%)

Neuromuscular/Skeletal
Asthenia / fatigue (51%)
Musculoskeletal pain (48%)

Ocular
Ocular adverse effect (24%)

Respiratory
Cough (33%)
Rhinitis / rhinosinusitis (see also sinusitis) (19%)
Upper respiratory tract infection (51%)

Other
Infection (78%)

LONCASTUXIMAB TESIRINE

Trade name: Zynlonta (ADC Therapeutics)
Indications: Treatment of relapsed or refractory large B-cell lymphoma
Class: Alkylating agent, Antibody-drug conjugate (ADC), Biologic, CD19-directed antibody-drug conjugate, Monoclonal antibody
Half-life: 21 days
Clinically important, potentially hazardous interactions with: none known
Pregnancy category: Can cause fetal harm when administered to pregnant women. Pregnancy testing is recommended for females of reproductive potential prior to initiating treatment. Advise women of reproductive potential to use effective contraception during treatment and for 9 months after the last dose.
Important contra-indications noted in the prescribing guidelines for: nursing mothers
Note: Loncastuximab tesirine is approved under accelerated approval based on overall response rate. Continued approval may be contingent upon verification and description of clinical benefit in a confirmatory trial(s). Loncastuximab tesirine is a CD19-directed antibody and alkylating agent conjugate consisting of a humanized IgG1 kappa monoclonal antibody conjugated to SG3199, a pyrrolobenzodiazepine dimer cytotoxic alkylating agent, through a protease-cleavable valine-alanine linker. Treatment-emergent adverse events considered likely to be related to the pyrrolobenzodiazepine moiety include pleural effusion, adverse skin reactions and elevated liver enzymes. Loncastuximab tesirine-lpvl is biosimiar.

Skin
Edema / fluid retention (28%)
Photosensitivity (10%)
Pigmentation (Skin) (includes hyperpigmentation) (4%)
Pruritus (itching) (12%)
Rash (30%)

Cardiovascular
Pericardial effusion (3%)

Endocrine/Metabolic
ALT increased (34%)
Appetite decreased (15%)
AST increased (41%)
GGT increased (21% grade 3/4) (57%)
Hyperglycemia (includes glucose increased) (8% grade 3/4) (48%)
Hypoalbuminemia / albumin decreased (37%)

Gastrointestinal/Hepatic
Abdominal pain (14%)
Constipation (12%)
Diarrhea (17%)
Nausea (23%)
Vomiting (13%)

Hematologic
Febrile neutropenia (3%)
Hemoglobin decreased (10% grade 3/4) (51%)
Neutropenia (neutrophils decreased) (30% grade 3/4) (52%)
Sepsis (2%)

Neuromuscular/Skeletal
Asthenia / fatigue (38%)
Musculoskeletal pain (23%)

Respiratory
Dyspnea / shortness of breath (13%)
Pleural effusion (10%)
Pneumonia (5%)
Upper respiratory tract infection (10%)

LOPERAMIDE

Trade names: Imodium (McNeil), Maalox (Novartis)
Indications: Diarrhea
Class: Opiate agonist
Half-life: 9–14 hours
Clinically important, potentially hazardous interactions with: lonafarnib, St John's wort
Important contra-indications noted in the prescribing guidelines for: nursing mothers; pediatric patients

---

Cardiovascular
Torsades de pointes [2]
Central Nervous System
Syncope / fainting [2]
Gastrointestinal/Hepatic
Abdominal pain [2]
Constipation [3]
Nausea [2]
Pancreatitis / acute pancreatitis [4]

LOPINAVIR

Trade name: Kaletra (AbbVie)
Indications: HIV-1 infected children above the age of 2 years and adults, in combination with other antiretroviral agents
Class: Antiretroviral, Covid-19 putative drug, HIV-1 protease inhibitor
Half-life: 5–6 hours
Clinically important, potentially hazardous interactions with: abacavir, alfuzosin, amiodarone, amprenavir, aripiprazole, artemether/lumefantrine, atazanavir, atorvastatin, atovaquone, bepridil, bosentan, brigatinib, bupropion, cabozantinib, carbamazepine, chlorpheniramine, cisapride, clarithromycin, colchicine, copanlisib, cyclosporine, darifenacin, darunavir, dasatinib, delavirdine, dexamethasone, didanosine, digoxin, disulfiram, efavirenz, elbasvir & grazoprevir, eltrombopag, eluxadoline, ergotamine, estradiol, felodipine, fentanyl, flecainide, fluticasone propionate, fosamprenavir, glecaprevir & pibrentasvir, indinavir, itraconazole, ketoconazole, lidocaine, lidocaine, lomitapide, lovastatin, maraviroc, methadone, methylergonovine, metronidazole, midazolam, midostaurin, mifepristone, nelfinavir, neratinib, nevirapine, nicardipine, nifedipine, nilotinib, olaparib, ombitasvir/paritaprevir/ritonavir, palbociclib, phenobarbital, phenytoin, pimozide, pitavastatin, ponatinib, primidone, quinidine, ranolazine, ribociclib, rifabutin, rifampin, rilpivirine, rivaroxaban, rosuvastatin, ruxolitinib, salmeterol, saquinavir, sildenafil, simeprevir, simvastatin, sirolimus, sofosbuvir/velpatasvir/voxilaprevir, St John's wort, tacrolimus, tadalafil, telithromycin, tenofovir disoproxil, tipranavir, tolterodine, trazodone, triazolam, vardenafil, venetoclax, vinblastine, vincristine, voriconazole, warfarin, zidovudine
Important contra-indications noted in the prescribing guidelines for: nursing mothers
Note: Kaletra is lopinavir and ritonavir.

Skin
Acneiform eruption / acneiform dermatitis / acneiform rash (<10%)
Lipodystrophy / acquired generalized lipodystrophy (<10%)
Rash (<10%) [5]
Hair
Alopecia / hair loss [3]
Central Nervous System
Vertigo / dizziness [2]
Gastrointestinal/Hepatic
Diarrhea (>10%) [5]
Flatulence (<10%)
Nausea (<10%) [4]
Pancreatitis / acute pancreatitis [2]
Vomiting (<10%) [3]
Neuromuscular/Skeletal
Asthenia / fatigue (<10%) [2]
Renal
Nephrolithiasis (kidney stones / renal calculi) [2]
Nephrotoxicity / kidney injury / acute kidney injury (AKI) / drug-induced kidney injury [3]

LORACARBEF

Trade name: Lorabid (Monarch)
Indications: Various infections caused by susceptible organisms
Class: Antibiotic, Antimicrobial, Cephalosporin, Cephalosporin; 2nd generation
Half-life: 1 hour
Clinically important, potentially hazardous interactions with: none known
Note: Penicillin and cephalosporins share a common beta-lactam structure. People who are allergic to penicillin are approximately 4 times more likely to develop an allergic reaction to a cephalosporin than those people who have no penicillin allergy. (From 5–16% of patients allergic to penicillin develop allergic reactions to cephalosporins).

Skin
Rash [3]
Central Nervous System
Headache [7]

LORATADINE

Trade names: Alavert (Wyeth), Claritin (Schering), Claritin-D (Schering)
Indications: Allergic rhinitis, urticaria
Class: Histamine H1 receptor antagonist
Half-life: 3–20 hours
Clinically important, potentially hazardous interactions with: amiodarone

---

Skin
Anaphylactoid reactions / anaphylaxis (includes anaphylactic shock) (>2%)
Angioedema (formerly named angioneurotic edema) (>2%)
Dermatitis (>2%)
Diaphoresis (>2%)
Erythema multiforme (>2%)
Fixed eruption / fixed drug eruption [3]
Flushing / rubefaction (>2%)
Peripheral edema (>2%)
Photosensitivity (>2%)
Pruritus (itching) (>2%)
Purpura (>2%)
Rash (>2%)
Urticaria / hives (>2%) [4]
Xerosis / xeroderma (>2%)
Hair
Alopecia / hair loss (>2%)
Dry hair (>2%)
Mucosal
Sialorrhea (ptyalism; hypersalivation) (>2%)
Stomatitis (oral mucositis) (>2%)
Xerostomia (dry mouth) (>10%) [9]
Cardiovascular
QT interval prolonged / QT prolongation [2]
Torsades de pointes [4]
Central Nervous System
Dysgeusia (taste perversion) (>2%)
Headache (12%) [3]
Hyperesthesia (>2%)
Paresthesias (>2%)
Somnolence (drowsiness) [2]
Endocrine/Metabolic
Gynecomastia (>2%)
Mastodynia (<10%)
Genitourinary
Vaginitis (includes vulvitis) (>2%)
Neuromuscular/Skeletal
Asthenia / fatigue (4%) [2]
Myalgia/Myopathy (>2%)
Respiratory
Pharyngitis (sore throat) [2]

LORAZEPAM

Trade name: Ativan (Valeant)
Indications: Anxiety, depression
Class: Benzodiazepine
Half-life: 10–20 hours
Clinically important, potentially hazardous interactions with: alcohol, amprenavir, barbiturates, chlorpheniramine, clarithromycin, clozapine, CNS depressants, cobicistat/elvitegravir/emtricitabine/tenofovir alafenamide, efavirenz, erythromycin, esomeprazole, eszopiclone, imatinib, MAO inhibitors, narcotics, nelfinavir, phenothiazines, valproate

---

Skin
Dermatitis (<10%)
Diaphoresis (>10%)
Pseudolymphoma / cutaneous pseudolymphoma [2]
Rash (>10%)
Mucosal
Nasal congestion (<10%)
Sialopenia (>10%)
Xerostomia (dry mouth) (>10%)
Cardiovascular
Hypotension [2]
Central Nervous System
Agitation [2]
Akathisia (<10%)
Amnesia (<10%) [18]
Catatonia [2]
Confusion (<10%)
Delirium [2]
Depression (<10%)
Hallucinations [2]
Headache (<10%)
Insomnia [2]
Somnolence (drowsiness) (<10%) [4]
Tremor (<10%)

Vertigo / dizziness (<10%) [2]

Local
Injection-site pain (>10%)
Injection-site phlebitis (>10%)

Ocular
Visual disturbances (<10%)

Respiratory
Apnea (<10%)
Hyperventilation (<10%)

Other
Adverse effects / adverse reactions [2]

LORCASERIN

Trade name: Belviq (Eisai)
Indications: Obesity in adults who have at least one weight-related health condition, such as high blood pressure, Type II diabetes, or high cholesterol
Class: Anti-obesity / weight loss pharmacotherapy, Serotonin receptor agonist
Half-life: ~11 hours
Clinically important, potentially hazardous interactions with: antipsychotics, bupropion, dextromethorphan, lithium, MAO inhibitors, SNRIs, SSRIs, St John's wort, tramadol, tricyclic antidepressants, triptans
Important contra-indications noted in the prescribing guidelines for: nursing mothers; pediatric patients
Note: On 2/13/2020, the U.S. Food and Drug Administration (FDA) requested that the manufacturer of lorcaserin (Belviq) voluntarily withdraw the weight-loss drug from the U.S. market because a safety clinical trial shows an increased occurrence of cancer. The drug manufacturer, Eisai, has submitted a request to voluntarily withdraw the drug.

Skin
Peripheral edema (5%)
Rash (2%)

Mucosal
Nasal congestion (3%)
Oropharyngeal pain (4%)
Xerostomia (dry mouth) (5%) [2]

Cardiovascular
Hypertension (5%)
Valvulopathy (2–3%) [5]

Central Nervous System
Anxiety (4%)
Cognitive impairment (2%) [2]
Depression (2%) [2]
Euphoria / elation [3]
Headache (15–17%) [12]
Insomnia (4%)
Vertigo / dizziness (7–9%) [10]

Endocrine/Metabolic
Appetite decreased (2%)
Diabetes mellitus (exacerbation) (3%)
Hypoglycemia (29%) [4]

Gastrointestinal/Hepatic
Constipation (6%)
Diarrhea (7%)
Gastroenteritis (3%)
Nausea (8–9%) [10]
Vomiting (4%)

Genitourinary
Urinary tract infection (7–9%)

Neuromuscular/Skeletal
Asthenia / fatigue (7%) [3]
Back pain (6–12%) [2]
Bone pain / joint pain (2%)
Muscle spasm (5%)

Respiratory
Cough (4%)
Nasopharyngitis (11–13%) [2]
Upper respiratory tract infection (14%)

Other
Toothache (odontalgia) (3%)

LORLATINIB

Trade name: Lorbrena (Pfizer)
Indications: indicated for the treatment of patients with anaplastic lymphoma kinase (ALK)-positive metastatic non-small cell lung cancer (NSCLC) whose disease has progressed on: crizotinib and at least one other ALK inhibitor for metastatic disease,
or alectinib as the first ALK inhibitor therapy for metastatic disease,
or ceritinib as the first ALK inhibitor therapy for metastatic disease.
Class: Anaplastic lymphoma kinase (ALK) inhibitor, Kinase inhibitor
Half-life: 24 hours
Clinically important, potentially hazardous interactions with: rifampin
Pregnancy category: can cause embryo-fetal harm
Important contra-indications noted in the prescribing guidelines for: nursing mothers

---

Skin
Edema / fluid retention (57%) [3]
Rash (14%)

Central Nervous System
Cognitive impairment (27%)
Fever (pyrexia) (includes hyperpyrexia) (12%)
Hallucinations (7%)
Headache (18%)
Mood changes (includes mood disorder) (23%)
Peripheral neuropathy (47%) [4]
Psychosis [3]
Sleep disturbances (10%)
Speech disorder (12%)
Vertigo / dizziness (16%)

Endocrine/Metabolic
ALP increased (24%)
ALT increased (28%)
AST increased (37%)
Hyperamylasemia (22%)
Hypercholesterolemia (96%) [6]
Hyperglycemia (includes glucose increased) (52%)
Hyperkalemia (21%)
Hyperlipasemia (24%)
Hypertriglyceridemia (includes triglycerides increased) (90%) [4]
Hypoalbuminemia / albumin decreased (33%)
Hypomagnesemia (21%)
Hypophosphatemia (21%)
Weight gain (24%) [2]

Gastrointestinal/Hepatic
Constipation (15%)
Diarrhea (22%)
Nausea (18%)
Vomiting (12%)

Hematologic
Anemia (52%)
Lymphopenia (lymphocytopenia) / lymphocytes decreased (22%)
Thrombocytopenia / platelets decreased (23%)

Neuromuscular/Skeletal
Arthralgia (23%)
Asthenia / fatigue (26%)
Back pain (13%)
Myalgia/Myopathy (17%)
Myasthenia gravis [2]
Pain in extremities (13%)

Ocular
Visual disturbances (15%)

Respiratory
Cough (18%)
Dyspnea / shortness of breath (27%)
Pulmonary hypertension [2]
Upper respiratory tract infection (12%)

Other
Adverse effects / adverse reactions [2]

LOSARTAN

Trade names: Cozaar (Merck), Hyzaar (Merck)
Indications: Hypertension
Class: Angiotensin receptor antagonist (blocker), Antihypertensive, Covid-19 putative drug
Half-life: 2 hours
Clinically important, potentially hazardous interactions with: aliskiren, rifampin, voriconazole
Pregnancy category: category C in first trimester; category D in second and third trimesters
Important contra-indications noted in the prescribing guidelines for: nursing mothers
Note: Hyzaar is losartan and hydrochlorothiazide. Hydrochlorothiazide is a sulfonamide and can be absorbed systemically. Sulfonamides can produce severe, possibly fatal, reactions such as toxic epidermal necrolysis and Stevens-Johnson syndrome.
Warning: CONTRA-INDICATED IN PREGNANCY

Skin
Anaphylactoid reactions / anaphylaxis (includes anaphylactic shock) [3]
Angioedema (formerly named angioneurotic edema) [17]
Henoch-Schönlein purpura / IgA vasculitis / immunoglobulin A vasculitis [2]
Photosensitivity [2]

Mucosal
Nasal congestion (2%)

Central Nervous System
Ageusia (taste loss) / taste disorder [2]
Vertigo / dizziness (3%)

Endocrine/Metabolic
Hyperkalemia [7]

Gastrointestinal/Hepatic
Hepatotoxicity / liver injury / acute liver injury / drug-induced liver injury (DILI) [6]

Neuromuscular/Skeletal
Back pain (2%)

Respiratory
Upper respiratory tract infection (8%)

Other
Adverse effects / adverse reactions [7]

LOTEPREDNOL

Trade names: Alrex (Bausch & Lomb), Lotemax (Bausch & Lomb)
Indications: Ophthalmic inflammation, seasonal allergic conjunctivitis, rhinitis
Class: Corticosteroid / Glucocorticoid, Corticosteroid, topical
Half-life: N/A
Clinically important, potentially hazardous interactions with: none known
Important contra-indications noted in the prescribing guidelines for: nursing mothers; pediatric patients
Note: Contra-indicated in most viral diseases of the cornea and conjunctiva including epithelial herpes simplex keratitis (dendritic keratitis), vaccinia, and varicella, and also in mycobacterial infection of the eye and fungal diseases of ocular structures.

Central Nervous System
Headache (<15%)

Ocular
Intraocular pressure increased [2]
Iritis (25%)

Respiratory
Rhinitis / rhinosinusitis (see also sinusitis) (<15%)

LOVASTATIN

Trade names: Advicor (Kos), Altoprev (Shionogi), Mevacor (Merck)
Indications: Hypercholesterolemia
Class: HMG-CoA reductase inhibitor / statin
Half-life: 1–2 hours
Clinically important, potentially hazardous interactions with: amprenavir, atazanavir, azithromycin, boceprevir, bosentan, cholestyramine, clarithromycin, cyclosporine, darunavir, delavirdine, efavirenz, elbasvir & grazoprevir, erythromycin, exenatide, fenofibrate, fosamprenavir, gemfibrozil, glecaprevir & pibrentasvir, grapefruit juice, imatinib, indinavir, itraconazole, letermovir, lomitapide, lonafarnib, lopinavir, mifepristone, nelfinavir, ombitasvir/paritaprevir/ritonavir, ombitasvir/paritaprevir/ritonavir and dasabuvir, paclitaxel, posaconazole, red rice yeast, tacrolimus, telaprevir, telithromycin, ticagrelor, tipranavir, tolvaptan, verapamil, viloxazine
Important contra-indications noted in the prescribing guidelines for: nursing mothers

---

Skin
Exanthems (<5%) [3]
Lupus erythematosus (subacute cutaneous lupus erythematosus (SCLE)) [4]
Pruritus (itching) (5%) [2]
Rash (5%) [3]

Central Nervous System
Parkinsonism [2]

Endocrine/Metabolic
Gynecomastia (<10%)

Gastrointestinal/Hepatic
Hepatotoxicity / liver injury / acute liver injury / drug-induced liver injury (DILI) [2]
Pancreatitis / acute pancreatitis [2]

Neuromuscular/Skeletal
Asthenia / fatigue [2]
Myalgia/Myopathy (<10%) [6]
Rhabdomyolysis [41]

LOXAPINE

Trade names: Adasuve (Teva), Loxitane (Watson)
Indications: Psychoses
Class: Antipsychotic
Half-life: 12–19 hours (terminal)
Clinically important, potentially hazardous interactions with: none known
Pregnancy category: May cause fetal harm based on animal studies
Important contra-indications noted in the prescribing guidelines for: the elderly; nursing mothers; pediatric patients
Warning: BRONCHOSPASM and INCREASED MORTALITY IN ELDERLY PATIENTS WITH DEMENTIA-RELATED PSYCHOSIS

Skin
Rash (<10%)

Mucosal
Xerostomia (dry mouth) (>10%)

Central Nervous System
Dysgeusia (taste perversion) (14%) [8]
Neuroleptic malignant syndrome [3]
Sedation (12%) [4]
Somnolence (drowsiness) [3]
Vertigo / dizziness [2]

Endocrine/Metabolic
Gynecomastia (<10%)

Gastrointestinal/Hepatic
Dysphagia [2]

Neuromuscular/Skeletal
Rhabdomyolysis [3]

Respiratory
Bronchospasm [3]
Pulmonary toxicity [3]

LUBIPROSTONE

Trade name: Amitiza (Takeda)
Indications: Constipation, irritable bowel syndrome
Class: Chloride channel activator
Half-life: 0–1.4 hours
Clinically important, potentially hazardous interactions with: none known
Important contra-indications noted in the prescribing guidelines for: nursing mothers; pediatric patients
Note: Contra-indicated in patients with known or suspected mechanical gastrointestinal obstruction.

Skin
Peripheral edema (4%)

Central Nervous System
Headache (13%) [7]

Gastrointestinal/Hepatic
Abdominal distension [5]
Abdominal pain (7%) [9]
Diarrhea [22]
Flatulence [3]
Nausea [24]
Vomiting [7]

Neuromuscular/Skeletal
Arthralgia (3%)
Asthenia / fatigue (2%)
Back pain (2%)

Respiratory
Dyspnea / shortness of breath [4]
Influenza- ('flu)-like syndrome (2%)
Sinusitis (see also rhinitis / rhinosinusitis) (5%)
Upper respiratory tract infection (4%)

Other
Adverse effects / adverse reactions [3]

LUMACAFTOR/ IVACAFTOR

Trade name: Orkambi (Vertex)
Indications: Cystic fibrosis in patients aged 12 years and older who are homozygous for the *F508del* mutation in the *CFTR* gene
Class: CFTR potentiator, CYP3A4 inducer
Half-life: 26 hours
Clinically important, potentially hazardous interactions with: rifampin, St John's wort
Important contra-indications noted in the prescribing guidelines for: nursing mothers; pediatric patients
Note: See also separate profile for ivacaftor.

Skin
Rash (7%) [3]

Mucosal
Rhinorrhea (6%) [2]

Endocrine/Metabolic
Creatine phosphokinase (CPK) / creatine kinase increased (hyperCKemia) (7%) [2]
Menstrual irregularities (10%)

Gastrointestinal/Hepatic
Diarrhea (12%)
Flatulence (7%)
Nausea (13%) [2]

Neuromuscular/Skeletal
Asthenia / fatigue (9%) [2]

Respiratory
Cough [2]
Dyspnea / shortness of breath (13%) [4]
Influenza (5%)
Nasopharyngitis (13%)
Upper respiratory tract infection (10%)

Other
Adverse effects / adverse reactions [2]

LUMATEPERONE

Trade name: Caplyta (Intra-Cellular Therapies)
Indications: Treatment of schizophrenia in adults
Class: Antipsychotic, Antipsychotic, atypical
Half-life: ~18 hours
Clinically important, potentially hazardous interactions with: amprenavir, aprepitant, armodafinil, carbamazepine, ciprofloxacin, clarithromycin, cyclosporine, CYP3A4 inducers, diltiazem, efavirenz, erythromycin, etravirine, fluconazole, fluvoxamine, grapefruit juice, itraconazole, modafinil, moderate or strong CYP3A4 inhibitors, nafcillin, nefazodone, nelfinavir, phenytoin, pioglitazone, prednisone, probenecid, rifampin, ritonavir, St John's wort, ugt inhibitors, valproic acid, verapamil, voriconazole
Pregnancy category: May cause extrapyramidal and/or withdrawal symptoms in neonates with

third trimester exposure. Breastfeeding is not recommended.
Important contra-indications noted in the prescribing guidelines for: nursing mothers
Note: Avoid use in patients with moderate or severe hepatic impairment (Child-Pugh B or C).
Warning:
INCREASED MORTALITY IN ELDERLY PATIENTS WITH DEMENTIA-RELATED PSYCHOSIS
ELDERLY PATIENTS WITH DEMENTIA-RELATED PSYCHOSIS TREATED WITH ANTIPSYCHOTIC DRUGS ARE AT AN INCREASED RISK OF DEATH.
LUMATEPERONE IS NOT APPROVED FOR THE TREATMENT OF PATIENTS WITH DEMENTIA-RELATED PSYCHOSIS.

Mucosal
Xerostomia (dry mouth) (6%) [4]
Central Nervous System
Headache [3]
Somnolence (drowsiness) (24%) [2]
Vertigo / dizziness (5%)
Endocrine/Metabolic
Appetite decreased (2%)
Creatine phosphokinase (CPK) / creatine kinase increased (hyperCKemia) (4%)
Hypertransaminasemia (hepatic transaminitis) / elevated transaminases (2%)
Gastrointestinal/Hepatic
Nausea (9%)
Vomiting (3%)
Neuromuscular/Skeletal
Asthenia / fatigue (3%)

LUMIRACOXIB

Trade names: Joicela (Novartis), Prexige (Novartis)
Indications: Osteoarthritis
Class: COX-2 selective inhibitor
Half-life: 4 hours
Clinically important, potentially hazardous interactions with: aspirin

---

Skin
Peripheral edema (2%)
Central Nervous System
Headache (8%)
Vertigo / dizziness (2%)
Gastrointestinal/Hepatic
Hepatotoxicity / liver injury / acute liver injury / drug-induced liver injury (DILI) [6]
Neuromuscular/Skeletal
Arthralgia (5%)
Asthenia / fatigue (2%)
Back pain (5%)
Myalgia/Myopathy (2%)
Respiratory
Cough (2%)
Nasopharyngitis (6%)

LURASIDONE

Trade name: Latuda (Sunovion)
Indications: Schizophrenia, depressive epidodes associated with bipolar I disorder
Class: Antipsychotic, Antipsychotic, atypical
Half-life: 18 hours
Clinically important, potentially hazardous interactions with: alcohol, amphetamines, CNS depressants, dasatinib, deferasirox, diltiazem, disopyramide, dopamine, dopamine agonists, droperidol, efavirenz, epinephrine, hydroxyzine, itraconazole, ketoconazole, levomepromazine, lithium, MAO inhibitors, methylphenidate, metoclopramide, ombitasvir/paritaprevir/ritonavir, ombitasvir/paritaprevir/ritonavir and dasabuvir, pimozide, procainamide, quinagolide, quinidine, rifampin, strong CYP3A4 inducers or inhibitors, tetrabenazine, tocilizumab, viloxazine
Important contra-indications noted in the prescribing guidelines for: the elderly; nursing mothers; pediatric patients
Warning: INCREASED MORTALITY IN ELDERLY PATIENTS WITH DEMENTIA-RELATED PSYCHOSIS

Mucosal
Sialorrhea (ptyalism; hypersalivation) (2%)
Central Nervous System
Agitation (5%)
Akathisia (13%) [26]
Anxiety (5%)
Extrapyramidal symptoms [3]
Headache [4]
Insomnia (10%) [4]
Parkinsonism (10%) [6]
Restlessness (2%) [2]
Sedation [10]
Somnolence (drowsiness) (17%) [20]
Tardive syndrome / tardive dyskinesia [3]
Vertigo / dizziness (4%) [4]
Endocrine/Metabolic
Hyperprolactinemia [2]
Weight gain (5%) [6]
Gastrointestinal/Hepatic
Dyspepsia / functional dyspepsia (indigestion) (see also gastroparesis) (6%)
Nausea (10%) [17]
Vomiting (8%) [4]
Neuromuscular/Skeletal
Dystonia (5%) [4]
Ocular
Oculogyric crisis / oculogyric dystonic reaction [2]
Other
Adverse effects / adverse reactions [4]

LYCOPENE

Scientific names: *All-Trans-Lycopene, Psi-Psi-Carotene*
Indications: Cancer (prevention), cardiovascular disease (prevention), asthma
Class: Antioxidant
Half-life: N/A
Clinically important, potentially hazardous interactions with: none known
Note: Cooking increases bioavailability of lycopene. Major dietary sources are tomato paste, juice, and ketchup.

Skin
Pigmentation (Skin) (includes hyperpigmentation) [2]
Other
Adverse effects / adverse reactions [2]

LYMECYCLINE

Trade name: Tetralysal (Galderma)
Indications: Various infections due to susceptible organisms
Class: Antibiotic, Antibiotic; tetracycline, Antimicrobial
Half-life: 10 hours
Clinically important, potentially hazardous interactions with: acitretin, aluminium, antacids, bismuth, coumarins, diuretics, ergotamine, kaolin, methysergide, oral contraceptives, oral iron, penicillins, phenindione, quinapril, retinoids, strontium ranelate, sucralfate, sulfonylureas, tripotassium dicitratobismuthate, zinc
Important contra-indications noted in the prescribing guidelines for: nursing mothers; pediatric patients

---

Nails
Photo-onycholysis [2]
Other
Adverse effects / adverse reactions [2]

MACITENTAN

Trade name: Opsumit (Actelion)
Indications: Pulmonary arterial hypertension
Class: Endothelin receptor (ETR) antagonist
Half-life: 16 hours
Clinically important, potentially hazardous interactions with: ketoconazole, rifampin, ritonavir, strong CYP3A4 inducers or inhibitors
Important contra-indications noted in the prescribing guidelines for: nursing mothers; pediatric patients
Note: Contra-indicated in pregnancy.
Warning: EMBRYO-FETAL TOXICITY

Skin
Peripheral edema [3]
Central Nervous System
Headache (14%) [8]
Gastrointestinal/Hepatic
Hepatotoxicity / liver injury / acute liver injury / drug-induced liver injury (DILI) [5]
Genitourinary
Urinary tract infection (9%)
Hematologic
Anemia (13%) [9]
Respiratory
Bronchitis (12%) [3]
Influenza (6%)
Nasopharyngitis (20%) [6]
Pharyngitis (sore throat) (20%)
Pulmonary hypertension [2]
Upper respiratory tract infection [2]
Other
Adverse effects / adverse reactions [3]

MARAVIROC

Trade names: Celsentri (ViiV), Selzentry (ViiV)
Indications: HIV infection
Class: Antiretroviral, CCR5 co-receptor antagonist
Half-life: 14–18 hours
Clinically important, potentially hazardous interactions with: atazanavir, clarithromycin, conivaptan, CYP3A4 inhibitors or inducers, darunavir, dasatinib, deferasirox, delavirdine, efavirenz, etravirine, indinavir, ketoconazole, lopinavir, nelfinavir, oxcarbazepine, rifampin, rifapentine, ritonavir, saquinavir, St John's wort, telithromycin, voriconazole
Important contra-indications noted in the prescribing guidelines for: the elderly; nursing mothers; pediatric patients
Warning: HEPATOTOXICITY

Skin
Dermatitis (5%)
Folliculitis (5%)
Lipodystrophy / acquired generalized lipodystrophy (5%)
Pruritus (itching) (6%) [2]
Rash (17%) [2]

Mucosal
Stomatitis (oral mucositis) (4%)

Cardiovascular
Postural hypotension [2]

Central Nervous System
Depression (6%)
Fever (pyrexia) (includes hyperpyrexia) (21%) [2]
Headache [3]
Pain (8%)
Paresthesias (8%)
Peripheral neuropathy (5%)
Sleep disturbances (12%)
Vertigo / dizziness (14%)

Gastrointestinal/Hepatic
Abdominal pain (14%)
Diarrhea [2]
Hepatotoxicity / liver injury / acute liver injury / drug-induced liver injury (DILI) [2]

Genitourinary
Urinary tract infection (4%)

Neuromuscular/Skeletal
Asthenia / fatigue [2]
Myalgia/Myopathy (5%)

Respiratory
Cough (22%) [2]
Influenza- ('flu)-like syndrome (3%)
Nasopharyngitis [2]
Pneumonia (4%)
Upper respiratory tract infection (37%) [2]

Other
Adverse effects / adverse reactions [6]

MARIHUANA

Synonyms: marijuana; grass; hashish; pot; cannabis
Indications: Nausea and vomiting, substance abuse drug
Class: Antiemetic, Cannabinoid, Hallucinogen
Half-life: N/A
Clinically important, potentially hazardous interactions with: atazanavir
Note: Marihuana is the popular name for the dried flowering leaves of the hemp plant, *cannabis sativa*. It contains tetrahydrocannabinols.

Mucosal
Xerostomia (dry mouth) [2]

Cardiovascular
Acute coronary syndrome [2]
Cardiomyopathy [3]
Cardiotoxicity [5]
Myocardial infarction [3]

Central Nervous System
Amnesia [2]
Catatonia [3]
Hallucinations [3]
Hallucinations, visual [2]
Mania [5]
Neurotoxicity [2]
Psychosis [5]
Schizophrenia [3]
Seizures [2]
Stroke / cerebrovascular accident [2]
Vertigo / dizziness [2]

Gastrointestinal/Hepatic
Pancreatitis / acute pancreatitis [4]

Genitourinary
Priapism [2]

Respiratory
Acute respiratory distress syndrome [2]

Other
Adverse effects / adverse reactions [2]

MAZINDOL

Indications: Obesity
Class: Anti-obesity / weight loss pharmacotherapy, Norepinephrine reuptake inhibitor
Half-life: 10 hours
Clinically important, potentially hazardous interactions with: cocaine, fenfluramine, fluoxetine, fluvoxamine, lithium, MAO inhibitors, paroxetine hydrochloride, phenelzine, sertraline, tranylcypromine

---

Mucosal
Xerostomia (dry mouth) [3]

Central Nervous System
Depression [2]

MDMA

Synonym: 3,4-methylenedioxymethamphetamine; ecstasy; E; X; molly; club drug
Indications: N/A
Class: Amphetamine, Enactogen / emathogen, Psychotomimetic
Half-life: N/A
Clinically important, potentially hazardous interactions with: none known
Pregnancy category: Not classified

Skin
Diaphoresis [4]

Mucosal
Xerostomia (dry mouth) [5]

Cardiovascular
Cardiotoxicity [2]
Myocardial infarction [2]

Central Nervous System
Amnesia [2]
Confusion [2]
Depression (37%) [14]
Hallucinations [4]
Hallucinations, visual [2]
Headache [2]
Hyperthermia [3]
Memory loss/memory impaired [3]
Neuroleptic malignant syndrome [4]
Neurotoxicity [5]
Parkinsonism [4]
Psychosis [4]
Seizures [3]
Serotonin syndrome [8]

Endocrine/Metabolic
Hyponatremia [7]
SIADH [8]

Gastrointestinal/Hepatic
Hepatitis [2]
Hepatotoxicity / liver injury / acute liver injury / drug-induced liver injury (DILI) [4]
Nausea [2]

Genitourinary
Priapism [2]

Hematologic
Coagulopathy / coagulation dysfunction / clotting factor deficiency (includes disseminated intravascular coagulation / DIC) [2]

Neuromuscular/Skeletal
Myalgia/Myopathy [2]
Rhabdomyolysis [36]

Renal
Nephrotoxicity / kidney injury / acute kidney injury (AKI) / drug-induced kidney injury [2]

Respiratory
Acute respiratory distress syndrome [2]

Other
Adverse effects / adverse reactions [2]
Bruxism (teeth grinding) [8]
Death [48]
Dipsia (thirst) / polydipsia [2]
Multiorgan failure [4]

MEADOWSWEET

Family: Rosaceae
Scientific names: *Filipendula ulmaria, Spiraea ulmaria*
Indications: Colds, fevers, cough, bronchitis, dyspepsia, heartburn, peptic ulcer, gout, rheumatic disorders
Class: Anti-inflammatory, Diuretic
Half-life: N/A
Clinically important, potentially hazardous interactions with: salicylates

MEBENDAZOLE

Trade name: Vermox (Janssen)
Indications: Parasitic worm infestations
Class: Anthelmintic, Antimicrobial
Half-life: 1–12 hours
Clinically important, potentially hazardous interactions with: aminophylline

---

Skin
Stevens-Johnson syndrome and toxic epidermal necrolysis (SJS/TEN) [2]

Hair
Alopecia / hair loss [3]
Central Nervous System
Headache [3]
Vertigo / dizziness [2]
Gastrointestinal/Hepatic
Abdominal pain [5]
Diarrhea [2]
Other
Adverse effects / adverse reactions [2]

MEBEVERINE

Trade name: Colofac (Solvay)
Indications: Irritable bowel syndrome
Class: Anticholinergic
Half-life: 1.5–1.87 hours
Clinically important, potentially hazardous interactions with: none known

MECHLORETHAMINE

Synonyms: mustine; nitrogen mustard
Indications: Hodgkin's disease, mycosis fungoides
Class: Alkylating agent
Half-life: <1 minute
Clinically important, potentially hazardous interactions with: aldesleukin, vaccines

---

Skin
Anaphylactoid reactions / anaphylaxis (includes anaphylactic shock) (<10%) [4]
Bullous dermatosis [3]
Dermatitis [28]
Herpes zoster (>10%)
Hypersensitivity (<10%)
Pigmentation (Skin) (includes hyperpigmentation) [10]
Pruritus (itching) [3]
Squamous cell carcinoma [3]
Urticaria / hives [3]
Hair
Alopecia / hair loss (<10%)
Central Nervous System
Dysgeusia (taste perversion) (<10%)
Local
Injection-site extravasation (<10%)
Injection-site thrombophlebitis (<10%) [2]

MECLIZINE

Trade name: Antivert (Pfizer)
Indications: Motion sickness
Class: Antiemetic, Histamine H1 receptor antagonist
Half-life: 5–6 hours
Clinically important, potentially hazardous interactions with: alcohol, barbiturates, chloral hydrate, ethchlorvynol, paraldehyde, phenothiazines, zolpidem
Important contra-indications noted in the prescribing guidelines for: nursing mothers; pediatric patients

---

Mucosal
Xerostomia (dry mouth) (<10%)
Central Nervous System
Somnolence (drowsiness) [3]

MEDROXY-PROGESTERONE

Trade names: Depo-Provera (Pfizer), Lunelle (Pfizer), Premphase (Wyeth), Prempro (Wyeth), Provera (Pfizer)
Indications: Secondary amenorrhea, renal or endometrial carcinoma
Class: Progestogen
Half-life: 30 days
Clinically important, potentially hazardous interactions with: acitretin, dofetilide

---

Skin
Acneiform eruption / acneiform dermatitis / acneiform rash (<5%)
Chloasma (<10%)
Diaphoresis (<31%)
Edema / fluid retention (>10%)
Flushing / rubefaction (12%)
Melasma (<10%)
Pruritus (itching) (<10%)
Rash (<5%)
Hair
Alopecia / hair loss (<5%)
Cardiovascular
Thrombophlebitis (<10%)
Endocrine/Metabolic
Amenorrhea [3]
Galactorrhea [2]
Mastodynia (<5%)
Weight gain [3]
Genitourinary
Vaginitis (includes vulvitis) (<5%)
Local
Injection-site pain (>10%)
Neuromuscular/Skeletal
Osteoporosis [2]

MEFLOQUINE

Trade name: Lariam (Roche)
Indications: Malaria
Class: Antimalarial, Antimicrobial, Antiprotozoal
Half-life: 21–22 days
Clinically important, potentially hazardous interactions with: acebutolol, artemether/lumefantrine, ethosuximide, halofantrine, ketoconazole, lacosamide, moxifloxacin, oxcarbazepine, quinine, tiagabine, typhoid vaccine, vigabatrin
Important contra-indications noted in the prescribing guidelines for: nursing mothers
Warning: NEUROPSYCHIATRIC ADVERSE REACTIONS

Skin
Anaphylactoid reactions / anaphylaxis (includes anaphylactic shock) [2]
Erythema [2]
Exanthems (30%)
Pruritus (itching) (4–10%) [2]
Psoriasis [2]
Rash (<10%)
Stevens-Johnson syndrome and toxic epidermal necrolysis (SJS/TEN) [3]
Vasculitis (angiitis) / cutaneous vasculitis (angiitis) [3]
Cardiovascular
Palpitation [3]
Tachycardia [2]
Central Nervous System
Abnormal dreams [3]
Aggression (includes anger) [2]
Amnesia [2]
Anorexia [2]
Anxiety [5]
Chills (<10%)
Confusion [2]
Delusions [2]
Depression [7]
Fever (pyrexia) (includes hyperpyrexia) (<10%) [2]
Hallucinations [3]
Headache (<10%) [5]
Insomnia [3]
Mania [4]
Neurotoxicity [8]
Psychosis [8]
Seizures [6]
Sleep disturbances [2]
Suicidal ideation [2]
Vertigo / dizziness (<10%) [21]
Gastrointestinal/Hepatic
Abdominal pain [4]
Diarrhea [4]
Nausea [8]
Vomiting [15]
Neuromuscular/Skeletal
Arthralgia [2]
Asthenia / fatigue (<10%) [2]
Myalgia/Myopathy (<10%) [2]
Ocular
Maculopathy [2]
Otic
Tinnitus (<10%)
Other
Adverse effects / adverse reactions [2]
Death [3]

MELATONIN

Family: None
Scientific name: *N-acetyl-5-methoxytryptamine*
Indications: Jet lag, sleep disorders, Alzheimer's disease, free radical scavenger, chemotherapy adjunct, tinnitus, depression, migraine, cluster headache, hypertension, hyperpigmentation, osteoporosis, antioxidant. Skin protectant against sunburn
Class: Hormone
Half-life: N/A
Clinically important, potentially hazardous interactions with: acetaminophen, NSAIDs, setraline

---

Skin
Fixed eruption / fixed drug eruption [2]
Central Nervous System
Somnolence (drowsiness) [2]

MELOXICAM

Trade name: Mobic (Boehringer Ingelheim)
Indications: Osteoarthritis
Class: COX-2 inhibitor, Non-steroidal anti-inflammatory (NSAID)
Half-life: 15–20 hours
Clinically important, potentially hazardous interactions with: ACE inhibitors, adrenergic neurone blockers, alcohol, aliskiren, alpha

blockers, angiotensin II receptor antagonists, anticoagulants, antidepressants, antiplatelet agents, aspirin, baclofen, beta blockers, bile acid sequestrants, calcium channel blockers, cardiac glycosides, cholestyramine, clonidine, clopidogrel, collagenase, conivaptan, corticosteroids, coumarins, cyclosporine, dabigatran, dasatinib, desmopressin, diazoxide, digoxin, diuretics, drotrecogin alfa, eplerenone, erlotinib, glucosamine, haloperidol, heparins, hydralazine, ibritumomab, iloprost, ketorolac, lithium, methotrexate, methyldopa, mifamurtide, minoxidil, moxonidine, nitrates, nitroprusside, NSAIDs, pemetrexed, penicillamine, pentosan, pentoxifylline, phenindione, pralatrexate, prasugrel, probenecid, prostacyclin analogues, quinolones, ritonavir, serotonin/norepinephrine reuptake inhibitors, SSRIs, sulfonylureas, tacrolimus, thrombolytic agents, tositumomab & iodine^{131}, treprostinil, vancomycin, venlafaxine, vitamin K antagonists, voriconazole, zidovudine
Pregnancy category: category D from 30 weeks gestation
Important contra-indications noted in the prescribing guidelines for: the elderly; nursing mothers
Note: NSAIDs may cause an increased risk of serious cardiovascular and gastrointestinal adverse events, which can be fatal. This risk may increase with duration of use.
Warning: CARDIOVASCULAR AND GASTROINTESTINAL RISKS

Skin
Anaphylactoid reactions / anaphylaxis (includes anaphylactic shock) (<2%)
Angioedema (formerly named angioneurotic edema) (<2%) [3]
Bullous dermatosis (<2%)
Edema / fluid retention (2–5%)
Erythema [2]
Erythema multiforme (<2%)
Exanthems (<2%)
Facial edema (<2%)
Hematoma / cutaneous hematoma [3]
Hot flashes / hot flushes (<2%)
Hyperhidrosis (<2%)
Hypersensitivity [2]
Photosensitivity (<2%)
Pruritus (itching) (<2%) [3]
Purpura (<2%)
Rash (<3%) [3]
Stevens-Johnson syndrome and toxic epidermal necrolysis (SJS/TEN) (<2%)
Urticaria / hives (<2%) [4]
Vasculitis (angiitis) / cutaneous vasculitis (angiitis) (<2%)

Hair
Alopecia / hair loss (<2%)

Mucosal
Ulcerative stomatitis (<2%)
Xerostomia (dry mouth) (<2%)

Cardiovascular
Angina (<2%)
Arrhythmias (<2%)
Cardiac failure (<2%)
Hypertension (<2%)
Hypotension (<2%)
Myocardial infarction (<2%)
Palpitation (<2%)
Tachycardia (<2%)

Central Nervous System
Abnormal dreams (<2%)
Anxiety (<2%)
Confusion (<2%)
Depression (<2%)
Dysgeusia (taste perversion) (<2%)
Fever (pyrexia) (includes hyperpyrexia) (<2%)
Headache (2–6%) [2]
Insomnia (<4%)
Nervousness (<2%)
Pain (4%)
Paresthesias (<2%)
Seizures (<2%)
Somnolence (drowsiness) (<2%)
Syncope / fainting (<2%)
Tremor (<2%)
Vertigo / dizziness (<3%)

Endocrine/Metabolic
ALT increased (<2%)
Appetite increased (<2%)
AST increased (<2%)
Dehydration (<2%)
GGT increased (<2%)
Weight gain (<2%)
Weight loss (<2%)

Gastrointestinal/Hepatic
Abdominal pain (2–5%) [2]
Black stools / melena (<2%)
Colitis (<2%)
Constipation (<3%) [2]
Diarrhea (2–6%) [2]
Dyspepsia / functional dyspepsia (indigestion) (see also gastroparesis) (4–10%) [2]
Eructation (belching) (<2%)
Esophagitis (<2%)
Flatulence (<3%)
Gastritis / pangastritis / gastric irritation (<2%)
Gastroesophageal reflux (<2%)
Gastrointestinal bleeding [2]
Gastrointestinal perforation / perforated colon / gastric perforation (<2%) [2]
Gastrointestinal ulceration (<2%) [3]
Hematemesis (<2%)
Hepatitis (<2%)
Hepatotoxicity / liver injury / acute liver injury / drug-induced liver injury (DILI) [6]
Nausea (3–7%) [4]
Pancreatitis / acute pancreatitis (<2%) [2]
Vomiting (<3%)

Genitourinary
Albuminuria (<2%)
Hematuria (<2%)
Urinary frequency (<2%)
Urinary tract infection (<7%)

Hematologic
Anemia (<4%)
Leukocytopenia (leukopenia) / leukocytes (white blood cells) decreased (<2%)

Neuromuscular/Skeletal
Arthralgia (<5%)
Asthenia / fatigue [2]
Back pain (<3%)
Bone pain / joint pain (2%)

Ocular
Abnormal vision (<2%)
Conjunctivitis (conjunctival inflammation) (<2%)

Otic
Tinnitus (<2%)

Renal
Nephrotoxicity / kidney injury / acute kidney injury (AKI) / drug-induced kidney injury [2]
Renal failure (<2%)

Respiratory
Asthma (<2%)
Bronchospasm (<2%)
Cough (<2%)
Dyspnea / shortness of breath (<2%)
Influenza- ('flu)-like syndrome (2–3%)
Upper respiratory tract infection (<8%)

Other
Adverse effects / adverse reactions (18%) [6]
Allergic reactions (<2%)

MELPHALAN

Trade names: Alkeran (GSK), Evomela (Spectrum)
Indications: Multiple myeloma, carcinomas
Class: Alkylating agent
Half-life: 90 minutes
Clinically important, potentially hazardous interactions with: aldesleukin, PEG-interferon, tasonermin
Important contra-indications noted in the prescribing guidelines for: the elderly; nursing mothers; pediatric patients
Warning: SEVERE BONE MARROW SUPPRESSION, HYPERSENSITIVITY, and LEUKEMOGENICITY

Skin
Anaphylactoid reactions / anaphylaxis (includes anaphylactic shock) [2]
Angioedema (formerly named angioneurotic edema) [2]
Cutaneous toxicity / skin toxicity [3]
Dermatitis [2]
Exanthems (4%) [4]
Hypersensitivity (<10%)
Pruritus (itching) (<10%)
Rash (<10%)
Urticaria / hives [3]
Vasculitis (angiitis) / cutaneous vasculitis (angiitis) (<10%)
Vesiculation (<10%)

Hair
Alopecia / hair loss (<10%) [2]

Nails
Beau's lines (transverse nail bands) [4]

Mucosal
Mucositis [8]
Stomatitis (oral mucositis) (<10%) [6]

Cardiovascular
Atrial fibrillation [2]

Central Nervous System
Peripheral neuropathy [3]

Gastrointestinal/Hepatic
Diarrhea [3]
Hepatotoxicity / liver injury / acute liver injury / drug-induced liver injury (DILI) [2]
Nausea [2]

Hematologic
Anemia [2]
Febrile neutropenia [3]
Hemotoxicity [2]
Neutropenia (neutrophils decreased) [6]
Thrombocytopenia / platelets decreased [6]

Neuromuscular/Skeletal
Rhabdomyolysis [2]

Ocular
Ocular adverse effect [2]

Other
Death [2]

MELPHALAN FLUFENAMIDE

Synonym: Melflufen
Trade name: Pepaxto (Oncopeptides)
Indications: Relapsed or refractory multiple myeloma (in combination with dexamethasone)
Class: Alkylating agent
Half-life: 70 minutes
Clinically important, potentially hazardous interactions with: none known
Pregnancy category: Based on its mechanism of action, melphalan flufenamide can cause fetal harm when administered to a pregnant woman. Advise pregnant women of the potential risk to a fetus
Note: Prodrug of melphalan .

Skin
- Hypersensitivity (in combination with dexamethasone) (7%)
- Peripheral edema (in combination with dexamethasone) (14%)

Central Nervous System
- Fever (pyrexia) (includes hyperpyrexia) (2% grade 3 or 4) (in combination with dexamethasone) (24%)
- Headache (in combination with dexamethasone) (13%)
- Insomnia (in combination with dexamethasone) (11%)
- Vertigo / dizziness (in combination with dexamethasone) (11%)

Endocrine/Metabolic
- Appetite decreased (in combination with dexamethasone) (14%)
- Hypocalcemia (in combination with dexamethasone) (10%)
- Hypokalemia (in combination with dexamethasone) (14%)
- Serum creatinine increased (in combination with dexamethasone) (68%)

Gastrointestinal/Hepatic
- Constipation (in combination with dexamethasone) (15%)
- Diarrhea (in combination with dexamethasone) (27%)
- Nausea (in combination with dexamethasone) (32%)
- Vomiting (in combination with dexamethasone) (13%)

Hematologic
- Febrile neutropenia (in combination with dexamethasone) (6%)
- Hemoglobin decreased (in combination with dexamethasone) (50%)
- Hemorrhage (grade 3 or 4) (in combination with dexamethasone) (4%)
- Leukocytopenia (leukopenia) / leukocytes (white blood cells) decreased (in combination with dexamethasone) (88%)
- Lymphopenia (lymphocytopenia) / lymphocytes decreased (in combination with dexamethasone) (95%)
- Neutropenia (neutrophils decreased) (in combination with dexamethasone) (82%)
- Sepsis (in combination with dexamethasone) (4%)

Neuromuscular/Skeletal
- Arthralgia (in combination with dexamethasone) (10%)
- Asthenia / fatigue (6% grade 3 or 4) (in combination with dexamethasone) (55%)
- Back pain (in combination with dexamethasone) (12%)
- Bone pain / joint pain (2% grade 3 or 4) (in combination with dexamethasone) (13%)
- Pain in extremities (2% grade 3 or 4) (in combination with dexamethasone) (13%)

Respiratory
- Cough (in combination with dexamethasone) (17%)
- Dyspnea / shortness of breath (in combination with dexamethasone) (11%)
- Pneumonia (11% grade 3 or 4) (in combination with dexamethasone) (13%)
- Respiratory tract infection (5% grade 3 or 4) (in combination with dexamethasone) (24%)

MEMANTINE

Trade names: Ebixa (Lundbeck), Namenda (Forest)
Indications: Alzheimer's disease, vascular dementia
Class: Adamantane, NMDA receptor antagonist
Half-life: 60–80 hours
Clinically important, potentially hazardous interactions with: amantadine, bromocriptine, darifenacin, dextromethorphan, ketamine, levodopa, levomepromazine, oxybutynin, risperidone, rotigotine, tiotropium, trimethoprim, trospium, zuclopenthixol
Important contra-indications noted in the prescribing guidelines for: nursing mothers; pediatric patients

---

Skin
- Peripheral edema (>2%)

Central Nervous System
- Agitation [2]
- Confusion [3]
- Depression (>2%)
- Gait instability / postural instability [3]
- Hallucinations, visual [2]
- Headache (6%) [3]
- Somnolence (drowsiness) [3]
- Vertigo / dizziness (7%) [7]

Gastrointestinal/Hepatic
- Constipation [2]
- Diarrhea [2]
- Vomiting [2]

Genitourinary
- Urinary tract infection [2]

Neuromuscular/Skeletal
- Arthralgia (>2%)
- Asthenia / fatigue (2%)
- Back pain (3%)
- Myoclonus (see also hypnic jerk) [2]

Respiratory
- Cough (4%)
- Influenza- ('flu)-like syndrome (>2%)
- Nasopharyngitis [2]

Other
- Adverse effects / adverse reactions [3]

MENADIONE

Synonym: vitamin K_3
Trade names: Menadione (Sigma-Aldrich) (Lilly), Synkavite (Roche)
Indications: Hemorrhage or threatened hemorrhage during severe hypoprothrombinemia, coagulation disorders
Class: Vitamin K
Half-life: 23–29 minutes
Clinically important, potentially hazardous interactions with: warfarin

MENINGOCOCCAL GROUP B VACCINE

Trade names: Bexsero (Novartis), Trumenba (Wyeth)
Indications: Immunization to prevent invasive disease caused by *Neisseria meningitidis* serogroup B
Class: Vaccine
Half-life: N/A
Clinically important, potentially hazardous interactions with: none known
Important contra-indications noted in the prescribing guidelines for: the elderly; nursing mothers; pediatric patients

---

Central Nervous System
- Chills (18–30%)
- Fever (pyrexia) (includes hyperpyrexia) (2–8%) [4]
- Headache (41–57%)

Gastrointestinal/Hepatic
- Diarrhea (9–15%)
- Vomiting (2–8%)

Local
- Injection-site edema (18–22%)
- Injection-site erythema (15–20%)
- Injection-site pain (85–93%) [3]
- Injection-site reaction [2]

Neuromuscular/Skeletal
- Arthralgia (16–22%)
- Asthenia / fatigue (44–65%)
- Myalgia/Myopathy (35–41%)

Respiratory
- Upper respiratory tract infection [2]

MEPENZOLATE

Indications: Peptic ulcer
Class: Muscarinic antagonist
Half-life: N/A
Clinically important, potentially hazardous interactions with: antacids, anticholinergics, arbutamine, digoxin, metoclopramide

MEPERIDINE

Synonym: pethidine
Trade name: Demerol (Sanofi-Aventis)
Indications: Pain
Class: Opiate agonist
Half-life: 3–4 hours
Clinically important, potentially hazardous interactions with: acyclovir, alcohol, amphetamines, barbiturates, CNS depressants, darunavir, duloxetine, fluoxetine, furazolidone, general anesthetics, glycopyrrolate,

glycopyrronium, indinavir, isocarboxazid, linezolid, lisdexamfetamine, lithium, MAO inhibitors, moclobemide, phenelzine, phenobarbital, phenothiazines, phenytoin, rasagiline, ritonavir, safinamide, selegiline, sibutramine, SSRIs, tipranavir, tranquilizers, tranylcypromine, tricyclic antidepressants, valacyclovir
Important contra-indications noted in the prescribing guidelines for: the elderly; nursing mothers; pediatric patients

---

Skin
Pruritus (itching) [3]
Mucosal
Xerostomia (dry mouth) (<10%)
Central Nervous System
Catatonia [2]
Delirium [2]
Seizures [2]
Serotonin syndrome [7]
Local
Injection-site erythema [2]
Injection-site pain (<10%)

MEPHENYTOIN

Trade name: Mesantoin (Novartis)
Indications: Partial seizures
Class: Anticonvulsant (see also antiepileptic (anti-seizure)), Antiepileptic; hydantoin
Half-life: 7 hours (for the active metabolite: 95–144 hours)
Clinically important, potentially hazardous interactions with: chloramphenicol, cyclosporine, disulfiram, dopamine, imatinib, itraconazole
Important contra-indications noted in the prescribing guidelines for: nursing mothers

---

Skin
Erythema multiforme [3]
Exanthems (8–10%) [5]
Lupus erythematosus (subacute cutaneous lupus erythematosus (SCLE)) [12]
Pigmentation (Skin) (includes hyperpigmentation) [4]
Stevens-Johnson syndrome and toxic epidermal necrolysis (SJS/TEN) [6]
Urticaria / hives [3]

MEPHOBARBITAL

Indications: Epilepsy, anxiety
Class: Barbiturate
Half-life: 34 hours
Clinically important, potentially hazardous interactions with: alcohol, anticoagulants, antihistamines, brompheniramine, buclizine, chlorpheniramine, dicumarol, ethanolamine, imatinib, warfarin

MEPIVACAINE

Trade names: Carbocaine (Hospira), Polocaine (AstraZeneca)
Indications: Local or regional analgesia and anesthesia by local infiltration, peripheral nerve block, central neural techniques including epidural and caudal blocks
Class: Anesthetic; local
Half-life: 1.9–3.2 hours (adults); 8.7–9 hours (neonates)
Clinically important, potentially hazardous interactions with: none known
Important contra-indications noted in the prescribing guidelines for: the elderly

---

Cardiovascular
Cardiac arrest [3]
Central Nervous System
Headache [3]
Horner's syndrome [2]
Seizures [2]

MEPOLIZUMAB

Trade name: Nucala (GSK)
Indications: Adjunctive treatment for severe eosinophilic asthma
Class: Interleukin-5 antagonist, Monoclonal antibody
Half-life: 16–22 days
Clinically important, potentially hazardous interactions with: none known
Pregnancy category: Insufficent evidence to inform drug-associated risk
Important contra-indications noted in the prescribing guidelines for: nursing mothers; pediatric patients

---

Skin
Eczema / eczematous reaction / eczematous eruption (3%)
Pruritus (itching) (3%)
Rash (>3%)
Mucosal
Nasal congestion (>3%)
Central Nervous System
Fever (pyrexia) (includes hyperpyrexia) (>3%)
Headache (19%) [6]
Vertigo / dizziness (>3%)
Gastrointestinal/Hepatic
Abdominal pain (3%)
Gastroenteritis (>3%)
Nausea (>3%) [3]
Vomiting (>3%)
Genitourinary
Cystitis (includes interstitial cystitis / bladder pain syndrome) (>3%)
Urinary tract infection (3%)
Local
Injection-site reaction (8%) [2]
Neuromuscular/Skeletal
Asthenia / fatigue (5%) [2]
Back pain (5%)
Bone pain / joint pain (>3%)
Muscle spasm (3%)
Otic
Ear infection (>3%)
Respiratory
Asthma [2]
Bronchitis (>3%) [3]
Dyspnea / shortness of breath (>3%)
Influenza (3%)
Nasopharyngitis (>3%) [3]
Pharyngitis (sore throat) (>3%)
Rhinitis / rhinosinusitis (see also sinusitis) (>3%)
Sinusitis (see also rhinitis / rhinosinusitis) [2]
Upper respiratory tract infection [2]
Other
Adverse effects / adverse reactions [5]
Infection (>3%) [2]
Toothache (odontalgia) (>3%)

MEPROBAMATE

Trade names: Equagesic (Women First), Miltown (MedPointe)
Indications: Anxiety, insomnia
Class: Anxiolytic, Central muscle relaxant
Half-life: 10 hours
Clinically important, potentially hazardous interactions with: carisoprodol
Important contra-indications noted in the prescribing guidelines for: the elderly; nursing mothers; pediatric patients

---

Skin
Angioedema (formerly named angioneurotic edema) [4]
Bullous dermatosis [2]
Erythema multiforme [2]
Exanthems (2%) [11]
Fixed eruption / fixed drug eruption [6]
Pruritus (itching) [6]
Purpura [13]
Rash (<10%)
Stevens-Johnson syndrome and toxic epidermal necrolysis (SJS/TEN) [3]
Urticaria / hives (2%) [10]
Vasculitis (angiitis) / cutaneous vasculitis (angiitis) [8]
Other
Side effects (2%) [2]

MEPTAZINOL

Trade name: Meptid (Wyeth)
Indications: Pain
Class: Analgesic; opioid
Half-life: 2–4 hours
Clinically important, potentially hazardous interactions with: antipsychotics, anxiolytics, cimetidine, ciprofloxacin, domperidone, hypnotics, MAO inhibitors, metoclopramide, ritonavir, tricyclic antidepressants

---

Central Nervous System
Dysphoria [2]
Vertigo / dizziness [2]
Gastrointestinal/Hepatic
Nausea [4]
Vomiting [2]
Respiratory
Respiratory depression [4]

MERCAPTOPURINE

Synonyms: 6-mercaptopurine; 6-MP
Trade name: Purinethol (Gate)
Indications: Leukemias
Class: Antimetabolite, Antineoplastic / anticancer agent (see also Immune checkpoint inhibitor)
Half-life: triphasic: 45 minutes; 2.5 hours; 10 hours
Clinically important, potentially hazardous interactions with: aldesleukin, allopurinol, balsalazide, febuxostat, influenza vaccine, mycophenolate, natalizumab, olsalazine, trimethoprim, typhoid vaccine, vaccines, yellow fever vaccine

---

Skin
Dermatitis (2%)
Hand–foot syndrome (palmar–plantar erythrodysesthesia) [3]
Hypersensitivity [2]
Peripheral edema [2]
Photosensitivity [2]
Pigmentation (Skin) (includes hyperpigmentation) (<10%)
Rash (<10%) [2]

Hair
Alopecia / hair loss [2]

Mucosal
Mucositis (<10%)
Oral lesions (<5%) [2]
Stomatitis (oral mucositis) (<10%)

Central Nervous System
Fever (pyrexia) (includes hyperpyrexia) [3]

Gastrointestinal/Hepatic
Hepatotoxicity / liver injury / acute liver injury / drug-induced liver injury (DILI) [6]
Nausea [2]
Pancreatitis / acute pancreatitis [10]

Hematologic
Leukocytopenia (leukopenia) / leukocytes (white blood cells) decreased [2]
Myelosuppression / bone marrow suppression / myelotoxicity [7]

Other
Death [2]
Neoplasms [2]

MEROPENEM

Trade name: Meronem (AstraZeneca)
Indications: Aerobic and anaerobic infections, febrile neutropenia
Class: Antibiotic, Antibiotic; carbapenem, Antimicrobial, Thienamycin
Half-life: 4–6 hours
Clinically important, potentially hazardous interactions with: oral contraceptives, probenecid, valproic acid

---

Skin
AGEP [2]
Hypersensitivity [3]
Rash (2%) [6]
Stevens-Johnson syndrome and toxic epidermal necrolysis (SJS/TEN) [2]

Central Nervous System
Encephalopathy (includes hepatic encephalopathy) [2]
Fever (pyrexia) (includes hyperpyrexia) [2]
Headache (2%)
Seizures [7]

Endocrine/Metabolic
ALT increased [3]
AST increased [3]

Gastrointestinal/Hepatic
Diarrhea [4]
Hepatotoxicity / liver injury / acute liver injury / drug-induced liver injury (DILI) [10]
Nausea [4]
Vomiting [2]

Hematologic
Neutropenia (neutrophils decreased) [2]

Local
Injection-site pain [3]

Renal
Nephrotoxicity / kidney injury / acute kidney injury (AKI) / drug-induced kidney injury [2]

Other
Adverse effects / adverse reactions [14]
Death [2]

MEROPENEM & VABORBACTAM

Trade name: Vabomere (Rempex)
Indications: Complicated urinary tract infections caused by susceptible bacteria
Class: Antibiotic, Antibiotic; carbapenem (meropenem), Antimicrobial, Beta-lactamase inhibitor (vaborbactam)
Half-life: 1–2 hours
Clinically important, potentially hazardous interactions with: probenecid, valproic acid
Pregnancy category: Potential risk to fetus based on animal studies
Important contra-indications noted in the prescribing guidelines for: pediatric patients
Note: See also separate entry for meropenem.

Skin
Hypersensitivity (2%)

Central Nervous System
Fever (pyrexia) (includes hyperpyrexia) (2%)
Headache (9%)

Endocrine/Metabolic
ALT increased (2%)
AST increased (2%)

Gastrointestinal/Hepatic
Diarrhea (3%)
Nausea (2%)

Local
Infusion-site reactions (4%)
Injection-site phlebitis (4%)

Other
Adverse effects / adverse reactions [2]

MESALAMINE

Synonyms: 5-aminosalicylic acid; 5-ASA; fisalamine; mesalazine
Trade names: Asacol (Procter & Gamble), Canasa (Aptalis), Lialda (Shire), Pentasa (Shire), Rowasa (Solvay)
Indications: Ulcerative colitis
Class: Aminosalicylate
Half-life: 0.5–1.5 hours
Clinically important, potentially hazardous interactions with: azathioprine, NSAIDs, pantoprazole
Important contra-indications noted in the prescribing guidelines for: the elderly; nursing mothers

---

Skin
Diaphoresis (3%)
DRESS syndrome (Drug-induced hypersensitivity syndrome) [3]
Exanthems [3]
Hypersensitivity [7]
Lupus erythematosus (subacute cutaneous lupus erythematosus (SCLE)) [2]
Lupus syndrome / drug-induced lupus (DIL) [3]
Photosensitivity [3]
Psoriasis [2]
Rash (3%) [6]

Hair
Alopecia / hair loss [6]

Cardiovascular
Bradycardia / sinus bradycardia [2]
Cardiotoxicity [4]
Kounis syndrome / allergic angina syndrome / allergic myocardial infarction [2]
Myocarditis [12]
Myopericarditis / perimyocarditis [8]
Pericarditis [10]
Pleuropericarditis [2]

Central Nervous System
Fever (pyrexia) (includes hyperpyrexia) (<6%) [6]
Headache (2–25%) [5]
Pain (14%)
Vertigo / dizziness (2–8%)

Gastrointestinal/Hepatic
Abdominal pain (<18%) [6]
Colitis (ulcerative / exacerbation) [4]
Diarrhea (2–8%) [4]
Eructation (belching) (16%)
Flatulence (<6%) [2]
Hepatitis [6]
Hepatotoxicity / liver injury / acute liver injury / drug-induced liver injury (DILI) [3]
Nausea (3–13%) [3]
Pancreatitis / acute pancreatitis [27]
Peptic ulceration (includes duodenal ulcer, esophageal ulcer) [3]
Vomiting (<5%) [2]

Hematologic
Anemia [2]
Eosinophilia / eosinophils increased [3]

Neuromuscular/Skeletal
Myalgia/Myopathy (3%)

Otic
Tinnitus (<3%)

Renal
Nephritis / interstitial nephritis / tubulointerstitial nephritis [13]
Nephrotoxicity / kidney injury / acute kidney injury (AKI) / drug-induced kidney injury [9]

Respiratory
Eosinophilic pneumonia [4]
Interstitial lung disease / interstitial pneumonitis / interstitial pneumonia (cryptogenic organizing pneumonia) / drug-induced interstitial lung disease [2]
Pharyngitis (sore throat) (11%)
Pneumonia [5]
Pneumonitis [2]
Pulmonary toxicity [10]

Other
Adverse effects / adverse reactions [13]
Allergic reactions [2]

MESORIDAZINE

Trade name: Serentil (Boehringer Ingelheim)
Indications: Schizophrenia
Class: Antipsychotic, Phenothiazine
Half-life: 24–48 hours
Clinically important, potentially hazardous interactions with: antihistamines, arsenic, chlorpheniramine, dofetilide, lithium, piperazine, quinolones, sparfloxacin
Important contra-indications noted in the prescribing guidelines for: pediatric patients

---

Skin
Photosensitivity (<10%)
Rash (<10%)
Endocrine/Metabolic
Mastodynia (<10%)

METAMIZOLE

Synonym: dipyrone
Trade name: Analgin (BPG)
Indications: Analgesic, antipyretic, anti-inflammatory
Class: Non-steroidal anti-inflammatory (NSAID)
Half-life: 2–10 hours
Clinically important, potentially hazardous interactions with: none known
Important contra-indications noted in the prescribing guidelines for: pediatric patients
Note: NSAIDs may cause an increased risk of serious cardiovascular and gastrointestinal adverse events, which can be fatal. This risk may increase with duration of use.
Parenteral administration of Analgin is contraindicated in infants <1 year old.
Metamizole is banned in more than 30 countries, including Japan, Australia, the UK and the USA.

Skin
AGEP [3]
Anaphylactoid reactions / anaphylaxis (includes anaphylactic shock) [12]
Erythema [2]
Exanthems [3]
Fixed eruption / fixed drug eruption [9]
Scrotal gangrene / Fournier's gangrene [2]
Stevens-Johnson syndrome and toxic epidermal necrolysis (SJS/TEN) [7]
Urticaria / hives [3]
Cardiovascular
Kounis syndrome / allergic angina syndrome / allergic myocardial infarction [3]
Central Nervous System
Fever (pyrexia) (includes hyperpyrexia) [3]
Somnolence (drowsiness) [2]
Gastrointestinal/Hepatic
Hepatotoxicity / liver injury / acute liver injury / drug-induced liver injury (DILI) [7]
Vomiting [2]
Hematologic
Agranulocytosis / severe selective neutropenia [21]
Anemia [2]
Neutropenia (neutrophils decreased) [3]
Ocular
Rhinoconjunctivitis [2]
Other
Adverse effects / adverse reactions [5]
Death [15]

METAXALONE

Trade name: Skelaxin (Elan)
Indications: Muscle spasm
Class: Central muscle relaxant
Half-life: 4–14 hours
Clinically important, potentially hazardous interactions with: alcohol, barbiturates, conivaptan, droperidol, interferon alfa, levomepromazine, St John's wort, tricyclic antidepressants
Important contra-indications noted in the prescribing guidelines for: nursing mothers; pediatric patients
Note: Contra-indicated in patients with known tendency to drug-induced, hemolytic, or other anemias, or significantly impaired renal or hepatic function.

Cardiovascular
Tachycardia [2]
Central Nervous System
Agitation [2]
Serotonin syndrome [3]
Somnolence (drowsiness) [3]
Vertigo / dizziness [3]
Gastrointestinal/Hepatic
Nausea [2]
Vomiting [2]

METFORMIN

Trade names: Avandamet (GSK), Fortamet (Andrx), Glucophage (Merck Serono), Glucovance (Merck Serono), Invokamet (Janssen), Janumet (Merck Sharpe & Dohme), Synjardy (Boehringer Ingelheim), Xigduo XR (AstraZeneca)
Indications: Diabetes
Class: Antidiabetic, Biguanide, Hypoglycemic (antihyperglycemic) agent
Half-life: 6 hours
Clinically important, potentially hazardous interactions with: ACE inhibitors, acetazolamide, alcohol, amiloride, anabolic steroids, beta blockers, bictegravir/emtricitabine/tenofovir alafenamide, calcium channel blockers, captopril, cephalexin, cilazapril, cimetidine, corticosteroids, diazoxide, dichlorphenamide, digoxin, disopyramide, diuretics, enalapril, estrogens, fosinopril, iodinated contrast agents, isoniazid, ketotifen, lanreotide, lisinopril, luteinizing hormone releasing hormone analogs, MAO inhibitors, morphine, nicotinic acid, octreotide, oral contraceptives, pegvisomant, phenothiazines, phenytoin, procainamide, progestogens, quinapril, quinidine, quinine, ramipril, ranitidine, risdiplam, somatropin, sotorasib, sympathomimetics, testosterone, thiazides, thyroid products, topiramate, trandolapril, triamterene, trilaciclib, trimethoprim, trospium, tucatinib, vancomycin, zonisamide
Important contra-indications noted in the prescribing guidelines for: the elderly; nursing mothers; pediatric patients
Note: Lactic acidosis is a rare, but serious, metabolic complication that can occur due to metformin accumulation.
Avandamet is metformin and rosiglitazone; Glucovance is metformin and glyburide; Invokamet is metformin and canagliflozin; Janumet is metformin and sitagliptin; Synjardy is metformin and empagliflozin; Xigduo XR is metformin and dapagliflozin.
Warning: LACTIC ACIDOSIS

Skin
Angioedema (formerly named angioneurotic edema) [2]
Bullous pemphigoid / pemphigoid [2]
Erythema (transient) [3]
Fixed eruption / fixed drug eruption [3]
Flushing / rubefaction (<10%)
Leukocytoclastic vasculitis (angiitis) [2]
Lichenoid eruption / lichenoid reaction [2]
Peripheral edema [5]
Photosensitivity (<10%)
Rash (<10%) [4]
Urticaria / hives (<10%) [4]
Vasculitis (angiitis) / cutaneous vasculitis (angiitis) [2]
Cardiovascular
Hypertension [3]
Palpitation (<10%)
Central Nervous System
Chills (<10%)
Dysgeusia (taste perversion) (3%)
Headache (6%) [10]
Nightmares [3]
Vertigo / dizziness (<10%) [6]
Endocrine/Metabolic
Acidosis (includes lactic acidosis) [24]
Appetite decreased [5]
Hypoglycemia [17]
Vitamin B-12 deficiency [6]
Weight gain [2]
Weight loss [5]
Gastrointestinal/Hepatic
Abdominal pain (6%) [5]
Constipation [3]
Diarrhea (10–35%) [33]
Dyspepsia / functional dyspepsia (indigestion) (see also gastroparesis) [5]
Flatulence [2]
Gastroenteritis [2]
Gastrointestinal adverse reaction [2]
Hepatitis [2]
Hepatotoxicity / liver injury / acute liver injury / drug-induced liver injury (DILI) [8]
Nausea (7–26%) [25]
Pancreatitis / acute pancreatitis [6]
Vomiting (7–26%) [12]
Genitourinary
Genital mycotic infection [9]
Pollakiuria [3]
Urinary tract infection [12]
Hematologic
Anemia [2]
Neuromuscular/Skeletal
Arthralgia [5]
Asthenia / fatigue (9%) [2]
Back pain [5]
Myalgia/Myopathy (<10%)

Renal
Nephrotoxicity / kidney injury / acute kidney injury (AKI) / drug-induced kidney injury [5]
Respiratory
Bronchitis [3]
Dyspnea / shortness of breath (<10%)
Influenza [2]
Nasopharyngitis [6]
Respiratory tract infection (<10%)
Sinusitis (see also rhinitis / rhinosinusitis) [2]
Upper respiratory tract infection [6]
Other
Adverse effects / adverse reactions [24]
Death [2]

METHADONE

Trade names: Dolophine (Roxane), Methadose (Mallinckrodt)
Indications: Pain, narcotic addiction
Class: Opiate agonist
Half-life: 15–25 hours
Clinically important, potentially hazardous interactions with: abacavir, amprenavir, boceprevir, citalopram, darunavir, delavirdine, diazepam, efavirenz, erythromycin, fluconazole, fluvoxamine, interferon alfa, itraconazole, ketoconazole, linezolid, lofexidine, lopinavir, nelfinavir, nilotinib, paroxetine hydrochloride, PEG-interferon, quetiapine, ribociclib, rifapentine, rilpivirine, safinamide, selegiline, St John's wort, tipranavir, vandetanib, voriconazole, zidovudine, zuclopenthixol
Important contra-indications noted in the prescribing guidelines for: pediatric patients
Note: Methadone is not licensed for use in children though it can be employed for the management of neonatal opiate withdrawal syndrome.

Skin
Diaphoresis (<48%) [4]
Pruritus (itching) [2]
Mucosal
Xerostomia (dry mouth) (<10%)
Cardiovascular
Arrhythmias [2]
QT interval prolonged / QT prolongation [37]
Torsades de pointes [27]
Ventricular arrhythmia [2]
Central Nervous System
Encephalopathy (includes hepatic encephalopathy) [2]
Hallucinations [2]
Hyperalgesia [2]
Neurotoxicity [2]
Serotonin syndrome [2]
Somnolence (drowsiness) [2]
Syncope / fainting [2]
Endocrine/Metabolic
Hypoglycemia [2]
Genitourinary
Sexual dysfunction [2]
Local
Injection-site pain (<10%)
Neuromuscular/Skeletal
Rhabdomyolysis [4]
Respiratory
Respiratory depression [4]
Other
Adverse effects / adverse reactions [2]
Death [15]

METHAMPHETAMINE

Trade name: Desoxyn (Recordati)
Indications: Attention deficit disorder, obesity
Class: Amphetamine, Anti-obesity / weight loss pharmacotherapy
Half-life: 4–5 hours
Clinically important, potentially hazardous interactions with: fluoxetine, fluvoxamine, MAO inhibitors, paroxetine hydrochloride, phenelzine, sertraline, tranylcypromine
Important contra-indications noted in the prescribing guidelines for: nursing mothers; pediatric patients
Warning: POTENTIAL FOR ABUSE

Skin
Diaphoresis (<10%)
Mucosal
Xerostomia (dry mouth) (<10%) [5]
Cardiovascular
Polyarteritis nodosa [2]
Central Nervous System
Depression [2]
Hallucinations [4]
Insomnia [2]
Neurotoxicity [6]
Paranoia [2]
Parkinsonism [2]
Psychosis [11]
Neuromuscular/Skeletal
Rhabdomyolysis (43%) [5]
Other
Bruxism (teeth grinding) [4]
Death [3]
Dental disease [2]
Tooth decay [2]

METHANTHELINE

Indications: Duodenal ulcer
Class: Muscarinic cholinergic agonist
Half-life: N/A
Clinically important, potentially hazardous interactions with: anticholinergics, arbutamine

---

Mucosal
Xerostomia (dry mouth) [4]

METHAZOLAMIDE

Indications: Glaucoma
Class: Carbonic anhydrase inhibitor, Diuretic
Half-life: ~14 hours
Clinically important, potentially hazardous interactions with: none known

---

Skin
Stevens-Johnson syndrome and toxic epidermal necrolysis (SJS/TEN) [7]
Central Nervous System
Depression [2]
Dysgeusia (taste perversion) (metallic taste) (>10%) [2]
Paresthesias [2]
Endocrine/Metabolic
Acidosis (includes lactic acidosis) [2]
Libido decreased [2]
Weight loss [2]
Gastrointestinal/Hepatic
Dyspepsia / functional dyspepsia (indigestion) (see also gastroparesis) [2]
Ocular
Glaucoma (includes acute angle-closure glaucoma) [2]
Myopia [3]
Renal
Nephrolithiasis (kidney stones / renal calculi) [2]

METHENAMINE

Trade name: Hiprex (Sanofi-Aventis)
Indications: Urinary tract infections
Class: Antibiotic, Antimicrobial
Half-life: 3–6 hours
Clinically important, potentially hazardous interactions with: lisdexamfetamine

---

Skin
Exanthems [2]
Rash (4%)

METHICILLIN

Indications: Various infections caused by susceptible organisms
Class: Antibiotic, Antibiotic; beta-lactam, Antibiotic; penicillin, Antimicrobial
Half-life: 30 minutes
Clinically important, potentially hazardous interactions with: anticoagulants, cyclosporine, imipenem/cilastatin, methotrexate, tetracycline

---

Skin
Exanthems (29%) [2]
Rash (<10%)

METHIMAZOLE

Synonym: thiamazole
Trade name: Tapazole (Paladin)
Indications: Hyperthyroidism
Class: Antithyroid, Antithyroid; hormone modifier
Half-life: 4–13 hours
Clinically important, potentially hazardous interactions with: anticoagulants, dicumarol, warfarin

---

Skin
Aplasia cutis congenita [4]
Exanthems (<15%) [5]
Hypersensitivity [3]
Lupus erythematosus (subacute cutaneous lupus erythematosus (SCLE)) (<10%) [13]
Pruritus (itching) (<5%) [4]
Rash (>10%)
Stevens-Johnson syndrome and toxic epidermal necrolysis (SJS/TEN) [2]
Urticaria / hives (>5%) [2]
Vasculitis (angiitis) / cutaneous vasculitis (angiitis) [6]
Mucosal
Gingival necrosis [3]
Parotitis [2]

Central Nervous System
- Ageusia (taste loss) / taste disorder (<10%)

Endocrine/Metabolic
- Hypoglycemia [2]
- Insulin autoimmune syndrome / insulin autoimmune hypoglycemia / Hirata's disease [6]

Gastrointestinal/Hepatic
- Cholestasis / cholestatic jaundice [5]
- Hepatotoxicity / liver injury / acute liver injury / drug-induced liver injury (DILI) [11]
- Pancreatitis / acute pancreatitis [6]

Hematologic
- Agranulocytosis / severe selective neutropenia [16]
- Neutropenia (neutrophils decreased) [2]
- Pancytopenia (includes bicytopenia) [4]

Neuromuscular/Skeletal
- Arthralgia [4]

Respiratory
- Pulmonary toxicity [2]

Other
- Death [2]
- Side effects (in high dosages) (28%) [2]
- Teratogenicity [2]

METHOCARBAMOL

Trade name: Robaxin (Baxter) (Elkins-Sinn)
Indications: Muscle spasm, tetanus
Class: Central muscle relaxant
Half-life: 1–2 hours
Clinically important, potentially hazardous interactions with: ethanol
Important contra-indications noted in the prescribing guidelines for: nursing mothers; pediatric patients

---

Skin
- Flushing / rubefaction (<10%)

Other
- Allergic reactions (<10%)

METHOHEXITAL

Synonym: Methohexitone
Trade name: Brevital (JHP Pharmaceuticals)
Indications: General anesthesia
Class: Barbiturate
Half-life: 4–8 minutes
Clinically important, potentially hazardous interactions with: none known

---

Skin
- Angioedema (formerly named angioneurotic edema) [2]
- Urticaria / hives [2]

Central Nervous System
- Seizures [3]

Gastrointestinal/Hepatic
- Vomiting [2]

Local
- Injection-site pain (18%)

Other
- Hiccups / singultus (13%) [5]

METHOTREXATE

Synonyms: amethopterin; MTX
Trade names: Rasuvo (Medac), Rheumatrex (Stada)
Indications: Carcinomas, leukemias, lymphomas, psoriasis, rheumatoid arthritis
Class: Antimetabolite, Antipsoriatic agent, Disease-modifying antirheumatic drug (DMARD), Folic acid antagonist
Half-life: 3–10 hours
Clinically important, potentially hazardous interactions with: acemetacin, acitretin, aldesleukin, aminoglycosides, amiodarone, amoxicillin, ampicillin, aspirin, bacampicillin, bismuth, carbenicillin, chloroquine, ciprofloxacin, cisplatin, cloxacillin, co-trimoxazole, cyclopenthiazide, dapsone, demeclocycline, dexamethasone, diclofenac, dicloxacillin, doxycycline, echinacea, etodolac, etoricoxib, etretinate, fenoprofen, flurbiprofen, folic acid antagonists, gadobenate, haloperidol, hydrocortisone, ibuprofen, indomethacin, infliximab, ketoprofen, ketorolac, leflunomide, magnesium trisalicylate, meclofenamate, mefenamic acid, meloxicam, methicillin, mezlocillin, minocycline, nabumetone, nafcillin, naproxen, natalizumab, NSAIDs, omeprazole, oxacillin, oxaprozin, oxtriphylline, oxytetracycline, pantoprazole, paromomycin, penicillin G, penicillin V, penicillins, phenylbutazone, piperacillin, piperacillin/tazobactam, piroxicam, polypeptide antibiotics, prednisolone, prednisone, pristinamycin, probenecid, procarbazine, rofecoxib, salicylates, salsalate, sapropterin, sulfadiazine, sulfamethoxazole, sulfapyridine, sulfasalazine, sulfisoxazole, sulindac, tafamidis meglumine, taxobactam, tenoxicam, tetracycline, ticarcillin, tolmetin, trimethoprim, vaccines
Important contra-indications noted in the prescribing guidelines for: the elderly; nursing mothers; pediatric patients
Note: August 2023: UK Medicines and Healthcare products Regulatory Agency Methotrexate: advise patients to take precautions in the sun to avoid photosensitivity reactions Photosensitivity reactions are known side effects of methotrexate treatment and can be severe. Patients should be advised to take precautions to protect their skin in the sun. .
Warning: SEVERE TOXIC REACTIONS, INCLUDING EMBRYOFETAL TOXICITY AND DEATH

Skin
- Abscess (peritoneal) [2]
- Acral erythema [14]
- Anaphylactoid reactions / anaphylaxis (includes anaphylactic shock) (<10%) [9]
- Bruise / bruising / contusion / ecchymosis (ecchymoses) [2]
- Bullous acral erythema [2]
- Bullous dermatosis [4]
- Capillaritis [2]
- Carcinoma [2]
- Cutaneous toxicity / skin toxicity [10]
- Dermatitis [2]
- Edema / fluid retention [2]
- Erosion of psoriatic plaques [8]
- Erythema (>10%)
- Erythema multiforme [4]
- Erythroderma [2]
- Exanthems (15%) [5]
- Folliculitis [2]
- Hand–foot syndrome (palmar–plantar erythrodysesthesia) [3]
- Herpes simplex [2]
- Herpes zoster [7]
- Hypersensitivity [5]
- Lymphoma [5]
- Lymphoproliferative disease / lymphoproliferative disorder [17]
- Malignant lymphoma [4]
- Molluscum contagiosum [2]
- Necrosis (skin necrosis) [8]
- Nodular eruption [15]
- Non-Hodgkin's lymphoma [2]
- Photosensitivity (5%) [9]
- Pigmentation (Skin) (includes hyperpigmentation) (<10%)
- Pruritus (itching) (<5%)
- Pseudolymphoma / cutaneous pseudolymphoma [10]
- Radiation recall dermatitis [8]
- Rash (<3%) [13]
- Squamous cell carcinoma [2]
- Stevens-Johnson syndrome and toxic epidermal necrolysis (SJS/TEN) [18]
- Sunburn (reactivation) [6]
- Ulceration of psoriatic plaques [4]
- Ulcerations [14]
- Urticaria / hives [4]
- Vasculitis (angiitis) / cutaneous vasculitis (angiitis) (>10%) [9]

Hair
- Alopecia / hair loss (<6%) [28]

Nails
- Nail pigmentation [2]
- Paronychia [2]

Mucosal
- Aphthous stomatitis / aphthous ulcer / aphtha (aphthae) [2]
- Gingivitis (>10%)
- Glossitis (inflammation of the tongue) (>10%)
- Mucocutaneous reactions [3]
- Mucositis [14]
- Nasal septal perforation [2]
- Oral ulceration [13]
- Stomatitis (oral mucositis) (3–10%) [29]

Cardiovascular
- Cardiotoxicity [2]
- Hypertension [2]
- Pericardial effusion [2]
- Pericarditis [5]

Central Nervous System
- Encephalopathy (includes hepatic encephalopathy) [6]
- Fever (pyrexia) (includes hyperpyrexia) [7]
- Headache [18]
- Leukoencephalopathy / posterior reversible encephalopathy syndrome (PRES) [65]
- Migraine [2]
- Myelopathy [9]
- Necrotizing myelopathy / necrotic myelopathy / subacute necrotic myelopathy [3]
- Neurotoxicity [14]
- Stroke / cerebrovascular accident [2]
- Vertigo / dizziness [3]

Endocrine/Metabolic
- ALT increased [7]
- AST increased [3]
- Diabetes mellitus [2]
- Gynecomastia [8]

Hypertransaminasemia (hepatic transaminitis) / elevated transaminases [3]
Hypoalbuminemia / albumin decreased [2]
Weight gain [2]

Gastrointestinal/Hepatic
Abdominal pain [9]
Colitis [2]
Diarrhea [13]
Dyspepsia / functional dyspepsia (indigestion) (see also gastroparesis) [3]
Gastroenteritis [2]
Hepatic failure [3]
Hepatic steatosis [2]
Hepatitis [3]
Hepatotoxicity / liver injury / acute liver injury / drug-induced liver injury (DILI) [62]
Nausea [32]
Vomiting [14]

Genitourinary
Urinary tract infection [4]

Hematologic
Anemia [10]
Febrile neutropenia [4]
Hemotoxicity [2]
Leukocytopenia (leukopenia) / leukocytes (white blood cells) decreased [11]
Myelosuppression / bone marrow suppression / myelotoxicity [13]
Neutropenia (neutrophils decreased) [12]
Pancytopenia (includes bicytopenia) [16]
Thrombocytopenia / platelets decreased [10]

Local
Injection-site reaction [3]

Neuromuscular/Skeletal
Arthralgia [5]
Asthenia / fatigue [16]
Back pain [2]
Bone pain / joint pain [2]

Ocular
Cotton wool spots [2]
Optic neuropathy [2]

Renal
Nephropathy [3]
Nephrotoxicity / kidney injury / acute kidney injury (AKI) / drug-induced kidney injury [34]
Renal failure [3]

Respiratory
Cough [3]
Nasopharyngitis [6]
Pharyngitis (sore throat) [2]
Pneumonia [8]
Pneumonitis [8]
Pulmonary toxicity [9]
Sinusitis (see also rhinitis / rhinosinusitis) [2]
Upper respiratory tract infection [9]

Other
Adverse effects / adverse reactions [45]
Death [19]
Hodgkin's disease (nodular sclerosing) [2]
Infection [25]
Malignancies [2]
Neoplasms [2]
Side effects [3]
Teratogenicity [3]

METHOXSALEN

Trade name: Oxsoralen (Valeant)
Indications: Psoriasis, vitiligo
Class: CYP1A2 inhibitor, Psoralen, Repigmenting agent
Half-life: 1.1 hours
Clinically important, potentially hazardous interactions with: caffeine, chloroquine, cyclosporine, fluoroquinolones, phenothiazines, sulfonamides
Important contra-indications noted in the prescribing guidelines for: pediatric patients
Note: Potential hazards of long-term therapy include the possibilities of carcinogenicity and cataractogenicity.

Skin
Anaphylactoid reactions / anaphylaxis (includes anaphylactic shock) [2]
Basal cell carcinoma [3]
Bullous dermatosis (with UVA) [4]
Burning / skin burning sensation (<10%) [3]
Carcinoma [5]
Dermatitis [4]
Edema / fluid retention (<10%)
Ephelides (freckles) (<10%) [5]
Erythema (<10%)
Exanthems [2]
Herpes zoster [2]
Hypomelanosis (<10%)
Lupus erythematosus (subacute cutaneous lupus erythematosus (SCLE)) [3]
Photosensitivity [9]
Phototoxicity [7]
Pigmentation (Skin) (includes hyperpigmentation) [3]
Porokeratosis (actinic) [3]
Pruritus (itching) (>10%)
Rash (<10%)
Squamous cell carcinoma [4]
Tumors [2]
Vitiligo [2]

Hair
Hypertrichosis [3]

Nails
Nail pigmentation [5]
Photo-onycholysis [5]

Mucosal
Cheilitis (inflammation of the lips) (<10%)

Central Nervous System
Pain [2]

Ocular
Ocular toxicity [2]

METHOXYFLURANE

Trade name: Penthrane (AbbVie) (Ger)
Indications: Anesthesia
Class: Anesthetic; inhalation
Half-life: N/A
Clinically important, potentially hazardous interactions with: cisatracurium, demeclocycline, doxacurium, doxycycline, gentamicin, kanamycin, minocycline, neomycin, oxytetracycline, pancuronium, rapacuronium, streptomycin, tetracycline

---

Gastrointestinal/Hepatic
Hepatotoxicity / liver injury / acute liver injury / drug-induced liver injury (DILI) [3]

Renal
Nephrotoxicity / kidney injury / acute kidney injury (AKI) / drug-induced kidney injury [4]

Other
Adverse effects / adverse reactions [2]

METHSUXIMIDE

Trade name: Celontin (Pfizer)
Indications: Absence (petit-mal) seizures
Class: Antiepileptic; succinimide
Half-life: 2–4 hours
Clinically important, potentially hazardous interactions with: phenobarbital, phenytoin
Note: Methsuximide should not be used in patients with a history of hypersensitivity to succinimides. Blood dyscrasias, including some with fatal outcome, have been reported to be associated with the use of succinimides; therefore, periodic blood counts should be performed.

Skin
Lupus erythematosus (subacute cutaneous lupus erythematosus (SCLE)) (>10%)
Stevens-Johnson syndrome and toxic epidermal necrolysis (SJS/TEN) (>10%)

METHYL SALICYLATE

Synonym: Oil of Wintergreen
Trade name: Salonpas (Hisamitsu)
Indications: Pain
Class: Analgesic, Non-steroidal anti-inflammatory (NSAID), Salicylate
Half-life: N/A
Clinically important, potentially hazardous interactions with: alcohol, anticoagulants, aspirin, ibuprofen, naproxen, triamcinolone, warfarin
Important contra-indications noted in the prescribing guidelines for: the elderly; pediatric patients
Note: Do not use in the last 3 months of pregnancy as it may cause problems in the unborn child or complications during delivery.
Salonpas contains menthol.

Skin
Cutaneous toxicity / skin toxicity [4]

METHYLDOPA

Trade name: Aldoclor (Merck)
Indications: Hypertension
Class: Adrenergic alpha-receptor agonist
Half-life: 1.7 hours
Clinically important, potentially hazardous interactions with: acebutolol, alfuzosin, bromocriptine, captopril, cilazapril, cyclopenthiazide, diclofenac, enalapril, ephedrine, fosinopril, irbesartan, levodopa, levomepromazine, linezolid, lisinopril, meloxicam, olmesartan, quinapril, ramipril, risperidone, rotigotine, trandolapril, triamcinolone, zuclopenthixol
Important contra-indications noted in the prescribing guidelines for: nursing mothers
Note: Aldoril is methyldopa and hydrochlorothiazide. Hydrochlorothiazide is a sulfonamide and can be absorbed systemically.

Sulfonamides can produce severe, possibly fatal, reactions such as toxic epidermal necrolysis and Stevens-Johnson syndrome.

Skin
- Eczema / eczematous reaction / eczematous eruption [3]
- Erythema multiforme [2]
- Exanthems (3%) [3]
- Lichen planus (includes hypertrophic lichen planus) [3]
- Lichenoid eruption / lichenoid reaction [9]
- Lupus erythematosus (subacute cutaneous lupus erythematosus (SCLE)) [14]
- Peripheral edema (>10%)
- Photosensitivity [2]
- Pigmentation (Skin) (includes hyperpigmentation) [3]
- Seborrheic dermatitis [3]
- Stevens-Johnson syndrome and toxic epidermal necrolysis (SJS/TEN) [3]
- Urticaria / hives [2]

Mucosal
- Oral lichenoid eruption [3]
- Oral ulceration [6]
- Xerostomia (dry mouth) (<10%)

Central Nervous System
- Anxiety (<10%)
- Depression (<10%)
- Dyskinesia [2]
- Fever (pyrexia) (includes hyperpyrexia) (<10%)
- Headache (<10%)
- Nightmares (<10%)
- Parkinsonism [2]

Endocrine/Metabolic
- Amenorrhea [2]
- Galactorrhea [4]

Gastrointestinal/Hepatic
- Hepatitis [3]
- Hepatotoxicity / liver injury / acute liver injury / drug-induced liver injury (DILI) [8]

Hematologic
- Hemolytic anemia [2]

METHYLERGONOVINE

Trade name: Methergine (Novartis)
Indications: Routine management after delivery of placenta, postpartum atony and hemorrhage, subinvolution
Class: Ergot alkaloid
Half-life: 1.5–12.7 hours
Clinically important, potentially hazardous interactions with: alkaloid drugs, amprenavir, boceprevir, clarithromycin, CYP3A4 inhibitors, delavirdine, dihydroergotamine, ergotamine, erythromycin, indinavir, itraconazole, ketoconazole, lopinavir, nefazodone, nelfinavir, ombitasvir/paritaprevir/ritonavir, ombitasvir/paritaprevir/ritonavir and dasabuvir, ritonavir, telaprevir, troleandomycin, voriconazole, zileuton
Important contra-indications noted in the prescribing guidelines for: nursing mothers

---

Cardiovascular
- Chest pain [2]

Gastrointestinal/Hepatic
- Nausea [3]
- Vomiting [3]

Respiratory
- Respiratory depression [2]

METHYLNALTREXONE

Trade name: Relistor (Wyeth)
Indications: Treatment of opioid-induced constipation in patients with advanced illness and receiving palliative care
Class: Opioid antagonist, Opioid receptor antagonist
Half-life: 8 hours
Clinically important, potentially hazardous interactions with: PEG-interferon
Important contra-indications noted in the prescribing guidelines for: nursing mothers; pediatric patients
Note: Contra-indicated in patients with known or suspected mechanical gastrointestinal obstruction.

Skin
- Hyperhidrosis (7%)

Cardiovascular
- Circulatory collapse [3]

Central Nervous System
- Vertigo / dizziness (7%) [2]

Endocrine/Metabolic
- Dehydration [3]

Gastrointestinal/Hepatic
- Abdominal pain (29%) [11]
- Diarrhea (6%) [5]
- Flatulence (13%) [4]
- Nausea (12%) [9]
- Vomiting [2]

METHYLPHENIDATE

Trade names: Concerta (Janssen), Metadate CD (Celltech), Methylin (Mallinckrodt), Ritalin (Novartis)
Indications: Attention deficit disorder, narcolepsy
Class: Amphetamine, Anti-attention deficit hyperactivity disorder (anti-ADHD)
Half-life: 2–4 hours
Clinically important, potentially hazardous interactions with: amitriptyline, benazepril, bupropion, captopril, citalopram, clevidipine, cyclosporine, enalapril, escitalopram, irbesartan, linezolid, lisinopril, lurasidone, MAO inhibitors, olmesartan, paliperidone, pantoprazole, paroxetine hydrochloride, phenylbutazone, pimozide, quinapril, safinamide, ziprasidone
Important contra-indications noted in the prescribing guidelines for: the elderly; nursing mothers
Warning: ABUSE AND DEPENDENCE

Skin
- Angioedema (formerly named angioneurotic edema) [2]
- Exanthems [2]
- Exfoliative dermatitis [2]
- Hypersensitivity (<10%)
- Leukoderma [2]

Mucosal
- Xerostomia (dry mouth) [7]

Cardiovascular
- Cardiotoxicity [3]
- Palpitation [4]
- QT interval prolonged / QT prolongation [2]
- Tachycardia [5]

Central Nervous System
- Agitation [2]
- Anorexia [8]
- Anxiety [7]
- Compulsions / obsessive-compulsive symptoms / obsessive-compulsive disorder [2]
- Depression [2]
- Fever (pyrexia) (includes hyperpyrexia) [2]
- Hallucinations [6]
- Hallucinations, visual [6]
- Headache [14]
- Insomnia [17]
- Irritability [6]
- Mood changes (includes mood disorder) [2]
- Nervousness [2]
- Neurotoxicity [3]
- Psychosis [3]
- Seizures [3]
- Somnolence (drowsiness) [3]
- Stuttering (dysphemia) / stammering [3]
- Suicidal ideation [2]
- Tic disorder [7]
- Tremor [2]
- Trichotillomania (hair-pulling disorder) [2]
- Vertigo / dizziness [5]
- Yawning [2]

Endocrine/Metabolic
- Appetite decreased [17]
- Weight loss [9]

Gastrointestinal/Hepatic
- Abdominal pain [13]
- Nausea [7]
- Vomiting [5]

Genitourinary
- Enuresis (urinary incontinence) [2]
- Menorrhagia [2]
- Priapism [5]

Neuromuscular/Skeletal
- Asthenia / fatigue [2]
- Dystonia [2]

Respiratory
- Cough [3]
- Nasopharyngitis [4]
- Upper respiratory tract infection [3]

Other
- Adverse effects / adverse reactions [8]
- Bruxism (teeth grinding) [2]

METHYL-PREDNISOLONE

Trade names: Advantan (Intendis), Medrol (Pharmacia), Solu-Medrol (Pharmacia)
Indications: Arthralgias, asthma, dermatoses, inflammatory ocular conditions, rhinitis
Class: Corticosteroid / Glucocorticoid, Corticosteroid, systemic, Covid-19 putative drug, Neuroprotectant
Half-life: 12–36 hours; 2–4 hours (plasma)
Clinically important, potentially hazardous interactions with: aminophylline, aprepitant, aspirin, carbamazepine, clarithromycin, conivaptan, cyclosporine, daclizumab, darunavir, delavirdine, erythromycin, indinavir, itraconazole, ketoconazole, live vaccines, oral contraceptives, phenobarbital, phenytoin, rifampin, telaprevir, telithromycin, troleandomycin, voriconazole, warfarin

Important contra-indications noted in the prescribing guidelines for: nursing mothers; pediatric patients

---

Skin
- Anaphylactoid reactions / anaphylaxis (includes anaphylactic shock) [15]
- Bruise / bruising / contusion / ecchymosis (ecchymoses) [2]
- Dermatitis [5]
- Flushing / rubefaction [2]
- Hypersensitivity [3]
- Pruritus (itching) [2]
- Rash [2]
- Urticaria / hives [5]

Cardiovascular
- Arrhythmias [2]
- Bradycardia / sinus bradycardia [13]
- Hypertension [7]
- Myocardial infarction [2]
- Myocardial toxicity [2]

Central Nervous System
- Depression [5]
- Dysgeusia (taste perversion) [4]
- Headache [2]
- Neurotoxicity [2]
- Psychosis [3]
- Seizures [3]
- Vertigo / dizziness [2]

Endocrine/Metabolic
- Diabetic ketoacidosis [2]
- Hyperglycemia (includes glucose increased) [5]
- Hypokalemia [2]

Gastrointestinal/Hepatic
- Abdominal pain [3]
- Gastrointestinal bleeding [2]
- Hepatotoxicity / liver injury / acute liver injury / drug-induced liver injury (DILI) [10]
- Pancreatitis / acute pancreatitis [3]

Neuromuscular/Skeletal
- Arthralgia [2]
- Myalgia/Myopathy [5]
- Osteonecrosis / avascular necrosis (includes steroid-induced osteonecrosis of the femoral head) [9]
- Osteoporosis [2]
- Tendinopathy/Tendon rupture [2]

Ocular
- Cataract [3]
- Glaucoma (includes acute angle-closure glaucoma) [2]

Respiratory
- Dysphonia (includes voice disorders / voice changes) [2]

Other
- Adverse effects / adverse reactions [7]
- Allergic reactions [3]
- Death [2]
- Hiccups / singultus [3]
- Infection [7]

METHYL-TESTOSTERONE

Trade names: Android (Valeant), Estratest (Solvay), Testred (Valeant)
Indications: Hypogonadism, impotence, metastatic breast cancer
Class: Androgen
Half-life: 2.5–3.5 hours
Clinically important, potentially hazardous interactions with: anticoagulants, cyclosporine, warfarin
Important contra-indications noted in the prescribing guidelines for: nursing mothers; pediatric patients

---

Skin
- Acneiform eruption / acneiform dermatitis / acneiform rash (>10%) [12]
- Edema / fluid retention (>10%)
- Flushing / rubefaction (<5%)

Hair
- Alopecia / hair loss [2]
- Hirsutism (in females) (<10%) [9]

Endocrine/Metabolic
- Mastodynia (>10%)

Genitourinary
- Priapism (>10%)

METHYSERGIDE

Trade name: Sansert (Novartis)
Indications: Vascular (migraine) headaches
Class: Hallucinogen, Psychotomimetic
Half-life: 10 hours
Clinically important, potentially hazardous interactions with: acebutolol, almotriptan, amprenavir, azithromycin, chlortetracycline, clarithromycin, delavirdine, demeclocycline, doxycycline, efavirenz, eletriptan, erythromycin, frovatriptan, indinavir, itraconazole, lymecycline, minocycline, naratriptan, nelfinavir, oxytetracycline, ritonavir, rizatriptan, saquinavir, sibutramine, sumatriptan, telithromycin, tetracycline, tigecycline, troleandomycin, voriconazole, zolmitriptan
Important contra-indications noted in the prescribing guidelines for: nursing mothers; pediatric patients

---

Skin
- Lupus erythematosus (subacute cutaneous lupus erythematosus (SCLE)) [2]
- Peripheral edema (<10%)
- Rash (<10%)
- Scleroderma [4]

Hair
- Alopecia / hair loss [4]

Cardiovascular
- Valvulopathy [3]

METIPRANOLOL

Trade name: OptiPranolol (Bausch & Lomb)
Indications: Open angle glaucoma, ocular hypertension
Class: Adrenergic beta-receptor antagonist
Half-life: N/A
Clinically important, potentially hazardous interactions with: beta blockers, calcium channel blockers, reserpine

---

Ocular
- Uveitis / anterior uveitis / posterior uveitis / panuveitis [14]

METOCLOPRAMIDE

Trade name: Reglan (Wyeth)
Indications: Gastroesophageal reflux
Class: Antiemetic, Dopamine receptor antagonist
Half-life: 4–6 hours
Clinically important, potentially hazardous interactions with: acetaminophen, amitriptyline, atovaquone, atovaquone/proguanil, bromocriptine, citalopram, darifenacin, hydromorphone, levodopa, levodopa, levomepromazine, lurasidone, mepenzolate, meptazinol, naratriptan, olanzapine, oxybutynin, paliperidone, posaconazole, propyphenazone, risperidone, rotigotine, safinamide, sertraline, tetrabenazine, tiotropium, trospium, venlafaxine, ziprasidone, zuclopenthixol
Warning: TARDIVE DYSKINESIA

Skin
- Anaphylactoid reactions / anaphylaxis (includes anaphylactic shock) [2]
- Angioedema (formerly named angioneurotic edema) [2]
- Exanthems [3]
- Rash (<10%)
- Urticaria / hives [2]

Mucosal
- Xerostomia (dry mouth) (<10%)

Cardiovascular
- QT interval prolonged / QT prolongation [2]
- Torsades de pointes [3]

Central Nervous System
- Akathisia [2]
- Depression [2]
- Encephalopathy (includes hepatic encephalopathy) [2]
- Extrapyramidal symptoms [7]
- Insomnia [2]
- Neuroleptic malignant syndrome [8]
- Parkinsonism [11]
- Psychosis [2]
- Sedation [2]
- Serotonin syndrome [2]
- Somnolence (drowsiness) [2]
- Tardive syndrome / tardive dyskinesia [12]

Endocrine/Metabolic
- Galactorrhea [4]
- Gynecomastia [2]
- Mastodynia (<10%)
- Porphyria [2]

Gastrointestinal/Hepatic
- Diarrhea [2]

Hematologic
- Sulfhemoglobinemia [2]

Multi-Organ and/or Multi-Metabolic Adverse Reactions
Pheochromocytoma crisis / paraganglioma crisis [3]

Neuromuscular/Skeletal
Dystonia [20]

Ocular
Oculogyric crisis / oculogyric dystonic reaction [7]

Respiratory
Respiratory failure [2]

Other
Adverse effects / adverse reactions [4]
Side effects [2]

METOLAZONE

Trade name: Zaroxolyn (Celltech)
Indications: Hypertension, edema
Class: Diuretic, thiazide
Half-life: 6–20 hours
Clinically important, potentially hazardous interactions with: digoxin, lithium
Note: Metolazone is a sulfonamide and can be absorbed systemically. Sulfonamides can produce severe, possibly fatal, reactions such as toxic epidermal necrolysis and Stevens-Johnson syndrome.

Skin
Anaphylactoid reactions / anaphylaxis (includes anaphylactic shock) (<2%)
Edema / fluid retention (<2%)
Photosensitivity (<2%)
Pruritus (itching) (<2%)
Rash (<2%)
Urticaria / hives (<2%)
Vasculitis (angiitis) / cutaneous vasculitis (angiitis) [2]
Xerosis / xeroderma (<2%)

Mucosal
Xerostomia (dry mouth) (<2%)

Central Nervous System
Chills (<10%)
Dysgeusia (taste perversion) (<2%)
Paresthesias (<2%)

Ocular
Dyschromatopsia (<2%)

METOPROLOL

Trade names: Lopressor (Novartis), Toprol XL (AstraZeneca)
Indications: Hypertension, angina pectoris
Class: Adrenergic beta-receptor agonist, Antiarrhythmic class II
Half-life: 3–4 hours
Clinically important, potentially hazardous interactions with: cinacalcet, clonidine, cobicistat/elvitegravir/emtricitabine/tenofovir alafenamide, cobicistat/elvitegravir/emtricitabine/tenofovir disoproxil, dronedarone, epinephrine, mirabegron, paroxetine hydrochloride, propoxyphene, tadalafil, telithromycin, tipranavir, venlafaxine, verapamil, viloxazine
Important contra-indications noted in the prescribing guidelines for: the elderly; pediatric patients
Note: Cutaneous side effects of beta-receptor blockers are clinically polymorphous. They apparently appear after several months of continuous therapy.

Skin
Eczema / eczematous reaction / eczematous eruption [2]
Erythroderma [2]
Lichenoid eruption / lichenoid reaction [4]
Pruritus (itching) (<5%)
Psoriasis (induction and aggravation of) [8]
Rash (<5%) [3]
Raynaud's phenomenon [3]

Cardiovascular
Arrhythmias [2]
Bradycardia / sinus bradycardia [8]
Hypotension [4]

Central Nervous System
Delirium [3]
Hallucinations [2]
Hallucinations, visual [3]
Sleep disturbances [2]

Gastrointestinal/Hepatic
Gastrointestinal disorder / discomfort [2]
Hepatotoxicity / liver injury / acute liver injury / drug-induced liver injury (DILI) [3]

Genitourinary
Peyronie's disease [5]

Neuromuscular/Skeletal
Asthenia / fatigue [2]

METRONIDAZOLE

Trade names: Flagyl (Pfizer), Metrocream (Galderma), MetroGel (Galderma), Metrolotion (Galderma), Noritate (Dermik), Vandazole (Upsher-Smith)
Indications: Various infections caused by susceptible organisms, rosacea
Class: Antibiotic, Antibiotic; nitroimidazole, Antimicrobial, Antiprotozoal
Half-life: 6–12 hours
Clinically important, potentially hazardous interactions with: alcohol, anisindione, anticoagulants, astemizole, barbiturates, busulfan, cimetidine, dicumarol, disulfiram, dronabinol, fluorouracil, lithium, lopinavir, mycophenolate, phenytoin, primidone, thalidomide, tipranavir, uracil/tegafur, warfarin
Pregnancy category: in patients with trichomoniasis, metronidazole is contra-indicated during the first trimester of pregnancy
Important contra-indications noted in the prescribing guidelines for: nursing mothers

---

Skin
AGEP [3]
Baboon syndrome / symmetrical drug-related intertriginous and flexural exanthema (SDRIFE) [2]
Dermatitis [2]
DRESS syndrome (Drug-induced hypersensitivity syndrome) [3]
Exanthems (<5%) [2]
Fixed eruption / fixed drug eruption [15]
Flushing / rubefaction [2]
Pruritus (itching) (<10%) [6]
Stevens-Johnson syndrome and toxic epidermal necrolysis (SJS/TEN) [8]
Urticaria / hives [4]

Mucosal
Glossitis (inflammation of the tongue) [2]
Tongue furry [2]
Xerostomia (dry mouth) [2]

Cardiovascular
Hypertension [2]
Torsades de pointes [2]

Central Nervous System
Cerebellar syndrome [7]
Dysarthria [3]
Dysgeusia (taste perversion) [8]
Encephalopathy (includes hepatic encephalopathy) [40]
Fever (pyrexia) (includes hyperpyrexia) [7]
Headache (7%) [7]
Leukoencephalopathy / posterior reversible encephalopathy syndrome (PRES) [8]
Neurotoxicity [17]
Paresthesias [2]
Peripheral neuropathy [5]
Psychosis [5]

Endocrine/Metabolic
ALT increased [3]
AST increased [3]

Gastrointestinal/Hepatic
Abdominal pain (5%) [8]
Diarrhea [15]
Hepatotoxicity / liver injury / acute liver injury / drug-induced liver injury (DILI) [6]
Nausea [19]
Pancreatitis / acute pancreatitis [7]
Vomiting [14]

Genitourinary
Vulvovaginal candidiasis [2]

Hematologic
Anemia [2]
Bleeding [2]

Neuromuscular/Skeletal
Ataxia [2]

Ocular
Vision loss [2]

Otic
Hearing loss (hypoacusis) [2]

Other
Adverse effects / adverse reactions [12]
Death [3]
Infection (fungal) (12%)

MEXILETINE

Trade name: Mexitil (Boehringer Ingelheim)
Indications: Ventricular arrhythmias
Class: Antiarrhythmic class Ib
Half-life: 10–12 hours
Clinically important, potentially hazardous interactions with: caffeine, citalopram, cobicistat/elvitegravir/emtricitabine/tenofovir alafenamide, cobicistat/elvitegravir/emtricitabine/tenofovir disoproxil, oxtriphylline
Important contra-indications noted in the prescribing guidelines for: nursing mothers
Warning: MORTALITY

Skin
Edema / fluid retention (4%)
Exanthems [9]
Hypersensitivity [5]
Pruritus (itching) [2]
Rash (4%)
Urticaria / hives [2]

Mucosal
Xerostomia (dry mouth) (3%)

Central Nervous System
Paresthesias (4%)

Trembling (<10%)
Tremor (13%)

Gastrointestinal/Hepatic
Gastrointestinal adverse reaction [2]
Peptic ulceration (includes duodenal ulcer, esophageal ulcer) [3]

Other
Adverse effects / adverse reactions [2]

MEZLOCILLIN

Indications: Various infections caused by susceptible organisms
Class: Antibiotic, Antibiotic; beta-lactam, Antibiotic; penicillin, Antimicrobial
Half-life: 0.8–1.0 hours
Clinically important, potentially hazardous interactions with: anticoagulants, cyclosporine, demeclocycline, doxycycline, imipenem/cilastatin, methotrexate, minocycline, oxytetracycline, tetracycline

---

Renal
Nephrotoxicity / kidney injury / acute kidney injury (AKI) / drug-induced kidney injury [2]

MIANSERIN

Trade names: Athimil (Hormoquimica), Bolvidon (Schering-Plough) (GSK), Lantanon (Schering-Plough), Lerivon (Schering-Plough), Miaxan (Orion), Norval (Schering-Plough) (GSK), Tetramide (Daiichi Sankyo), Tolvon (Schering-Plough)
Indications: Depression
Class: Antidepressant; tetracyclic
Half-life: 10 hours
Clinically important, potentially hazardous interactions with: codeine, diazepam, morphine, temazepam, zopiclone
Note: Not available in the US.

Cardiovascular
Ventricular tachycardia [2]

Central Nervous System
Restless legs syndrome / Willis-Ekbom disease (includes restless arms syndrome variant) [4]

MICAFUNGIN

Trade name: Mycamine (Astellas)
Indications: Invasive candidiasis, esophageal candidiasis
Class: Antifungal / antimycotic, Antimicrobial, Antimycobacterial; echinocandin
Half-life: 11–21 hours
Clinically important, potentially hazardous interactions with: amphotericin B, conivaptan, cyclosporine, itraconazole, nifedipine, sirolimus
Important contra-indications noted in the prescribing guidelines for: nursing mothers; pediatric patients

---

Skin
Anaphylactoid reactions / anaphylaxis (includes anaphylactic shock) [2]
Peripheral edema (7%)
Pruritus (itching) (6%)
Rash (9%) [6]
Ulcerations (5%)

Mucosal
Epistaxis (nosebleed) (6%) [2]
Mucosal inflammation (14%)

Cardiovascular
Bradycardia / sinus bradycardia (3%)
Hypertension (7%) [2]
Hypotension (9%)
Phlebitis (6%)
Shock (8%)
Tachycardia (8%)

Central Nervous System
Anorexia (6%)
Anxiety (6%)
Fever (pyrexia) (includes hyperpyrexia) (20%) [6]
Headache (16%) [3]
Insomnia (10%)
Rigors (9%)

Endocrine/Metabolic
ALP increased (5%) [2]
ALT increased (5%) [6]
AST increased (6%) [4]
Hyperbilirubinemia [3]
Hyperglycemia (includes glucose increased) (6%)
Hyperkalemia (5%)
Hypernatremia (5%)
Hypocalcemia (7%)
Hypoglycemia (6%)
Hypokalemia (18%) [3]
Hypomagnesemia (13%)

Gastrointestinal/Hepatic
Abdominal pain (10%) [3]
Constipation (11%)
Diarrhea (23%) [8]
Dyspepsia / functional dyspepsia (indigestion) (see also gastroparesis) (6%)
Hepatotoxicity / liver injury / acute liver injury / drug-induced liver injury (DILI) [9]
Nausea (22%) [6]
Vomiting (22%) [5]

Hematologic
Anemia (10%) [3]
Febrile neutropenia (6%)
Hemolysis [3]
Neutropenia (neutrophils decreased) (14%)
Sepsis (5%)
Thrombocytopenia / platelets decreased (15%) [3]

Local
Infusion-related reactions [2]

Neuromuscular/Skeletal
Asthenia / fatigue (6%)
Back pain (5%)

Respiratory
Cough (8%)
Dyspnea / shortness of breath (6%)
Pneumonia (2%)

Other
Adverse effects / adverse reactions [5]
Infection (40%)

MICONAZOLE

Trade names: Monistat (Janssen), Oravig (Dara)
Indications: Fungal infections, oropharyngeal candidiasis
Class: Antifungal / antimycotic, Antifungal; imidazole, Antimicrobial
Half-life: initial: 40 minutes; terminal: 24 hours
Clinically important, potentially hazardous interactions with: anisindione, anticoagulants, astemizole, clopidogrel, dicumarol, gliclazide, simvastatin, thioridazine, tolvaptan, vinblastine, vincristine, warfarin
Important contra-indications noted in the prescribing guidelines for: nursing mothers; pediatric patients

---

Skin
Angioedema (formerly named angioneurotic edema) (2%)
Contact dermatitis [2]
Cutaneous toxicity / skin toxicity [2]
Dermatitis [11]
Exanthems (2–87%) [5]
Flushing / rubefaction (<2%) [2]
Pruritus (itching) (2–36%) [3]
Purpura (3–8%)
Rash (9%)
Urticaria / hives (2%)

Cardiovascular
Phlebitis (5–79%) [3]

Central Nervous System
Chills (>5%)

Gastrointestinal/Hepatic
Nausea [2]

Local
Injection-site pain (10%)

Other
Adverse effects / adverse reactions [2]

MIDAZOLAM

Trade name: Versed (Roche)
Indications: Preoperative sedation
Class: Benzodiazepine
Half-life: 1–4 hours
Clinically important, potentially hazardous interactions with: amprenavir, aprepitant, atazanavir, atorvastatin, boceprevir, carbamazepine, chlorpheniramine, cimetidine, clarithromycin, clorazepate, CNS depressants, cobicistat/elvitegravir/emtricitabine/tenofovir alafenamide, cobicistat/elvitegravir/emtricitabine/tenofovir disoproxil, conivaptan, darunavir, delavirdine, dexamethasone, efavirenz, enzalutamide, erythromycin, esomeprazole, fluconazole, fluoxetine, fosamprenavir, grapefruit juice, griseofulvin, imatinib, indinavir, itraconazole, ivermectin, ketoconazole, letermovir, lonafarnib, lopinavir, nelfinavir, nevirapine, nilotinib, ombitasvir/paritaprevir/ritonavir, ombitasvir/paritaprevir/ritonavir and dasabuvir, phenobarbital, phenytoin, posaconazole, primidone, ribociclib, rifabutin, rifampin, ritonavir, roxithromycin, saquinavir, selpercatinib, St John's wort, telaprevir, telithromycin, tibolone, tipranavir, tucatinib, viloxazine, voriconazole, voxelotor

---

Skin
Edema / fluid retention [2]

Pruritus (itching) [3]
Urticaria / hives [2]

Cardiovascular
Bradycardia / sinus bradycardia [3]
Hypotension [10]

Central Nervous System
Agitation [3]
Amnesia [39]
Dysphoria [2]
Extrapyramidal symptoms [2]
Hallucinations [2]
Sedation [2]
Vertigo / dizziness [2]

Gastrointestinal/Hepatic
Vomiting [4]

Local
Injection-site pain (>10%)
Injection-site reaction (>10%)

Respiratory
Apnea [2]
Hypoxia [2]
Respiratory depression [2]

Other
Adverse effects / adverse reactions [8]
Hiccups / singultus [4]

MIDODRINE

Trade name: Proamatine (Shire)
Indications: Orthostatic hypotension, urinary incontinence
Class: Adrenergic alpha-receptor agonist
Half-life: ~3–4 hours
Clinically important, potentially hazardous interactions with: none known
Important contra-indications noted in the prescribing guidelines for: nursing mothers; pediatric patients

---

Skin
Flushing / rubefaction (<10%)
Pruritus (itching) (13%) [3]
Rash (2%)
Xerosis / xeroderma (2%)

Hair
Pili torti [2]

Mucosal
Xerostomia (dry mouth) (<10%)

Central Nervous System
Chills (5%)
Dysgeusia (taste perversion) [2]
Pain (5%)
Paresthesias (13–18%) [3]

MIDOSTAURIN

Trade name: Rydapt (Novartis)
Indications: Aggressive systemic mastocytosis, systemic mastocytosis with associated hematological neoplasm, or mast cell leukemia, acute myeloid leukemia (FLT3 mutation-positive) in combination with cytarabine and daunorubicin induction and cytarabine consolidation
Class: Multikinase inhibitor
Half-life: 21 hours
Clinically important, potentially hazardous interactions with: boceprevir, carbamazepine, clarithromycin, cobicistat, conivaptan, danoprevir, diltiazem, elvitegravir, enzalutamide, grapefruit juice, idelalisib, indinavir, itraconazole, ketoconazole, lopinavir, mitotane, nefazodone, nelfinavir, ombitasvir/paritaprevir/ritonavir, ombitasvir/paritaprevir/ritonavir and dasabuvir, phenytoin, posaconazole, rifampin, ritonavir, saquinavir, St John's wort, stong CYP3A inducers and inhibitors, tipranavir, troleandomycin, voriconazole
Pregnancy category: May cause fetal toxicity based on findings in animal studies
Important contra-indications noted in the prescribing guidelines for: the elderly; nursing mothers; pediatric patients

---

Skin
Cellulitis and pseudocellulitis (5%)
Desquamation [2]
Edema / fluid retention (40%)
Erysipelas (5%)
Hematoma / cutaneous hematoma (6%)
Herpes zoster (10%)
Hypersensitivity (4%)
Rash (14%) [4]
Sweet's syndrome [2]

Mucosal
Epistaxis (nosebleed) (12%)
Mucositis [2]
Oropharyngeal pain (4%)
Stomatitis (oral mucositis) [2]

Cardiovascular
Cardiac failure (6%)
Cardiotoxicity [2]
Hypotension (9%)
Myocardial infarction (4%)
Myocardial ischemia (4%)
QT interval prolonged / QT prolongation (11%) [3]

Central Nervous System
Chills (5%)
Fever (pyrexia) (includes hyperpyrexia) (27%) [2]
Headache (26%) [2]
Impaired concentration (7%)
Insomnia (11%)
Mental status changes (4%)
Pain [2]
Tremor (6%)
Vertigo / dizziness (13%)

Endocrine/Metabolic
ALP increased (39%)
ALT increased (31%) [2]
AST increased (32%)
GGT increased (35%)
Hyperamylasemia (20%)
Hyperbilirubinemia (29%) [2]
Hyperglycemia (includes glucose increased) (80%) [3]
Hyperkalemia (23%)
Hyperlipasemia (37%)
Hyperuricemia (37%)
Hypoalbuminemia / albumin decreased (27%)
Hypocalcemia (39%)
Hypokalemia (25%) [4]
Hypomagnesemia (20%)
Hyponatremia (34%) [2]
Hypophosphatemia (22%)
Serum creatinine increased (25%)
Weight gain (6%)

Gastrointestinal/Hepatic
Abdominal pain (34%)
Constipation (29%) [3]
Diarrhea (54%) [8]
Dyspepsia / functional dyspepsia (indigestion) (see also gastroparesis) (6%)
Gastritis / pangastritis / gastric irritation (3%)
Gastrointestinal bleeding (14%)
Nausea (82%) [13]
Vomiting (68%) [11]

Genitourinary
Urinary tract infection (16%)

Hematologic
Anemia (60%) [4]
Febrile neutropenia (8%) [4]
Leukocytopenia (leukopenia) / leukocytes (white blood cells) decreased (61%) [2]
Lymphopenia (lymphocytopenia) / lymphocytes decreased (66%) [2]
Neutropenia (neutrophils decreased) (49%) [3]
Sepsis (9%)
Thrombocytopenia / platelets decreased (50%) [3]

Neuromuscular/Skeletal
Arthralgia (19%)
Asthenia / fatigue (34%) [6]
Bone pain / joint pain (35%)

Renal
Nephrotoxicity / kidney injury / acute kidney injury (AKI) / drug-induced kidney injury (11%)

Respiratory
Bronchitis (6%)
Cough (18%) [2]
Dyspnea / shortness of breath (23%)
Pleural effusion (13%)
Pneumonia (10%) [2]
Pneumonitis (2%) [2]
Pulmonary edema (cardiogenic / non-cardiogenic) (3%)
Upper respiratory tract infection (30%)

Other
Infection [3]

MIFEPRISTONE

Trade names: Korlym (Corcept), Mifeprex (Danco)
Indications: Medical termination of intrauterine pregnancy (Mifeprex), Cushing's syndrome in patients with Type II diabetes (Korlym)
Class: Corticosteroid antagonist, CYP3A4 inhibitor, Progestogen antagonist
Half-life: 85 hours
Clinically important, potentially hazardous interactions with: amprenavir, aprepitant, atazanavir, boceprevir, bupropion, carbamazepine, ciclesonide, ciprofloxacin, clarithromycin, conivaptan, cyclosporine, darunavir, dihydroergotamine, diltiazem, efavirenz, ergotamine, erythromycin, fentanyl, fluconazole, fluvastatin, fosamprenavir, grapefruit juice, imatinib, indinavir, itraconazole, lopinavir, lovastatin, mibefradil, nefazodone, nelfinavir, NSAIDs, oral contraceptives, phenobarbital, phenytoin, pimozide, posaconazole, quinidine, repaglinide, rifabutin, rifampin, rifapentine, ritonavir, ritonavir, saquinavir, simvastatin, sirolimus, St John's wort, tacrolimus, telaprevir, telithromycin, tenoxicam, triamcinolone, verapamil, voriconazole, warfarin
Important contra-indications noted in the prescribing guidelines for: nursing mothers; pediatric patients
Note: Contra-indicated in pregnancy, with concurrent use of simvastatin or lovastatin and CYP3A substrates with narrow therapeutic range

or long-term corticosteroid use, and in women with a history of unexplained vaginal bleeding or with endometrial hyperplasia with atypia or endometrial carcinoma.
Warning: TERMINATION OF PREGNANCY

Skin
Edema / fluid retention (5–10%)
Peripheral edema (26%)
Pruritus (itching) (4%)
Rash (4%)

Mucosal
Xerostomia (dry mouth) (18%)

Cardiovascular
Chest pain (5–10%)
Hypertension (24%)

Central Nervous System
Anorexia (10%)
Anxiety (10%)
Chills (3–38%)
Fever (pyrexia) (includes hyperpyrexia) (4%)
Headache (2–44%)
Insomnia (5–10%)
Pain (14%)
Somnolence (drowsiness) (10%)
Vertigo / dizziness (<22%)

Endocrine/Metabolic
Adrenal insufficiency (hypoadrenalism) / Addisonian crisis (includes Addison's disease) (4%)
Appetite decreased (20%)
Hypoglycemia (5–10%)
Hypokalemia (44%) [2]
Menstrual irregularities [2]

Gastrointestinal/Hepatic
Abdominal pain (5–89%) [2]
Constipation (10%)
Diarrhea (12–20%)
Gastroesophageal reflux (5–10%)
Nausea (43–61%)
Vomiting (16–26%)

Genitourinary
Metrorrhagia (5–10%)
Uterine pain (83%)
Vaginal bleeding (5–10%)
Vaginitis (includes vulvitis) (3%)

Neuromuscular/Skeletal
Arthralgia (30%)
Asthenia / fatigue (<48%)
Back pain (9–16%)
Myalgia/Myopathy (14%)
Pain in extremities (12%)

Respiratory
Dyspnea / shortness of breath (16%)
Nasopharyngitis (12%)
Sinusitis (see also rhinitis / rhinosinusitis) (14%)

Other
Dipsia (thirst) / polydipsia (5–10%)
Infection [3]

MIGLITOL

Trade name: Glyset (Pfizer)
Indications: Non-insulin dependent diabetes Type II
Class: Alpha-glucosidase inhibitor, Antidiabetic, Hypoglycemic (antihyperglycemic) agent
Half-life: ~2 hours
Clinically important, potentially hazardous interactions with: pramlintide
Important contra-indications noted in the prescribing guidelines for: nursing mothers

---

Skin
Rash (4%)

Endocrine/Metabolic
Hypoglycemia [2]

Gastrointestinal/Hepatic
Abdominal pain (12%) [5]
Diarrhea (29%) [3]
Flatulence (42%) [2]

Other
Adverse effects / adverse reactions [2]

MIGLUSTAT

Trade name: Zavesca (Actelion)
Indications: Gaucher disease, Niemann-Pick disease
Class: Glucosylceramide synthase inhibitor
Half-life: 6–7 hours
Clinically important, potentially hazardous interactions with: imiglucerase
Important contra-indications noted in the prescribing guidelines for: nursing mothers; pediatric patients

---

Mucosal
Xerostomia (dry mouth) (8%)

Central Nervous System
Headache (22%)
Paresthesias (7%)
Tremor (~30%) [4]
Vertigo / dizziness (11%)

Endocrine/Metabolic
Weight loss [5]

Gastrointestinal/Hepatic
Abdominal pain (50%) [3]
Diarrhea [6]
Flatulence [4]

Neuromuscular/Skeletal
Back pain (8%)
Leg cramps (11%)

Other
Adverse effects / adverse reactions [3]

MILK THISTLE

Family: Asteraceae; Compositae
Scientific names: *Carduus marainum, Silibum marianum*
Indications: Dyspepsia, liver protectant, hepatitis, loss of appetite, spleen diseases, supportive treatment for mushroom poisoning
Class: Immunomodulator
Half-life: N/A
Clinically important, potentially hazardous interactions with: simeprevir
Note: Seed as opposed to the "above-ground parts".

Other
Adverse effects / adverse reactions [3]

MILNACIPRAN

Trade name: Savella (Forest)
Indications: Fibromyalgia
Class: Antidepressant, Selective norepinepherine reuptake inhibitor
Half-life: 6–8 hours
Clinically important, potentially hazardous interactions with: alcohol, alpha / beta argonists, antipsychotics, aspirin, clomipramine, clonidine, CNS-active drugs, digoxin, droperidol, epinephrine, levomepromazine, lithium, MAO inhibitors, norepinephrine, NSAIDs, serotonergic drugs, sibutramine, St John's wort, tryptophan, vitamin K antagonists
Important contra-indications noted in the prescribing guidelines for: the elderly; nursing mothers; pediatric patients
Note: Contra-indicated in patients with uncontrolled narrow-angle glaucoma.
Warning: SUICIDALITY AND ANTIDEPRESSANT DRUGS

Skin
Flushing / rubefaction (4%)
Hot flashes / hot flushes (12%)
Hyperhidrosis (9%) [6]
Pruritus (itching) (2%)
Rash (4%)

Mucosal
Xerostomia (dry mouth) (5%)

Cardiovascular
Chest pain (2%)
Hypertension (4%) [4]
Palpitation (7%)
Tachycardia (2%) [2]

Central Nervous System
Anxiety (3%)
Chills (2%)
Headache (17%) [7]
Hypoesthesia / hypesthesia (numbness) (2%)
Insomnia (12%) [2]
Migraine (4%)
Paresthesias (3%)
Serotonin syndrome [2]
Tremor (2%)
Vertigo / dizziness (10%) [3]

Endocrine/Metabolic
Appetite decreased (2%)

Gastrointestinal/Hepatic
Abdominal pain (3%)
Constipation (15%) [6]
Nausea (39%) [17]
Vomiting (7%)

Genitourinary
Dysuria (>2%) [2]
Ejaculatory dysfunction (>2%) [2]

Ocular
Vision blurred (2%)

Respiratory
Dyspnea / shortness of breath (2%)
Upper respiratory tract infection (6%)

Other
Adverse effects / adverse reactions [3]

MILRINONE

Trade name: Primacor (Sanofi-Aventis)
Indications: Severe congestive heart failure unresponsive to conventional maintenance therapy, acute heart failure, including low output states following cardiac surgery
Class: Phosphodiesterase inhibitor
Half-life: 2.3 hours
Clinically important, potentially hazardous interactions with: anagrelide
Important contra-indications noted in the prescribing guidelines for: nursing mothers; pediatric patients

---

Cardiovascular
Arrhythmias [2]
Hypotension (<10%) [7]
Supraventricular arrhythmias (<10%)
Vasodilation [2]
Ventricular tachycardia (<10%)

Central Nervous System
Headache (<10%)

MILTEFOSINE

Trade name: Impavido (Paladin)
Indications: Leishmaniasis, skin cancer, breast cancer
Class: Membrane integrity antagonist
Half-life: ~6–8 days
Clinically important, potentially hazardous interactions with: none known
Important contra-indications noted in the prescribing guidelines for: nursing mothers; pediatric patients
Note: Contraindicated in patients with Sjogren-Larsson-Syndrome.
Warning: EMBRYO-FETAL TOXICITY

Skin
Abscess (<2%)
Cellulitis and pseudocellulitis (<2%)
Lymphadenopathy (<2%)
Pruritus (itching) (5–6%) [2]
Pyoderma (<2%)
Rash (<2%) [2]
Stevens-Johnson syndrome and toxic epidermal necrolysis (SJS/TEN) (<2%)
Urticaria / hives (<2%)

Central Nervous System
Anorexia [2]
Fever (pyrexia) (includes hyperpyrexia) (6%) [2]
Headache (28%) [2]
Paresthesias (<2%)
Somnolence (drowsiness) (3%)
Vertigo / dizziness (5–13%)

Endocrine/Metabolic
ALT increased [2]
Appetite decreased (23%) [2]
AST increased [3]
Hypertransaminasemia (hepatic transaminitis) / elevated transaminases [2]
Serum creatinine increased [5]

Gastrointestinal/Hepatic
Abdominal distension (<2%)
Abdominal pain (8–11%) [4]
Constipation (<2%)
Diarrhea (8–20%) [14]
Dysphagia (<2%)
Flatulence (<2%)
Nausea (36–42%) [7]
Vomiting (5–38%) [14]

Genitourinary
Ejaculatory dysfunction [2]
Testicular pain / orchialgia / orchidalgia (<2%)

Hematologic
Anemia (<2%)

Neuromuscular/Skeletal
Arthralgia [3]
Asthenia / fatigue (3–6%)
Myalgia/Myopathy [3]

Other
Adverse effects / adverse reactions [4]

MINOCYCLINE

Trade names: Dynacin (Medicis), Minocin (Wyeth), Solodyn (Medicis)
Indications: Various infections caused by susceptible organisms
Class: Antibiotic, Antibiotic; tetracycline, Antimicrobial, Disease-modifying antirheumatic drug (DMARD)
Half-life: 11–23 hours
Clinically important, potentially hazardous interactions with: acitretin, aluminum, amoxicillin, ampicillin, antacids, bacampicillin, BCG vaccine, bismuth, carbenicillin, cloxacillin, coumarins, digoxin, ergotamine, estradiol, estrogens, isotretinoin, kaolin, magnesium salts, methotrexate, methoxyflurane, methysergide, mezlocillin, nafcillin, oral iron, oral typhoid vaccine, oxacillin, penicillin G, penicillin V, penicillins, phenindione, piperacillin, quinapril, retinoids, St John's wort, strontium ranelate, sucralfate, sulfonylureas, ticarcillin, tripotassium dicitratobismuthate, vitamin A, zinc
Important contra-indications noted in the prescribing guidelines for: nursing mothers; pediatric patients

---

Skin
Anaphylactoid reactions / anaphylaxis (includes anaphylactic shock) [3]
Angioedema (formerly named angioneurotic edema) [2]
Candidiasis / candidosis [2]
Cellulitis and pseudocellulitis [2]
Cutaneous polyarteritis nodosa [7]
DRESS syndrome (Drug-induced hypersensitivity syndrome) [19]
Erythema multiforme [2]
Erythema nodosum [2]
Exanthems [5]
Exfoliative dermatitis [3]
Fixed eruption / fixed drug eruption [8]
Folliculitis [2]
Hypersensitivity [25]
Livedo reticularis / livedo racemosa [3]
Lupus erythematosus (subacute cutaneous lupus erythematosus (SCLE)) [50]
Lupus syndrome / drug-induced lupus (DIL) [3]
Lymphocytic thrombophilic arteritis [2]
Ochronosis [2]
Photosensitivity (<10%) [9]
Pigmentation (Skin) (includes hyperpigmentation) [126]
Pruritus (itching) [7]
Purpura [4]
Rash [9]
Raynaud's phenomenon [2]
Serum sickness [4]
Serum sickness-like reaction (3–5%) [6]
Stevens-Johnson syndrome and toxic epidermal necrolysis (SJS/TEN) [4]
Sweet's syndrome [4]
Thrombocytopenic purpura [2]
Urticaria / hives [9]
Vasculitis (angiitis) / cutaneous vasculitis (angiitis) [13]

Hair
Alopecia / hair loss [2]

Nails
Nail pigmentation (<5%) [20]
Photo-onycholysis [3]

Mucosal
Black tongue / black hairy tongue (lingua villosa nigra) [4]
Gingival pigmentation (8%) [2]
Oral pigmentation (7%) [23]

Cardiovascular
Polyarteritis nodosa [5]

Central Nervous System
Fever (pyrexia) (includes hyperpyrexia) [2]
Headache [6]
Intracranial pressure increased (intracranial hypertension) [6]
Pseudotumor cerebri [15]
Vertigo / dizziness [8]

Endocrine/Metabolic
Black thyroid syndrome [5]
Galactorrhea (black) [2]
Thyroid dysfunction [2]

Gastrointestinal/Hepatic
Abdominal pain [2]
Diarrhea [2]
Hepatitis [11]
Hepatotoxicity / liver injury / acute liver injury / drug-induced liver injury (DILI) [22]
Nausea [6]
Pancreatitis / acute pancreatitis [2]
Vomiting [3]

Hematologic
Thrombocytopenia / platelets decreased [2]

Neuromuscular/Skeletal
Arthralgia [6]
Asthenia / fatigue [4]
Black bone disease [11]
Myalgia/Myopathy [7]

Ocular
Conjunctival pigmentation [2]
Diplopia (double vision) [2]
Papilledema [3]
Scleral pigmentation [6]

Otic
Tinnitus [2]

Respiratory
Eosinophilic pneumonia [5]
Pneumonitis [2]

Other
Adverse effects / adverse reactions [6]
Death [2]
Tooth pigmentation / discoloration (primarily in children) (>10%) [23]

MINOXIDIL

Trade names: Loniten (Par), Rogaine (Pfizer) (topical)
Indications: Hypertension, androgenetic alopecia
Class: Vasodilator
Half-life: 4.2 hours
Clinically important, potentially hazardous interactions with: acebutolol, alcohol, alfuzosin, captopril, cilazapril, diclofenac, enalapril, fosinopril, guanethidine, levodopa, levomepromazine, lisinopril, meloxicam, olmesartan, quinapril, ramipril, trandolapril, triamcinolone, trifluoperazine
Note: Topical [T].

Skin
- Bullous dermatosis [2]
- Dermatitis [T] (7%) [18]
- Eczema / eczematous reaction / eczematous eruption [2]
- Edema / fluid retention [T] (>10%) [4]
- Exanthems [4]
- Irritation (skin) [2]
- Lupus erythematosus (subacute cutaneous lupus erythematosus (SCLE)) [3]
- Peripheral edema (7%)
- Pruritus (itching) [T] [10]
- Stevens-Johnson syndrome and toxic epidermal necrolysis (SJS/TEN) [3]
- Xerosis / xeroderma [2]

Hair
- Alopecia / hair loss [T] [2]
- Hair pigmentation [2]
- Hirsutism (in women) (100%) [4]
- Hypertrichosis (80–100%) [28]

Cardiovascular
- Palpitation [3]
- Pericardial effusion [2]
- Postural hypotension [2]

Central Nervous System
- Headache [3]
- Vertigo / dizziness [2]

Respiratory
- Pleural effusion [2]

Other
- Adverse effects / adverse reactions [4]

MIRABEGRON

Trade name: Myrbetriq (Astellas)
Indications: Overactive bladder
Class: Beta-3 adrenergic agonist
Half-life: 50 hours
Clinically important, potentially hazardous interactions with: antimuscarinics, desipramine, digoxin, flecainide, metoprolol, propafenone, thioridazine
Important contra-indications noted in the prescribing guidelines for: nursing mothers; pediatric patients
Note: Mirabegron alone or in combination with solifenacin succinate 5 mg can increase blood pressure. Periodic blood pressure determinations are recommended, especially in hypertensive patients. Mirabegron is not recommended for use in severe uncontrolled hypertensive patients.

Mucosal
- Xerostomia (dry mouth) (3%) [8]

Cardiovascular
- Hypertension (8–11%) [9]
- Tachycardia (<2%) [3]

Central Nervous System
- Headache (2–4%) [5]
- Vertigo / dizziness (3%) [2]

Gastrointestinal/Hepatic
- Constipation (2–3%) [6]
- Diarrhea (<2%)
- Gastrointestinal disorder / discomfort [2]

Genitourinary
- Cystitis (includes interstitial cystitis / bladder pain syndrome) (2%)
- Dysuria [2]
- Urinary tract infection (3–6%) [5]

Neuromuscular/Skeletal
- Arthralgia (<2%)
- Back pain (3%)

Respiratory
- Influenza (3%)
- Nasopharyngitis (4%) [4]
- Sinusitis (see also rhinitis / rhinosinusitis) (<3%)
- Upper respiratory tract infection (2%)

Other
- Adverse effects / adverse reactions [5]

MIRTAZAPINE

Synonyms: Esmirtazapine [(S)-(+)-enantiomer of mirtazapine]
Trade name: Remeron (Organon)
Indications: Depression
Class: Adrenergic alpha-receptor agonist, Antidepressant; tetracyclic
Half-life: 20–40 hours
Clinically important, potentially hazardous interactions with: dacomitinib, linezolid, tapentadol, venlafaxine
Warning: SUICIDALITY AND ANTIDEPRESSANT DRUGS

Skin
- Diaphoresis [2]
- Edema / fluid retention (<10%) [2]
- Peripheral edema (<10%)
- Pigmentation (Skin) (includes hyperpigmentation) [2]
- Rash (<10%)

Mucosal
- Glossitis (inflammation of the tongue) (<10%)
- Xerostomia (dry mouth) (25%) [4]

Cardiovascular
- QT interval prolonged / QT prolongation [2]

Central Nervous System
- Abnormal dreams (4%)
- Anorexia (<10%)
- Cognitive impairment [2]
- Dyskinesia [2]
- Headache [2]
- Mania [3]
- Neurotoxicity [3]
- Nightmares [3]
- Restless legs syndrome / Willis-Ekbom disease (includes restless arms syndrome variant) [10]
- Sedation [4]
- Seizures [3]
- Serotonin syndrome [7]
- Sleep-related eating disorder (SRED) [2]
- Somnolence (drowsiness) (54%) [11]
- Tremor (<10%) [2]
- Vertigo / dizziness (7%) [2]

Endocrine/Metabolic
- ALT increased (2%)
- Appetite increased (12%) [2]
- Galactorrhea [2]
- Gynecomastia [2]
- Weight gain (12%) [11]

Gastrointestinal/Hepatic
- Abdominal pain (<10%)
- Constipation (<10%) [2]
- Hepatotoxicity / liver injury / acute liver injury / drug-induced liver injury (DILI) [3]
- Pancreatitis / acute pancreatitis [8]
- Vomiting (<10%)

Neuromuscular/Skeletal
- Arthralgia [4]
- Asthenia / fatigue [7]
- Myalgia/Myopathy (<10%)
- Rhabdomyolysis [5]

Ocular
- Glaucoma (includes acute angle-closure glaucoma) [2]

Respiratory
- Influenza- ('flu)-like syndrome (<10%)

Other
- Adverse effects / adverse reactions [2]

MISTLETOE

Family: Loranthacae; Viscaceae
Scientific names: *Phoradendron flavescens, Phoradendron leucarpum, Phoradendron macrophyllum, Phoradendron rubrum, Phoradendron serotinum, Phoradendron tomentosum, Viscum album*
Indications: Injected: adjuvant tumor therapy. **Oral:** abortifacient, arteriosclerosis, arthritis, asthma, colds, depression, headache, HIV infection, hypertension, hypotension, hysteria, labor pain, lumbago, metrorrhagia, muscle spasms, otitis, whooping cough, hemorrhoids, internal bleeding, gout, sleep disorders, amenorrhea, liver and gallbladder conditions
Class: Immunomodulator
Half-life: N/A
Clinically important, potentially hazardous interactions with: bepridil, clevidipine, corticosteroids, immunosuppressants, MAO inhibitors, squill
Note: Purified extracts injected intramuscularly, subcutaneously or by intravenous infusion. Unless otherwise indicated, side effects listed are from injected preparations. The FDA considers *Viscum album* unsafe.
The well-known mistletoe is an evergreen parasitic plant, growing on the branches of some tree species. Shakespeare calls it "the baleful mistletoe," an illusion to the Scandinavian legend that Balder, the god of Peace, was slain with an arrow made of mistletoe.

Skin
- Anaphylactoid reactions / anaphylaxis (includes anaphylactic shock) (28%) [3]
- Erythema [3]
- Pruritus (itching) [2]

Mucosal
- Gingivitis [2]

Cardiovascular
Hypertension [2]
Central Nervous System
Chills [4]
Fever (pyrexia) (includes hyperpyrexia) [6]
Headache [2]
Gastrointestinal/Hepatic
Hepatotoxicity / liver injury / acute liver injury / drug-induced liver injury (DILI) [3]
Nausea [2]
Local
Injection-site edema [2]
Injection-site inflammation [8]
Injection-site reaction [5]
Respiratory
Influenza- ('flu)-like syndrome [3]
Other
Adverse effects / adverse reactions [8]
Allergic reactions [4]
Death (low incidence – accidental ingestion) [4]

MITAPIVAT

Trade name: Pyrukynd (Agios Pharmaceuticals Inc)
Indications: Treatment of hemolytic anemia in adults with pyruvate kinase deficiency
Class: Pyruvate kinase activator
Half-life: 3–5 hours
Clinically important, potentially hazardous interactions with: CYP2B6 substrates, cyp2c substrates, CYP3A inducers, CYP3A inhibitors, CYP3A substrates, ethinyl estradiol, hormonal contraceptives, P-gp substrates, UGT1A1 substrates
Pregnancy category: Insufficient evidence to evaluate for a drug-associated risk of major birth defects, miscarriage or other adverse maternal or fetal outcomes in normal pregnancies. (Untreated pyruvate kinase deficiency in pregnant women may precipitate acute hemolysis, pre-term labor, miscarriage and severe anemia requiring frequent transfusion. Additionally, preeclampsia and severe hypertension have been reported).
Note: Acute Hemolysis: Avoid abrupt interruption or abrupt discontinuation of mitapivat to minimize the risk of acute hemolysis. A gradual reduction in dosing rather than abrupt cessation is recommended when possible. In a clinical trial with male patients with pyruvate kinase deficiency receiving mitapivat, increases in serum testosterone and decreases in serum estrone and estradiol were observed. These changes in hormones persisted throughout the study period. In patients who discontinued mitapivat and had follow-up hormone measurements, the hormone changes returned close to the baseline levels 28 days after discontinuing mitapivat.

Skin
Hot flashes / hot flushes (8%)
Mucosal
Oropharyngeal pain (8%)
Xerostomia (dry mouth) (5%)
Cardiovascular
Arrhythmias (5%)
Hypertension (5% ≥ grade 3) (5%)
Central Nervous System
Headache [2]
Paresthesias (5%)
Endocrine/Metabolic
Hypertriglyceridemia (includes triglycerides increased) (5% ≥ grade 3) (8%)
Hyperuricemia (15%)
Gastrointestinal/Hepatic
Constipation (5%)
Gastroenteritis (3% ≥ grade 3) (8%)
Nausea [2]
Neuromuscular/Skeletal
Arthralgia (10%)
Back pain (15%)
Breast disorder / breast discomfort (5%)

MITOMYCIN

Synonyms: mitomycin-C; MTC
Trade name: Mutamycin (Bristol-Myers Squibb)
Indications: Carcinomas
Class: Alkylating agent, Antibiotic, Antibiotic; anthracycline, Antimicrobial
Half-life: 23–78 minutes
Clinically important, potentially hazardous interactions with: aldesleukin
Important contra-indications noted in the prescribing guidelines for: nursing mothers; pediatric patients

---

Skin
Dermatitis [9]
Erythema multiforme [2]
Exanthems [2]
Exfoliative dermatitis [2]
Hand–foot syndrome (palmar–plantar erythrodysesthesia) [2]
Thrombocytopenic purpura [2]
Hair
Alopecia / hair loss (<10%) [2]
Nails
Nail pigmentation (purple) (<10%)
Mucosal
Oral lesions (2–8%) [4]
Oral ulceration (<10%)
Stomatitis (oral mucositis) (>10%)
Cardiovascular
Congestive heart failure (3–15%)
Veno-occlusive disease [3]
Central Nervous System
Anorexia (14%)
Fever (pyrexia) (includes hyperpyrexia) (14%)
Paresthesias (<10%)
Gastrointestinal/Hepatic
Nausea (14%)
Vomiting (14%)
Hematologic
Anemia (19–24%)
Hemolytic uremic syndrome [41]
Neutropenia (neutrophils decreased) [2]
Local
Injection-site cellulitis (>10%)
Injection-site necrosis (>10%) [3]
Neuromuscular/Skeletal
Asthenia / fatigue [2]
Ocular
Epiphora [2]
Keratitis (ocular keratitis) / corneal inflammation) [3]
Limbal stem cell deficiency [3]
Ocular toxicity [3]
Renal
Nephrotoxicity / kidney injury / acute kidney injury (AKI) / drug-induced kidney injury [2]
Respiratory
Cough (7%)
Pneumonitis [3]
Other
Adverse effects / adverse reactions [2]

MITOTANE

Indications: Inoperable adrenocortical carcinoma
Class: Antineoplastic / anticancer agent (see also Immune checkpoint inhibitor)
Half-life: 18–159 days
Clinically important, potentially hazardous interactions with: aldesleukin, betamethasone, copanlisib, doravirine, doravirine/lamiduvine/tenofovir disoproxil, fostemsavir, midostaurin, neratinib, spironolactone, triamcinolone

---

Skin
Acral erythema [2]
Erythema multiforme [2]
Exanthems (9–16%) [2]
Flushing / rubefaction (<10%)
Pigmentation (Skin) (includes hyperpigmentation) (16%) [2]
Rash (15%)
Hair
Alopecia / hair loss (16%) [2]
Central Nervous System
Encephalopathy (includes hepatic encephalopathy) [3]
Neurotoxicity [2]
Neuromuscular/Skeletal
Myalgia/Myopathy (<10%)
Other
Adverse effects / adverse reactions [2]
Side effects (13–17%) [2]

MITOXANTRONE

Trade name: Novantrone (OSI)
Indications: Acute myelogenous leukemia, multiple sclerosis, prostate cancer
Class: Antibiotic, Antibiotic; anthracycline, Antimicrobial, Antineoplastic / anticancer agent (see also Immune checkpoint inhibitor)
Half-life: median terminal: 75 hours
Clinically important, potentially hazardous interactions with: aldesleukin, safinamide
Important contra-indications noted in the prescribing guidelines for: nursing mothers; pediatric patients

---

Skin
Bruise / bruising / contusion / ecchymosis (ecchymoses) (7%)
Diaphoresis (<10%)
Edema / fluid retention (>10%)
Fungal dermatitis (>15%)
Peripheral edema [2]
Petechiae (>10%)
Purpura (>10%)
Hair
Alopecia / hair loss (20–60%) [7]
Cardiovascular
Cardiac failure [2]
Cardiotoxicity [4]

Congestive heart failure [3]

Central Nervous System
Chills (<10%)

Endocrine/Metabolic
Amenorrhea [4]
Menstrual irregularities [2]

Gastrointestinal/Hepatic
Diarrhea [2]
Nausea [6]
Vomiting [3]

Genitourinary
Urinary tract infection [2]

Hematologic
Anemia [2]
Febrile neutropenia [2]
Leukemia [4]
Leukocytopenia (leukopenia) / leukocytes (white blood cells) decreased [4]
Neutropenia (neutrophils decreased) [6]
Thrombocytopenia / platelets decreased [2]

Other
Adverse effects / adverse reactions [2]
Death [2]
Infection (>66%) [4]

MIVACURIUM

Trade name: Mivacron (GSK)
Indications: Adjunct to general anesthesia
Class: Nicotinic antagonist
Half-life: 1.8–2 hours
Clinically important, potentially hazardous interactions with: acetazolamide, aminoglycosides, anticholinesterases, bambuterol, calcium channel blockers, chloroquine, chlorpromazine, clindamycin, d-penicillamine, ecothiophate iodide, enflurane, furosemide, halothane, hexomethonium, isoflurane, ketamine, lidocaine, lincomycin, lithium salts, magnesium salts, mannitol, MAO inhibitors, organophosphates, pancuronium, phenytoin, polymyxins, procainamide, quinidine, sevoflurane, spectinomycin, tetracyclines
Important contra-indications noted in the prescribing guidelines for: nursing mothers; pediatric patients

---

Skin
Anaphylactoid reactions / anaphylaxis (includes anaphylactic shock) [3]
Erythema [4]
Flushing / rubefaction (16%) [6]

Cardiovascular
Hypotension [5]

Central Nervous System
Paralysis / paraplegia [8]

Neuromuscular/Skeletal
Muscular paralysis [7]

Respiratory
Bronchospasm [3]

MIZOLASTINE

Trade name: Mizollen (Sanofi-Aventis)
Indications: Allergic rhinoconjunctivitis, urticaria
Class: Histamine H1 receptor antagonist
Half-life: 13 hours
Clinically important, potentially hazardous interactions with: azithromycin, cimetidine, cyclosporine, erythromycin, itraconazole, ketoconazole, moxifloxacin, nifedipine, sotalol

---

Skin
Anaphylactoid reactions / anaphylaxis (includes anaphylactic shock) [2]

Mucosal
Xerostomia (dry mouth) [3]

Central Nervous System
Somnolence (drowsiness) [3]

Neuromuscular/Skeletal
Asthenia / fatigue [2]

MIZORIBINE

Trade name: Bredinin (Asahi Kasei Pharma)
Indications: Rheumatoid arthritis, systemic lupus erythematosus, prevention of rejection in renal transplantation, lupus nephritis, nephrotic syndrome
Class: Immunosuppressant
Half-life: 6 hours
Clinically important, potentially hazardous interactions with: none known

---

Skin
Stevens-Johnson syndrome and toxic epidermal necrolysis (SJS/TEN) [2]

Hair
Alopecia / hair loss [2]

Endocrine/Metabolic
Hyperuricemia [8]

Renal
Nephrotoxicity / kidney injury / acute kidney injury (AKI) / drug-induced kidney injury [2]

Other
Infection [2]

MOBOCERTINIB

Trade name: Exkivity (Takeda)
Indications: Non-small cell lung cancer where the disease has progressed on or after platinum-based chemotherapy
Class: Epidermal growth factor receptor (EGFR) inhibitor / antagonist, Kinase inhibitor, Tyrosine kinase inhibitor
Half-life: 18 hours
Clinically important, potentially hazardous interactions with: CYP3A inducers, CYP3A inhibitors, CYP3A substrates, efavirenz, itraconazole, ketoconazole, rifampin
Pregnancy category: Mobocertinib can cause fetal harm when administered to a pregnant woman. Advise females of reproductive potential to use effective non-hormonal contraception during treatment with mobocertinib and for 1 month after the last dose. Advise males with female partners of reproductive potential to use effective contraception during treatment with mobocertinib and for 1 week after the last dose.
Important contra-indications noted in the prescribing guidelines for: nursing mothers
Warning: MOBOCERTINIB CAN CAUSE LIFE-THREATENING HEART RATE-CORRECTED QT (QTC) PROLONGATION, INCLUDING TORSADES DE POINTES, WHICH CAN BE FATAL, AND REQUIRES MONITORING OF QTC AND ELECTROLYTES AT BASELINE AND PERIODICALLY DURING TREATMENT. INCREASE MONITORING FREQUENCY IN PATIENTS WITH RISK FACTORS FOR QTC PROLONGATION AVOID USE OF CONCOMITANT DRUGS WHICH ARE KNOWN TO PROLONG THE QTC INTERVAL AND THE USE OF STRONG OR MODERATE CYP3A INHIBITORS WITH MOBOCERTINIB, WHICH MAY FURTHER PROLONG THE QTC. WITHHOLD, REDUCE THE DOSE, OR PERMANENTLY DISCONTINUE MOBOCERTINIB BASED ON THE SEVERITY OF QTC PROLONGATION.

Skin
Acneiform eruption / acneiform dermatitis / acneiform rash [3]
Dry skin (32%) [3]
Edema / fluid retention (9%)
Hand–foot syndrome (palmar–plantar erythrodysesthesia) (4%)
Maculopapular rash / morbilliform rash [2]
Pruritus (itching) (24%) [3]
Rash (2% grade 3) (78%) [2]

Hair
Alopecia / hair loss (19%)

Nails
Paronychia (39%) [3]

Mucosal
Rhinorrhea (13%)
Stomatitis (oral mucositis) (4% grade 3) (46%) [3]

Cardiovascular
Cardiac failure (3%)
Hypertension (4% grade 3) (10%)
QT interval prolonged / QT prolongation (4% grade 3 or 4) (10%)

Central Nervous System
Headache (10%)
Peripheral neuropathy (7%)

Endocrine/Metabolic
ALP increased (2% grade 3 or 4) (25%)
ALT increased (3% grade or 4) (22%)
Appetite decreased (39%) [3]
AST increased (2% grade 3 or 4) (21%)
Hyperamylasemia (13% grade or 4) (40%)
Hyperlipasemia (10% grade or 4) (35%) [3]
Hypoalbuminemia / albumin decreased (2% grade or 4) (23%)
Hypokalemia (5% grade 3 or 4) (29%)
Hypomagnesemia (3% grade 3 or 4) (23%)
Hyponatremia (20%)
Serum creatinine increased (3% grade 3 or 4) (52%) [2]
Weight loss (21%) [2]

Gastrointestinal/Hepatic
Abdominal pain (2% grade 3) (18%)
Diarrhea (22% grade 3 or 4) (92%) [4]
Dyspepsia / functional dyspepsia (indigestion) (see also gastroparesis) (11%)
Gastroesophageal reflux (15%)
Nausea (4% grade 3) (37%) [4]
Vomiting (3% grade 3) (40%) [3]

Hematologic
Anemia (4% grade 3 or 4) (59%) [3]
Leukocytopenia (leukopenia) / leukocytes (white blood cells) decreased (25%)
Lymphopenia (lymphocytopenia) / lymphocytes decreased (15% grade 3 or 4) (52%)
Thrombocytopenia / platelets decreased (26%)

Neuromuscular/Skeletal
Asthenia / fatigue (4% grade 3) (29%) [3]
Musculoskeletal pain (3% grade 3) (34%)

Ocular
Ocular toxicity (11%)

Renal
Nephrotoxicity / kidney injury / acute kidney injury (AKI) / drug-induced kidney injury (8%)

Respiratory
Cough (24%)
Dyspnea / shortness of breath (4% grade 3 or 4) (15%)
Pneumonitis (3%)
Upper respiratory tract infection (16%)

MOCLOBEMIDE

Trade names: Aurorix (Roche), Manerix (Roche)
Indications: Depression, social anxiety
Class: Antidepressant
Half-life: 2–4 hours
Clinically important, potentially hazardous interactions with: amitriptyline, benzodiazepines, cimetidine, citalopram, clomipramine, clopidogrel, clorazepate, dextromethorphan, duloxetine, fluoxetine, hydromorphone, levodopa, meperidine, paroxetine hydrochloride, pethidine, selegiline, tyramine, venlafaxine, zolmitriptan
Pregnancy category: not recommended in pregnancy
Important contra-indications noted in the prescribing guidelines for: nursing mothers; pediatric patients

---

Central Nervous System
Insomnia [2]
Serotonin syndrome [5]
Vertigo / dizziness [2]

MODAFINIL

Trade name: Provigil (Cephalon)
Indications: Narcolepsy
Class: Analeptic, CNS stimulant, CYP1A2 inducer, CYP3A4 inducer
Half-life: ~15 hours
Clinically important, potentially hazardous interactions with: elbasvir & grazoprevir, enzalutamide, lemborexant, lumateperone, neratinib, olaparib, oral contraceptives, palbociclib, sonidegib, thalidomide, venetoclax
Important contra-indications noted in the prescribing guidelines for: the elderly; nursing mothers; pediatric patients

---

Skin
Fixed eruption / fixed drug eruption [2]

Mucosal
Xerostomia (dry mouth) (5%)

Cardiovascular
Hypertension [2]
Palpitation [2]

Central Nervous System
Agitation [2]
Chills (2%)
Hallucinations [2]
Hallucinations, visual [2]
Headache (28%) [14]
Insomnia (5%) [6]
Nervousness [2]
Paresthesias (3%)
Psychosis [3]
Vertigo / dizziness (5%) [3]

Gastrointestinal/Hepatic
Abdominal pain [2]
Diarrhea (6%) [3]
Nausea (11%) [7]

Neuromuscular/Skeletal
Back pain (6%)

Respiratory
Rhinitis / rhinosinusitis (see also sinusitis) (7%)

Other
Adverse effects / adverse reactions [3]

MOLINDONE

Trade name: Moban (Endo)
Indications: Schizophrenia
Class: Antipsychotic
Half-life: 1.5 hours
Clinically important, potentially hazardous interactions with: paroxetine hydrochloride
Important contra-indications noted in the prescribing guidelines for: the elderly; nursing mothers; pediatric patients
Warning: INCREASED MORTALITY IN ELDERLY PATIENTS WITH DEMENTIA-RELATED PSYCHOSIS

Mucosal
Xerostomia (dry mouth) (>10%)

Central Nervous System
Neuroleptic malignant syndrome [2]
Tardive syndrome / tardive dyskinesia [4]

Endocrine/Metabolic
Galactorrhea [2]
Gynecomastia (<10%)

MOMETASONE

Trade names: Asmanex (MSD), Dulera (Merck), Elocon (Merck), Nasonex (Merck)
Indications: Dermatoses, rhinitis, asthma
Class: Corticosteroid / Glucocorticoid, Corticosteroid, inhaled, Corticosteroid, topical
Half-life: 7 hours
Clinically important, potentially hazardous interactions with: conivaptan, darunavir, delavirdine, indinavir, ketoconazole, live vaccines, telithromycin, voriconazole
Important contra-indications noted in the prescribing guidelines for: nursing mothers; pediatric patients
Note: Dulera is mometasone and formoterol.

Skin
Atrophy / Skin atrophy [2]
Burning / skin burning sensation [4]
Erythema [2]
Pruritus (itching) [2]
Stinging [2]
Telangiectasia [2]

Mucosal
Epistaxis (nosebleed) [2]
Oral candidiasis [3]

Central Nervous System
Headache [6]

Respiratory
Pharyngitis (sore throat) [2]
Rhinitis / rhinosinusitis (see also sinusitis) [2]
Upper respiratory tract infection [2]

MONOSODIUM GLUTAMATE

Family: N/A
Scientific name: *Monosodium glutamate*
Indications: Food additive, flavor enhancer
Class: Food additive
Half-life: N/A
Clinically important, potentially hazardous interactions with: BCG vaccine, MAO inhibitors
Note: The US Food & Drug Administration has determined that MSG is a safe food ingredient if used in moderation. Only a very small subset of individuals is allergic to MSG.
The etiologic agent of Chinese Restaurant Syndrome.

Skin
Anaphylactoid reactions / anaphylaxis (includes anaphylactic shock) [2]
Angioedema (formerly named angioneurotic edema) [5]
Atopic dermatitis [2]
Churg-Strauss syndrome [2]
Sensitivity [2]
Urticaria / hives [5]

Central Nervous System
Headache [6]
Hypoesthesia / hypesthesia (numbness) [2]
Paresthesias [2]

MONTELUKAST

Trade name: Singulair (Merck)
Indications: Asthma
Class: Leukotriene receptor antagonist
Half-life: 2.7–5.5 hours
Clinically important, potentially hazardous interactions with: prednisone
Important contra-indications noted in the prescribing guidelines for: nursing mothers
Note: April 2024, UK MHRA – Montelukast: reminder of the risk of neuropsychiatric reactions. Healthcare professionals prescribing montelukast should be alert to the risk of neuropsychiatric reactions in all patients including children and adolescents. Reported neuropsychiatric reactions include sleep disorders, hallucinations, anxiety and depression, as well as changes in behaviour and mood. Healthcare professionals should advise patients and their caregivers to be alert to these risks and seek medical advice as soon as possible if neuropsychiatric reactions occur. New boxed warnings are being added to the patient information leaflet supplied for montelukast in the UK.
Warning: SERIOUS NEUROPSYCHIATRIC EVENTS HAVE BEEN REPORTED IN PATIENTS TAKING MONTELUKAST.
DISCUSS BENEFITS AND RISKS OF MONTELUKAST WITH PATIENTS AND CAREGIVERS.
MONITOR FOR NEUROPSYCHIATRIC SYMPTOMS IN PATIENTS TAKING MONTELUKAST.
DISCONTINUE MONTELUKAST IMMEDIATELY IF NEUROPSYCHIATRIC SYMPTOMS OCCUR.
BECAUSE THE BENEFITS OF MONTELUKAST MAY NOT OUTWEIGH THE POTENTIAL RISK

OF NEUROPSYCHIATRIC SYMPTOMS IN PATIENTS WITH ALLERGIC RHINITIS, RESERVE USE FOR PATIENTS WHO HAVE AN INADEQUATE RESPONSE OR INTOLERANCE TO ALTERNATIVE THERAPIES

Skin
- Angioedema (formerly named angioneurotic edema) [3]
- Churg-Strauss syndrome [29]
- Rash (2%) [2]
- Urticaria / hives (2%)

Central Nervous System
- Aggression (includes anger) [3]
- Anxiety [2]
- Behavioral disturbances / personality changes [2]
- Depression [3]
- Hallucinations [2]
- Headache [4]
- Irritability [2]
- Neuropsychiatric / neuropsychological adverse effect [3]
- Neurotoxicity [5]
- Nightmares [3]
- Psychiatric adverse effect [3]
- Sleep disturbances [3]
- Suicidal ideation [2]

Gastrointestinal/Hepatic
- Abdominal pain [2]
- Hepatotoxicity / liver injury / acute liver injury / drug-induced liver injury (DILI) [3]

Respiratory
- Cough [2]
- Influenza- ('flu)-like syndrome (<10%)

Other
- Adverse effects / adverse reactions [3]

MORICIZINE

Trade name: Ethmozine (Shire)
Indications: Ventricular arrhythmias
Class: Antiarrhythmic class Ic
Half-life: 3–4 hours
Clinically important, potentially hazardous interactions with: diltiazem, oxtriphylline, warfarin

---

Skin
- Diaphoresis (2–5%)
- Pruritus (itching) (<2%)
- Urticaria / hives (<2%)
- Xerosis / xeroderma (<2%)

Mucosal
- Tongue edema (<2%)
- Xerostomia (dry mouth) (2–5%) [2]

Cardiovascular
- Arrhythmias [3]
- Tachycardia [3]
- Thrombophlebitis (<2%)

Central Nervous System
- Dysgeusia (taste perversion) (<2%)
- Hyperesthesia (2–5%)
- Paresthesias (2–5%)

Ocular
- Periorbital edema (<10%)

Other
- Death [3]

MORPHINE

Trade names: Avinza (Ligand), Duramorph (Baxter) (Elkins-Sinn), Infumorph (Baxter), Kadian (aaiPharma), Morphabond (Inspirion), MS Contin (Purdue), MSIR Oral (Purdue), Roxanol (aaiPharma)
Indications: Severe pain, acute myocardial infarction
Class: Opiate agonist
Half-life: 2–4 hours
Clinically important, potentially hazardous interactions with: buprenorphine, cimetidine, furazolidone, MAO inhibitors, metformin, mianserin, pentazocine, rifapentine, trospium
Important contra-indications noted in the prescribing guidelines for: nursing mothers; pediatric patients
Warning: ADDICTION, ABUSE, AND MISUSE; LIFE-THREATENING RESPIRATORY DEPRESSION; ACCIDENTAL INGESTION; NEONATAL OPIOID WITHDRAWAL SYNDROME; and INTERACTION WITH ALCOHOL

Skin
- AGEP [3]
- Edema / fluid retention [2]
- Pruritus (itching) (5–65%) [40]

Mucosal
- Xerostomia (dry mouth) (>10%) [8]

Cardiovascular
- Cardiotoxicity [3]
- Hypotension [5]

Central Nervous System
- Allodynia [4]
- Confusion [2]
- Fever (pyrexia) (includes hyperpyrexia) [2]
- Hallucinations [4]
- Hyperalgesia [10]
- Hypothermia [2]
- Sedation [2]
- Somnolence (drowsiness) [5]
- Trembling (<10%)
- Vertigo / dizziness [5]

Endocrine/Metabolic
- Adrenal insufficiency (hypoadrenalism) / Addisonian crisis (includes Addison's disease) [2]
- Amenorrhea [2]

Gastrointestinal/Hepatic
- Constipation [7]
- Nausea [16]
- Vomiting [13]

Genitourinary
- Urinary retention [2]

Local
- Injection-site pain (>10%)

Neuromuscular/Skeletal
- Myoclonus (see also hypnic jerk) [5]
- Rhabdomyolysis [2]

Respiratory
- Respiratory depression [6]

Other
- Adverse effects / adverse reactions [2]
- Death [3]
- Hiccups / singultus [3]

MOXIFLOXACIN

Trade names: Avelox (Bayer), Moxeza (Alcon)
Indications: Various infections caused by susceptible organisms
Class: Antibiotic, Antibiotic; fluoroquinolone, Antimicrobial, Drug-resistant antituberculosis agent
Half-life: 12 hours
Clinically important, potentially hazardous interactions with: alfuzosin, aminophylline, amiodarone, amitriptyline, antacids, arsenic, artemether/lumefantrine, asenapine, atomoxetine, BCG vaccine, benperidol, bepridil, bretylium, chloroquine, ciprofloxacin, corticosteroids, cyclosporine, degarelix, didanosine, disopyramide, dronedarone, droperidol, erythromycin, gadobutrol, haloperidol, hydroxychloroquine, insulin, lanthanum, levomepromazine, magnesium salts, mefloquine, mizolastine, mycophenolate, nilotinib, NSAIDs, oral iron, oral typhoid vaccine, pentamidine, phenothiazines, pimavanserin, pimozide, probenecid, procainamide, QT prolonging agents, quinapril, quinidine, quinine, ribociclib, sevelamer, sotalol, strontium ranelate, sucralfate, sulfonylureas, tetrabenazine, thioridazine, tricyclic antidepressants, vandetanib, vitamin K antagonists, warfarin, zinc, ziprasidone, zolmitriptan, zuclopenthixol
Important contra-indications noted in the prescribing guidelines for: the elderly; nursing mothers; pediatric patients
Note: Fluoroquinolones are associated with an increased risk of tendinitis and tendon rupture in all ages. This risk is further increased in older patients usually over 60 years of age, in patients taking corticosteroid drugs, and in patients with kidney, heart or lung transplants. Fluoroquinolones may exacerbate muscle weakness in persons with myasthenia gravis. Moxeza is for topical ophthalmic use only.
Warning: SERIOUS ADVERSE REACTIONS INCLUDING TENDINITIS, TENDON RUPTURE, PERIPHERAL NEUROPATHY, CENTRAL NERVOUS SYSTEM EFFECTS and EXACERBATION OF MYASTHENIA GRAVIS

Skin
- AGEP [2]
- Anaphylactoid reactions / anaphylaxis (includes anaphylactic shock) [5]
- Bullous dermatosis [2]
- DRESS syndrome (Drug-induced hypersensitivity syndrome) [4]
- Hypersensitivity [5]
- Photosensitivity [5]
- Pruritus (itching) [3]
- Rash [4]
- Stevens-Johnson syndrome and toxic epidermal necrolysis (SJS/TEN) [2]
- Thrombocytopenic purpura [2]
- Urticaria / hives [3]

Cardiovascular
- Phlebitis [2]
- QT interval prolonged / QT prolongation [15]
- Torsades de pointes [9]

Central Nervous System
- Delirium [2]
- Dysgeusia (taste perversion) [3]
- Hallucinations [3]

Headache (4%) [5]
Seizures [2]
Somnolence (drowsiness) [2]
Vertigo / dizziness (3%) [7]

Endocrine/Metabolic
Hyperglycemia (includes glucose increased) [2]

Gastrointestinal/Hepatic
Abdominal pain [5]
Diarrhea (6%) [6]
Gastrointestinal disorder / discomfort [2]
Hepatotoxicity / liver injury / acute liver injury / drug-induced liver injury (DILI) [3]
Nausea (7%) [10]
Vomiting [6]

Hematologic
Neutropenia (neutrophils decreased) [5]

Local
Injection-site reaction [2]

Neuromuscular/Skeletal
Asthenia / fatigue [2]
Myasthenia gravis (exacerbation) [2]
Tendinopathy/Tendon rupture [3]

Otic
Tinnitus [2]

Other
Adverse effects / adverse reactions [8]
Hiccups / singultus [2]

MOXISYLYTE

Synonym: Thymoxamine (British Approved Name)
Trade name: Opilon (Concord)
Indications: Impotence, primary Raynaud's phenomenon
Class: Alpha-adrenergic channel blocker
Half-life: 1–2 hours
Clinically important, potentially hazardous interactions with: acebutolol, alfuzosin, captopril, cilazapril, enalapril, fosinopril, indoramin, irbesartan, lisinopril, olmesartan, quinapril, ramipril, trandolapril, tricyclic antidepressants

---

Gastrointestinal/Hepatic
Hepatotoxicity / liver injury / acute liver injury / drug-induced liver injury (DILI) [5]

MOXONIDINE

Trade name: Physiotens (Solvay)
Indications: Hypertension
Class: Antihypertensive, Imidazoline receptor agonist
Half-life: 2–3 hours
Clinically important, potentially hazardous interactions with: acebutolol, alfuzosin, amitriptyline, antihypertensives, captopril, clobazam, diclofenac, enalapril, fosinopril, hypnotics, irbesartan, levodopa, levomepromazine, lisinopril, meloxicam, olmesartan, quinapril, ramipril, sedatives, trandolapril, triamcinolone, trifluoperazine

---

Mucosal
Xerostomia (dry mouth) [3]

Central Nervous System
Headache [2]
Somnolence (drowsiness) [2]
Vertigo / dizziness [2]

Other
Death [3]

MYCOPHENOLATE

Synonyms: mycophenolate mofetil, mycophenolate sodium, mycophenolic acid
Trade names: CellCept (Roche), Myfortic (Novartis)
Indications: Prophylaxis of organ rejection
Class: Immunosuppressant
Half-life: 18 hours
Clinically important, potentially hazardous interactions with: antacids, azathioprine, basiliximab, belatacept, cholestyramine, ciprofloxacin, corticosteroids, cyclophosphamide, cyclosporine, daclizumab, gemifloxacin, Hemophilus B vaccine, levofloxacin, mercaptopurine, metronidazole, moxifloxacin, norfloxacin, ofloxacin, pantoprazole, rifapentine, sevelamer, tacrolimus, vaccines
Important contra-indications noted in the prescribing guidelines for: the elderly; nursing mothers; pediatric patients
Warning: EMBRYOFETAL TOXICITY, MALIGNANCIES AND SERIOUS INFECTIONS

Skin
Acneiform eruption / acneiform dermatitis / acneiform rash (>10%) [4]
Carcinoma (non-melanoma) (4%)
Cutaneous toxicity / skin toxicity [2]
Edema / fluid retention (12%)
Herpes simplex [3]
Herpes zoster [8]
Peripheral edema (29%)
Rash (8%) [2]
Verrucae vulgaris / warts / verrucae [2]

Hair
Alopecia / hair loss [4]

Nails
Onychomycosis [2]

Mucosal
Gingival hyperplasia / gingival hypertrophy / gingival enlargement / gingival overgrowth [2]
Oral candidiasis (10%)
Oral ulceration [7]

Cardiovascular
Hypertension [4]
Thrombophlebitis (<10%)

Central Nervous System
Encephalopathy (includes hepatic encephalopathy) [2]
Fever (pyrexia) (includes hyperpyrexia) [3]
Headache (>20%) [5]
Insomnia [4]
Leukoencephalopathy / posterior reversible encephalopathy syndrome (PRES) [4]
Neurotoxicity [2]
Pain (>20%)
Primary central nervous system lymphoma (PCNSL) [3]
Tremor (11%)

Endocrine/Metabolic
ALT increased [3]
Dyslipidemia [2]
Hyperglycemia (includes glucose increased) [4]
Hyperlipidemia / lipids elevated [3]

Gastrointestinal/Hepatic
Abdominal distension [2]
Abdominal pain [6]
Colitis [11]
Diarrhea [17]
Hepatotoxicity / liver injury / acute liver injury / drug-induced liver injury (DILI) [6]
Nausea [6]
Vomiting [6]

Genitourinary
Urinary tract infection [3]

Hematologic
Anemia (>20%) [2]
Leukocytopenia (leukopenia) / leukocytes (white blood cells) decreased [6]
Lymphopenia (lymphocytopenia) / lymphocytes decreased [3]
Myelosuppression / bone marrow suppression / myelotoxicity [3]
Neutropenia (neutrophils decreased) [4]
Thrombocytopenia / platelets decreased [4]

Neuromuscular/Skeletal
Arthralgia [4]
Asthenia / fatigue [6]
Back pain (6%)
Myalgia/Myopathy [4]

Renal
Nephrotoxicity / kidney injury / acute kidney injury (AKI) / drug-induced kidney injury [3]

Respiratory
Bronchitis [2]
Cough [2]
Upper respiratory tract infection [3]

Other
Adverse effects / adverse reactions [22]
Death [2]
Infection (12–20%) [19]
Teratogenicity [4]

MYRRH

Family: Burseraceae
Scientific names: *Commiphora abyssinica, Commiphora erythraea, Commiphora habessinica, Commiphora kataf, Commiphora madagascariensis, Commiphora molmol, Commiphora myrrh*
Indications: Fascioliasis, schistosomiasis, ulcers, eczema, catarrh, amenorrhea, gum disease, aphthous stomatitis
Class: Anthelmintic, Anti-inflammatory
Half-life: N/A
Clinically important, potentially hazardous interactions with: none known

---

Skin
Dermatitis [5]

Gastrointestinal/Hepatic
Abdominal pain (2%)

Neuromuscular/Skeletal
Asthenia / fatigue (2%)

NABUMETONE

Trade name: Relafen (GSK)
Indications: Arthritis
Class: Non-steroidal anti-inflammatory (NSAID)
Half-life: 22.5–30 hours
Clinically important, potentially hazardous interactions with: methotrexate

Important contra-indications noted in the prescribing guidelines for: nursing mothers; pediatric patients
Note: NSAIDs may cause an increased risk of serious cardiovascular and gastrointestinal adverse events, which can be fatal. This risk may increase with duration of use.
Warning: CARDIOVASCULAR AND GASTROINTESTINAL RISKS

Skin
Diaphoresis (<3%)
Edema / fluid retention (3–9%)
Erythema [2]
Hypersensitivity [3]
Photosensitivity [2]
Pruritus (itching) (3–9%) [2]
Pseudoporphyria [8]
Rash (3–9%) [4]

Mucosal
Stomatitis (oral mucositis) (<3%)
Xerostomia (dry mouth) (<3%)

Central Nervous System
Headache (3–9%) [2]
Insomnia (3–9%)
Nervousness (3–9%)
Somnolence (drowsiness) (3–9%)
Vertigo / dizziness (3–9%)

Gastrointestinal/Hepatic
Abdominal pain (12%) [5]
Constipation (3–9%)
Diarrhea (14%) [5]
Dyspepsia / functional dyspepsia (indigestion) (see also gastroparesis) (13%) [4]
Flatulence (3–9%)
Gastrointestinal ulceration [3]
Hepatotoxicity / liver injury / acute liver injury / drug-induced liver injury (DILI) [2]
Nausea (3–9%) [2]
Vomiting (3–9%)

Otic
Tinnitus (<10%)

Renal
Nephrotoxicity / kidney injury / acute kidney injury (AKI) / drug-induced kidney injury [2]

Other
Adverse effects / adverse reactions [6]

NADOLOL

Trade name: Corzide (Monarch)
Indications: Hypertension, angina pectoris
Class: Adrenergic beta-receptor antagonist, Antiarrhythmic class II
Half-life: 10–24 hours
Clinically important, potentially hazardous interactions with: clonidine, epinephrine, verapamil
Important contra-indications noted in the prescribing guidelines for: nursing mothers; pediatric patients
Note: Corzide is nadolol and bendroflumethiazide. Cutaneous side effects of beta-receptor blockers are clinically polymorphous. They apparently appear after several months of continuous therapy. Contra-indicated in patients with bronchial asthma, sinus bradycardia and greater than first degree conduction block, cardiogenic shock, and overt cardiac failure.

Skin
Edema / fluid retention (<5%)
Psoriasis [4]
Raynaud's phenomenon (2%) [2]

Cardiovascular
Bradycardia / sinus bradycardia (2%)

Central Nervous System
Hypoesthesia / hypesthesia (numbness) (fingers and toes) (>5%)
Paresthesias (>5%)
Vertigo / dizziness (2%)

Neuromuscular/Skeletal
Asthenia / fatigue (2%)

Other
Adverse effects / adverse reactions [4]

NAFCILLIN

Trade name: Nafcil (Merz)
Indications: Various infections caused by susceptible organisms
Class: Antibiotic, Antibiotic; beta-lactam, Antibiotic; penicillin, Antimicrobial, CYP1A2 inducer
Half-life: 0.5–1.5 hours
Clinically important, potentially hazardous interactions with: anticoagulants, cyclosporine, demeclocycline, doxycycline, elbasvir & grazoprevir, enzalutamide, imipenem/cilastatin, lumateperone, methotrexate, minocycline, olaparib, oxytetracycline, palbociclib, tetracycline, venetoclax, warfarin
Important contra-indications noted in the prescribing guidelines for: nursing mothers; pediatric patients

---

Skin
Exanthems (10%)
Rash (<32%)

Gastrointestinal/Hepatic
Hepatotoxicity / liver injury / acute liver injury / drug-induced liver injury (DILI) [4]

Local
Injection-site necrosis [2]

Renal
Nephrotoxicity / kidney injury / acute kidney injury (AKI) / drug-induced kidney injury [5]

NALBUPHINE

Trade name: Nubain (Endo)
Indications: Moderate to severe pain
Class: Opiate agonist
Half-life: 5 hours
Clinically important, potentially hazardous interactions with: CNS depressants, diazepam, hydrocodone, hydromorphone, oliceridine, oxymorphone, pentobarbital, promethazine, tapentadol
Note: Nalbuphine contains sulfites.

Skin
Clammy skin (9%)
Diaphoresis (9%)

Mucosal
Xerostomia (dry mouth) (4%)

Central Nervous System
Vertigo / dizziness (5%)

Local
Injection-site pain [4]

NALDEMEDINE

Trade name: Symproic (Shionogi)
Indications: Opioid-induced constipation in adult patients with chronic non-cancer pain
Class: Opioid antagonist, Opioid receptor antagonist
Half-life: 11 hours
Clinically important, potentially hazardous interactions with: amiodarone, aprepitant, atazanavir, captopril, carbamazepine, clarithromycin, cyclosporine, diltiazem, erythromycin, fluconazole, itraconazole, ketoconazole, moderate or strong CYP3A inhibitors, other opioid antagonists, P-gp inhibitors, phenytoin, quercetin, quinidine, rifampin, ritonavir, saquinavir, St John's wort, strong CYP3A inducers, verapamil
Pregnancy category: Potential for opioid withdrawal in fetus
Important contra-indications noted in the prescribing guidelines for: nursing mothers; pediatric patients
Note: Contra-indicated in patients with known or suspected gastrointestinal obstruction. Opioid withdrawal symptoms have occurred in patients treated with naldemedine.

Skin
Hypersensitivity (<2%)
Rash (<2%)

Central Nervous System
Psychiatric adverse effect [2]

Gastrointestinal/Hepatic
Abdominal pain (8–11%) [4]
Diarrhea (7%) [12]
Gastroenteritis (2–3%)
Gastrointestinal disorder / discomfort [4]
Nausea (4–6%)
Vomiting (3%)

Respiratory
Bronchospasm (<2%)

Other
Adverse effects / adverse reactions [4]

NALMEFENE

Trade name: Revex (Baxter)
Indications: Reversal of opioid depression. Also used for alcohol dependence, impulse control disorders such as pathological gambling, pruritus of cholestasis
Class: Antidote, Opioid antagonist
Half-life: 10.8 hours
Clinically important, potentially hazardous interactions with: flumazenil
Important contra-indications noted in the prescribing guidelines for: the elderly; nursing mothers; pediatric patients
Note: As an antidote, it is difficult to differentiate side effects due to the drug from those due to the effects of the poison.

Cardiovascular
Hypertension (5%)
Tachycardia (5%)

Central Nervous System
Fever (pyrexia) (includes hyperpyrexia) (3%)
Insomnia [4]
Pain (postoperative) (4%)
Somnolence (drowsiness) [3]

Vertigo / dizziness (3%) [7]

Gastrointestinal/Hepatic

Nausea (18%) [2]
Vomiting (9%) [2]

Neuromuscular/Skeletal

Asthenia / fatigue [4]

Respiratory

Nasopharyngitis [2]

NALOXEGOL

Trade name: Movantik (AstraZeneca)
Indications: Opioid-induced constipation
Class: Opioid receptor antagonist
Half-life: 6–11 hours
Clinically important, potentially hazardous interactions with: diltiazem, erythromycin, grapefruit juice, verapamil, viloxazine
Important contra-indications noted in the prescribing guidelines for: nursing mothers; pediatric patients
Note: Contra-indicated in patients with known or suspected gastrointestinal obstruction, patients at increased risk of recurrent gastrointestinal obstruction, and patients concomitantly using strong CYP3A4 inhibitors.

Skin

Hyperhidrosis (<3%)

Central Nervous System

Headache (4%) [3]

Gastrointestinal/Hepatic

Abdominal pain (12–21%) [5]
Diarrhea (6–9%) [5]
Flatulence (3–6%) [2]
Nausea (7–8%) [5]
Vomiting (3–5%)

Other

Adverse effects / adverse reactions [2]

NALOXONE

Trade names: Suboxone (Reckitt Benckiser), Talwin-NX (Sanofi-Aventis), Targiniq (Purdue)
Indications: Narcotic overdose
Class: Opioid antagonist
Half-life: <1.5 hours
Clinically important, potentially hazardous interactions with: cobicistat/elvitegravir/emtricitabine/tenofovir alafenamide, cobicistat/elvitegravir/emtricitabine/tenofovir disoproxil, thioridazine
Important contra-indications noted in the prescribing guidelines for: nursing mothers
Note: Suboxone is buprenorphine and naloxone. Targiniq is naloxone and oxycodone.

Skin

Diaphoresis (<10%)
Pruritus (itching) [2]
Rash (<10%)

Mucosal

Xerostomia (dry mouth) [2]

Cardiovascular

Arrhythmias [2]
Bradycardia / sinus bradycardia [2]
Hypertension [8]
Hypotension [2]

Central Nervous System

Headache [4]
Seizures [5]
Somnolence (drowsiness) [3]

Gastrointestinal/Hepatic

Constipation [8]
Nausea [4]
Vomiting [2]

Neuromuscular/Skeletal

Asthenia / fatigue [3]
Myoclonus (see also hypnic jerk) [2]

Respiratory

Pulmonary edema (cardiogenic / non-cardiogenic) [6]

Other

Adverse effects / adverse reactions [5]
Death [2]

NALTREXONE

Trade names: Contrave (Takeda), Depade (Mallinckrodt), Nalorex (Bristol-Myers Squibb), Opizone (Genus), ReVia (Meda), Troxyca (Pfizer), Vivitrex (Alkermes), Vivitrol (Alkermes)
Indications: Substance abuse, opioid dependence, alcohol dependence.
Adjunct for the treatment of obesity and for weight loss management in defined populations and health conditions.

Class: Anti-obesity / weight loss pharmacotherapy, Opioid antagonist
Half-life: 4 hours
Clinically important, potentially hazardous interactions with: bremelanotide, lofexidine, opioid analgesics, opioid containing medications
Important contra-indications noted in the prescribing guidelines for: nursing mothers; pediatric patients
Note: Naltrexone has the capacity to cause hepatocellular injury when given in excessive doses.
Troxyca is naltrexone and oxycodone. Contra-indicated in acute hepatitis or liver failure; patients receiving opioid analgesics, with current physiologic opioid dependence, or in acute opioid withdrawal. Contrave, a combination of naltrexone and bupropion, has been approved by the FDA for chronic weight management.

Skin

AGEP [2]
Nicolau syndrome [2]
Pruritus (itching) [2]
Rash (<10%)

Cardiovascular

Hypertension [4]

Central Nervous System

Anxiety [2]
Chills (<10%)
Compulsions / obsessive-compulsive symptoms / obsessive-compulsive disorder [2]
Depression [2]
Headache [5]
Insomnia [5]
Seizures [2]
Somnolence (drowsiness) [2]
Vertigo / dizziness [5]

Gastrointestinal/Hepatic

Constipation [6]
Diarrhea [3]
Hepatotoxicity / liver injury / acute liver injury / drug-induced liver injury (DILI) [5]
Nausea [10]
Vomiting [6]

Local

Injection-site pain [2]
Injection-site reaction [5]

Neuromuscular/Skeletal

Arthralgia (>10%)
Asthenia / fatigue [4]

Respiratory

Eosinophilic pneumonia [2]
Influenza [2]
Nasopharyngitis [2]

Other

Adverse effects / adverse reactions [3]

NANDROLONE

Trade name: Deca-Durabolin (Organon)
Indications: Anemia of renal insufficiency, control of metastatic breast cancer, osteoporosis in post-menopausal women
Class: Anabolic steroid
Half-life: 6–14 days
Clinically important, potentially hazardous interactions with: acenocoumarol, anisindione, anticoagulants, dabigatran, danaparoid, fondaparinux, heparin, warfarin
Important contra-indications noted in the prescribing guidelines for: nursing mothers; pediatric patients
Note: Deca Durabolin contains Arachis oil (peanut oil) and should not be taken / applied by patients known to be allergic to peanut.

Hair

Hirsutism [3]

Other

Adverse effects / adverse reactions [2]

NAPHAZOLINE

Trade name: Albalon (Allergan)
Indications: Ocular irritation and/or congestion, allergic, inflammatory ocular conditions
Class: Sympathomimetic
Half-life: N/A
Clinically important, potentially hazardous interactions with: MAO inhibitors, maprotiline, tricyclic antidepressants
Important contra-indications noted in the prescribing guidelines for: nursing mothers; pediatric patients
Note: Contra-indicated in narrow angle glaucoma.

Skin

Diaphoresis [2]

Cardiovascular

Bradycardia / sinus bradycardia [2]
Hypertension [2]

Respiratory

Pulmonary edema (cardiogenic / non-cardiogenic) [3]

NAPROXEN

Trade names: Aleve (Bayer), Naprosyn (Roche), Synflex (Roche)
Indications: Pain, arthritis
Class: Covid-19 putative drug, Non-steroidal anti-inflammatory (NSAID)
Half-life: 15 hours
Clinically important, potentially hazardous interactions with: methotrexate, methyl salicylate, prednisolone
Important contra-indications noted in the prescribing guidelines for: the elderly; nursing mothers; pediatric patients
Note: NSAIDs may cause an increased risk of serious cardiovascular and gastrointestinal adverse events, which can be fatal. This risk may increase with duration of use.

Skin
- Anaphylactoid reactions / anaphylaxis (includes anaphylactic shock) [2]
- Angioedema (formerly named angioneurotic edema) [5]
- Bruise / bruising / contusion / ecchymosis (ecchymoses) (3–9%)
- Bullous dermatosis [5]
- Diaphoresis (<3%) [3]
- DRESS syndrome (Drug-induced hypersensitivity syndrome) [4]
- Edema / fluid retention (<9%)
- Erythema multiforme [2]
- Exanthems (<14%) [9]
- Fixed eruption / fixed drug eruption [26]
- Hypersensitivity [2]
- Lichen planus (includes hypertrophic lichen planus) [3]
- Lichenoid eruption / lichenoid reaction [3]
- Lupus erythematosus (subacute cutaneous lupus erythematosus (SCLE)) [2]
- Photosensitivity [16]
- Pruritus (itching) (3–17%) [5]
- Pseudoporphyria [29]
- Purpura (<3%) [4]
- Pustules / pustular eruption [2]
- Rash (3–9%) [2]
- Stevens-Johnson syndrome and toxic epidermal necrolysis (SJS/TEN) [5]
- Urticaria / hives (<5%) [6]
- Vasculitis (angiitis) / cutaneous vasculitis (angiitis) [9]

Hair
- Alopecia / hair loss [3]

Mucosal
- Stomatitis (oral mucositis) (<3%)
- Xerostomia (dry mouth) [2]

Cardiovascular
- Chest pain [2]
- Myocardial infarction [2]

Central Nervous System
- Somnolence (drowsiness) [2]
- Vertigo / dizziness [6]

Gastrointestinal/Hepatic
- Abdominal pain [4]
- Constipation [2]
- Diarrhea [3]
- Dyspepsia / functional dyspepsia (indigestion) (see also gastroparesis) [10]
- Gastrointestinal disorder / discomfort [2]
- Hepatotoxicity / liver injury / acute liver injury / drug-induced liver injury (DILI) [4]
- Nausea [10]

Hematologic
- Thrombocytopenia / platelets decreased [2]

Neuromuscular/Skeletal
- Leg cramps [2]

Otic
- Tinnitus [2]

Renal
- Nephrotoxicity / kidney injury / acute kidney injury (AKI) / drug-induced kidney injury [3]

Respiratory
- Nasopharyngitis [2]

Other
- Adverse effects / adverse reactions [12]
- Death [2]
- Side effects (5–9%) [3]

NARATRIPTAN

Trade names: Amerge (GSK), Naramig (GSK)
Indications: Acute migraine attacks
Class: 5-HT1 agonist, Serotonin receptor antagonist, Triptan
Half-life: 6 hours
Clinically important, potentially hazardous interactions with: 5-ht$_1$ agonists, dihydroergotamine, duloxetine, ergotamine, methysergide, metoclopramide, oral contraceptives, rizatriptan, selegiline, sibutramine, SNRIs, SSRIs, St John's wort, sumatriptan, triptans, venlafaxine, zolmitriptan
Important contra-indications noted in the prescribing guidelines for: the elderly; nursing mothers; pediatric patients
Note: Contra-indicated in patients with history, symptoms, or signs of ischemic cardiac, cerebrovascular, or peripheral vascular syndromes.

Central Nervous System
- Neurotoxicity (4–7%) [2]
- Pain (2–4%)
- Paresthesias (<2%)
- Somnolence (drowsiness) (<2%)
- Vertigo / dizziness (<2%)

Gastrointestinal/Hepatic
- Colitis [5]
- Gastrointestinal disorder / discomfort (6–7%)
- Nausea (4–5%) [3]

Neuromuscular/Skeletal
- Asthenia / fatigue (<2%)

Other
- Adverse effects / adverse reactions [6]

NATALIZUMAB

Synonym: antegren
Trade name: Tysabri (Biogen)
Indications: Multiple sclerosis, Crohn's disease
Class: Immunomodulator, Monoclonal antibody
Half-life: 11 days
Clinically important, potentially hazardous interactions with: abatacept, alefacept, azacitidine, azathioprine, betamethasone, cabazitaxel, certolizumab, cortocosteroids, cyclosporine, denileukin, docetaxel, fingolimod, gefitinib, leflunomide, lenalidomide, mercaptopurine, methotrexate, oxaliplatin, pazopanib, pemetrexed, pralatrexate, rilonacept, temsirolimus, triamcinolone, vedolizumab
Important contra-indications noted in the prescribing guidelines for: nursing mothers; pediatric patients
Note: Contra-indicated in patients who have or have had progressive multifocal leukoencephalopathy. Natalizumab-sztn (Tyruko) is biosimilar to Natalizumab (Tysabri). Approved 08/24/2023.
Warning: PROGRESSIVE MULTIFOCAL LEUKOENCEPHALOPATHY

Skin
- Dermatitis (6%)
- Eosinophilic fasciitis (Shulman syndrome / Shulman disease) [2]
- Herpes simplex [2]
- Hypersensitivity [6]
- Pruritus (itching) (4%)
- Rash (9%)

Central Nervous System
- Depression (17%)
- Headache (35%) [3]
- Leukoencephalopathy / posterior reversible encephalopathy syndrome (PRES) [79]
- Tremor (3%)

Gastrointestinal/Hepatic
- Hepatotoxicity / liver injury / acute liver injury / drug-induced liver injury (DILI) [5]

Genitourinary
- Vaginitis (includes vulvitis) (8%)

Hematologic
- Eosinophilia / eosinophils increased [4]

Local
- Application-site reactions (22%)
- Infusion-related reactions [3]
- Infusion-site reactions [2]

Neuromuscular/Skeletal
- Asthenia / fatigue (24%) [4]

Respiratory
- Pneumonitis [2]

Other
- Adverse effects / adverse reactions [6]
- Allergic reactions (7%) [4]
- Death [7]
- Infection (2%) [5]

NEBIVOLOL

Trade names: Bystolic (Forest), Byvalson (Forest), Nebilet (Menarini)
Indications: Hypertension
Class: Adrenergic beta-receptor antagonist, Beta blocker
Half-life: 8 hours
Clinically important, potentially hazardous interactions with: beta blockers, cinacalcet, clonidine, CYP2D6 inhibitors, delavirdine, digitalis glycosides, duloxetine, terbinafine, tipranavir, viloxazine
Important contra-indications noted in the prescribing guidelines for: nursing mothers; pediatric patients
Note: Byvalson is nebivolol and valsartan.
Warning: Byvalson: FETAL TOXICITY

Cardiovascular
- Bradycardia / sinus bradycardia [3]
- Hypotension [2]

Central Nervous System
- Headache (6–9%) [10]
- Vertigo / dizziness (2–4%) [6]

Gastrointestinal/Hepatic
Diarrhea (<2%)
Nausea (<3%)
Neuromuscular/Skeletal
Asthenia / fatigue (2–5%) [4]
Respiratory
Nasopharyngitis [3]
Upper respiratory tract infection [3]
Other
Adverse effects / adverse reactions [4]

NEDOCROMIL

Trade names: Alocril (Allergan), Tilade (Monarch)
Indications: Bronchial asthma, pruritus of allergic conjunctivitis
Class: Mast cell stabilizer
Half-life: 3.3 hours
Clinically important, potentially hazardous interactions with: none known
Important contra-indications noted in the prescribing guidelines for: nursing mothers

---

Central Nervous System
Dysgeusia (taste perversion) (<12%) [4]
Gastrointestinal/Hepatic
Abdominal pain (2%)
Ocular
Ocular burning (<3%) [2]
Ocular stinging [2]
Respiratory
Cough (9%)
Rhinitis / rhinosinusitis (see also sinusitis) (7%)
Upper respiratory tract infection (7%)

NEFAZODONE

Trade name: Serzone (Bristol-Myers Squibb)
Indications: Depression
Class: Antidepressant, CYP3A4 inhibitor, Norepinephrine reuptake inhibitor
Half-life: 2–4 hours
Clinically important, potentially hazardous interactions with: abiraterone, aprepitant, astemizole, atorvastatin, avanafil, buspirone, cabozantinib, calcifediol, ceritinib, copanlisib, crizotinib, darunavir, dasatinib, dronedarone, eletriptan, erlotinib, eszopiclone, fesoterodine, flibanserin, fluticasone propionate, indinavir, isocarboxazid, ivabradine, ixabepilone, lapatinib, lomitapide, lumateperone, MAO inhibitors, methylergonovine, midostaurin, mifepristone, neratinib, olaparib, osimertinib, paclitaxel, palbociclib, phenelzine, pimozide, ponatinib, rimonabant, romidepsin, ruxolitinib, selegiline, sibutramine, simvastatin, solifenacin, sonidegib, St John's wort, sumatriptan, sunitinib, temsirolimus, ticagrelor, tipranavir, tolvaptan, tramadol, tranylcypromine, trazodone, ulipristal, vemurafenib, vorapaxar
Important contra-indications noted in the prescribing guidelines for: nursing mothers; pediatric patients
Note: This drug has been withdrawn.
Warning: SUICIDALITY AND ANTIDEPRESSANT DRUGS and HEPATOTOXICITY

Skin
Flushing / rubefaction (4%)
Peripheral edema (3%)
Pruritus (itching) (2%)
Rash (2%)
Mucosal
Xerostomia (dry mouth) (25%)
Central Nervous System
Dysgeusia (taste perversion) (2%)
Paresthesias (4%)
Gastrointestinal/Hepatic
Hepatotoxicity / liver injury / acute liver injury / drug-induced liver injury (DILI) [5]
Genitourinary
Vaginitis (includes vulvitis) (2%)
Neuromuscular/Skeletal
Asthenia / fatigue [2]
Rhabdomyolysis [3]
Respiratory
Influenza- ('flu)-like syndrome (<10%)
Other
Infection (8%)

NELARABINE

Trade name: Arranon (GSK)
Indications: T-cell acute lymphoblastic leukemia, T-cell lymphoblastic lymphoma
Class: Antimetabolite, Antineoplastic / anticancer agent (see also Immune checkpoint inhibitor), Purine analog
Half-life: 0.5–3 hours
Clinically important, potentially hazardous interactions with: pentostatin
Important contra-indications noted in the prescribing guidelines for: the elderly; nursing mothers
Note: Nelarabine is a pro-drug of Ara-G.

Skin
Edema / fluid retention (11%)
Peripheral edema (15%)
Petechiae (12%)
Mucosal
Epistaxis (nosebleed) (8%)
Stomatitis (oral mucositis) (8%)
Cardiovascular
Chest pain (5%)
Hypotension (8%)
Tachycardia (8%)
Central Nervous System
Amnesia (3%)
Balance disorder (2%)
Confusion (8%)
Depression (6%)
Dysgeusia (taste perversion) (3%)
Fever (pyrexia) (includes hyperpyrexia) (23%)
Gait instability / postural instability (6%)
Headache (17%)
Hypoesthesia / hypesthesia (numbness) (17%)
Insomnia (7%)
Myelopathy [8]
Neurotoxicity [14]
Pain (11%)
Paralysis / paraplegia [2]
Paresthesias (4%) [2]
Peripheral neuropathy (21%) [5]
Rigors (8%)
Seizures (6%) [2]
Somnolence (drowsiness) (23%) [3]
Tremor (4%)
Vertigo / dizziness (21%)
Endocrine/Metabolic
AST increased (6%)
Dehydration (7%)
Hyperglycemia (includes glucose increased) (6%)
Gastrointestinal/Hepatic
Abdominal distension (6%)
Abdominal pain (9%)
Constipation (21%)
Diarrhea (22%)
Hepatotoxicity / liver injury / acute liver injury / drug-induced liver injury (DILI) [2]
Nausea (41%)
Vomiting (22%)
Hematologic
Anemia (99%)
Febrile neutropenia (12%)
Hemotoxicity [2]
Myelosuppression / bone marrow suppression / myelotoxicity [3]
Neutropenia (neutrophils decreased) (81%) [2]
Thrombocytopenia / platelets decreased (86%) [2]
Neuromuscular/Skeletal
Arthralgia (9%)
Asthenia / fatigue (17–50%)
Ataxia (9%)
Back pain (8%)
Myalgia/Myopathy (13%)
Pain in extremities (7%)
Ocular
Vision blurred (4%)
Respiratory
Cough (25%)
Dyspnea / shortness of breath (7–20%)
Pleural effusion (10%)
Pneumonia (8%)
Sinusitis (see also rhinitis / rhinosinusitis) (7%)
Wheezing (5%)
Other
Adverse effects / adverse reactions [5]
Death [2]
Infection (9%)

NELFINAVIR

Trade name: Viracept (ViiV)
Indications: HIV infection
Class: Antiretroviral, Covid-19 putative drug, CYP3A4 inhibitor, HIV-1 protease inhibitor
Half-life: 3.5–5 hours
Clinically important, potentially hazardous interactions with: abiraterone, afatinib, alfuzosin, amiodarone, amprenavir, aripiprazole, artemether/lumefantrine, atorvastatin, avanafil, barbiturates, benzodiazepines, brigatinib, cabazitaxel, cabozantinib, calcifediol, carbamazepine, chlordiazepoxide, ciclesonide, cisapride, clonazepam, clorazepate, copanlisib, crizotinib, cyclosporine, darifenacin, dasatinib, delavirdine, diazepam, dihydroergotamine, eletriptan, eplerenone, ergot alkaloids, ergotamine, erlotinib, estrogens, eszopiclone, etravirine, eucalyptus, everolimus, fentanyl, fesoterodine, flibanserin, flurazepam, fluticasone propionate, indinavir, ivabradine, ixabepilone, lapatinib, lomitapide, lopinavir, lorazepam,

lovastatin, lumateperone, maraviroc, methadone, methylergonovine, methysergide, midazolam, midostaurin, mifepristone, neratinib, olaparib, omeprazole, oral contraceptives, oxazepam, paclitaxel, palbociclib, pantoprazole, pazopanib, phenytoin, pimozide, ponatinib, primidone, progestogens, quazepam, quinidine, quinine, ranolazine, rifabutin, rifampin, rilpivirine, ritonavir, rivaroxaban, romidepsin, rosuvastatin, ruxolitinib, saquinavir, sildenafil, simeprevir, simvastatin, solifenacin, St John's wort, sunitinib, tacrolimus, tadalafil, telithromycin, temazepam, temsirolimus, ticagrelor, tolterodine, tolvaptan, triazolam, vardenafil, vemurafenib, vorapaxar
Important contra-indications noted in the prescribing guidelines for: nursing mothers
Note: Protease inhibitors cause dyslipidemia which includes elevated triglycerides and cholesterol and redistribution of body fat centrally to produce the so-called 'protease paunch', breast enlargement, facial atrophy, and 'buffalo hump'.

Skin
Rash (<10%) [4]
Gastrointestinal/Hepatic
Diarrhea [3]
Hepatotoxicity / liver injury / acute liver injury / drug-induced liver injury (DILI) [3]
Genitourinary
Urolithiasis / ureteral stones / urinary calculi [2]
Hematologic
Lymphopenia (lymphocytopenia) / lymphocytes decreased [2]

NEOMYCIN

Trade names: Maxitrol (Falcon), Neosporin (Monarch)
Indications: Various infections caused by susceptible organisms
Class: Antibiotic, Antibiotic; aminoglycoside, Antimicrobial
Half-life: 3 hours
Clinically important, potentially hazardous interactions with: acarbose, aldesleukin, aminoglycosides, atracurium, bacitracin, bumetanide, doxacurium, ethacrynic acid, furosemide, methoxyflurane, neostigmine, pancuronium, penicillin V, polypeptide antibiotics, rocuronium, sorafenib, succinylcholine, teicoplanin, torsemide, vecuronium
Important contra-indications noted in the prescribing guidelines for: nursing mothers; pediatric patients
Note: Aminoglycosides may cause neurotoxicity and/or nephrotoxicity.

Skin
Anaphylactoid reactions / anaphylaxis (includes anaphylactic shock) [2]
Contact dermatitis (<10%) [70]
Eczema / eczematous reaction / eczematous eruption [2]
Exanthems [2]
Rash (<10%)
Stevens-Johnson syndrome and toxic epidermal necrolysis (SJS/TEN) [2]
Urticaria / hives (<10%)
Otic
Hearing loss (hypoacusis) [3]

NEOSTIGMINE

Trade name: Prostigmin (Valeant)
Indications: Myasthenia gravis
Class: Acetylcholinesterase inhibitor, Cholinesterase inhibitor, Parasympathomimetic
Half-life: 52 minutes
Clinically important, potentially hazardous interactions with: aminoglycosides, antiarrhythmics, anticholinergics, chloroquine, clindamycin, hydroxychloroquine, kanamycin, lithium, local and general anesthetics, neomycin, non-depolarising muscle relaxants, polymixins, propafenone, propranolol, streptomycin, succinylcholine
Pregnancy category: Anticholinesterase drugs may cause uterine irritability and induce premature labor when given intravenously to pregnant women near term
Important contra-indications noted in the prescribing guidelines for: nursing mothers; pediatric patients
Note: Neostigmine bromide is given orally; neostigmine methylsulfate is given parenterally. Contra-indicated in patients with a previous history of reaction to bromides, or those with peritonitis or mechanical obstruction of the intestinal or urinary tract.

Skin
Anaphylactoid reactions / anaphylaxis (includes anaphylactic shock) [3]
Cardiovascular
Atrioventricular block [3]
Bradycardia / sinus bradycardia [4]
Cardiac arrest [3]
Tachycardia [2]
Central Nervous System
Anxiety [2]
Sedation [2]
Gastrointestinal/Hepatic
Abdominal pain [3]
Diarrhea [2]
Nausea [14]
Vomiting [12]
Respiratory
Bronchospasm [3]
Pulmonary edema (cardiogenic / non-cardiogenic) [4]

NERATINIB

Trade name: Nerlynx (Puma)
Indications: Early stage HER2-overexpressed/amplified breast cancer, to follow adjuvant trastuzumab-based therapy
Class: Epidermal growth factor receptor (EGFR) inhibitor / antagonist, Kinase inhibitor, Tyrosine kinase inhibitor
Half-life: 7–17 hours
Clinically important, potentially hazardous interactions with: aprepitant, boceprevir, bosentan, carbamazepine, cimetidine, ciprofloxacin, clarithromycin, clotrimazole, cobicistat, conivaptan, crizotinib, cyclosporine, dabigatran, digoxin, diltiazem, dronedarone, efavirenz, enzalutamide, erythromycin, etravirine, fexofenadine, fluconazole, fluvoxamine, grapefruit juice, H2-receptor antagonists, idelalisib, imatinib, indinavir, itraconazole, ketoconazole, lansoprazole, lopinavir, mitotane, modafinil, nefazodone, nelfinavir, ombitasvir/paritaprevir/ritonavir, ombitasvir/paritaprevir/ritonavir and dasabuvir, phenytoin, posaconazole, rifampin, ritonavir, saquinavir, St John's wort, strong or moderate CYP3A4 inhibitors or inducers, tipranavir, tofisopam, troleandomycin, verapamil, voriconazole
Pregnancy category: Can cause fetal harm
Important contra-indications noted in the prescribing guidelines for: nursing mothers; pediatric patients

---

Skin
Fissures (2%)
Rash (18%)
Xerosis / xeroderma (6%)
Nails
Nail disorder (8%)
Mucosal
Epistaxis (nosebleed) (5%)
Stomatitis (oral mucositis) (14%) [2]
Xerostomia (dry mouth) (3%)
Cardiovascular
Cardiotoxicity [2]
Central Nervous System
Anorexia [5]
Peripheral neuropathy [2]
Endocrine/Metabolic
ALT increased (9%)
Appetite decreased (12%)
AST increased (7%)
Dehydration (4%)
Weight loss (5%)
Gastrointestinal/Hepatic
Abdominal distension (5%)
Abdominal pain (36%) [3]
Constipation [2]
Diarrhea (95%) [18]
Dyspepsia / functional dyspepsia (indigestion) (see also gastroparesis) (10%)
Hepatotoxicity / liver injury / acute liver injury / drug-induced liver injury (DILI) (<2%)
Nausea (43%) [12]
Vomiting (26%) [8]
Genitourinary
Urinary tract infection (5%)
Hematologic
Anemia [2]
Leukocytopenia (leukopenia) / leukocytes (white blood cells) decreased [2]
Neutropenia (neutrophils decreased) [3]
Neuromuscular/Skeletal
Asthenia / fatigue (27%) [7]
Muscle spasm (11%)

NETARSUDIL

Trade name: Rhopressa (Aerie)
Indications: Reduction of elevated intraocular pressure in open angle glaucoma or ocular hypertension
Class: Rho kinase inhibitor
Half-life: N/A
Clinically important, potentially hazardous interactions with: none known
Pregnancy category: No available data to inform drug-associated risk

Important contra-indications noted in the prescribing guidelines for: nursing mothers; pediatric patients

---

Local
Application-site erythema (5–10%)
Application-site pain (~20%)

Ocular
Conjunctival hemorrhage (~20%)
Conjunctival hyperemia / conjunctival injection (53%) [6]
Corneal deposits (~20%)
Corneal staining (5–10%)
Eyelid erythema (5–10%)
Lacrimation (5–10%)
Reduced visual acuity (5–10%)
Vision blurred (5–10%)

NETUPITANT & PALONOSETRON

Synonym: NEPA
Trade name: Akynzeo (Helsinn)
Indications: Acute and delayed nausea and vomiting associated with cancer chemotherapy
Class: Neurokinin 1 receptor antagonist (netupitant), Serotonin type 3 receptor antagonist (palonosetron)
Half-life: 40 hours
Clinically important, potentially hazardous interactions with: rifampin
Important contra-indications noted in the prescribing guidelines for: nursing mothers; pediatric patients

---

Skin
Erythema (3%)

Central Nervous System
Headache (9%) [7]

Gastrointestinal/Hepatic
Constipation (3%) [7]
Dyspepsia / functional dyspepsia (indigestion) (see also gastroparesis) (4%) [2]

Neuromuscular/Skeletal
Asthenia / fatigue (4–8%)

Other
Adverse effects / adverse reactions [2]
Hiccups / singultus [2]

NEVIRAPINE

Trade name: Viramune (Boehringer Ingelheim)
Indications: HIV infection
Class: Antiretroviral, CYP3A4 inducer, Non-nucleoside reverse transcriptase inhibitor
Half-life: 45 hours
Clinically important, potentially hazardous interactions with: amiodarone, amprenavir, atazanavir, carbamazepine, caspofungin, clarithromycin, clonazepam, cyclosporine, diltiazem, disopyramide, doravirine, efavirenz, ethosuximide, etravirine, fentanyl, fluconazole, fosamprenavir, indinavir, itraconazole, ketoconazole, levonorgestrel, lidocaine, lopinavir, midazolam, nifedipine, rifampin, rilpivirine, simeprevir, St John's wort, verapamil
Important contra-indications noted in the prescribing guidelines for: nursing mothers
Warning: LIFE-THREATENING (INCLUDING FATAL) HEPATOTOXICITY and SKIN REACTIONS

Skin
Angioedema (formerly named angioneurotic edema) [2]
Cutaneous toxicity / skin toxicity [3]
DRESS syndrome (Drug-induced hypersensitivity syndrome) [12]
Exanthems [6]
Hypersensitivity [15]
Lipodystrophy / acquired generalized lipodystrophy [2]
Rash (<48%) [31]
Stevens-Johnson syndrome and toxic epidermal necrolysis (SJS/TEN) [45]

Mucosal
Gingivitis (<3%)
Ulcerative stomatitis (4%)

Central Nervous System
Fever (pyrexia) (includes hyperpyrexia) [2]
Paresthesias (2%)
Peripheral neuropathy [2]

Endocrine/Metabolic
Acidosis (includes lactic acidosis) [2]

Gastrointestinal/Hepatic
Hepatic failure [2]
Hepatotoxicity / liver injury / acute liver injury / drug-induced liver injury (DILI) [33]

Hematologic
Anemia [2]
Neutropenia (neutrophils decreased) [2]

Neuromuscular/Skeletal
Myalgia/Myopathy (<10%)

Other
Adverse effects / adverse reactions [7]
Death [3]

NIACIN

Synonyms: nicotinic acid; vitamin B_3
Trade names: Advicor (Kos), Niacor (Upsher-Smith), Niaspan (Merck), Simcor (AbbVie), Slo-Niacin (Upsher-Smith)
Indications: Hyperlipidemia
Class: Vitamin
Half-life: 45 minutes
Clinically important, potentially hazardous interactions with: antihypertensives, atorvastatin, bile acid sequestrants, insulin aspart, insulin degludec, insulin detemir, insulin glargine, insulin glulisine, pitavastatin, rosuvastatin, selenium
Pregnancy category: Where niacin is co-administered with a statin, refer to the pregnancy category for the statin
Important contra-indications noted in the prescribing guidelines for: nursing mothers; pediatric patients
Note: Contra-indicated in patients with active liver or peptic ulcer disease, or arterial bleeding. Simcor is niacin and simvastatin.

Skin
Acanthosis nigricans (8%) [14]
Exanthems (<3%)
Flushing / rubefaction (<30%) [34]
Pruritus (itching) (<5%) [9]
Rash [5]

Central Nervous System
Paresthesias (<10%) [2]
Syncope / fainting [2]

Endocrine/Metabolic
Hyperglycemia (includes glucose increased) [2]

Gastrointestinal/Hepatic
Hepatic failure [4]
Hepatotoxicity / liver injury / acute liver injury / drug-induced liver injury (DILI) [6]
Nausea [2]

Neuromuscular/Skeletal
Myalgia/Myopathy [5]

Ocular
Maculopathy [3]

NIACINAMIDE

Synonyms: nicotinamide; vitamin B_3
Indications: Prophylaxis and treatment of pellagra
Class: Vitamin
Half-life: 45 minutes
Clinically important, potentially hazardous interactions with: atorvastatin, primidone, rosuvastatin
Pregnancy category: the pregnancy category will be C if used in doses above the RDA

Skin
Pruritus (itching) (<5%) [2]

Central Nervous System
Paresthesias (<10%)

Gastrointestinal/Hepatic
Hepatotoxicity / liver injury / acute liver injury / drug-induced liver injury (DILI) [2]

Hematologic
Thrombocytopenia / platelets decreased [2]

NICARDIPINE

Trade name: Cardene (Roche)
Indications: Angina, hypertension
Class: Calcium channel blocker
Half-life: 2–4 hours
Clinically important, potentially hazardous interactions with: amprenavir, atazanavir, boceprevir, cobicistat/elvitegravir/emtricitabine/tenofovir alafenamide, cobicistat/elvitegravir/emtricitabine/tenofovir disoproxil, delavirdine, epirubicin, imatinib, indinavir, lopinavir, posaconazole, propranolol, telaprevir
Important contra-indications noted in the prescribing guidelines for: the elderly; pediatric patients

---

Skin
Erythromelalgia / erythermalgia [4]
Flushing / rubefaction (6%) [2]
Peripheral edema (7%) [2]
Rash [3]
Urticaria / hives [3]

Mucosal
Gingival hyperplasia / gingival hypertrophy / gingival enlargement / gingival overgrowth [2]

Endocrine/Metabolic
Gynecomastia [2]

Local
Injection-site phlebitis [2]

Respiratory
Pulmonary edema (cardiogenic / non-cardiogenic) [5]

Other
Adverse effects / adverse reactions [2]
Side effects [2]

NICORANDIL

Trade names: Corflo (Wockhardt), Korandil (Sun Pharma), Nicoran (Torrent), Zynicor (Cadila Healthcare)
Indications: Angina pectoris
Class: Potassium channel activator
Half-life: N/A
Clinically important, potentially hazardous interactions with: amitriptyline, sildenafil, tadalafil, vardenafil

---

Skin
Leg ulceration [2]
Ulcerations [9]

Mucosal
Aphthous stomatitis / aphthous ulcer / aphtha (aphthae) [7]
Mucocutaneous reactions [2]
Oral ulceration [26]
Perianal ulcerations [16]
Tongue ulceration [3]

Central Nervous System
Cranial neuropathy (includes types of palsy) [3]
Headache [10]
Vertigo / dizziness [2]

Gastrointestinal/Hepatic
Gastrointestinal fistula [3]
Gastrointestinal ulceration [2]

Genitourinary
Penile ulceration [2]

Hematologic
Methemoglobinemia [2]

Ocular
Corneal ulceration (see also corneal melting) [2]

NICOTINE

Trade names: Habitrol Patch (Novartis), Nicoderm (GSK), Nicorette (GSK), Nicotrol (Pfizer)
Indications: Aid to smoking cessation
Class: Alkaloid
Half-life: varies with the delivery system
Clinically important, potentially hazardous interactions with: adenosine, bendamustine, heparin, horsetail
Important contra-indications noted in the prescribing guidelines for: nursing mothers; pediatric patients
Note: Smoking cessation therapy has various delivery systems. These include: transdermal patches, chewing gum, nasal spray, inhaler, and oral forms.

Skin
Acneiform eruption / acneiform dermatitis / acneiform rash (3%)
Diaphoresis (<3%)
Erythema (>10%)
Pigmentation (Skin) (includes hyperpigmentation) [3]
Pruritus (itching) (>10%)

Mucosal
Sialorrhea (ptyalism; hypersalivation) (>10%)
Stomatitis (oral mucositis) (>10%)
Xerostomia (dry mouth) (<3%)

Central Nervous System
Headache (18–26%)

Gastrointestinal/Hepatic
Dyspepsia / functional dyspepsia (indigestion) (see also gastroparesis) (18%)
Flatulence (4%)
Pancreatitis / acute pancreatitis [2]
Throat irritation/pain (66%)

Neuromuscular/Skeletal
Arthralgia (5%)
Back pain (6%)
Myalgia/Myopathy (<10%)

Respiratory
Cough (32%) [2]
Rhinitis / rhinosinusitis (see also sinusitis) (23%)

Other
Death [2]
Hiccups / singultus [2]

NIFEDIPINE

Trade names: Adalat (Bayer), Coracten (UCB), Procardia (Pfizer), Tenif (AstraZeneca), Tensipine MR (Genus), Valni XL (Winthrop)
Indications: Angina, hypertension
Class: Calcium channel blocker
Half-life: 2–5 hours (immediate release products)
Clinically important, potentially hazardous interactions with: acebutolol, amprenavir, atazanavir, beta blockers, boceprevir, carbamazepine, cobicistat/elvitegravir/emtricitabine/tenofovir alafenamide, cobicistat/elvitegravir/emtricitabine/tenofovir disoproxil, cyclosporine, delavirdine, digoxin, diltiazem, dronedarone, efavirenz, epirubicin, fentanyl, fluoxetine, grapefruit juice, imatinib, indinavir, insulin, lopinavir, micafungin, mizolastine, nevirapine, oxcarbazepine, parenteral magnesium, phenytoin, posaconazole, propranolol, rifampin, ritonavir, St John's wort, tacrolimus, vardenafil, vincristine
Important contra-indications noted in the prescribing guidelines for: the elderly; nursing mothers; pediatric patients
Note: Although not approved for this purpose, immediate-release nifedipine capsules have been used (orally and sublingually) for acute reduction of blood pressure. The literature reports several cases of profound hypotension, myocardial infarction, and death when immediate-release nifedipine was used in this way. Immediate-release nifedipine capsules should not be used for the acute reduction of blood pressure.
Tenif is atenolol and nifedipine.

Skin
AGEP [3]
Angioedema (formerly named angioneurotic edema) [2]
Bullous dermatosis [2]
Dermatitis (<2%)
Diaphoresis (<2%) [2]
Edema / fluid retention [3]
Erysipelas [2]
Erythema [2]
Erythema multiforme [5]
Erythema nodosum [2]
Erythromelalgia / erythermalgia [6]
Exanthems [9]
Exfoliative dermatitis [5]
Fixed eruption / fixed drug eruption [2]
Flushing / rubefaction (3–25%) [9]
Lichenoid eruption / lichenoid reaction [3]
Lupus erythematosus (subacute cutaneous lupus erythematosus (SCLE)) [3]
Peripheral edema [12]
Photosensitivity [5]
Pruritus (itching) (<2%) [3]
Purpura (<2%) [3]
Rash (<3%) [2]
Stevens-Johnson syndrome and toxic epidermal necrolysis (SJS/TEN) [5]
Telangiectasia [2]
Urticaria / hives [7]
Vasculitis (angiitis) / cutaneous vasculitis (angiitis) [4]

Hair
Alopecia / hair loss [4]

Mucosal
Gingival hyperplasia / gingival hypertrophy / gingival enlargement / gingival overgrowth (6–10%) [76]
Xerostomia (dry mouth) (<3%)

Cardiovascular
Hypotension [10]
Tachycardia [4]

Central Nervous System
Chills (2%)
Headache (19%) [8]
Paresthesias (<3%)
Tremor (2–8%)
Vertigo / dizziness [5]

Endocrine/Metabolic
Gynecomastia [6]

Gastrointestinal/Hepatic
Hepatotoxicity / liver injury / acute liver injury / drug-induced liver injury (DILI) [3]
Nausea (2%) [2]

Neuromuscular/Skeletal
Asthenia / fatigue (4%)

Respiratory
Pulmonary edema (cardiogenic / non-cardiogenic) [3]

Other
Adverse effects / adverse reactions [4]
Side effects [3]

NILOTINIB

Trade name: Tasigna (Novartis)
Indications: Chronic myelogenous leukemia
Class: Antineoplastic / anticancer agent (see also Immune checkpoint inhibitor), Bcr-Abl tyrosine kinase inhibitor / (Breakpoint cluster region Abelson (Bcr-Abl) tyrosine kinase inhibitor, Tyrosine kinase inhibitor, Vascular endothelial growth factor (VEGF) inhibitor / antagonist
Half-life: 17 hours
Clinically important, potentially hazardous interactions with: amiodarone, amitriptyline, amoxapine, arsenic, astemizole, bepridil, carbamazepine, chloroquine, cisapride, citalopram, clarithromycin, clozapine, conivaptan, darunavir, dasatinib, degarelix, delavirdine, digoxin, dihydroergotamine, disopyramide, dolasetron, efavirenz, ergotamine, grapefruit juice, halofantrine, haloperidol, indinavir, itraconazole, ketoconazole, lapatinib,

levofloxacin, lopinavir, methadone, midazolam, moxifloxacin, oxcarbazepine, pazopanib, phenobarbital, phenytoin, pimozide, procainamide, quinidine, rifampin, rifapentine, ritonavir, sotalol, St John's wort, telavancin, telithromycin, terfenadine, voriconazole, vorinostat, ziprasidone
Important contra-indications noted in the prescribing guidelines for: nursing mothers; pediatric patients
Note: Contra-indicated in patients with hypokalemia, hypomagnesemia, or long QT syndrome.
Warning: QT PROLONGATION AND SUDDEN DEATHS

Skin
- Acneiform eruption / acneiform dermatitis / acneiform rash (<10%)
- Cutaneous toxicity / skin toxicity [8]
- Dermatitis (<10%)
- Eczema / eczematous reaction / eczematous eruption (<10%)
- Edema / fluid retention [3]
- Erythema (<10%) [2]
- Exanthems [2]
- Flushing / rubefaction (<10%)
- Folliculitis (<10%)
- Hematoma / cutaneous hematoma (<10%)
- Hyperhidrosis (<10%)
- Peripheral edema (<10%)
- Pruritus (itching) (<10%) [18]
- Rash (<10%) [19]
- Sweet's syndrome [3]
- Urticaria / hives (<10%)
- Xerosis / xeroderma [2]

Hair
- Alopecia / hair loss (<10%) [5]

Cardiovascular
- Angina (<10%)
- Arrhythmias (<10%) [2]
- Arterial occlusion [5]
- Atrial fibrillation (<10%) [2]
- Atrioventricular block (<10%)
- Bradycardia / sinus bradycardia (<10%)
- Cardiotoxicity [5]
- Chest pain (<10%)
- Extrasystoles (<10%)
- Hypertension (<10%)
- Myocardial infarction [3]
- Palpitation (<10%)
- Pericardial effusion [2]
- QT interval prolonged / QT prolongation (<10%) [8]

Central Nervous System
- Anorexia (<10%) [2]
- Carotid artery stenosis [2]
- Cerebrovascular adverse event [2]
- Depression (<10%) [2]
- Fever (pyrexia) (includes hyperpyrexia) (<10%) [3]
- Headache (~10%) [16]
- Hypoesthesia / hypesthesia (numbness) (<10%)
- Insomnia (<10%)
- Pain [2]
- Paresthesias (<10%)
- Stroke / cerebrovascular accident [2]
- Vertigo / dizziness (<10%) [2]

Endocrine/Metabolic
- ALP increased [2]
- ALT increased (4%) [7]
- AST increased (<3%) [4]
- Diabetes mellitus (<10%) [2]
- Hyperamylasemia [3]
- Hyperbilirubinemia [14]
- Hypercalcemia (<10%)
- Hypercholesterolemia (<10%) [2]
- Hyperglycemia (includes glucose increased) (6–12%) [6]
- Hyperkalemia (2–6%)
- Hyperlipasemia [5]
- Hyperlipidemia / lipids elevated (<10%)
- Hypocalcemia (<10%)
- Hypokalemia (<10%) [2]
- Hypomagnesemia (<10%)
- Hyponatremia (<10%)
- Hypophosphatemia (5–17%) [4]
- Hypothyroidism [2]
- Weight gain (<10%)
- Weight loss (<10%)

Gastrointestinal/Hepatic
- Abdominal distension (<10%)
- Abdominal pain (<10%) [2]
- Constipation (~10%) [3]
- Diarrhea (~10%) [5]
- Dyspepsia / functional dyspepsia (indigestion) (see also gastroparesis) (<10%)
- Flatulence (<10%)
- Hepatotoxicity / liver injury / acute liver injury / drug-induced liver injury (DILI) [7]
- Nausea (~10%) [8]
- Pancreatitis / acute pancreatitis (<10%) [4]
- Vomiting (~10%)

Genitourinary
- Pollakiuria (<10%)

Hematologic
- Anemia (4–27%) [10]
- Febrile neutropenia (<10%)
- Leukocytopenia (leukopenia) / leukocytes (white blood cells) decreased [4]
- Lymphopenia (lymphocytopenia) / lymphocytes decreased (<10%) [2]
- Neutropenia (neutrophils decreased) (12–42%) [9]
- Pancytopenia (includes bicytopenia) (<10%)
- Thrombocytopenia / platelets decreased (10–42%) [14]

Neuromuscular/Skeletal
- Arthralgia (<10%) [3]
- Asthenia / fatigue (<10%) [10]
- Bone pain / joint pain (<10%)
- Muscle spasm [3]
- Myalgia/Myopathy (<10%) [5]
- Neck pain (<10%)

Ocular
- Conjunctivitis (conjunctival inflammation) (<10%)
- Ocular hemorrhage (<10%)
- Periorbital edema (<10%)
- Xerophthalmia (dry eyes) (<10%)

Respiratory
- Cough (<10%)
- Dysphonia (includes voice disorders / voice changes) (<10%)
- Dyspnea / shortness of breath (<10%) [2]
- Nasopharyngitis [2]
- Pleural effusion [2]
- Pulmonary hypertension [3]
- Upper respiratory tract infection [2]

Other
- Adverse effects / adverse reactions [3]
- Death [3]
- Side effects [3]

NILUTAMIDE

Trade names: Anandron (Sanofi-Aventis), Nilandron (Concordia)
Indications: Metastatic prostate cancer, androgen-independent prostate cancer
Class: Androgen antagonist, Antineoplastic / anticancer agent (see also Immune checkpoint inhibitor)
Half-life: N/A
Clinically important, potentially hazardous interactions with: alcohol, aminophylline, aspirin, chlordiazepoxide, diazepam, lidocaine, phenytoin, propranolol, warfarin

---

Skin
- Diaphoresis (6%)
- Edema / fluid retention (2%)
- Hot flashes / hot flushes (28%)
- Peripheral edema (<2%)
- Pruritus (itching) (2%)
- Rash (5%)
- Xerosis / xeroderma (5%)

Mucosal
- Xerostomia (dry mouth) (2%)

Cardiovascular
- Angina (2%)
- Cardiac failure (3%)
- Chest pain (<10%)
- Hypertension (5%)

Central Nervous System
- Depression (9%)
- Fever (pyrexia) (includes hyperpyrexia) (<10%) [3]
- Headache (<3%)
- Hyperesthesia (5%)
- Pain (27%)
- Paresthesias (3%)
- Syncope / fainting (2%)
- Vertigo / dizziness (10%)

Endocrine/Metabolic
- Gynecomastia (10%)

Gastrointestinal/Hepatic
- Abdominal pain (10%)
- Hepatotoxicity / liver injury / acute liver injury / drug-induced liver injury (DILI) [7]

Genitourinary
- Impotence (11%)

Neuromuscular/Skeletal
- Arthralgia (2%)
- Asthenia / fatigue (19%)
- Bone pain / joint pain (6%)

Ocular
- Cataract (2%)
- Ocular toxicity [2]
- Photophobia (2%)
- Visual disturbances [11]

Respiratory
- Cough (2%) [3]
- Dyspnea / shortness of breath [3]
- Influenza- ('flu)-like syndrome (7%)
- Pneumonia [8]
- Upper respiratory tract infection (8%)

Other
- Death [3]

NIMESULIDE

Trade name: Sulide (Novartis)
Indications: Pain, arthopathies
Class: COX-2 inhibitor, Non-steroidal anti-inflammatory (NSAID), Sulfonamide
Half-life: N/A
Clinically important, potentially hazardous interactions with: none known
Important contra-indications noted in the prescribing guidelines for: nursing mothers
Note: Nimesulide is a sulfonamide and can be absorbed systemically. Sulfonamides can produce severe, possibly fatal, reactions such as toxic epidermal necrolysis and Stevens-Johnson syndrome. NSAIDs may cause an increased risk of serious cardiovascular and gastrointestinal adverse events, which can be fatal. This risk may increase with duration of use.

Skin
- Anaphylactoid reactions / anaphylaxis (includes anaphylactic shock) [2]
- Angioedema (formerly named angioneurotic edema) [2]
- Fixed eruption / fixed drug eruption [6]
- Purpura [2]
- Stevens-Johnson syndrome and toxic epidermal necrolysis (SJS/TEN) [4]
- Urticaria / hives [6]

Gastrointestinal/Hepatic
- Hepatotoxicity / liver injury / acute liver injury / drug-induced liver injury (DILI) [36]

Renal
- Nephrotoxicity / kidney injury / acute kidney injury (AKI) / drug-induced kidney injury [5]

Respiratory
- Respiratory distress [2]

Other
- Adverse effects / adverse reactions [7]
- Death [4]

NIMODIPINE

Trade name: Nimotop (Bayer)
Indications: Subarachnoid hemorrhage
Class: Calcium channel blocker
Half-life: 3 hours
Clinically important, potentially hazardous interactions with: amprenavir, delavirdine, epirubicin, imatinib

---

Skin
- Edema / fluid retention (2%)
- Exanthems (2%) [2]
- Flushing / rubefaction (2%)
- Rash (3%)

Cardiovascular
- Bradycardia / sinus bradycardia [2]
- Hypotension [3]

Hematologic
- Hypoxemia [2]

NINTEDANIB

Trade name: Ofev (Boehringer Ingelheim)
Indications: Idiopathic pulmonary fibrosis
Class: Angiogenesis inhibitor / antiangiogenic agent, Tyrosine kinase inhibitor
Half-life: 9.5 hours
Clinically important, potentially hazardous interactions with: anticoagulants, carbamazepine, erythromycin, phenytoin, St John's wort
Important contra-indications noted in the prescribing guidelines for: nursing mothers; pediatric patients

---

Skin
- Hand–foot syndrome (palmar–plantar erythrodysesthesia) [2]
- Rash [4]

Hair
- Alopecia / hair loss [2]

Mucosal
- Epistaxis (nosebleed) [2]

Cardiovascular
- Cardiotoxicity [2]
- Hypertension (5%) [7]
- Myocardial infarction (2%)

Central Nervous System
- Anorexia [8]
- Headache (8%)
- Peripheral neuropathy [2]

Endocrine/Metabolic
- ALT increased [12]
- Appetite decreased (11%) [6]
- AST increased [10]
- Hypertransaminasemia (hepatic transaminitis) / elevated transaminases [2]
- Weight loss (10%) [5]

Gastrointestinal/Hepatic
- Abdominal pain (15%) [6]
- Diarrhea (62%) [50]
- Gastrointestinal adverse reaction [3]
- Gastrointestinal disorder / discomfort [6]
- Hepatotoxicity / liver injury / acute liver injury / drug-induced liver injury (DILI) (14%) [10]
- Nausea (24%) [30]
- Pneumatosis intestinalis / pneumatosis cystoides intestinalis [4]
- Vomiting (12%) [22]

Hematologic
- Anemia [3]
- Bleeding (10%) [3]
- Leukocytopenia (leukopenia) / leukocytes (white blood cells) decreased [2]
- Neutropenia (neutrophils decreased) [4]
- Thrombocytopenia / platelets decreased [3]
- Thrombotic microangiopathy [2]

Neuromuscular/Skeletal
- Asthenia / fatigue [16]

Respiratory
- Bronchitis [3]
- Cough [3]
- Dyspnea / shortness of breath [4]
- Nasopharyngitis [3]
- Pneumonia [3]
- Upper respiratory tract infection [2]

Other
- Adverse effects / adverse reactions [9]
- Death [4]

NIRAPARIB

Trade name: Zejula (Tesaro)
Indications: Maintenance treatment of adult patients with recurrent epithelial ovarian, fallopian tube, or primary peritoneal cancer who are in a complete or partial response to platinum-based chemotherapy
Class: Poly (ADP-ribose) polymerase (PARP) inhibitor
Half-life: 36 hours
Clinically important, potentially hazardous interactions with: none known
Pregnancy category: Can cause fetal harm
Important contra-indications noted in the prescribing guidelines for: nursing mothers; pediatric patients

---

Skin
- Peripheral edema (<10%)
- Rash (21%)

Mucosal
- Epistaxis (nosebleed) (<10%)
- Mucositis (20%)
- Stomatitis (oral mucositis) (20%)
- Xerostomia (dry mouth) (10%)

Cardiovascular
- Hypertension (20%) [3]
- Palpitation (10%)
- Tachycardia (<10%)

Central Nervous System
- Anxiety (11%)
- Depression (<10%)
- Dysgeusia (taste perversion) (10%)
- Headache (26%)
- Insomnia (27%)
- Vertigo / dizziness (18%)

Endocrine/Metabolic
- ALT increased (10%)
- Appetite decreased (25%) [3]
- AST increased (10%)
- Creatine phosphokinase (CPK) / creatine kinase increased (hyperCKemia) (<10%)
- GGT increased (<10%)
- Hypokalemia (<10%)
- Serum creatinine increased (<10%)
- Weight loss (<10%)

Gastrointestinal/Hepatic
- Abdominal distension (33%)
- Abdominal pain (33%)
- Constipation (40%)
- Diarrhea (20%)
- Dyspepsia / functional dyspepsia (indigestion) (see also gastroparesis) (18%)
- Nausea (74%) [6]
- Vomiting (34%) [3]

Genitourinary
- Urinary tract infection (13%)

Hematologic
- Anemia (50%) [11]
- Leukocytopenia (leukopenia) / leukocytes (white blood cells) decreased (17%)
- Neutropenia (neutrophils decreased) (30%) [9]
- Thrombocytopenia / platelets decreased (61%) [16]

Neuromuscular/Skeletal
- Arthralgia (13%)
- Asthenia / fatigue (57%) [3]
- Back pain (18%)
- Myalgia/Myopathy (19%)

Ocular
Conjunctivitis (conjunctival inflammation) (<10%)

Respiratory
Bronchitis (<10%)
Dyspnea / shortness of breath (20%)
Nasopharyngitis (23%)

Other
Adverse effects / adverse reactions [4]

NISOLDIPINE

Trade name: Sular (First Horizon)
Indications: Hypertension
Class: Calcium channel blocker
Half-life: 7–12 hours
Clinically important, potentially hazardous interactions with: amprenavir, conivaptan, cyclosporine, darunavir, delavirdine, efavirenz, epirubicin, grapefruit juice, imatinib, indinavir, itraconazole, ketoconazole, oxcarbazepine, propranolol, telaprevir, telithromycin, viloxazine, voriconazole

---

Skin
Peripheral edema (22%) [6]
Rash (2%)

Central Nervous System
Headache [4]

Endocrine/Metabolic
Gynecomastia [2]

NITAZOXANIDE

Trade name: Alinia (Romark)
Indications: Diarrhea caused by *Cryptosporidium parvum* or *Giardia lamblia* (in children)
Class: Antimicrobial, Antiprotozoal
Half-life: N/A
Clinically important, potentially hazardous interactions with: none known

---

Central Nervous System
Headache [2]

Gastrointestinal/Hepatic
Abdominal pain [3]
Diarrhea [2]

Other
Adverse effects / adverse reactions [2]

NITRAZEPAM

Trade name: Mogadon (Roche)
Indications: Insomnia
Class: Benzodiazepine, CNS depressant
Half-life: 14–48 hours
Clinically important, potentially hazardous interactions with: erythromycin

---

Mucosal
Sialorrhea (ptyalism; hypersalivation) [2]

NITROFURANTOIN

Trade names: Furadantin (First Horizon), Macrobid (Procter & Gamble), Macrodantin (Procter & Gamble)
Indications: Various urinary tract infections caused by susceptible organisms
Class: Antibiotic, Antimicrobial
Half-life: 1–2 minutes
Clinically important, potentially hazardous interactions with: norfloxacin
Important contra-indications noted in the prescribing guidelines for: nursing mothers; pediatric patients

---

Skin
Anaphylactoid reactions / anaphylaxis (includes anaphylactic shock) [2]
Angioedema (formerly named angioneurotic edema) [4]
Dermatitis [3]
DRESS syndrome (Drug-induced hypersensitivity syndrome) [4]
Eczema / eczematous reaction / eczematous eruption [2]
Erythema multiforme [3]
Exanthems (<5%) [9]
Exfoliative dermatitis [3]
Lupus erythematosus (subacute cutaneous lupus erythematosus (SCLE)) [8]
Purpura [2]
Rash [2]
Stevens-Johnson syndrome and toxic epidermal necrolysis (SJS/TEN) [7]
Urticaria / hives [8]

Hair
Alopecia / hair loss [5]

Central Nervous System
Neurotoxicity [2]
Paresthesias (<10%)

Gastrointestinal/Hepatic
Hepatitis [2]
Hepatotoxicity / liver injury / acute liver injury / drug-induced liver injury (DILI) [15]

Hematologic
Agranulocytosis / severe selective neutropenia [3]
Hemolysis [2]
Hemolytic anemia [4]

Respiratory
Interstitial lung disease / interstitial pneumonitis / interstitial pneumonia (cryptogenic organizing pneumonia) / drug-induced interstitial lung disease [3]
Pneumonitis [3]
Pulmonary toxicity [15]

Other
Adverse effects / adverse reactions [3]
Death [3]

NITROGLYCERIN

Synonyms: glyceryl trinitrate; nitroglycerol; NTG
Trade names: Minitran (3M), Nitrodur (Schering) (Key), Nitrolingual (First Horizon), Nitrostat (Pfizer)
Indications: Acute angina
Class: Nitrate, Vasodilator
Half-life: 1–4 minutes
Clinically important, potentially hazardous interactions with: acetylcysteine, alteplase, heparin, sildenafil, tadalafil, vardenafil
Important contra-indications noted in the prescribing guidelines for: nursing mothers; pediatric patients

---

Skin
Dermatitis (to topical systems) [25]
Eczema / eczematous reaction / eczematous eruption [2]
Erythema (to transdermal delivery system) [2]
Exfoliative dermatitis (<10%)
Flushing / rubefaction (>10%)
Purpura [2]
Rash (<10%)
Urticaria / hives [2]

Cardiovascular
Bradycardia / sinus bradycardia [2]
Hypotension [6]

Central Nervous System
Headache [15]
Migraine [2]

NITROPRUSSIDE

Trade names: Nipride (Exela), Nitropress (Hospira)
Indications: Hypertensive crises, congestive heart failure, erectile dysfunction, schizophrenia
Class: Vasodilator
Half-life: 1–2 minutes
Clinically important, potentially hazardous interactions with: acebutolol, alfuzosin, captopril, cilazapril, clevidipine, diclofenac, enalapril, fosinopril, levomepromazine, lisinopril, meloxicam, olmesartan, quinapril, ramipril, riociguat, tadalafil, trandolapril, triamcinolone, trifluoperazine, vardenafil
Pregnancy category: May cause fetal harm
Warning: Nipride: EXCESSIVE HYPOTENSION; CYANIDE TOXICITY

Skin
Cutaneous toxicity / skin toxicity (cyanide) [2]
Diaphoresis (<10%)

Cardiovascular
Hypertension [2]
Hypotension [3]

Central Nervous System
Headache (<10%)

Neuromuscular/Skeletal
Asthenia / fatigue (<10%)

Otic
Tinnitus (<10%)

Other
Death [2]

NIVOLUMAB

Trade name: Opdivo (Bristol-Myers Squibb)
Indications: Metastatic squamous non-small cell lung cancer with progression on or after platinum-based chemotherapy, unresectable or metastatic melanoma and disease progression following ipilimumab and, if BRAF V600 mutation positive, a BRAF inhibitor, advanced renal cell carcinoma with prior anti-angiogenic therapy, Hodgkin lymphoma that has relapsed or progressed after autologous hematopoietic stem cell transplantation and post-transplantation brentuximab vedotin, head and neck cancer, colon cancer, liver cancer
Class: Antineoplastic / anticancer agent (see also Immune checkpoint inhibitor), Biologic, Immune checkpoint inhibitor (incl. programmed death receptor-1 (PD-1) inhibitor), Monoclonal antibody
Half-life: 27 days
Clinically important, potentially hazardous interactions with: none known
Pregnancy category: Can cause fetal harm
Important contra-indications noted in the prescribing guidelines for: nursing mothers; pediatric patients
Note: In a review (May 2021) of the adverse reactions associated with nivolumab and ipilimumab, respectively, Health Canada concluded that there may be a link between nivolumab used alone or in combination with ipilimumab and the risks of autoimmune hemolytic anemia, aplastic anemia, cytokine release syndrome and tumor lysis syndrome. The Canadian product safety information (Canadian Product Monograph) for nivolumab has been updated to include a warning for the risk of autoimmune hemolytic anemia. Health Canada is working with the manufacturer of nivolumab to also include the risks of aplastic anemia, cytokine release syndrome, and tumor lysis syndrome in the Canadian Product Monograph (CPM).

Skin

Bullous pemphigoid / pemphigoid [13]
Contact dermatitis [2]
Cutaneous toxicity / skin toxicity [7]
Dermatitis [3]
Dermatomyositis [7]
DRESS syndrome (Drug-induced hypersensitivity syndrome) [3]
Eczema / eczematous reaction / eczematous eruption [2]
Edema / fluid retention (17%) [4]
Eosinophilic fasciitis (Shulman syndrome / Shulman disease) [6]
Erythema [5]
Erythema multiforme (<10%) [2]
Exanthems [3]
Exfoliative dermatitis (<10%)
Granuloma annulare [2]
Granulomatous reaction [2]
Henoch-Schönlein purpura / IgA vasculitis / immunoglobulin A vasculitis [3]
Hidradenitis suppurativa (acne inversa) [3]
Hypersensitivity [3]
Keratoacanthoma (Grzybowski syndrome) [3]
Lichen planus (includes hypertrophic lichen planus) [4]
Lichen planus pemphigoides [4]
Lichen sclerosus [4]
Lichenoid dermatitis [4]
Lichenoid eruption / lichenoid reaction [6]
Lipodystrophy / acquired generalized lipodystrophy [5]
Lupus erythematosus (subacute cutaneous lupus erythematosus (SCLE)) [5]
Lymphadenopathy [3]
Morphea / localized scleroderma [4]
Pruritus (itching) (11–19%) [30]
Psoriasiform dermatitis [2]
Psoriasis (<10%) [10]
Rash (16–21%) [47]
Sarcoidosis / sarcoid-like reaction (cutaneous sarcoidosis) [10]
Scleroderma [5]
Stevens-Johnson syndrome and toxic epidermal necrolysis (SJS/TEN) [11]
Thrombocytopenic purpura [2]
Thrombotic thrombocytopenic purpura [4]
Transient acantholytic dermatosis (Grover's disease) [2]
Urticaria / hives [2]
Vasculitis (angiitis) / cutaneous vasculitis (angiitis) [3]
Vitiligo (<10%) [15]

Hair

Alopecia areata [3]
Lichen planopilaris [3]

Nails

Onycholysis [2]

Mucosal

Lichenoid stomatitis [2]
Sialadenitis [2]
Sjögren's syndrome (see also sicca syndrome) [2]
Stomatitis (oral mucositis) (<10%) [2]
Xerostomia (dry mouth) [3]

Cardiovascular

Aortitis / periaortitis [3]
Capillary leak syndrome [4]
Cardiac tamponade / pericardial tamponade [2]
Cardiomyopathy [3]
Chest pain (13%)
Large-vessel vasculitis (includes giant cell arteritis) [2]
Myocarditis [22]
Myocarditis, myositis and myasthenia gravis overlap syndrome (Triple-M Syndrome / 3M Syndrome) [6]
Pericardial effusion [2]
Pericarditis [5]
Takotsubo syndrome [2]
Ventricular arrhythmia (<10%)
Ventricular tachycardia [2]

Central Nervous System

Antiphospholipid antibody syndrome [2]
Cerebellitis [2]
Encephalitis [10]
Encephalopathy (includes hepatic encephalopathy) [12]
Fever (pyrexia) (includes hyperpyrexia) (17%) [12]
Guillain-Barré syndrome / acute inflammatory demyelinating polyradiculoneuropathy / acute motor axonal neuropathy [10]
Headache [2]
Leukoencephalopathy / posterior reversible encephalopathy syndrome (PRES) [3]
Meningoencephalitis [4]
Myelitis / myeloradiculitis [2]
Neuromyelitis optica [3]
Neurotoxicity [7]
Pain (10%)
Paraneoplastic neurological syndromes [2]
Paresis [2]
Peripheral neuropathy (<10%) [3]
Vertigo / dizziness (<10%)

Endocrine/Metabolic

Adrenal insufficiency (hypoadrenalism) / Addisonian crisis (includes Addison's disease) [19]
Adrenocorticotropic hormone (corticotropin; ACTH) deficiency [6]
ALP increased (14–22%)
ALT increased (12–16%) [11]
Appetite decreased (35%) [10]
AST increased (16–28%) [9]
Autosplenectomy [2]
Diabetes insipidus [2]
Diabetes mellitus [28]
Diabetic ketoacidosis [9]
Hyperamylasemia [4]
Hypercalcemia (20%)
Hyperkalemia (15–18%)
Hyperlipasemia [8]
Hyperthyroidism (includes 'thyroid storm') [12]
Hypocalcemia (18%)
Hypokalemia (20%) [2]
Hypomagnesemia (20%)
Hyponatremia (25–38%)
Hypophosphatemia [2]
Hypophysitis [31]
Hypothyroidism [34]
Serum creatinine increased (22%) [2]
Thyroid dysfunction [17]
Thyroiditis [15]
Thyrotoxicosis [3]
Weight loss (13%)

Gastrointestinal/Hepatic

Abdominal pain (16%)
Cholangitis / sclerosing cholangitis [10]
Colitis [43]
Constipation (24%) [2]
Diarrhea (18%) [41]
Duodenitis [3]
Enteritis [3]
Enterocolitis [4]
Enteropathy [2]
Esophagitis [4]
Gastritis / pangastritis / gastric irritation [9]
Gastrointestinal perforation / perforated colon / gastric perforation [2]
Hemorrhagic gastritis [2]
Hepatic (liver) disorder / hepatobiliary disorder / hepatic (liver) dysfunction [3]
Hepatitis [17]
Hepatotoxicity / liver injury / acute liver injury / drug-induced liver injury (DILI) [23]
Intestinal pseudo-obstruction (Ogilvie syndrome) [2]
Nausea (29%) [16]
Pancreatic insufficiency [2]
Pancreatitis / acute pancreatitis [8]
Vomiting (19%) [3]

Genitourinary

Cystitis (includes interstitial cystitis / bladder pain syndrome) [9]
Penile ulceration [2]

Hematologic

Anemia (28%) [10]
Aplastic anemia [5]
Coagulopathy / coagulation dysfunction / clotting factor deficiency (includes

disseminated intravascular coagulation / DIC) [2]
Cryoglobulinemia [2]
Cytopenia [2]
Eosinophilia / eosinophils increased [5]
Hemolytic anemia [8]
Hemophagocytic lymphohistiocytosis / hemophagocytic syndrome [4]
Lymphopenia (lymphocytopenia) / lymphocytes decreased (47%) [4]
Neutropenia (neutrophils decreased) [13]
Pancytopenia (includes bicytopenia) [2]
Pure red cell aplasia [4]
Thrombocytopenia / platelets decreased (14%) [14]

Local
Infusion-related reactions (<10%) [8]

Neuromuscular/Skeletal
Arthralgia (13%) [11]
Arthritis / polyarthritis [2]
Asthenia / fatigue (19–50%) [40]
Ataxia [2]
Bone pain / joint pain (36%)
Inflammatory arthritis [4]
Lambert-Eaton myasthenic syndrome [5]
Myalgia/Myopathy [24]
Myasthenia gravis [25]
Osteonecrosis / avascular necrosis (includes steroid-induced osteonecrosis of the femoral head) [2]
Polymyalgia rheumatica [8]
Polymyositis [2]
Rhabdomyolysis [6]
Synovial effusions [3]

Ocular
Iridocyclitis (<10%)
Ocular adverse effect [2]
Uveitis / anterior uveitis / posterior uveitis / panuveitis [7]

Renal
Glomerulonephritis (includes membranous nephropathy) [4]
Immunoglobulin A (IgA) nephropathy (Berger's disease) [2]
Nephritis / interstitial nephritis / tubulointerstitial nephritis [5]
Nephrotoxicity / kidney injury / acute kidney injury (AKI) / drug-induced kidney injury [10]
Renal failure [5]
Renal tubular acidosis [2]
Tumor lysis syndrome (TLS) [3]

Respiratory
Bronchitis (<10%)
Cough (17–32%) [2]
Dyspnea / shortness of breath (38%) [3]
Eosinophilic pneumonia [3]
Interstitial lung disease / interstitial pneumonitis / interstitial pneumonia (cryptogenic organizing pneumonia) / drug-induced interstitial lung disease [9]
Pneumonia (10%) [5]
Pneumonitis [40]
Pneumothorax [2]
Pulmonary granuloma [4]
Pulmonary toxicity [3]
Upper respiratory tract infection (11%)

Other
Adverse effects / adverse reactions [47]
Cytokine release syndrome / cytokine storm [8]
Death [41]
Immune-related adverse effect [9]
Serositis / polyserositis [2]
Side effects [2]
Vocal cord / vocal fold paralysis (vocal cord / vocal fold palsy) [2]
Vogt-Koyanagi-Harada syndrome [10]

NIZATIDINE

Trade name: Axid (Reliant)
Indications: Duodenal ulcer, gastroesophageal reflux disease (GERD)
Class: Histamine H2 receptor antagonist
Half-life: 1–2 hours
Clinically important, potentially hazardous interactions with: delavirdine, rilpivirine
Important contra-indications noted in the prescribing guidelines for: the elderly; nursing mothers; pediatric patients

---

Skin
Diaphoresis [2]
Pruritus (itching) (2%) [2]
Rash (2%)
Urticaria / hives [2]

Cardiovascular
Chest pain (2%)

Central Nervous System
Abnormal dreams (2%)
Anxiety (2%)
Fever (pyrexia) (includes hyperpyrexia) (2%)
Headache (17%)
Insomnia (3%)
Pain (4%)
Somnolence (drowsiness) (2%)
Vertigo / dizziness (5%)

Gastrointestinal/Hepatic
Abdominal pain (8%)
Constipation (3%)
Diarrhea (7%)
Dyspepsia / functional dyspepsia (indigestion) (see also gastroparesis) (4%)
Flatulence (5%)
Nausea (5%)
Vomiting (4%)

Neuromuscular/Skeletal
Asthenia / fatigue (3%)
Back pain (2%)
Myalgia/Myopathy (2%)

Respiratory
Cough (2%)
Pharyngitis (sore throat) (3%)
Rhinitis / rhinosinusitis (see also sinusitis) (9%)
Sinusitis (see also rhinitis / rhinosinusitis) (2%)

Other
Infection (2%)

NORFLOXACIN

Trade names: Chibroxin (Merck), Noroxin (Merck)
Indications: Various urinary tract infections caused by susceptible organisms, conjunctivitis
Class: Antibiotic, Antibiotic; fluoroquinolone, Antimicrobial, CYP3A4 inhibitor
Half-life: 3–4 hours
Clinically important, potentially hazardous interactions with: aminophylline, amiodarone, antacids, arsenic, artemether/lumefantrine, bepridil, bretylium, caffeine, ciprofibrate, clozapine, cyclosporine, dairy products, didanosine, disopyramide, erythromycin, glyburide, lanthanum, mycophenolate, nitrofurantoin, NSAIDs, oral iron, oral typhoid vaccine, oxtriphylline, phenothiazines, probenecid, procainamide, quinidine, ropinirole, sotalol, strontium ranelate, sucralfate, tacrine, tamoxifen, tizanidine, tricyclic antidepressants, warfarin, zinc, zolmitriptan
Important contra-indications noted in the prescribing guidelines for: the elderly; nursing mothers; pediatric patients
Note: Fluoroquinolones are associated with an increased risk of tendinitis and tendon rupture in all ages. This risk is further increased in older patients usually over 60 years of age, in patients taking corticosteroid drugs, and in patients with kidney, heart or lung transplants.
Fluoroquinolones may exacerbate muscle weakness in persons with myasthenia gravis.

Skin
Erythema [2]
Exanthems [2]
Fixed eruption / fixed drug eruption [3]
Phototoxicity [4]
Stevens-Johnson syndrome and toxic epidermal necrolysis (SJS/TEN) [4]

Nails
Photo-onycholysis [2]

Neuromuscular/Skeletal
Rhabdomyolysis [2]
Tendinopathy/Tendon rupture [4]

Other
Adverse effects / adverse reactions [2]

NORTRIPTYLINE

Trade names: Aventyl (Ranbaxy), Pamelor (Mallinckrodt)
Indications: Depression
Class: Antidepressant; tricyclic
Half-life: 28–31 hours
Clinically important, potentially hazardous interactions with: amprenavir, arbutamine, clonidine, cobicistat/elvitegravir/emtricitabine/tenofovir alafenamide, cobicistat/elvitegravir/emtricitabine/tenofovir disoproxil, epinephrine, fluoxetine, formoterol, guanethidine, isocarboxazid, linezolid, MAO inhibitors, phenelzine, quinolones, sparfloxacin, tranylcypromine, viloxazine
Important contra-indications noted in the prescribing guidelines for: pediatric patients
Warning: SUICIDALITY AND ANTIDEPRESSANT DRUGS

Skin
Diaphoresis (<10%)
Photosensitivity [2]

Mucosal
Xerostomia (dry mouth) (>10%) [9]

Central Nervous System
Dysgeusia (taste perversion) (>10%)
Parkinsonism (<10%)
Vertigo / dizziness [2]

Other
Adverse effects / adverse reactions [2]

OBETICHOLIC ACID

Trade name: Ocaliva (Intercept)
Indications: Primary biliary cholangitis
Class: Farnesoid X receptor (FXR) agonist
Half-life: N/A
Clinically important, potentially hazardous interactions with: aminophylline, tizanidine, warfarin
Pregnancy category: Insufficient evidence to inform drug-associated risk
Important contra-indications noted in the prescribing guidelines for: nursing mothers; pediatric patients
Note: Contra-indicated in patients with complete biliary obstruction.

Skin
Eczema / eczematous reaction / eczematous eruption (3–6%)
Peripheral edema (3–7%)
Pruritus (itching) (56–70%) [9]
Rash (7–10%)
Urticaria / hives (<10%)

Mucosal
Oropharyngeal pain (7–8%)

Cardiovascular
Palpitation (3–7%)

Central Nervous System
Fever (pyrexia) (includes hyperpyrexia) (<7%)
Syncope / fainting (<7%)
Vertigo / dizziness (7%)

Endocrine/Metabolic
Thyroid dysfunction (4–6%)

Gastrointestinal/Hepatic
Abdominal pain (10–19%)
Constipation (7%)

Neuromuscular/Skeletal
Arthralgia (6–10%)
Asthenia / fatigue (19–25%)

OBINUTUZUMAB

Trade name: Gazyva (Genentech)
Indications: Chronic lymphocytic leukemia (in combination with chlorambucil), follicular lymphoma (firstly with bendamustine then as monotherapy)
Class: CD20-directed cytolytic monoclonal antibody, Monoclonal antibody
Half-life: 28 days
Clinically important, potentially hazardous interactions with: live vaccines
Pregnancy category: Insufficient evidence to inform drug-associated risk
Important contra-indications noted in the prescribing guidelines for: nursing mothers; pediatric patients
Warning: HEPATITIS B VIRUS REACTIVATION AND PROGRESSIVE MULTIFOCAL LEUKOENCEPHALOPATHY

Central Nervous System
Fever (pyrexia) (includes hyperpyrexia) (10%) [5]
Headache [2]
Leukoencephalopathy / posterior reversible encephalopathy syndrome (PRES) [2]

Endocrine/Metabolic
ALP increased (16%)
AST increased (25%)
Hyperkalemia (31%)
Hypoalbuminemia / albumin decreased (22%)
Hypocalcemia (32%)
Hypokalemia (13%)

Gastrointestinal/Hepatic
Nausea [3]

Hematologic
Anemia (12%) [6]
Leukocytopenia (leukopenia) / leukocytes (white blood cells) decreased (7%)
Neutropenia (neutrophils decreased) (40%) [18]
Thrombocytopenia / platelets decreased (15%) [16]

Local
Infusion-related reactions (69%) [16]

Renal
Tumor lysis syndrome (TLS) [5]

Respiratory
Cough (10%) [2]

Other
Death [2]
Infection (38%) [8]

OCRELIZUMAB

Trade name: Ocrevus (Genentech)
Indications: Relapsing or primary progressive forms of multiple sclerosis
Class: CD20-directed cytolytic monoclonal antibody, Monoclonal antibody
Half-life: 26 days
Clinically important, potentially hazardous interactions with: none known
Pregnancy category: May cause fetal toxicity based on findings in animal studies
Important contra-indications noted in the prescribing guidelines for: nursing mothers; pediatric patients
Note: Contra-indicated in active hepatitis B virus infection. Immune-mediated colitis, which can present as a severe and acute-onset form of colitis, has been reported in patients receiving ocrelizumab in the postmarketing setting. Some cases of colitis were serious, requiring hospitalization, with a few patients requiring surgical intervention. Systemic corticosteroids were required in many of these patients. The time from treatment initiation to onset of symptoms in these cases ranged from a few weeks to years. Monitor patients for immune-mediated colitis during ocrelizumab treatment, and evaluate promptly if signs and symptoms that may indicate immune-mediated colitis, such as new or persistent diarrhea or other gastrointestinal signs and symptoms, occur.

Central Nervous System
Depression (8%)
Headache [2]

Gastrointestinal/Hepatic
Colitis [9]

Genitourinary
Urinary tract infection [2]

Hematologic
Hypogammaglobulinemia [3]
Neutropenia (neutrophils decreased) (13%) [6]

Local
Infusion-related reactions (34–40%) [9]

Neuromuscular/Skeletal
Back pain (6%)
Pain in extremities (5%)

Respiratory
Interstitial lung disease / interstitial pneumonitis / interstitial pneumonia (cryptogenic organizing pneumonia) / drug-induced interstitial lung disease [4]
Upper respiratory tract infection (40–49%) [3]

Other
Infection (58%) [9]

OCTREOTIDE

Trade name: Sandostatin (Novartis)
Indications: Diarrhea, sulfonylurea poisoning
Class: Somatostatin analog
Half-life: 1.5 hours
Clinically important, potentially hazardous interactions with: bromocriptine, insulin aspart, insulin degludec, metformin
Important contra-indications noted in the prescribing guidelines for: the elderly; nursing mothers; pediatric patients

---

Skin
Cellulitis and pseudocellulitis (<4%)
Diaphoresis (5–15%)
Edema / fluid retention (<10%)
Flushing / rubefaction (<4%)
Petechiae (<4%)
Pruritus (itching) (18%)
Purpura (<4%)
Rash (5–15%)
Raynaud's phenomenon (<4%)
Urticaria / hives (<4%)

Hair
Alopecia / hair loss (~13%) [4]

Cardiovascular
Arrhythmias (3–9%)
Bradycardia / sinus bradycardia (19–25%) [4]
Chest pain (20%)
Hypertension (13%) [3]
QT interval prolonged / QT prolongation [2]
Thrombophlebitis (<4%)

Central Nervous System
Anorexia (4–6%)
Headache [3]
Pain (4–6%)
Rigors (5–15%)
Vertigo / dizziness [2]

Endocrine/Metabolic
Galactorrhea (<4%)
Gynecomastia (<4%)
Hyperglycemia (includes glucose increased) [8]
Hypoglycemia [2]
Hypothyroidism (12%)

Gastrointestinal/Hepatic
Abdominal pain (5–61%) [5]
Diarrhea (34–58%) [5]
Flatulence (38%) [2]
Gastrointestinal disorder / discomfort [2]
Hepatotoxicity / liver injury / acute liver injury / drug-induced liver injury (DILI) [5]
Loose stools / soft feces [2]
Nausea (5–61%) [6]
Pancreatitis / acute pancreatitis [2]
Vomiting (4–21%)

Genitourinary
- Vaginitis (includes vulvitis) (<4%)

Hematologic
- Anemia (15%)
- Neutropenia (neutrophils decreased) [2]
- Thrombocytopenia / platelets decreased [3]

Local
- Injection-site granuloma [2]
- Injection-site pain (8%) [2]

Neuromuscular/Skeletal
- Arthralgia (5–15%)
- Asthenia / fatigue [5]
- Myalgia/Myopathy (5–15%) [2]

Otic
- Ear pain (5–15%)

Respiratory
- Cough (5–15%)
- Pharyngitis (sore throat) (5–15%)
- Rhinitis / rhinosinusitis (see also sinusitis) (5–15%)
- Sinusitis (see also rhinitis / rhinosinusitis) (5–15%)

OFATUMUMAB

Trade name: Arzerra (Novartis)
Indications: Chronic lymphocytic leukemia
Class: CD20-directed cytolytic monoclonal antibody, Monoclonal antibody
Half-life: 14 days
Clinically important, potentially hazardous interactions with: live vaccines
Pregnancy category: May cause fetal B-cell depletion
Important contra-indications noted in the prescribing guidelines for: nursing mothers; pediatric patients
Warning: HEPATITIS B VIRUS REACTIVATION AND PROGRESSIVE MULTIFOCAL LEUKOENCEPHALOPATHY

Skin
- Cutaneous toxicity / skin toxicity [3]
- Herpes (6%)
- Hyperhidrosis (5%)
- Peripheral edema (9%)
- Rash (14%) [2]
- Urticaria / hives (8%)

Cardiovascular
- Angina [2]
- Hypertension (5%)
- Hypotension (5%)
- Tachycardia (5%)

Central Nervous System
- Chills (8%)
- Fever (pyrexia) (includes hyperpyrexia) (20%) [2]
- Headache (6%)
- Insomnia (7%)
- Peripheral neuropathy [2]

Gastrointestinal/Hepatic
- Diarrhea (18%) [2]
- Nausea (11%) [3]

Hematologic
- Anemia (16%) [4]
- Hemolysis [2]
- Hemolytic anemia [2]
- Leukocytopenia (leukopenia) / leukocytes (white blood cells) decreased [2]
- Lymphopenia (lymphocytopenia) / lymphocytes decreased [3]
- Neutropenia (neutrophils decreased) (>10%) [13]
- Sepsis (8%)
- Thrombocytopenia / platelets decreased [5]

Local
- Infusion-related reactions [10]
- Infusion-site reactions [3]

Neuromuscular/Skeletal
- Asthenia / fatigue (15%) [4]
- Back pain (8%)

Respiratory
- Bronchitis (11%)
- Cough (19%)
- Dyspnea / shortness of breath (14%)
- Nasopharyngitis (8%)
- Pneumonia (23%)
- Pulmonary toxicity [3]
- Upper respiratory tract infection (11%)

Other
- Adverse effects / adverse reactions [3]
- Infection (70%) [10]

OFLOXACIN

Trade names: Floxin (Ortho-McNeil), Ocuflox (Allergan), Taravid (Sanofi-Aventis)
Indications: Various infections caused by susceptible organisms
Class: Antibiotic, Antibiotic; fluoroquinolone, Antibiotic; quinolone, Antimicrobial
Half-life: 4–8 hours
Clinically important, potentially hazardous interactions with: aminophylline, amiodarone, antacids, arsenic, artemether/lumefantrine, BCG vaccine, bendamustine, bepridil, bretylium, calcium salts, clozapine, corticosteroids, cyclosporine, CYP1A2 substrates, didanosine, disopyramide, erythromycin, insulin, lanthanum, magnesiuim salts, mycophenolate, NSAIDs, oral iron, oral typhoid vaccine, oxtriphylline, phenothiazines, probenecid, procainamide, quinapril, quinidine, sevelamer, sotalol, St John's wort, strontium ranelate, sucralfate, sulfonylureas, tricyclic antidepressants, vitamin K antagonists, warfarin, zinc, zolmitriptan
Important contra-indications noted in the prescribing guidelines for: the elderly; nursing mothers; pediatric patients
Note: Fluoroquinolones are associated with an increased risk of tendinitis and tendon rupture in all ages. This risk is further increased in older patients usually over 60 years of age, in patients taking corticosteroid drugs, and in patients with kidney, heart or lung transplants.
Fluoroquinolones may exacerbate muscle weakness in persons with myasthenia gravis.
Ofloxacin is a racemate. See Levofloxacin for the adverse reactions of the (S)-isomer.
Warning: SERIOUS ADVERSE REACTIONS INCLUDING TENDINITIS, TENDON RUPTURE, PERIPHERAL NEUROPATHY, CENTRIAL NERVOUS SYSTEM EFFECTS and EXACERBATION OF MYASTHENIA GRAVIS

Skin
- Anaphylactoid reactions / anaphylaxis (includes anaphylactic shock) [4]
- Angioedema (formerly named angioneurotic edema) [3]
- Exanthems [3]
- Fixed eruption / fixed drug eruption [5]
- Hypersensitivity [2]
- Photosensitivity [8]
- Phototoxicity [3]
- Pruritus (itching) (<3%) [5]
- Pruritus ani et vulvae (<3%)
- Rash (<10%) [5]
- Stevens-Johnson syndrome and toxic epidermal necrolysis (SJS/TEN) [8]
- Urticaria / hives [3]
- Vasculitis (angiitis) / cutaneous vasculitis (angiitis) [4]

Nails
- Photo-onycholysis [3]

Mucosal
- Oral mucosal eruption [3]
- Xerostomia (dry mouth) (<3%)

Cardiovascular
- QT interval prolonged / QT prolongation [3]

Central Nervous System
- Dysgeusia (taste perversion) (<3%) [2]
- Hallucinations [3]
- Headache [3]
- Insomnia [2]
- Peripheral neuropathy [2]
- Psychosis [2]
- Seizures [2]
- Vertigo / dizziness [3]

Gastrointestinal/Hepatic
- Abdominal pain [3]
- Diarrhea [2]
- Nausea [4]
- Pancreatitis / acute pancreatitis [2]
- Vomiting [2]

Genitourinary
- Vaginitis (includes vulvitis) (<10%)

Local
- Injection-site pain (<10%)

Neuromuscular/Skeletal
- Arthralgia [2]
- Arthropathy [2]
- Asthenia / fatigue [2]
- Myalgia/Myopathy [2]
- Rhabdomyolysis [2]
- Tendinopathy/Tendon rupture [7]

Other
- Adverse effects / adverse reactions [10]
- Death [3]
- Side effects [2]

OLANZAPINE

Trade names: Symbyax (Lilly), Zyprexa (Lilly), Zyprexa Relprevv (Lilly)
Indications: Schizophrenia, bipolar I disorder
Class: Antipsychotic, Antipsychotic, atypical, Muscarinic antagonist
Half-life: 21–54 hours
Clinically important, potentially hazardous interactions with: alcohol, antihypertensive agents, carbamazepine, ciprofloxacin, CNS acting drugs, diazepam, dopamine agonists, eszopiclone, fluoxetine, fluvoxamine, insulin degludec, insulin detemir, insulin glargine, levodopa, lithium, metoclopramide, tetrabenazine, valproic acid
Important contra-indications noted in the prescribing guidelines for: the elderly; nursing mothers; pediatric patients
Note: Can cause DRESS and other serious skin reactions.
Symbyax is olanzapine and fluoxetine; Zypraxa Relprevv is olanzapine pamoate.
Warning: INCREASED MORTALITY IN ELDERLY PATIENTS WITH DEMENTIA-

RELATED PSYCHOSIS
Zyprexa Relprevv: POST-INJECTION DELIRIUM/SEDATION SYNDROME

Skin
AGEP [2]
Angioedema (formerly named angioneurotic edema) [2]
Edema / fluid retention [3]
Hypersensitivity [2]
Peripheral edema (<10%) [5]
Psoriasis [3]
Purpura (<10%)
Rash (>2%) [2]
Vesiculobullous eruption (2%)
Xanthomas [2]

Hair
Alopecia / hair loss [3]

Mucosal
Black tongue / black hairy tongue (lingua villosa nigra) [4]
Epistaxis (nosebleed) (<10%)
Sialorrhea (ptyalism; hypersalivation) [4]
Xerostomia (dry mouth) (13%) [13]

Cardiovascular
Bradycardia / sinus bradycardia [2]
Cardiomyopathy [2]
Hypertension (<10%)
Hypotension (<10%) [5]
Myocarditis [2]
Orthostatic hypotension [3]
QT interval prolonged / QT prolongation [6]
Tachycardia (<10%)
Torsades de pointes [3]
Venous thromboembolism [4]

Central Nervous System
Akathisia (<10%) [9]
Amnesia [2]
Anxiety [3]
Compulsions / obsessive-compulsive symptoms / obsessive-compulsive disorder [2]
Confusion [2]
Delirium [6]
Extrapyramidal symptoms [5]
Fever (pyrexia) (includes hyperpyrexia) [2]
Hallucinations [2]
Headache (17%) [7]
Insomnia (12%) [3]
Myokymia / twitching / fasciculation (2%)
Neuroleptic malignant syndrome [36]
Parkinsonism (<10%) [8]
Psychosis [2]
Restless legs syndrome / Willis-Ekbom disease (includes restless arms syndrome variant) [10]
Restlessness [2]
Sedation [20]
Seizures [8]
Serotonin syndrome [2]
Somnambulism (sleepwalking; noctambulism) [2]
Somnolence (drowsiness) (20–39%) [21]
Stroke / cerebrovascular accident [2]
Stuttering (dysphemia) / stammering [4]
Suicidal ideation [2]
Tardive syndrome / tardive dyskinesia [6]
Tremor (<10%) [5]
Vertigo / dizziness [8]

Endocrine/Metabolic
ALT increased [2]
Appetite increased [2]
AST increased [2]
Diabetes mellitus [7]
Diabetic ketoacidosis [2]
Dyslipidemia [5]
Galactorrhea [2]
Glucose dysregulation [3]
Gynecomastia [2]
Hypercholesterolemia [3]
Hyperglycemia (includes glucose increased) [7]
Hyperprolactinemia [3]
Hyponatremia [2]
Metabolic syndrome (includes metabolic disorder) [13]
Weight gain (5–40%) [65]

Gastrointestinal/Hepatic
Abdominal pain (<10%)
Constipation (9–11%) [8]
Diarrhea (<10%) [2]
Dyspepsia / functional dyspepsia (indigestion) (see also gastroparesis) (7–11%)
Flatulence (<10%)
Hepatotoxicity / liver injury / acute liver injury / drug-induced liver injury (DILI) [7]
Nausea (<10%) [2]
Pancreatitis / acute pancreatitis [8]
Vomiting (<10%)

Genitourinary
Enuresis (urinary incontinence) (<10%)
Priapism [19]
Sexual dysfunction [2]
Urinary tract infection (<10%)

Hematologic
Agranulocytosis / severe selective neutropenia [2]
Eosinophilia / eosinophils increased [2]
Leukocytopenia (leukopenia) / leukocytes (white blood cells) decreased [3]
Neutropenia (neutrophils decreased) [4]
Pancytopenia (includes bicytopenia) [2]
Thrombocytopenia / platelets decreased [2]

Neuromuscular/Skeletal
Asthenia / fatigue (8–20%) [5]
Back pain (<10%)
Dystonia [7]
Myalgia/Myopathy [2]
Pisa syndrome (pleurothotonus) [3]
Rhabdomyolysis [16]

Ocular
Amblyopia (<10%)
Oculogyric crisis / oculogyric dystonic reaction [8]
Vision blurred [2]

Respiratory
Cough (<10%)
Nasopharyngitis [3]
Pharyngitis (sore throat) (<10%)
Pneumonia [2]
Pulmonary embolism [3]
Rhinitis / rhinosinusitis (see also sinusitis) (<10%)
Sinusitis (see also rhinitis / rhinosinusitis) (<10%)

Other
Adverse effects / adverse reactions [10]
Death [8]

OLAPARIB

Trade name: Lynparza (AstraZeneca)
Indications: BRCA-mutated ovarian cancer
Class: Poly (ADP-ribose) polymerase (PARP) inhibitor
Half-life: 7–17 hours
Clinically important, potentially hazardous interactions with: amprenavir, aprepitant, atazanavir, boceprevir, bosentan, carbamazepine, ciprofloxacin, clarithromycin, crizotinib, darunavir, diltiazem, efavirenz, erythromycin, etravirine, fluconazole, fosamprenavir, grapefruit juice, imatinib, indinavir, itraconazole, ketoconazole, lopinavir, modafinil, nafcillin, nefazodone, nelfinavir, phenytoin, posaconazole, rifampin, ritonavir, saquinavir, St John's wort, strong and moderate CYP3A inhibitors, telaprevir, telithromycin, verapamil, voriconazole
Important contra-indications noted in the prescribing guidelines for: nursing mothers; pediatric patients

---

Skin
Cutaneous toxicity / skin toxicity [2]
Eczema / eczematous reaction / eczematous eruption (<10%)
Hot flashes / hot flushes (<10%)
Peripheral edema (10–20%)
Pruritus (itching) (<10%)
Rash (25%) [2]
Vasculitis (angiitis) / cutaneous vasculitis (angiitis) [2]
Xerosis / xeroderma (<10%)

Hair
Alopecia / hair loss [2]

Mucosal
Stomatitis (oral mucositis) (<10%)

Cardiovascular
Hypertension (<10%) [2]
Venous thromboembolism (<10%)

Central Nervous System
Anxiety (<10%)
Depression (<10%)
Dysgeusia (taste perversion) (21%) [3]
Fever (pyrexia) (includes hyperpyrexia) (<10%)
Headache (25%) [4]
Insomnia (<10%)
Peripheral neuropathy (<10%) [2]

Endocrine/Metabolic
ALT increased [3]
Appetite decreased (22–25%) [4]
Creatine phosphokinase (CPK) / creatine kinase increased (hyperCKemia) (26–30%)
Folic acid (folate) deficiency / vitamin B9 deficiency / hypofolatemia [2]
Hyperglycemia (includes glucose increased) (<10%) [2]
Hypomagnesemia (<10%)

Gastrointestinal/Hepatic
Abdominal pain (43–47%) [3]
Constipation (10–20%) [2]
Diarrhea (28–31%) [10]
Dyspepsia / functional dyspepsia (indigestion) (see also gastroparesis) (25%) [3]
Gastrointestinal obstruction / gastrointestinal stricture [2]
Hepatotoxicity / liver injury / acute liver injury / drug-induced liver injury (DILI) [2]
Nausea (64–75%) [18]
Vomiting (32–43%) [12]

Genitourinary
Dysuria (<10%)
Enuresis (urinary incontinence) (<10%)
Urinary tract infection (10–20%)

Hematologic
Anemia (25–34%) [24]
Febrile neutropenia [2]
Leukocytopenia (leukopenia) / leukocytes (white blood cells) decreased (<10%) [3]
Lymphopenia (lymphocytopenia) / lymphocytes decreased (56%)
Myelodysplastic syndrome [2]
Myeloid leukemia [2]
Neutropenia (neutrophils decreased) (25–32%) [13]
Thrombocytopenia / platelets decreased (26–30%) [9]

Neuromuscular/Skeletal
Arthralgia (21–32%)
Asthenia / fatigue (66–68%) [21]
Back pain (25%)
Myalgia/Myopathy (22–25%)

Respiratory
Cough (21%) [2]
Dyspnea / shortness of breath (10–20%)
Interstitial lung disease / interstitial pneumonitis / interstitial pneumonia (cryptogenic organizing pneumonia) / drug-induced interstitial lung disease [5]
Nasopharyngitis (26–43%)
Pharyngitis (sore throat) (43%)
Pulmonary embolism (<10%)
Upper respiratory tract infection (26–43%)

Other
Adverse effects / adverse reactions [9]
Death [3]

OLICERIDINE

Trade name: Olinvyk (Trevena)
Indications: Analgesic for management of acute pain
Class: Opioid agonist
Half-life: 1.3–3 hours (unmetabolized); ~44 hours (metabolites)
Clinically important, potentially hazardous interactions with: buprenorphine, bupropion, butorphanol, carbamazepine, central nervous system depressants, CYP2D6 inhibitors, CYP3A4 inducers, CYP3A4 inhibitors, erythromycin, fluoxetine, ketoconazole, nalbuphine, paroxetine hydrochloride, pentazocine, phenytoin, quinidine, rifampin, ritonavir, serotonergic agents
Pregnancy category: May cause fetal harm.
Note: It is not known whether oliceridine is present in human milk. The effects of oliceridine on a breastfeeding infant and on milk production have not been evaluated.
Warning: OLICERIDINE EXPOSES PATIENTS AND OTHER USERS TO THE RISKS OF OPIOID ADDICTION, ABUSE, AND MISUSE, WHICH CAN LEAD TO OVERDOSE AND DEATH. ASSESS EACH PATIENT'S RISK BEFORE PRESCRIBING, AND MONITOR REGULARLY FOR THE DEVELOPMENT OF BEHAVIORS OR CONDITIONS.
SERIOUS, LIFE-THREATENING, OR FATAL RESPIRATORY DEPRESSION MAY OCCUR. MONITOR FOR RESPIRATORY DEPRESSION, ESPECIALLY DURING INITIATION OR FOLLOWING A DOSE INCREASE.
PROLONGED USE OF OLICERIDINE DURING PREGNANCY CAN RESULT IN NEONATAL OPIOID WITHDRAWAL SYNDROME, WHICH MAY BE LIFE-THREATENING IF NOT RECOGNIZED AND TREATED. IF PROLONGED OPIOID USE IS REQUIRED IN A PREGNANT WOMAN, ADVISE THE PATIENT OF THE RISK OF NEONATAL OPIOID WITHDRAWAL SYNDROME AND ENSURE THAT APPROPRIATE TREATMENT WILL BE AVAILABLE.
CONCOMITANT USE OF OLICERIDINE WITH BENZODIAZEPINES OR OTHER CNS DEPRESSANTS, INCLUDING ALCOHOL, MAY RESULT IN PROFOUND SEDATION, RESPIRATORY DEPRESSION, COMA, AND DEATH. RESERVE CONCOMITANT PRESCRIBING FOR USE IN PATIENTS FOR WHOM ALTERNATIVE TREATMENT OPTIONS ARE INADEQUATE; LIMIT DOSAGES AND DURATIONS TO THE MINIMUM REQUIRED; AND FOLLOW PATIENTS FOR SIGNS AND SYMPTOMS OF RESPIRATORY DEPRESSION AND SEDATION.

Skin
Flushing / rubefaction (4–7%)
Pruritus (itching) (9–14%)

Central Nervous System
Headache (26%)
Sedation (7%)
Somnolence (drowsiness) (6–10%)
Vertigo / dizziness (18–27%)

Gastrointestinal/Hepatic
Constipation (12–14%)
Nausea (52–66%)
Vomiting (26–42%)

Neuromuscular/Skeletal
Back pain (4–6%)

Respiratory
Hypoxia (6–12%)

OLMESARTAN

Trade names: Benicar (Sankyo), Olmetec (Daiichi Sankyo)
Indications: Hypertension
Class: Angiotensin receptor antagonist (blocker), Antihypertensive
Half-life: ~13 hours
Clinically important, potentially hazardous interactions with: ACE inhibitors, adrenergic neurone blockers, aldesleukin, aliskiren, alprostadil, amifostine, antihypertensives, antipsychotics, anxiolytics and hypnotics, baclofen, beta blockers, calcium channel blockers, clonidine, colesevelam, corticosteroids, cyclosporine, diazoxide, diuretics, eltrombopag, eplerenone, estrogens, general anesthetics, heparins, hydralazine, levodopa, lithium, MAO inhibitors, methyldopa, methylphenidate, minoxidil, moxisylyte, moxonidine, nitrates, nitroprusside, NSAIDs, pentoxifylline, phosphodiesterase 5 inhibitors, potassium salts, quinine, rituximab, tacrolimus, tizanidine, tolvaptan, trimethoprim
Pregnancy category: category C in first trimester; category D in second and third trimesters
Important contra-indications noted in the prescribing guidelines for: nursing mothers; pediatric patients
Note: Contra-indicated in patients with diabetes.
Warning: FETAL TOXICITY

Skin
Angioedema (formerly named angioneurotic edema) [3]
Edema / fluid retention [2]
Peripheral edema [2]

Cardiovascular
Hypotension [2]

Central Nervous System
Vertigo / dizziness (3%) [9]

Endocrine/Metabolic
Hyperkalemia [3]

Gastrointestinal/Hepatic
Colitis [2]
Diarrhea [4]
Enteropathy [33]
Gastritis / pangastritis / gastric irritation [6]
Gastrointestinal disorder / discomfort [6]

Neuromuscular/Skeletal
Asthenia / fatigue [2]

Respiratory
Upper respiratory tract infection [2]

Other
Adverse effects / adverse reactions [6]

OLODATEROL

Trade names: Stiolto Respimat (Boehringer Ingelheim), Striverdi Respimat (Boehringer Ingelheim)
Indications: Chronic obstructive pulmonary disease including chronic bronchitis and emphysema
Class: Beta-2 adrenergic agonist
Half-life: 8 hours
Clinically important, potentially hazardous interactions with: adrenergics, beta blockers, diuretics, MAO inhibitors, QT interval prolonging agents, steroids, tricyclic antidepressants, xanthine derivatives
Important contra-indications noted in the prescribing guidelines for: nursing mothers; pediatric patients
Note: Stiolto Respimat is olodaterol and tiotropium.
Warning: ASTHMA-RELATED DEATH

Skin
Rash (2%)

Cardiovascular
Extrasystoles [2]
Hypertension [3]

Central Nervous System
Fever (pyrexia) (includes hyperpyrexia) (>2%)
Headache [4]
Vertigo / dizziness (2%) [3]

Gastrointestinal/Hepatic
Constipation (>2%)
Diarrhea (3%) [3]
Nausea [2]

Genitourinary
Urinary tract infection (3%) [3]

Neuromuscular/Skeletal
Arthralgia (2%) [3]
Back pain (4%) [4]
Myalgia/Myopathy [2]

Respiratory
Bronchitis (5%) [4]

COPD [2]
Cough (4%) [4]
Dyspnea / shortness of breath [3]
Nasopharyngitis (11%) [5]
Pneumonia (>2%) [3]
Upper respiratory tract infection (8%) [4]

Other
Adverse effects / adverse reactions [2]

OLOPATADINE

Trade names: Pataday (Alcon), Patanol (Alcon)
Indications: Pruritus due to allergic conjunctivitis, rhinitis
Class: Histamine H1 receptor antagonist
Half-life: 3 hours
Clinically important, potentially hazardous interactions with: none known
Important contra-indications noted in the prescribing guidelines for: nursing mothers; pediatric patients

---

Central Nervous System
Headache (7%) [2]

Ocular
Eyelid burning (<5%)
Eyelid edema / palpebral edema / blepharedema (<5%)
Eyelid stinging (<5%)

OLSALAZINE

Trade name: Dipentum (Celltech)
Indications: Ulcerative colitis
Class: Aminosalicylate
Half-life: 0.9 hours
Clinically important, potentially hazardous interactions with: azathioprine, mercaptopurine

---

Skin
Rash (2%) [2]
Urticaria / hives (4%)

OMALIZUMAB

Trade name: Xolair (Genentech)
Indications: Asthma
Class: IgE-targeting monoclonal antibody, Monoclonal antibody
Half-life: 26 days
Clinically important, potentially hazardous interactions with: none known
Important contra-indications noted in the prescribing guidelines for: nursing mothers
Warning: ANAPHYLAXIS

Skin
Anaphylactoid reactions / anaphylaxis (includes anaphylactic shock) [11]
Angioedema (formerly named angioneurotic edema) [3]
Churg-Strauss syndrome [14]
Dermatitis (2%)
Hypersensitivity [2]
Pityriasis rosea [2]
Pruritus (itching) (2%)
Rash [2]
Serum sickness [2]
Serum sickness-like reaction [2]
Urticaria / hives (7%) [5]

Central Nervous System
Fever (pyrexia) (includes hyperpyrexia) [2]
Headache (15%) [8]
Pain (7%)
Vertigo / dizziness (3%)

Gastrointestinal/Hepatic
Abdominal pain [3]
Diarrhea [3]
Nausea [3]

Local
Injection-site pain [2]
Injection-site reaction (45%) [8]

Neuromuscular/Skeletal
Arthralgia (8%) [3]
Asthenia / fatigue (3%) [3]
Myalgia/Myopathy [3]

Ocular
Ocular myasthenia gravis [2]

Respiratory
Cough [2]
Nasopharyngitis [4]
Sinusitis (see also rhinitis / rhinosinusitis) (16%) [4]
Upper respiratory tract infection (20%) [5]

Other
Adverse effects / adverse reactions [10]
Infection [2]

OMBITASVIR/ PARITAPREVIR/ RITONAVIR

Trade names: Technivie (AbbVie), Viekira Pak (AbbVie), Viekirax (AbbVie)
Indications: Genotype 4 chronic hepatitis C virus infection in patients without cirrhosis (in combination with ribavirin)
Class: CYP3A4 inhibitor (ritonavir), Direct-acting antiviral, Hepatitis C virus NS3/4A protease inhibitor (paritaprevir), Hepatitis C virus NS5A inhibitor (ombitasvir)
Half-life: 21–25 hours (ombitasvir); 6 hours (paritaprevir); 4 hours (ritonavir)
Clinically important, potentially hazardous interactions with: atazanavir, carbamazepine, cisapride, colchicine, dihydroergotamine, dronedarone, efavirenz, ergotamine, ethinyl estradiol-containing medications, lopinavir, lovastatin, lurasidone, methylergonovine, midazolam, midostaurin, neratinib, phenobarbital, phenytoin, pimozide, ranolazine, rifampin, rilpivirine, salmeterol, sildenafil, simvastatin, St John's wort, triazolam, voriconazole
Pregnancy category: pregnancy category will be X when administered with ribavirin
Important contra-indications noted in the prescribing guidelines for: nursing mothers; pediatric patients
Note: Contra-indicated in patients with moderate or severe hepatic impairment or with known hypersensitivity to ritonavir (see separate entry). See also separate entry for ribavirin. Viekira Pak is ombitasvir/paritaprevir/ritonavir co-packaged with dasabuvir. See also Ombitasvir/ Paritaprevir/Ritonavir and Dasabuvir (Viekira XR).

Skin
Dermatitis (<5%)
Eczema / eczematous reaction / eczematous eruption (<5%)
Erythema (<5%)
Exfoliative dermatitis (<5%)
Photosensitivity (<5%)
Pruritus (itching) (5%) [9]
Psoriasis (<5%)
Rash (<5%) [4]
Ulcerations (<5%)
Urticaria / hives (<5%)
Xerosis / xeroderma [2]

Central Nervous System
Headache [20]
Insomnia (5%) [13]
Irritability [3]
Vertigo / dizziness [2]

Endocrine/Metabolic
Acidosis (includes lactic acidosis) [2]
ALT increased [4]
AST increased [4]

Gastrointestinal/Hepatic
Diarrhea [12]
Nausea (9%) [15]
Vomiting [2]

Hematologic
Anemia [8]
Hemoglobin decreased [2]

Neuromuscular/Skeletal
Arthralgia [2]
Asthenia / fatigue (7–25%) [20]
Myalgia/Myopathy [2]

Respiratory
Cough [3]
Dyspnea / shortness of breath [3]
Nasopharyngitis [2]

Other
Adverse effects / adverse reactions [4]
Death [2]

OMBITASVIR/PARITA-PREVIR/RITONAVIR AND DASABUVIR

Trade name: Viekira XR (AbbVie)
Indications: Genotype 1a chronic hepatitis C virus with or without cirrhosis, genotype 1b chronic hepatitis C virus with or without cirrhosis in combination with ribavirin
Class: CYP3A4 inhibitor (ritonavir), Direct-acting antiviral, Hepatitis C virus non-nucleoside NS5B palm polymerase inhibitor (dasabuvir), Hepatitis C virus NS3/4A protease inhibitor (paritaprevir), Hepatitis C virus NS5A inhibitor (ombitasvir)
Half-life: 6 hours (dasabuvir); 21–25 hours (ombitasvir); 6 hours (paritaprevir); 4 hours (ritonavir)
Clinically important, potentially hazardous interactions with: alfuzosin, carbamazepine, cisapride, copanlisib, dihydroergotamine, dronedarone, efavirenz, ergotamine, ethinyl estradiol-containing medications, gemfibrozil, lovastatin, lurasidone, methylergonovine, midazolam, midostaurin, neratinib, phenobarbital, phenytoin, pimozide, ranolazine, rifampin, sildenafil, simvastatin, St John's wort, triazolam
Pregnancy category: Insufficient evidence to inform drug-associated risk; contra-indicated in pregnancy when given with ribavirin

Important contra-indications noted in the prescribing guidelines for: nursing mothers; pediatric patients
Note: Contra-indicated in patients with moderate to severe hepatic impairment. Viekira XR is a combined ombitasvir, paritaprevir, ritonavir and dasabuvir extended release tablet. In May 2018, the FDA announced the discontinuation of Viekira XR with an estimated product availability through until January 1, 2019. See also separate entries for Ombitasvir/ Paritaprevir/Ritonavir (co-packaged with Dasabuvir as Viekira Pak) and Ribavirin.

Skin
Pruritus (itching) (7%) [5]
Rash (7%)

Central Nervous System
Headache [3]
Insomnia (5%) [4]

Endocrine/Metabolic
ALT increased [3]
AST increased [2]
Hyperbilirubinemia (2%) [4]

Gastrointestinal/Hepatic
Hepatotoxicity / liver injury / acute liver injury / drug-induced liver injury (DILI) [2]
Nausea (8%) [2]

Neuromuscular/Skeletal
Asthenia / fatigue (4%) [8]

OMEGA-3 FATTY ACIDS

Family: N/A
Scientific names: *docosahexaenoic acid (DHA), eicosapentaenoic acid (EPA), Lovaza (GSK), Omega-3 fatty acids, Omtryg*
Indications: Albuminuria, anorexia nervosa, hypertension, lupus erythematosus, macular degeneration, osteoarthritis, otitis media, psoriasis
Class: Anti-inflammatory, Lipid regulator
Half-life: N/A
Clinically important, potentially hazardous interactions with: abciximab, clopidogrel
Important contra-indications noted in the prescribing guidelines for: pediatric patients
Note: More than 25 mL or 3 g per day can increase the risk of bleeding. Fish oils contain a significant amount of vitamins A and D and high doses may be toxic.

Central Nervous System
Dysgeusia (taste perversion) (4%) [4]

Gastrointestinal/Hepatic
Diarrhea [4]
Dyspepsia / functional dyspepsia (indigestion) (see also gastroparesis) (3%)
Eructation (belching) (4%)
Nausea [2]

Other
Adverse effects / adverse reactions [3]

OMEPRAZOLE

Trade names: Prilosec (AstraZeneca), Yosprala (Aralez)
Indications: Duodenal ulcer, gastric ulcer, gastroesophageal reflux disease (GERD), erosive esophagitis
Class: CYP1A2 inducer, Proton pump inhibitor (PPI)
Half-life: 0.5–1 hour
Clinically important, potentially hazardous interactions with: amoxicillin, atazanavir, bendamustine, benzodiazepines, cilostazol, clarithromycin, clobazam, clopidogrel, clozapine, coumarins, cyclosporine, dasatinib, delavirdine, diazepam, digoxin, disulfiram, emtricitabine/ rilpivirine/tenofovir alafenamide, enzalutamide, erlotinib, escitalopram, itraconazole, ketoconazole, lapatinib, letermovir, methotrexate, nelfinavir, phenytoin, posaconazole, prednisone, raltegravir, rilpivirine, saquinavir, selpercatinib, sofosbuvir & velpatasvir, sotorasib, St John's wort, tacrolimus, tipranavir, ulipristal, voriconazole, warfarin
Important contra-indications noted in the prescribing guidelines for: nursing mothers; pediatric patients
Note: Yosprala is omeprazole and aspirin.

Skin
AGEP [2]
Anaphylactoid reactions / anaphylaxis (includes anaphylactic shock) [7]
Angioedema (formerly named angioneurotic edema) [5]
Baboon syndrome / symmetrical drug-related intertriginous and flexural exanthema (SDRIFE) [3]
Bullous pemphigoid / pemphigoid [2]
Contact dermatitis [2]
Eczema / eczematous reaction / eczematous eruption [2]
Edema / fluid retention (<10%) [2]
Erythroderma [2]
Exfoliative dermatitis [3]
Hypersensitivity [2]
Lichen planus (includes hypertrophic lichen planus) [2]
Lichen spinulosus [2]
Lichenoid eruption / lichenoid reaction [2]
Lupus erythematosus (subacute cutaneous lupus erythematosus (SCLE)) [5]
Pemphigus (exacerbation) [2]
Peripheral edema [2]
Pruritus (itching) (<10%) [8]
Rash (2%) [6]
Stevens-Johnson syndrome and toxic epidermal necrolysis (SJS/TEN) [5]
Urticaria / hives (<10%) [9]
Vasculitis (angiitis) / cutaneous vasculitis (angiitis) [2]
Xerosis / xeroderma [2]

Hair
Alopecia / hair loss [2]

Mucosal
Oral candidiasis [3]
Xerostomia (dry mouth) (<10%) [2]

Central Nervous System
Anorexia [3]
Delirium [3]
Dysgeusia (taste perversion) (<10%) [4]
Headache (7%) [2]
Paresthesias [2]
Somnolence (drowsiness) [2]
Vertigo / dizziness (2%)

Endocrine/Metabolic
Electrolyte imbalance / electrolyte disorder / electrolyte abnormalities / dyselectrolytemia [3]
Galactorrhea [2]
Gynecomastia [11]
Hypocalcemia [2]
Hypomagnesemia [13]
Hyponatremia [2]

Gastrointestinal/Hepatic
Abdominal distension [2]
Abdominal pain (5%) [4]
Constipation [3]
Diarrhea (4%) [9]
Flatulence (3%)
Hepatitis [4]
Hepatotoxicity / liver injury / acute liver injury / drug-induced liver injury (DILI) [4]
Nausea (4%) [7]
Pancreatitis / acute pancreatitis [2]
Vomiting (3%) [6]

Hematologic
Agranulocytosis / severe selective neutropenia [3]
Hemolytic anemia [2]
Leukocytopenia (leukopenia) / leukocytes (white blood cells) decreased [3]
Neutropenia (neutrophils decreased) [3]

Neuromuscular/Skeletal
Asthenia / fatigue [2]
Myalgia/Myopathy (<10%)
Rhabdomyolysis [3]

Ocular
Visual disturbances [2]

Renal
Nephrotoxicity / kidney injury / acute kidney injury (AKI) / drug-induced kidney injury [9]

Respiratory
Cough [2]
Upper respiratory tract infection (2%)

Other
Adverse effects / adverse reactions [9]

ONDANSETRON

Trade names: Zofran (GSK), Zuplenz (Par)
Indications: Nausea and vomiting
Class: 5-HT3 antagonist, Antiemetic, Serotonin type 3 receptor antagonist
Half-life: 3–6 hours
Clinically important, potentially hazardous interactions with: amisulpride, apomorphine, carbamazepine, phenytoin, ribociclib, rifampin, tramadol
Important contra-indications noted in the prescribing guidelines for: nursing mothers; pediatric patients

---

Skin
Anaphylactoid reactions / anaphylaxis (includes anaphylactic shock) [11]
Fixed eruption / fixed drug eruption [2]
Flushing / rubefaction [2]
Hypersensitivity [2]
Pruritus (itching) (5%)

Mucosal
Sialopenia (<5%)
Xerostomia (dry mouth) (<10%) [3]

Cardiovascular
Bradycardia / sinus bradycardia [2]
Hypotension [3]
Kounis syndrome / allergic angina syndrome / allergic myocardial infarction [2]
Myocardial ischemia [2]
QT interval prolonged / QT prolongation [14]
Torsades de pointes [3]
Ventricular tachycardia [2]

Central Nervous System
Anxiety (6%)
Chills (5–10%)
Fever (pyrexia) (includes hyperpyrexia) (2–8%)
Headache (17–25%) [15]
Leukoencephalopathy / posterior reversible encephalopathy syndrome (PRES) [2]
Paresthesias (2%)
Seizures [3]
Somnolence (drowsiness) (8%) [5]
Vertigo / dizziness (4–7%) [9]

Endocrine/Metabolic
ALT increased [2]

Gastrointestinal/Hepatic
Abdominal pain [2]
Constipation (6–11%) [7]
Diarrhea (8–16%) [3]

Local
Injection-site reaction (4%)

Neuromuscular/Skeletal
Asthenia / fatigue (9–13%)

Ocular
Blindness [2]
Oculogyric crisis / oculogyric dystonic reaction [2]

Respiratory
Hypoxia (9%)

Other
Adverse effects / adverse reactions [3]
Death [3]
Hiccups / singultus [2]

OPICAPONE

Trade name: Ongentys (Neurocrine Biosciences)
Indications: Adjunctive treatment to levodopa/carbidopa in patients with Parkinson's disease experiencing "off" episodes. (Given concomitantly with levodopa/carbidopa)
Class: Catechol-O-methyl transferase inhibitor
Half-life: 1–2 hours
Clinically important, potentially hazardous interactions with: isocarboxazid, phenelzine, tranylcypromine
Pregnancy category: No adequate data on the developmental risk associated with use in pregnant women.

Mucosal
Xerostomia (dry mouth) (with levodopa and a DOPA decarboxylase inhibitor) (3%)

Cardiovascular
Hypertension (with levodopa and a DOPA decarboxylase inhibitor) (3%)
Hypotension (with levodopa and a DOPA decarboxylase inhibitor) (5%)

Central Nervous System
Dyskinesia (with levodopa and a DOPA decarboxylase inhibitor) (20%) [3]
Hallucinations (with levodopa and a DOPA decarboxylase inhibitor) (3%)
Insomnia (with levodopa and a DOPA decarboxylase inhibitor) (3%)
Syncope / fainting (with levodopa and a DOPA decarboxylase inhibitor) (5%)
Vertigo / dizziness (with levodopa and a DOPA decarboxylase inhibitor) (3%)

Endocrine/Metabolic
Serum creatinine increased (with levodopa and a DOPA decarboxylase inhibitor) (5%)
Weight loss (with levodopa and a DOPA decarboxylase inhibitor) (4%)

Gastrointestinal/Hepatic
Constipation (with levodopa and a DOPA decarboxylase inhibitor) (6%)

Other
Adverse effects / adverse reactions [2]

ORAL CONTRACEPTIVES

Trade names: Alesse (Wyeth), Aviane (Barr), Brevicon (Watson), Demulen (Pfizer), Desogen (Organon), Estrostep (Pfizer), Evra (Johnson & Johnson), Levlen (Bayer), Levlite (Bayer), Levora (Watson), Lo/Ovral (Wyeth), Loestrin (Barr), Lunelle (Pfizer), Mircette (Organon), Modicon (Ortho), Necon (Watson), Nordette (Monarch), Norinyl (Watson), Ortho Tri-Cyclen (Ortho-McNeil), Ortho-Cept (Ortho-McNeil), Ortho-Cyclen (Ortho-McNeil), Ortho-Novum (Ortho-McNeil), Ovcon (Warner Chilcott), Ovral (Wyeth), Tri-Levlen (Bayer), Tri-Norinyl (Watson), Triphasil (Wyeth), Trivora (Watson), Yasmin (Bayer), Yaz (Bayer), Zovia (Watson)
Indications: Prevention of pregnancy
Class: Hormone
Half-life: N/A
Clinically important, potentially hazardous interactions with: aminophylline, amprenavir, anticonvulsants, aprepitant, atazanavir, atorvastatin, beclomethasone, bexarotene, bosentan, budesonide, cenobamate, cigarette smoking, danazol, doxycycline, efavirenz, eslicarbazepine, exenatide, flucloxacillin, flunisolide, fluticasone propionate, glecaprevir & pibrentasvir, hydrocortisone, insulin aspart, insulin degludec, insulin detemir, insulin glargine, insulin glulisine, isotretinoin, lamotrigine, lomitapide, lymecycline, meropenem, metformin, methylprednisolone, mifepristone, modafinil, naratriptan, nelfinavir, oxcarbazepine, perampanel, prednisolone, prednisone, rifabutin, rifampin, ritonavir, roflumilast, selegiline, St John's wort, teriflunomide, ticarcillin, tigecycline, triamcinolone, troleandomycin, tuberculostatics, ursodiol, zolmitriptan
Warning: CIGARETTE SMOKING AND SERIOUS CARDIOVASCULAR EVENTS

Skin
Acneiform eruption / acneiform dermatitis / acneiform rash [17]
Angioedema (formerly named angioneurotic edema) [4]
Candidiasis / candidosis [9]
Chloasma [13]
Erythema multiforme [2]
Erythema nodosum [18]
Exanthems [2]
Herpes gestationis [3]
Lupus erythematosus (subacute cutaneous lupus erythematosus (SCLE)) [29]
Melanoma [5]
Melasma [8]
Perioral dermatitis [8]
Photosensitivity [12]
Pigmentation (Skin) (includes hyperpigmentation) [18]
Pruritus (itching) [5]
Purpura [3]
Seborrhea [3]
Spider angioma [2]
Sweet's syndrome [2]
Telangiectasia [6]
Urticaria / hives [2]

Hair
Alopecia / hair loss [19]
Alopecia areata [4]
Hirsutism [12]

Mucosal
Gingival hyperplasia / gingival hypertrophy / gingival enlargement / gingival overgrowth [2]

Cardiovascular
Thrombophlebitis [2]
Venous thromboembolism [6]

Central Nervous System
Chorea [2]
Depression [2]
Headache [3]

Endocrine/Metabolic
Acute intermittent porphyria [5]
Galactorrhea [2]
Mastodynia [3]
Porphyria cutanea tarda [28]
Porphyria variegata [2]

Gastrointestinal/Hepatic
Colitis [3]
Nausea [5]

Genitourinary
Vaginal bleeding [4]

Local
Application-site reactions (92%) [2]

Other
Adverse effects / adverse reactions [5]

ORITAVANCIN

Trade name: Orbactiv (Medicines Co)
Indications: Acute bacterial skin and skin structure infections caused or suspected to be caused by susceptible isolates of designated Gram-positive microorganisms
Class: Antibiotic, Antibiotic; lipoglycopeptide, Antimicrobial
Half-life: 245 hours
Clinically important, potentially hazardous interactions with: warfarin
Important contra-indications noted in the prescribing guidelines for: nursing mothers; pediatric patients

---

Skin
Abscess (4%) [3]
Angioedema (formerly named angioneurotic edema) (<2%)
Cellulitis and pseudocellulitis [4]
Erythema multiforme (<2%)
Hypersensitivity (<2%)
Leukocytoclastic vasculitis (angiitis) (<2%)
Pruritus (itching) (<2%) [3]

Rash (<2%)
Urticaria / hives (<2%)

Cardiovascular
Phlebitis [2]
Tachycardia (3%)

Central Nervous System
Fever (pyrexia) (includes hyperpyrexia) [4]
Headache (7%) [7]
Vertigo / dizziness (3%) [4]

Endocrine/Metabolic
ALT increased (3%) [4]
AST increased (2%) [2]
Hyperuricemia (<2%)
Hypoglycemia (<2%)

Gastrointestinal/Hepatic
Constipation [5]
Diarrhea (4%) [6]
Nausea (10%) [8]
Vomiting (5%) [6]

Hematologic
Anemia (<2%)
Eosinophilia / eosinophils increased (<2%)

Local
Infusion-site reactions (2%) [3]
Injection-site extravasation [3]
Injection-site phlebitis [3]
Injection-site reaction [2]

Neuromuscular/Skeletal
Myalgia/Myopathy (<2%)
Osteomyelitis (<2%)

Respiratory
Bronchospasm (<2%)
Wheezing (<2%)

ORLISTAT

Trade names: Alli (GSK), Xenical (Roche)
Indications: Obesity, weight reduction. Adjunct for the treatment of obesity and for weight loss management in defined populations and health conditions.

Class: Anti-obesity / weight loss pharmacotherapy, Lipase inhibitor
Half-life: 1–2 hours
Clinically important, potentially hazardous interactions with: acarbose, amiodarone, antiepileptics, coumarins, cyclosporine, ergocalciferol, ethosuximide, lacosamide, levothyroxine, oxcarbazepine, paricalcitol, phytonadione, tiagabine, vigabatrin, vitamin A, vitamin E, warfarin
Important contra-indications noted in the prescribing guidelines for: nursing mothers; pediatric patients
Note: Contra-indicated in organ transplant recipients. Orlistat interferes with the medicines used to prevent transplant rejection.

Skin
Lichenoid eruption / lichenoid reaction [2]
Peripheral edema (3%)
Rash (4%)
Xerosis / xeroderma (2%)

Mucosal
Gingivitis (2–4%)

Central Nervous System
Anxiety (3–5%)
Depression (3%)
Headache (31%) [2]
Sleep-related disorder (4%)
Vertigo / dizziness (5%)

Endocrine/Metabolic
Hypoglycemia (in diabetic patients) [2]
Menstrual irregularities (10%)

Gastrointestinal/Hepatic
Abdominal pain (26%) [4]
Cholelithiasis (gallstones in the gall bladder or the bile duct) (3%)
Defecation (increased) (3–11%) [3]
Fecal incontinence (2–8%) [2]
Fecal urgency (3–23%) [3]
Flatulence (with discharge) (2–24%) [4]
Hepatic failure [2]
Hepatitis [3]
Hepatotoxicity / liver injury / acute liver injury / drug-induced liver injury (DILI) [5]
Nausea (4–8%)
Pancreatitis / acute pancreatitis [5]
Vomiting (4%)

Genitourinary
Urinary tract infection (6–8%)
Vaginitis (includes vulvitis) (3–4%)

Neuromuscular/Skeletal
Arthralgia (5%)
Asthenia / fatigue (3–7%)
Back pain (14%)
Bone pain / joint pain (2%)
Myalgia/Myopathy (4%)
Tendinitis (2%)

Otic
Otitis (otitis externa, otitis media, otitis interna) (3–4%)

Renal
Nephrotoxicity / kidney injury / acute kidney injury (AKI) / drug-induced kidney injury [11]
Renal failure [2]

Respiratory
Influenza (40%)
Upper respiratory tract infection (26–38%) [2]

Other
Adverse effects / adverse reactions [7]
Tooth disorder (3–4%)

ORPHENADRINE

Trade names: Banflex (Forest), Norflex (3M)
Indications: Painful musculoskeletal conditions
Class: Central muscle relaxant, Muscarinic antagonist
Half-life: 14 hours
Clinically important, potentially hazardous interactions with: none known
Important contra-indications noted in the prescribing guidelines for: the elderly

---

Skin
Flushing / rubefaction (<10%)
Rash (<10%)

Cardiovascular
Tachycardia [2]

OSELTAMIVIR

Trade name: Tamiflu (Roche)
Indications: Influenza infection
Class: Antiviral, Covid-19 putative drug, Neuraminidase inhibitor
Half-life: 6–10 hours
Clinically important, potentially hazardous interactions with: none known

---

Skin
Rash [5]
Stevens-Johnson syndrome and toxic epidermal necrolysis (SJS/TEN) [6]

Central Nervous System
Delirium [5]
Hallucinations [3]
Headache [3]
Insomnia [2]
Mania [2]
Neuropsychiatric / neuropsychological adverse effect [4]
Neurotoxicity [5]
Seizures [2]
Suicidal ideation [2]

Gastrointestinal/Hepatic
Abdominal pain (2–5%) [2]
Diarrhea (<3%) [12]
Hemorrhagic colitis [7]
Hepatotoxicity / liver injury / acute liver injury / drug-induced liver injury (DILI) [2]
Nausea (4–10%) [17]
Vomiting (2–15%) [19]

Hematologic
Thrombocytopenia / platelets decreased [2]

Ocular
Glaucoma (includes acute angle-closure glaucoma) [2]

Respiratory
Respiratory failure [2]
Upper respiratory tract infection [2]

Other
Adverse effects / adverse reactions [8]

OSILODROSTAT

Trade name: Isturisa (Novartis)
Indications: Treatment of adult patients with Cushing's disease
Class: Cortisol synthesis inhibitor
Half-life: ~ 4 hours
Clinically important, potentially hazardous interactions with: carbamazepine, clarithromycin, CYP3A4 inhibitors, CYP3A4 inducers, CYP2B6 inducers, itraconazole, phenobarbital, phenobarbital, rifampin
Pregnancy category: No available data in pregnant women to evaluate a drug-associated risk of major birth defects, miscarriage, or adverse maternal or fetal outcomes.
Important contra-indications noted in the prescribing guidelines for: nursing mothers
Note: Osilodrostat blocks cortisol synthesis and may increase circulating levels of cortisol and aldosterone precursors (11-deoxy cortisol and 11-deoxycorticosterone) and androgens. Hypertension and hypokalemia were the most common adrenal hormone precursor-related adverse reactions observed in clinical trials.

Skin
Acne vulgaris ('acne') (9%)
Edema / fluid retention (21%)
Rash (15%)

Hair
Alopecia / hair loss (6%)
Hirsutism (10%)

Cardiovascular
Hypertension (10%)
Hypotension (12%)
QT interval prolonged / QT prolongation (4%)
Tachycardia (7%)

Central Nervous System
Anxiety (7%)
Depression (7%)
Fever (pyrexia) (includes hyperpyrexia) (11%)
Headache (31%)
Insomnia (8%)
Malaise (7%)
Syncope / fainting (2%)
Vertigo / dizziness (14%)

Endocrine/Metabolic
Adrenal insufficiency (hypoadrenalism) / Addisonian crisis (includes Addison's disease) (43%) [2]
Adrenocorticotropic hormone (corticotropin; ACTH) increased (14%)
Appetite decreased (12%)
Hypertransaminasemia (hepatic transaminitis) / elevated transaminases (4%)
Hypocortisolism (see also adrenal insufficiency) (18–31%)
Hypokalemia (12%)

Gastrointestinal/Hepatic
Abdominal pain (13%)
Diarrhea (15%)
Dyspepsia / functional dyspepsia (indigestion) (see also gastroparesis) (8%)
Gastroenteritis (7%)
Nausea (37%) [2]
Vomiting (19%)

Genitourinary
Urinary tract infection (12%)

Hematologic
Anemia (10%)

Neuromuscular/Skeletal
Arthralgia (18%)
Asthenia / fatigue (39%)
Back pain (15%)
Myalgia/Myopathy (12%)

Respiratory
Cough (10%)
Influenza (10%)
Nasopharyngitis (20%)

OSIMERTINIB

Synonyms: AZD9291; mereletinib
Trade name: Tagrisso (AstraZeneca)
Indications: Metastatic epidermal growth factor receptor T790M mutation-positive non-small cell lung cancer
Class: Epidermal growth factor receptor (EGFR) inhibitor / antagonist, Kinase inhibitor, Tyrosine kinase inhibitor
Half-life: 48 hours
Clinically important, potentially hazardous interactions with: carbamazepine, cyclosporine, ergot alkaloids, fentanyl, itraconazole, nefazodone, phenytoin, quinidine, rifampin, ritonavir, St John's wort, strong CYP3A inhibitors or inducers, telithromycin
Pregnancy category: Can cause fetal harm
Important contra-indications noted in the prescribing guidelines for: nursing mothers; pediatric patients

---

Skin
Cutaneous toxicity / skin toxicity [2]
Dry skin [4]
Rash (41%) [17]
Stevens-Johnson syndrome and toxic epidermal necrolysis (SJS/TEN) [6]
Vasculitis (angiitis) / cutaneous vasculitis (angiitis) [4]
Xerosis / xeroderma (31%) [4]

Nails
Nail toxicity (25%) [3]
Paronychia [9]

Mucosal
Stomatitis (oral mucositis) (12%) [4]

Cardiovascular
Cardiac failure [2]
Cardiomyopathy [4]
Cardiotoxicity [5]
Congestive heart failure [3]
Hypertension [2]
QT interval prolonged / QT prolongation (3%) [3]
Torsades de pointes [2]
Venous thromboembolism (7%)

Central Nervous System
Headache (10%)
Stroke / cerebrovascular accident (3%)

Endocrine/Metabolic
Appetite decreased (16%) [5]
Creatine phosphokinase (CPK) / creatine kinase increased (hyperCKemia) [2]
Hypermagnesemia (20%)
Hyponatremia (26%)

Gastrointestinal/Hepatic
Constipation (15%)
Diarrhea (42%) [18]
Hepatotoxicity / liver injury / acute liver injury / drug-induced liver injury (DILI) [2]
Nausea (17%) [3]

Hematologic
Anemia (44%) [2]
Lymphopenia (lymphocytopenia) / lymphocytes decreased (63%)
Neutropenia (neutrophils decreased) (33%)
Thrombocytopenia / platelets decreased (54%) [4]

Neuromuscular/Skeletal
Asthenia / fatigue (14%) [5]
Back pain (13%)
Myalgia/Myopathy [4]

Ocular
Ocular adverse effect (18%)

Respiratory
Alveolar hemorrhage (pulmonary) [2]
Cough (14%)
Dyspnea / shortness of breath [3]
Eosinophilic pneumonia [2]
Interstitial lung disease / interstitial pneumonitis / interstitial pneumonia (cryptogenic organizing pneumonia) / drug-induced interstitial lung disease [17]
Pneumonia (4%)
Pneumonitis (3%) [5]
Pulmonary toxicity [6]

Other
Adverse effects / adverse reactions [4]
Death [3]

OSPEMIFENE

Trade name: Osphena (Shionogi)
Indications: Dyspareunia due to menopausal vulvar and vaginal atrophy
Class: Estrogen agonist, Estrogen antagonist, Selective estrogen receptor modulator (SERM)
Half-life: 26 hours
Clinically important, potentially hazardous interactions with: fluconazole, ketoconazole, other estrogen agonists or antagonists, rifampin
Important contra-indications noted in the prescribing guidelines for: nursing mothers; pediatric patients
Note: Contra-indicated in patients with undiagnosed abnormal genital bleeding, known or suspected estrogen-dependent neoplasia, active DVT or pulmonary embolism, or active arterial thromboembolic disease.
Warning: ENDOMETRIAL CANCER AND CARDIOVASCULAR DISORDERS

Skin
Hot flashes / hot flushes (8%) [8]
Hyperhidrosis (2%)

Genitourinary
Urinary tract infection [3]
Vaginal discharge (4%)

Neuromuscular/Skeletal
Muscle spasm (3%)

OXACILLIN

Indications: Various infections caused by susceptible organisms
Class: Antibiotic, Antibiotic; beta-lactam, Antibiotic; penicillin, Antimicrobial
Half-life: 23–60 minutes
Clinically important, potentially hazardous interactions with: anticoagulants, cyclosporine, demeclocycline, doxycycline, imipenem/cilastatin, methotrexate, minocycline, oxytetracycline, tetracycline
Important contra-indications noted in the prescribing guidelines for: the elderly; nursing mothers; pediatric patients

---

Skin
Exanthems [2]
Leukocytoclastic vasculitis (angiitis) [2]
Rash (<22%)

Other
Adverse effects / adverse reactions [2]

OXALIPLATIN

Trade name: Eloxatin (Sanofi-Aventis)
Indications: Metastatic carcinoma of the colon or rectum (in combination with fluorouracil/leucovorin (FOLFOX, mFOLFOX6)). Advanced pancreatic cancer (in combination with irinotecan/fluorouracil/leucovorin (FOLFIRINOX or FOLFOXIRI))
Class: Alkylating agent, Antineoplastic / anticancer agent (see also Immune checkpoint inhibitor), Platinum-based antineoplastic
Half-life: 391 hours
Clinically important, potentially hazardous interactions with: aminoglycosides, BCG vaccine, capreomycin, cardiac glycosides, clozapine, denosumab, diuretics, leflunomide, natalizumab, pimecrolimus, polymyxins, sipuleucel-T, tacrolimus, taxanes, topotecan, trastuzumab, vaccines, vitamin K antagonists
Important contra-indications noted in the prescribing guidelines for: nursing mothers; pediatric patients
Note: CapeOX (also called XELOX) is a combination of capecitabine and oxaliplatin.
Warning: ANAPHYLACTIC REACTIONS

Skin
- Anaphylactoid reactions / anaphylaxis (includes anaphylactic shock) [11]
- Cutaneous toxicity / skin toxicity [3]
- Diaphoresis (5%) [2]
- Edema / fluid retention (13–15%) [2]
- Erythema [4]
- Exanthems (2–5%)
- Flushing / rubefaction (2–7%) [3]
- Hand–foot syndrome (palmar–plantar erythrodysesthesia) (7–13%) [14]
- Hot flashes / hot flushes (2–5%)
- Hypersensitivity (12%) [31]
- Peripheral edema (11%)
- Pruritus (itching) (6%) [6]
- Purpura (2–5%)
- Radiation recall dermatitis [3]
- Rash (5–11%) [11]
- Thrombocytopenic purpura [2]
- Urticaria / hives [3]
- Xerosis / xeroderma (6%)

Hair
- Alopecia / hair loss (3–38%) [4]

Mucosal
- Epistaxis (nosebleed) (<16%)
- Gingivitis (2–5%)
- Mucositis (10%) [6]
- Stomatitis (oral mucositis) (32–42%) [6]
- Xerostomia (dry mouth) (5%)

Cardiovascular
- Chest pain (4%) [2]
- Coronary vasospasm [2]
- Extravasation [2]
- Hypertension [6]
- Hypotension (5%) [2]
- Tachycardia [3]
- Takotsubo syndrome [3]
- Thromboembolism (4%)
- Vascular trauma [2]

Central Nervous System
- Anorexia (13–35%) [7]
- Anxiety (5%)
- Chills [3]
- Depression (9%)
- Dysesthesia (often cold-induced or cold-exacerbated) (38%) [7]
- Dysgeusia (taste perversion) (<14%)
- Dysphasia (5%)
- Fever (pyrexia) (includes hyperpyrexia) (16–27%) [9]
- Headache (7–13%)
- Hyperalgesia [2]
- Hypoesthesia / hypesthesia (numbness) [2]
- Insomnia (4–13%)
- Ischemic stroke / cerebral infarction (includes transient ischemic attack) [2]
- Leukoencephalopathy / posterior reversible encephalopathy syndrome (PRES) [4]
- Neurotoxicity (48%) [38]
- Pain (5–9%) [2]
- Paresthesias (77%) [7]
- Peripheral neuropathy (92%) [60]
- Rigors (8%)
- Sensory disturbances (8%)
- Vertigo / dizziness (7–8%)

Endocrine/Metabolic
- ALP increased (42%)
- ALT increased (57%)
- AST increased [2]
- Dehydration (9%)
- Hyperammonemia [2]
- Hyperglycemia (includes glucose increased) (14%)
- Hypoalbuminemia / albumin decreased (8%)
- Hypocalcemia (7%)
- Hypokalemia (11%)
- Hyponatremia (8%) [2]
- Serum creatinine increased (4%) [2]
- Weight gain (10%)
- Weight loss (11%)

Gastrointestinal/Hepatic
- Abdominal pain (18–31%) [4]
- Constipation (22–32%) [2]
- Diarrhea (44–56%) [47]
- Dyspepsia / functional dyspepsia (indigestion) (see also gastroparesis) (8–12%)
- Flatulence (6–9%)
- Gastroesophageal reflux (3%)
- Hepatotoxicity / liver injury / acute liver injury / drug-induced liver injury (DILI) [8]
- Nausea (59–74%) [29]
- Non-cirrhotic portal hypertension [5]
- Sinusoidal obstruction syndrome / hepatic sinusoidal obstruction syndrome [4]
- Vomiting (27–47%) [22]

Genitourinary
- Urinary frequency (5%)

Hematologic
- Anemia (27–76%) [26]
- Evans' syndrome [2]
- Febrile neutropenia (<4%) [12]
- Hemolytic anemia [4]
- Leukocytopenia (leukopenia) / leukocytes (white blood cells) decreased (34–85%) [16]
- Lymphopenia (lymphocytopenia) / lymphocytes decreased (6%)
- Myelosuppression / bone marrow suppression / myelotoxicity [4]
- Neutropenia (neutrophils decreased) (25–81%) [64]
- Thrombocytopenia / platelets decreased (20–77%) [42]
- Thrombosis (6%) [2]

Local
- Injection-site reaction (5–11%) [2]

Neuromuscular/Skeletal
- Arthralgia (5–10%)
- Asthenia / fatigue (44–70%) [24]
- Ataxia [2]
- Back pain (11–16%)
- Digital ischemia [2]
- Myalgia/Myopathy (14%)

Ocular
- Abnormal vision (5%)
- Conjunctivitis (conjunctival inflammation) (9%)
- Epiphora [3]
- Lacrimation (4–9%)
- Transient vision loss (amaurosis fugax) [3]
- Vision blurred [2]

Otic
- Hearing loss (hypoacusis) [4]

Renal
- Nephrotoxicity / kidney injury / acute kidney injury (AKI) / drug-induced kidney injury [3]
- Proteinuria [2]

Respiratory
- Cough (9–35%)
- Dyspnea / shortness of breath (5–18%) [2]
- Pharyngitis (sore throat) (10%)
- Pneumonia [2]
- Pulmonary embolism [2]
- Pulmonary fibrosis [2]
- Pulmonary toxicity [2]
- Rhinitis / rhinosinusitis (see also sinusitis) (4–10%)
- Upper respiratory tract infection (4%)

Other
- Adverse effects / adverse reactions [5]
- Allergic reactions (3%) [4]
- Death [4]
- Hiccups / singultus (5%)
- Infection (8–25%) [3]

OXAPROZIN

Trade name: Daypro (Pfizer)
Indications: Arthritis
Class: Non-steroidal anti-inflammatory (NSAID)
Half-life: 42–50 hours
Clinically important, potentially hazardous interactions with: methotrexate
Important contra-indications noted in the prescribing guidelines for: nursing mothers; pediatric patients
Note: NSAIDs may cause an increased risk of serious cardiovascular and gastrointestinal adverse events, which can be fatal. This risk may increase with duration of use.

Skin
- Pruritus (itching) (<10%)
- Pseudoporphyria [3]
- Rash (>10%) [2]
- Stevens-Johnson syndrome and toxic epidermal necrolysis (SJS/TEN) [5]

Gastrointestinal/Hepatic
- Hepatotoxicity / liver injury / acute liver injury / drug-induced liver injury (DILI) [3]

Renal
- Nephrotoxicity / kidney injury / acute kidney injury (AKI) / drug-induced kidney injury [2]

Other
- Adverse effects / adverse reactions [3]

OXAZEPAM

Trade name: Serax (Mayne Pharma)
Indications: Anxiety, depression
Class: Benzodiazepine
Half-life: 3–6 hours
Clinically important, potentially hazardous interactions with: amprenavir, chlorpheniramine, clarithromycin, efavirenz, esomeprazole, imatinib, nelfinavir
Important contra-indications noted in the prescribing guidelines for: pediatric patients

---

Skin
- Dermatitis (<10%)
- Diaphoresis (>10%)
- Rash (>10%)

Mucosal
- Sialopenia (>10%)
- Sialorrhea (ptyalism; hypersalivation) (<10%)
- Xerostomia (dry mouth) (>10%)

OXCARBAZEPINE

Trade names: Oxtellar XR (Supernus), Trileptal (Novartis)
Indications: Partial epileptic seizures
Class: Anticonvulsant (see also antiepileptic (anti-seizure)), CYP3A4 inducer, Mood stabilizer
Half-life: 1–2.5 hours
Clinically important, potentially hazardous interactions with: alcohol, antipsychotics, bictegravir/emtricitabine/tenofovir alafenamide, carbamazepine, chloroquine, clopidogrel, cobicistat/elvitegravir/emtricitabine/tenofovir alafenamide, cobicistat/elvitegravir/emtricitabine/tenofovir disoproxil, cyclosporine, CYP3A4 substrates, doravirine, doravirine/lamiduvine/tenofovir disoproxil, dronedarone, emtricitabine/rilpivirine/tenofovir alafenamide, eslicarbazepine, everolimus, exemestane, guanfacine, hydroxychloroquine, imatinib, ixabepilone, ledipasvir & sofosbuvir, levomepromazine, levonorgestrel, MAO inhibitors, maraviroc, mefloquine, nifedipine, nilotinib, nisoldipine, oral contraceptives, orlistat, pazopanib, perampanel, phenobarbital, phenytoin, praziquantel, ranolazine, rilpivirine, risperidone, romidepsin, saxagliptin, selegiline, simeprevir, sofosbuvir, sofosbuvir & velpatasvir, sofosbuvir/velpatasvir/voxilaprevir, sorafenib, SSRIs, St John's wort, tadalafil, tenofovir alafenamide, thiazide diuretics, tolvaptan, tricyclic antidepressants, ulipristal, valproic acid, zuclopenthixol
Important contra-indications noted in the prescribing guidelines for: nursing mothers; pediatric patients

---

Skin
- Acneiform eruption / acneiform dermatitis / acneiform rash (<2%)
- Angioedema (formerly named angioneurotic edema) [2]
- Bruise / bruising / contusion / ecchymosis (ecchymoses) (4%)
- Diaphoresis (3%)
- DRESS syndrome (Drug-induced hypersensitivity syndrome) [8]
- Edema / fluid retention (<2%)
- Exanthems [4]
- Hot flashes / hot flushes (<2%)
- Hyperhidrosis (3%)
- Hypersensitivity [6]
- Lupus erythematosus (subacute cutaneous lupus erythematosus (SCLE)) [2]
- Lymphadenopathy (2%)
- Purpura (2%)
- Rash (<6%) [12]
- Stevens-Johnson syndrome and toxic epidermal necrolysis (SJS/TEN) [15]

Mucosal
- Epistaxis (nosebleed) (4%)
- Rectal hemorrhage / rectal bleeding (2%)
- Xerostomia (dry mouth) (3%)

Cardiovascular
- Chest pain (2%)
- Hypotension (<3%)

Central Nervous System
- Agitation (<2%)
- Amnesia (4%)
- Anorexia (3–5%)
- Anxiety (5–7%)
- Coma [2]
- Confusion (<7%)
- Dysgeusia (taste perversion) (5%)
- Emotional lability (2–3%)
- Fever (pyrexia) (includes hyperpyrexia) (3%)
- Gait instability / postural instability (5–17%)
- Headache (13–32%) [8]
- Hyperesthesia (3%)
- Hypoesthesia / hypesthesia (numbness) (<3%)
- Incoordination (<4%)
- Insomnia (2–6%)
- Nervousness (2–4%)
- Seizures (2–5%) [5]
- Somnolence (drowsiness) (5–36%) [5]
- Speech disorder (<3%)
- Tremor (3–16%) [2]
- Vertigo / dizziness (3–49%) [12]

Endocrine/Metabolic
- Hyponatremia (<5%) [19]
- SIADH [3]
- Weight gain (<2%)

Gastrointestinal/Hepatic
- Abdominal pain (3–13%)
- Constipation (2–6%)
- Diarrhea (5–7%)
- Dyspepsia / functional dyspepsia (indigestion) (see also gastroparesis) (5–6%)
- Gastritis / pangastritis / gastric irritation (<2%)
- Nausea (15–29%) [8]
- Vomiting (13–36%) [4]

Genitourinary
- Ejaculatory dysfunction [3]
- Urinary frequency (<2%)
- Urinary tract infection (<5%)
- Vaginitis (includes vulvitis) (2%)

Hematologic
- Leukocytopenia (leukopenia) / leukocytes (white blood cells) decreased [3]
- Thrombocytopenia / platelets decreased [2]

Neuromuscular/Skeletal
- Asthenia / fatigue (3–15%) [5]
- Ataxia (<31%) [2]
- Back pain (4%)
- Myoclonus (see also hypnic jerk) [3]
- Osteoporosis [2]

Ocular
- Abnormal vision (2–14%)
- Accommodation disorder (<3%)
- Diplopia (double vision) (<40%) [10]
- Nystagmus (2–26%)

Otic
- Ear pain (<2%)

Respiratory
- Cough (5%)
- Pharyngitis (sore throat) (3%)
- Pneumonia (2%)
- Rhinitis / rhinosinusitis (see also sinusitis) (2–5%)
- Sinusitis (see also rhinitis / rhinosinusitis) (4%)
- Upper respiratory tract infection (5–10%)

Other
- Adverse effects / adverse reactions [8]
- Allergic reactions (2%) [3]
- Dipsia (thirst) / polydipsia (2%)
- Infection (2–7%)
- Teratogenicity [3]
- Toothache (odontalgia) (2%)

OXERUTINS

Trade name: Paroven (Novartis)
Indications: Edema associated with chronic venous insufficiency
Class: Benzypyrone
Half-life: 10–25 hours
Clinically important, potentially hazardous interactions with: none known

OXPRENOLOL

Trade name: Trasicor (Amdipharm)
Indications: Angina pectoris, hypertension, disturbances of cardiac rhythm
Class: Antihypertensive
Half-life: 1–2 hours
Clinically important, potentially hazardous interactions with: alcohol, amiodarone, beta blockers, cimetidine, clonidine, digoxin, diltiazem, disopyramide, ephedrine, epinephrine, ergot alkaloids, guanethidine, halothane, isoprenaline, lidocaine, noradrenaline, NSAIDs, phenylephrine, quinidine, reserpine, verapamil
Important contra-indications noted in the prescribing guidelines for: nursing mothers

---

Skin
- Dermatitis [3]
- Psoriasis [3]
- Rash [3]

Mucosal
- Xerostomia (dry mouth) (10%)

Cardiovascular
- Bradycardia / sinus bradycardia (<10%)
- Cardiac failure (<10%)
- Hypotension (<10%)

Central Nervous System
- Depression (<10%)
- Headache (<10%)
- Paresthesias (<10%)
- Vertigo / dizziness (<10%)

Gastrointestinal/Hepatic
- Constipation (<10%)
- Nausea (<10%)

Neuromuscular/Skeletal
- Asthenia / fatigue (<10%)

Respiratory
- Dyspnea / shortness of breath (<10%)

Other
- Death [4]

OXTRIPHYLLINE

Trade names: Choledyl (Pfizer), Choledyl SA (Warner Chilcott)
Indications: Asthma, chronic bronchitis, emphysema, bronchospastic disorders
Class: Bronchodilator
Half-life: 1–9 hours in pediatric patients; 3–15 hours in non-smoking adults; 4–5 hours in cigarette smokers
Clinically important, potentially hazardous interactions with: aminoglutethimide, carbamazepine, cimetidine, ciprofloxacin, clarithromycin, disulfiram, enoxacin, erythromycin, estradiol, estrogens, febuxostat, fluvoxamine, isoproterenol, methotrexate, mexiletine, moricizine, norfloxacin, ofloxacin, phenobarbital, phenytoin, propranolol, rifampin, sucralfate, tacrine, ticlopidine, verapamil

---

Other
Adverse effects / adverse reactions [2]

OXYBUTYNIN

Trade names: Cystrin (Sanofi-Aventis), Ditropan (Ortho-McNeil), Lyrinel (Janssen-Cilag)
Indications: Neurogenic bladder, urinary incontinence, palmar and axillary hyperhidrosis
Class: Anticholinergic, Muscarinic antagonist
Half-life: 2–3 hours
Clinically important, potentially hazardous interactions with: alcohol, anticholinergics, antihistamines, arbutamine, cannabinoids, clozapine, conivaptan, diphenoxylate, disopyramide, domperidone, haloperidol, ketoconazole, levodopa, MAO inhibitors, memantine, metoclopramide, nefopam, nitrates, parasympathomimetics, pramlintide, secretin, tricyclic antidepressants
Important contra-indications noted in the prescribing guidelines for: nursing mothers
Note: Contra-indicated in patients with urinary retention, gastric retention and other severe decreased gastrointestinal motility conditions, uncontrolled narrow-angle glaucoma and in patients who are at risk for these conditions.

Skin
Hot flashes / hot flushes (<10%)
Pruritus (itching) [2]
Rash (<10%)

Mucosal
Sialopenia [2]
Xerostomia (dry mouth) (71%) [31]

Central Nervous System
Cognitive impairment [4]
Headache (8%) [2]
Insomnia (6%)
Nervousness (7%)
Somnolence (drowsiness) (14%)
Vertigo / dizziness (17%) [2]

Gastrointestinal/Hepatic
Constipation (15%) [4]
Dyspepsia / functional dyspepsia (indigestion) (see also gastroparesis) (6%)
Nausea [3]

Genitourinary
Urinary retention (6%)
Urinary tract infection (7%)

Ocular
Blindness [2]
Vision blurred (10%)

Other
Adverse effects / adverse reactions [4]
Allergic reactions [2]

OXYCODONE

Trade names: OxyContin (Purdue), OxyIR (Purdue), Percocet (Endo), Roxicodone (aaiPharma), Targiniq (Purdue), Troxyca (Pfizer), Tylox (Ortho-McNeil), Xtampza ER (Collegium)
Indications: Pain
Class: Opiate agonist
Half-life: 4.6 hours
Clinically important, potentially hazardous interactions with: cimetidine, clonazepam, telithromycin, voriconazole
Important contra-indications noted in the prescribing guidelines for: the elderly; nursing mothers; pediatric patients
Note: Oxycodone is often combined with acetaminophen (Percocet, Roxicet, Tylox) or aspirin (Percodan, Roxiprin); Targiniq is oxycodone and naloxone; Troxyca is oxycodone and naltrexone. Contra-indicated in patients with significant respiratory depression, acute or severe bronchial asthma, or with known or suspected gastrointestinal obstruction, including paralytic ileus.
Warning: ADDICTION, ABUSE and MISUSE; LIFE-THREATENING RESPIRATORY DEPRESSION; ACCIDENTAL INGESTION; NEONATAL OPIOID WITHDRAWAL SYNDROME; and CYTOCHROME P450 3A4 INTERACTION

Skin
Pruritus (itching) [8]

Mucosal
Xerostomia (dry mouth) [2]

Cardiovascular
Bradycardia / sinus bradycardia [2]

Central Nervous System
Fever (pyrexia) (includes hyperpyrexia) [2]
Hallucinations, visual [2]
Headache [6]
Insomnia [3]
Neurotoxicity [2]
Sedation [2]
Serotonin syndrome [2]
Somnolence (drowsiness) [15]
Vertigo / dizziness [9]

Gastrointestinal/Hepatic
Abdominal pain [3]
Constipation [16]
Diarrhea [2]
Ileus / adynamic ileus / paralytic ileus [2]
Nausea [26]
Vomiting [20]

Genitourinary
Urinary retention [2]

Local
Injection-site pain (<10%)

Neuromuscular/Skeletal
Asthenia / fatigue [9]

Other
Adverse effects / adverse reactions [11]
Death [3]
Tooth disorder [2]

OXYMORPHONE

Trade name: Opana (Endo)
Indications: Pain (moderate to severe)
Class: Analgesic, Opiate agonist
Half-life: 7–9 hours
Clinically important, potentially hazardous interactions with: anticholinergics, buprenorphine, butorphanol, cimetidine, CNS depressants, MAO inhibitors, nalbuphine, pentazocine
Important contra-indications noted in the prescribing guidelines for: the elderly; nursing mothers; pediatric patients
Note: Contra-indicated in patients with a known hypersensitivity to morphine analogs such as codeine; in patients with respiratory depression, except in monitored settings and in the presence of resuscitative equipment; in patients with acute or severe bronchial asthma or hypercarbia; in any patient who has or is suspected of having paralytic ileus; and in patients with moderate or severe hepatic impairment.

Skin
Hyperhidrosis (<10%)
Pruritus (itching) (8%) [2]

Mucosal
Xerostomia (dry mouth) (<10%)

Cardiovascular
Hypotension (<10%)
Tachycardia (<10%)

Central Nervous System
Anxiety (<10%)
Confusion (3%)
Fever (pyrexia) (includes hyperpyrexia) (14%)
Headache (7%)
Sedation (<10%)
Somnolence (drowsiness) (9%) [2]
Vertigo / dizziness (7%)

Gastrointestinal/Hepatic
Abdominal distension (<10%)
Constipation (4%) [3]
Flatulence (<10%)
Nausea (19%) [4]
Vomiting (9%) [2]

Local
Injection-site reaction (<10%)

Respiratory
Hypoxia (<10%)

OXYTETRACYCLINE

Trade name: Terramycin (Pfizer)
Indications: Various infections caused by susceptible organisms
Class: Antibiotic, Antibiotic; tetracycline, Antimicrobial
Half-life: 6–10 hours
Clinically important, potentially hazardous interactions with: acitretin, amoxicillin, ampicillin, antacids, bacampicillin, calcium salts, carbenicillin, cloxacillin, coumarins, dairy products, digoxin, ergotamine, kaolin, methotrexate, methoxyflurane, methysergide, mezlocillin, nafcillin, oral iron, oral typhoid vaccine, oxacillin, penicillins, phenindione, piperacillin, quinapril, retinoids, strontium ranelate, sucralfate, sulfonylureas, ticarcillin, tripotassium dicitratobismuthate, zinc

Skin
- Dermatitis [3]
- Fixed eruption / fixed drug eruption [5]
- Photosensitivity (<10%) [4]

Other
- Tooth pigmentation / discoloration (in children) (>10%)

OXYTOCIN

Trade name: Pitocin (Par)
Indications: Induction of labor
Class: Oxytocic
Half-life: N/A
Clinically important, potentially hazardous interactions with: cyclopropane, gemeprost, halothane, prostaglandins

Skin
- Anaphylactoid reactions / anaphylaxis (includes anaphylactic shock) [7]

Mucosal
- Xerostomia (dry mouth) [3]

Cardiovascular
- Bradycardia / sinus bradycardia [2]

Central Nervous System
- Fever (pyrexia) (includes hyperpyrexia) [2]
- Shivering [2]

Genitourinary
- Urinary frequency [3]
- Uterine hyperstimulation [3]

Respiratory
- Hypoxia [2]
- Pulmonary edema (cardiogenic / non-cardiogenic) [5]

OZANIMOD

Trade name: Zeposia (Celgene)
Indications: Treatment of relapsing forms of multiple sclerosis
Class: Sphingosine1-phosphate receptor modulator
Half-life: ~21 hours
Clinically important, potentially hazardous interactions with: cyclosporine, CYP2C8 inhibitors, breast cancer resistance protein (bcrp) inhibitors, CYP2C8 inducers, MAO inhibitors, adrenergic and serotonergic drugs, opioid drugs, gemfibrozil, linezolid, phenelzine, rifampin, selegiline
Pregnancy category: No adequate data on the developmental risk associated with the use of ozanimod in pregnant women.

Cardiovascular
- Hypertension (4%)
- Orthostatic hypotension (4%)

Central Nervous System
- Headache [2]

Endocrine/Metabolic
- Hypertransaminasemia (hepatic transaminitis) / elevated transaminases (10%)

Gastrointestinal/Hepatic
- Abdominal pain (2%)

Genitourinary
- Urinary tract infection (4%)

Neuromuscular/Skeletal
- Back pain (4%)

Respiratory
- Nasopharyngitis [2]
- Upper respiratory tract infection (26%)

PACLITAXEL

Trade name: Taxol (Bristol-Myers Squibb)
Indications: Breast cancer and metastatic carcinoma of the ovary
Class: Antineoplastic / anticancer agent (see also Immune checkpoint inhibitor), Taxane
Half-life: 5–17 hours
Clinically important, potentially hazardous interactions with: atazanavir, bexarotene, buspirone, carbamazepine, cisplatin, clarithromycin, delavirdine, doxorubicin, efavirenz, eletriptan, felodipine, gadobenate, gemfibrozil, indinavir, itraconazole, ketoconazole, lapatinib, lovastatin, nefazodone, nelfinavir, repaglinide, rifampin, ritonavir, rosiglitazone, saquinavir, sildenafil, simvastatin, telithromycin, teriflunomide, thalidomide, trastuzumab, triazolam
Important contra-indications noted in the prescribing guidelines for: the elderly; nursing mothers; pediatric patients
Note: Nab-paclitaxel (Abraxane) is nanoparticle albumin–bound paclitaxel. Studies have shown that elderly patients have an increased risk of severe myelosuppression, severe neuropathy and a higher incidence of cardiovascular events.

Skin
- Acneiform eruption / acneiform dermatitis / acneiform rash [6]
- Acral erythema [4]
- Anaphylactoid reactions / anaphylaxis (includes anaphylactic shock) [3]
- Cutaneous toxicity / skin toxicity [10]
- Dermatitis [2]
- Desquamation (7%)
- Edema / fluid retention (21%) [2]
- Erythema [6]
- Exanthems [2]
- Fixed eruption / fixed drug eruption [2]
- Flushing / rubefaction (28%) [3]
- Folliculitis [2]
- Hand–foot syndrome (palmar–plantar erythrodysesthesia) [21]
- Hypersensitivity (31–45%) [26]
- Lupus erythematosus (subacute cutaneous lupus erythematosus (SCLE)) [5]
- Photosensitivity [4]
- Pigmentation (Skin) (includes hyperpigmentation) [3]
- Pruritus (itching) [6]
- Pustules / pustular eruption [2]
- Radiation recall dermatitis [11]
- Rash (12%) [19]
- Recall reaction [2]
- Scleroderma [9]
- Stevens-Johnson syndrome and toxic epidermal necrolysis (SJS/TEN) [3]
- Urticaria / hives (2–4%) [4]

Hair
- Alopecia / hair loss (87–100%) [52]

Nails
- Leukonychia striata (Mees' lines) [2]
- Nail changes (2%) [6]
- Nail pigmentation (2%) [4]
- Onycholysis [11]
- Onychomadesis [2]
- Pyogenic granuloma [2]

Mucosal
- Epistaxis (nosebleed) [2]
- Mucosal inflammation [3]
- Mucositis (17–35%) [16]
- Oral lesions (3–8%)
- Stomatitis (oral mucositis) (2–39%) [11]

Cardiovascular
- Atrial fibrillation [2]
- Bradycardia / sinus bradycardia (3%)
- Capillary leak syndrome [2]
- Cardiotoxicity [3]
- Congestive heart failure [3]
- Hypertension [17]
- Hypotension (4–12%)
- Kounis syndrome / allergic angina syndrome / allergic myocardial infarction [2]
- Myocardial infarction [6]
- Tachycardia (2%)

Central Nervous System
- Anorexia [8]
- Dysgeusia (taste perversion) [3]
- Fever (pyrexia) (includes hyperpyrexia) [4]
- Headache [2]
- Insomnia [2]
- Neurotoxicity [42]
- Pain [9]
- Paresthesias (>10%) [5]
- Peripheral neuropathy (42–70%) [59]
- Seizures [2]
- Vertigo / dizziness [7]

Endocrine/Metabolic
- ALP increased [2]
- ALT increased [11]
- Appetite decreased [5]
- AST increased [8]
- Hyperbilirubinemia [2]
- Hyperglycemia (includes glucose increased) [4]
- SIADH [3]

Gastrointestinal/Hepatic
- Abdominal pain (>10%) [2]
- Constipation [8]
- Diarrhea (38%) [42]
- Dyspepsia / functional dyspepsia (indigestion) (see also gastroparesis) [2]
- Gastrointestinal bleeding [2]
- Gastrointestinal disorder / discomfort [2]
- Gastrointestinal fistula [2]
- Gastrointestinal perforation / perforated colon / gastric perforation [5]
- Hepatotoxicity / liver injury / acute liver injury / drug-induced liver injury (DILI) [7]
- Nausea (52%) [36]
- Pancreatitis / acute pancreatitis [4]
- Vomiting [28]

Hematologic
- Anemia (47%) [44]
- Bleeding [3]
- Febrile neutropenia [29]
- Hematological adverse effect [2]
- Hemotoxicity [11]
- Leukocytopenia (leukopenia) / leukocytes (white blood cells) decreased (90%) [39]
- Lymphopenia (lymphocytopenia) / lymphocytes decreased [2]
- Myelosuppression / bone marrow suppression / myelotoxicity [8]
- Neutropenia (neutrophils decreased) (78–98%) [113]
- Thrombocytopenia / platelets decreased (4–20%) [32]

Local
- Injection-site cellulitis (>10%)

Injection-site extravasation (>10%) [4]
Injection-site pain (>10%)
Injection-site reaction (13%) [2]

Neuromuscular/Skeletal
Arthralgia (60%) [16]
Asthenia / fatigue (17%) [61]
Bone pain / joint pain [3]
Myalgia/Myopathy (19–60%) [24]

Ocular
Macular edema [14]
Maculopathy [2]

Renal
Proteinuria [6]
Tumor lysis syndrome (TLS) [2]

Respiratory
Cough [3]
Dyspnea / shortness of breath (2%) [4]
Interstitial lung disease / interstitial pneumonitis / interstitial pneumonia (cryptogenic organizing pneumonia) / drug-induced interstitial lung disease [6]
Pneumonia [5]
Pneumonitis [5]
Pulmonary toxicity [6]

Other
Adverse effects / adverse reactions [10]
Allergic reactions (15%) [8]
Death [16]
Infection (3–22%) [16]

PACRITINIB

Trade name: Vonjo (CTI Biopharma)
Indications: Primary or secondary (post-polycythemia vera or post-essential thrombocythemia) myelofibrosis with a platelet count below 50 10^9/L

Class: Janus kinase (JAK) inhibitor, Janus kinase-2 inhibitor, Kinase inhibitor
Half-life: 28 hours
Clinically important, potentially hazardous interactions with: clarithromycin, CYP3A4 inducers, CYP3A4 inhibitors, rifampin
Pregnancy category: No available data on use in pregnant women to evaluate for a drug-associated risk of major birth defects, miscarriage, or adverse maternal or fetal outcomes.

Skin
Peripheral edema (20%)
Pruritus (itching) (10%)

Mucosal
Epistaxis (nosebleed) (5% ≥ grade 3) (12%)

Central Nervous System
Fever (pyrexia) (includes hyperpyrexia) (15%)
Vertigo / dizziness (15%)

Gastrointestinal/Hepatic
Diarrhea (48%) [2]
Nausea (32%)
Vomiting (19%)

Hematologic
Anemia (22% ≥ grade 3) (24%)
Thrombocytopenia / platelets decreased (32% ≥ grade 3) (34%)

Respiratory
Cough (8%)
Dyspnea / shortness of breath (10%)
Upper respiratory tract infection (10%)

PALBOCICLIB

Trade name: Ibrance (Pfizer)
Indications: Treatment of postmenopausal women with estrogen receptor (ER)-positive, human epidermal growth factor receptor 2 (HER2)-negative advanced breast cancer (in combination with letrozole)
Class: Cyclin-dependent kinase (CDK) 4/6 inhibitor
Half-life: 29 hours
Clinically important, potentially hazardous interactions with: bosentan, carbamazepine, clarithromycin, efavirenz, etravirine, grapefruit juice, indinavir, itraconazole, ketoconazole, lopinavir, modafinil, nafcillin, nefazodone, nelfinavir, phenytoin, posaconazole, rifampin, ritonavir, saquinavir, St John's wort, telaprevir, telithromycin, verapamil, voriconazole
Pregnancy category: Can cause fetal harm
Important contra-indications noted in the prescribing guidelines for: nursing mothers; pediatric patients

---

Skin
Peripheral edema [2]
Rash [5]
Vitiligo [2]

Hair
Alopecia / hair loss (22%) [2]

Mucosal
Epistaxis (nosebleed) (11%) [2]
Stomatitis (oral mucositis) (25%) [5]

Central Nervous System
Fever (pyrexia) (includes hyperpyrexia) [2]
Headache [2]
Peripheral neuropathy (13%)

Endocrine/Metabolic
Appetite decreased (16%)

Gastrointestinal/Hepatic
Constipation [2]
Diarrhea (21%) [8]
Hepatotoxicity / liver injury / acute liver injury / drug-induced liver injury (DILI) [3]
Nausea (25%) [9]
Vomiting (15%) [4]

Hematologic
Anemia (35%) [12]
Febrile neutropenia [11]
Leukocytopenia (leukopenia) / leukocytes (white blood cells) decreased (43%) [16]
Lymphopenia (lymphocytopenia) / lymphocytes decreased [2]
Neutropenia (neutrophils decreased) (75%) [39]
Thrombocytopenia / platelets decreased (17%) [10]

Neuromuscular/Skeletal
Asthenia / fatigue (13–41%) [13]

Respiratory
Dyspnea / shortness of breath [2]
Pneumonitis [4]
Upper respiratory tract infection (31%)

Other
Adverse effects / adverse reactions [3]
Death [3]
Infection [4]

PALIPERIDONE

Trade name: Invega (Janssen)
Indications: Schizophrenia
Class: Antipsychotic, Antipsychotic, atypical
Half-life: ~23 hours
Clinically important, potentially hazardous interactions with: ACE inhibitors, alcohol, alpha blockers, amphetamines, angiotensin II receptor antagonists, carbamazepine, CNS depressants, dopamine agonists, droperidol, general anesthetics, itraconazole, levodopa, levomepromazine, lithium, methylphenidate, metoclopramide, myleosuppressives, P-glycoprotein inhibitors or inducers, quinagolide, risperidone, tetrabenazine, valproic acid
Important contra-indications noted in the prescribing guidelines for: the elderly; nursing mothers; pediatric patients
Note: Invega is not recommended for patients with creatinine clearance below 10 mL/min. Paliperidone is the active metabolite of risperidone (see separate entry).
Warning: INCREASED MORTALITY IN ELDERLY PATIENTS WITH DEMENTIA-RELATED PSYCHOSIS

Skin
Anaphylactoid reactions / anaphylaxis (includes anaphylactic shock) (<2%)
Angioedema (formerly named angioneurotic edema) [3]
Edema / fluid retention (<2%)
Peripheral edema [4]
Pruritic rash [2]
Pruritus (itching) (<2%)
Rash (<2%)

Mucosal
Nasal congestion (<2%)
Sialorrhea (ptyalism; hypersalivation) (<6%) [3]
Tongue edema (3%)
Xerostomia (dry mouth) (<4%)

Cardiovascular
Arrhythmias (<2%)
Atrioventricular block (<2%)
Bradycardia / sinus bradycardia (<2%) [2]
Bundle branch block (<3%)
Hypertension (<2%)
Palpitation (<2%) [2]
Tachycardia (<14%) [6]

Central Nervous System
Agitation (<2%) [6]
Akathisia (3–17%) [25]
Anxiety (2–9%) [9]
Depression [2]
Dysarthria (<4%) [2]
Extrapyramidal symptoms (4–23%) [17]
Headache (4–14%) [18]
Insomnia (<2%) [24]
Neuroleptic malignant syndrome [10]
Nightmares (<2%)
Parkinsonism [6]
Psychosis [3]
Restlessness [2]
Schizophrenia [7]
Sleep-related disorder (2–3%)
Somnolence (drowsiness) (6–26%) [13]
Tardive syndrome / tardive dyskinesia [3]
Tremor [7]
Vertigo / dizziness (2–6%) [3]

Endocrine/Metabolic
ALT increased (<2%)
Amenorrhea (6%) [3]
Appetite decreased (<2%)
Appetite increased (2–3%)
AST increased (<2%)
Galactorrhea (4%) [5]
Gynecomastia (3%)
Hyperprolactinemia [12]
Hyponatremia [2]
Hypothyroidism [2]
Menstrual irregularities (<2%)
Weight gain (2–7%) [21]

Gastrointestinal/Hepatic
Abdominal pain (<3%)
Constipation (4–5%) [4]
Diarrhea [2]
Dyspepsia / functional dyspepsia (indigestion) (see also gastroparesis) (5–6%)
Flatulence (<2%)
Nausea [3]
Vomiting (3–11%)

Genitourinary
Ejaculatory dysfunction (<2%)
Erectile dysfunction [2]
Sexual dysfunction [3]
Urinary tract infection (<2%)

Hematologic
Leukocytopenia (leukopenia) / leukocytes (white blood cells) decreased [2]
Neutropenia (neutrophils decreased) [3]

Local
Injection-site pain [11]

Neuromuscular/Skeletal
Asthenia / fatigue (<4%) [4]
Bone pain / joint pain [2]
Dystonia [7]
Hyperkinesia [2]
Rhabdomyolysis [5]

Ocular
Vision blurred (3%)

Respiratory
Cough (<3%)
Nasopharyngitis (2–5%) [6]
Pharyngolaryngeal pain (<2%)
Pulmonary embolism [2]
Rhinitis / rhinosinusitis (see also sinusitis) (<3%)
Upper respiratory tract infection [2]

Other
Adverse effects / adverse reactions [8]
Death [4]

PALONOSETRON

Trade name: Aloxi (MGI)
Indications: Antiemetic (for cancer chemotherapy)
Class: 5-HT3 antagonist, Antiemetic, Serotonin type 3 receptor antagonist
Half-life: 40 hours
Clinically important, potentially hazardous interactions with: apomorphine
Note: See also the fixed drug combination Netupitant & Palonosetron (separate entry).

Skin
Hot flashes / hot flushes (<15)
Pruritus (itching) (8–22%)
Rash (6%)

Central Nervous System
Anorexia [2]
Fever (pyrexia) (includes hyperpyrexia) [2]
Headache (9%) [14]
Vertigo / dizziness [4]

Endocrine/Metabolic
AST increased [2]

Gastrointestinal/Hepatic
Abdominal pain [2]
Constipation [11]
Diarrhea [4]

Neuromuscular/Skeletal
Asthenia / fatigue [4]
Osteonecrosis / avascular necrosis (includes steroid-induced osteonecrosis of the femoral head) (jaw) [13]

Renal
Nephrotoxicity / kidney injury / acute kidney injury (AKI) / drug-induced kidney injury [3]

Other
Hiccups / singultus [4]

PAMIDRONATE

Trade name: Aredia (Novartis)
Indications: Hypercalcemia, Paget's disease, osteogenesis imperfecta
Class: Bisphosphonate
Half-life: 1.6 hours
Clinically important, potentially hazardous interactions with: none known
Important contra-indications noted in the prescribing guidelines for: nursing mothers; pediatric patients

---

Skin
Candidiasis / candidosis (6%)

Cardiovascular
Atrial fibrillation (6%)
Hypertension (6%)
Tachycardia (6%)

Central Nervous System
Anorexia (26%)
Fever (pyrexia) (includes hyperpyrexia) (18–39%) [8]
Headache (26%)
Insomnia (22%)
Somnolence (drowsiness) (6%)

Endocrine/Metabolic
Hypocalcemia [10]
Hypophosphatemia [2]
Hypothyroidism (6%)

Gastrointestinal/Hepatic
Abdominal pain (23%)
Constipation (6%)
Dyspepsia / functional dyspepsia (indigestion) (see also gastroparesis) (23%)
Nausea (54%)
Vomiting (36%) [2]

Genitourinary
Azotemia (prerenal) (4%)
Urinary tract infection (19%)

Hematologic
Anemia (43%)
Granulocytopenia (20%)

Local
Injection-site reaction (18%)

Neuromuscular/Skeletal
Arthralgia (14%) [2]
Asthenia / fatigue (37%) [2]
Bone pain / joint pain [3]
Fractures [3]
Myalgia/Myopathy [3]
Osteonecrosis / avascular necrosis (includes steroid-induced osteonecrosis of the femoral head) [20]

Ocular
Conjunctivitis (conjunctival inflammation) [5]
Episcleritis [2]
Orbital inflammation [2]
Scleritis [4]
Uveitis / anterior uveitis / posterior uveitis / panuveitis [12]
Vision blurred [2]

Renal
Nephrotoxicity / kidney injury / acute kidney injury (AKI) / drug-induced kidney injury [11]

Respiratory
Cough (26%)
Influenza- ('flu)-like syndrome [3]
Rhinitis / rhinosinusitis (see also sinusitis) (6%)
Sinusitis (see also rhinitis / rhinosinusitis) (16%)

PANCRELIPASE

Trade names: Cotazym (Janssen), Creon (AbbVie), Ultrasa (Aptalis), Viokace (Aptalis), Zenpep (Aptalis)
Indications: Pancreatic insufficiency, steatorrhea
Class: Enzyme
Half-life: N/A
Clinically important, potentially hazardous interactions with: ferrous sulfate
Important contra-indications noted in the prescribing guidelines for: nursing mothers; pediatric patients

---

Skin
Lymphadenopathy (11%)
Peripheral edema (3%)
Pruritus ani et vulvae (7%)
Rash (3%)

Mucosal
Epistaxis (nosebleed) (7%)
Nasal congestion (14%)

Central Nervous System
Headache (3–15%)
Vertigo / dizziness (4%)

Endocrine/Metabolic
Hyperglycemia (includes glucose increased) (8%)
Hypoglycemia (4%)
Weight loss (6%)

Gastrointestinal/Hepatic
Abdominal pain (3–18%)
Ascites (3%)
Flatulence (3–6%)
Vomiting (6%)

Hematologic
Anemia (3%)

Neuromuscular/Skeletal
Neck pain (14%)

Otic
Ear pain (11%)

Renal
Nephrolithiasis (kidney stones / renal calculi) (7%)

Respiratory
Cough (4–6%)
Nasopharyngitis (4%)
Pharyngolaryngeal pain (7%)

Other
Adverse effects / adverse reactions [2]
Infection (3%)

PANCURONIUM

Indications: Anesthesia adjunct, neuromuscular blockade, muscle relaxant
Class: Non-depolarizing neuromuscular blocker
Half-life: 89–161 minutes
Clinically important, potentially hazardous interactions with: aminoglycosides, cortisone, cyclopropane, deflazacort, enflurane, gentamicin, halothane, hydrocortisone, isoflurane, kanamycin, methoxyflurane, mivacurium, neomycin, piperacillin, prednisolone, prednisone, streptomycin, tobramycin, triamcinolone, trospium

---

Skin
Anaphylactoid reactions / anaphylaxis (includes anaphylactic shock) [9]

Neuromuscular/Skeletal
Myalgia/Myopathy [3]

PANITUMUMAB

Trade name: Vectibix (Amgen)
Indications: Metastatic colorectal carcinoma progression
Class: Antineoplastic / anticancer agent (see also Immune checkpoint inhibitor), Biologic, Epidermal growth factor receptor (EGFR) inhibitor / antagonist, Monoclonal antibody
Half-life: ~7.5 days
Clinically important, potentially hazardous interactions with: none known
Important contra-indications noted in the prescribing guidelines for: nursing mothers; pediatric patients
Warning: DERMATOLOGIC TOXICITY and INFUSION REACTIONS

Skin
Acneiform eruption / acneiform dermatitis / acneiform rash (57%) [18]
Cutaneous toxicity / skin toxicity (90%) [26]
Desquamation [3]
Eczema / eczematous reaction / eczematous eruption [2]
Erythema (65%) [5]
Exfoliative dermatitis (25%) [2]
Fissures (20%) [5]
Folliculitis [3]
Hand–foot syndrome (palmar–plantar erythrodysesthesia) [3]
Papulopustular eruption [5]
Peripheral edema (12%)
Pruritus (itching) (57%) [10]
Rash (22%) [33]
Xerosis / xeroderma (10%) [12]

Hair
Alopecia / hair loss [3]
Hair changes (9%) [2]

Nails
Nail changes (9–29%) [2]
Paronychia (25%) [14]

Mucosal
Mucosal inflammation (6%)
Mucositis [4]
Stomatitis (oral mucositis) (7%) [4]

Cardiovascular
Arrhythmias [2]

Central Nervous System
Anorexia [4]
Fever (pyrexia) (includes hyperpyrexia) [2]
Neurotoxicity [2]

Endocrine/Metabolic
Dehydration [3]
Hypocalcemia [4]
Hypokalemia [6]
Hypomagnesemia [21]

Gastrointestinal/Hepatic
Abdominal pain (25%) [3]
Constipation (21%) [4]
Diarrhea (21%) [21]
Nausea (23%) [9]
Vomiting (19%) [9]

Hematologic
Anemia [2]
Febrile neutropenia [2]
Leukocytopenia (leukopenia) / leukocytes (white blood cells) decreased [2]
Neutropenia (neutrophils decreased) [7]
Thrombocytopenia / platelets decreased [5]

Local
Infusion-related reactions (3%) [5]
Injection-site reaction (4%)

Neuromuscular/Skeletal
Asthenia / fatigue (26%) [18]

Ocular
Conjunctivitis (conjunctival inflammation) (4%) [2]
Corneal perforation [2]
Eyelashes – hypertrichosis (eyelash megalotrichosis) (6%)
Lacrimation (2%)
Ocular toxicity (15%) [2]
Trichomegaly [3]

Respiratory
Cough (14%)
Dyspnea / shortness of breath [3]
Pulmonary embolism [3]
Pulmonary fibrosis [3]
Pulmonary toxicity [7]

Other
Adverse effects / adverse reactions [5]
Death [2]
Infection [3]

PANTOPRAZOLE

Trade names: Protium (Nycomed), Protonix (Wyeth)
Indications: Esophagitis associated with gastroesophageal reflux disease (GERD), Zollinger-Ellison syndrome, erosive esophagitis
Class: Proton pump inhibitor (PPI)
Half-life: 1 hour
Clinically important, potentially hazardous interactions with: alcohol, allopurinol, atazanavir, cefditoren, clopidogrel, conivaptan, CYP2C19 inducers and substrates, dabigatran, dasatinib, delavirdine, dexmethylphenidate, digoxin, emtricitabine/rilpivirine/tenofovir alafenamide, erlotinib, eucalyptus, fluconazole, indinavir, iron salts, itraconazole, ketoconazole, lapatinib, letermovir, mesalamine, methotrexate, methylphenidate, mycophenolate, nelfinavir, PEG-interferon, posaconazole, raltegravir, rilpivirine, saquinavir, tipranavir, topotecan, ulipristal, voriconazole, warfarin
Important contra-indications noted in the prescribing guidelines for: nursing mothers

---

Skin
Anaphylactoid reactions / anaphylaxis (includes anaphylactic shock) [13]
Baboon syndrome / symmetrical drug-related intertriginous and flexural exanthema (SDRIFE) [2]
Edema / fluid retention (<2%)
Facial edema (<4%)
Hypersensitivity [2]
Lupus erythematosus (subacute cutaneous lupus erythematosus (SCLE)) (discoid) [3]
Peripheral edema [2]
Photosensitivity (<2%)
Pruritus (itching) (<2%)
Rash (<2%) [3]
Urticaria / hives (<4%) [2]

Mucosal
Xerostomia (dry mouth) (<2%)

Cardiovascular
Kounis syndrome / allergic angina syndrome / allergic myocardial infarction [2]

Central Nervous System
Depression (<2%)
Fever (pyrexia) (includes hyperpyrexia) (>4%) [3]
Headache (12%) [3]
Seizures [3]
Vertigo / dizziness (3%)

Endocrine/Metabolic
Creatine phosphokinase (CPK) / creatine kinase increased (hyperCKemia) (<2%)
Hypomagnesemia [7]

Gastrointestinal/Hepatic
Abdominal pain (6%)
Constipation (<4%) [2]
Diarrhea (9%)
Flatulence (<4%)
Hepatitis (<2%) [5]
Nausea (7%) [2]
Vomiting (4%)

Hematologic
Leukocytopenia (leukopenia) / leukocytes (white blood cells) decreased (<2%)
Thrombocytopenia / platelets decreased (<2%) [7]

Neuromuscular/Skeletal
Arthralgia (<4%)
Myalgia/Myopathy (<4%)

Ocular
Vision blurred (<2%)

Renal
Nephrotoxicity / kidney injury / acute kidney injury (AKI) / drug-induced kidney injury [4]

Respiratory
Influenza- ('flu)-like syndrome (<10%)
Upper respiratory tract infection (>4%)

Other
Adverse effects / adverse reactions [2]
Allergic reactions (<4%)
Infection (<10%)

PAPAVERINE

Indications: Peripheral and cerebral ischemia
Class: Opium alkaloid, Vasodilator, peripheral
Half-life: 0.5–2 hours
Clinically important, potentially hazardous interactions with: levodopa, reboxetine

Important contra-indications noted in the prescribing guidelines for: nursing mothers; pediatric patients

Cardiovascular
Hypotension [2]

Genitourinary
Priapism (11%) [16]

PARICALCITOL

Trade name: Zemplar (AbbVie)
Indications: Secondary hyperparathyroidism associated with renal failure
Class: Vitamin D receptor agonist
Half-life: 4–7 hours
Clinically important, potentially hazardous interactions with: bile acid sequestrants, cardiac glycosides, conivaptan, danazol, darunavir, delavirdine, digitalis (with overdose of paricalcitol), digoxin, ergocalciferol, indinavir, ketoconazole, orlistat, orlistat, strong CYP3A4 inhibitors, sucralfate, telithromycin, thiazide diuretics, tocilizumab, voriconazole
Important contra-indications noted in the prescribing guidelines for: nursing mothers
Note: Contra-indicated in patients with evidence of vitamin D toxicity or hypercalcemia.

Skin
Burning / skin burning sensation (<2%)
Edema / fluid retention (7%)
Hyperhidrosis (<2%)
Lymphadenopathy (<2%)
Peripheral edema (<2%)
Pruritus (itching) (<2%)

Hair
Alopecia / hair loss (<2%)
Hirsutism (<2%)

Mucosal
Rectal hemorrhage / rectal bleeding (<2%)
Xerostomia (dry mouth) (3%)

Cardiovascular
Arrhythmias (<2%)
Atrial flutter (<2%)
Cardiac arrest (<2%)
Hypertension (<2%)
Hypotension (<2%)
Palpitation (3%)

Central Nervous System
Agitation (<2%)
Chills (5%)
Confusion (<2%)
Delirium (<2%)
Dysgeusia (taste perversion) (<2%)
Fever (pyrexia) (includes hyperpyrexia) (5%)
Gait instability / postural instability (<2%)
Headache (<2%)
Hypoesthesia / hypesthesia (numbness) (<2%)
Insomnia (<2%)
Nervousness (<2%)
Pain (<2%)
Paresthesias (<2%)
Restlessness (<2%)
Stroke / cerebrovascular accident (<2%)
Syncope / fainting (<2%)
Vertigo / dizziness (<2%)

Endocrine/Metabolic
Appetite decreased (<2%)
AST increased (<2%)
Hypercalcemia (<2%) [5]
Hyperkalemia (<2%)
Hyperparathyroidism (<2%)
Hyperphosphatemia (<2%)
Hypocalcemia (<2%)
Hypoparathyroidism (<2%)
Mastodynia (<2%)
Weight loss (<2%)

Gastrointestinal/Hepatic
Abdominal pain (<2%)
Constipation (<2%)
Diarrhea (<2%)
Dysphagia (<2%)
Gastritis / pangastritis / gastric irritation (<2%)
Gastrointestinal bleeding (5%)
Hepatotoxicity / liver injury / acute liver injury / drug-induced liver injury (DILI) (<2%)
Nausea (13%) [2]
Vomiting (8%) [2]

Genitourinary
Erectile dysfunction (<2%)

Hematologic
Anemia (<2%)
Prothrombin time (INR) increased (<2%)
Sepsis (5%)

Local
Injection-site extravasation (<2%)
Injection-site pain (<2%)

Neuromuscular/Skeletal
Arthralgia (5%)
Asthenia / fatigue (3%)
Myalgia/Myopathy (<2%)

Ocular
Conjunctivitis (conjunctival inflammation) (<2%)
Glaucoma (includes acute angle-closure glaucoma) (<2%)
Ocular hyperemia (<2%)

Respiratory
Cough (<2%)
Dyspnea / shortness of breath (<2%)
Influenza (5%)
Nasopharyngitis (<2%)
Pneumonia (5%)
Pulmonary edema (cardiogenic / non-cardiogenic) (<2%)
Upper respiratory tract infection (<2%)
Wheezing (<2%)

Other
Cancer (breast) (<2%)
Dipsia (thirst) / polydipsia (<2%)

PAROMOMYCIN

Trade name: Humatin (Pfizer)
Indications: Intestinal amebiasis
Class: Antibiotic, Antibiotic; aminoglycoside, Antimicrobial
Half-life: N/A
Clinically important, potentially hazardous interactions with: methotrexate, succinylcholine

Skin
Pruritus (itching) [2]

Central Nervous System
Pain [2]

Gastrointestinal/Hepatic
Abdominal pain [2]

Local
Injection-site pain [3]

PAROXETINE HYDROCHLORIDE

Trade names: Paxil (GSK), Paxil CR (GSK), Seroxat (GSK)
Indications: Depression, obsessive-compulsive disorder, panic disorder, social and generalized anxiety disorders, post-traumatic stress disorder
Class: Antidepressant, Selective serotonin reuptake inhibitor (SSRI)
Half-life: 21 hours
Clinically important, potentially hazardous interactions with: alcohol, amitriptyline, amphetamines, antiepileptics, aprepitant, aripiprazole, artemether/lumefantrine, asenapine, aspirin, astemizole, atomoxetine, barbiturates, clarithromycin, clozapine, cobicistat/elvitegravir/emtricitabine/tenofovir alafenamide, cobicistat/elvitegravir/emtricitabine/tenofovir disoproxil, coumarins, cyproheptadine, darifenacin, darunavir, deutetrabenazine, dexibuprofen, dextroamphetamine, diethylpropion, digitalis, digoxin, duloxetine, eluxadoline, entacapone, erythromycin, galantamine, iloperidone, isocarboxazid, linezolid, lithium, MAO inhibitors, mazindol, methadone, methamphetamine, methylene blue, methylphenidate, metoprolol, moclobemide, molindone, NSAIDs, oliceridine, perphenazine, phendimetrazine, phenelzine, phenobarbital, phentermine, phenylpropanolamine, phenytoin, pimozide, primidone, procyclidine, propafenone, propranolol, pseudoephedrine, ranolazine, rasagiline, risperidone, ritonavir, selegiline, sibutramine, St John's wort, sumatriptan, sympathomimetics, tamoxifen, tamsulosin, tetrabenazine, thioridazine, tramadol, tranylcypromine, trazodone, tricyclic antidepressants, troleandomycin, tryptophan, valbenazine, vortioxetine
Important contra-indications noted in the prescribing guidelines for: nursing mothers; pediatric patients
Note: For menopausal indications see separate entry for paroxetine mesylate.
Warning: SUICIDALITY AND ANTIDEPRESSANT DRUGS

Skin
Bruise / bruising / contusion / ecchymosis (ecchymoses) [2]
Diaphoresis (11%) [10]
Exanthems [2]
Hyperhidrosis [2]
Photosensitivity [3]
Pruritus (itching) [3]
Rash (2%)
Vasculitis (angiitis) / cutaneous vasculitis (angiitis) [2]

Mucosal
Xerostomia (dry mouth) (18%) [17]

Cardiovascular
QT interval prolonged / QT prolongation [2]
Venous thromboembolism [2]

Central Nervous System
Abnormal dreams (3–4%)
Agitation (3–6%)
Akathisia [3]

Anxiety (5%) [2]
Chills (2%) [2]
Delirium [3]
Depression [3]
Dysarthria [2]
Dysgeusia (taste perversion) (2%)
Extrapyramidal symptoms [2]
Hallucinations, auditory [5]
Hallucinations, visual [2]
Headache (17–28%) [12]
Insomnia (11–24%) [5]
Irritability [2]
Mania [2]
Nervousness (4–9%)
Neuroleptic malignant syndrome [4]
Paresthesias (4%)
Parkinsonism [3]
Restless legs syndrome / Willis-Ekbom disease (includes restless arms syndrome variant) [7]
Serotonin syndrome [20]
Sleep disturbances [2]
Somnolence (drowsiness) (15–24%) [5]
Suicidal ideation [4]
Tic disorder [3]
Tremor (4–11%) [5]
Vertigo / dizziness (6–14%) [7]
Yawning (2–4%)

Endocrine/Metabolic
Galactorrhea [6]
Gynecomastia [2]
Libido decreased (3–15%)
SIADH [18]
Weight gain [9]

Gastrointestinal/Hepatic
Abdominal pain (4%) [2]
Constipation (5–18%) [2]
Diarrhea (9–12%) [3]
Nausea (26%) [8]
Vomiting [3]

Genitourinary
Ejaculatory dysfunction (13–28%)
Erectile dysfunction [2]
Priapism [4]
Sexual dysfunction [8]

Neuromuscular/Skeletal
Asthenia / fatigue [4]
Myalgia/Myopathy (<10%)

Ocular
Glaucoma (includes acute angle-closure glaucoma) [2]
Vision impaired [2]

Respiratory
Pharyngitis (sore throat) (4%)
Rhinitis / rhinosinusitis (see also sinusitis) (3%)
Sinusitis (see also rhinitis / rhinosinusitis) (4%)

Other
Adverse effects / adverse reactions [4]
Bruxism (teeth grinding) [4]
Congenital malformations [2]
Death [2]
Infection (5–6%)

PAROXETINE MESYLATE

Trade name: Brisdelle (Noven)
Indications: Vasomotor symptoms associated with the menopause
Class: Selective serotonin reuptake inhibitor (SSRI)
Half-life: N/A
Clinically important, potentially hazardous interactions with: eluxadoline, linezolid, MAO inhibitors, methylene blue, pimozide, tamoxifen, thioridazine
Important contra-indications noted in the prescribing guidelines for: the elderly; nursing mothers; pediatric patients
Note: Brisdelle contains a low dose of paroxetine and is not indicated for psychiatric conditions. Paroxetine mesylate is also available as Pexeva. For psychiatric indications see separate entry for paroxetine hydrochloride.
Warning: SUICIDAL THOUGHTS AND BEHAVIORS

Central Nervous System
Headache (6%)

Gastrointestinal/Hepatic
Nausea (4%) [2]
Vomiting (4%)

Neuromuscular/Skeletal
Asthenia / fatigue (5%)

Other
Adverse effects / adverse reactions [2]

PASIREOTIDE

Trade name: Signifor (Novartis)
Indications: Cushing's disease
Class: Somatostatin analog
Half-life: 12 hours
Clinically important, potentially hazardous interactions with: antiarrhythmics, bromocriptine, cyclosporine, drugs prolonging the QT interval
Important contra-indications noted in the prescribing guidelines for: nursing mothers; pediatric patients

---

Skin
Peripheral edema (10%)
Pruritus (itching) (8%)
Xerosis / xeroderma (6%)

Hair
Alopecia / hair loss (12%)

Cardiovascular
Bradycardia / sinus bradycardia [2]
Hypertension (10%)
Hypotension (7%)
QT interval prolonged / QT prolongation (6%)

Central Nervous System
Anorexia [2]
Anxiety (9%)
Headache (28%) [4]
Insomnia (9%)
Vertigo / dizziness (6–9%) [2]

Endocrine/Metabolic
ALT increased (10%)
Appetite decreased (10%)
AST increased (6%)
Diabetes mellitus (18%) [7]
GGT increased (10%)
Hypercholesterolemia (10%)
Hyperglycemia (includes glucose increased) (40%) [36]
Hypoglycemia (9%) [2]
Hypokalemia (6%)
Weight loss [2]

Gastrointestinal/Hepatic
Abdominal distension (6%)
Abdominal pain (10–24%) [6]
Cholelithiasis (gallstones in the gall bladder or the bile duct) (30%) [7]
Constipation (7%)
Diarrhea (58%) [17]
Gastrointestinal disorder / discomfort [3]
Hepatotoxicity / liver injury / acute liver injury / drug-induced liver injury (DILI) [2]
Nausea (52%) [12]
Vomiting (7%)

Hematologic
Anemia (4%)
Prothrombin time (INR) increased (2%)

Local
Injection-site reaction (17%) [3]

Neuromuscular/Skeletal
Arthralgia (8%)
Asthenia / fatigue (11–19%) [3]
Back pain (6%)
Myalgia/Myopathy (9%)
Pain in extremities (6%)

Respiratory
Influenza (9%)
Nasopharyngitis (13%) [2]

Other
Adverse effects / adverse reactions [7]

PATISIRAN

Trade name: Onpattro (Alnylam Pharma Inc)
Indications: indicated for the treatment of the polyneuropathy of hereditary transthyretin-mediated amyloidosis in adults
Class: Small interfering RNA (siRNA), Transthyretin-directed small interfering RNA
Half-life: 1.8–3.2 days
Clinically important, potentially hazardous interactions with: none known
Pregnancy category: no available data

Skin
Erythema (7%)
Facial edema (1–19%)
Facial erythema (1–19%)
Flushing / rubefaction (1–19%)
Rash (1–19%)

Cardiovascular
Atrioventricular block (3%)
Chest pain (1–19%)
Hypertension (1–19%)
Hypotension (1–19%)
Tachycardia (1–19%)

Central Nervous System
Chills (1–19%)
Headache (1–19%)
Pain (1–19%)
Vertigo / dizziness (5%)

Gastrointestinal/Hepatic
Abdominal pain (1–19%)
Dyspepsia / functional dyspepsia (indigestion) (see also gastroparesis) (8%)
Nausea (1–19%)

Neuromuscular/Skeletal
Arthralgia (7%)
Asthenia / fatigue (1–19%)
Back pain (1–19%)
Muscle spasm (8%)
Neck pain (1–19%)

Ocular
Keratoconjunctivitis (5%)
Vision blurred (3%)
Vitreous floaters / floaters / myodesopsia / myiodesopsia / muscae volitantes (2%)

Respiratory
Bronchitis (7%)
Cough (1–19%)
Dyspnea / shortness of breath (8%)
Nasopharyngitis (1–29%)
Pharyngitis (sore throat) (1–29%)
Respiratory tract infection (1–29%)
Rhinitis / rhinosinusitis (see also sinusitis) (1–29%)
Sinusitis (see also rhinitis / rhinosinusitis) (1–29%)
Upper respiratory tract infection (1–29%)

Other
Adverse effects / adverse reactions [2]

PAZOPANIB

Trade name: Votrient (Novartis)
Indications: Advanced renal cell carcinoma
Class: Angiogenesis inhibitor / antiangiogenic agent, Antineoplastic / anticancer agent (see also Immune checkpoint inhibitor), Tyrosine kinase inhibitor, Vascular endothelial growth factor (VEGF) inhibitor / antagonist
Half-life: 31 hours
Clinically important, potentially hazardous interactions with: alfuzosin, artemether/lumefantrine, atazanavir, BCG vaccine, boceprevir, cardiac glycosides, chloroquine, ciprofloxacin, clarithromycin, clozapine, conivaptan, CYP3A4 inducers or inhibitors, cyproterone, darunavir, deferasirox, delavirdine, denosumab, dronedarone, efavirenz, gadobutrol, grapefruit juice, indacaterol, indinavir, itraconazole, ketoconazole, lapatinib, leflunomide, natalizumab, nelfinavir, nilotinib, oxcarbazepine, P-glycoprotein inhibitors, pimecrolimus, pimozide, QT prolonging agents, quetiapine, quinine, rifampin, rifapentine, ritonavir, roflumilast, saquinavir, simvastatin, sipuleucel-T, St John's wort, tacrolimus, telithromycin, tetrabenazine, thioridazine, tocilizumab, toremifene, trastuzumab, vaccines, vandetanib, vemurafenib, vitamin K antagonists, voriconazole, ziprasidone
Important contra-indications noted in the prescribing guidelines for: nursing mothers; pediatric patients
Warning: HEPATOTOXICITY

Skin
Cutaneous toxicity / skin toxicity [5]
Depigmentation (3%)
Hand–foot syndrome (palmar–plantar erythrodysesthesia) (6%) [12]
Pigmentation (Skin) (includes hyperpigmentation) [7]
Pruritus (itching) [3]
Rash (8%) [6]

Hair
Alopecia / hair loss (8%) [2]
Hair changes (38%)
Hair pigmentation [9]

Mucosal
Epistaxis (nosebleed) [2]
Stomatitis (oral mucositis) [5]

Cardiovascular
Cardiac failure [2]
Chest pain (5%)
Hypertension (47%) [34]
Myocardial infarction [2]
QT interval prolonged / QT prolongation (<2%)
Thromboembolism [2]

Central Nervous System
Anorexia (22%) [6]
Dysgeusia (taste perversion) [3]
Headache (10%) [3]

Endocrine/Metabolic
ALT increased (53%) [9]
Appetite decreased [3]
AST increased (53%) [10]
Hypothyroidism (7%) [5]
Weight loss (9%) [2]

Gastrointestinal/Hepatic
Abdominal pain (11%) [2]
Diarrhea (52%) [29]
Dyspepsia / functional dyspepsia (indigestion) (see also gastroparesis) (5%) [2]
Gastrointestinal disorder / discomfort [2]
Gastrointestinal perforation / perforated colon / gastric perforation [2]
Hepatic (liver) disorder / hepatobiliary disorder / hepatic (liver) dysfunction [2]
Hepatotoxicity / liver injury / acute liver injury / drug-induced liver injury (DILI) [18]
Intestinal lymphangiectasia / intestinal lymphangiectasis [2]
Nausea (26%) [17]
Pancreatitis / acute pancreatitis [6]
Vomiting (21%) [10]

Hematologic
Anemia [5]
Hemorrhage [2]
Leukocytopenia (leukopenia) / leukocytes (white blood cells) decreased (37%) [2]
Lymphopenia (lymphocytopenia) / lymphocytes decreased (31%)
Myelosuppression / bone marrow suppression / myelotoxicity [2]
Neutropenia (neutrophils decreased) (34%) [7]
Thrombocytopenia / platelets decreased (32%) [10]

Neuromuscular/Skeletal
Asthenia / fatigue (14%) [27]

Renal
Proteinuria (9%) [5]

Respiratory
Hemoptysis (2%)
Pneumothorax [4]
Pulmonary embolism [2]

Other
Adverse effects / adverse reactions [14]
Death [6]

PEG-INTERFERON

Trade names: PegIntron (Schering), Sylatron (Schering)
Indications: Chronic hepatitis C, melanoma
Class: Immunomodulator, Interferon
Half-life: ~40 hours
Clinically important, potentially hazardous interactions with: ACE inhibitors, acetaminophen, aldesleukin, bupivacaine, cilostazol, cinacalcet, CYP2C9 substrates, CYP2D6 substrates, delavirdine, duloxetine, estradiol, fesoterodine, fingolimod, fluoxetine, indinavir, melphalan, methadone, methylnaltrexone, pantoprazole, pegloticase, ribavirin, sildenafil, tapentadol, telbivudine, theophylline, theophylline derivatives, tiotropium, trimethoprim, voriconazole, warfarin, zidovudine
Pregnancy category: pregnancy category will be X when used in combination with ribavirin
Important contra-indications noted in the prescribing guidelines for: nursing mothers; pediatric patients
Note: PEG-interferon is commonly administered with ribavirin and many of the reactions listed below are in combination therapy with this drug. Contra-indicated in patients with known hypersensitivity reactions, such as urticaria, angioedema, bronchoconstriction, anaphylaxis, Stevens-Johnson syndrome, and toxic epidermal necrolysis to interferon alpha or any other product component; or with autoimmune hepatitis.
Warning: RISK OF SERIOUS DISORDERS AND RIBAVIRIN-ASSOCIATED EFFECTS and DEPRESSION AND OTHER NEUROPSYCHIATRIC DISORDERS

Skin
Cutaneous toxicity / skin toxicity [3]
Dermatitis (7%)
Diaphoresis (6%)
DRESS syndrome (Drug-induced hypersensitivity syndrome) [2]
Eczema / eczematous reaction / eczematous eruption [2]
Exanthems [5]
Fixed eruption / fixed drug eruption [2]
Flushing / rubefaction (6%)
Lupus erythematosus (subacute cutaneous lupus erythematosus (SCLE)) [3]
Nummular eczema [2]
Photosensitivity [4]
Pruritus (itching) (12%) [11]
Psoriasis [4]
Rash (6%) [24]
Rosacea fulminans [2]
Sarcoidosis / sarcoid-like reaction (cutaneous sarcoidosis) [9]
Stevens-Johnson syndrome and toxic epidermal necrolysis (SJS/TEN) [2]
Vasculitis (angiitis) / cutaneous vasculitis (angiitis) [2]
Vitiligo [3]
Xerosis / xeroderma (11%) [2]

Hair
Alopecia / hair loss (22%) [5]
Alopecia areata [2]

Central Nervous System
Anorexia (17%) [2]
Chills [2]
Cognitive impairment [2]
Depression (16–29%) [10]

Dysgeusia (taste perversion) (<10%) [5]
Fever (pyrexia) (includes hyperpyrexia) (37%) [8]
Headache (54%) [16]
Insomnia (19%) [4]
Irritability [2]
Neurotoxicity [2]
Pain (12%)
Parkinsonism [2]
Psychosis [2]
Vertigo / dizziness (16%) [3]

Endocrine/Metabolic
ALT increased [3]
Appetite decreased [2]
AST increased [3]
Diabetes mellitus [2]
Thyroid dysfunction [2]
Weight loss (16%) [3]

Gastrointestinal/Hepatic
Abdominal pain (15%)
Diarrhea (16%) [4]
Hepatotoxicity / liver injury / acute liver injury / drug-induced liver injury (DILI) [5]
Nausea (24%) [12]
Pancreatitis / acute pancreatitis [4]
Vomiting (24%) [2]

Genitourinary
Urinary tract infection [2]

Hematologic
Anemia (14%) [44]
Hemotoxicity [2]
Leukocytopenia (leukopenia) / leukocytes (white blood cells) decreased [6]
Lymphopenia (lymphocytopenia) / lymphocytes decreased (14%) [3]
Neutropenia (neutrophils decreased) (21%) [20]
Sepsis [2]
Thrombocytopenia / platelets decreased (5%) [16]

Local
Injection-site pain (2%)
Injection-site reaction (22%) [4]

Neuromuscular/Skeletal
Arthralgia (28%) [2]
Asthenia / fatigue (56%) [24]
Back pain (9%)
Myalgia/Myopathy (38–42%) [4]

Ocular
Retinopathy [7]
Vision blurred (4%)

Otic
Hearing loss (hypoacusis) [2]
Tinnitus [2]

Renal
Nephrotoxicity / kidney injury / acute kidney injury (AKI) / drug-induced kidney injury [4]

Respiratory
Cough (6%)
Dyspnea / shortness of breath (13%) [2]
Influenza- ('flu)-like syndrome (46%) [11]
Pneumonitis [2]

Other
Adverse effects / adverse reactions [27]
Death [2]
Infection (3%) [4]

PEGAPTANIB

Trade name: Macugen (Valeant)
Indications: Neovascular (wet) age-related macular degeneration
Class: Angiogenesis inhibitor / antiangiogenic agent, Vascular endothelial growth factor (VEGF) inhibitor / antagonist
Half-life: 6–14 days
Clinically important, potentially hazardous interactions with: none known
Important contra-indications noted in the prescribing guidelines for: nursing mothers; pediatric patients
Note: Contra-indicated in patients with ocular or periocular infections.

Skin
Dermatitis (<5%)

Cardiovascular
Arterial occlusion (carotid) (<5%)
Chest pain (<5%)
Hypertension (10–40%)
Myocardial ischemia (transient) (<5%)

Central Nervous System
Headache (6–10%)
Ischemic injury (transient) (<5%)
Stroke / cerebrovascular accident (<5%)
Vertigo / dizziness (<10%)

Endocrine/Metabolic
Diabetes mellitus (<5%)

Gastrointestinal/Hepatic
Diarrhea (6–10%)
Nausea (6–10%)
Vomiting (<5%)

Genitourinary
Urinary retention (<5%)
Urinary tract infection (6–10%)

Neuromuscular/Skeletal
Arthralgia (<5%)

Ocular
Blepharitis (6–10%)
Cataract (10–40%) [2]
Conjunctival edema (<5%)
Conjunctival hemorrhage (10–40%)
Conjunctivitis (conjunctival inflammation) (<10%)
Corneal abnormalities (<5%)
Corneal deposits (<5%)
Corneal edema (10–40%)
Endophthalmitis (<5%) [4]
Eyelid irritation (<5%)
Intraocular pressure increased (10–40%)
Meibomianitis (<5%)
Mydriasis (<5%)
Ocular edema (eye edema) (<5%)
Ocular hypertension (10–40%)
Ocular inflammation (<5%) [2]
Ocular pain (10–40%)
Ocular stinging (10–40%)
Ophthalmitis (<5%)
Periorbital hematoma (<5%)
Photopsia (6–10%)
Punctate keratitis (10–40%)
Reduced visual acuity (10–40%)
Retinal detachment (<10%) [5]
Retinal edema (<5%)
Vision blurred (10–40%)
Visual disturbances (10–40%)
Vitreous floaters / floaters / myodesopsia / myiodesopsia / muscae volitantes (10–40%)

Otic
Hearing loss (hypoacusis) (<5%)
Otitis (otitis externa, otitis media, otitis interna) (<5%)

Respiratory
Bronchitis (6–10%)
Pleural effusion (<5%)

PEGINESATIDE

Trade name: Omontys (Affymax)
Indications: Anemia due to chronic kidney disease in adult patients on dialysis
Class: Erythropoiesis-stimulating agent (ESA)
Half-life: 17–33 hours (following intravenous administration)
Clinically important, potentially hazardous interactions with: none known
Important contra-indications noted in the prescribing guidelines for: nursing mothers; pediatric patients
Note: Contra-indicated in patients with uncontrolled hypertension.
This drug has been recalled.
Warning: ERYTHROPOIESIS-STIMULATING AGENTS (ESAs) INCREASE THE RISK OF DEATH, MYOCARDIAL INFARCTION, STROKE, VENOUS THROMBOEMBOLISM, THROMBOSIS OF VASCULAR ACCESS AND TUMOR PROGRESSION OR RECURRENCE

Cardiovascular
Hypertension (13%) [3]
Hypotension (14%) [2]

Central Nervous System
Fever (pyrexia) (includes hyperpyrexia) (12%)
Headache (15%) [3]
Vertigo / dizziness [3]

Endocrine/Metabolic
Hyperkalemia (11%)

Gastrointestinal/Hepatic
Constipation [2]
Diarrhea (18%) [2]
Nausea (17%) [3]
Vomiting (15%) [2]

Local
Infusion-site reactions (11–16%)

Neuromuscular/Skeletal
Arthralgia (11%) [2]
Back pain (11%)
Muscle spasm (15%)
Pain in extremities (11%)

Respiratory
Cough (16%) [2]
Dyspnea / shortness of breath (18%)
Upper respiratory tract infection (11%) [2]

Other
Adverse effects / adverse reactions [3]

PEGVISOMANT

Trade name: Somavert (Pfizer)
Indications: Acromegaly
Class: Growth hormone analog
Half-life: 6 days
Clinically important, potentially hazardous interactions with: acarbose, exenatide, hydromorphone, insulin, latex, metformin, opioids, oral hypoglycemics, pioglitazone, saxagliptin, tapentadol

Important contra-indications noted in the prescribing guidelines for: the elderly; nursing mothers; pediatric patients

---

Skin
Lipohypertrophy (<5%) [2]
Peripheral edema (4–8%)

Cardiovascular
Chest pain (4–8%)
Hypertension (8%)

Central Nervous System
Pain (4–14%)
Paresthesias (7%)
Vertigo / dizziness (4–8%)

Gastrointestinal/Hepatic
Diarrhea (4–14%)
Hepatitis [2]
Hepatotoxicity / liver injury / acute liver injury / drug-induced liver injury (DILI) [6]
Nausea (8–14%)

Local
Injection-site reaction (8–11%) [4]

Neuromuscular/Skeletal
Back pain (4–8%)

Respiratory
Influenza- ('flu)-like syndrome (4–12%)
Sinusitis (see also rhinitis / rhinosinusitis) (4–8%)

Other
Adverse effects / adverse reactions [4]
Infection (23%)

PEMBROLIZUMAB

Synonym: Lambrolizumab
Trade name: Keytruda (Merck Sharpe & Dohme)
Indications: Unresectable or metastatic melanoma and disease progression following ipilimumab and, if BRAF V600 mutation positive, a BRAF inhibitor
Class: Antineoplastic / anticancer agent (see also Immune checkpoint inhibitor), Immune checkpoint inhibitor (incl. programmed death receptor-1 (PD-1) inhibitor), Monoclonal antibody
Half-life: 26 days
Clinically important, potentially hazardous interactions with: none known
Important contra-indications noted in the prescribing guidelines for: nursing mothers; pediatric patients

---

Skin
Bullous pemphigoid / pemphigoid [21]
Cutaneous toxicity / skin toxicity [7]
Dermatitis [6]
Dermatomyositis [5]
Eczema / eczematous reaction / eczematous eruption [2]
Edema / fluid retention [2]
Eosinophilic fasciitis (Shulman syndrome / Shulman disease) [5]
Erythema [3]
Erythema multiforme [3]
Exanthems [4]
Granuloma annulare [2]
Keratoacanthoma (Grzybowski syndrome) [2]
Lichen planus (includes hypertrophic lichen planus) [7]
Lichen planus pemphigoides [7]
Lichenoid dermatitis [4]
Lichenoid eruption / lichenoid reaction [7]
Lipodystrophy / acquired generalized lipodystrophy [6]
Lupus erythematosus (subacute cutaneous lupus erythematosus (SCLE)) [3]
Maculopapular rash / morbilliform rash [2]
Morphea / localized scleroderma [4]
Panniculitis [2]
Peripheral edema (17%)
Pruritus (itching) (30%) [21]
Psoriasiform dermatitis [3]
Psoriasis [9]
Radiation recall dermatitis [4]
Rash (29%) [26]
Sarcoidosis / sarcoid-like reaction (cutaneous sarcoidosis) [12]
Scleroderma [8]
Stevens-Johnson syndrome and toxic epidermal necrolysis (SJS/TEN) [20]
Transient acantholytic dermatosis (Grover's disease) [2]
Vasculitis (angiitis) / cutaneous vasculitis (angiitis) [5]
Vitiligo (11%) [14]

Hair
Alopecia / hair loss [2]
Alopecia areata [3]
Lichen planopilaris [2]

Mucosal
Mucositis [2]
Mucous membrane pemphigoid [3]
Sjögren's syndrome (see also sicca syndrome) [3]
Stomatitis (oral mucositis) [4]
Xerostomia (dry mouth) [2]

Cardiovascular
Aortitis / periaortitis [3]
Atrioventricular block [2]
Capillary leak syndrome [3]
Cardiac tamponade / pericardial tamponade [8]
Cardiotoxicity [4]
Hypertension [4]
Myocarditis [24]
Myocarditis, myositis and myasthenia gravis overlap syndrome (Triple-M Syndrome / 3M Syndrome) [9]
Pericardial effusion [3]
Takotsubo syndrome [4]

Central Nervous System
Antiphospholipid antibody syndrome [3]
Aseptic meningitis [4]
Chills (14%)
Cranial neuropathy (includes types of palsy) [2]
Encephalitis [16]
Encephalopathy (includes hepatic encephalopathy) [4]
Fever (pyrexia) (includes hyperpyrexia) (11%) [6]
Guillain-Barré syndrome / acute inflammatory demyelinating polyradiculoneuropathy / acute motor axonal neuropathy [5]
Headache (16%) [3]
Insomnia (14%)
Leukoencephalopathy / posterior reversible encephalopathy syndrome (PRES) [3]
Meningoencephalitis [2]
Myelitis / myeloradiculitis [3]
Neurological adverse effect / neurological deficit [2]
Neuromyelitis optica [2]
Neurotoxicity [3]
Pain [2]
Peripheral neuropathy [6]
Seizures [2]
Vertigo / dizziness (11%)

Endocrine/Metabolic
Adrenal insufficiency (hypoadrenalism) / Addisonian crisis (includes Addison's disease) [13]
Adrenocorticotropic hormone (corticotropin; ACTH) deficiency [5]
ALT increased [10]
Appetite decreased (26%) [11]
AST increased (24%) [7]
Diabetes mellitus [16]
Diabetic ketoacidosis [8]
Endocrine-related adverse effect / endocrinopathy [2]
Hyperlipasemia [2]
Hyperthyroidism (includes 'thyroid storm') [11]
Hypertransaminasemia (hepatic transaminitis) / elevated transaminases [2]
Hypertriglyceridemia (includes triglycerides increased) (25%) [4]
Hypoalbuminemia / albumin decreased (34%)
Hypocalcemia (24%)
Hyponatremia (35%) [6]
Hypophysitis [19]
Hypothyroidism (8%) [31]
Thyroid dysfunction [6]
Thyroiditis [10]
Thyrotoxicosis [2]

Gastrointestinal/Hepatic
Abdominal pain (12%) [2]
Cholangiopathy [2]
Cholangitis / sclerosing cholangitis [8]
Colitis [25]
Constipation (21%)
Diarrhea (20%) [25]
Duodenitis [3]
Enteritis [3]
Gastritis / pangastritis / gastric irritation [9]
Gastrointestinal perforation / perforated colon / gastric perforation [2]
Hemorrhagic gastritis [4]
Hepatitis [20]
Hepatotoxicity / liver injury / acute liver injury / drug-induced liver injury (DILI) [7]
Intestinal pseudo-obstruction (Ogilvie syndrome) [3]
Nausea (30%) [14]
Pancreatic insufficiency [3]
Pancreatitis / acute pancreatitis [18]
Peptic ulceration (includes duodenal ulcer, esophageal ulcer) [2]
Vomiting (16%) [3]

Hematologic
Agranulocytosis / severe selective neutropenia [4]
Anemia (14–55%) [8]
Aplastic anemia [2]
Eosinophilia / eosinophils increased [2]
Hemolytic anemia [6]
Hemophagocytic lymphohistiocytosis / hemophagocytic syndrome [9]
Lymphopenia (lymphocytopenia) / lymphocytes decreased [3]
Neutropenia (neutrophils decreased) [10]
Pancytopenia (includes bicytopenia) [3]
Pure red cell aplasia [4]
Sepsis (<10%) [2]

Thrombocytopenia / platelets decreased [10]

Local

Infusion-related reactions [3]

Neuromuscular/Skeletal

Arthralgia (20%) [12]
Asthenia / fatigue (47%) [34]
Back pain (12%)
Inflammatory arthritis [5]
Lambert-Eaton myasthenic syndrome [2]
Myalgia/Myopathy (14%) [25]
Myasthenia gravis [29]
Necrotizing myopathy / immune-mediated necrotizing myopathy [2]
Pain in extremities (18%)
Psoriatic arthralgia / psoriatic arthritis [2]

Ocular

Eyelid ptosis / blepharoptosis [3]
Hypotony [2]
Iridocyclitis [2]
Ocular adverse effect [2]
Ocular myasthenia gravis [8]
Optic neuritis / papillitis [2]
Orbital (ocular) myositis [3]
Uveitis / anterior uveitis / posterior uveitis / panuveitis [8]

Renal

Glomerulonephritis (includes membranous nephropathy) [4]
Nephritis / interstitial nephritis / tubulointerstitial nephritis [2]
Nephrotoxicity / kidney injury / acute kidney injury (AKI) / drug-induced kidney injury [9]
Renal failure [3]

Respiratory

Asthma [2]
Cough (30%) [6]
Dyspnea / shortness of breath (18%) [4]
Eosinophilic pneumonia [2]
Interstitial lung disease / interstitial pneumonitis / interstitial pneumonia (cryptogenic organizing pneumonia) / drug-induced interstitial lung disease [3]
Pneumonia [8]
Pneumonitis (3%) [32]
Pulmonary fibrosis [2]
Pulmonary sarcoidosis [3]
Rhinitis / rhinosinusitis (see also sinusitis) [2]
Upper respiratory tract infection (11%)

Other

Adverse effects / adverse reactions [34]
Cytokine release syndrome / cytokine storm [8]
Death [29]
Immune-related adverse effect [3]
Infection [2]
Remitting seronegative symmetrical synovitis with pitting edema syndrome [2]
Side effects [3]
Vogt-Koyanagi-Harada syndrome [3]

PEMETREXED

Trade name: Alimta (Lilly)
Indications: Non-squamous non-small cell lung cancer, mesothelioma (in combination with cisplatin)
Class: Antimetabolite, Folic acid antagonist
Half-life: 3.5 hours
Clinically important, potentially hazardous interactions with: clozapine, digoxin, leflunomide, meloxicam, natalizumab, nephrotoxic drugs, NSAIDs, phenytoin, pimecrolimus, probenecid, pyrimethamine, sipuleucel-T, tacrolimus, trastuzumab, vaccines
Important contra-indications noted in the prescribing guidelines for: nursing mothers; pediatric patients

---

Skin

AGEP [4]
Anaphylactoid reactions / anaphylaxis (includes anaphylactic shock) [2]
Cellulitis and pseudocellulitis [6]
Cutaneous toxicity / skin toxicity [2]
Desquamation (10–14%)
Edema / fluid retention (<5%)
Erythema multiforme (<5%)
Hypersensitivity (<5%)
Peripheral edema [4]
Pruritus (itching) (<7%)
Radiation recall dermatitis [7]
Rash (10–14%) [22]
Stevens-Johnson syndrome and toxic epidermal necrolysis (SJS/TEN) [5]
Urticaria / hives [3]
Vasculitis (angiitis) / cutaneous vasculitis (angiitis) [2]

Hair

Alopecia / hair loss (<6%) [5]

Mucosal

Epistaxis (nosebleed) [2]
Mucositis (7%) [6]
Stomatitis (oral mucositis) (7–15%) [6]

Cardiovascular

Hypertension [8]
Venous thromboembolism [2]

Central Nervous System

Anorexia (19–22%) [9]
Depression (14%)
Dysgeusia (taste perversion) [2]
Fever (pyrexia) (includes hyperpyrexia) (<8%) [2]
Headache [4]
Insomnia [2]
Neurotoxicity (<9%)
Peripheral neuropathy [3]

Endocrine/Metabolic

ALT increased (8–10%) [4]
Appetite decreased [6]
AST increased (7–8%) [4]
Creatine phosphokinase (CPK) / creatine kinase increased (hyperCKemia) (<5%) [3]
Hyperglycemia (includes glucose increased) [2]
Hyperkalemia [2]
Hypokalemia [2]
Hypomagnesemia [3]
Hyponatremia [3]

Gastrointestinal/Hepatic

Abdominal pain (<5%)
Constipation (<6%) [5]
Diarrhea (5–13%) [13]
Gastrointestinal disorder / discomfort [2]
Hepatotoxicity / liver injury / acute liver injury / drug-induced liver injury (DILI) [7]
Nausea (19–31%) [20]
Vomiting (9–16%) [10]

Hematologic

Anemia (15–19%) [26]
Febrile neutropenia (<5%) [12]
Hemotoxicity [4]
Leukocytopenia (leukopenia) / leukocytes (white blood cells) decreased (6–12%) [15]
Lymphopenia (lymphocytopenia) / lymphocytes decreased [3]
Myelosuppression / bone marrow suppression / myelotoxicity [4]
Neutropenia (neutrophils decreased) (6–11%) [27]
Pancytopenia (includes bicytopenia) [2]
Sepsis [2]
Thrombocytopenia / platelets decreased (<8%) [18]
Thrombotic complications [2]

Neuromuscular/Skeletal

Asthenia / fatigue (25–34%) [34]

Ocular

Conjunctivitis (conjunctival inflammation) (<5%)
Eyelid edema / palpebral edema / blepharedema [3]
Lacrimation (<5%)

Renal

Nephrogenic diabetes insipidus / arginine vasopressin resistance [2]
Nephrotoxicity / kidney injury / acute kidney injury (AKI) / drug-induced kidney injury [4]
Proteinuria [2]
Renal failure [2]

Respiratory

Cough [2]
Dysphonia (includes voice disorders / voice changes) [2]
Dyspnea / shortness of breath [4]
Hemoptysis [2]
Pharyngitis (sore throat) (15%)
Pneumonia [2]
Pneumonitis [2]
Pulmonary toxicity [2]

Other

Adverse effects / adverse reactions (53%) [16]
Allergic reactions (<5%)
Death [5]
Hiccups / singultus [2]
Infection (<5%) [7]

PEMIGATINIB

Trade name: Pemazyre (Incyte)
Indications: Unresectable locally advanced or metastatic cholangiocarcinoma with a fibroblast growth factor receptor 2 (FGFR2) fusion or other rearrangement
Class: Fibroblast growth factor receptor inhibitor, Kinase inhibitor
Half-life: 15.4 hours
Clinically important, potentially hazardous interactions with: CYP3A inducers, CYP3A inhibitors, itraconazole, rifampin
Pregnancy category: Can cause fetal harm. Advise patients of reproductive potential of the potential risk to the fetus and use effective contraception.
Note: Pemigatinib can cause retinal pigment epithelial detachment. Perform ophthalmological examination including optical coherence tomography prior to initiation of therapy, every 2 months for the first 6 months of treatment and every 3 months thereafter, and urgently at any time for visual symptoms.

Skin

Dry skin (20%)
Hand–foot syndrome (palmar–plantar erythrodysesthesia) (15%)
Peripheral edema (18%)

Hair
Alopecia / hair loss (49%)
Nails
Nail toxicity (43%)
Mucosal
Stomatitis (oral mucositis) (35%)
Xerostomia (dry mouth) (34%)
Central Nervous System
Dysgeusia (taste perversion) (40%)
Headache (16%)
Endocrine/Metabolic
ALP increased (41%)
ALT increased (43%)
Appetite decreased (33%)
AST increased (43%)
Dehydration (15%)
Hyperbilirubinemia (26%)
Hypercalcemia (43%)
Hyperglycemia (includes glucose increased) (36%)
Hyperkalemia (12%)
Hyperphosphatemia (60%) [3]
Hyperuricemia (30%)
Hypoalbuminemia / albumin decreased (34%)
Hypocalcemia (17%)
Hypoglycemia (11%)
Hypokalemia (26%)
Hyponatremia (39%)
Hypophosphatemia (23%)
Serum creatinine increased (41%)
Weight loss (16%)
Gastrointestinal/Hepatic
Abdominal pain (23%)
Constipation (35%)
Diarrhea (47%) [2]
Nausea (40%)
Vomiting (27%)
Genitourinary
Urinary tract infection (16%)
Hematologic
Hemoglobin decreased (43%)
Leukocytopenia (leukopenia) / leukocytes (white blood cells) decreased (18%)
Leukocytosis (elevated white blood cell (WBC) count) (27%)
Lymphopenia (lymphocytopenia) / lymphocytes decreased (36%)
Thrombocytopenia / platelets decreased (28%)
Neuromuscular/Skeletal
Arthralgia (25%)
Asthenia / fatigue (42%) [2]
Back pain (20%)
Pain in extremities (19%)
Ocular
Dry eye (keratoconjunctivitis sicca) (35%)
Retinopathy [2]
Serous retinopathy [2]

PEMIROLAST

Trade name: Alamast (Johnson & Johnson)
Indications: Pruritus of allergic conjunctivitis
Class: Mast cell stabilizer
Half-life: 4.5 hours
Clinically important, potentially hazardous interactions with: none known

---

Neuromuscular/Skeletal
Back pain (<5%)
Ocular
Ocular stinging (<5%)
Respiratory
Influenza- ('flu)-like syndrome (10–25%)

PEMOLINE

Trade name: Cylert (AbbVie)
Indications: Attention deficit disorder, narcolepsy
Class: Amphetamine
Half-life: 9–14 hours
Clinically important, potentially hazardous interactions with: pimozide
Note: This drug has been withdrawn.

Skin
Rash (>10%)
Central Nervous System
Choreoathetosis [7]
Tic disorder [2]
Tourette's syndrome [3]
Gastrointestinal/Hepatic
Hepatotoxicity / liver injury / acute liver injury / drug-induced liver injury (DILI) [18]

PENBUTOLOL

Trade name: Levatol (Schwarz)
Indications: Hypertension
Class: Adrenergic beta-receptor antagonist
Half-life: 5 hours
Clinically important, potentially hazardous interactions with: clonidine, epinephrine, verapamil
Note: Cutaneous side effects of beta-receptor blockers are clinically polymorphous. They apparently appear after several months of continuous therapy.

Skin
Diaphoresis (2%)
Exanthems (<5%)
Flushing / rubefaction (<5%)
Other
Allergic reactions (<5%)

PENICILLAMINE

Trade name: Depen (MedPointe)
Indications: Wilson's disease, rheumatoid arthritis
Class: Antidote, Chelator, Disease-modifying antirheumatic drug (DMARD)
Half-life: 1.7–3.2 hours
Clinically important, potentially hazardous interactions with: aluminum, antacids, ascorbic acid, bone marrow suppressants, chloroquine, clozapine, cytotoxic agents, diclofenac, ferrous sulfate, food, gold & gold compounds, hydroxychloroquine, iron, magnesium, meloxicam, primaquine, probenecid, sodium picosulfate
Important contra-indications noted in the prescribing guidelines for: nursing mothers; pediatric patients
Note: In the treatment of Wilson's disease, it is sometimes difficult to differentiate side effects due to the drug from those due to the effects of the disease.

Skin
Bullous dermatosis [3]
Bullous pemphigoid / pemphigoid [6]
Cicatricial pemphigoid [2]
Cutis laxa / elastolysis [14]
Dermatitis [4]
Dermatomyositis [14]
Edema of lip (<10%)
Ehlers–Danlos syndrome [2]
Elastosis perforans serpiginosa [45]
Epidermolysis bullosa [4]
Epidermolysis bullosa acquisita [2]
Erythema multiforme (<5%)
Exanthems [8]
Hypersensitivity [3]
Lichen planus (includes hypertrophic lichen planus) [4]
Lichenoid eruption / lichenoid reaction [7]
Lupus erythematosus (subacute cutaneous lupus erythematosus (SCLE)) [44]
Morphea / localized scleroderma [2]
Pemphigus [76]
Pemphigus erythematodes (pemphigus erythematosus) (Senear-Usher syndrome) (Senear–Usher) [10]
Pemphigus foliaceus [16]
Pemphigus herpetiformis [3]
Pemphigus vulgaris [2]
Penicillamine-induced degenerative dermopathy [3]
Peripheral edema (<10%)
Pruritus (itching) (44–50%) [2]
Pseudoxanthoma elasticum [16]
Psoriasis [4]
Purpura [5]
Rash (44–50%) [6]
Scleroderma [7]
Skin fragility [2]
Stevens-Johnson syndrome and toxic epidermal necrolysis (SJS/TEN) [4]
Urticaria / hives (44–50%) [2]
Vasculitis (angiitis) / cutaneous vasculitis (angiitis) [7]
Hair
Alopecia / hair loss [3]
Hirsutism [2]
Nails
Yellow nail syndrome [3]
Mucosal
Aphthous stomatitis / aphthous ulcer / aphtha (aphthae) [2]
Mucosal lesions (pemphigus-like) [2]
Oral ulceration [5]
Stomatitis (oral mucositis) [6]
Central Nervous System
Ageusia (taste loss) / taste disorder (12%) [2]
Dysgeusia (taste perversion) (metallic taste) [8]
Hypogeusia (25–33%) [2]
Endocrine/Metabolic
Gynecomastia [5]
Gastrointestinal/Hepatic
Hepatotoxicity / liver injury / acute liver injury / drug-induced liver injury (DILI) [3]
Hematologic
Hemotoxicity [2]
Myelosuppression / bone marrow suppression / myelotoxicity [3]
Neuromuscular/Skeletal
Dystonia [3]
Myasthenia gravis [75]
Polymyositis [8]

Ocular
Ocular myasthenia gravis [2]

Renal
Glomerulonephritis (includes membranous nephropathy) [3]
Nephrotoxicity / kidney injury / acute kidney injury (AKI) / drug-induced kidney injury [5]
Proteinuria [2]

Respiratory
Pulmonary toxicity [2]

Other
Adverse effects / adverse reactions [2]
Death [2]

PENICILLIN G

Trade name: Crystapen (Britannia)
Indications: Anthrax, cellulitis, endocarditis, infections, otitis media, rheumatic fever, respiratory infections, septicemia
Class: Antibiotic, Antibiotic; beta-lactam, Antibiotic; penicillin, Antimicrobial
Half-life: 4 hours
Clinically important, potentially hazardous interactions with: estrogens, imipenem/cilastatin, imipenem/cilastatin, methotrexate, minocycline, phenindione, probenecid, sulfinpyrazone, warfarin
Important contra-indications noted in the prescribing guidelines for: nursing mothers

---

Skin
Anaphylactoid reactions / anaphylaxis (includes anaphylactic shock) [5]
Dermatitis [2]
Hypersensitivity [4]
Jarisch–Herxheimer reaction [22]
Nicolau syndrome [2]
Rash [4]
Serum sickness-like reaction [2]

Central Nervous System
Seizures [2]

Gastrointestinal/Hepatic
Hepatotoxicity / liver injury / acute liver injury / drug-induced liver injury (DILI) [2]

Genitourinary
Cystitis (includes interstitial cystitis / bladder pain syndrome) [4]

Hematologic
Thrombosis [2]

Renal
Nephrotoxicity / kidney injury / acute kidney injury (AKI) / drug-induced kidney injury [2]

Other
Hoigne's syndrome [16]

PENICILLIN V

Trade name: V-cillin K (Lilly)
Indications: Cellulitis, endocarditis, erysipelas, oral infections, otitis media, rheumatic fever, scarlet fever, tonsillitis
Class: Antibiotic, Antibiotic; beta-lactam, Antibiotic; penicillin, Antimicrobial
Half-life: 4 hours
Clinically important, potentially hazardous interactions with: estrogens, imipenem/cilastatin, methotrexate, minocycline, neomycin, phenindione, probenecid, sulfinpyrazone, warfarin

---

Skin
Anaphylactoid reactions / anaphylaxis (includes anaphylactic shock) [2]
DRESS syndrome (Drug-induced hypersensitivity syndrome) [2]
Hypersensitivity [3]
Serum sickness [2]
Serum sickness-like reaction [2]
Urticaria / hives [3]

Central Nervous System
Fever (pyrexia) (includes hyperpyrexia) [3]

Gastrointestinal/Hepatic
Diarrhea [2]

Neuromuscular/Skeletal
Arthralgia [2]

PENTAMIDINE

Trade names: NebuPent (Astellas), Pentacarinat (Sanofi-Aventis), Pentam 300 (Astellas)
Indications: *Pneumocystis jiroveci* infection, trypanosomiasis, leishmaniasis
Class: Antimicrobial, Antiprotozoal
Half-life: 9.1–13.2 hours (intramuscular); 6.5 hours (intravenous)
Clinically important, potentially hazardous interactions with: adefovir, aminoglycosides, amiodarone, amisulpride, amitriptyline, amphotericin B, cisplatin, droperidol, erythromycin, foscarnet, insulin aspart, insulin degludec, insulin detemir, insulin glargine, insulin glulisine, ivabradine, levomepromazine, moxifloxacin, phenothiazines, saquinavir, sparfloxacin, sulpiride / levosulpiride, tricyclic antidepressants, trifluoperazine, vancomycin
Important contra-indications noted in the prescribing guidelines for: nursing mothers; pediatric patients
Note: The rate of adverse side effects is increased in patients with AIDS.

Skin
Exanthems (<15%) [10]
Pruritus (itching) [2]
Rash (<47%) [4]
Stevens-Johnson syndrome and toxic epidermal necrolysis (SJS/TEN) [3]
Urticaria / hives [3]

Cardiovascular
QT interval prolonged / QT prolongation [8]
Torsades de pointes [4]

Central Nervous System
Dysgeusia (taste perversion) (metallic taste) (2%)
Paresthesias [2]
Vertigo / dizziness [2]

Gastrointestinal/Hepatic
Pancreatitis / acute pancreatitis [6]

Local
Injection-site irritation [2]
Injection-site pain [2]
Injection-site reaction (>10%)

Neuromuscular/Skeletal
Myalgia/Myopathy (<5%)
Rhabdomyolysis [4]

Other
Adverse effects / adverse reactions [6]

PENTAZOCINE

Trade name: Talwin (Hospira)
Indications: Pain
Class: Opiate agonist
Half-life: 2–3 hours
Clinically important, potentially hazardous interactions with: cimetidine, hydrocodone, hydromorphone, morphine, oliceridine, oxymorphone, tapentadol

---

Skin
Rash (<10%)
Scleroderma [2]
Sclerosis [3]
Stevens-Johnson syndrome and toxic epidermal necrolysis (SJS/TEN) [2]
Ulcerations [9]

Mucosal
Xerostomia (dry mouth) (<10%)

Central Nervous System
Hallucinations [2]

Local
Injection-site calcification [2]
Injection-site granuloma [3]
Injection-site induration [8]

Neuromuscular/Skeletal
Fibromyalgia [2]

PENTOBARBITAL

Indications: Insomnia, sedation
Class: Barbiturate
Half-life: 15–50 hours
Clinically important, potentially hazardous interactions with: alcohol, anticoagulants, antihistamines, brompheniramine, buclizine, chlorpheniramine, dicumarol, ethanolamine, imatinib, nalbuphine, pizotifen, warfarin

---

Skin
Lupus erythematosus (subacute cutaneous lupus erythematosus (SCLE)) [2]

Local
Injection-site pain (<10%)

PENTOSAN

Synonym: PPS
Trade name: Elmiron (Ortho-McNeil)
Indications: Bladder pain, interstitial cystitis
Class: Analgesic; urinary
Half-life: 4.8 hours
Clinically important, potentially hazardous interactions with: abciximab, argatroban, cilostazol, clopidogrel, dabigatran, meloxicam, tinzaparin

---

Skin
Rash (<10%)

Hair
Alopecia / hair loss (<10%)

Ocular
Maculopathy [3]

PENTOSTATIN

Synonym: deoxycoformycin
Trade name: Nipent (SuperGen)
Indications: Hairy-cell leukemia
Class: Antimetabolite, Antineoplastic / anticancer agent (see also Immune checkpoint inhibitor)
Half-life: 5–15 hours
Clinically important, potentially hazardous interactions with: aldesleukin, clofazimine, cyclophosphamide, fludarabine, nelarabine

---

Skin
- Acneiform eruption / acneiform dermatitis / acneiform rash (<3%)
- Anaphylactoid reactions / anaphylaxis (includes anaphylactic shock) (<3%)
- Bruise / bruising / contusion / ecchymosis (ecchymoses) (3–10%)
- Bullous dermatosis (3–10%)
- Candidiasis / candidosis (<3%)
- Cutaneous toxicity / skin toxicity [2]
- Diaphoresis (3–10%)
- Eczema / eczematous reaction / eczematous eruption (3–10%)
- Exanthems (3–10%) [2]
- Exfoliative dermatitis (<3%)
- Facial edema (<3%)
- Flushing / rubefaction (<3%)
- Herpes simplex (3–10%)
- Herpes zoster (3–10%) [3]
- Peripheral edema (3–10%)
- Petechiae (3–10%)
- Photosensitivity (<3%)
- Pigmentation (Skin) (includes hyperpigmentation) (3–10%)
- Pruritus (itching) (3–10%)
- Psoriasis (<3%)
- Purpura (<3%)
- Rash (26%) [2]
- Recall reaction [2]
- Seborrhea (3–10%)
- Xerosis / xeroderma (3–10%)

Hair
- Alopecia / hair loss (<3%)

Mucosal
- Gingivitis (<3%)
- Leukoplakia (<3%)
- Stomatitis (oral mucositis) (<10%)

Cardiovascular
- Thrombophlebitis (3–10%)

Central Nervous System
- Dysgeusia (taste perversion) (<3%)
- Fever (pyrexia) (includes hyperpyrexia) [5]
- Paresthesias (3–10%)

Endocrine/Metabolic
- Gynecomastia (<3%)

Gastrointestinal/Hepatic
- Hepatotoxicity / liver injury / acute liver injury / drug-induced liver injury (DILI) [4]

Genitourinary
- Vaginitis (includes vulvitis) (<3%)

Hematologic
- Hemolytic uremic syndrome [2]

Local
- Injection-site bleeding (<3%)
- Injection-site inflammation (<3%)

Neuromuscular/Skeletal
- Myalgia/Myopathy (>10%)

Other
- Adverse effects / adverse reactions (17%)
- Allergic reactions (>10%)
- Infection [6]

PENTOXIFYLLINE

Trade names: Pentoxil (Upsher-Smith), Trental (Sanofi-Aventis)
Indications: Peripheral vascular disease, intermittent claudication
Class: Vasodilator, peripheral, Xanthine alkaloid
Half-life: 0.4–0.8 hours
Clinically important, potentially hazardous interactions with: abciximab, benazepril, captopril, ceftobiprole, cilostazol, ciprofloxacin, citalopram, clevidipine, clopidogrel, diclofenac, enalapril, eptifibatide, fosinopril, insulin degludec, insulin glargine, insulin glulisine, irbesartan, lisinopril, meloxicam, olmesartan, quinapril, ramipril, tinzaparin

---

Skin
- Flushing / rubefaction (2%) [2]

Mucosal
- Xerostomia (dry mouth) [2]

PEPPERMINT

Family: Labiatae
Scientific name: *Mentha piperita*
Indications: Dyspepsia, regress pancreatic, mammary, and liver tumors, irritable bowel syndrome, colonic spasm, colic, nausea, vomiting, biliary disorders, common cold, dysmenorrhoea, anxiolytic. **Topical:** pain, itching, inflammations, headaches, toothache, pruritus, urticaria, mosquito repellant. **Vapor:** bronchial catarrh, fever, influenza. Flavoring, cosmetics, toothpaste, mouthwash
Class: Analgesic, Antiemetic, Carminative, Vasodilator, peripheral
Half-life: N/A
Clinically important, potentially hazardous interactions with: cisapride

---

Skin
- Burning / skin burning sensation (anal) [3]
- Contact dermatitis [5]
- Dermatitis [5]
- Hypersensitivity [2]
- Sensitivity [2]

Mucosal
- Cheilitis (inflammation of the lips) [3]
- Oral ulceration [2]
- Stomatitis (oral mucositis) [2]

Gastrointestinal/Hepatic
- Dyspepsia / functional dyspepsia (indigestion) (see also gastroparesis) [3]
- Hepatotoxicity / liver injury / acute liver injury / drug-induced liver injury (DILI) [2]
- Nausea [2]
- Vomiting [2]

Other
- Adverse effects / adverse reactions [6]
- Allergic reactions [2]
- Side effects [3]

PERAMIVIR

Trade name: Rapivab (BioCryst)
Indications: Influenza
Class: Antiviral, Neuraminidase inhibitor
Half-life: ~20 hours
Clinically important, potentially hazardous interactions with: live attenuated influenza vaccine
Important contra-indications noted in the prescribing guidelines for: nursing mothers; pediatric patients

---

Skin
- Rash [2]

Cardiovascular
- Hypertension (2%)

Central Nervous System
- Behavioral disturbances / personality changes [2]
- Insomnia (3%)

Endocrine/Metabolic
- ALT increased (3%)
- AST increased (3%)
- Creatine phosphokinase (CPK) / creatine kinase increased (hyperCKemia) (4%)
- Hyperglycemia (includes glucose increased) (5%)

Gastrointestinal/Hepatic
- Constipation (4%)
- Diarrhea (8%) [6]
- Nausea [4]
- Vomiting [4]

Hematologic
- Leukocytopenia (leukopenia) / leukocytes (white blood cells) decreased [2]
- Neutropenia (neutrophils decreased) (8%) [4]
- Thrombocytopenia / platelets decreased [2]

PERAMPANEL

Trade name: Fycompa (Eisai)
Indications: Partial-onset seizures, primary generalized tonic-clonic seizures
Class: AMPA glutamate receptor antagonist, Anticonvulsant (see also antiepileptic (anti-seizure)), Antiepileptic (anti-seizure)
Half-life: ~105 hours
Clinically important, potentially hazardous interactions with: alcohol, carbamazepine, oral contraceptives, oxcarbazepine, phenobarbital, phenytoin, primidone, rifampin, St John's wort
Important contra-indications noted in the prescribing guidelines for: the elderly; nursing mothers; pediatric patients
Warning: SERIOUS PSYCHIATRIC AND BEHAVIORAL REACTIONS

Skin
- Peripheral edema (<2%)
- Rash [2]

Mucosal
- Oropharyngeal pain (2%)

Central Nervous System
- Aggression (includes anger) (<3%) [15]
- Anxiety (2–4%) [2]
- Balance disorder (<5%) [2]
- Behavioral disturbances / personality changes [9]
- Cognitive impairment [2]

Confusion (<2%) [2]
Depression [3]
Dysarthria (<4%)
Euphoria / elation (<2%)
Fall [3]
Gait instability / postural instability (<4%) [14]
Headache (11–13%) [22]
Hypersomnia (<3%)
Hypoesthesia / hypesthesia (numbness) (<3%)
Incoordination (<2%)
Irritability (4–12%) [31]
Memory loss/memory impaired (<2%)
Mood changes (includes mood disorder) (<2%)
Neurotoxicity [2]
Paresthesias (<2%)
Psychiatric adverse effect [3]
Psychosis [2]
Sedation [3]
Seizures [3]
Somnolence (drowsiness) (9–18%) [52]
Suicidal ideation [3]
Vertigo / dizziness (16–43%) [65]

Endocrine/Metabolic
Hyponatremia (<2%)
Weight gain (4%) [12]

Gastrointestinal/Hepatic
Constipation (2–3%)
Nausea (3–8%) [8]
Vomiting (2–4%) [2]

Neuromuscular/Skeletal
Arthralgia (<3%)
Asthenia / fatigue (<12%) [25]
Ataxia (<8%) [9]
Back pain (2–5%)
Bone pain / joint pain (<2%)
Myalgia/Myopathy (<3%)
Pain in extremities (<3%)

Ocular
Diplopia (double vision) (<3%)
Vision blurred (<4%)

Respiratory
Cough (<4%)
Nasopharyngitis [8]
Upper respiratory tract infection (3–4%) [3]

Other
Adverse effects / adverse reactions [13]

PERICYAZINE

Trade name: Neulactil (Winthrop)
Indications: Schizophrenia, anxiety, psychomotor agitation, violent/impulsive behaviour
Class: Neuroleptic
Half-life: 12.4 hours
Clinically important, potentially hazardous interactions with: adrenaline, alcohol, alpha adrenoceptor blocking agents, amfetamines, antiarrhythmics, anticholinergic drugs, antidepressants, antipsychotics, barbiturates, clonidine, deferoxamine, guanethidine, levodopa, lithium, prochlorperazine
Note: Not available in the USA.

Hematologic
Leukocytopenia (leukopenia) / leukocytes (white blood cells) decreased (30%)

PERINDOPRIL

Trade names: Aceon (Solvay), Prestalia (Symplmed)
Indications: Hypertension, coronary disease
Class: Angiotensin-converting enzyme (ACE) inhibitor, Antihypertensive
Half-life: 1.5–3 hours
Clinically important, potentially hazardous interactions with: none known
Pregnancy category: category C in first trimester; category D in second and third trimesters
Important contra-indications noted in the prescribing guidelines for: nursing mothers; pediatric patients
Note: Prestalia is perindopril and amlodipine.
Warning: FETAL TOXICITY

Skin
Angioedema (formerly named angioneurotic edema) [6]
Edema / fluid retention (4%)
Peripheral edema [4]
Pruritus (itching) (<10%)
Rash (<10%)

Mucosal
Tongue edema [2]

Central Nervous System
Paresthesias (2%)
Vertigo / dizziness [4]

Gastrointestinal/Hepatic
Intestinal angioedema [3]

Neuromuscular/Skeletal
Back pain (6%)

Respiratory
Cough (12%) [18]

Other
Adverse effects / adverse reactions [2]

PERPHENAZINE

Trade names: Decentan (Merck), Fentazin (Goldshield), Trilafon (Schering)
Indications: Psychotic disorders, nausea and vomiting
Class: Antiemetic, Antipsychotic, Phenothiazine
Half-life: 9 hours
Clinically important, potentially hazardous interactions with: cobicistat/elvitegravir/emtricitabine/tenofovir alafenamide, cobicistat/elvitegravir/emtricitabine/tenofovir disoproxil, paroxetine hydrochloride, sparfloxacin, viloxazine
Note: Perphenazine is also used in combination with amitriptyline.

Skin
Exanthems [2]
Lupus erythematosus (subacute cutaneous lupus erythematosus (SCLE)) [4]
Rash (<10%)

Central Nervous System
Tardive syndrome / tardive dyskinesia [2]

Endocrine/Metabolic
Mastodynia (<10%)

Genitourinary
Priapism [2]

Neuromuscular/Skeletal
Rhabdomyolysis [2]

PERTUZUMAB

Trade name: Perjeta (Genentech)
Indications: HER2-positive metastatic breast cancer (in combination with trastuzumab and docetaxel)
Class: HER2/neu receptor antagonist (HER2 receptor antagonist), Monoclonal antibody
Half-life: 18 days
Clinically important, potentially hazardous interactions with: none known
Important contra-indications noted in the prescribing guidelines for: nursing mothers; pediatric patients
Warning: EMBRYO-FETAL TOXICITY

Skin
Hypersensitivity (10%)
Peripheral edema (23%)
Pruritus (itching) (14%)
Rash (34%) [9]
Xerosis / xeroderma (11%)

Hair
Alopecia / hair loss (61%)

Nails
Nail disorder (23%)
Paronychia (7%)

Mucosal
Mucosal inflammation (28%)
Stomatitis (oral mucositis) (19%)

Cardiovascular
Cardiotoxicity (left ventricular dysfunction) (4%) [2]

Central Nervous System
Dysgeusia (taste perversion) (18%)
Fever (pyrexia) (includes hyperpyrexia) (19%)
Headache (21%)
Insomnia (13%)
Peripheral neuropathy (32%) [3]
Vertigo / dizziness (13%)

Endocrine/Metabolic
ALT increased [3]
Appetite decreased (29%)
AST increased [2]

Gastrointestinal/Hepatic
Constipation (15%)
Diarrhea (67%) [19]
Nausea (42%) [5]
Vomiting (24%)

Hematologic
Anemia (23%) [2]
Febrile neutropenia (14%) [7]
Leukocytopenia (leukopenia) / leukocytes (white blood cells) decreased (18%) [2]
Neutropenia (neutrophils decreased) (53%) [12]
Thrombocytopenia / platelets decreased [3]

Neuromuscular/Skeletal
Arthralgia (16%)
Asthenia / fatigue (26–38%) [6]
Myalgia/Myopathy (23%)

Ocular
Lacrimation (14%)

Respiratory
Nasopharyngitis (12%)
Pleural effusion (5%)
Upper respiratory tract infection (17%) [2]

Other
Adverse effects / adverse reactions [5]
Allergic reactions [2]

PHELLODENDRON

Family: Rutaceae
Scientific names: *Phellodendron amurense, Phellodendron chinense, Phellodendron wilsonii*
Indications: Anti-inflammatory, muscle and joint pain, gastroenteritis, abdominal pain, diarrhea, gastric ulcers, thrush, cholera, night sweats, fever, nocturnal emissions, dysentery, jaundice, leukorrhea, weakness and edema of legs, consumptive fever. **Topical:** sores, skin infection with local redness and swelling, eczema with itching, periodontal disease (in dentifrice)
Class: COX-2 selective inhibitor, Immunosuppressant
Half-life: N/A
Clinically important, potentially hazardous interactions with: aspirin, NSAIDs
Note: Contra-indicated in patients with impaired renal function, impaired heart function, or hypertension.

PHENACEMIDE

Trade name: Phenurone (AbbVie)
Indications: Epilepsy
Class: Anticonvulsant (see also antiepileptic (anti-seizure))
Half-life: 22–25 hours
Clinically important, potentially hazardous interactions with: ethotoin

PHENAZOPYRIDINE

Trade name: Pyridium (Warner Chilcott)
Indications: Urinary urgency, dysuria
Class: Analgesic; urinary
Half-life: N/A
Clinically important, potentially hazardous interactions with: none known
Important contra-indications noted in the prescribing guidelines for: nursing mothers; pediatric patients

---

Skin
Pigmentation (Skin) (includes hyperpigmentation) [2]

Hematologic
Methemoglobinemia [10]
Sulfhemoglobinemia [5]

PHENDIMETRAZINE

Trade name: Bontril (Amarin)
Indications: Obesity
Class: Amphetamine, Anti-obesity / weight loss pharmacotherapy
Half-life: 5–12.5 hours
Clinically important, potentially hazardous interactions with: cyclobenzaprine, fluoxetine, fluvoxamine, MAO inhibitors, paroxetine hydrochloride, phenelzine, sertraline, tranylcypromine
Note: Phendimetrazine has been withdrawn in the European Union and some other countries.

Mucosal
Xerostomia (dry mouth) [2]

Central Nervous System
Headache [2]
Insomnia [2]

Gastrointestinal/Hepatic
Constipation [2]

PHENELZINE

Trade name: Nardil (Pfizer)
Indications: Depression
Class: Antidepressant, Monoamine oxidase (MAO) inhibitor, Muscarinic antagonist
Half-life: 12 hours
Clinically important, potentially hazardous interactions with: amitriptyline, amoxapine, amphetamines, bupropion, citalopram, clomipramine, cyproheptadine, desipramine, dextroamphetamine, dextromethorphan, diethylpropion, dopamine, doxepin, entacapone, ephedra, ephedrine, epinephrine, fluoxetine, fluvoxamine, ginseng, imipramine, isoetharine, levodopa, mazindol, meperidine, methamphetamine, nefazodone, nortriptyline, opicapone, ozanimod, paroxetine hydrochloride, phendimetrazine, phentermine, phenylephrine, pizotifen, propoxyphene, protriptyline, pseudoephedrine, rizatriptan, sertraline, sibutramine, sumatriptan, sympathomimetics, tramadol, tricyclic antidepressants, trimipramine, tryptophan, valbenazine, venlafaxine, viloxazine, zolmitriptan
Important contra-indications noted in the prescribing guidelines for: the elderly; nursing mothers; pediatric patients
Warning: SUICIDALITY AND ANTIDEPRESSANT DRUGS

Skin
Lupus erythematosus (subacute cutaneous lupus erythematosus (SCLE)) [2]
Peripheral edema [2]
Photosensitivity [2]
Pruritus (itching) (13%)

Mucosal
Xerostomia (dry mouth) (<10%)

Central Nervous System
Hallucinations [2]
Mania [2]
Psychosis [3]
Serotonin syndrome [3]

PHENINDAMINE

Indications: Allergic rhinitis, urticaria, angioedema
Class: Histamine H1 receptor antagonist
Half-life: N/A
Clinically important, potentially hazardous interactions with: none known

PHENOBARBITAL

Synonyms: phenobarbitone; phenylethylmalonylurea
Trade name: Luminal (Sanofi-Aventis)
Indications: Insomnia, seizures
Class: Anticonvulsant (see also antiepileptic (anti-seizure)), Barbiturate, CYP3A4 inducer
Half-life: 2–6 days
Clinically important, potentially hazardous interactions with: abacavir, abiraterone, afatinib, alcohol, amprenavir, anticoagulants, antihistamines, apremilast, aprepitant, betamethasone, bictegravir/emtricitabine/tenofovir alafenamide, boceprevir, brompheniramine, buclizine, buprenorphine, cabazitaxel, cabozantinib, caffeine, calcifediol, cenobamate, chlorpheniramine, cobicistat/elvitegravir/emtricitabine/tenofovir disoproxil, crizotinib, darunavir, dasatinib, deferasirox, delavirdine, dexamethasone, dicumarol, doravirine, doravirine/lamiduvine/tenofovir disoproxil, doxercalciferol, dronedarone, eliglustat, emtricitabine/rilpivirine/tenofovir alafenamide, enzalutamide, erlotinib, estradiol, ethanolamine, ethosuximide, etravirine, fesoterodine, flibanserin, fluconazole, flunisolide, fosamprenavir, gefitinib, hydrocortisone, imatinib, indinavir, influenza vaccine, itraconazole, ixabepilone, lacosamide, lapatinib, ledipasvir & sofosbuvir, lisdexamfetamine, lopinavir, meperidine, methsuximide, methylprednisolone, midazolam, mifepristone, nilotinib, ombitasvir/paritaprevir/ritonavir, ombitasvir/paritaprevir/ritonavir and dasabuvir, osilodrostat, osilodrostat, oxcarbazepine, oxtriphylline, paroxetine hydrochloride, perampanel, piracetam, pizotifen, prednisolone, prednisone, propranolol, ranolazine, regorafenib, rilpivirine, riociguat, rivaroxaban, roflumilast, romidepsin, rufinamide, simeprevir, sodium oxybate, sofosbuvir, sofosbuvir & velpatasvir, sofosbuvir/velpatasvir/voxilaprevir, solifenacin, sonidegib, sorafenib, sunitinib, telaprevir, telithromycin, temsirolimus, teniposide, tenofovir alafenamide, tezacaftor/ivacaftor, tiagabine, ticagrelor, tipranavir, trabectedin, triamcinolone, ulipristal, vandetanib, vemurafenib, voriconazole, warfarin
Important contra-indications noted in the prescribing guidelines for: the elderly; nursing mothers
Note: Aromatic antiepileptic drugs, phenytoin, phenobarbital, carbamazepine and primidone, are a frequent cause of severe cutaneous adverse reactions. A strong genetic association between HLA-B*1502 and phenobarbital-induced Stevens-Johnson syndrome and toxic epidermal necrolysis has been shown in Han Chinese patients.

Skin
Bullous dermatosis [5]
DRESS syndrome (Drug-induced hypersensitivity syndrome) [24]
Erythema multiforme [7]
Erythroderma [2]
Exanthems [13]
Exfoliative dermatitis [6]
Fibromatosis [includes palmar fibromatosis (Dupuytren's contracture / Dupuytren's disease), plantar fibromatosis (Ledderhose disease) and penile fibromatosis (Peyronie disease)] [2]
Fixed eruption / fixed drug eruption [9]
Hypersensitivity [12]
Lupus erythematosus (subacute cutaneous lupus erythematosus (SCLE)) [2]
Pellagra [2]
Purpura [2]
Rash [4]
Stevens-Johnson syndrome and toxic epidermal necrolysis (SJS/TEN) [40]

Nails
Nail hypoplasia [2]

Mucosal
Gingival hyperplasia / gingival hypertrophy / gingival enlargement / gingival overgrowth [4]

Central Nervous System
Behavioral disturbances / personality changes [3]
Somnolence (drowsiness) [2]
Vertigo / dizziness [2]

Gastrointestinal/Hepatic
Hepatotoxicity / liver injury / acute liver injury / drug-induced liver injury (DILI) [2]

Local
Injection-site pain (>10%)
Injection-site thrombophlebitis (>10%)

Neuromuscular/Skeletal
Asthenia / fatigue [2]
Hypoplasia of phalanges [2]

Other
Allergic reactions [2]
Death [2]
Side effects [2]
Teratogenicity [5]

PHENOLPHTHALEIN

Trade name: Ex-Lax (Novartis)
Indications: Constipation
Class: Stimulant laxative
Half-life: N/A
Clinically important, potentially hazardous interactions with: none known

---

Skin
Erythema multiforme [2]
Exanthems [2]
Fixed eruption / fixed drug eruption [17]
Stevens-Johnson syndrome and toxic epidermal necrolysis (SJS/TEN) [9]

PHENOXY-BENZAMINE

Trade name: Dibenzyline (Wellspring)
Indications: Pheochromocytoma
Class: Adrenergic alpha-receptor antagonist
Half-life: 24 hours
Clinically important, potentially hazardous interactions with: epinephrine

---

Skin
Dermatitis [2]

Mucosal
Xerostomia (dry mouth) (<10%)

Cardiovascular
Hypotension [3]

Central Nervous System
Vertigo / dizziness [2]

Genitourinary
Impotence [2]

PHENTERMINE

Trade names: Adipex-P (Teva), Ionamin (Celltech), Lomaira (Avanthi), Qsymia (Vivus)
Indications: Obesity.
Adjunct for the treatment of obesity and for weight loss management in defined populations and health conditions.

Class: Amphetamine, Anti-obesity / weight loss pharmacotherapy
Half-life: 19–24 hours
Clinically important, potentially hazardous interactions with: fluoxetine, fluvoxamine, MAO inhibitors, paroxetine hydrochloride, phenelzine, sertraline, tranylcypromine
Important contra-indications noted in the prescribing guidelines for: the elderly; nursing mothers; pediatric patients
Note: Qsymia, a combination of phentermine and topiramate, has been approved by the FDA for chronic weight management.

Mucosal
Xerostomia (dry mouth) [8]

Cardiovascular
Cardiotoxicity [3]
Hypertension [11]
Palpitation [3]
Tachycardia [5]
Valvulopathy [17]

Central Nervous System
Anxiety [2]
Cognitive impairment [4]
Depression [3]
Dysgeusia (taste perversion) [6]
Headache [2]
Insomnia [8]
Irritability [2]
Paresthesias [8]
Vertigo / dizziness [6]

Endocrine/Metabolic
Acidosis (includes lactic acidosis) [3]

Gastrointestinal/Hepatic
Constipation [7]

Renal
Nephrotoxicity / kidney injury / acute kidney injury (AKI) / drug-induced kidney injury [2]

Other
Death [4]
Teratogenicity [2]

PHENTOLAMINE

Trade name: Regitine (Novartis)
Indications: Hypertensive episodes in pheochromocytoma
Class: Adrenergic alpha-receptor antagonist
Half-life: 19 minutes
Clinically important, potentially hazardous interactions with: none known
Important contra-indications noted in the prescribing guidelines for: nursing mothers

---

Skin
Flushing / rubefaction (<10%) [2]

Central Nervous System
Headache [2]

Genitourinary
Priapism [4]

PHENYLBUTAZONE

Indications: Ankylosing spondylitis, gouty arthritis, osteoarthritis, rheumatoid arthritis
Class: Non-steroidal anti-inflammatory (NSAID)
Half-life: 54–99 hours
Clinically important, potentially hazardous interactions with: anticoagulants, antidiabetics, barbiturates, chlorpheniramine, corticosteroids, digoxin, gliclazide, lithium, methotrexate, methylphenidate, phenytoin, rifampin, sulfonamides
Note: NSAIDs may cause an increased risk of serious cardiovascular and gastrointestinal adverse events, which can be fatal. This risk may increase with duration of use.

Skin
Angioedema (formerly named angioneurotic edema) [3]
Contact dermatitis [6]
DRESS syndrome (Drug-induced hypersensitivity syndrome) [2]
Erythema multiforme [4]
Exfoliative dermatitis [2]
Fixed eruption / fixed drug eruption [4]
Hypersensitivity [2]
Lupus erythematosus (subacute cutaneous lupus erythematosus (SCLE)) [4]
Stevens-Johnson syndrome and toxic epidermal necrolysis (SJS/TEN) [11]
Urticaria / hives [3]
Vasculitis (angiitis) / cutaneous vasculitis (angiitis) [2]

Mucosal
Sialadenitis [3]

PHENYLEPHRINE

Trade names: Rynatan (MedPointe), Tussi-12D (MedPointe)
Indications: Nasal congestion, glaucoma, hypotension
Class: Adrenergic alpha-receptor agonist, Sympathomimetic
Half-life: 2.5 hours
Clinically important, potentially hazardous interactions with: epinephrine, furazolidone, iobenguane, MAO inhibitors, oxprenolol, phenelzine, tranylcypromine
Important contra-indications noted in the prescribing guidelines for: nursing mothers; pediatric patients

---

Skin
Dermatitis [16]
Hypersensitivity [2]
Stinging (from nasal or ophthalmic preparations) (<10%)

Cardiovascular
Bradycardia / sinus bradycardia [3]
Hypertension [2]

Ocular
Blepharoconjunctivitis [4]
Periorbital dermatitis [4]

Other
Adverse effects / adverse reactions [2]

PHENYL-PROPANOLAMINE

Synonym: PPA
Trade name: St. Joseph Aspirin-Free Cold Tablets (McNeil)
Indications: Nasal decongestion, anorexiant
Class: Adrenergic alpha-receptor agonist
Half-life: 3–4 hours
Clinically important, potentially hazardous interactions with: caffeine, ephedrine, fluoxetine, fluvoxamine, furazolidone, iobenguane, paroxetine hydrochloride, sertraline, tranylcypromine

---

Neuromuscular/Skeletal
Rhabdomyolysis [4]
Other
Death [2]

PHENYTOIN

Synonyms: diphenylhydantoin; DPH; phenytoin sodium
Trade name: Dilantin (Pfizer)
Indications: Grand mal seizures
Class: Antiarrhythmic class Ib, Anticonvulsant (see also antiepileptic (anti-seizure)), Antiepileptic; hydantoin, CYP3A4 inducer
Half-life: 7–42 hours (dose dependent)
Clinically important, potentially hazardous interactions with: abacavir, abiraterone, acitretin, afatinib, amiodarone, amitriptyline, amlodipine, amprenavir, apixaban, apremilast, aprepitant, artemether/lumefantrine, beclomethasone, bictegravir/emtricitabine/tenofovir alafenamide, boceprevir, brigatinib, brivaracetam, buprenorphine, cabazitaxel, cabozantinib, caffeine, calcium, capecitabine, caspofungin, cefazolin, cenobamate, ceritinib, chloramphenicol, cimetidine, ciprofloxacin, citalopram, clobazam, clorazepate, cobicistat/elvitegravir/emtricitabine/tenofovir disoproxil, cobimetinib, colesevelam, copanlisib, crizotinib, cyclosporine, cyproterone, dabigatran, daclatasvir, darunavir, dasatinib, deferasirox, deflazacort, delavirdine, dexamethasone, diazoxide, disulfiram, dopamine, doravirine, doravirine/lamiduvine/tenofovir disoproxil, doxycycline, dronedarone, efavirenz, elbasvir & grazoprevir, eliglustat, emtricitabine/rilpivirine/tenofovir alafenamide, enzalutamide, erlotinib, eslicarbazepine, ethosuximide, etravirine, everolimus, ezogabine, fesoterodine, flibanserin, floxuridine, fluconazole, flunisolide, fluoxetine, fosamprenavir, fostemsavir, gefitinib, gold & gold compounds, hydrocortisone, ibrexafungerp, ibrexafungerp, ibrutinib, idelalisib, imatinib, indinavir, influenza vaccine, isoniazid, isotretinoin, isradipine, itraconazole, ivabradine, ixabepilone, ixazomib, lacosamide, lapatinib, ledipasvir & sofosbuvir, leflunomide, letermovir, levodopa, levomepromazine, levonorgestrel, lisdexamfetamine, lomustine, lopinavir, lumateperone, meperidine, metformin, methsuximide, methylprednisolone, metronidazole, midazolam, midostaurin, mifepristone, mivacurium, naldemedine, nelfinavir, neratinib, nifedipine, nilotinib, nilutamide, nintedanib, olaparib, oliceridine, ombitasvir/paritaprevir/ritonavir, ombitasvir/paritaprevir/ritonavir and dasabuvir, omeprazole, ondansetron, osimertinib, oxcarbazepine, oxtriphylline, palbociclib, paroxetine hydrochloride, pemetrexed, perampanel, phenylbutazone, pimavanserin, piracetam, ponatinib, ponesimod, ponesimod, posaconazole, prednisolone, prednisone, propranolol, regorafenib, rifapentine, rilpivirine, riociguat, risperidone, ritonavir, rivaroxaban, roflumilast, romidepsin, saquinavir, simeprevir, sofosbuvir, sofosbuvir & velpatasvir, sofosbuvir/velpatasvir/voxilaprevir, solifenacin, sonidegib, sorafenib, St John's wort, sucralfate, sunitinib, tegafur/gimeracil/oteracil, telaprevir, telithromycin, temsirolimus, teniposide, tenofovir alafenamide, tezacaftor/ivacaftor, thalidomide, tiagabine, ticagrelor, ticlopidine, tinidazole, tipranavir, tizanidine, tolvaptan, triamcinolone, trimethoprim, ubrogepant, ulipristal, uracil/tegafur, valbenazine, vandetanib, vemurafenib, venetoclax, vigabatrin, vorapaxar, voriconazole, vortioxetine, zidovudine, zuclopenthixol
Note: Aromatic antiepileptic drugs, phenytoin, phenobarbital, carbamazepine and primidone, are a frequent cause of severe cutaneous adverse reactions. A strong genetic association between HLA-B*1502 and phenytoin-induced Stevens-Johnson syndrome and toxic epidermal necrolysis has been shown in Han Chinese patients. Children whose mothers receive phenytoin during pregnancy are born with fetal hydantoin syndrome. The main features of this syndrome are mental and growth retardation, unusual facies, digital and nail hypoplasia, and coarse scalp hair. Occasionally neonatal acne will be present.

Skin
Acne keloid [2]
Acneiform eruption / acneiform dermatitis / acneiform rash [8]
AGEP [5]
Angioedema (formerly named angioneurotic edema) [2]
Coarse facies [4]
Cutaneous adverse reaction (includes severe cutaneous adverse drug reaction (SCAR)) [5]
Dermatomyositis [2]
DRESS syndrome (Drug-induced hypersensitivity syndrome) [47]
Erythema multiforme [11]
Erythroderma [9]
Exanthems (6–71%) [22]
Exfoliative dermatitis [15]
Fixed eruption / fixed drug eruption [5]
Hypersensitivity [47]
Kaposi's varicelliform eruption [2]
Linear IgA bullous dermatosis [8]
Lupus erythematosus (subacute cutaneous lupus erythematosus (SCLE)) [19]
Lymphoma [6]
Mycosis fungoides [7]
Pemphigus [2]
Pigmentation (Skin) (includes hyperpigmentation) [4]
Pruritus (itching) [5]
Pseudolymphoma / cutaneous pseudolymphoma [31]
Purple glove syndrome [10]
Purpura [4]
Pustules / pustular eruption [3]
Rash (<10%) [13]
Reticular hyperplasia [2]
Serum sickness-like reaction [2]
Stevens-Johnson syndrome and toxic epidermal necrolysis (SJS/TEN) (14%) [106]
Urticaria / hives [5]
Vasculitis (angiitis) / cutaneous vasculitis (angiitis) (2%) [11]
Hair
Alopecia / hair loss [3]
Hirsutism [8]
Nails
Nail changes [2]
Nail hypoplasia [3]
Mucosal
Gingival hyperplasia / gingival hypertrophy / gingival enlargement / gingival overgrowth (>10%) [61]
Mucocutaneous eruption (includes fixed eruption) [2]
Cardiovascular
Bradycardia / sinus bradycardia [4]
Hypotension [3]
Polyarteritis nodosa [2]
Central Nervous System
Ageusia (taste loss) / taste disorder [2]
Brain atrophy / cerebral atrophy / cerebellar atrophy [5]
Chorea [2]
Dyskinesia [2]
Fetal hydantoin syndrome [8]
Hallucinations [2]
Hallucinations, visual [2]
Hypothermia [2]
Neurotoxicity [2]
Paresthesias [2]
Restless legs syndrome / Willis-Ekbom disease (includes restless arms syndrome variant) [2]
Gastrointestinal/Hepatic
Hepatotoxicity / liver injury / acute liver injury / drug-induced liver injury (DILI) [10]
Hematologic
Agranulocytosis / severe selective neutropenia [2]
Thrombocytopenia / platelets decreased [5]
Local
Injection-site extravasation [2]
Injection-site necrosis [2]
Neuromuscular/Skeletal
Ataxia [3]
Digital malformations [4]
Dystonia [2]
Myalgia/Myopathy [2]
Myasthenia gravis [2]
Osteoporosis [2]
Rhabdomyolysis [6]
Respiratory
Cough [2]
Other
Adverse effects / adverse reactions [4]
Death [4]
Hiccups / singultus [2]
Teratogenicity [3]

PHYSOSTIGMINE

Synonym: eserine
Indications: Miotic in glaucoma treatment, reverses toxic CNS effects caused by anticholinergic drugs
Class: Cholinesterase inhibitor
Half-life: 15–40 minutes
Clinically important, potentially hazardous interactions with: bethanechol, corticosteroids, galantamine, methacholine, succinylcholine
Important contra-indications noted in the prescribing guidelines for: nursing mothers
Note: Antilirium is a derivative of the Calabar bean, and its active moiety, physostigmine, is also known as eserine. Physostigmine is used to reverse the effect upon the nervous system caused by clinical or toxic dosages of drugs and herbs capable of producing the anticholinergic syndrome. Some of the drugs responsible are: amitriptyline, amoxapine, atropine, benztropine, biperiden, clidinium, cyclobenzaprine, desipramine, doxepin, hyoscyamine, imipramine, lorazepam, maprotiline, nortriptyline, protriptyline, propantheline, scopolamine, trimipramine. Some herbals that can elicit the anticholinergic syndrome are black henbane, deadly nightshade, Devil's apple, Jimson weed, Loco seeds or weeds, Matrimony vine, night blooming jessamine, stinkweed.

Skin
Diaphoresis (>10%)
Erythema (<10%)
Mucosal
Sialorrhea (ptyalism; hypersalivation) (>10%)
Cardiovascular
Atrial fibrillation [2]
Bradycardia / sinus bradycardia [3]
Central Nervous System
Myokymia / twitching / fasciculation (<10%)
Seizures (<10%) [4]
Gastrointestinal/Hepatic
Nausea [4]
Vomiting [3]
Ocular
Epiphora (>10%)
Ocular burning (<10%)
Ocular stinging (>10%)

PHYTONADIONE

Synonym: vitamin K_1
Trade names: Mephyton (Valeant), Vitamin K (AbbVie)
Indications: Coagulation disorders
Class: Vitamin
Half-life: 2–4 hours
Clinically important, potentially hazardous interactions with: cholestyramine, orlistat, warfarin
Important contra-indications noted in the prescribing guidelines for: nursing mothers; pediatric patients

---

Skin
Anaphylactoid reactions / anaphylaxis (includes anaphylactic shock) [4]
Dermatitis [9]
Eczema / eczematous reaction / eczematous eruption [2]
Nicolau syndrome [2]
Scleroderma [12]
Urticaria / hives [4]
Local
Injection-site eczematous eruption [10]
Injection-site erythema [2]
Injection-site induration [15]
Other
Allergic reactions [2]

PILOCARPINE

Trade names: Ocusert Pilo (Akorn), Pilopine (Alcon), Salagen (MGI)
Indications: Glaucoma, miosis induction, xerostomia
Class: Miotic, Muscarinic cholinergic agonist
Half-life: N/A
Clinically important, potentially hazardous interactions with: acebutolol, galantamine
Important contra-indications noted in the prescribing guidelines for: nursing mothers; pediatric patients

---

Skin
Burning / skin burning sensation (<10%)
Dermatitis [4]
Diaphoresis [6]
Edema / fluid retention (4%)
Hyperhidrosis [2]
Hypersensitivity (<10%)
Stinging (<10%)
Central Nervous System
Dysgeusia (taste perversion) (2%)
Headache [2]
Ocular
Cataract [2]

PIMAVANSERIN

Trade name: Nuplazid (Acadia)
Indications: Hallucinations and delusions associated with Parkinson's disease psychosis
Class: Antipsychotic, Antipsychotic, atypical
Half-life: 57 hours
Clinically important, potentially hazardous interactions with: amiodarone, carbamazepine, chlorpromazine, clarithromycin, disopyramide, drugs known to prolong the QT interval, gatifloxacin, indinavir, itraconazole, ketoconazole, moxifloxacin, phenytoin, procainamide, quinidine, rifampin, sotalol, St John's wort, strong CYP3A4 inhibitors and inducers, thioridazine, ziprasidone
Pregnancy category: No available data to inform drug-associated risk
Important contra-indications noted in the prescribing guidelines for: the elderly; nursing mothers; pediatric patients
Warning: INCREASED MORTALITY IN ELDERLY PATIENTS WITH DEMENTIA-RELATED PSYCHOSIS

Skin
Peripheral edema (7%) [5]
Cardiovascular
QT interval prolonged / QT prolongation [3]
Central Nervous System
Confusion (6%) [4]
Gait instability / postural instability (2%) [6]
Hallucinations (5%) [4]
Headache [2]
Gastrointestinal/Hepatic
Constipation (4%)
Nausea (7%) [2]
Genitourinary
Urinary tract infection [6]

PIMECROLIMUS

Trade name: Elidel (Valeant)
Indications: Second-line therapy for the short-term and non-continuous chronic treatment of mild to moderate atopic dermatitis
Class: Immunomodulator, Macrolactam
Half-life: N/A
Clinically important, potentially hazardous interactions with: abatacept, alcohol, alefacept, aprepitant, azacitidine, betamethasone, cabazitaxel, calcium channel blockers, cimetidine, conivaptan, CYP3A4 inhibitors, darunavir, delavirdine, denileukin, docetaxel, efavirenz, erythromycin, fingolimod, fluconazole, gefitinib, immunosuppressants, indinavir, itraconazole, ketoconazole, lapatinib, leflunomide, lenalidomide, oxaliplatin, pazopanib, pemetrexed, pralatrexate, telithromycin, temsirolimus, triamcinolone, voriconazole
Important contra-indications noted in the prescribing guidelines for: nursing mothers; pediatric patients
Warning: LONG-TERM SAFETY OF TOPICAL CALCINEURIN INHIBITORS HAS NOT BEEN ESTABLISHED.

Skin
Burning / skin burning sensation [5]
Dermatitis [2]
Peripheral edema [3]
Pruritus (itching) [2]
Rosacea [5]
Tinea [3]
Cardiovascular
Cardiac arrest [2]
Local
Application-site burning (8–26%)
Application-site reactions (2%)
Respiratory
Upper respiratory tract infection (19%)
Other
Infection (5%) [2]

PIMOZIDE

Trade name: Orap (Teva)
Indications: Tourette's syndrome, schizophrenia
Class: Antipsychotic
Half-life: 50 hours
Clinically important, potentially hazardous interactions with: amitriptyline, amoxapine, amphetamines, amprenavir, aprepitant, arsenic, artemether/lumefantrine, astemizole, atazanavir, azithromycin, azole antifungals, boceprevir, ceritinib, citalopram, clarithromycin, crizotinib, darunavir, dasatinib, degarelix, delavirdine, dirithromycin, dolasetron, droperidol, efavirenz, eluxadoline, enzalutamide, erythromycin, fluoxetine, fosamprenavir, grapefruit juice, imatinib, indinavir, itraconazole, ketoconazole, lapatinib, letermovir, levofloxacin, levomepromazine, lopinavir, lurasidone,

methylphenidate, mifepristone, moxifloxacin, nefazodone, nelfinavir, nilotinib, ombitasvir/paritaprevir/ritonavir, ombitasvir/paritaprevir/ritonavir and dasabuvir, paroxetine hydrochloride, paroxetine mesylate, paroxetine mesylate, pazopanib, pemoline, phenothiazines, posaconazole, protease inhibitors, quinidine, quinine, ribociclib, ritonavir, saquinavir, sertraline, sotalol, sparfloxacin, sulpiride / levosulpiride, telaprevir, telavancin, telithromycin, thioridazine, tipranavir, tricyclic antidepressants, trifluoperazine, troleandomycin, vandetanib, voriconazole, vorinostat, zileuton, ziprasidone
Important contra-indications noted in the prescribing guidelines for: nursing mothers; pediatric patients

---

Skin
- Facial edema (<10%)
- Rash (8%)

Mucosal
- Sialorrhea (ptyalism; hypersalivation) (14%)
- Xerostomia (dry mouth) (>10%) [3]

Cardiovascular
- QT interval prolonged / QT prolongation [4]

Endocrine/Metabolic
- Gynecomastia (>10%)

Neuromuscular/Skeletal
- Myalgia/Myopathy (3%)

PINDOLOL

Trade name: Visken (Novartis)
Indications: Hypertension
Class: Adrenergic beta-receptor antagonist
Half-life: 3–4 hours
Clinically important, potentially hazardous interactions with: clonidine, epinephrine, verapamil
Note: Cutaneous side effects of beta-receptor blockers are clinically polymorphous. They apparently appear after several months of continuous therapy.

Skin
- Diaphoresis (2%)
- Edema / fluid retention (6%)
- Lichenoid eruption / lichenoid reaction [2]
- Lupus erythematosus (subacute cutaneous lupus erythematosus (SCLE)) [2]
- Pruritus (itching) (<5%)
- Psoriasis [5]
- Rash (<10%)
- Raynaud's phenomenon [2]

Central Nervous System
- Paresthesias (3%)

PIOGLITAZONE

Trade name: Actos (Takeda)
Indications: Type II diabetes
Class: Antidiabetic, CYP3A4 inducer, Hypoglycemic (antihyperglycemic) agent, Thiazolidinedione
Half-life: 3–7 hours
Clinically important, potentially hazardous interactions with: alcohol, conivaptan, corticosteroids, CYP2C8 inhibitors and inducers, dapagliflozin, deferasirox, gemfibrozil, insulin, lumateperone, lumateperone, pegvisomant, pregabalin, rifampin, saxagliptin, somatropin, teriflunomide, trimethoprim
Important contra-indications noted in the prescribing guidelines for: nursing mothers; pediatric patients
Note: National regulators in Australia and the United Kingdom (UK) have issued safety advisories on the association between pioglitazone use and bladder cancer. The Australian advisory noted that males were at higher risk of bladder cancer than females, while the UK advisory highlighted a new recommendation, suggest careful consideration in the elderly due to increasing risk with age. In an updated review in 2016, the U.S. Food and Drug Administration (FDA) concluded that use of pioglitazone may be linked to an increased risk of bladder cancer. The FDA advised that pioglitazone should not be used in patients with active bladder cancer, and should carefully consider the benefits and risks before using pioglitazone in patients with a history of bladder cancer.
Contra-indicated in patients with established NYHA Class III or IV heart failure.
Warning: CONGESTIVE HEART FAILURE

Skin
- Edema / fluid retention (4–11%) [30]
- Peripheral edema [12]

Cardiovascular
- Cardiac failure (<10%) [14]
- Cardiomyopathy [3]
- Cardiotoxicity [2]
- Myocardial infarction [3]

Central Nervous System
- Headache (9%) [4]
- Stroke / cerebrovascular accident [2]

Endocrine/Metabolic
- Hypoglycemia [11]
- Weight gain [20]

Gastrointestinal/Hepatic
- Diarrhea [4]
- Hepatotoxicity / liver injury / acute liver injury / drug-induced liver injury (DILI) [8]
- Nausea [3]
- Vomiting [2]

Genitourinary
- Bladder cancer [8]

Hematologic
- Anemia (<2%) [2]
- Pancytopenia (includes bicytopenia) [2]

Neuromuscular/Skeletal
- Asthenia / fatigue (4%)
- Bone loss / bone disorder [4]
- Fractures [10]
- Myalgia/Myopathy (5%)

Ocular
- Macular edema [2]

Respiratory
- Nasopharyngitis [3]
- Pharyngitis (sore throat) (5%)
- Sinusitis (see also rhinitis / rhinosinusitis) (6%)
- Upper respiratory tract infection (13%)

Other
- Adverse effects / adverse reactions [5]
- Death [3]
- Tooth disorder (5%)

PIPECURONIUM

Trade name: Arduan (Organon)
Indications: Adjunct to general anesthesia
Class: Non-depolarizing neuromuscular blocker
Half-life: 2–3 hours
Clinically important, potentially hazardous interactions with: anesthetics (inhalational), antibiotics, gentamicin, magnesium salts, quinidine, succinylcholine

PIPERACILLIN

Trade names: Pipracil (Wyeth), Zosyn (Wyeth)
Indications: Various infections caused by susceptible organisms
Class: Antibiotic, Antibiotic, Antibiotic; beta-lactam, Antibiotic; penicillin, Antimicrobial
Half-life: 0.6–1.2 hours
Clinically important, potentially hazardous interactions with: anisindione, anticoagulants, atracurium, cisatracurium, demeclocycline, dicumarol, doxacurium, doxycycline, imipenem/cilastatin, methotrexate, minocycline, non-depolarizing muscle relaxants, oxytetracycline, pancuronium, rapacuronium, reteplase, tetracycline, warfarin
Note: Zosyn is piperacillin and tazobactam - see separate profile.

Skin
- AGEP [3]
- Anaphylactoid reactions / anaphylaxis (includes anaphylactic shock) [2]
- Exanthems (56%) [5]
- Hypersensitivity [4]
- Urticaria / hives [4]

Central Nervous System
- Seizures [3]

Hematologic
- Hemolytic anemia [5]
- Myelosuppression / bone marrow suppression / myelotoxicity [2]
- Thrombocytopenia / platelets decreased [4]

Local
- Injection-site pain (2%)
- Injection-site phlebitis (2%)

Renal
- Nephrotoxicity / kidney injury / acute kidney injury (AKI) / drug-induced kidney injury [2]

Other
- Allergic reactions (2–4%) [2]

PIPERACILLIN/TAZOBACTAM

Trade name: Zosyn (Wyeth)
Indications: Moderate to severe infections
Class: Antibiotic, Antimicrobial
Half-life: 0.7–1.2 hours
Clinically important, potentially hazardous interactions with: heparin, methotrexate
Important contra-indications noted in the prescribing guidelines for: nursing mothers

---

Skin
- AGEP [3]
- DRESS syndrome (Drug-induced hypersensitivity syndrome) [5]
- Hypersensitivity [2]

Linear IgA bullous dermatosis [3]
Rash [5]

Central Nervous System
Fever (pyrexia) (includes hyperpyrexia) [5]
Neurotoxicity [2]

Endocrine/Metabolic
Hypokalemia [3]

Gastrointestinal/Hepatic
Diarrhea [4]
Hepatotoxicity / liver injury / acute liver injury / drug-induced liver injury (DILI) [4]
Nausea [2]
Vomiting [2]

Hematologic
Hemolytic anemia [6]
Hemotoxicity [2]
Neutropenia (neutrophils decreased) [2]
Thrombocytopenia / platelets decreased [9]

Renal
Nephrotoxicity / kidney injury / acute kidney injury (AKI) / drug-induced kidney injury [6]

Other
Adverse effects / adverse reactions [5]

PIRACETAM

Trade name: Nootropil (UCB)
Indications: Psycho-organic syndromes or cognitive decline and cortical myclonus
Class: Neuroprotectant, Nootropics
Half-life: 5 hours
Clinically important, potentially hazardous interactions with: carbamazepine, clonazepam, phenobarbital, phenytoin, sodium valproate

---

Central Nervous System
Depression [2]
Nervousness (<10%)
Vertigo / dizziness [2]

Endocrine/Metabolic
Weight gain (<10%)

Neuromuscular/Skeletal
Hyperkinesia (<10%)

PIRBUTEROL

Trade name: Maxair (3M)
Indications: Asthma, bronchospasm
Class: Beta-2 adrenergic agonist, Bronchodilator
Half-life: 2–3 hours
Clinically important, potentially hazardous interactions with: none known
Important contra-indications noted in the prescribing guidelines for: nursing mothers

---

Central Nervous System
Dysgeusia (taste perversion) (<10%)
Trembling (>10%)

PIRFENIDONE

Trade name: Esbriet (Intermune)
Indications: Idiopathic pulmonary fibrosis
Class: Immunosuppressant, Pyridone
Half-life: 3 hours
Clinically important, potentially hazardous interactions with: ciprofloxacin, fluvoxamine, viloxazine
Important contra-indications noted in the prescribing guidelines for: nursing mothers; pediatric patients

---

Skin
Lichenoid eruption / lichenoid reaction [2]
Photosensitivity (9%) [27]
Phototoxicity [2]
Pruritus (itching) (8%) [3]
Rash (30%) [15]

Cardiovascular
Chest pain (5%) [3]

Central Nervous System
Anorexia (13%) [11]
Dysgeusia (taste perversion) (6%)
Headache (22%) [4]
Insomnia (10%)
Sedation [2]
Vertigo / dizziness (18%) [7]

Endocrine/Metabolic
ALT increased [5]
Appetite decreased (8%) [5]
AST increased [5]
Hyponatremia [3]
Weight loss (10%) [4]

Gastrointestinal/Hepatic
Abdominal pain (24%) [7]
Diarrhea (26%) [14]
Dyspepsia / functional dyspepsia (indigestion) (see also gastroparesis) (19%) [10]
Gastroesophageal reflux (11%) [6]
Gastrointestinal adverse reaction [2]
Gastrointestinal disorder / discomfort [4]
Hepatotoxicity / liver injury / acute liver injury / drug-induced liver injury (DILI) [6]
Nausea (36%) [24]
Vomiting (13%) [7]

Neuromuscular/Skeletal
Arthralgia (10%)
Asthenia / fatigue (6–26%) [12]

Respiratory
Bronchitis [2]
Cough [4]
Dyspnea / shortness of breath [4]
Nasopharyngitis [2]
Sinusitis (see also rhinitis / rhinosinusitis) (11%)
Upper respiratory tract infection (27%) [4]

Other
Adverse effects / adverse reactions [11]

PIROXICAM

Trade name: Feldene (Pfizer)
Indications: Arthritis
Class: Non-steroidal anti-inflammatory (NSAID)
Half-life: 50 hours
Clinically important, potentially hazardous interactions with: ACE inhibitors, aspirin, furosemide, lithium, methotrexate, ritonavir, warfarin
Pregnancy category: pregnancy category C prior to 30 weeks gestation; category D starting at 30 weeks gestation
Important contra-indications noted in the prescribing guidelines for: the elderly; nursing mothers
Note: NSAIDs may cause an increased risk of serious cardiovascular and gastrointestinal adverse events, which can be fatal. This risk may increase with duration of use. Elderly patients are at greater risk for serious gastrointestinal events.
Warning: CARDIOVASCULAR AND GASTROINTESTINAL RISKS

Skin
AGEP [2]
Angioedema (formerly named angioneurotic edema) [3]
Dermatitis [5]
Erythema multiforme [12]
Erythroderma [2]
Exanthems (>5%) [8]
Fixed eruption / fixed drug eruption [15]
Lichenoid eruption / lichenoid reaction [5]
Linear IgA bullous dermatosis [3]
Pemphigus [3]
Photosensitivity [40]
Pruritus (itching) (<10%) [6]
Purpura [2]
Rash (>10%)
Stevens-Johnson syndrome and toxic epidermal necrolysis (SJS/TEN) [13]
Urticaria / hives [7]
Vasculitis (angiitis) / cutaneous vasculitis (angiitis) [3]
Vesiculation [2]

Hair
Alopecia / hair loss [3]

Mucosal
Aphthous stomatitis / aphthous ulcer / aphtha (aphthae) [4]

Central Nervous System
Anorexia (<10%)
Vertigo / dizziness (<10%)

Gastrointestinal/Hepatic
Abdominal pain (<10%)
Constipation (<10%)
Diarrhea (<10%)
Dyspepsia / functional dyspepsia (indigestion) (see also gastroparesis) (<10%)
Flatulence (<10%)
Gastrointestinal ulceration (<10%)
Nausea (<10%)
Vomiting (<10%)

Otic
Hearing loss (hypoacusis) [2]
Tinnitus [2]

Renal
Renal function abnormal / renal dysfunction (<10%)

Other
Adverse effects / adverse reactions [2]
Side effects (47%)

PITAVASTATIN

Trade name: Livalo (Kowa)
Indications: Primary hyperlipidemia, mixed dyslipidemia
Class: HMG-CoA reductase inhibitor / statin
Half-life: 12 hours
Clinically important, potentially hazardous interactions with: alcohol, cyclosporine, erythromycin, gemfibrozil, letermovir, lopinavir, niacin, rifampin, ritonavir, sofosbuvir/velpatasvir/voxilaprevir
Important contra-indications noted in the prescribing guidelines for: nursing mothers; pediatric patients
Note: Contra-indicated in patients with active liver disease.

Skin
Hypersensitivity (<2%)
Rash (<2%)
Urticaria / hives (<2%)
Central Nervous System
Headache (<2%)
Endocrine/Metabolic
ALT increased [2]
AST increased [2]
Creatine phosphokinase (CPK) / creatine kinase increased (hyperCKemia) [2]
Gastrointestinal/Hepatic
Constipation (2–4%)
Diarrhea (2–3%)
Neuromuscular/Skeletal
Arthralgia (<2%)
Back pain (2–4%)
Myalgia/Myopathy (2–3%) [6]
Pain in extremities (<2%)
Respiratory
Influenza (<2%)
Nasopharyngitis (<2%) [2]
Other
Adverse effects / adverse reactions [6]

PITOLISANT HYDROCHLORIDE

Trade name: Wakix (Bioprojet)
Indications: Treatment of excessive daytime sleepiness in patients with narcolepsy
Class: Histamine H3 receptor antagonist, Histamine H3 receptor inverse agonist
Half-life: ~20 hours
Clinically important, potentially hazardous interactions with: CYP2D6 inhibitors, CYP3A4 inducers, CYP3A4 substrates
Pregnancy category: Pitolisant may reduce the effectiveness of hormonal contraceptives.
Note: Pitolisant prolongs the QT interval. Its use should be avoided in patients with known QT prolongation or in combination with other drugs known to prolong QT interval. Pitolisant should also be avoided in patients with a history of cardiac arrhythmias. The risk of QT prolongation may be greater in patients with hepatic or renal impairment due to higher concentrations of pitolisant.

Skin
Rash (2%)
Mucosal
Xerostomia (dry mouth) (2%)
Cardiovascular
Tachycardia (3%)
Central Nervous System
Anxiety (5%) [2]
Cataplexy (2%)
Hallucinations (3%)
Headache (18%) [3]
Insomnia (6%) [2]
Irritability (3%)
Sleep disturbances (3%)
Endocrine/Metabolic
Appetite decreased (3%)
Gastrointestinal/Hepatic
Abdominal pain (3%)
Nausea (6%) [2]
Neuromuscular/Skeletal
Musculoskeletal pain (5%)
Respiratory
Upper respiratory tract infection (5%)

PIZOTIFEN

Trade name: Sanomigran (Novartis)
Indications: Recurrent vascular headaches, including classical migraine, common migraine and cluster headaches
Class: 5-Hydroxytryptamine antagonist
Half-life: 23 hours
Clinically important, potentially hazardous interactions with: adrenergic neurone blockers, alcohol, antihistamines, butalbital, hypnotics, isocarboxazid, pentobarbital, phenelzine, phenobarbital, primidone, sedatives, tranylcypromine, zolpidem
Important contra-indications noted in the prescribing guidelines for: nursing mothers

---

Mucosal
Xerostomia (dry mouth) (<10%)
Central Nervous System
Somnolence (drowsiness) (<10%) [4]
Vertigo / dizziness (<10%)
Endocrine/Metabolic
Appetite increased (<10%)
Weight gain (>10%) [8]
Gastrointestinal/Hepatic
Nausea (<10%)
Neuromuscular/Skeletal
Asthenia / fatigue (<10%)

PLAZOMICIN

Trade name: Zemdri (Achaogen Inc)
Indications: treatment of patients 18 years of age or older with Complicated Urinary Tract Infections (cUTI) including Pyelonephritis
Class: Antibiotic, Antibiotic; aminoglycoside, Antimicrobial
Half-life: 3.5 hours
Clinically important, potentially hazardous interactions with: none known
Pregnancy category: Aminoglycosides can cause fetal harm, however, there are no available data on the use of Plazomicin in pregnant women to inform a drug associated risk of adverse developmental outcomes.
Warning: NEPHROTOXICITY, OTOTOXICITY, NEUROMUSCULAR BLOCKADE and FETAL HARM

Cardiovascular
Hypertension (2%)
Endocrine/Metabolic
Serum creatinine increased (7%)
Gastrointestinal/Hepatic
Diarrhea (2%)
Renal
Renal function abnormal / renal dysfunction (4%)

PLICAMYCIN

Synonym: Mithramycin
Indications: Paget's disease, malignant testicular tumors
Class: Antibiotic, Antimicrobial
Half-life: 1 hour
Clinically important, potentially hazardous interactions with: aldesleukin, ceftobiprole
Important contra-indications noted in the prescribing guidelines for: nursing mothers

---

Skin
Flushing / rubefaction (<35%) [3]
Petechiae (<10%)
Purpura (10%)
Mucosal
Oral lesions (<15%) [2]
Stomatitis (oral mucositis) (>10%)
Gastrointestinal/Hepatic
Vomiting [2]
Local
Injection-site cellulitis (<10%)
Injection-site erythema (<10%)
Injection-site pain (<10%)

POLYPODIUM LEUCOTOMOS

Family: Polypodiaceae
Scientific names: *Anapsos, Calagualine, Calagula, Difur, Fernblock, Heliocare, Polypodium leucotomos*
Indications: Oral and topical photoprotection, vitiligo, psoriasis, dermatitis, arthritis
Class: Anti-inflammatory, Antioxidant
Half-life: N/A
Clinically important, potentially hazardous interactions with: none known
Note: It is the first oral agent effective in reducing side effects of PUVA treatment.

POLYTHIAZIDE

Trade names: Minizide (Pfizer), Renese (Pfizer)
Indications: Hypertension, edema
Class: Adrenergic alpha-receptor agonist, Diuretic, thiazide
Half-life: N/A
Clinically important, potentially hazardous interactions with: digoxin, lithium
Note: Polythiazide is a sulfonamide and can be absorbed systemically. Sulfonamides can produce severe, possibly fatal, reactions such as toxic epidermal necrolysis and Stevens-Johnson syndrome.
Minizide is polythiazide and prazosin.

POMALIDOMIDE

Trade name: Pomalyst (Celgene)
Indications: Multiple myeloma in patients who have received at least two prior therapies including lenalidomide and bortezomib
Class: Immunomodulator, Thalidomide analog
Half-life: 7.5–9.5 hours
Clinically important, potentially hazardous interactions with: ketoconazole, P-glycoprotein, rifampin

Important contra-indications noted in the prescribing guidelines for: nursing mothers; pediatric patients
Warning: EMBRYO-FETAL TOXICITY and VENOUS AND ARTERIAL THROMBOEMBOLISM

Skin
Edema / fluid retention [4]
Hyperhidrosis (6%)
Peripheral edema (23%)
Pruritus (itching) (15%)
Rash (22%) [2]
Xerosis / xeroderma (9%)
Mucosal
Epistaxis (nosebleed) (15%)
Cardiovascular
Chest pain (22%)
Venous thromboembolism [8]
Central Nervous System
Anorexia [2]
Anxiety (11%)
Chills (9%)
Confusion (10%)
Fever (pyrexia) (includes hyperpyrexia) (19%) [3]
Headache (13%)
Insomnia (7%)
Neurotoxicity (18%) [3]
Pain (6%)
Peripheral neuropathy (10%) [3]
Tremor (9%) [2]
Vertigo / dizziness (20%)
Endocrine/Metabolic
Appetite decreased (22%)
Dehydration [2]
Hypercalcemia (21%)
Hyperglycemia (includes glucose increased) (12%) [2]
Hypocalcemia (6%)
Hypokalemia (10%)
Hyponatremia (10%)
Hypothyroidism [2]
Serum creatinine increased (15%)
Weight loss (14%)
Gastrointestinal/Hepatic
Constipation (36%) [2]
Diarrhea (34%) [2]
Nausea (36%)
Vomiting (14%)
Genitourinary
Urinary tract infection (8%)
Hematologic
Anemia (38%) [18]
Febrile neutropenia [3]
Leukocytopenia (leukopenia) / leukocytes (white blood cells) decreased (11%) [3]
Lymphopenia (lymphocytopenia) / lymphocytes decreased (4%) [2]
Myelosuppression / bone marrow suppression / myelotoxicity [4]
Neutropenia (neutrophils decreased) (52%) [29]
Sepsis [2]
Thrombocytopenia / platelets decreased (25%) [18]
Neuromuscular/Skeletal
Arthralgia (16%)
Asthenia / fatigue (12–55%) [12]
Back pain (32%) [3]
Bone pain / joint pain (11–12%) [2]
Muscle spasm (19%)
Myalgia/Myopathy [2]
Pain in extremities (5%)
Renal
Renal failure (15%)
Respiratory
Cough (14%)
Dyspnea / shortness of breath (34%) [5]
Pneumonia (23%) [7]
Pulmonary toxicity [4]
Upper respiratory tract infection (32%)
Other
Death [3]
Infection [12]

PONATINIB

Trade name: Iclusig (Ariad)
Indications: Chronic myeloid leukemia or Philadelphia chromosome positive acute lymphoblastic leukemia that is resistant or intolerant to prior tyrosine kinase inhibitor therapy
Class: Angiogenesis inhibitor / antiangiogenic agent, Bcr-Abl tyrosine kinase inhibitor / (Breakpoint cluster region Abelson (Bcr-Abl) tyrosine kinase inhibitor, Tyrosine kinase inhibitor
Half-life: 24 hours
Clinically important, potentially hazardous interactions with: antacids, boceprevir, carbamazepine, clarithromycin, conivaptan, grapefruit juice, histamine H_2 antagonists, indinavir, itraconazole, ketoconazole, lopinavir, nefazodone, nelfinavir, phenytoin, posaconazole, proton pump inhibitors, rifampin, ritonavir, saquinavir, St John's wort, strong CYP3A inhibitors or inducers, telaprevir, telithromycin, voriconazole
Important contra-indications noted in the prescribing guidelines for: nursing mothers; pediatric patients
Warning: VASCULAR OCCLUSION, HEART FAILURE, and HEPATOTOXICITY

Skin
Cellulitis and pseudocellulitis (<11%)
Edema / fluid retention (23%) [2]
Ichthyosis [7]
Peripheral edema (13–22%)
Pityriasis rubra pilaris [3]
Rash (34–54%) [10]
Xerosis / xeroderma (24–39%) [6]
Mucosal
Stomatitis (oral mucositis) (9–23%)
Cardiovascular
Atrial fibrillation [2]
Cardiac failure (6–15%)
Cardiotoxicity [3]
Congestive heart failure (4%)
Hypertension (53–71%) [6]
Myocardial infarction (5%)
Pericardial effusion (<3%)
Supraventricular arrhythmias (5%)
Central Nervous System
Cerebral hemorrhage (2%)
Chills (7–13%)
Fever (pyrexia) (includes hyperpyrexia) (23–32%)
Headache (25–39%) [4]
Insomnia (7–12%)
Pain (6–16%)
Peripheral neuropathy (6–13%)
Vertigo / dizziness (3–11%)
Endocrine/Metabolic
ALT increased (56%)
Appetite decreased (8–31%)
AST increased (56%)
Hyperlipasemia [2]
Weight loss (5–13%)
Gastrointestinal/Hepatic
Abdominal pain (34–49%) [6]
Constipation (24–47%) [3]
Diarrhea (13–26%)
Gastrointestinal bleeding (2–11%)
Hepatotoxicity / liver injury / acute liver injury / drug-induced liver injury (DILI) [4]
Nausea (22–32%) [2]
Pancreatitis / acute pancreatitis (6%) [6]
Genitourinary
Urinary tract infection (<12%)
Hematologic
Anemia (9–55%) [2]
Bleeding (24%)
Febrile neutropenia (<25%)
Leukocytopenia (leukopenia) / leukocytes (white blood cells) decreased (14–63%) [2]
Lymphopenia (lymphocytopenia) / lymphocytes decreased (10–37%)
Myelosuppression / bone marrow suppression / myelotoxicity (48%) [4]
Neutropenia (neutrophils decreased) (24–63%) [4]
Sepsis (<22%)
Thrombocytopenia / platelets decreased (36–57%) [7]
Thrombosis [5]
Neuromuscular/Skeletal
Arthralgia (13–31%) [2]
Asthenia / fatigue (31–39%) [2]
Back pain (11–16%)
Bone pain / joint pain (9–12%)
Muscle spasm (5–13%)
Myalgia/Myopathy (6–22%) [2]
Pain in extremities (9–17%)
Ocular
Vision blurred (6%)
Respiratory
Cough (6–18%)
Nasopharyngitis (3–12%)
Pleural effusion (3–19%)
Upper respiratory tract infection (<11%)
Other
Adverse effects / adverse reactions [2]

PONESIMOD

Trade name: Ponvory (Janssen)
Indications: Treatment of relapsing forms of multiple sclerosis
Class: Sphingosine1-phosphate receptor modulator
Half-life: ~33 hours
Clinically important, potentially hazardous interactions with: alemtuzumab, amiodarone, anti-arrhythmic drugs, QT prolonging drugs, drugs that may decrease heart rate, attenuated vaccines, beta-blockers, carbamazepine, carbamazepine, CYP3A4 and UGT1A1 inducers, digoxin, diltiazem, phenytoin, procainamide, quinidine, rifampin, sotalol, verapamil
Pregnancy category: May cause fetal harm. Contraception is advised.
Important contra-indications noted in the prescribing guidelines for: nursing mothers

---

Cardiovascular
Hypertension (10%)

Central Nervous System
Fever (pyrexia) (includes hyperpyrexia) (2%)
Somnolence (drowsiness) (3%)
Vertigo / dizziness (5%)

Endocrine/Metabolic
C-reactive protein (CRP) increased (2%)
Hypercholesterolemia (2%)
Hypertransaminasemia (hepatic transaminitis) / elevated transaminases (23%)

Genitourinary
Urinary tract infection (6%)

Neuromuscular/Skeletal
Pain in extremities (4%)

Respiratory
Cough (4%)
Dyspnea / shortness of breath (5%)
Upper respiratory tract infection (37%)

POSACONAZOLE

Trade name: Noxafil (Schering)
Indications: *Aspergillus* and *Candida* infection prophylaxis in immunocompromised patients
Class: Antifungal / antimycotic, Antifungal; triazole, Antimicrobial
Half-life: 35 hours
Clinically important, potentially hazardous interactions with: alprazolam, atazanavir, atorvastatin, boceprevir, brigatinib, cabozantinib, calcium channel blockers, cimetidine, copanlisib, cyclosporine, digoxin, dihydroergotamine, diltiazem, dronedarone, efavirenz, ergotamine, esomeprazole, everolimus, felodipine, flibanserin, fosamprenavir, HMG-CoA reductase inhibitors, ibrutinib, lapatinib, lomitapide, lovastatin, metoclopramide, midazolam, midostaurin, mifepristone, neratinib, nicardipine, nifedipine, olaparib, omeprazole, palbociclib, pantoprazole, phenytoin, pimozide, ponatinib, quinidine, regorafenib, rifabutin, rilpivirine, ritonavir, rivaroxaban, ruxolitinib, simeprevir, simvastatin, sirolimus, sonidegib, tacrolimus, telaprevir, temsirolimus, tezacaftor/ivacaftor, triazolam, venetoclax, verapamil, vinblastine, vincristine, vorapaxar
Important contra-indications noted in the prescribing guidelines for: nursing mothers; pediatric patients

---

Skin
Edema / fluid retention (9%)
Herpes (14%)
Herpes simplex (3–15%)
Hyperhidrosis (2–10%)
Jaundice (see also cholestasis / cholestatic jaundice) (<5%)
Peripheral edema (15%)
Petechiae (11%)
Pruritus (itching) (11%)
Rash (3–19%) [3]
Thrombocytopenic purpura (<5%)

Mucosal
Epistaxis (nosebleed) (14%)
Mucositis (17%)
Oral candidiasis (<12%)

Cardiovascular
Hypertension (18%)
Hypotension (14%)
QT interval prolonged / QT prolongation [3]
Tachycardia (12%)
Torsades de pointes (<5%)

Central Nervous System
Anorexia (2–19%)
Anxiety (9%)
Dysgeusia (taste perversion) (~2%)
Fever (pyrexia) (includes hyperpyrexia) (6–45%)
Headache (8–28%) [6]
Insomnia (<17%)
Neurotoxicity [2]
Paresthesias (<5%)
Rigors (<20%)
Tremor (~2%)
Vertigo / dizziness (11%) [4]

Endocrine/Metabolic
Adrenal insufficiency (hypoadrenalism) / Addisonian crisis (includes Addison's disease) (<5%)
ALP increased (3–13%)
ALT increased (3–11%) [2]
AST increased (6–17%) [2]
Dehydration (<11%)
Hyperbilirubinemia [2]
Hyperglycemia (includes glucose increased) (11%)
Hypocalcemia (9%)
Hypokalemia (30%)
Hypomagnesemia (18%)
Mineralocorticoid excess / apparent mineralocorticoid excess [3]
Weight loss (<14%)

Gastrointestinal/Hepatic
Abdominal pain (5–27%) [3]
Constipation (21%)
Diarrhea (10–42%) [6]
Dyspepsia / functional dyspepsia (indigestion) (see also gastroparesis) (10%)
Flatulence [2]
Hepatitis (<5%)
Hepatomegaly (<5%)
Hepatotoxicity / liver injury / acute liver injury / drug-induced liver injury (DILI) (<5%) [7]
Nausea (9–38%) [14]
Vomiting (7–29%) [7]

Genitourinary
Vaginal bleeding (10%)

Hematologic
Anemia (2–25%)
Febrile neutropenia (20%)
Hemolytic uremic syndrome (<5%)
Neutropenia (neutrophils decreased) (4–23%) [2]
Thrombocytopenia / platelets decreased (29%) [2]

Neuromuscular/Skeletal
Arthralgia (11%)
Asthenia / fatigue (3–17%) [3]
Back pain (10%)
Bone pain / joint pain (16%)
Myalgia/Myopathy (16%)

Ocular
Vision blurred (~2%)

Renal
Renal failure (<5%)

Respiratory
Cough (3–25%)
Dyspnea / shortness of breath (<20%)
Pharyngitis (sore throat) (12%)
Pneumonia (3–10%)
Pulmonary embolism (<5%)
Upper respiratory tract infection (7%)

Other
Adverse effects / adverse reactions [11]
Allergic reactions (<5%)
Infection (18%)

POTASSIUM IODIDE

Synonyms: KI; Lugol's solution
Trade name: SSKI (Upsher-Smith)
Indications: Hyperthyroidism, erythema nodosum, sporotrichosis
Class: Antihyperthyroid, Antimycobacterial (including antitubercular)
Half-life: N/A
Clinically important, potentially hazardous interactions with: ACE inhibitors, potassium-sparing diuretics, spironolactone, triamterene
Important contra-indications noted in the prescribing guidelines for: nursing mothers

---

Skin
Acneiform eruption / acneiform dermatitis / acneiform rash (<10%) [3]
Angioedema (formerly named angioneurotic edema) (<10%)
Bullous pemphigoid / pemphigoid [2]
Dermatitis herpetiformis [2]
Iododerma [17]
Psoriasis [2]
Urticaria / hives (<10%)
Vasculitis (angiitis) / cutaneous vasculitis (angiitis) [3]

Central Nervous System
Dysgeusia (taste perversion) (<10%) [2]

Endocrine/Metabolic
Hypothyroidism [2]

Gastrointestinal/Hepatic
Gastrointestinal disorder / discomfort [2]

PRALATREXATE

Trade name: Folotyn (Allos)
Indications: Relapsed or refractory peripheral T-cell lymphoma
Class: Folate analogue metabolic inhibitor
Half-life: 12–18 hours
Clinically important, potentially hazardous interactions with: BCG vaccine, cardiac glycosides, denosumab, echinacea, leflunomide, meloxicam, natalizumab, NSAIDs, pimecrolimus, probenecid, roflumilast, salicylates, sapropterin, sipuleucel-T, sulfamethoxazole, tacrolimus, trastuzumab, trimethoprim, vaccines, vitamin K antagonists
Important contra-indications noted in the prescribing guidelines for: nursing mothers; pediatric patients

---

Skin
Edema / fluid retention (30%)
Pruritus (itching) (14%)
Rash (15%)

Mucosal
Epistaxis (nosebleed) (26%)
Mucositis (70%) [6]

Cardiovascular
Tachycardia (10%)

Central Nervous System
Anorexia (15%)

Fever (pyrexia) (includes hyperpyrexia) (32%)

Endocrine/Metabolic
ALT increased (13%)
AST increased (13%)
Hypokalemia (15%)

Gastrointestinal/Hepatic
Abdominal pain (12%)
Constipation (33%)
Diarrhea (21%)
Nausea (40%)
Vomiting (25%)

Hematologic
Anemia (34%) [2]
Leukocytopenia (leukopenia) / leukocytes (white blood cells) decreased (11%)
Neutropenia (neutrophils decreased) (24%) [3]
Thrombocytopenia / platelets decreased (41%) [3]

Neuromuscular/Skeletal
Asthenia / fatigue (10–36%) [2]
Back pain (11%)

Respiratory
Cough (28%)
Dyspnea / shortness of breath (19%)
Upper respiratory tract infection (10%)

PRAMIPEXOLE

Trade name: Mirapex (Boehringer Ingelheim)
Indications: Parkinsonism, restless legs syndrome
Class: Dopamine receptor agonist
Half-life: ~8 hours
Clinically important, potentially hazardous interactions with: levomepromazine, risperidone, zuclopenthixol
Important contra-indications noted in the prescribing guidelines for: nursing mothers; pediatric patients

---

Skin
Edema / fluid retention (5%)
Peripheral edema (5%) [4]

Mucosal
Xerostomia (dry mouth) (7%) [3]

Cardiovascular
Chest pain (3%)
Hypotension (~53%) [2]
Orthostatic hypotension [2]

Central Nervous System
Abnormal dreams (11%)
Akathisia (2–3%)
Amnesia (4–6%)
Anorexia (<5%)
Compulsions / obsessive-compulsive symptoms / obsessive-compulsive disorder [6]
Confusion [2]
Depression (2%)
Dyskinesia (17–47%) [4]
Hallucinations (5–17%) [6]
Headache (4–7%) [3]
Hyperesthesia (3%)
Hypersexuality [4]
Impulse control disorder / impulsivity / drug-induced impulsivity [13]
Insomnia (4–27%) [2]
Myokymia / twitching / fasciculation (2%)
Othello syndrome [2]
Restless legs syndrome / Willis-Ekbom disease (includes restless arms syndrome variant) [2]
Somnolence (drowsiness) (9–36%) [10]
Tremor (4%)
Vertigo / dizziness (2–26%) [7]

Gastrointestinal/Hepatic
Constipation [5]
Nausea [10]
Vomiting (4%) [3]

Genitourinary
Urinary frequency (6%)
Urinary tract infection (4%)

Neuromuscular/Skeletal
Arthralgia (4%)
Asthenia / fatigue (<14%) [2]
Cervical dystonia / antecollis / spasmodic torticollis [2]

Respiratory
Cough (3%)
Dyspnea / shortness of breath (4%)
Rhinitis / rhinosinusitis (see also sinusitis) (3%)

Other
Adverse effects / adverse reactions (2%) [5]
Hiccups / singultus [2]

PRAMLINTIDE

Trade name: Symlin (Amylin)
Indications: Diabetes, adjunct to insulin treatment
Class: Amylinomimetic, Antidiabetic, Protein analog
Half-life: 48 minutes
Clinically important, potentially hazardous interactions with: acarbose, acetaminophen, alcohol, amitriptyline, anticholinergics, atropine, cyclobenzaprine, fesoterodine, insulin aspart, insulin degludec, insulin glargine, insulin glulisine, miglitol, oxybutynin, tiotropium, trospium
Important contra-indications noted in the prescribing guidelines for: nursing mothers; pediatric patients
Note: Contra-indicated in patients with a confirmed diagnosis of gastroparesis; or with hypoglycemia unawareness.

Central Nervous System
Anorexia (9–17%) [4]
Headache (5–13%)
Vertigo / dizziness (2–6%)

Endocrine/Metabolic
Hypoglycemia [6]
Weight loss [3]

Gastrointestinal/Hepatic
Abdominal pain (2–8%)
Nausea (28–48%) [11]
Vomiting (7–11%) [3]

Neuromuscular/Skeletal
Arthralgia (2–7%)
Asthenia / fatigue (3–7%)

Respiratory
Cough (2–6%)
Pharyngitis (sore throat) (3–5%)

Other
Allergic reactions (6%)

PRASUGREL

Trade name: Effient (Lilly)
Indications: Acute coronary syndrome in patients who are to be managed with percutaneous coronary intervention
Class: Antiplatelet; thienopyridine
Half-life: 2–15 hours
Clinically important, potentially hazardous interactions with: cangrelor, clopidogrel, conivaptan, coumarins, darunavir, delavirdine, diclofenac, indinavir, inotersen, meloxicam, NSAIDs, phenindione, telithromycin, voriconazole, warfarin
Important contra-indications noted in the prescribing guidelines for: the elderly; nursing mothers; pediatric patients
Note: Contra-indicated in patients with active pathological bleeding, prior transient ischemic attack or stroke.
Warning: BLEEDING RISK

Skin
Hypersensitivity [2]
Peripheral edema (3%)
Rash (3%) [4]

Mucosal
Epistaxis (nosebleed) (6%)

Cardiovascular
Atrial fibrillation (3%)
Bradycardia / sinus bradycardia (3%)
Chest pain (3%)
Hypertension (8%)
Hypotension (4%)

Central Nervous System
Fever (pyrexia) (includes hyperpyrexia) (3%)
Headache (6%)
Vertigo / dizziness (4%)

Endocrine/Metabolic
Hypercholesterolemia (7%)
Hyperlipidemia / lipids elevated (7%)

Gastrointestinal/Hepatic
Diarrhea (3%)
Gastrointestinal bleeding (2%)
Nausea (5%)

Hematologic
Anemia (2%)
Bleeding (<14%) [27]
Hemorrhage [2]
Leukocytopenia (leukopenia) / leukocytes (white blood cells) decreased (3%)

Neuromuscular/Skeletal
Asthenia / fatigue (4%)
Back pain (5%)
Pain in extremities (3%)

Respiratory
Cough (4%)
Dyspnea / shortness of breath (5%)
Respiratory distress [2]

Other
Adverse effects / adverse reactions [2]
Malignant neoplasms (2%)

PRAVASTATIN

Trade names: Lipostat (Bristol-Myers Squibb), Pravachol (Bristol-Myers Squibb)
Indications: Hypercholesterolemia
Class: HMG-CoA reductase inhibitor / statin
Half-life: ~2–3 hours
Clinically important, potentially hazardous interactions with: azithromycin, bempedoic acid, ciprofibrate, clarithromycin, colchicine, cyclosporine, darunavir, efavirenz, erythromycin, gemfibrozil, imatinib, letermovir, red rice yeast, telithromycin
Important contra-indications noted in the prescribing guidelines for: nursing mothers

---

Skin
- Dermatomyositis [2]
- Eczema / eczematous reaction / eczematous eruption (generalized) [2]
- Edema / fluid retention (3%)
- Lichenoid eruption / lichenoid reaction [2]
- Pruritus (itching) [2]
- Rash (5–7%) [7]

Cardiovascular
- Angina (5%)
- Chest pain (3–10%)

Central Nervous System
- Anxiety (5%)
- Fever (pyrexia) (includes hyperpyrexia) (2%)
- Headache (6%)
- Nervousness (5%)
- Paresthesias (3%)
- Sleep disturbances (3%)
- Vertigo / dizziness (4–7%)

Endocrine/Metabolic
- ALT increased (3%)
- Creatine phosphokinase (CPK) / creatine kinase increased (hyperCKemia) (4%) [3]
- GGT increased (2%)
- Weight gain (4%)
- Weight loss (3%)

Gastrointestinal/Hepatic
- Abdominal distension (2%)
- Diarrhea (7%)
- Dyspepsia / functional dyspepsia (indigestion) (see also gastroparesis) (3%)
- Flatulence (3%)
- Nausea (7%)
- Pancreatitis / acute pancreatitis [4]
- Vomiting (7%)

Genitourinary
- Urinary tract infection (3%)

Neuromuscular/Skeletal
- Asthenia / fatigue (3–8%)
- Bone pain / joint pain (25%)
- Cramps (5%)
- Myalgia/Myopathy (2–3%) [10]
- Rhabdomyolysis [24]

Ocular
- Diplopia (double vision) (3%)
- Vision blurred (3%)

Renal
- Renal failure [2]

Respiratory
- Bronchitis (3%)
- Cough (3–8%)
- Influenza (9%)
- Pharyngitis (sore throat) (2%)
- Pulmonary toxicity (4%)
- Rhinitis / rhinosinusitis (see also sinusitis) (4%)
- Upper respiratory tract infection (6–21%)

Other
- Adverse effects / adverse reactions [3]
- Infection (3%)

PRAZIQUANTEL

Synonym: Arpraziquantel
Trade name: Biltricide (Bayer)
Indications: Helmintic infections
Class: Anthelmintic
Half-life: 0.8–1.5 hours
Clinically important, potentially hazardous interactions with: dexamethasone, efavirenz, oxcarbazepine, rifampin, rifapentine
Important contra-indications noted in the prescribing guidelines for: nursing mothers
Note: Arpraziquantel is the (R)-form.

Skin
- Diaphoresis (<10%)
- Edema / fluid retention [2]
- Pruritus (itching) [3]
- Rash [2]
- Urticaria / hives [5]

Central Nervous System
- Fever (pyrexia) (includes hyperpyrexia) [2]
- Headache [9]
- Seizures [2]
- Somnolence (drowsiness) [3]
- Vertigo / dizziness [7]

Gastrointestinal/Hepatic
- Abdominal pain [13]
- Diarrhea [8]
- Nausea [6]
- Vomiting [9]

Neuromuscular/Skeletal
- Asthenia / fatigue [3]

Other
- Adverse effects / adverse reactions [4]
- Allergic reactions [2]

PRAZOSIN

Trade names: Minipress (Pfizer), Minizide (Pfizer)
Indications: Hypertension
Class: Adrenergic alpha-receptor antagonist
Half-life: 2–4 hours
Clinically important, potentially hazardous interactions with: acebutolol, epinephrine
Note: Minizide is prazosin and polythiazide.

Skin
- Anaphylactoid reactions / anaphylaxis (includes anaphylactic shock) [2]
- Diaphoresis [2]
- Edema / fluid retention (<4%)
- Exanthems (<5%)
- Lupus erythematosus (subacute cutaneous lupus erythematosus (SCLE)) [3]
- Rash (<4%) [2]

Mucosal
- Xerostomia (dry mouth) (<4%) [3]

Central Nervous System
- Vertigo / dizziness [2]

Genitourinary
- Priapism [8]

PREDNISOLONE

Trade names: Blephamide (Allergan), Delta-Cortef (Pharmacia), Hydeltrasol (Merck), Inflamase (Novartis), Pediapred (UCB), Prelone (Teva)
Indications: Arthralgias, asthma, dermatoses, inflammatory ocular conditions
Class: Corticosteroid / Glucocorticoid, Corticosteroid, systemic
Half-life: 2–4 hours
Clinically important, potentially hazardous interactions with: aluminum, aminophylline, carbamazepine, carbimazole, cyclosporine, daclizumab, diuretics, etoposide, etretinate, grapefruit juice, indomethacin, isoniazid, itraconazole, ketoconazole, live vaccines, methotrexate, naproxen, oral contraceptives, pancuronium, phenobarbital, phenytoin, rifampin, troleandomycin

---

Skin
- Acneiform eruption / acneiform dermatitis / acneiform rash [4]
- AGEP [2]
- Candidiasis / candidosis [2]
- Cushingoid features [2]
- Cutaneous toxicity / skin toxicity [3]
- Dermatitis [3]
- Edema / fluid retention [7]
- Erythema [2]
- Erythema multiforme [2]
- Exanthems [3]
- Flushing / rubefaction [2]
- Kaposi's sarcoma [3]
- Pruritus (itching) [2]
- Stevens-Johnson syndrome and toxic epidermal necrolysis (SJS/TEN) [3]

Hair
- Alopecia / hair loss [3]

Cardiovascular
- Atrial fibrillation [2]
- Cardiotoxicity [4]
- Hypertension [14]
- Tachycardia [2]

Central Nervous System
- Behavioral disturbances / personality changes [2]
- Depression [4]
- Psychosis [4]

Endocrine/Metabolic
- ALT increased [2]
- Cushing's syndrome [4]
- Diabetes mellitus [5]
- Hyperglycemia (includes glucose increased) [4]
- Hypokalemia [7]
- Weight gain [2]

Gastrointestinal/Hepatic
- Constipation [3]
- Diarrhea [2]
- Hepatotoxicity / liver injury / acute liver injury / drug-induced liver injury (DILI) [6]
- Nausea [2]
- Pancreatitis / acute pancreatitis [4]

Hematologic
- Anemia [3]
- Febrile neutropenia [3]
- Neutropenia (neutrophils decreased) [4]
- Thrombocytopenia / platelets decreased [2]

Neuromuscular/Skeletal
- Arthralgia [4]

Asthenia / fatigue [5]
Back pain [4]
Bone pain / joint pain [5]
Myalgia/Myopathy [2]
Osteonecrosis / avascular necrosis (includes steroid-induced osteonecrosis of the femoral head) [5]
Osteoporosis [33]

Ocular
Cataract [6]
Chorioretinopathy [2]
Glaucoma (includes acute angle-closure glaucoma) [3]
Intraocular pressure increased [4]

Respiratory
Upper respiratory tract infection [2]

Other
Adverse effects / adverse reactions [12]
Allergic reactions [2]
Death [3]
Infection [18]
Side effects [4]

PREDNISONE

Trade names: Deltasone (Pharmacia), Meticorten (Schering)
Indications: Arthralgias, asthma, dermatoses, inflammatory ocular conditions
Class: Corticosteroid / Glucocorticoid, Corticosteroid, systemic
Half-life: N/A
Clinically important, potentially hazardous interactions with: aluminum, aminophylline, aspirin, chlorambucil, cimetidine, clarithromycin, cyclophosphamide, cyclosporine, dicumarol, diuretics, docetaxel, estrogens, grapefruit juice, indomethacin, influenza vaccine, itraconazole, ketoconazole, lansoprazole, live vaccines, lumateperone, lumateperone, methotrexate, montelukast, omeprazole, oral contraceptives, pancuronium, phenobarbital, phenytoin, ranitidine, rifampin, timolol, tolbutamide, vitamin A, yellow fever vaccine
Important contra-indications noted in the prescribing guidelines for: the elderly; nursing mothers

---

Skin
Bruise / bruising / contusion / ecchymosis (ecchymoses) [3]
Cutaneous toxicity / skin toxicity [2]
Dermatitis [4]
Erythema [3]
Hot flashes / hot flushes [2]
Kaposi's sarcoma [7]
Squamous cell carcinoma [2]
Thinning [2]

Hair
Alopecia / hair loss [2]

Mucosal
Stomatitis (oral mucositis) [2]

Cardiovascular
Cardiotoxicity [3]
Hypertension [9]

Central Nervous System
Headache [3]
Leukoencephalopathy / posterior reversible encephalopathy syndrome (PRES) [3]
Mania [4]
Peripheral neuropathy [4]
Psychosis [2]

Endocrine/Metabolic
ALT increased [3]
Diabetes mellitus [3]
Hyperglycemia (includes glucose increased) [5]
Hypokalemia [3]
Weight gain [4]

Gastrointestinal/Hepatic
Constipation [3]
Diarrhea [4]
Nausea [4]
Vomiting [2]

Hematologic
Anemia [5]
Febrile neutropenia [3]
Leukocytopenia (leukopenia) / leukocytes (white blood cells) decreased [3]
Lymphopenia (lymphocytopenia) / lymphocytes decreased [3]
Neutropenia (neutrophils decreased) [15]
Thrombocytopenia / platelets decreased [10]

Neuromuscular/Skeletal
Arthralgia [2]
Asthenia / fatigue [7]
Back pain [2]
Bone pain / joint pain [2]
Fractures [3]
Myalgia/Myopathy [5]
Osteonecrosis / avascular necrosis (includes steroid-induced osteonecrosis of the femoral head) [4]
Osteoporosis [23]

Ocular
Cataract [3]

Respiratory
Cough [2]
Nasopharyngitis [2]
Upper respiratory tract infection [2]

Other
Adverse effects / adverse reactions [10]
Death [3]
Infection [12]
Side effects [3]

PREGABALIN

Trade name: Lyrica (Pfizer)
Indications: Neuropathy, post-herpetic neuralgia, partial epilepsy, fibromyalgia
Class: Anticonvulsant (see also antiepileptic (anti-seizure)), GABA analog, Gabapentinoid
Half-life: 6 hours
Clinically important, potentially hazardous interactions with: lacosamide, pioglitazone
Pregnancy category: Pregabalin may slightly increase the risk of major congenital malformations if used in pregnancy. Patients should continue to use effective contraception during treatment and avoid use in pregnancy unless clearly necessary.
Important contra-indications noted in the prescribing guidelines for: nursing mothers; pediatric patients
Note: Pregabalin (Lyrica) and risk of abuse and dependence: new scheduling requirements from 1 April 2019 (UK) As of 1 April 2019 in the UK, pregabalin is controlled under the Misuse of Drugs Act 1971 as a Class C substance and scheduled under the Misuse of Drugs Regulations 2001 as Schedule 3. Patients should be evaluated carefully for a history of drug abuse before prescribing pregabalin and patients should be observed for development of signs of abuse and dependence. .

Skin
Edema / fluid retention (2%) [10]
Hypersensitivity [2]
Peripheral edema (9%) [16]

Mucosal
Xerostomia (dry mouth) (5%) [11]

Cardiovascular
Cardiac failure [4]
Chest pain (2%)

Central Nervous System
Anorgasmia [3]
Confusion [2]
Depression [2]
Gait instability / postural instability [4]
Hallucinations [3]
Headache (7%) [9]
Impaired concentration [2]
Insomnia [3]
Memory loss/memory impaired [2]
Neurotoxicity [4]
Pain (5%)
Psychosis [3]
Sedation [6]
Somnolence (drowsiness) [50]
Suicidal ideation [4]
Tremor [2]
Vertigo / dizziness (4%) [63]

Endocrine/Metabolic
Appetite increased [2]
Hypoglycemia [3]
Weight gain [23]

Gastrointestinal/Hepatic
Constipation [7]
Diarrhea [2]
Hepatotoxicity / liver injury / acute liver injury / drug-induced liver injury (DILI) [2]
Nausea [9]
Vomiting [3]

Genitourinary
Erectile dysfunction [3]
Priapism [2]
Sexual dysfunction [4]

Neuromuscular/Skeletal
Asthenia / fatigue (5%) [10]
Ataxia [8]
Back pain (2%)
Muscle spasm [2]
Myalgia/Myopathy [2]
Myoclonus (see also hypnic jerk) [4]
Rhabdomyolysis [7]

Ocular
Diplopia (double vision) (9%) [2]
Ocular edema (eye edema) [2]
Vision blurred (6%) [8]

Respiratory
Respiratory depression [2]
Upper respiratory tract infection [2]

Other
Adverse effects / adverse reactions [8]
Congenital malformations [2]
Dipsia (thirst) / polydipsia [2]
Infection (7%)
Side effects [2]

PRETOMANID

Trade name: PA-824 (TB Alliance)
Indications: Part of a combination regimen with **bedaquiline** and **linezolid** for the<br / >treatment of adults with pulmonary extensively drug resistant, treatment-intolerant or nonresponsive multidrug-resistant tuberculosis
Class: Antimycobacterial (including antitubercular)
Half-life: 17 hours
Clinically important, potentially hazardous interactions with: organic anion transporter-3 substrates, strong or moderate CYP3A4 inducers
Pregnancy category: There are no studies or available data on pretomanid use in pregnant women to inform any drug-associated risks. Breastfeeding is not recommended during treatment with pretomanid or with combination therapies.
Important contra-indications noted in the prescribing guidelines for: nursing mothers
Note: Pretomanid is indicated for use in a limited and specific population of patients.

Skin
- Acneiform eruption / acneiform dermatitis / acneiform rash (with bedaquiline and linezolid) (39%)
- Dry skin (with bedaquiline and linezolid) (7%)
- Pruritus (itching) (with bedaquiline and linezolid) (20%)
- Rash (with bedaquiline and linezolid) (21%)

Cardiovascular
- Hypertension (with bedaquiline and linezolid) (7%)
- QT interval prolonged / QT prolongation (with bedaquiline and linezolid) (6%)

Central Nervous System
- Dysgeusia (taste perversion) (with bedaquiline and linezolid) (<5%)
- Headache (with bedaquiline and linezolid) (28%)
- Insomnia (with bedaquiline and linezolid) (6%)
- Peripheral neuropathy (with bedaquiline and linezolid) (81%)
- Seizures (with bedaquiline and linezolid) (<5%)
- Vertigo / dizziness (with bedaquiline and linezolid) (<5%)

Endocrine/Metabolic
- ALP increased (with bedaquiline and linezolid) (<5%)
- Appetite decreased (with bedaquiline and linezolid) (22%)
- Creatine phosphokinase (CPK) / creatine kinase increased (hyperCKemia) (with bedaquiline and linezolid) (<5%)
- GGT increased (with bedaquiline and linezolid) (17%)
- Hyperamylasemia (with bedaquiline and linezolid) (14%)
- Hyperglycemia (includes glucose increased) (with bedaquiline and linezolid) (<5%)
- Hyperkalemia (with bedaquiline and linezolid) (<5%)
- Hyperlipasemia (with bedaquiline and linezolid) (6%)
- Hypertransaminasemia (hepatic transaminitis) / elevated transaminases (with bedaquiline and linezolid) (28%)
- Hypoglycemia (with bedaquiline and linezolid) (11%)
- Hypokalemia (with bedaquiline and linezolid) (<5%)
- Hypomagnesemia (with bedaquiline and linezolid) (<5%)
- Hyponatremia (with bedaquiline and linezolid) (<5%)
- Serum creatinine increased (with bedaquiline and linezolid) (<5%)
- Weight loss (with bedaquiline and linezolid) (10%)

Gastrointestinal/Hepatic
- Abdominal pain (with bedaquiline and linezolid) (19%)
- Constipation (with bedaquiline and linezolid) (8%)
- Diarrhea (with bedaquiline and linezolid) (10%)
- Dyspepsia / functional dyspepsia (indigestion) (see also gastroparesis) (with bedaquiline and linezolid) (24%)
- Gastritis / pangastritis / gastric irritation (with bedaquiline and linezolid) (8%)
- Nausea (with bedaquiline and linezolid) (37%)
- Pancreatitis / acute pancreatitis (with bedaquiline and linezolid) (<5%)
- Vomiting (with bedaquiline and linezolid) (34%)

Hematologic
- Anemia (with bedaquiline and linezolid) (serious / 2 cases) (37%)
- Leukocytopenia (leukopenia) / leukocytes (white blood cells) decreased (with bedaquiline and linezolid) (<5%)
- Neutropenia (neutrophils decreased) (with bedaquiline and linezolid) (serious / 1 case) (8%)
- Thrombocytopenia / platelets decreased (with bedaquiline and linezolid) (6%)

Neuromuscular/Skeletal
- Musculoskeletal pain (with bedaquiline and linezolid) (29%)
- Pleuritic pain (with bedaquiline and linezolid) (19%)

Ocular
- Optic neuropathy (with bedaquiline and linezolid) (serious / 2 cases) (2%)
- Vision impaired (with bedaquiline and linezolid) (12%)

Respiratory
- Cough (with bedaquiline and linezolid) (12%)
- Hemoptysis (with bedaquiline and linezolid) (13%)
- Lower respiratory tract infection (with bedaquiline and linezolid) (15%)

PRILOCAINE

Trade name: Citanest (AstraZeneca)
Indications: Local anesthetic
Class: Membrane integrity antagonist, Potassium channel antagonist, Sodium channel antagonist
Half-life: 2 hours
Clinically important, potentially hazardous interactions with: adenosine, amide-type anesthetics, antimalarials, co-trimoxazole, dronedarone, nitric compounds, sulfonamides
Important contra-indications noted in the prescribing guidelines for: nursing mothers; pediatric patients

---

Skin
- Angioedema (formerly named angioneurotic edema) [3]
- Contact dermatitis [3]
- Hypersensitivity [2]
- Petechiae [3]
- Purpura [3]

Central Nervous System
- Coma [4]
- Paresthesias [3]
- Seizures [2]

Hematologic
- Methemoglobinemia [12]

Other
- Adverse effects / adverse reactions [2]

PRIMAQUINE

Trade name: Primaquine (Sanofi-Aventis)
Indications: Malaria
Class: Antimalarial, Antimicrobial, Antiprotozoal
Half-life: 4–10 hours
Clinically important, potentially hazardous interactions with: penicillamine

---

Skin
- Exanthems (5%)

Hematologic
- Hemolysis [2]

PRIMIDONE

Trade name: Mysoline (Xcel)
Indications: Seizures
Class: Anticonvulsant (see also antiepileptic (anti-seizure)), Barbiturate
Half-life: 10–12 hours
Clinically important, potentially hazardous interactions with: alcohol, amitriptyline, amlodipine, anticoagulants, antihistamines, betamethasone, brompheniramine, buclizine, chlorpheniramine, dexamethasone, dichlorphenamide, dicumarol, doxycycline, ethanolamine, ethosuximide, imatinib, levomepromazine, lopinavir, metronidazole, midazolam, nelfinavir, niacinamide, paroxetine hydrochloride, perampanel, pizotifen, risperidone, rufinamide, telithromycin, triamcinolone, warfarin, zafirlukast, zuclopenthixol
Note: Aromatic antiepileptic drugs, phenytoin, phenobarbital, carbamazepine and primidone, are a frequent cause of severe cutaneous adverse reactions. A strong genetic association between HLA-B*1502 and primidone-induced Stevens-Johnson syndrome and toxic epidermal necrolysis has been shown in Han Chinese patients.

Skin
- Erythema multiforme [2]
- Exanthems (<5%)
- Hypersensitivity [2]
- Lupus erythematosus (subacute cutaneous lupus erythematosus (SCLE)) [7]
- Rash [2]
- Stevens-Johnson syndrome and toxic epidermal necrolysis (SJS/TEN) [5]

PRISTINAMYCIN

Trade name: Pyostacine (Sanofi-Aventis)
Indications: Staphylococcal and streptococcal infections
Class: Antibiotic, Antibiotic; streptogramin, Antimicrobial
Half-life: 4.03±2.77 hours
Clinically important, potentially hazardous interactions with: calcium channel blockers, cyclosporine, methotrexate, quinidine, trimetrexate

---

Skin
AGEP [8]
Baboon syndrome / symmetrical drug-related intertriginous and flexural exanthema (SDRIFE) [2]
Exanthems [2]
Pruritus (itching) (2%)
Rash (3%) [2]
Stevens-Johnson syndrome and toxic epidermal necrolysis (SJS/TEN) [3]

Central Nervous System
Headache (2%)
Pain (2%)

Local
Injection-site edema (17%)
Injection-site inflammation (40%)
Injection-site pain (42%)

Neuromuscular/Skeletal
Arthralgia (~47%)
Myalgia/Myopathy (~47%)

PROBENECID

Indications: Gouty arthritis
Class: Uricosuric
Half-life: 6–12 hours (dose-dependent)
Clinically important, potentially hazardous interactions with: acemetacin, acetaminophen, amphotericin B, ampicillin/sulbactam, benzodiazepines, captopril, cefazolin, cefditoren, cefixime, ceftaroline fosamil, ceftazidime & avibactam, ceftriaxone, ciprofloxacin, deferiprone, doripenem, ertapenem, flucloxacillin, furosemide, gemifloxacin, glibenclamide, ketoprofen, ketorolac, levodopa, levofloxacin, lumateperone, meloxicam, meropenem, meropenem & vaborbactam, methotrexate, moxifloxacin, norfloxacin, NSAIDs, ofloxacin, pemetrexed, penicillamine, penicillin G, penicillin V, pralatrexate, salicylates, sulfamethoxazole, sulfonamides, ticarcillin, torsemide, zidovudine
Important contra-indications noted in the prescribing guidelines for: nursing mothers; pediatric patients

---

Skin
Flushing / rubefaction (<10%)
Pruritus (itching) (<10%)
Rash (<10%)
Urticaria / hives (<5%)

Mucosal
Gingivitis (<10%)

Hematologic
Thrombocytopenia / platelets decreased [2]

Renal
Nephrotoxicity / kidney injury / acute kidney injury (AKI) / drug-induced kidney injury [3]

PROCAINAMIDE

Trade names: Procan (Pfizer), Procanbid (Pfizer)
Indications: Ventricular arrhythmias
Class: Antiarrhythmic, Antiarrhythmic class Ia
Half-life: 2.5–4.5 hours
Clinically important, potentially hazardous interactions with: abarelix, amiodarone, amisulpride, arsenic, artemether/lumefantrine, asenapine, astemizole, ciprofloxacin, enoxacin, ethoxzolamide, gatifloxacin, glycopyrrolate, glycopyrronium, imidapril, lomefloxacin, lurasidone, metformin, mivacurium, moxifloxacin, nilotinib, norfloxacin, ofloxacin, pimavanserin, ponesimod, quinine, quinolones, ribociclib, rocuronium, sotalol, sparfloxacin, tetrabenazine, trimethoprim, trospium, vandetanib, zofenopril
Important contra-indications noted in the prescribing guidelines for: nursing mothers; pediatric patients

---

Skin
Dermatitis (6%)
Exanthems (<8%) [5]
Hypersensitivity [2]
Lupus erythematosus (subacute cutaneous lupus erythematosus (SCLE)) (>10%) [176]
Purpura [3]
Urticaria / hives (<5%)
Vasculitis (angiitis) / cutaneous vasculitis (angiitis) [5]

Mucosal
Oral mucosal eruption (2%)

Cardiovascular
Hypotension [2]
QT interval prolonged / QT prolongation [5]
Torsades de pointes [3]

Central Nervous System
Dysgeusia (taste perversion) (3–4%)
Psychosis [2]

Gastrointestinal/Hepatic
Hepatotoxicity / liver injury / acute liver injury / drug-induced liver injury (DILI) [3]
Nausea [3]

Hematologic
Agranulocytosis / severe selective neutropenia [4]
Neutropenia (neutrophils decreased) [3]
Pancytopenia (includes bicytopenia) [2]
Pure red cell aplasia [3]

Neuromuscular/Skeletal
Myalgia/Myopathy [2]
Myasthenia gravis [3]

Respiratory
Pulmonary toxicity [2]

PROCARBAZINE

Trade name: Matulane (Sigma-Tau)
Indications: Hodgkin's disease, lymphomas
Class: Alkylating agent
Half-life: 1 hour
Clinically important, potentially hazardous interactions with: aldesleukin, methotrexate

---

Skin
Exanthems (4–9%) [5]
Flushing / rubefaction [2]
Hypersensitivity (2%) [2]
Pigmentation (Skin) (includes hyperpigmentation) (<10%)
Stevens-Johnson syndrome and toxic epidermal necrolysis (SJS/TEN) [3]
Urticaria / hives (9%) [3]

Hair
Alopecia / hair loss (<10%) [2]

Mucosal
Oral lesions (<5%) [2]
Stomatitis (oral mucositis) (>10%)

Central Nervous System
Neurotoxicity [2]
Paresthesias (>10%)

Gastrointestinal/Hepatic
Hepatotoxicity / liver injury / acute liver injury / drug-induced liver injury (DILI) [2]

Hematologic
Neutropenia (neutrophils decreased) [2]
Thrombocytopenia / platelets decreased [3]

PROCHLORPERAZINE

Trade name: Compazine (GSK)
Indications: Psychotic disorders, control of severe nausea and vomiting
Class: Antiemetic, Antipsychotic, Muscarinic antagonist, Phenothiazine
Half-life: 23 hours
Clinically important, potentially hazardous interactions with: antihistamines, arsenic, chlorpheniramine, dofetilide, pericyazine, piperazine, quinine, quinolones, sparfloxacin
Important contra-indications noted in the prescribing guidelines for: the elderly; nursing mothers; pediatric patients

---

Skin
Anaphylactoid reactions / anaphylaxis (includes anaphylactic shock) (<10%)
Fixed eruption / fixed drug eruption [3]
Photosensitivity (<10%) [3]
Pruritus (itching) (<10%)
Rash (<10%)
Stevens-Johnson syndrome and toxic epidermal necrolysis (SJS/TEN) [2]

Mucosal
Xerostomia (dry mouth) (>10%)

Central Nervous System
Akathisia [15]
Extrapyramidal symptoms [3]
Neuroleptic malignant syndrome [4]
Parkinsonism [4]
Somnolence (drowsiness) [2]

Endocrine/Metabolic
Gynecomastia (<10%)

Neuromuscular/Skeletal
Dystonia [7]

PROCYCLIDINE

Trade name: Kemadrin (Monarch)
Indications: Parkinsonism
Class: Muscarinic antagonist
Half-life: N/A
Clinically important, potentially hazardous interactions with: anticholinergics, arbutamine, paroxetine hydrochloride

---

Skin
Photosensitivity (<10%)
Xerosis / xeroderma (>10%)

Mucosal
Xerostomia (dry mouth) (>10%)

PROGESTINS

Trade names: Aygestin (Barr), Megace (Bristol-Myers Squibb), Micronor (Ortho), Ovrette (Wyeth), Provera (Pfizer)
Indications: Prevention of pregnancy
Class: Progestogen
Half-life: N/A
Clinically important, potentially hazardous interactions with: acitretin, aprepitant, dofetilide, rosuvastatin, voriconazole

Skin
Acneiform eruption / acneiform dermatitis / acneiform rash [3]
Dermatitis [4]
Diaphoresis (31%)
Erythema multiforme [2]
Flushing / rubefaction (12%)
Urticaria / hives [2]
Endocrine/Metabolic
Amenorrhea [2]

PROMAZINE

Indications: Psychotic disorders, schizophrenia
Class: Antipsychotic, Phenothiazine
Half-life: 24 hours
Clinically important, potentially hazardous interactions with: sparfloxacin

Skin
Exanthems [2]
Photosensitivity (<10%)
Phototoxicity [3]
Rash (<10%)
Cardiovascular
Hypotension [2]
Endocrine/Metabolic
Mastodynia (<10%)

PROMETHAZINE

Trade name: Phenergan (Wyeth)
Indications: Allergic rhinitis, urticaria
Class: Histamine H1 receptor antagonist
Half-life: 10–14 hours
Clinically important, potentially hazardous interactions with: antihistamines, arsenic, chlorpheniramine, dofetilide, nalbuphine, piperazine, quinolones, sparfloxacin, zaleplon
Important contra-indications noted in the prescribing guidelines for: the elderly; nursing mothers; pediatric patients
Note: Not for intra-arterial or subcutaneous injection and contra-indicated in comatose states.
Warning: RESPIRATORY DEPRESSION and SEVERE TISSUE INJURY, INCLUDING GANGRENE

Skin
Dermatitis [3]
Erythema multiforme [2]
Lupus erythematosus (subacute cutaneous lupus erythematosus (SCLE)) [2]
Photosensitivity [12]
Purpura [2]
Stevens-Johnson syndrome and toxic epidermal necrolysis (SJS/TEN) [2]
Urticaria / hives [3]
Mucosal
Xerostomia (dry mouth) (<10%) [2]
Cardiovascular
QT interval prolonged / QT prolongation [2]
Central Nervous System
Delirium [2]
Neuroleptic malignant syndrome [2]
Seizures [2]
Somnolence (drowsiness) [3]

PROPAFENONE

Trade name: Rythmol (Reliant)
Indications: Ventricular arrhythmias
Class: Antiarrhythmic, Antiarrhythmic class Ic
Half-life: 10–32 hours
Clinically important, potentially hazardous interactions with: amitriptyline, boceprevir, carvedilol, clozapine, cobicistat/elvitegravir/emtricitabine/tenofovir alafenamide, cobicistat/elvitegravir/emtricitabine/tenofovir disoproxil, delavirdine, digoxin, efavirenz, fosamprenavir, grapefruit juice, mirabegron, neostigmine, paroxetine hydrochloride, propranolol, pyridostigmine, rifapentine, ritonavir, telaprevir, tipranavir
Important contra-indications noted in the prescribing guidelines for: nursing mothers; pediatric patients

Skin
Lupus erythematosus (subacute cutaneous lupus erythematosus (SCLE)) [3]
Psoriasis [2]
Rash (<3%)
Mucosal
Oral lesions (>5%)
Xerostomia (dry mouth) (2%)
Cardiovascular
Bradycardia / sinus bradycardia [3]
Brugada syndrome [7]
Cardiotoxicity [3]
Congestive heart failure [2]
Hypotension [3]
Central Nervous System
Dysgeusia (taste perversion) (3–23%)
Seizures [3]
Syncope / fainting [2]
Gastrointestinal/Hepatic
Hepatotoxicity / liver injury / acute liver injury / drug-induced liver injury (DILI) [8]
Local
Injection-site pain (28–90%) [4]

PROPOFOL

Trade name: Diprivan (AstraZeneca)
Indications: Induction and maintenance of anesthesia
Class: Anesthetic; general
Half-life: initial: 40 minutes; terminal: 3 days
Clinically important, potentially hazardous interactions with: zinc
Important contra-indications noted in the prescribing guidelines for: nursing mothers; pediatric patients
Note: Fospropofol disodium a prodrug of propofol was withdrawn in 2012.

Skin
Anaphylactoid reactions / anaphylaxis (includes anaphylactic shock) (<10%) [10]
Angioedema (formerly named angioneurotic edema) [2]
Exanthems (6%) [2]
Rash (5%)
Urticaria / hives [2]
Hair
Hair pigmentation [3]
Cardiovascular
Bradycardia / sinus bradycardia [16]
Brugada syndrome [2]
Cardiac failure [2]
Hypotension [23]
Tachycardia [2]
Central Nervous System
Amnesia [10]
Hallucinations [3]
Myokymia / twitching / fasciculation (<10%)
Neurological adverse effect / neurological deficit [2]
Sedation [2]
Seizures [10]
Shivering [2]
Endocrine/Metabolic
Acidosis (includes lactic acidosis) [3]
Hypertriglyceridemia (includes triglycerides increased) [3]
Gastrointestinal/Hepatic
Nausea [4]
Pancreatitis / acute pancreatitis [9]
Vomiting [5]
Hematologic
Hypoxemia [2]
Local
Infusion-related reactions [3]
Injection-site pain (>10%) [38]
Neuromuscular/Skeletal
Ataxia [2]
Myoclonus (see also hypnic jerk) [3]
Opisthotonus [3]
Rhabdomyolysis [10]
Renal
Green urine [8]
Respiratory
Apnea [4]
Cough [2]
Hypoxia [7]
Respiratory depression [4]
Other
Adverse effects / adverse reactions [6]
Death [9]
Hiccups / singultus [3]

PROPOLIS

Family: None
Scientific name: *Propolis*
Indications: Tuberculosis, bacterial, fungal and protozoal infections, nasopharyngeal carcinoma, duodenal ulcer, *Helicobacter pylori* infection, cold, wound cleansing, mouth rinse, genital herpes. Ingredient in cosmetics
Class: Immunomodulator
Half-life: N/A
Clinically important, potentially hazardous interactions with: none known

Skin
Contact dermatitis [3]

Dermatitis [39]
Hypersensitivity [4]
Sensitivity [4]

Mucosal
Cheilitis (inflammation of the lips) [2]

Other
Allergic reactions [8]

PROPOXYPHENE

Trade names: Darvocet-N (Xanodyne), Darvon (Xanodyne), Darvon Compound (Xanodyne)
Indications: Pain
Class: Opiate agonist
Half-life: 8–24 hours
Clinically important, potentially hazardous interactions with: alcohol, alprazolam, amitriptyline, carbamazepine, insulin aspart, insulin degludec, insulin glargine, insulin glulisine, linezolid, lisdexamfetamine, metoprolol, phenelzine, ritonavir, safinamide, selegiline, warfarin
Pregnancy category: category D with prolonged use
Note: Darvocet is propoxyphene and acetaminophen; Darvon Compound is propoxyphene and aspirin.
This drug has been withdrawn from the European market. Xanodyne has voluntarily removed its products from the US market. The FDA is advising healthcare professionals to stop prescribing propoxyphene to their patients.

Mucosal
Xerostomia (dry mouth) (<10%)

Central Nervous System
Vertigo / dizziness [2]

Local
Injection-site pain (<10%)

PROPRANOLOL

Trade names: Hemangeol (Pierre Fabre), Inderal (Wyeth)
Indications: Hypertension, angina pectoris, atrial fibrillation, myocardial infarction, migraine, tremor, infantile hemangioma
Class: Antiarrhythmic, Antiarrhythmic class II, Beta adrenergic blocker, Beta blocker
Half-life: 2–6 hours
Clinically important, potentially hazardous interactions with: alcohol, aluminum hydroxide, aminophylline, amiodarone, barbiturates, bupivacaine, chlorpromazine, cholestyramine, cimetidine, ciprofloxacin, clonidine, colestipol, delavirdine, diazepam, dronedarone, epinephrine, ethanol, fluconazole, fluoxetine, fluvoxamine, haloperidol, imipramine, insulin, insulin detemir, insulin glargine, insulin glulisine, isoniazid, levothyroxine, lidocaine, neostigmine, nicardipine, nifedipine, nilutamide, nisoldipine, oxtriphylline, paroxetine hydrochloride, phenobarbital, phenytoin, propafenone, pyridostigmine, quinidine, rifampin, ritonavir, rizatriptan, sodium iodide I-131, teniposide, terbutaline, tolbutamide, verapamil, warfarin, zileuton, zolmitriptan
Important contra-indications noted in the prescribing guidelines for: nursing mothers; pediatric patients
Note: Cutaneous side effects of beta-receptor blockers are clinically polymorphous. They apparently appear after several months of continuous therapy.

Skin
Acneiform eruption / acneiform dermatitis / acneiform rash [2]
Angioedema (formerly named angioneurotic edema) [2]
Cold extremities [7]
Dermatitis [2]
Eczema / eczematous reaction / eczematous eruption [2]
Exanthems [4]
Flushing / rubefaction [2]
Lichenoid eruption / lichenoid reaction [3]
Lupus erythematosus (subacute cutaneous lupus erythematosus (SCLE)) [2]
Necrosis (skin necrosis) [3]
Pemphigus [2]
Psoriasis [21]
Rash (<10%) [3]
Raynaud's phenomenon [3]
Stevens-Johnson syndrome and toxic epidermal necrolysis (SJS/TEN) [3]
Urticaria / hives [3]

Hair
Alopecia / hair loss [6]

Nails
Nail thickening [2]

Cardiovascular
Bradycardia / sinus bradycardia [22]
Cardiac arrest [2]
Hypertension [2]
Hypotension [22]

Central Nervous System
Agitation [2]
Amnesia [2]
Confusion [2]
Delirium [3]
Hallucinations [5]
Hallucinations, visual [4]
Headache [2]
Insomnia [2]
Irritability [2]
Nightmares [2]
Psychosis [3]
Sleep disturbances [10]
Sleep-related disorder [3]
Somnambulism (sleepwalking; noctambulism) [2]
Somnolence (drowsiness) [4]
Vertigo / dizziness [4]

Endocrine/Metabolic
Hyperkalemia [4]
Hypoglycemia [17]
Weight gain [2]

Gastrointestinal/Hepatic
Constipation [2]
Diarrhea [6]
Gastroesophageal reflux [2]
Nausea [2]

Genitourinary
Peyronie's disease [6]

Neuromuscular/Skeletal
Asthenia / fatigue [6]
Myalgia/Myopathy [3]

Respiratory
Bronchospasm [4]
Upper respiratory tract infection [2]
Wheezing [3]

Other
Adverse effects / adverse reactions [13]
Death [3]
Side effects [2]
Tooth decay [2]

PROPYLTHIOURACIL

Trade name: Propyl-Thyracil (Paladin)
Indications: Hyperthyroidism
Class: Antithyroid, Antithyroid; hormone modifier
Half-life: <5 hours
Clinically important, potentially hazardous interactions with: anticoagulants, dicumarol, warfarin
Warning: SEVERE LIVER INJURY and ACUTE LIVER FAILURE

Skin
Angioedema (formerly named angioneurotic edema) [3]
Anti-neutrophil cytoplasmic antibody (ANCA) vasculitis (angiitis) [6]
DRESS syndrome (Drug-induced hypersensitivity syndrome) [5]
Erythema nodosum [2]
Exanthems (3–5%) [6]
Hypersensitivity [4]
Lupus erythematosus (subacute cutaneous lupus erythematosus (SCLE)) (<20%) [16]
Lupus syndrome / drug-induced lupus (DIL) [3]
Pruritus (itching) [2]
Purpura [2]
Pyoderma gangrenosum [6]
Rash (>10%)
Sweet's syndrome [3]
Ulcerations [2]
Urticaria / hives [3]
Vasculitis (angiitis) / cutaneous vasculitis (angiitis) [54]
Vesiculation (in newborn) [2]

Hair
Alopecia / hair loss [3]

Mucosal
Oral ulceration [3]

Central Nervous System
Ageusia (taste loss) / taste disorder (1–10%)
Dysgeusia (taste perversion) (metallic taste) (<10%) [2]
Fever (pyrexia) (includes hyperpyrexia) [2]

Gastrointestinal/Hepatic
Hepatotoxicity / liver injury / acute liver injury / drug-induced liver injury (DILI) [8]

Hematologic
Agranulocytosis / severe selective neutropenia [6]

Otic
Otitis (otitis externa, otitis media, otitis interna) [2]

Renal
Nephrotoxicity / kidney injury / acute kidney injury (AKI) / drug-induced kidney injury [6]

Respiratory
Cough [2]
Pneumonia [4]

Other
Death [4]

PROPYPHENAZONE

Trade names: Migradon (Trenka), Saridon (Bayer)
Indications: Pain and fever
Class: Analgesic, Antipyretic
Half-life: 1–2 hours
Clinically important, potentially hazardous interactions with: alcohol, anticoagulants, antiepileptics, chloramphenicol, ergotamine, metoclopramide, rifampin, sedatives

---

Skin
Anaphylactoid reactions / anaphylaxis (includes anaphylactic shock) [2]

PROTRIPTYLINE

Trade name: Vivactil (Odyssey)
Indications: Depression
Class: Antidepressant; tricyclic
Half-life: 54–92 hours
Clinically important, potentially hazardous interactions with: amprenavir, arbutamine, clonidine, epinephrine, formoterol, guanethidine, isocarboxazid, linezolid, MAO inhibitors, phenelzine, quinolones, sparfloxacin, tranylcypromine
Important contra-indications noted in the prescribing guidelines for: the elderly; nursing mothers; pediatric patients
Warning: SUICIDALITY AND ANTIDEPRESSANT DRUGS

Skin
Dermatitis (3%)
Diaphoresis (<10%)
Pruritus (itching) (<5%)
Mucosal
Xerostomia (dry mouth) (>10%)
Central Nervous System
Dysgeusia (taste perversion) (>10%)
Parkinsonism (<10%)

PRUCALOPRIDE

Trade name: Motegrity (Shire)
Indications: indicated for the treatment of chronic idiopathic constipation (CIC) in adults
Class: Serotonin type 4 receptor agonist
Half-life: ~1 day
Clinically important, potentially hazardous interactions with: none known
Pregnancy category: insufficient data to identify any drug-associated risks

---

Central Nervous System
Headache (19%) [16]
Migraine (<2%)
Suicidal ideation [2]
Vertigo / dizziness (4%)
Endocrine/Metabolic
Appetite decreased (<2%)
Gastrointestinal/Hepatic
Abdominal distension (5%)
Abdominal pain (16%) [11]
Diarrhea (13%) [10]
Flatulence (3%)
Nausea (14%) [8]
Vomiting (3%)
Genitourinary
Pollakiuria (<2%)

PSEUDOEPHEDRINE

Trade names: Allegra-D (Sanofi-Aventis), Benadryl (Pfizer), Bromfed (Muro), Entex (Andrx), Robitussin-CF (Wyeth), Sudafed (Pfizer), Trinalin (Schering)
Indications: Nasal congestion
Class: Adrenergic alpha-receptor agonist
Half-life: 9–16 hours
Clinically important, potentially hazardous interactions with: bromocriptine, fluoxetine, fluvoxamine, furazolidone, iobenguane, MAO inhibitors, paroxetine hydrochloride, phenelzine, rasagiline, sertraline, tranylcypromine
Note: (February 2023) The European Medicines Agency has started a review of medicines containing pseudoephedrine following concerns about the risk of posterior reversible encephalopathy syndrome (PRES) and reversible cerebral vasoconstriction syndrome (RCVS) from the use of over-the-counter decongestants containing pseudoephedrine.

Skin
AGEP [3]
Baboon syndrome / symmetrical drug-related intertriginous and flexural exanthema (SDRIFE) [2]
Dermatitis [3]
Diaphoresis (<10%)
Erythroderma [2]
Exanthems [4]
Fixed eruption / fixed drug eruption [15]
Cardiovascular
Myocardial infarction [2]
Palpitation [2]
Central Nervous System
Hallucinations, visual [2]
Leukoencephalopathy / posterior reversible encephalopathy syndrome (PRES) [3]
Somnolence (drowsiness) [2]

PSORALENS

Trade names: Oxsoralen (Valeant), Trisoralen (Valeant)
Indications: Psoriasis, eczema, vitiligo, cutaneous T-cell lymphoma
Class: Psoralen
Half-life: 2 hours
Clinically important, potentially hazardous interactions with: none known

---

Skin
Anaphylactoid reactions / anaphylaxis (includes anaphylactic shock) [2]
Basal cell carcinoma [3]
Bullous pemphigoid / pemphigoid (with UVA) [14]
Burning / skin burning sensation (<10%) [3]
Dermatitis [11]
Eczema / eczematous reaction / eczematous eruption [2]
Edema / fluid retention (<10%)
Ephelides (freckles) (<10%) [5]
Erythema [2]
Herpes simplex [2]
Herpes zoster [2]
Hypomelanosis (<10%)
Lupus erythematosus (subacute cutaneous lupus erythematosus (SCLE)) [5]
Melanoma [3]
Photosensitivity [14]
Phototoxicity [15]
Pigmentation (Skin) (includes hyperpigmentation) [9]
Porokeratosis (actinic) [3]
Pruritus (itching) (>10%) [4]
Rash (<10%)
Squamous cell carcinoma [4]
Tumors (for the most part malignant) [18]
Vesiculation [2]
Vitiligo [2]
Hair
Hypertrichosis [4]
Nails
Nail pigmentation [4]
Photo-onycholysis [4]
Mucosal
Cheilitis (inflammation of the lips) (<10%)
Central Nervous System
Pain [3]

PYRAZINAMIDE

Trade names: Pyrazinamide (Clonmel), Rifater (Sanofi-Aventis)
Indications: Tuberculosis
Class: Antibiotic, Antimicrobial, Antimycobacterial (including antitubercular)
Half-life: 9–10 hours
Clinically important, potentially hazardous interactions with: rifampin

---

Skin
Anaphylactoid reactions / anaphylaxis (includes anaphylactic shock) [2]
DRESS syndrome (Drug-induced hypersensitivity syndrome) [4]
Rash [5]
Stevens-Johnson syndrome and toxic epidermal necrolysis (SJS/TEN) [2]
Endocrine/Metabolic
Hyperuricemia [5]
Gastrointestinal/Hepatic
Hepatotoxicity / liver injury / acute liver injury / drug-induced liver injury (DILI) [21]
Hematologic
Sideroblastic anemia / acquired sideroblastic anemia [2]
Neuromuscular/Skeletal
Myalgia/Myopathy (<10%) [3]
Other
Adverse effects / adverse reactions [4]
Death [7]

PYRIDOSTIGMINE

Trade names: Mestinon (Valeant), Regonol (Novartis)
Indications: Myasthenia gravis
Class: Acetylcholinesterase inhibitor
Half-life: ~2 hours
Clinically important, potentially hazardous interactions with: aminoglycosides, bacitracin, clindamycin, colistin, edrophonium, polymyxin B, propafenone, propranolol, quinidine, tetracyclines

Important contra-indications noted in the prescribing guidelines for: nursing mothers; pediatric patients

---

Cardiovascular
Atrioventricular block [2]
Myocardial infarction [2]

Central Nervous System
Neurotoxicity [3]
Parkinsonism [2]

Gastrointestinal/Hepatic
Abdominal pain [5]
Diarrhea [2]
Nausea [3]

Other
Adverse effects / adverse reactions [2]
Side effects [2]

PYRIDOXINE

Synonym: vitamin B_6
Indications: Pyridoxine deficiency
Class: Vitamin
Half-life: 15–20 days
Clinically important, potentially hazardous interactions with: levodopa
Pregnancy category: the pregnancy category will be C if used in doses above the RDA

Skin
Acneiform eruption / acneiform dermatitis / acneiform rash [3]
Dermatitis [4]
Photosensitivity [4]

PYRIMETHAMINE

Trade names: Daraprim (GSK), Fansidar (Roche)
Indications: Malaria
Class: Antimalarial, Antimicrobial, Antiprotozoal
Half-life: 80–95 hours
Clinically important, potentially hazardous interactions with: dapsone, pemetrexed, trimethoprim, zidovudine
Important contra-indications noted in the prescribing guidelines for: the elderly; nursing mothers
Note: Fansidar is pyrimethamine and sulfadoxine. Sulfadoxine is a sulfonamide and can be absorbed systemically. Sulfonamides can produce severe, possibly fatal, reactions such as toxic epidermal necrolysis and Stevens-Johnson syndrome.

Skin
Angioedema (formerly named angioneurotic edema) [2]
Bullous dermatosis [2]
DRESS syndrome (Drug-induced hypersensitivity syndrome) [2]
Erythema multiforme [4]
Exanthems [3]
Exfoliative dermatitis [2]
Fixed eruption / fixed drug eruption [3]
Hypersensitivity (>10%)
Lichenoid eruption / lichenoid reaction [2]
Photosensitivity (>10%) [3]
Pigmentation (Skin) (includes hyperpigmentation) [5]
Pruritus (itching) [2]
Stevens-Johnson syndrome and toxic epidermal necrolysis (SJS/TEN) (<10%) [33]

Central Nervous System
Vertigo / dizziness [2]

Gastrointestinal/Hepatic
Diarrhea [2]
Nausea [2]
Vomiting [2]

Neuromuscular/Skeletal
Asthenia / fatigue [2]

Other
Adverse effects / adverse reactions [2]
Death [4]

QUAZEPAM

Trade name: Doral (MedPointe)
Indications: Insomnia
Class: Benzodiazepine
Half-life: 25–41 hours
Clinically important, potentially hazardous interactions with: amprenavir, chlorpheniramine, clarithromycin, efavirenz, esomeprazole, imatinib, indinavir, nelfinavir, ritonavir

---

Skin
Dermatitis (<10%)
Diaphoresis (>10%)
Rash (>10%)

Mucosal
Sialopenia (>10%)
Sialorrhea (ptyalism; hypersalivation) (<10%)
Xerostomia (dry mouth) (<5%)

QUETIAPINE

Trade name: Seroquel (AstraZeneca)
Indications: Schizophrenia, bipolar I disorder
Class: Antipsychotic, Antipsychotic, atypical, Mood stabilizer
Half-life: ~6 hours
Clinically important, potentially hazardous interactions with: alcohol, amoxapine, antihypertensive agents, arsenic, atazanavir, azithromycin, CNS acting drugs, darunavir, dolasetron, dopamine, drugs known to cause electrolyte imbalance or increase QT interval, erythromycin, fluconazole, hepatic enzyme inducers, itraconazole, ketoconazole, levodopa, methadone, P4503A inhibitors, pazopanib, telavancin, tipranavir, tricyclic antidepressants, voriconazole
Important contra-indications noted in the prescribing guidelines for: the elderly; nursing mothers; pediatric patients
Note: Elderly patients with dementia-related psychosis treated with antipsychotic drugs are at an increased risk of death. Quetiapine is not approved for the treatment of patients with dementia-related psychosis.
Warning: INCREASED MORTALITY IN ELDERLY PATIENTS WITH DEMENTIA-RELATED PSYCHOSIS and SUICIDALITY AND ANTIDEPRESSANT DRUGS

Skin
Diaphoresis (<10%)
DRESS syndrome (Drug-induced hypersensitivity syndrome) [3]
Edema / fluid retention [2]
Hyperhidrosis (2%)
Peripheral edema [6]
Rash (4%)
Thrombocytopenic purpura [3]

Mucosal
Sialorrhea (ptyalism; hypersalivation) [3]
Xerostomia (dry mouth) (9%) [22]

Cardiovascular
Bradycardia / sinus bradycardia [2]
Hypertension (41%)
Hypotension [8]
Myocarditis [2]
Postural hypotension [2]
QT interval prolonged / QT prolongation [7]
Tachycardia (6%) [3]

Central Nervous System
Abnormal dreams (2–3%)
Agitation (20%) [3]
Akathisia (8%) [6]
Anxiety (2–4%)
Catatonia [3]
Compulsions / obsessive-compulsive symptoms / obsessive-compulsive disorder [3]
Confusion [2]
Delirium [3]
Depression (3%) [3]
Extrapyramidal symptoms [4]
Headache (21%) [6]
Hypoesthesia / hypesthesia (numbness) (2%)
Hypomania [3]
Impulse control disorder / impulsivity / drug-induced impulsivity [2]
Insomnia (9%) [2]
Mania [3]
Neuroleptic malignant syndrome [19]
Pain (7%)
Paresthesias (3%)
Parkinsonism (4%) [5]
Psychosis [3]
Restless legs syndrome / Willis-Ekbom disease (includes restless arms syndrome variant) [7]
Sedation [15]
Seizures [7]
Serotonin syndrome [3]
Sleep-related disorder [2]
Somnambulism (sleepwalking; noctambulism) [2]
Somnolence (drowsiness) (18%) [23]
Suicidal ideation [3]
Tardive syndrome / tardive dyskinesia (5%) [3]
Tic disorder [3]
Tremor [3]
Vertigo / dizziness (11%) [14]

Endocrine/Metabolic
ALT increased (5%)
Appetite increased [3]
Diabetes mellitus [3]
Galactorrhea [2]
Hyperglycemia (includes glucose increased) [3]
Hypertriglyceridemia (includes triglycerides increased) [4]
Hyponatremia [3]
Hypothyroidism [7]
Libido decreased (2%)
Metabolic syndrome (includes metabolic disorder) [2]
SIADH [5]
Thyroid dysfunction [2]
Weight gain (5%) [23]

Gastrointestinal/Hepatic
Abdominal pain (4–7%)
Colitis [3]
Constipation (8%) [6]
Dyspepsia / functional dyspepsia (indigestion) (see also gastroparesis) (5%)
Hepatotoxicity / liver injury / acute liver injury / drug-induced liver injury (DILI) [2]
Nausea (7%)
Pancreatitis / acute pancreatitis [6]
Vomiting (6%)

Genitourinary
Priapism [14]
Sexual dysfunction [2]
Urinary retention [2]

Hematologic
Leukocytopenia (leukopenia) / leukocytes (white blood cells) decreased [3]
Neutropenia (neutrophils decreased) [2]
Thrombocytopenia / platelets decreased [3]

Neuromuscular/Skeletal
Asthenia / fatigue (5%) [5]
Ataxia (2%)
Dystonia [2]
Myoclonus (see also hypnic jerk) [4]
Pisa syndrome (pleurothotonus) [3]
Rhabdomyolysis [6]

Ocular
Amblyopia (2–3%)
Vision blurred (<4%)

Renal
Renal failure [2]

Respiratory
Pneumonia [2]

Other
Adverse effects / adverse reactions [11]
Death [9]
Toothache (odontalgia) (2–3%)

QUINACRINE

Synonym: mepacrine
Trade name: Atabrine (Winthrop)
Indications: Various infections caused by susceptible helminths
Class: Antibiotic, Antimalarial, Antimicrobial
Half-life: 4–10 hours
Clinically important, potentially hazardous interactions with: none known

---

Skin
Exanthems [3]
Exfoliative dermatitis (8%) [3]
Fixed eruption / fixed drug eruption [3]
Lichenoid eruption / lichenoid reaction (12%) [6]
Ochronosis [2]
Pigmentation (Skin) (includes hyperpigmentation) [9]
Squamous cell carcinoma [2]

Hair
Alopecia / hair loss (80%) [2]

Nails
Nail pigmentation (ala nasi) (blue-gray) [2]

Mucosal
Oral pigmentation [4]

Central Nervous System
Psychiatric adverse effect [4]
Psychosis [9]

Gastrointestinal/Hepatic
Nausea [2]
Vomiting [2]

QUINAGOLIDE

Trade name: Norprolac (Ferring)
Indications: Hyperprolactinemia
Class: Antiprolactin, Dopamine receptor agonist
Half-life: 11.5 hours
Clinically important, potentially hazardous interactions with: alcohol, lurasidone, paliperidone, ziprasidone

---

Skin
Edema / fluid retention (<10%)
Flushing / rubefaction (<10%)

Mucosal
Nasal congestion (>10%)

Central Nervous System
Anorexia (<10%)
Headache (>10%)
Insomnia (<10%)
Vertigo / dizziness (>10%)

Gastrointestinal/Hepatic
Abdominal pain (<10%)
Constipation (<10%)
Diarrhea (<10%)
Nausea (>10%)
Vomiting (>10%)

Neuromuscular/Skeletal
Asthenia / fatigue (>10%)

QUINAPRIL

Trade names: Accupril (Pfizer), Accupro (Pfizer), Accuretic (Pfizer)
Indications: Hypertension, heart failure
Class: Angiotensin-converting enzyme (ACE) inhibitor, Antihypertensive, Vasodilator
Half-life: 2 hours
Clinically important, potentially hazardous interactions with: alcohol, aldesleukin, allopurinol, alpha blockers, alprostadil, amifostine, amiloride, angiotensin II receptor antagonists, antacids, antidiabetics, antihypertensives, antipsychotics, anxiolytics and hypnotics, aprotinin, azathioprine, baclofen, beta blockers, calcium channel blockers, chlortetracycline, ciprofloxacin, clonidine, corticosteroids, cyclosporine, demeclocycline, diazoxide, diuretics, doxycycline, eplerenone, estrogens, everolimus, gemifloxacin, general anesthetics, gold & gold compounds, heparins, hydralazine, insulin, levodopa, lithium, lymecycline, MAO inhibitors, metformin, methyldopa, methylphenidate, minocycline, minoxidil, moxifloxacin, moxisylyte, moxonidine, nitrates, nitroprusside, NSAIDs, ofloxacin, oxytetracycline, pentoxifylline, phosphodiesterase 5 inhibitors, potassium salts, prostacyclin analogues, quinine, quinolones, rituximab, salicylates, sirolimus, spironolactone, sulfonylureas, temsirolimus, tetracycline, tetracyclines, tigecycline, tizanidine, tolvaptan, triamterene, trimethoprim
Pregnancy category: category C in first trimester; category D in second and third trimesters
Important contra-indications noted in the prescribing guidelines for: nursing mothers; pediatric patients
Note: Contra-indicated in patients with a history of angioedema related to previous treatment with an ACE inhibitor.
Warning: FETAL TOXICITY
WHEN USED IN PREGNANCY DURING THE SECOND AND THIRD TRIMESTERS, ACE INHIBITORS CAN CAUSE INJURY AND EVEN DEATH TO THE DEVELOPING FETUS. WHEN PREGNANCY IS DETECTED, QUINAPRIL SHOULD BE DISCONTINUED AS SOON AS POSSIBLE.
See full prescribing information for complete boxed warning.

Skin
Angioedema (formerly named angioneurotic edema) [10]
Diaphoresis [3]
Edema / fluid retention [4]
Peripheral edema [3]
Photosensitivity [2]
Pruritus (itching) [7]
Rash [5]

Central Nervous System
Dysgeusia (taste perversion) [3]

Neuromuscular/Skeletal
Myalgia/Myopathy (2%)

Respiratory
Cough [9]

Other
Adverse effects / adverse reactions [2]

QUINETHAZONE

Indications: Hypertension, edema
Class: Diuretic, thiazide
Half-life: N/A
Clinically important, potentially hazardous interactions with: digoxin, lithium
Note: Quinethazone is a sulfonamide and can be absorbed systemically. Sulfonamides can produce severe, possibly fatal, reactions such as toxic epidermal necrolysis and Stevens-Johnson syndrome.

Skin
Photosensitivity [2]

QUINIDINE

Indications: Tachycardia, atrial fibrillation
Class: Antiarrhythmic, Antiarrhythmic class Ia, Antimalarial, Antimicrobial, Antiprotozoal
Half-life: 6–8 hours
Clinically important, potentially hazardous interactions with: abarelix, afatinib, amiloride, amiodarone, amisulpride, amitriptyline, amprenavir, anisindione, anticoagulants, aripiprazole, arsenic, artemether/lumefantrine, asenapine, astemizole, atazanavir, boceprevir, celiprolol, ceritinib, ciprofloxacin, clevidipine, clozapine, cobicistat/elvitegravir/emtricitabine/tenofovir alafenamide, cobicistat/elvitegravir/emtricitabine/tenofovir disoproxil, crizotinib, dabigatran, darunavir, dasatinib, degarelix, delavirdine, deutetrabenazine, dicumarol, digoxin, duloxetine, eluxadoline, enoxacin, enzalutamide, ethoxzolamide, fosamprenavir, gatifloxacin,

glycopyrrolate, glycopyrronium, indinavir, itraconazole, ketoconazole, letermovir, lomefloxacin, lopinavir, lurasidone, metformin, mifepristone, mivacurium, moxifloxacin, naldemedine, nelfinavir, nilotinib, norfloxacin, ofloxacin, oliceridine, osimertinib, oxprenolol, pimavanserin, pimozide, pipecuronium, ponesimod, posaconazole, pristinamycin, propranolol, pyridostigmine, quinine, quinolones, ranolazine, ribociclib, rifapentine, ritonavir, rocuronium, sertindole, sotalol, sparfloxacin, sulpiride / levosulpiride, telaprevir, telithromycin, tetrabenazine, tipranavir, tramadol, valbenazine, vecuronium, venetoclax, verapamil, voriconazole, vortioxetine, warfarin, zuclopenthixol
Important contra-indications noted in the prescribing guidelines for: nursing mothers; pediatric patients

---

Skin
Acneiform eruption / acneiform dermatitis / acneiform rash [2]
AGEP [2]
Dermatitis [4]
Exanthems [6]
Exfoliative dermatitis [5]
Fixed eruption / fixed drug eruption [2]
Flushing / rubefaction [2]
Lichen planus (includes hypertrophic lichen planus) [7]
Lichenoid eruption / lichenoid reaction [6]
Livedo reticularis / livedo racemosa [6]
Lupus erythematosus (subacute cutaneous lupus erythematosus (SCLE)) [35]
Photosensitivity [21]
Pigmentation (Skin) (includes hyperpigmentation) [3]
Pruritus (itching) [3]
Psoriasis [5]
Purpura [13]
Rash (<10%)
Stevens-Johnson syndrome and toxic epidermal necrolysis (SJS/TEN) [2]
Vasculitis (angiitis) / cutaneous vasculitis (angiitis) [5]

Mucosal
Oral mucosal eruption [2]

Cardiovascular
Congestive heart failure [2]
QT interval prolonged / QT prolongation [9]
Torsades de pointes [13]

Central Nervous System
Dysgeusia (taste perversion) (>10%)
Headache (<10%) [2]
Syncope / fainting [2]
Tremor (2%)
Vertigo / dizziness [2]

Gastrointestinal/Hepatic
Diarrhea (>10%) [7]

Genitourinary
Urinary tract infection [2]

Hematologic
Thrombocytopenia / platelets decreased [2]

QUININE

Trade name: Qualaquin (URL Pharma)
Indications: Malaria
Class: Antimalarial, Antimicrobial, Antiprotozoal
Half-life: 8–14 hours
Clinically important, potentially hazardous interactions with: amantadine, amiodarone, amitriptyline, amoxapine, anisindione, anticoagulants, arsenic, artemether/lumefantrine, astemizole, atazanavir, atorvastatin, cimetidine, cisapride, citalopram, class Ia or III antiarrhythmics, clevidipine, CYP3A4 and CYP2D6 substrates, CYP3A4 inducers or inhibitors, darunavir, dasatinib, degarelix, dicumarol, digoxin, disopyramide, dofetilide, dolasetron, droperidol, enalapril, flecainide, fosamprenavir, halofantrine, haloperidol, histamine, indinavir, lapatinib, levofloxacin, mefloquine, metformin, moxifloxacin, nelfinavir, neuromuscular blocking agents, olmesartan, oral typhoid vaccine, pazopanib, pimozide, procainamide, prochlorperazine, quinapril, quinidine, ramipril, rifampin, ritonavir, saquinavir, sotalol, succinylcholine, telavancin, telithromycin, terfenadine, tipranavir, voriconazole, vorinostat, warfarin, ziprasidone
Important contra-indications noted in the prescribing guidelines for: nursing mothers; pediatric patients
Note: Qualaquin (quinine sulfate) is not indicated for the prevention or treatment of nocturnal leg cramps.
Contra-indicated in patients with prolongation of QT interval, G6PD deficiency, myasthenia gravis, or optic neuritis.

Skin
Acneiform eruption / acneiform dermatitis / acneiform rash [2]
Acral necrosis [2]
Dermatitis [6]
Erythema multiforme [2]
Exanthems (<5%) [3]
Exfoliative dermatitis [2]
Fixed eruption / fixed drug eruption [12]
Lichen planus (includes hypertrophic lichen planus) [3]
Lichenoid eruption / lichenoid reaction [3]
Livedo reticularis / livedo racemosa (photosensitive) [3]
Photosensitivity [19]
Pigmentation (Skin) (includes hyperpigmentation) [6]
Purpura [13]
Raynaud's phenomenon [2]
Stevens-Johnson syndrome and toxic epidermal necrolysis (SJS/TEN) [5]
Thrombocytopenic purpura [8]
Urticaria / hives [2]
Vasculitis (angiitis) / cutaneous vasculitis (angiitis) [5]

Cardiovascular
Cardiotoxicity [2]

Endocrine/Metabolic
Hypoglycemia [3]

Hematologic
Hemolytic anemia [2]
Hemolytic uremic syndrome [16]
Thrombocytopenia / platelets decreased [11]
Thrombotic microangiopathy [2]

Neuromuscular/Skeletal
Leg cramps [2]
Rhabdomyolysis [2]

Ocular
Amblyopia [8]

Otic
Hearing loss (hypoacusis) [4]
Ototoxicity [2]
Tinnitus [9]

Renal
Nephrotoxicity / kidney injury / acute kidney injury (AKI) / drug-induced kidney injury [2]

Other
Adverse effects / adverse reactions [3]
Death [2]

RABEPRAZOLE

Trade name: Aciphex (Eisai) (Janssen)
Indications: Gastroesophageal reflux disease (GERD), duodenal ulcers, Zollinger-Ellison syndrome
Class: Proton pump inhibitor (PPI)
Half-life: 1–2 hours
Clinically important, potentially hazardous interactions with: atazanavir, capmatinib, clopidogrel, cyclosporine, digoxin, emtricitabine/rilpivirine/tenofovir alafenamide, ketoconazole, rilpivirine, simvastatin, warfarin
Important contra-indications noted in the prescribing guidelines for: nursing mothers

---

Skin
Pruritus (itching) [2]
Rash [3]

Central Nervous System
Dysgeusia (taste perversion) [2]
Headache (2–5%) [4]
Pain (3%)
Vertigo / dizziness [4]

Endocrine/Metabolic
Galactorrhea [2]
Hypomagnesemia [2]

Gastrointestinal/Hepatic
Abdominal pain [6]
Constipation (2%)
Diarrhea (3%) [8]
Dyspepsia / functional dyspepsia (indigestion) (see also gastroparesis) [3]
Flatulence [2]
Gastrointestinal bleeding [2]
Nausea [5]
Vomiting [5]

Neuromuscular/Skeletal
Asthenia / fatigue [3]

Renal
Nephrotoxicity / kidney injury / acute kidney injury (AKI) / drug-induced kidney injury [2]

Respiratory
Cough [3]
Upper respiratory tract infection [2]

Other
Adverse effects / adverse reactions [4]

RALOXIFENE

Trade name: Evista (Lilly)
Indications: Osteoporosis, reduction in risk of invasive breast cancer in postmenopausal women with osteoporosis or at high risk for invasive breast cancer
Class: Selective estrogen receptor modulator (SERM)
Half-life: 27.7 hours
Clinically important, potentially hazardous interactions with: cholestyramine, levothyroxine
Important contra-indications noted in the prescribing guidelines for: nursing mothers; pediatric patients
Warning: INCREASED RISK OF VENOUS THROMBOEMBOLISM AND DEATH FROM STROKE

Skin
Diaphoresis (3%)
Hot flashes / hot flushes (8–29%) [14]
Peripheral edema (3–5%) [4]
Rash (6%)

Cardiovascular
Chest pain (3%)
Venous thromboembolism [5]

Central Nervous System
Insomnia (6%)
Stroke / cerebrovascular accident [4]

Endocrine/Metabolic
Mastodynia (4%) [2]
Weight gain (9%)

Gastrointestinal/Hepatic
Abdominal pain (7%)
Vomiting (5%)

Genitourinary
Vaginal bleeding (6%)
Vaginitis (includes vulvitis) (4%)

Hematologic
Thrombosis [2]

Neuromuscular/Skeletal
Arthralgia (11–16%)
Leg cramps (6–12%) [5]
Myalgia/Myopathy (8%)

Respiratory
Bronchitis (10%)
Influenza- ('flu)-like syndrome (~2%)
Pharyngitis (sore throat) (8%)
Pneumonia (3%)
Sinusitis (see also rhinitis / rhinosinusitis) (10%)

Other
Adverse effects / adverse reactions [2]
Infection (11%)

RALTEGRAVIR

Trade name: Isentress (Merck)
Indications: HIV-1 infection
Class: Antiretroviral, Integrase strand transfer inhibitor
Half-life: 9 hours
Clinically important, potentially hazardous interactions with: atazanavir, efavirenz, histamine H_2 antagonists, omeprazole, pantoprazole, proton pump inhibitors, rifampin, St John's wort, strong UGT inducers, tipranavir
Important contra-indications noted in the prescribing guidelines for: nursing mothers; pediatric patients

---

Skin
DRESS syndrome (Drug-induced hypersensitivity syndrome) [4]
Herpes zoster (<2%)
Hypersensitivity (<2%) [7]
Pruritus (itching) (4%)
Rash [9]

Central Nervous System
Depression (<2%) [2]
Headache (2%) [10]
Insomnia (4%) [4]
Neurotoxicity [2]
Vertigo / dizziness (<2%) [2]

Endocrine/Metabolic
ALT increased [3]
Creatine phosphokinase (CPK) / creatine kinase increased (hyperCKemia) [2]
Serum creatinine increased [2]

Gastrointestinal/Hepatic
Abdominal pain (<2%) [2]
Diarrhea [8]
Dyspepsia / functional dyspepsia (indigestion) (see also gastroparesis) (<2%)
Gastritis / pangastritis / gastric irritation (<2%)
Hepatitis [2]
Hepatotoxicity / liver injury / acute liver injury / drug-induced liver injury (DILI) (<2%) [3]
Nausea (<2%) [9]
Vomiting (<2%) [2]

Neuromuscular/Skeletal
Asthenia / fatigue (<2%) [4]
Myalgia/Myopathy [3]
Rhabdomyolysis [8]

Renal
Nephrolithiasis (kidney stones / renal calculi) (<2%)
Renal failure (<2%)

Other
Adverse effects / adverse reactions [6]

RAMELTEON

Trade name: Rozerem (Takeda)
Indications: Insomnia
Class: Hypnotic, Melatonin receptor agonist
Half-life: 1–2.6 hours
Clinically important, potentially hazardous interactions with: alcohol, antifungals, CNS depressants, conivaptan, CYP1A2 inhibitors, donepezil, doxepin, droperidol, fluconazole, fluvoxamine, food, ketoconazole, levomepromazine, rifampin, rifapentine, St John's wort, viloxazine, voriconazole, zolpidem
Important contra-indications noted in the prescribing guidelines for: nursing mothers; pediatric patients

---

Central Nervous System
Depression (2%)
Dysgeusia (taste perversion) (2%)
Headache (7%) [8]
Insomnia (exacerbation) (3%)
Somnolence (drowsiness) (3%) [9]
Vertigo / dizziness (4%) [6]

Gastrointestinal/Hepatic
Nausea (3%) [3]

Genitourinary
Urinary tract infection [2]

Neuromuscular/Skeletal
Arthralgia (2%)
Asthenia / fatigue (3%) [4]
Myalgia/Myopathy (2%)

Respiratory
Upper respiratory tract infection (3%)

Other
Adverse effects / adverse reactions [7]

RAMIPRIL

Trade names: Altace (Monarch), Tritace (Sanofi-Aventis)
Indications: Hypertension
Class: Angiotensin-converting enzyme (ACE) inhibitor, Antihypertensive, Vasodilator
Half-life: 2–17 hours
Clinically important, potentially hazardous interactions with: alcohol, aldesleukin, allopurinol, alpha blockers, alprostadil, amifostine, amiloride, angiotensin II receptor antagonists, antacids, antihypertensives, antipsychotics, azathioprine, baclofen, beta blockers, calcium channel blockers, clonidine, corticosteroids, cyclosporine, diazoxide, diuretics, eplerenone, estrogens, everolimus, general anesthetics, gold & gold compounds, heparins, hydralazine, hypotensives, insulin, levodopa, lithium, MAO inhibitors, metformin, methyldopa, minoxidil, moxisylyte, moxonidine, nitrates, nitroprusside, NSAIDs, pentoxifylline, phosphodiasterase 5 inhibitors, potassium salts, prostacyclin analogues, quinine, rituximab, sirolimus, spironolactone, sulfonylureas, telmisartan, temsirolimus, tizanidine, tolvaptan, triamterene, trimethoprim
Pregnancy category: category C in first trimester; category D in second and third trimesters
Important contra-indications noted in the prescribing guidelines for: nursing mothers; pediatric patients
Note: Contra-indicated in patients with a history of angioedema related to previous treatment with an ACE inhibitor, or a history of hereditary or idiopathic angioedema.
Warning: FETAL TOXICITY

Skin
Angioedema (formerly named angioneurotic edema) [14]
Diaphoresis [2]
Flushing / rubefaction [2]
Lichen planus pemphigoides [3]
Photosensitivity [2]
Pruritus (itching) [3]
Rash [4]
Stevens-Johnson syndrome and toxic epidermal necrolysis (SJS/TEN) [2]

Hair
Alopecia / hair loss (<10%)

Cardiovascular
Angina (3%)
Hypotension (11%) [3]
Postural hypotension (2%)

Central Nervous System
Headache (5%) [2]
Syncope / fainting (2%)
Vertigo / dizziness (2–4%) [4]

Endocrine/Metabolic
Hyperkalemia [2]

Gastrointestinal/Hepatic
Hepatotoxicity / liver injury / acute liver injury / drug-induced liver injury (DILI) [3]
Intestinal angioedema [2]
Nausea (2%)
Pancreatitis / acute pancreatitis [2]
Vomiting (2%)

Neuromuscular/Skeletal
Asthenia / fatigue (2%)

Respiratory
Cough (8–12%) [22]

Other
Adverse effects / adverse reactions [4]

RAMUCIRUMAB

Trade name: Cyramza (Lilly)
Indications: Gastric cancer
Class: Angiogenesis inhibitor / antiangiogenic agent, Monoclonal antibody
Half-life: 15 days
Clinically important, potentially hazardous interactions with: none known
Important contra-indications noted in the prescribing guidelines for: nursing mothers; pediatric patients
Warning: HEMORRHAGE, GASTROINSTINAL PERFORATION, AND IMPAIRED WOUND HEALING

Skin
Peripheral edema [3]
Rash (4%)

Mucosal
Epistaxis (nosebleed) (5%) [2]
Stomatitis (oral mucositis) [5]

Cardiovascular
Hypertension (16%) [33]
Thromboembolism (2%) [2]
Venous thromboembolism [2]

Central Nervous System
Anorexia [3]
Headache (9%) [3]

Endocrine/Metabolic
Appetite decreased [8]
AST increased [3]
Dehydration [2]
Hyperbilirubinemia [2]
Hyponatremia (6%)

Gastrointestinal/Hepatic
Abdominal pain [2]
Ascites [3]
Constipation [3]
Diarrhea (14%) [12]
Gastrointestinal obstruction / gastrointestinal stricture (2%)
Gastrointestinal perforation / perforated colon / gastric perforation [6]
Hepatotoxicity / liver injury / acute liver injury / drug-induced liver injury (DILI) [2]
Nausea [5]
Vomiting [4]

Hematologic
Anemia [10]
Bleeding [7]
Febrile neutropenia [14]
Hematological adverse effect [2]
Hemorrhage [4]
Leukocytopenia (leukopenia) / leukocytes (white blood cells) decreased [10]
Neutropenia (neutrophils decreased) (5%) [23]
Thrombocytopenia / platelets decreased [7]

Local
Infusion-related reactions [4]

Neuromuscular/Skeletal
Asthenia / fatigue [17]

Renal
Nephrotoxicity / kidney injury / acute kidney injury (AKI) / drug-induced kidney injury [2]
Proteinuria [16]

Respiratory
Dyspnea / shortness of breath [3]

Other
Adverse effects / adverse reactions [2]
Death [4]

RANIBIZUMAB

Trade name: Lucentis (Genentech)
Indications: Neovascular (wet) age-related macular degeneration, macular edema (following retinal vein occlusion)
Class: Angiogenesis inhibitor / antiangiogenic agent, Monoclonal antibody, Vascular endothelial growth factor (VEGF) inhibitor / antagonist
Half-life: 9 days
Clinically important, potentially hazardous interactions with: none known
Important contra-indications noted in the prescribing guidelines for: nursing mothers; pediatric patients
Note: Contra-indicated in patients with ocular or periocular infections. Ranibizumab-nuna (Byooviz) is biosimilar to Ranibizumab. Approved 09/17/2021 Ranibizumab-Eqrn (Cimerli) is biosimilar to Ranibizumab. Approved 08/02/2022.

Cardiovascular
Atrial fibrillation (<5%)
Hypertension [4]
Myocardial infarction [2]
Thromboembolism [3]

Central Nervous System
Anxiety (<4%)
Guillain-Barré syndrome / acute inflammatory demyelinating polyradiculoneuropathy / acute motor axonal neuropathy [2]
Hallucinations, visual [2]
Headache (3–12%)
Insomnia (<5%)
Stroke / cerebrovascular accident [4]

Endocrine/Metabolic
Hypercholesterolemia (<5%)

Gastrointestinal/Hepatic
Gastroenteritis (<4%)
Nausea (<9%)

Genitourinary
Urinary tract infection (<9%)

Hematologic
Anemia (<8%)

Local
Injection-site bleeding (<6%)

Neuromuscular/Skeletal
Arthralgia (2–11%)
Pain in extremities (<5%)

Ocular
Blepharitis (<13%)
Cataract (2–17%) [4]
Conjunctival hemorrhage (48–74%) [4]
Conjunctival hyperemia / conjunctival injection (<8%)
Endophthalmitis [9]
Glaucoma (includes acute angle-closure glaucoma) [3]
Intraocular inflammation (<18%) [5]
Intraocular pressure increased (7–24%) [8]
Iridocyclitis [3]
Lacrimation (increased) (2–14%)
Maculopathy (6–11%)
Ocular adverse effect [6]
Ocular hemorrhage [6]
Ocular hyperemia (5–11%)
Ocular itching / ocular pruritus (<12%)
Ocular pain (17–35%) [4]
Ocular stinging (7–15%)
Posterior capsule opacification (<8%)
Retinal atrophy [2]
Retinal detachment [2]
Retinal vein occlusion [2]
Vision blurred (5–18%)
Visual disturbances (5–18%)
Vitreous detachment (4–21%)
Vitreous floaters / floaters / myodesopsia / myiodesopsia / muscae volitantes (7–27%) [2]
Xerophthalmia (dry eyes) (3–12%)

Respiratory
Bronchitis (<12%)
COPD (<7%)
Cough (2–9%)
Dyspnea / shortness of breath (<5%)
Influenza (3–7%)
Nasopharyngitis (5–16%) [2]
Sinusitis (see also rhinitis / rhinosinusitis) (3–8%)
Upper respiratory tract infection (2–9%)

Other
Adverse effects / adverse reactions [6]
Systemic reactions [2]

RANITIDINE

Trade name: Zantac (Concordia)
Indications: Duodenal ulcer
Class: Histamine H2 receptor antagonist
Half-life: 2.5 hours
Clinically important, potentially hazardous interactions with: acalabrutinib, alfentanil, delavirdine, fentanyl, gefitinib, lemborexant, metformin, prednisone, rilpivirine, risperidone
Important contra-indications noted in the prescribing guidelines for: nursing mothers

---

Skin
AGEP [2]
Anaphylactoid reactions / anaphylaxis (includes anaphylactic shock) [18]
Dermatitis [6]
Eczema / eczematous reaction / eczematous eruption [2]
Exanthems [5]
Hypersensitivity [2]
Photosensitivity [2]
Pseudolymphoma / cutaneous pseudolymphoma [2]
Purpura [2]
Rash (<10%)

Stevens-Johnson syndrome and toxic epidermal necrolysis (SJS/TEN) [2]
Urticaria / hives [4]

Central Nervous System
Confusion [2]
Somnolence (drowsiness) [2]

Endocrine/Metabolic
Gynecomastia [3]
Porphyria [3]

Hematologic
Thrombocytopenia / platelets decreased [2]

Respiratory
Pneumonia [2]

Other
Adverse effects / adverse reactions [3]
Cancer [2]

RANOLAZINE

Trade name: Ranexa (CV Therapeutics)
Indications: Angina
Class: Anti-ischemic, Fatty acid oxidation inhibitor
Half-life: 7 hours
Clinically important, potentially hazardous interactions with: aprepitant, atazanavir, clarithromycin, conivaptan, cyclosporine, CYP3A inducers, CYP3A inhibitors, darunavir, delavirdine, diltiazem, dofetilide, efavirenz, erythromycin, grapefruit juice, indinavir, itraconazole, ketoconazole, lopinavir, nelfinavir, ombitasvir/paritaprevir/ritonavir, ombitasvir/paritaprevir/ritonavir and dasabuvir, oxcarbazepine, paroxetine hydrochloride, phenobarbital, quinidine, rifampin, rifapentine, ritonavir, simvastatin, sotalol, telithromycin, thioridazine, tipranavir, venetoclax, verapamil, voriconazole, ziprasidone
Important contra-indications noted in the prescribing guidelines for: nursing mothers
Note: Contra-indicated in patients with existing QT prolongation, and in patients with liver disease.

Mucosal
Xerostomia (dry mouth) (<2%)

Cardiovascular
Palpitation (<2%)
QT interval prolonged / QT prolongation [7]
Torsades de pointes [2]

Central Nervous System
Headache (3%) [4]
Vertigo / dizziness [10]

Gastrointestinal/Hepatic
Abdominal pain (<2%)
Constipation [8]
Nausea [9]
Vomiting [2]

Neuromuscular/Skeletal
Asthenia / fatigue [3]
Myalgia/Myopathy [4]

Otic
Tinnitus (<2%)

RASAGILINE

Trade name: Azilect (Teva)
Indications: Parkinsonism
Class: Monoamine oxidase B inhibitor, Neuroprotectant
Half-life: 0.6–2.0 hours
Clinically important, potentially hazardous interactions with: aminophylline, amitriptyline, ciprofloxacin, citalopram, dextromethorphan, entacapone, fluoxetine, fluvoxamine, MAO inhibitors, meperidine, paroxetine hydrochloride, pethidine, pseudoephedrine, SSRIs, viloxazine
Important contra-indications noted in the prescribing guidelines for: nursing mothers; pediatric patients

---

Skin
Bruise / bruising / contusion / ecchymosis (ecchymoses) (2%)

Mucosal
Xerostomia (dry mouth) (3%)

Cardiovascular
Hypotension (5%)

Central Nervous System
Depression (5%) [2]
Dyskinesia (>10%) [3]
Fever (pyrexia) (includes hyperpyrexia) (3%)
Gait instability / postural instability (5%)
Headache (14%) [2]
Paresthesias (2%)
Somnolence (drowsiness) [3]
Vertigo / dizziness (2%) [3]

Gastrointestinal/Hepatic
Dyspepsia / functional dyspepsia (indigestion) (see also gastroparesis) (7%)
Gastroenteritis (3%)
Nausea [2]

Neuromuscular/Skeletal
Arthralgia (7%) [2]
Asthenia / fatigue (2%)
Dystonia (2%)
Neck pain (2%)

Ocular
Conjunctivitis (conjunctival inflammation) (3%)

Respiratory
Influenza- ('flu)-like syndrome (5%)
Nasopharyngitis [2]
Rhinitis / rhinosinusitis (see also sinusitis) (3%)

RASBURICASE

Trade name: Elitek (Sanofi-Aventis)
Indications: Hyperuricemia (associated with tumor lysis syndrome)
Class: Antimetabolite, Urate oxidase
Half-life: 18 hours
Clinically important, potentially hazardous interactions with: none known
Important contra-indications noted in the prescribing guidelines for: nursing mothers
Note: Since the FDA's approval of rasburicase use for the treatment of tumor lysis syndrome, multiple cases of rasburicase-induced methemoglobinemia and hemolytic anemia have been reported among patients with glucose-6-phosphate dehydrogenase (G6PD) deficiency.
Warning: ANAPHYLAXIS, HEMOLYSIS, METHEMOGLOBINEMIA, AND INTERFERENCE WITH URIC ACID MEASUREMENTS

Skin
Hypersensitivity [7]
Rash (13%) [6]

Mucosal
Mucositis (2–15%)

Central Nervous System
Fever (pyrexia) (includes hyperpyrexia) (46%)

Gastrointestinal/Hepatic
Abdominal pain (20%)

Hematologic
Anemia [2]
Hemolysis [7]
Hemolytic anemia [6]
Methemoglobinemia [16]

Other
Death [2]

RASPBERRY LEAF

Family: Rosaceae
Scientific name: *Rubus idaeus*
Indications: Astringent, stimulant, gargle for sore throat, mouth ulcers, bleeding gums, diarrhea, morning sickness, to shorten labor, menstrual complaints, respiratory tract infections, fever, dysmenorrhea, menorrhagia, rash
Class: Food supplement
Half-life: N/A
Clinically important, potentially hazardous interactions with: aminophylline, atropine

REBOXETINE

Trade name: Edronax (Pfizer)
Indications: Clinical depression, panic disorder
Class: Antidepressant, Noradrenaline reuptake inhibitor
Half-life: 13 hours
Clinically important, potentially hazardous interactions with: azithromycin, bosentan, itraconazole, ketoconazole, MAO inhibitors, papaverine, voriconazole
Pregnancy category: not recommended in pregnancy
Important contra-indications noted in the prescribing guidelines for: the elderly; nursing mothers; pediatric patients

---

Skin
Diaphoresis [8]

Mucosal
Xerostomia (dry mouth) [12]

Central Nervous System
Headache [5]
Insomnia [9]
Somnolence (drowsiness) [2]

Genitourinary
Ejaculatory dysfunction [2]

RED CLOVER

Family: Leguminosae
Scientific name: *Trifolium pratense*
Indications: Menopausal symptoms, hot flashes, muscle spasms, hypercholesterolemia, breast pain, osteoporosis, diuretic, expectorant, mild antispasmodic, sedative, blood purifier, bladder infections, liver disorders. Ointment for acne, eczema, psoriasis and other rashes
Class: Phytoestrogen
Half-life: N/A
Clinically important, potentially hazardous interactions with: conjugated estrogens
Note: Red clover contains phytoestrogens that bind to estrogen and progesterone receptors, potentially adversely affecting breast tissue.

RED RICE YEAST

Family: Monascaceae
Scientific name: *Monascus purpureus*
Indications: Hypercholesterolemia, indigestion, diarrhea, improved circulation. In foodstuff
Class: HMG-CoA reductase inhibitor / statin
Half-life: N/A
Clinically important, potentially hazardous interactions with: atorvastatin, cerivastatin, fluvastatin, grapefruit juice, levothyroxine, lovastatin, pravastatin, simvastatin, St John's wort
Note: Red yeast rice is derived from the fermentation of rice with the yeast Monascus purpureus, yielding a series of cholesterol-lowering monacolins. The monacolin in highest concentration in red yeast rice is monacolin K, also known as lovastatin, the first FDA-approved HMG-CoA reductase inhibitor. Red yeast that is not fermented correctly may contain the nephrotoxin, citrinin.

Gastrointestinal/Hepatic
Hepatitis [2]

Neuromuscular/Skeletal
Myalgia/Myopathy [5]
Rhabdomyolysis [3]

REGADENOSON

Trade name: Lexiscan (Astellas)
Indications: Radionuclide myocardial perfusion imaging
Class: Adenosine A2A receptor agonist, Diagnostic aid
Half-life: immediate: 30 minutes; terminal: 2 hours
Clinically important, potentially hazardous interactions with: caffeine, dipyridamole, theophylline
Important contra-indications noted in the prescribing guidelines for: nursing mothers; pediatric patients
Note: Contra-indicated in patients with second- or third-degree AV block or sinus node dysfunction.

Skin
Flushing / rubefaction (16%) [7]
Hot flashes / hot flushes (5%)

Mucosal
Xerostomia (dry mouth) [3]

Cardiovascular
Angina (12%)
Atrioventricular block [2]
Chest pain (7–13%) [9]
Hypotension (7%)
Myocardial infarction [2]
Premature atrial contractions (7%)
Tachycardia (66%)

Central Nervous System
Dysgeusia (taste perversion) (5%)
Fever (pyrexia) (includes hyperpyrexia) (5%)
Headache (26%) [13]
Syncope / fainting [2]
Vertigo / dizziness (8%) [8]

Gastrointestinal/Hepatic
Abdominal pain (5%) [2]
Diarrhea [3]
Nausea (6%) [3]

Neuromuscular/Skeletal
Asthenia / fatigue [2]

Respiratory
Dyspnea / shortness of breath (11–28%) [14]
Wheezing (3%)

Other
Adverse effects / adverse reactions [9]

REGORAFENIB

Trade name: Stivarga (Bayer)
Indications: Metastatic colorectal cancer, gastrointestinal stomal tumors
Class: Angiogenesis inhibitor / antiangiogenic agent, Tyrosine kinase inhibitor, Vascular endothelial growth factor (VEGF) inhibitor / antagonist
Half-life: 28 hours
Clinically important, potentially hazardous interactions with: carbamazepine, clarithromycin, CYP3A4 inducers and inhibitors, grapefruit juice, itraconazole, ketoconazole, phenobarbital, phenytoin, posaconazole, rifampin, St John's wort, telithromycin, voriconazole
Important contra-indications noted in the prescribing guidelines for: nursing mothers; pediatric patients
Warning: HEPATOTOXICITY

Skin
Cutaneous toxicity / skin toxicity [5]
Desquamation [4]
Hand–foot syndrome (palmar–plantar erythrodysesthesia) (45%) [65]
Nevi (naevi) [2]
Rash (26%) [17]

Hair
Alopecia / hair loss (8%)

Mucosal
Mucositis (33%) [11]
Stomatitis (oral mucositis) [5]
Xerostomia (dry mouth) (5%)

Cardiovascular
Cardiac failure [2]
Chest pain [2]
Hypertension (30%) [57]
Myocardial infarction [2]

Central Nervous System
Anorexia [13]
Fever (pyrexia) (includes hyperpyrexia) (28%) [4]
Headache (10%)
Leukoencephalopathy / posterior reversible encephalopathy syndrome (PRES) [2]
Pain (29%) [3]
Tremor (2%)

Endocrine/Metabolic
ALT increased (45%) [6]
Appetite decreased (47%)
AST increased (65%) [6]
Hyperammonemia [2]
Hyperbilirubinemia [8]
Hyperlipasemia [2]
Hypertransaminasemia (hepatic transaminitis) / elevated transaminases [3]
Hypocalcemia (59%)
Hypokalemia (26%)
Hyponatremia (30%)
Hypophosphatemia (57%) [8]
Hypothyroidism (4%) [7]
Weight loss (32%) [7]

Gastrointestinal/Hepatic
Abdominal pain [4]
Diarrhea (43%) [37]
Gastrointestinal perforation / perforated colon / gastric perforation [3]
Hepatic (liver) disorder / hepatobiliary disorder / hepatic (liver) dysfunction [2]
Hepatotoxicity / liver injury / acute liver injury / drug-induced liver injury (DILI) [15]
Nausea [6]
Vomiting [2]

Hematologic
Anemia (79%) [8]
Hemorrhage (21%) [2]
Leukocytopenia (leukopenia) / leukocytes (white blood cells) decreased [4]
Lymphopenia (lymphocytopenia) / lymphocytes decreased (54%)
Neutropenia (neutrophils decreased) (3%) [4]
Thrombocytopenia / platelets decreased (41%) [11]

Neuromuscular/Skeletal
Asthenia / fatigue [52]

Renal
Proteinuria (60%) [4]

Respiratory
Dysphonia (includes voice disorders / voice changes) (30%) [6]
Hoarseness [2]
Interstitial lung disease / interstitial pneumonitis / interstitial pneumonia (cryptogenic organizing pneumonia) / drug-induced interstitial lung disease [2]

Other
Adverse effects / adverse reactions [11]
Death [4]
Infection (31%)

RELUGOLIX

Trade name: Orgovyx (Myovant Sciences)
Indications: Treatment of adult patients with advanced prostate cancer
Class: Gonadotropin-releasing hormone (GnRH) antagonist
Half-life: 25 hours
Clinically important, potentially hazardous interactions with: CYP3A inducers, erythromycin, P-gp inhibitors, rifampin
Pregnancy category: Relugolix can cause fetal harm. Advise males with female partners of

reproductive potential to use effective contraception.
Note: Androgen deprivation therapy, such as Relugolix, may prolong the QT/QTc interval.

Skin
Hot flashes / hot flushes (54%) [2]
Endocrine/Metabolic
ALT increased (27%)
AST increased (18%)
Hyperglycemia (includes glucose increased) (44%)
Hypertriglyceridemia (includes triglycerides increased) (35%)
Gastrointestinal/Hepatic
Constipation (12%)
Diarrhea (12%) [2]
Hematologic
Hemoglobin decreased (28%)
Neuromuscular/Skeletal
Asthenia / fatigue (26%) [2]
Musculoskeletal pain (30%)

REMDESIVIR

Trade names: GS-5734 (Gilead), Veklury (Gilead)
Indications: Treatment of coronavirus disease 2019 (Covid-19) requiring hospitalization
Class: Antiviral, Antiviral; nucleotide analog, Covid-19 putative drug, RNA polymerase inhibitor
Half-life: 1 hour
Clinically important, potentially hazardous interactions with: clinical drug-drug interaction studies have not been performed with remdesivir.
Pregnancy category: Insufficient data to evaluate a drug-associated risk of major birth defects, miscarriage, or adverse maternal or fetal outcomes.
Note: Because transaminase elevations have been reported as a clinical feature of Covid-19, and the incidence was similar in patients receiving placebo versus remdesivir in clinical trials of remdesivir, discerning the contribution of remdesivir to transaminase elevations in patients with Covid-19 can be challenging.
Co-administration of remdesivir with chloroquine phosphate or hydroxychloroquine sulfate is not recommended.

Skin
Rash [2]
Cardiovascular
Bradycardia / sinus bradycardia [3]
Endocrine/Metabolic
ALT increased (in subjects with mild, moderate or severe Covid-19) (2–6%)
AST increased (in subjects with mild, moderate or severe Covid-19) (6–7%)
Hyperbilirubinemia (2%)
Hyperglycemia (includes glucose increased) (in subjects with mild, moderate or severe Covid-19) (4–12%)
Hypertransaminasemia (hepatic transaminitis) / elevated transaminases [3]
Serum creatinine increased (in subjects with mild, moderate or severe Covid-19) (5–15%)
Gastrointestinal/Hepatic
Nausea (in subjects with mild, moderate or severe Covid-19) (3–7%)
Hematologic
Hemoglobin decreased (in subjects with mild, moderate or severe Covid-19) (3–15%)
Lymphopenia (lymphocytopenia) / lymphocytes decreased (in subjects with mild, moderate or severe Covid-19) (11%)
Prothrombin time (INR) increased (in subjects with mild, moderate or severe Covid-19) (9%)
Renal
Nephrotoxicity / kidney injury / acute kidney injury (AKI) / drug-induced kidney injury [2]
Other
Adverse effects / adverse reactions (17–20%) [4]

REMIMAZOLAM

Synonym: Remimazolam besylate
Trade name: Byfavo (Acacia Pharma)
Indications: Induction and maintenance of procedural sedation in adults undergoing procedures lasting 30 minutes or less (intravenous administration)
Class: Benzodiazepine
Half-life: 37–53 minutes (terminal elimination half-life from plasma)
Clinically important, potentially hazardous interactions with: none known
Pregnancy category: Benzodiazepines cross the placenta and may produce respiratory depression and sedation in neonates.
Important contra-indications noted in the prescribing guidelines for: the elderly; nursing mothers; pediatric patients
Note: Remimazolam should not be used in patients less than 18 years of age. Remimazolam may cause confusion and over-sedation in the elderly; elderly patients generally should be observed closely.
A case of intravenous line occlusion has been reported when using Acetated Ringer's solution and remimazolam (https://doi.org/10.1016/j.jclinane.2021.110190).
Warning: REMIMAZOLAM HAS BEEN ASSOCIATED WITH HYPOXIA, BRADYCARDIA, AND HYPOTENSION. CONCOMITANT USE OF BENZODIAZEPINES WITH OPIOID ANALGESICS MAY RESULT IN PROFOUND SEDATION, RESPIRATORY DEPRESSION, COMA, AND DEATH. THE SEDATIVE EFFECT OF INTRAVENOUS REMIMAZOLAM CAN BE ACCENTUATED BY CONCOMITANTLY ADMINISTERED CNS DEPRESSANT MEDICATIONS, INCLUDING OTHER BENZODIAZEPINES AND PROPOFOL.

Skin
Anaphylactoid reactions / anaphylaxis (includes anaphylactic shock) [8]
Cardiovascular
Blood pressure variations (with prior administration of fentanyl) (3%)
Bradycardia / sinus bradycardia (with prior administration of fentanyl) (3–11%)
Hypertension (5–22% systolic hypertension; 10–25% diastolic hypertension) (with prior administration of fentanyl) (20–42%)
Hypotension (3–14% diastolic hypotension) (with prior administration of fentanyl) (33–58%)
Tachycardia (with prior administration of fentanyl) (8%)
Central Nervous System
Fever (pyrexia) (includes hyperpyrexia) (with prior administration of fentanyl) (4%)
Headache (with prior administration of fentanyl) (3%)
Gastrointestinal/Hepatic
Nausea (with prior administration of fentanyl) (4%)
Respiratory
Bradypnea / respiratory rate decreased (with prior administration of fentanyl) (3%)
Hypoxia (with prior administration of fentanyl) (22%)
Respiratory tract infection (with prior administration of fentanyl) (3%)
Tachypnea / respiratory rate increased (with prior administration of fentanyl) (14%)

REPAGLINIDE

Trade name: Prandin (Novo Nordisk)
Indications: Non-insulin dependent diabetes Type II
Class: Antidiabetic, Hypoglycemic (antihyperglycemic) agent, Meglitinide
Half-life: 1 hour
Clinically important, potentially hazardous interactions with: clarithromycin, co-trimoxazole, deferasirox, erythromycin, gemfibrozil, grapefruit juice, itraconazole, lanreotide, lapatinib, letermovir, mifepristone, paclitaxel, rifapentine, selpercatinib, telithromycin, teriflunomide, trimethoprim, tucatinib, voriconazole
Important contra-indications noted in the prescribing guidelines for: nursing mothers; pediatric patients

---

Central Nervous System
Headache [2]
Paresthesias (3%)
Endocrine/Metabolic
Hypoglycemia [2]
Gastrointestinal/Hepatic
Hepatotoxicity / liver injury / acute liver injury / drug-induced liver injury (DILI) [4]
Other
Allergic reactions (2%)

RESERPINE

Trade names: Ser-Ap-Es (Novartis), Serpasil (Novartis)
Indications: Hypertension
Class: Rauwolfia alkaloid
Half-life: 50–100 hours
Clinically important, potentially hazardous interactions with: atenolol, bisoprolol, insulin degludec, insulin detemir, insulin glargine, insulin glulisine, iobenguane, linezolid, metipranolol, oxprenolol, sotalol, St John's wort, tetrabenazine
Note: Ser-Ap-Es is reserpine, hydralazine and hydrochlorothiazide.

Skin
Peripheral edema (<10%)

Mucosal
Xerostomia (dry mouth) (>10%)

Cardiovascular
Bradycardia / sinus bradycardia [2]

Central Nervous System
Parkinsonism [2]

RESVERATROL

Family: N/A
Scientific names: *3,4',5-trihydroxystilbene, trans-resveratrol-3-O-glucuronide, trans-resveratrol-3-sulfate*
Indications: Cancers, dermal wound healing, atherosclerosis, herpes simplex, cholesterol-lowering, heart disease, skin cancers
Class: Immunomodulator, Phytoestrogen
Half-life: N/A
Clinically important, potentially hazardous interactions with: aspirin, warfarin
Note: Resveratrol is extracted from: *Vitis vinifera* "grape seed and skin", *Polygonium cuspidatum*, and nuts. Red wine is associated with the so-called French paradox – low incidence of heart disease among French people who drink moderate quantities of red wine. A glass of red wine contains approximately 640 micrograms of resveratrol.

RETEPLASE

Trade name: Retavase (Centocor)
Indications: Acute myocardial infarction
Class: Fibrinolytic
Half-life: 13–16 minutes
Clinically important, potentially hazardous interactions with: abciximab, aspirin, bivalirudin, dipyridamole, piperacillin, salicylates

---

Local
Injection-site bleeding (<10%)

RIBAVIRIN

Trade names: Copegus (Roche), Rebetol (Schering-Plough), Rebetron (Schering), Virazole (Valeant)
Indications: Respiratory syncytial viral infections
Class: Antiviral; nucleoside analog
Half-life: 24 hours
Clinically important, potentially hazardous interactions with: abacavir, azathioprine, didanosine, emtricitabine, interferon alfa, PEG-interferon, stavudine, zidovudine
Important contra-indications noted in the prescribing guidelines for: nursing mothers
Note: [INH] = Inhalation; [O] = Oral. Rebetron is ribavirin and interferon.
Warning: RISK OF SERIOUS DISORDERS AND RIBAVIRIN-ASSOCIATED EFFECTS

Skin
Cutaneous toxicity / skin toxicity [2]
Dermatitis [O] (16%)
DRESS syndrome (Drug-induced hypersensitivity syndrome) [2]
Eczema / eczematous reaction / eczematous eruption [O] (4–5%) [3]
Exanthems [5]
Flushing / rubefaction [O] (4%)
Lichenoid eruption / lichenoid reaction [2]
Nummular eczema [2]
Peripheral edema [2]
Photosensitivity [7]
Pruritus (itching) [O] (13–29%) [28]
Psoriasis [2]
Rash [O] (5–28%) [39]
Sarcoidosis / sarcoid-like reaction (cutaneous sarcoidosis) [16]
Stevens-Johnson syndrome and toxic epidermal necrolysis (SJS/TEN) [2]
Vasculitis (angiitis) / cutaneous vasculitis (angiitis) [2]
Vitiligo [2]
Xerosis / xeroderma [O] (10–24%) [2]

Hair
Alopecia / hair loss [O] (27–36%) [5]
Alopecia areata [2]

Central Nervous System
Depression [O] (20–36%) [10]
Dysgeusia (taste perversion) [O] (4–9%) [4]
Fever (pyrexia) (includes hyperpyrexia) [O] (32–55%) [8]
Headache [INH] (Insomnia [O] (25–41%) [30]
Irritability [10]
Neurotoxicity [2]
Pain [O] (10%)
Rigors [O] (25–48%)
Suicidal ideation [O] (2%) [2]
Vertigo / dizziness [O] (14–26%) [7]

Endocrine/Metabolic
ALT increased [6]
Appetite decreased [2]
AST increased [5]
Diabetes mellitus [2]
Hyperbilirubinemia [4]
Hyperuricemia [O] (33–38%)
Thyroid dysfunction [2]
Weight loss [O] (10–29%) [2]

Gastrointestinal/Hepatic
Diarrhea [17]
Dyspepsia / functional dyspepsia (indigestion) (see also gastroparesis) [2]
Hepatotoxicity / liver injury / acute liver injury / drug-induced liver injury (DILI) [6]
Nausea [INH] (<10%) [40]
Pancreatitis / acute pancreatitis [5]
Vomiting [O] (9–25%) [3]

Genitourinary
Erectile dysfunction [2]

Hematologic
Anemia [INH] (<10%) [82]
Hemoglobin decreased [4]
Hemolytic anemia [2]
Hemotoxicity [2]
Leukocytopenia (leukopenia) / leukocytes (white blood cells) decreased [O] (6–45%) [3]
Lymphopenia (lymphocytopenia) / lymphocytes decreased [O] (12–14%) [2]
Neutropenia (neutrophils decreased) [O] (8–42%) [18]
Thrombocytopenia / platelets decreased [INH] (<15%) [11]

Local
Injection-site reaction [2]

Neuromuscular/Skeletal
Arthralgia [INH] (22–34%) [7]
Asthenia / fatigue [65]
Muscle spasm [3]
Myalgia/Myopathy [INH] (40–64%) [5]

Ocular
Retinopathy [6]

Otic
Hearing loss (hypoacusis) [2]
Tinnitus [2]

Renal
Nephrotoxicity / kidney injury / acute kidney injury (AKI) / drug-induced kidney injury [5]

Respiratory
Cough [O] (7–23%) [9]
Dyspnea / shortness of breath [O] (13–26%) [7]
Influenza- ('flu)-like syndrome [O] (13–18%) [9]
Nasopharyngitis [3]
Pneumonitis [2]
Rhinitis / rhinosinusitis (see also sinusitis) [O] (8%)
Upper respiratory tract infection [3]

Other
Adverse effects / adverse reactions [27]
Death [4]
Infection [INH] [4]
Vogt-Koyanagi-Harada syndrome [6]

RIBOCICLIB

Trade name: Kisqali (Novartis)
Indications: Treatment of postmenopausal women with hormone receptor (HR)-positive, human epidermal growth factor receptor 2 (HER2)-negative advanced or metastatic breast cancer (in combination with an aromatase inhibitor)
Class: Cyclin-dependent kinase (CDK) 4/6 inhibitor
Half-life: 30–55 hours
Clinically important, potentially hazardous interactions with: alfentanil, amiodarone, bepridil, boceprevir, chloroquine, clarithromycin, conivaptan, cyclosporine, CYP3A4 substrates, dihydroergotamine, disopyramide, ergotamine, everolimus, fentanyl, grapefruit juice, halofantrine, haloperidol, indinavir, itraconazole, ketoconazole, lopinavir, metformin, methadone, midazolam, moxifloxacin, ondansetron, pimozide, procainamide, QT prolonging drugs, quinidine, rifampin, ritonavir, rosuvastatin, saquinavir, simvastatin, sirolimus, sotalol, strong CYP3A4 inducers and inhibitors, tacrolimus, voriconazole
Pregnancy category: Can cause fetal harm
Important contra-indications noted in the prescribing guidelines for: nursing mothers; pediatric patients

---

Skin
Peripheral edema (12%)
Phototoxicity [2]
Pruritus (itching) (14%)
Rash (17%) [2]
Stevens-Johnson syndrome and toxic epidermal necrolysis (SJS/TEN) [3]
Vitiligo [6]

Hair
Alopecia / hair loss (33%) [3]

Mucosal
Stomatitis (oral mucositis) (12%)

Cardiovascular
Hypertension [2]

Central Nervous System
Fever (pyrexia) (includes hyperpyrexia) (13%)
Headache (22%) [2]
Insomnia (12%)

Endocrine/Metabolic
ALT increased (46%) [4]
Appetite decreased (19%)
AST increased (44%) [5]
Hyperbilirubinemia (18%)
Serum creatinine increased (20%)

Gastrointestinal/Hepatic
Abdominal pain (11%)
Constipation (25%) [2]
Diarrhea (35%) [3]
Hepatotoxicity / liver injury / acute liver injury / drug-induced liver injury (DILI) [7]
Nausea (52%) [9]
Vomiting (29%) [5]

Genitourinary
Urinary tract infection (11%)

Hematologic
Anemia (18%) [3]
Febrile neutropenia [2]
Leukocytopenia (leukopenia) / leukocytes (white blood cells) decreased (33%) [9]
Lymphopenia (lymphocytopenia) / lymphocytes decreased (11%) [3]
Neutropenia (neutrophils decreased) (75%) [15]
Thrombocytopenia / platelets decreased [3]

Neuromuscular/Skeletal
Arthralgia [2]
Asthenia / fatigue (37%) [7]
Back pain (20%) [2]
Rhabdomyolysis [3]

Ocular
Cornea verticillata / vortex keratopathy / whorl keratopathy [2]

Respiratory
Dyspnea / shortness of breath (12%)
Interstitial lung disease / interstitial pneumonitis / interstitial pneumonia (cryptogenic organizing pneumonia) / drug-induced interstitial lung disease [2]

Other
Infection [2]

RIFABUTIN

Trade name: Mycobutin (Pfizer)
Indications: Disseminated *Mycobacterium avium* infection
Class: Antibiotic, Antibiotic; rifamycin, Antimicrobial, CYP3A4 inducer
Half-life: 45 hours
Clinically important, potentially hazardous interactions with: abiraterone, amiodarone, amprenavir, anisindione, anticoagulants, atazanavir, atovaquone, atovaquone/proguanil, azithromycin, bedaquiline, bictegravir/emtricitabine/tenofovir alafenamide, boceprevir, cabazitaxel, cabozantinib, cobicistat/elvitegravir/emtricitabine/tenofovir alafenamide, cobicistat/elvitegravir/emtricitabine/tenofovir disoproxil, corticosteroids, crizotinib, cyclosporine, dapsone, darunavir, delavirdine, dicumarol, doravirine, doravirine/lamiduvine/tenofovir disoproxil, efavirenz, enzalutamide, erlotinib, etravirine, flibanserin, fosamprenavir, indinavir, itraconazole, ixabepilone, lapatinib, ledipasvir & sofosbuvir, levonorgestrel, lopinavir, midazolam, mifepristone, nelfinavir, oral contraceptives, posaconazole, rilpivirine, ritonavir, romidepsin, simeprevir, sofosbuvir, sofosbuvir & velpatasvir, sofosbuvir/velpatasvir/voxilaprevir, solifenacin, sonidegib, sorafenib, sunitinib, tacrolimus, temsirolimus, tenofovir alafenamide, tezacaftor/ivacaftor, thalidomide, tipranavir, tolvaptan, vandetanib, vemurafenib, voriconazole
Important contra-indications noted in the prescribing guidelines for: the elderly; nursing mothers; pediatric patients

---

Skin
Lupus erythematosus (subacute cutaneous lupus erythematosus (SCLE)) [2]
Pigmentation (Skin) (includes hyperpigmentation) [2]
Rash (11%) [2]

Central Nervous System
Anorexia (2%)
Dysgeusia (taste perversion) (3%)
Fever (pyrexia) (includes hyperpyrexia) (2%)
Headache (3%)

Gastrointestinal/Hepatic
Abdominal pain (4%)
Diarrhea (3%) [2]
Dyspepsia / functional dyspepsia (indigestion) (see also gastroparesis) (3%)
Eructation (belching) (3%)
Flatulence (2%)
Hepatotoxicity / liver injury / acute liver injury / drug-induced liver injury (DILI) [2]
Nausea (6%)

Neuromuscular/Skeletal
Arthralgia [6]
Myalgia/Myopathy (2%)

Ocular
Intraocular inflammation [2]
Ocular toxicity [2]
Uveitis / anterior uveitis / posterior uveitis / panuveitis [31]
Visual disturbances [2]

RIFAMPIN

Synonym: rifampicin
Trade names: Rifadin (Sanofi-Aventis), Rimactane (Novartis)
Indications: Tuberculosis
Class: Antibiotic, Antibiotic; rifamycin, Antimicrobial, Antimycobacterial (including antitubercular), CYP1A2 inducer, CYP3A4 inducer
Half-life: 3–5 hours
Clinically important, potentially hazardous interactions with: abacavir, abiraterone, acalabrutinib, afatinib, amiodarone, amprenavir, anisindione, antacids, anticoagulants, apixaban, apremilast, aprepitant, artemether/lumefantrine, atazanavir, atorvastatin, atovaquone, atovaquone/proguanil, axitinib, beclomethasone, bedaquiline, berotralstat, betamethasone, bictegravir/emtricitabine/tenofovir alafenamide, bisoprolol, boceprevir, bosentan, brentuximab vedotin, brigatinib, brivaracetam, buprenorphine, cabazitaxel, cabozantinib, canagliflozin, capmatinib, caspofungin, ceritinib, clobazam, clozapine, cobimetinib, copanlisib, corticosteroids, cortisone, crizotinib, cyclosporine, cyproterone, dabigatran, daclatasvir, dapsone, darunavir, dasatinib, deferasirox, deflazacort, delavirdine, dexamethasone, diclofenac, dicumarol, digoxin, doravirine, doravirine/lamiduvine/tenofovir disoproxil, doxycycline, dronedarone, edoxaban, efavirenz, elbasvir & grazoprevir, eliglustat, eluxadoline, emtricitabine/rilpivirine/tenofovir alafenamide, enzalutamide, erlotinib, esomeprazole, estradiol, eszopiclone, etoricoxib, etravirine, everolimus, fesoterodine, flibanserin, fludrocortisone, flunisolide, fosamprenavir, fostemsavir, gadoxetate, gefitinib, gestrinone, glecaprevir & pibrentasvir, halothane, hydrocortisone, ibrexafungerp, ibrutinib, idelalisib, imatinib, indinavir, infigratinib, isavuconazonium sulfate, isoniazid, itraconazole, ivabradine, ivacaftor, ixabepilone, ixazomib, ketoconazole, lapatinib, ledipasvir & sofosbuvir, leflunomide, lemborexant, lesinurad, letermovir, levodopa, levonorgestrel, linagliptin, linezolid, lopinavir, lorcainide, lorlatinib, losartan, lumacaftor/ivacaftor, lumateperone, lurasidone, macitentan, maraviroc, methylprednisolone, midazolam, midostaurin, mifepristone, naldemedine, nelfinavir, neratinib, netupitant & palonosetron, nevirapine, nifedipine, nilotinib, olaparib, oliceridine, ombitasvir/paritaprevir/ritonavir, ombitasvir/paritaprevir/ritonavir and dasabuvir, ondansetron, oral contraceptives, osilodrostat, osimertinib, ospemifene, oxtriphylline, ozanimod, paclitaxel, palbociclib, pazopanib, pemigatinib, perampanel, phenylbutazone, pimavanserin, pioglitazone, pitavastatin, pomalidomide, ponatinib, ponesimod, pralsetinib, praziquantel, prednisolone, prednisone, propranolol, propyphenazone, protease inhibitors, pyrazinamide, quinine, raltegravir, ramelteon, ranolazine, regorafenib, relugolix, ribociclib, rilpivirine, rimegepant, riociguat, ritonavir, rivaroxaban, roflumilast, romidepsin, rosiglitazone, saquinavir, selpercatinib, simeprevir, simvastatin, sofosbuvir, sofosbuvir & velpatasvir, sofosbuvir/velpatasvir/voxilaprevir, solifenacin, sonidegib, sorafenib, sotorasib, sunitinib, tacrolimus, tadalafil, tasimelteon, telaprevir, telithromycin, temsirolimus, tenofovir alafenamide, terbinafine, tezacaftor/ivacaftor, thalidomide, ticagrelor, tipranavir, tofacitinib, tolvaptan, trabectedin, treprostinil, triamcinolone, triazolam, trimethoprim, troleandomycin, tucatinib, ubrogepant, ulipristal, upadacitinib hemihydrate, valbenazine, vandetanib, vemurafenib, venetoclax, vorapaxar, voriconazole, vortioxetine, warfarin, zaleplon, zidovudine, zolpidem

---

Skin
Acneiform eruption / acneiform dermatitis / acneiform rash [3]
AGEP [2]
Anaphylactoid reactions / anaphylaxis (includes anaphylactic shock) [8]
Dermatitis [3]
Diaphoresis (<10%)
DRESS syndrome (Drug-induced hypersensitivity syndrome) [5]
Erythema multiforme [4]
Exanthems (<5%) [6]
Fixed eruption / fixed drug eruption [6]
Flushing / rubefaction (7%) [8]
Hypersensitivity [5]
Lichenoid eruption / lichenoid reaction [3]
Linear IgA bullous dermatosis [3]
Pemphigus [9]

Pruritus (itching) (<62%) [9]
Purpura [6]
Rash (<5%) [6]
Red man syndrome / flushing syndrome [7]
Serum sickness-like reaction [2]
Stevens-Johnson syndrome and toxic epidermal necrolysis (SJS/TEN) [9]
Thrombocytopenic purpura [2]
Urticaria / hives [8]
Vasculitis (angiitis) / cutaneous vasculitis (angiitis) [5]

Cardiovascular
Shock [2]

Central Nervous System
Fever (pyrexia) (includes hyperpyrexia) [2]
Seizures [3]
Vertigo / dizziness [2]

Endocrine/Metabolic
Amenorrhea [2]
Porphyria [2]

Gastrointestinal/Hepatic
Abdominal pain [3]
Diarrhea [2]
Hepatitis [3]
Hepatotoxicity / liver injury / acute liver injury / drug-induced liver injury (DILI) [19]
Nausea [4]
Vomiting [2]

Hematologic
Agranulocytosis / severe selective neutropenia [2]
Anemia [3]
Hemolysis [3]
Thrombocytopenia / platelets decreased [11]

Neuromuscular/Skeletal
Asthenia / fatigue [3]

Renal
Nephritis / interstitial nephritis / tubulointerstitial nephritis [3]
Nephrotoxicity / kidney injury / acute kidney injury (AKI) / drug-induced kidney injury [14]
Renal failure [3]

Respiratory
Pneumonitis [2]

Other
Adverse effects / adverse reactions [13]
Death [7]
Side effects (5%)

RIFAPENTINE

Trade name: Priftin (Sanofi-Aventis)
Indications: Tuberculosis (in combination with one or more antituberculosis drugs)
Class: Antibiotic, Antibiotic; rifamycin, Antimicrobial, Antimycobacterial (including antitubercular)
Half-life: 14–17 hours
Clinically important, potentially hazardous interactions with: abiraterone, alfentanil, amiodarone, angiotensin II receptor blockers, anisindione, antiarrhythmics, anticoagulants, antifungals, aprepitant, atovaquone, barbiturates, bedaquiline, benzodiazepines, beta blockers, bictegravir/emtricitabine/tenofovir alafenamide, buspirone, cabozantinib, calcium channel blockers, clopidogrel, cobicistat/elvitegravir/emtricitabine/tenofovir alafenamide, cobicistat/elvitegravir/emtricitabine/tenofovir disoproxil, corticosteroids, cyclosporine, CYP2C8 substrates, CYP2C9 substrates, CYP3A4 substrates, dapsone, delavirdine, dicumarol, disopyramide, doravirine, doravirine/lamiduvine/tenofovir disoproxil, dronedarone, emtricitabine/rilpivirine/tenofovir alafenamide, enzalutamide, erlotinib, etravirine, everolimus, exemestane, fentanyl, flibanserin, fluconazole, food, gefitinib, guanfacine, hormonal contraceptives, imatinib, indinavir, isoniazid, ixabepilone, ledipasvir & sofosbuvir, maraviroc, methadone, mifepristone, morphine, mycophenolate, mycophenolate, nilotinib, pazopanib, phenytoin, praziquantel, propafenone, protease inhibitors, quinidine, ramelteon, ranolazine, repaglinide, reverse transcriptase inhibitors, rilpivirine, ritonavir, romidepsin, saxagliptin, simeprevir, sofosbuvir, sofosbuvir & velpatasvir, sofosbuvir/velpatasvir/voxilaprevir, solifenacin, sorafenib, sunitinib, tacrolimus, tadalafil, tamoxifen, temsirolimus, tenofovir alafenamide, terbinafine, tolvaptan, treprostinil, ulipristal, vandetanib, vemurafenib, vitamin K antagonists, voriconazole, warfarin, zaleplon, zidovudine, zolpidem
Important contra-indications noted in the prescribing guidelines for: nursing mothers; pediatric patients

---

Skin
Acneiform eruption / acneiform dermatitis / acneiform rash (3%)
Hyperhidrosis (6%)
Pruritus (itching) (4%)
Rash (6%)

Cardiovascular
Chest pain (6%)
Hypertension (2%)

Central Nervous System
Anorexia (6%)
Headache (4%)
Pain (6%)
Vertigo / dizziness (2%)

Endocrine/Metabolic
ALT increased (7%)
AST increased (6%)
Hyperglycemia (includes glucose increased) (4%)
Hyperkalemia (9%)
Hyperuricemia (with pyrazinamide) (32%)
Hypoglycemia (10%)

Gastrointestinal/Hepatic
Abdominal pain (2%)
Constipation (2%)
Diarrhea (2%)
Dyspepsia / functional dyspepsia (indigestion) (see also gastroparesis) (3%)
Hepatotoxicity / liver injury / acute liver injury / drug-induced liver injury (DILI) [2]
Nausea (3%)
Vomiting (2%)

Genitourinary
Cystitis (includes interstitial cystitis / bladder pain syndrome) (2%)
Hematuria (18%)
Pyuria (22%)
Urinary casts (8%)
Urinary tract infection (13%)

Hematologic
Anemia (12%)
Leukocytopenia (leukopenia) / leukocytes (white blood cells) decreased (7%)
Leukocytosis (elevated white blood cell (WBC) count) (3%)
Lymphopenia (lymphocytopenia) / lymphocytes decreased (12%)
Neutropenia (neutrophils decreased) (13%)
Polycythemia / erythrocytosis (2%)
Thrombocytopenia / platelets decreased (3%)

Neuromuscular/Skeletal
Arthralgia (4%)
Back pain (7%)

Ocular
Conjunctivitis (conjunctival inflammation) (3%)

Renal
Proteinuria (13%)

Respiratory
Bronchitis (3%)
Cough (8%)
Hemoptysis (8%)
Influenza (8%)
Influenza- ('flu)-like syndrome [2]
Pharyngitis (sore throat) (2%)
Upper respiratory tract infection (5%)

Other
Adverse effects / adverse reactions [4]

RIFAXIMIN

Trade names: Xifaxan (Salix), Xifaxanta (Norgine)
Indications: Diarrhea in travelers (caused by non-invasive strains of *E. coli*), reduction in risk of overt hepatic encephalopathy recurrence (in adults)
Class: Antibiotic, Antibiotic; rifamycin, Antimicrobial
Half-life: 2–5 hours
Clinically important, potentially hazardous interactions with: BCG vaccine
Important contra-indications noted in the prescribing guidelines for: nursing mothers; pediatric patients

---

Skin
Cellulitis and pseudocellulitis (2–5%)
Clammy skin (<2%)
Diaphoresis (<2%)
Edema / fluid retention (2–5%)
Hot flashes / hot flushes (<2%)
Hyperhidrosis (<2%)
Peripheral edema (15%) [2]
Pruritus (itching) (9%)
Rash (<5%)
Sunburn (<2%)

Mucosal
Epistaxis (nosebleed) (2–5%)
Gingival lesions (<2%)
Rhinorrhea (<2%)
Xerostomia (dry mouth) (2–5%)

Cardiovascular
Chest pain (<5%) [2]
Hypotension (2–5%)

Central Nervous System
Abnormal dreams (<2%)
Ageusia (taste loss) / taste disorder (<2%)
Amnesia (2–5%)
Anorexia (<5%)
Confusion (2–5%)
Depression (7%)
Dysgeusia (taste perversion) (<2%) [2]
Fever (pyrexia) (includes hyperpyrexia) (3–6%)
Headache (10%) [8]

Hypoesthesia / hypesthesia (numbness) (2–5%)
Impaired concentration (2–5%)
Insomnia (<7%)
Migraine (<2%)
Pain (<5%)
Syncope / fainting (<2%)
Tremor (2–5%)
Vertigo / dizziness (<13%) [3]

Endocrine/Metabolic
AST increased (<2%)
Dehydration (<5%)
Hyperglycemia (includes glucose increased) (2–5%)
Hyperkalemia (2–5%)
Hypoglycemia (2–5%)
Hyponatremia (2–5%)
Weight gain (2–5%)

Gastrointestinal/Hepatic
Abdominal distension (<8%)
Abdominal pain (2–9%) [10]
Ascites (11%)
Black stools / melena (<2%)
Constipation (4–6%)
Diarrhea (<2%) [6]
Fecal urgency (6%)
Flatulence (11%) [2]
Hernia (<2%)
Nausea (5–14%) [8]
Tenesmus (7%)
Vomiting (2%) [3]

Genitourinary
Dysuria (<2%)
Hematuria (<2%)
Polyuria (includes polyuric syndrome) (<2%)
Urinary frequency (<2%)

Hematologic
Anemia (8%)
Lymphocytosis / lymphocytes increased (<2%)
Monocytosis (<2%)
Neutropenia (neutrophils decreased) (<2%)

Neuromuscular/Skeletal
Arthralgia (<6%)
Asthenia / fatigue (<12%) [3]
Back pain (6%)
Muscle spasm (<9%)
Myalgia/Myopathy (<5%)
Neck pain (<2%)
Pain in extremities (2–5%)
Rhabdomyolysis [3]

Otic
Ear pain (<2%)
Tinnitus (<2%)

Renal
Proteinuria (<2%)

Respiratory
Cough (7%)
Dyspnea / shortness of breath (<6%)
Influenza- ('flu)-like syndrome (2–5%)
Nasopharyngitis (<7%) [4]
Pharyngitis (sore throat) (<2%)
Pharyngolaryngeal pain (<2%)
Pneumonia (2–5%)
Rhinitis / rhinosinusitis (see also sinusitis) (<5%)
Sinusitis (see also rhinitis / rhinosinusitis) [2]
Upper respiratory tract infection (2–5%) [6]

Other
Adverse effects / adverse reactions [3]
Breast cancer [2]

RILONACEPT

Trade name: Arcalyst (Regeneron)
Indications: Cryopyrin-associated periodic syndromes (CAPS) including familial cold autoinflammatory syndrome (FCAS), Muckle-Wells syndrome (MWS)
Class: Fusion protein, Interleukin-1 inhibitor
Half-life: N/A
Clinically important, potentially hazardous interactions with: anti-TNF agents, lenalidomide, live vaccines, natalizumab
Note: Cryopyrin-associated periodic syndromes (CAPS) are characterized by life-long, recurrent symptoms of rash, fever/chills, joint pain, eye redness/pain, and fatigue. Intermittent, disruptive exacerbations or flares can be triggered at any time by exposure to cooling temperatures, stress, exercise, or other unknown stimuli.

Central Nervous System
Hyperesthesia (9%)

Local
Injection-site reaction (48%) [3]

Respiratory
Cough (9%)
Sinusitis (see also rhinitis / rhinosinusitis) (9%)
Upper respiratory tract infection (26%)

RILPIVIRINE

Trade names: Complera (Gilead), Edurant (Centocor), Juluca (ViiV)
Indications: HIV-1 infection
Class: Antiretroviral, Non-nucleoside reverse transcriptase inhibitor
Half-life: 50 hours
Clinically important, potentially hazardous interactions with: antacids, atazanavir, carbamazepine, cimetidine, clarithromycin, darunavir, delavirdine, dexamethasone, efavirenz, erythromycin, esomeprazole, etravirine, famotidine, fluconazole, fosamprenavir, indinavir, itraconazole, ketoconazole, lansoprazole, lopinavir, methadone, nelfinavir, nevirapine, nizatidine, ombitasvir/paritaprevir/ritonavir, omeprazole, oxcarbazepine, pantoprazole, phenobarbital, phenytoin, posaconazole, QT prolonging agents, rabeprazole, ranitidine, rifabutin, rifampin, rifapentine, ritonavir, saquinavir, St John's wort, tipranavir, troleandomycin, voriconazole
Important contra-indications noted in the prescribing guidelines for: the elderly; nursing mothers; pediatric patients
Note: Complera is rilpivirine, emtricitabine and tenofovir; Juluca is rilpivirine and dolutegravir.

Skin
Rash (3%) [10]

Central Nervous System
Abnormal dreams [2]
Depression [4]
Headache (3%) [3]
Insomnia (3%) [2]
Neurotoxicity [3]
Nightmares [2]
Sleep-related disorder [2]
Vertigo / dizziness [5]

Endocrine/Metabolic
Serum creatinine increased [2]

Gastrointestinal/Hepatic
Hepatotoxicity / liver injury / acute liver injury / drug-induced liver injury (DILI) [4]

Local
Injection-site reaction [2]

Other
Adverse effects / adverse reactions [2]

RILUZOLE

Trade name: Rilutek (Sanofi-Aventis)
Indications: Amyotrophic lateral sclerosis
Class: Neuromuscular blocker (in ALS), Neuroprotectant
Half-life: N/A
Clinically important, potentially hazardous interactions with: none known
Pregnancy category: May cause fetal toxicity based on findings in animal studies
Important contra-indications noted in the prescribing guidelines for: nursing mothers; pediatric patients

---

Skin
Eczema / eczematous reaction / eczematous eruption (2%)
Peripheral edema (3%)

Mucosal
Xerostomia (dry mouth) (4%)

Central Nervous System
Paresthesias (circumoral) [3]
Vertigo / dizziness [5]

Gastrointestinal/Hepatic
Abdominal pain (2%) [2]
Hepatotoxicity / liver injury / acute liver injury / drug-induced liver injury (DILI) [2]
Pancreatitis / acute pancreatitis [6]

Neuromuscular/Skeletal
Asthenia / fatigue (5%) [12]

Other
Adverse effects / adverse reactions [2]

RIMANTADINE

Trade name: Flumadine (Forest)
Indications: Various infections caused by influenza virus
Class: Adamantane, Antiviral
Half-life: 25–30 hours
Clinically important, potentially hazardous interactions with: none known

---

Skin
Edema / fluid retention (pedal) (<10%)

Mucosal
Xerostomia (dry mouth) (2%)

RIMEGEPANT

Trade name: Nurtec ODT (Biohaven Pharma)
Indications: Treatment of migraine
Class: Calcitonin gene-related peptide (CGRP) receptor antagonist
Half-life: ~11 hours
Clinically important, potentially hazardous interactions with: fluconazole, itraconazole, rifampin, strong CYP3A4 inhibitors; moderate

CYP3A4 inhibitors; strong and moderate CYP3A inducers; inhibitors of P-gp or bcrp
Pregnancy category: No adequate data on the developmental risk associated with use in pregnant women.

Gastrointestinal/Hepatic
Nausea [2]
Genitourinary
Urinary tract infection [2]

RIMONABANT

Trade name: Acomplia (Sanofi-Aventis)
Indications: Obesity
Class: Anti-obesity / weight loss pharmacotherapy, CB1 Cannabinoid receptor antagonist
Half-life: N/A
Clinically important, potentially hazardous interactions with: clarithromycin, itraconazole, ketoconazole, nefazodone, ritonavir, telithromycin
Note: This drug has been withdrawn.

Central Nervous System
Anxiety [5]
Depression [7]
Mood changes (includes mood disorder) [2]
Neurotoxicity [2]
Vertigo / dizziness [4]
Gastrointestinal/Hepatic
Nausea [2]
Other
Adverse effects / adverse reactions [3]

RIOCIGUAT

Trade name: Adempas (Bayer)
Indications: Pulmonary hypertension
Class: Soluble guanylate cyclase (sGC) stimulator
Half-life: 7–12 hours
Clinically important, potentially hazardous interactions with: antacids, carbamazepine, dipyridamole, nitrates or nitric oxide donors, nitroprusside, phenobarbital, phenytoin, rifampin, sildenafil, St John's wort, tadalafil, theophylline, vardenafil
Important contra-indications noted in the prescribing guidelines for: nursing mothers; pediatric patients
Warning: EMBRYO-FETAL TOXICITY

Skin
Peripheral edema [5]
Cardiovascular
Cardiac failure [2]
Hypotension (10%) [7]
Central Nervous System
Headache (27%) [4]
Syncope / fainting [3]
Vertigo / dizziness (20%) [4]
Gastrointestinal/Hepatic
Constipation (5%)
Diarrhea (12%)
Dyspepsia / functional dyspepsia (indigestion) (see also gastroparesis) (21%) [3]
Gastroesophageal reflux (5%)
Nausea (14%)
Vomiting (10%)
Hematologic
Anemia (7%)
Bleeding (2%) [2]
Respiratory
Pneumonia [2]
Other
Adverse effects / adverse reactions [6]

RISANKIZUMAB

Trade name: Skyrizi (AbbVie)
Indications: Moderate-to-severe plaque psoriasis in adults who are candidates for systemic therapy or phototherapy
Class: Interleukin-17 (IL-17) antagonist / interleukin-17 inhibitor, Interleukin-23 inhibitor, Monoclonal antibody
Half-life: ~ 28 days
Clinically important, potentially hazardous interactions with: live vaccines
Pregnancy category: Limited available data in pregnant women to evaluate a drug associated risk of major birth defects, miscarriage, or adverse maternal or fetal outcome. Risankizumab may be transmitted from the mother to the developing fetus.
Note: May increase the risk of infection. Evaluate for TB prior to initiating treatment with risankizumab.
Risankizumab-Rzaa is a biosimilar to Risankizumab.

Central Nervous System
Headache (4%)
Local
Injection-site reaction (2%)
Neuromuscular/Skeletal
Asthenia / fatigue (3%)
Respiratory
Upper respiratory tract infection (13%)
Other
Infection (22%)

RISEDRONATE

Trade names: Actonel (Procter & Gamble), Atelvia (Warner Chilcott)
Indications: Paget's disease of bone, osteoporosis
Class: Bisphosphonate
Half-life: terminal: 220 hours
Clinically important, potentially hazardous interactions with: antacids, calcium supplements, iron preparations, laxatives, magnesium-based supplements
Important contra-indications noted in the prescribing guidelines for: nursing mothers; pediatric patients

---

Skin
Bruise / bruising / contusion / ecchymosis (ecchymoses) (4%)
Peripheral edema (8%)
Pruritus (itching) (3%)
Rash (8%)
Cardiovascular
Chest pain (5%)
Hypertension (11%)
Central Nervous System
Depression (7%)
Fever (pyrexia) (includes hyperpyrexia) [2]
Headache (10%) [3]
Insomnia (5%)
Pain (14%)
Paresthesias (2%)
Vertigo / dizziness (7%)
Endocrine/Metabolic
Hypocalcemia [2]
Gastrointestinal/Hepatic
Abdominal pain (12%) [3]
Constipation (13%) [3]
Diarrhea (11%) [4]
Dyspepsia / functional dyspepsia (indigestion) (see also gastroparesis) (11%) [2]
Esophagitis [2]
Gastrointestinal disorder / discomfort [4]
Hepatotoxicity / liver injury / acute liver injury / drug-induced liver injury (DILI) [6]
Nausea (11%) [2]
Genitourinary
Urinary tract infection (11%)
Neuromuscular/Skeletal
Arthralgia (10–24%) [7]
Asthenia / fatigue (5%)
Back pain (28%) [5]
Bone pain / joint pain (7%) [5]
Fractures (9%) [9]
Myalgia/Myopathy (7%) [3]
Neck pain (5%) [3]
Osteonecrosis / avascular necrosis (includes steroid-induced osteonecrosis of the femoral head) [6]
Tendinopathy/Tendon rupture (3%)
Ocular
Cataract (7%)
Ocular adverse effect [3]
Scleritis [2]
Respiratory
Bronchitis (10%)
Cough (6%)
Influenza [3]
Influenza- ('flu)-like syndrome (11%) [2]
Nasopharyngitis [3]
Pharyngitis (sore throat) (6%)
Rhinitis / rhinosinusitis (see also sinusitis) (6%)
Sinusitis (see also rhinitis / rhinosinusitis) (9%)
Other
Adverse effects / adverse reactions [6]
Allergic reactions (4%)
Infection (31%) [3]
Tooth disorder (2%)

RISPERIDONE

Trade names: Risperdal (Ortho-McNeil) (Janssen), Risperdal Consta (Ortho-McNeil) (Janssen)
Indications: Schizophrenia, bipolar mania, irritability associated with autistic disorder
Class: Antipsychotic, Antipsychotic, atypical, Mood stabilizer
Half-life: 3–30 hours
Clinically important, potentially hazardous interactions with: ACE inhibitors, alcohol, alpha blockers, amantadine, angiotensin II receptor antagonists, anxiolytics and hypnotics, apomorphine, artemether/lumefantrine, barbiturates, bromocriptine, cabergoline, calcium channel blockers, carbamazepine, cimetidine, citalopram, clozapine, cobicistat/elvitegravir/

emtricitabine/tenofovir alafenamide, cobicistat/elvitegravir/emtricitabine/tenofovir disoproxil, ethosuximide, fluoxetine, general anesthetics, histamine, levodopa, memantine, methyldopa, metoclopramide, opioid analgesics, oxcarbazepine, paliperidone, paroxetine hydrochloride, pergolide, phenytoin, pramipexole, primidone, ranitidine, ritonavir, ropinirole, rotigotine, sodium oxybate, sympathomimetics, tetrabenazine, tramadol, tricyclics, valproic acid, viloxazine
Important contra-indications noted in the prescribing guidelines for: nursing mothers; pediatric patients
Note: Safety and effectiveness have not been established for pediatric patients with schizophrenia <13 years of age, for bipolar mania <10 years of age, and for autistic disorder <5 years of age. [C] = in children.
Warning: INCREASED MORTALITY IN ELDERLY PATIENTS WITH DEMENTIA-RELATED PSYCHOSIS

Skin
Angioedema (formerly named angioneurotic edema) [9]
Bullous pemphigoid / pemphigoid [3]
Edema / fluid retention [3]
Peripheral edema (16%) [4]
Photosensitivity (<10%) [2]
Rash [C] (11%) (2–4%) [2]
Seborrhea (2%)
Urticaria / hives [2]
Xerosis / xeroderma (2%)

Hair
Alopecia / hair loss [2]

Mucosal
Sialopenia (5%)
Sialorrhea (ptyalism; hypersalivation) [C] (22%) (<3%) [12]
Xerostomia (dry mouth) [C] (13%) (4%) [7]

Cardiovascular
Bradycardia / sinus bradycardia [2]
Cardiotoxicity [2]
Hypotension [3]
QT interval prolonged / QT prolongation [4]
Tachycardia [C] (7%) (<5%)
Venous thromboembolism [6]
Ventricular arrhythmia [2]

Central Nervous System
Agitation [2]
Akathisia [C] (16%) (5–9%) [20]
Anorexia [C] (8%) (2%)
Anxiety [C] (16%) (2–16%) [5]
Catatonia [2]
Compulsions / obsessive-compulsive symptoms / obsessive-compulsive disorder [3]
Depression (14%) [7]
Extrapyramidal symptoms [20]
Fever (pyrexia) (includes hyperpyrexia) [C] (20%) (<2%)
Headache [11]
Hypothermia [2]
Insomnia [9]
Neuroleptic malignant syndrome [27]
Neurotoxicity [2]
Parkinsonism [C] (2–16%) (12–20%) [9]
Psychosis [3]
Rabbit syndrome (oral vertical dyskinesia) [6]
Restless legs syndrome / Willis-Ekbom disease (includes restless arms syndrome variant) [2]
Schizophrenia [2]
Sedation [4]
Seizures [3]
Serotonin syndrome [3]
Somnolence (drowsiness) [C] (12–67%) (5–14%) [16]
Stuttering (dysphemia) / stammering [2]
Suicidal ideation [3]
Tardive syndrome / tardive dyskinesia [6]
Tic disorder [2]
Tremor [C] (10–12%) (6%) [7]
Vertigo / dizziness [C] (7–16%) (4–10%) [5]

Endocrine/Metabolic
Amenorrhea [6]
Appetite decreased [2]
Appetite increased [C] (49%) [4]
Diabetes mellitus [2]
Galactorrhea (<10%) [14]
Gynecomastia (<10%) [6]
Hyperprolactinemia [27]
Metabolic syndrome (includes metabolic disorder) [5]
Weight gain [C] (5%) [36]

Gastrointestinal/Hepatic
Abdominal pain [C] (15–18%) (3–4%)
Constipation [C] (21%) (8–9%) [5]
Diarrhea [C] (7%) (73%)
Dyspepsia / functional dyspepsia (indigestion) (see also gastroparesis) [C] (5–16%) (4–10%)
Dysphagia [2]
Nausea [C] (8–16%) (4–9%) [4]
Pancreatitis / acute pancreatitis [2]
Vomiting [C] (10–25%)

Genitourinary
Enuresis (urinary incontinence) [C] (5–22%) (2%) [6]
Priapism (<10%) [29]
Sexual dysfunction [6]
Urinary retention [2]
Urinary tract infection (3%)

Hematologic
Leukocytopenia (leukopenia) / leukocytes (white blood cells) decreased [3]
Neutropenia (neutrophils decreased) [4]

Local
Injection-site pain [3]

Neuromuscular/Skeletal
Arthralgia (2–3%)
Asthenia / fatigue [C] (18–42%) (<3%) [5]
Back pain (2–3%)
Dystonia [C] (9–18%) (5–11%) [5]
Pisa syndrome (pleurothotonus) [4]
Rhabdomyolysis [7]

Ocular
Abnormal vision [C] (4–7%) (<3%)
Oculogyric crisis / oculogyric dystonic reaction [5]
Periorbital edema [2]
Vision blurred [3]

Respiratory
Cough [C] (34%) (3%)
Dyspnea / shortness of breath [C] (2–5%) (2%)
Laryngospasm (laryngeal dystonia / spasmodic dysphonia) [2]
Pneumonia [2]
Pulmonary embolism [3]
Respiratory depression [3]
Rhinitis / rhinosinusitis (see also sinusitis) [C] (13–36%) (7–11%)
Upper respiratory tract infection [C] (34%) (2–3%) [2]

Other
Adverse effects / adverse reactions [11]
Death [3]
Tooth disorder (<3%)

RITODRINE

Indications: Preterm labor
Class: Beta-2 adrenergic agonist, Tocolytic
Half-life: 1.3–12 hours
Clinically important, potentially hazardous interactions with: glycopyrrolate

---

Skin
Anaphylactoid reactions / anaphylaxis (includes anaphylactic shock) (<3%)
Diaphoresis (<14%)
Erythema (10–15%) [2]
Pustules / pustular eruption [2]
Rash (<3%)
Stevens-Johnson syndrome and toxic epidermal necrolysis (SJS/TEN) [2]
Vasculitis (angiitis) / cutaneous vasculitis (angiitis) [2]

Cardiovascular
Chest pain [2]
Myocardial ischemia [2]

Central Nervous System
Chills (3–10%)
Tremor (>10%)

Endocrine/Metabolic
Hypokalemia [2]

Gastrointestinal/Hepatic
Hepatotoxicity / liver injury / acute liver injury / drug-induced liver injury (DILI) [3]

Neuromuscular/Skeletal
Rhabdomyolysis [4]

Ocular
Glaucoma (includes acute angle-closure glaucoma) [2]

Respiratory
Pulmonary edema (cardiogenic / non-cardiogenic) [3]

Other
Adverse effects / adverse reactions [4]
Fetal adverse effect [3]

RITONAVIR

Trade names: Kaletra (AbbVie), Norvir (AbbVie)
Indications: HIV infection
Class: Antiretroviral, CYP3A4 inhibitor, HIV-1 protease inhibitor
Half-life: 3–5 hours
Clinically important, potentially hazardous interactions with: abiraterone, afatinib, alfentanil, alfuzosin, alprazolam, amiodarone, amitriptyline, amprenavir, aprepitant, astemizole, atazanavir, atorvastatin, atovaquone, atovaquone/proguanil, avanafil, azithromycin, bepridil, boceprevir, bosentan, brigatinib, buprenorphine, bupropion, buspirone, cabazitaxel, cabozantinib, calcifediol, carbamazepine, ceritinib, chlordiazepoxide, ciclesonide, citalopram, clozapine, cobicistat/elvitegravir/emtricitabine/tenofovir disoproxil, colchicine, conivaptan, copanlisib, crizotinib, cyclosporine, cyproterone, darifenacin, dasatinib, deferasirox, delavirdine, diazepam, diclofenac, dihydroergotamine, docetaxel, dronedarone, dutasteride, efavirenz, eletriptan, eluxadoline, ergot alkaloids,

ergotamine, erlotinib, estazolam, estradiol, eszopiclone, etravirine, everolimus, ezetimibe, fentanyl, fesoterodine, flecainide, flibanserin, flurazepam, fluticasone propionate, fosamprenavir, glecaprevir & pibrentasvir, halazepam, indacaterol, isavuconazonium sulfate, itraconazole, ivabradine, ixabepilone, ketoconazole, lapatinib, ledipasvir & sofosbuvir, levomepromazine, levothyroxine, lomitapide, lumateperone, macitentan, maraviroc, meloxicam, meperidine, meptazinol, methylergonovine, methysergide, midazolam, midostaurin, mifepristone, naldemedine, nelfinavir, neratinib, nifedipine, nilotinib, olaparib, oliceridine, oral contraceptives, osimertinib, paclitaxel, palbociclib, paroxetine hydrochloride, pazopanib, phenytoin, pimozide, piroxicam, pitavastatin, ponatinib, posaconazole, propafenone, propoxyphene, propranolol, quazepam, quinidine, quinine, ranolazine, ribociclib, rifabutin, rifampin, rifapentine, rilpivirine, rimonabant, risperidone, rivaroxaban, romidepsin, rosuvastatin, ruxolitinib, saquinavir, sildenafil, silodosin, simeprevir, simvastatin, sofosbuvir, sofosbuvir/velpatasvir/voxilaprevir, solifenacin, St John's wort, sunitinib, tadalafil, telaprevir, telithromycin, temsirolimus, tenofovir disoproxil, ticagrelor, tolvaptan, trabectedin, triazolam, ulipristal, vardenafil, vemurafenib, venetoclax, vorapaxar, voriconazole, zolpidem, zuclopenthixol

Important contra-indications noted in the prescribing guidelines for: nursing mothers

Note: Protease inhibitors cause dyslipidemia which includes elevated triglycerides and cholesterol and redistribution of body fat centrally to produce the so-called 'protease paunch', breast enlargement, facial atrophy, and 'buffalo hump'. Kaletra is ritonavir and lopinavir. See also separate entry for ombitasvir/paritaprevir/ritonavir.

Paxlovid is ritonavir and nirmatrelvir.

Warning: DRUG-DRUG INTERACTIONS LEADING TO POTENTIALLY SERIOUS AND/OR LIFE-THREATENING REACTIONS

Skin

- Acneiform eruption / acneiform dermatitis / acneiform rash (4%)
- Bruise / bruising / contusion / ecchymosis (ecchymoses) (<2%)
- Bullous dermatosis (<2%)
- Cutaneous toxicity / skin toxicity [2]
- Dermatitis (<2%)
- Diaphoresis (<10%)
- Eczema / eczematous reaction / eczematous eruption (<2%)
- Edema / fluid retention (6%)
- Exanthems (<2%) [2]
- Facial edema (8%)
- Flushing / rubefaction (13%)
- Folliculitis (<2%)
- Hypersensitivity (8%)
- Jaundice (see also cholestasis / cholestatic jaundice) [3]
- Lipodystrophy / acquired generalized lipodystrophy [4]
- Peripheral edema (6%)
- Photosensitivity (<2%)
- Pruritus (itching) (12%)
- Psoriasis (<2%)
- Rash (27%) [12]
- Seborrhea (<2%)
- Urticaria / hives (8%)
- Xanthomas [2]
- Xerosis / xeroderma (<2%)

Hair

- Alopecia / hair loss [2]

Mucosal

- Cheilitis (inflammation of the lips) (<2%)
- Gingivitis (<2%)
- Oral candidiasis (<2%)
- Oral ulceration (<2%)
- Oropharyngeal pain (16%)
- Xerostomia (dry mouth) (<2%)

Cardiovascular

- Bradycardia / sinus bradycardia [3]
- Cardiotoxicity [2]
- Hypertension (3%)
- Hypotension (2%)
- Orthostatic hypotension (2%)

Central Nervous System

- Ageusia (taste loss) / taste disorder (<2%)
- Confusion (3%)
- Dysgeusia (taste perversion) (16%)
- Headache [8]
- Hyperesthesia (<2%)
- Impaired concentration (3%)
- Insomnia [2]
- Neurotoxicity [2]
- Paresthesias (51%)
- Parosmia (<2%)
- Peripheral neuropathy (10%)
- Syncope / fainting (3%)
- Vertigo / dizziness (16%) [2]

Endocrine/Metabolic

- ALT increased [3]
- Cushing's syndrome [7]
- Gynecomastia [2]
- Hyperbilirubinemia [6]
- Hypercholesterolemia (3%) [2]
- Hyperlipidemia / lipids elevated [2]
- Hypertriglyceridemia (includes triglycerides increased) (9%) [3]

Gastrointestinal/Hepatic

- Abdominal pain (26%) [2]
- Diarrhea (68%) [14]
- Dyspepsia / functional dyspepsia (indigestion) (see also gastroparesis) (12%)
- Flatulence (8%)
- Gastrointestinal bleeding (2%)
- Gastrointestinal disorder / discomfort [5]
- Hepatotoxicity / liver injury / acute liver injury / drug-induced liver injury (DILI) (9%) [6]
- Nausea (57%) [13]
- Vomiting (32%) [7]

Genitourinary

- Urinary frequency (4%)

Neuromuscular/Skeletal

- Arthralgia (19%)
- Asthenia / fatigue (46%) [3]
- Back pain (19%)
- Myalgia/Myopathy (4–9%)
- Rhabdomyolysis [2]

Ocular

- Vision blurred (6%)

Renal

- Fanconi syndrome (proximal tubular dysfunction) [4]
- Nephrolithiasis (kidney stones / renal calculi) [3]
- Nephrotoxicity / kidney injury / acute kidney injury (AKI) / drug-induced kidney injury [3]
- Renal failure [2]

Respiratory

- Cough (22%)
- Nasopharyngitis [2]
- Upper respiratory tract infection [2]

Other

- Adverse effects / adverse reactions [10]
- Allergic reactions (<2%)

RITUXIMAB

Trade names: MabThera (Roche), Rituxan (Genentech)

Indications: Non-Hodgkin's lymphoma, chronic lymphocytic leukemia, rhematoid arthritis (in combination with methotrexate), granulomatosis with polyangiitis and mycroscopic polyangiitis (in combination with glucocorticoids)

Class: Biologic, Biologic disease-modifying antirheumatic drug (bDMARD), CD20-directed cytolytic monoclonal antibody, Disease-modifying antirheumatic drug (DMARD), Immunosuppressant, Monoclonal antibody

Half-life: 60 hours (after first infusion)

Clinically important, potentially hazardous interactions with: benazepril, captopril, certolizumab, cisplatin, clevidipine, enalapril, fosinopril, irbesartan, lisinopril, olmesartan, quinapril, ramipril

Important contra-indications noted in the prescribing guidelines for: nursing mothers; pediatric patients

Note: Rituximab-Abbs (Truxima) is a biosimilar to Rituximab (Rituxan). Approved 11/28/2018

Rituximab-pvvr (Ruxience) is a biosimilar to Rituximab (Rituxan). Approved 07/23/2019

Rituximab-arrx (Riabni) is a biosimilar to Rituximab (Rituxan). Approved 12/17/2020.

Warning: FATAL INFUSION REACTIONS, SEVERE MUCOCUTANEOUS REACTIONS, HEPATITIS B VIRUS REACTIVATION and PROGRESSIVE MULTIFOCAL LEUKOENCEPHALOPATHY

Skin

- Anaphylactoid reactions / anaphylaxis (includes anaphylactic shock) [8]
- Angioedema (formerly named angioneurotic edema) (11%) [4]
- Cutaneous toxicity / skin toxicity [3]
- Dermatitis [2]
- Diaphoresis (15%) [2]
- Erythema [2]
- Flushing / rubefaction (5%)
- Herpes simplex [2]
- Herpes zoster [7]
- Hypersensitivity [6]
- Kaposi's sarcoma [3]
- Palmoplantar pustulosis [4]
- Paraneoplastic pemphigus [2]
- Peripheral edema (8%)
- Pruritus (itching) (14%) [8]
- Psoriasis [4]
- Pyoderma gangrenosum [6]
- Rash (15%) [13]
- Sarcoidosis / sarcoid-like reaction (cutaneous sarcoidosis) [3]
- Serum sickness [28]
- Serum sickness-like reaction [6]
- Stevens-Johnson syndrome and toxic epidermal necrolysis (SJS/TEN) [6]
- Urticaria / hives (8%) [5]
- Vasculitis (angiitis) / cutaneous vasculitis (angiitis) [5]

Mucosal
Mucocutaneous reactions [2]
Stomatitis (oral mucositis) [2]

Cardiovascular
Atrial fibrillation [2]
Capillary leak syndrome [3]
Cardiotoxicity [5]
Hypertension (6%) [3]
Hypotension (10%) [10]
Myocardial infarction [2]
Ventricular tachycardia [3]

Central Nervous System
Anxiety (5%)
Chills (33%) [15]
Encephalitis [3]
Encephalopathy (includes hepatic encephalopathy) [2]
Fever (pyrexia) (includes hyperpyrexia) (53%) [23]
Headache (19%) [4]
Leukoencephalopathy / posterior reversible encephalopathy syndrome (PRES) [27]
Neurotoxicity [4]
Pain (12%)
Peripheral neuropathy [6]
Rigors [4]
Vertigo / dizziness (10%)

Endocrine/Metabolic
ALT increased [3]
AST increased [3]
Hyperglycemia (includes glucose increased) (9%)
Hypokalemia [2]
Hyponatremia [2]

Gastrointestinal/Hepatic
Abdominal pain (14%)
Colitis [5]
Constipation [2]
Diarrhea (10%) [11]
Hepatitis [4]
Hepatotoxicity / liver injury / acute liver injury / drug-induced liver injury (DILI) [7]
Nausea (23%) [14]
Pancreatitis / acute pancreatitis [3]
Vomiting (10%) [8]

Genitourinary
Urinary tract infection [9]

Hematologic
Anemia (8%) [15]
Cytopenia [4]
Febrile neutropenia [18]
Hemotoxicity [3]
Hypogammaglobulinemia [11]
Leukocytopenia (leukopenia) / leukocytes (white blood cells) decreased (14%) [15]
Lymphopenia (lymphocytopenia) / lymphocytes decreased (48%) [14]
Myelosuppression / bone marrow suppression / myelotoxicity [7]
Neutropenia (neutrophils decreased) (14%) [62]
Sepsis [4]
Thrombocytopenia / platelets decreased (12%) [45]
Thrombosis [2]

Local
Application-site reactions [4]
Infusion-related reactions [39]
Infusion-site reactions [13]
Injection-site pain [2]
Injection-site reaction [5]

Neuromuscular/Skeletal
Arthralgia (10%) [3]
Asthenia / fatigue (26%) [18]
Back pain (10%)
Myalgia/Myopathy (10%) [2]

Ocular
Macular edema [6]

Renal
Nephrotoxicity / kidney injury / acute kidney injury (AKI) / drug-induced kidney injury [3]
Tumor lysis syndrome (TLS) [4]

Respiratory
Acute respiratory distress syndrome [3]
Bronchospasm (8%) [6]
Cough (increased) (13%) [6]
Dyspnea / shortness of breath (7%) [7]
Influenza- ('flu)-like syndrome [3]
Interstitial lung disease / interstitial pneumonitis / interstitial pneumonia (cryptogenic organizing pneumonia) / drug-induced interstitial lung disease [4]
Lung injury [2]
Nasopharyngitis [3]
Pneumonia [24]
Pneumonitis [2]
Pulmonary toxicity [16]
Rhinitis / rhinosinusitis (see also sinusitis) (12%) [2]
Sinusitis (see also rhinitis / rhinosinusitis) (6%) [5]
Upper respiratory tract infection [10]

Other
Adverse effects / adverse reactions [38]
Allergic reactions [4]
Death [34]
Infection (31%) [65]

RIVAROXABAN

Trade name: Xarelto (Janssen)
Indications: Prevention of venous thromboembolism in patients undergoing knee or hip replacement surgery, treatment of deep vein thrombosis and pulmonary embolism
Class: Anticoagulant (antithrombotic), Direct factor Xa inhibitor
Half-life: 5–9 hours
Clinically important, potentially hazardous interactions with: anticoagulants, aspirin, atazanavir, atorvastatin, carbamazepine, clarithromycin, clopidogrel, combined P-glycoprotein and strong CYP3A4 inhibitors and inducers, conivaptan, dabigatran, darunavir, delavirdine, diclofenac, efavirenz, enoxaparin, erythromycin, fosamprenavir, HIV protease inhibitors, indinavir, itraconazole, ketoconazole, ketorolac, lapatinib, lopinavir, nelfinavir, phenobarbital, phenytoin, posaconazole, rifampin, ritonavir, saquinavir, St John's wort, telithromycin, tipranavir, voriconazole
Important contra-indications noted in the prescribing guidelines for: nursing mothers; pediatric patients
Note: Contra-indicated in patients with active pathological bleeding.
Warning: PREMATURE DISCONTINUATION OF XARELTO INCREASES THE RISK OF THROMBOTIC EVENTS and SPINAL/ EPIDURAL HEMATOMA

Skin
Anaphylactoid reactions / anaphylaxis (includes anaphylactic shock) [2]
Angioedema (formerly named angioneurotic edema) [2]
Hematoma / cutaneous hematoma [3]
Hypersensitivity [4]
Leukocytoclastic vasculitis (angiitis) [2]
Pruritus (itching) (2%)
Rash [3]

Mucosal
Epistaxis (nosebleed) [7]
Gingival bleeding [2]

Cardiovascular
Cardiac tamponade / pericardial tamponade [3]
Congestive heart failure [2]
Hypertension [2]
Myocardial infarction [2]

Central Nervous System
Stroke / cerebrovascular accident [2]

Gastrointestinal/Hepatic
Abdominal pain [2]
Black stools / melena [2]
Diarrhea [2]
Gastrointestinal bleeding [3]
Hepatotoxicity / liver injury / acute liver injury / drug-induced liver injury (DILI) [6]

Genitourinary
Hematuria [5]

Hematologic
Anemia (3%)
Bleeding [15]
Hemorrhage [5]

Neuromuscular/Skeletal
Spinal epidural hematoma [5]

Renal
Nephritis / interstitial nephritis / tubulointerstitial nephritis [2]

Other
Adverse effects / adverse reactions [4]

RIVASTIGMINE

Trade name: Exelon (Novartis)
Indications: Alzheimer's disease and dementia
Class: Acetylcholinesterase inhibitor, Cholinesterase inhibitor, Neuroprotectant
Half-life: 1–2 hours
Clinically important, potentially hazardous interactions with: galantamine
Important contra-indications noted in the prescribing guidelines for: nursing mothers; pediatric patients

---

Skin
Dermatitis [2]
Diaphoresis (10%)
Exanthems [2]
Hyperhidrosis (4%)
Peripheral edema (>2%)
Rash (>2%) [2]

Cardiovascular
Bradycardia / sinus bradycardia [5]
Chest pain (>2%)
Hypertension (3%) [2]
QT interval prolonged / QT prolongation [2]
Thrombophlebitis (<2%)

Central Nervous System
Aggression (includes anger) (3%)
Agitation (>2%)
Anorexia (6–17%) [4]
Anxiety (4–5%)
Confusion (8%) [2]

Delusions of parasitosis (>2%)
Depression (6%)
Hallucinations (4%)
Headache (4–17%) [3]
Insomnia (3–9%)
Nervousness (>2%)
Pain (>2%)
Parkinsonism (2%)
Restlessness [2]
Somnolence (drowsiness) (3–5%)
Syncope / fainting (3%) [4]
Tremor (4–10%) [3]
Vertigo / dizziness (6–21%) [6]

Endocrine/Metabolic
Dehydration (2%)
Weight loss (3%) [3]

Gastrointestinal/Hepatic
Abdominal pain (4–13%) [2]
Constipation (5%) [2]
Diarrhea (7–19%) [8]
Dyspepsia / functional dyspepsia (indigestion) (see also gastroparesis) (9%)
Eructation (belching) (2%)
Flatulence (4%)
Nausea (29–47%) [15]
Vomiting (17–31%) [15]

Genitourinary
Enuresis (urinary incontinence) (>2%)
Urinary tract infection (7%)

Local
Application-site erythema [2]
Application-site pruritus [3]
Application-site reactions [3]

Neuromuscular/Skeletal
Arthralgia (>2%)
Asthenia / fatigue (2–9%)
Back pain (>2%)
Dystonia [2]
Fractures (>2%)
Myalgia/Myopathy (20%)
Pisa syndrome (pleurothotonus) [3]

Respiratory
Bronchitis (>2%)
Cough (>2%)
Influenza- ('flu)-like syndrome (3%)
Pharyngitis (sore throat) (>2%)
Rhinitis / rhinosinusitis (see also sinusitis) (4%)

Other
Adverse effects / adverse reactions [6]
Death [2]
Infection (>2%)

RIZATRIPTAN

Trade name: Maxalt (Merck)
Indications: Migraine
Class: 5-HT1 agonist, Serotonin receptor agonist, Triptan
Half-life: 2–3 hours
Clinically important, potentially hazardous interactions with: dihydroergotamine, ergot-containing drugs, isocarboxazid, MAO inhibitors, methysergide, naratriptan, phenelzine, propranolol, sibutramine, SSRIs, St John's wort, sumatriptan, tranylcypromine, zolmitriptan
Important contra-indications noted in the prescribing guidelines for: nursing mothers

---

Mucosal
Xerostomia (dry mouth) (3%)

Cardiovascular
Chest pain (<3%) [2]

Central Nervous System
Headache (<2%)
Neurotoxicity [2]
Pain (3%)
Paresthesias (3–4%)
Somnolence (drowsiness) (4–6%)
Vertigo / dizziness (4–9%) [10]

Gastrointestinal/Hepatic
Nausea (4–6%)

Neuromuscular/Skeletal
Asthenia / fatigue (4–7%) [9]
Jaw pain (<2%)
Neck pain (<2%)

Other
Adverse effects / adverse reactions [4]

ROCURONIUM

Trade name: Zemuron (Organon)
Indications: Adjunct to general anesthesia
Class: Non-depolarizing neuromuscular blocker
Half-life: 1–2 minutes
Clinically important, potentially hazardous interactions with: aminoglycosides, bacitracin, cisatracurium, cisatracurium, clindamycin, gentamicin, kanamycin, lithium, neomycin, neomycin, procainamide, quinidine, streptomycin, streptomycin, tetracycline, tobramycin, tobramycin, vancomycin

---

Skin
Anaphylactoid reactions / anaphylaxis (includes anaphylactic shock) [46]

Local
Injection-site pain [15]

ROFECOXIB

Trade name: Vioxx (Merck)
Indications: Osteoarthritis, acute pain
Class: COX-2 inhibitor, Non-steroidal anti-inflammatory (NSAID)
Half-life: 17 hours
Clinically important, potentially hazardous interactions with: anisindione, anticoagulants, dicumarol, lithium, methotrexate, tizanidine, warfarin
Note: NSAIDs may cause an increased risk of serious cardiovascular and gastrointestinal adverse events, which can be fatal. This risk may increase with duration of use.
This drug has been withdrawn.
Warning: CARDIOVASCULAR AND GASTROINTESTINAL RISKS

Skin
Abrasion (<2%)
Angioedema (formerly named angioneurotic edema) [5]
Atopic dermatitis (<2%)
Basal cell carcinoma (<2%)
Bullous dermatosis (<2%)
Cellulitis and pseudocellulitis (<2%)
Dermatitis (<2%)
Diaphoresis (<2%)
Edema / fluid retention (4%) [3]
Erythema (<2%)
Fixed eruption / fixed drug eruption [2]
Flushing / rubefaction (<2%)
Fungal dermatitis (<2%)
Herpes simplex (<2%)
Herpes zoster (<2%)
Peripheral edema (6%) [3]
Pruritus (itching) (<2%)
Psoriasis [2]
Rash (<2%)
Stevens-Johnson syndrome and toxic epidermal necrolysis (SJS/TEN) [5]
Urticaria / hives (<2%) [3]
Vasculitis (angiitis) / cutaneous vasculitis (angiitis) [2]
Xerosis / xeroderma (<2%)

Hair
Alopecia / hair loss (<2%)

Nails
Nail changes (<2%)

Mucosal
Aphthous stomatitis / aphthous ulcer / aphtha (aphthae) (<2%)
Oral ulceration (<2%)
Xerostomia (dry mouth) (<2%)

Cardiovascular
Cardiotoxicity [3]
Hypertension [4]
Myocardial infarction [12]

Central Nervous System
Hyperesthesia (<2%)
Paresthesias (<2%)
Vertigo / dizziness (2%) [2]

Gastrointestinal/Hepatic
Abdominal pain [2]
Dyspepsia / functional dyspepsia (indigestion) (see also gastroparesis) [2]
Gastrointestinal bleeding [3]
Nausea [3]

Hematologic
Thrombosis [2]

Neuromuscular/Skeletal
Myalgia/Myopathy (<2%)
Tendinopathy/Tendon rupture (<2%)

Renal
Nephrotoxicity / kidney injury / acute kidney injury (AKI) / drug-induced kidney injury [4]

Respiratory
Influenza- ('flu)-like syndrome (3%)

Other
Allergic reactions (<2%)
Death [3]

ROFLUMILAST

Trade names: Daliresp (Takeda), Daxas (Takeda)
Indications: To reduce the risk of COPD exacerbations in patients with severe COPD associated with chronic bronchitis and a history of exacerbations
Class: Anti-inflammatory, Phosphodiesterase inhibitor, Phosphodiesterase type 4 (PDE4) inhibitor
Half-life: 17 hours
Clinically important, potentially hazardous interactions with: aminophylline, carbamazepine, cimetidine, denileukin, efavirenz, enoxacin, erythromycin, fingolimod, fluvoxamine, ketoconazole, oral contraceptives, pazopanib, phenobarbital, phenytoin, pralatrexate, rifampin

Important contra-indications noted in the prescribing guidelines for: nursing mothers; pediatric patients
Note: Contra-indicated in patients with moderate to severe liver impairment (Child-Pugh B or C class).

Cardiovascular
Cardiotoxicity [2]
Hypertension [3]
Central Nervous System
Anorexia [3]
Anxiety (<2%) [2]
Depression (<2%)
Headache (4%) [22]
Insomnia (2%) [7]
Neurotoxicity [3]
Suicidal ideation [2]
Tremor (<2%)
Vertigo / dizziness [4]
Endocrine/Metabolic
Appetite decreased (2%) [7]
Weight loss (8%) [27]
Gastrointestinal/Hepatic
Abdominal pain (<2%) [3]
Diarrhea (10%) [26]
Dyspepsia / functional dyspepsia (indigestion) (see also gastroparesis) (<2%)
Gastritis / pangastritis / gastric irritation (<2%) [2]
Nausea (5%) [26]
Vomiting (<2%) [2]
Genitourinary
Urinary tract infection (<2%)
Neuromuscular/Skeletal
Back pain (3%) [4]
Muscle spasm (<2%)
Respiratory
Bronchitis [3]
COPD [4]
Dyspnea / shortness of breath [3]
Influenza (3%) [3]
Nasopharyngitis [4]
Pneumonia [3]
Rhinitis / rhinosinusitis (see also sinusitis) (<2%)
Sinusitis (see also rhinitis / rhinosinusitis) (<2%)
Upper respiratory tract infection [5]
Other
Adverse effects / adverse reactions [6]

ROLAPITANT

Trade name: Varubi (Tesaro)
Indications: Delayed nausea and vomiting from chemotherapy, in combination with dexamethasone and a 5HT3-receptor antagonist
Class: Antiemetic, Neurokinin 1 receptor antagonist
Half-life: ~7 days
Clinically important, potentially hazardous interactions with: thioridazine
Pregnancy category: A teratogen in animal studies. Drug usage in pregnant women should be conducted only after necessary studies and approvals from regulatory agencies.
Important contra-indications noted in the prescribing guidelines for: nursing mothers; pediatric patients
Note: Based on its teratogenic properties in developed chick embryos, it is recommended that rolapitant should be taken only when a valid diagnosis has been established and only at the recommended dose, not at a larger dose or for an extended period of time. Drug usage in pregnant women should be conducted after necessary studies and approvals from regulatory agencies. (Cureus, 2022 Aug 17;14(8):e28097, doi: 10.7759/cureus.28097).

Mucosal
Stomatitis (oral mucositis) (4%)
Central Nervous System
Headache [6]
Vertigo / dizziness (6%) [2]
Endocrine/Metabolic
Appetite decreased (9%)
Gastrointestinal/Hepatic
Abdominal pain (3%)
Constipation [6]
Dyspepsia / functional dyspepsia (indigestion) (see also gastroparesis) (4%) [3]
Genitourinary
Urinary tract infection (4%)
Hematologic
Anemia (3%)
Neutropenia (neutrophils decreased) (7–9%) [2]
Neuromuscular/Skeletal
Asthenia / fatigue [5]
Other
Hiccups / singultus (5%) [3]

ROMIDEPSIN

Trade name: Istodax (Celgene)
Indications: Cutaneous T-cell lymphoma (CTCL)
Class: Histone deacetylase (HDAC) inhibitor
Half-life: 3 hours
Clinically important, potentially hazardous interactions with: atazanavir, carbamazepine, clarithromycin, conivaptan, coumadin derivatives, CYP3A4 inhibitors and inducers, darunavir, delavirdine, dexamethasone, efavirenz, indinavir, itraconazole, ketoconazole, nefazodone, nelfinavir, oxcarbazepine, phenobarbital, phenytoin, rifabutin, rifampin, rifapentine, ritonavir, saquinavir, St John's wort, telithromycin, voriconazole, warfarin
Important contra-indications noted in the prescribing guidelines for: nursing mothers; pediatric patients

---

Skin
Dermatitis (4–27%)
Edema / fluid retention (>2%)
Exfoliative dermatitis (4–27%)
Peripheral edema (6–10%)
Pruritus (itching) (7–31%)
Mucosal
Stomatitis (oral mucositis) (6–10%)
Cardiovascular
Hypotension (7–23%)
Supraventricular arrhythmias (>2%)
Tachycardia (10%)
Ventricular arrhythmia (>2%)
Central Nervous System
Anorexia (23–54%) [5]
Chills (11–17%)
Dysgeusia (taste perversion) (15–40%)
Fever (pyrexia) (includes hyperpyrexia) (20–47%)
Headache (15–34%)
Endocrine/Metabolic
ALT increased (3–22%)
AST increased (3–28%)
Hyperglycemia (includes glucose increased) (2–51%)
Hypermagnesemia (27%)
Hyperuricemia (33%)
Hypoalbuminemia / albumin decreased (3–48%)
Hypocalcemia (4–52%)
Hypokalemia (6–20%)
Hypomagnesemia (22–28%)
Hyponatremia (<20%)
Hypophosphatemia (27%)
Weight loss (10–15%)
Gastrointestinal/Hepatic
Abdominal pain (13–14%)
Constipation (12–40%)
Diarrhea (20–36%)
Nausea (56–86%) [9]
Vomiting (34–52%) [5]
Hematologic
Anemia (19–72%) [3]
Leukocytopenia (leukopenia) / leukocytes (white blood cells) decreased (4–55%) [2]
Lymphopenia (lymphocytopenia) / lymphocytes decreased (4–57%) [2]
Neutropenia (neutrophils decreased) (11–66%) [5]
Sepsis (>2%)
Thrombocytopenia / platelets decreased (17–72%) [8]
Neuromuscular/Skeletal
Asthenia / fatigue (53–77%) [10]
Respiratory
Cough (18–21%)
Dyspnea / shortness of breath (13–21%)
Other
Adverse effects / adverse reactions [2]
Infection (46–54%) [2]

ROPINIROLE

Trade name: Requip (GSK)
Indications: Parkinsonism
Class: Dopamine receptor agonist
Half-life: ~6 hours
Clinically important, potentially hazardous interactions with: ciprofloxacin, estradiol, levomepromazine, norfloxacin, risperidone, warfarin, zuclopenthixol
Important contra-indications noted in the prescribing guidelines for: nursing mothers; pediatric patients

---

Skin
Diaphoresis (3–6%)
Flushing / rubefaction (3%)
Herpes simplex (5%)
Hyperhidrosis (3%)
Peripheral edema (2–7%) [2]
Rash [2]
Mucosal
Xerostomia (dry mouth) (5%)
Cardiovascular
Cardiotoxicity [2]
Chest pain (4%)
Hypotension [2]
Orthostatic hypotension [4]
Central Nervous System
Amnesia (3%)

Dyskinesia [9]
Hallucinations (<5%) [7]
Headache (6%) [6]
Hyperesthesia (4%)
Impulse control disorder / impulsivity / drug-induced impulsivity [3]
Insomnia [2]
Pain (3–8%)
Paresthesias (5%)
Psychosis [5]
Sleep-related disorder [2]
Somnolence (drowsiness) (11–40%) [13]
Syncope / fainting (<12%) [3]
Tremor (6%)
Vertigo / dizziness (6–40%) [17]
Yawning (3%)

Gastrointestinal/Hepatic
Abdominal pain (3–7%) [2]
Constipation [2]
Diarrhea (5%)
Dyspepsia / functional dyspepsia (indigestion) (see also gastroparesis) (4–10%) [3]
Nausea (40–60%) [20]
Vomiting (11%) [5]

Genitourinary
Impotence (3%)
Urinary tract infection (5%)

Neuromuscular/Skeletal
Arthralgia (4%)
Asthenia / fatigue (8–11%) [4]
Back pain [2]
Myalgia/Myopathy (3%)

Ocular
Abnormal vision (6%)
Xerophthalmia (dry eyes) (2%)

Respiratory
Cough (3%)
Dyspnea / shortness of breath (3%)
Influenza- ('flu)-like syndrome (3%)
Pharyngitis (sore throat) (6–9%)
Rhinitis / rhinosinusitis (see also sinusitis) (4%)
Sinusitis (see also rhinitis / rhinosinusitis) (4%)

Other
Adverse effects / adverse reactions [5]
Hiccups / singultus [2]
Infection (viral) (11%)

ROPIVACAINE

Trade name: Naropin (AstraZeneca)
Indications: Surgical anesthesia, acute pain management
Class: Anesthetic; local
Half-life: 1.1–2.5 hours after intravascular administration; 3.2–5.2 hours after epidural administration
Clinically important, potentially hazardous interactions with: adenosine, aminophylline, amiodarone, ciprofloxacin, dronedarone, fluvoxamine, imipramine, ketoconazole
Important contra-indications noted in the prescribing guidelines for: nursing mothers

---

Skin
Pruritus (itching) (5%) [2]

Cardiovascular
Bradycardia / sinus bradycardia (9%)
Cardiac arrest [8]
Hypotension (37%)

Central Nervous System
Fever (pyrexia) (includes hyperpyrexia) (9%)
Headache (5%)
Neurotoxicity [2]
Pain (8%)
Paresthesias (6%)
Seizures [4]
Vertigo / dizziness [2]

Gastrointestinal/Hepatic
Nausea (25%) [3]
Vomiting (12%) [3]

Hematologic
Anemia (6%)

Neuromuscular/Skeletal
Back pain (5%)

ROSEMARY

Family: Lamiaceae; Labiatae
Scientific name: *Rosmarinus officinalis*
Indications: Oral: dyspepsia, flatulence, gout, cough, headache, loss of appetite, high blood pressure. **Topical:** alopecia areata, circulatory disturbances, toothache, eczema, musculoskeletal pain. Culinary spice, fragrance component, insect repellent
Class: Antibacterial, Antifungal / antimycotic, Antimicrobial
Half-life: N/A
Clinically important, potentially hazardous interactions with: none known
Note: Oils from rosemary, thyme, lavender and cedarwood, used to treat alopecia areata, improved hair growth by 44% in 7 months (1998 *Arch Dermatol* 134:1349).

Skin
Dermatitis [5]

Other
Adverse effects / adverse reactions [2]

ROSIGLITAZONE

Trade names: Avandamet (GSK), Avandaryl (GSK), Avandia (GSK)
Indications: Type II diabetes
Class: Antidiabetic, Hypoglycemic (antihyperglycemic) agent, Thiazolidinedione
Half-life: 3–4 hours
Clinically important, potentially hazardous interactions with: CYP2C8 inhibitors and inducers, gemfibrozil, grapefruit juice, letermovir, paclitaxel, rifampin, teriflunomide
Important contra-indications noted in the prescribing guidelines for: nursing mothers
Note: Thiazolidinediones, including rosiglitazone, cause or exacerbate congestive heart failure in some patients.
Contra-indicated in patients with established NYHA Class III or IV heart failure. Avandaryl is rosiglitazone and glimepiride; Avandamet is rosiglitazone and metformin.
Warning: CONGESTIVE HEART FAILURE

Skin
Edema / fluid retention (5%) [12]
Peripheral edema [11]

Cardiovascular
Cardiac failure [13]
Congestive heart failure [2]
Myocardial infarction [9]
Myocardial ischemia [3]

Central Nervous System
Headache (6%)
Stroke / cerebrovascular accident [2]

Endocrine/Metabolic
Weight gain [4]

Gastrointestinal/Hepatic
Hepatotoxicity / liver injury / acute liver injury / drug-induced liver injury (DILI) [9]
Nausea [2]

Genitourinary
Bladder disorder [2]

Hematologic
Anemia [2]

Neuromuscular/Skeletal
Arthralgia (5%)
Back pain (4%)
Fractures [5]

Ocular
Macular edema [8]
Proptosis [2]

Respiratory
Dyspnea / shortness of breath [2]
Nasopharyngitis (6%)
Respiratory tract infection (10%)

Other
Adverse effects / adverse reactions [3]
Death [6]

ROSUVASTATIN

Trade name: Crestor (AstraZeneca)
Indications: Hypercholesterolemia, mixed dyslipidemia
Class: HMG-CoA reductase inhibitor / statin
Half-life: ~19 hours
Clinically important, potentially hazardous interactions with: alcohol, amiodarone, antacids, atazanavir, ciprofibrate, colchicine, conivaptan, coumarins, cyclosporine, daptomycin, darunavir, dronedarone, elbasvir & grazoprevir, eltrombopag, eluxadoline, erythromycin, ethinylestradiol, fenofibrate, fibrates, fosamprenavir, fusidic acid, gemfibrozil, indinavir, ledipasvir & sofosbuvir, letermovir, lopinavir, nelfinavir, niacin, niacinamide, phenindione, progestins, protease inhibitors, ritonavir, safinamide, saquinavir, sofosbuvir/velpatasvir/voxilaprevir, tafamidis meglumine, tipranavir, trabectedin, vitamin K antagonists, warfarin
Important contra-indications noted in the prescribing guidelines for: nursing mothers

---

Skin
Peripheral edema (>2%)
Rash (>2%)

Central Nervous System
Depression (>2%)
Headache (6%)
Insomnia [2]
Pain (>2%)
Paresthesias (>2%)
Vertigo / dizziness (4%) [4]

Endocrine/Metabolic
Creatine phosphokinase (CPK) / creatine kinase increased (hyperCKemia) [2]
Diabetes mellitus [3]

Gastrointestinal/Hepatic
Abdominal pain (>2%)
Constipation (2%)
Hepatitis [2]

Hepatotoxicity / liver injury / acute liver injury / drug-induced liver injury (DILI) [5]
Nausea (3%)
Pancreatitis / acute pancreatitis [2]

Neuromuscular/Skeletal
Arthralgia (>2%)
Asthenia / fatigue (3%) [2]
Back pain (3%)
Myalgia/Myopathy (3%) [20]
Rhabdomyolysis [28]

Renal
Nephrotoxicity / kidney injury / acute kidney injury (AKI) / drug-induced kidney injury [6]
Renal failure [3]

Respiratory
Cough (>2%)
Influenza- ('flu)-like syndrome (2%)
Rhinitis / rhinosinusitis (see also sinusitis) (2%)
Sinusitis (see also rhinitis / rhinosinusitis) (2%)

Other
Adverse effects / adverse reactions [8]

ROTIGOTINE

Trade name: Neupro (Schwarz)
Indications: Parkinsonism, restless legs syndrome
Class: Dopamine receptor agonist
Half-life: 5–7 hours
Clinically important, potentially hazardous interactions with: antipsychotics, levomepromazine, memantine, methyldopa, metoclopramide, risperidone, zuclopenthixol
Important contra-indications noted in the prescribing guidelines for: nursing mothers; pediatric patients
Note: Neupro contains sodium metabisulfite which is capable of causing anaphylactoid reactions in patients with sulfite allergy.

Skin
Diaphoresis (4%)
Erythema (2%)
Peripheral edema (7%) [3]
Rash (2%) [3]

Mucosal
Xerostomia (dry mouth) (3%) [3]

Cardiovascular
Chest pain (>2%)
Hypertension (3%)
Hypotension [2]

Central Nervous System
Abnormal dreams (3%)
Anorexia (3%)
Anxiety (>2%)
Depression (>2%)
Dyskinesia [4]
Gait instability / postural instability [2]
Hallucinations (2%) [3]
Hallucinations, visual (2%) [2]
Headache (14%) [8]
Impulse control disorder / impulsivity / drug-induced impulsivity [4]
Insomnia (10%) [3]
Somnolence (drowsiness) (25%) [16]
Tremor (>2%) [2]
Vertigo / dizziness (3–18%) [7]

Gastrointestinal/Hepatic
Abdominal pain (>2%)
Constipation (5%)
Diarrhea (>2%)
Dyspepsia / functional dyspepsia (indigestion) (see also gastroparesis) (4%)
Gastrointestinal disorder / discomfort [2]
Nausea (38%) [24]
Vomiting (13%) [6]

Genitourinary
Urinary frequency (>2%)
Urinary tract infection (3%)

Local
Application-site erythema [4]
Application-site pruritus [4]
Application-site reactions (37%) [31]

Neuromuscular/Skeletal
Arthralgia (4%)
Asthenia / fatigue (8%) [10]
Back pain (6%)
Myalgia/Myopathy (2%)

Ocular
Abnormal vision (3%)
Visual disturbances (3%)

Respiratory
Cough (>2%)
Influenza- ('flu)-like syndrome (>2%)
Rhinitis / rhinosinusitis (see also sinusitis) (>2%)
Sinusitis (see also rhinitis / rhinosinusitis) (3%)
Upper respiratory tract infection (>2%)

Other
Adverse effects / adverse reactions [6]

ROXATIDINE

Trade name: Roxit (Noristan)
Indications: Gastric and duodenal ulcers
Class: Histamine H2 receptor antagonist
Half-life: 5–6 hours
Clinically important, potentially hazardous interactions with: none known
Important contra-indications noted in the prescribing guidelines for: nursing mothers; pediatric patients

---

Skin
Lichenoid eruption / lichenoid reaction [2]
Rash [2]

Central Nervous System
Headache (27%)
Vertigo / dizziness (27%)

ROXITHROMYCIN

Trade names: Biaxsig (Aventis), Romicin (Pacific), Rulid (Roussel-Uclaf)
Indications: Respiratory tract, urinary and soft tissue infections
Class: Antibiotic, Antibiotic; macrolide, Antimicrobial
Half-life: 8–15 hours
Clinically important, potentially hazardous interactions with: aminophylline, digoxin, disopyramide, ergot alkaloids, gemfibrozil, midazolam, simvastatin, terfenadine, warfarin

---

Skin
Rash [2]
Urticaria / hives [2]

Cardiovascular
QT interval prolonged / QT prolongation [2]

Gastrointestinal/Hepatic
Abdominal pain [2]
Hepatotoxicity / liver injury / acute liver injury / drug-induced liver injury (DILI) [2]

Other
Adverse effects / adverse reactions [7]

RUE

Family: Rutaceae
Scientific names: *Ruta chalepensis, Ruta corsica, Ruta graveolens, Ruta montana*
Indications: Hysteria, coughs, croup, colic, flatulence, mild stomachic, insomnia, abdominal cramps, nervous headache, giddiness, hysteria, palpitation, abortifacient, cysticide, vermifuge, insecticide. **Topical:** irritant, rubefacient for eczemas, psoriasis and rheumatic pain, sciatica, headache, chronic bronchitis. Flavoring in alcoholic beverages, salads, meats and cheeses
Class: Antispasmodic
Half-life: N/A
Clinically important, potentially hazardous interactions with: none known

---

Skin
Bullous dermatosis [2]
Erythema [2]
Photosensitivity [11]
Vesiculation [2]

RUFINAMIDE

Trade names: Banzel (Eisai), Inovelon (Eisai)
Indications: Epilepsy, Lennox-Gastaut syndrome
Class: Anticonvulsant (see also antiepileptic (anti-seizure)), Antiepileptic (anti-seizure)
Half-life: 6–10 hours
Clinically important, potentially hazardous interactions with: carbamazepine, lamotrigine, phenobarbital, primidone, topiramate, valproic acid, vigabatrin
Important contra-indications noted in the prescribing guidelines for: the elderly; nursing mothers
Note: Contra-indicated in patients with familial short QT syndrome.

Skin
Acneiform eruption / acneiform dermatitis / acneiform rash (<10%)
Pruritus (itching) (3%)
Rash (4%)

Mucosal
Epistaxis (nosebleed) (<10%)

Cardiovascular
QT interval shortening [2]

Central Nervous System
Aggression (includes anger) (3%)
Anxiety (3%)
Fever (pyrexia) (includes hyperpyrexia) [2]
Gait instability / postural instability (3%)
Headache (16–27%) [8]
Impaired concentration (3%)
Irritability [2]
Seizures (aggravation) [2]
Somnolence (drowsiness) (11–17%) [19]
Status epilepticus (<10%)
Tremor (6%)
Vertigo / dizziness (3–19%) [10]

Endocrine/Metabolic
Appetite decreased (5%) [7]
Oligomenorrhea (<10%)
Weight loss [2]

Gastrointestinal/Hepatic
Abdominal pain (3%)
Constipation (3%)
Dyspepsia / functional dyspepsia (indigestion) (see also gastroparesis) (3%)
Nausea (7–12%) [8]
Vomiting (5–17%) [16]

Neuromuscular/Skeletal
Asthenia / fatigue (9–16%) [15]
Ataxia (4%) [2]
Back pain (3%)
Psychomotor hyperactivity (<10%)

Ocular
Diplopia (double vision) (4–9%) [6]
Nystagmus (6%)
Vision blurred (5%)

Otic
Ear infection (3%)

Respiratory
Bronchitis (3%)
Influenza (5%)
Nasopharyngitis (5%)
Pneumonia (<10%)
Rhinitis / rhinosinusitis (see also sinusitis) (<10%)
Sinusitis (see also rhinitis / rhinosinusitis) (3%)

Other
Adverse effects / adverse reactions [8]

RUPATADINE

Trade name: Rupafin (GSK)
Indications: Allergic rhinitis and chronic idiopathic urticaria
Class: Histamine H1 receptor antagonist
Half-life: 5.9 hours
Clinically important, potentially hazardous interactions with: alcohol, CNS depressants, erythromycin, grapefruit juice, ketoconazole, statins

---

Mucosal
Xerostomia (dry mouth) (<10%)

Cardiovascular
Torsades de pointes [2]

Central Nervous System
Headache (<10%) [4]
Somnolence (drowsiness) (<10%) [9]
Vertigo / dizziness (<10%)

Gastrointestinal/Hepatic
Diarrhea [2]

Neuromuscular/Skeletal
Asthenia / fatigue (<10%)

RUXOLITINIB

Trade name: Jakafi (Incyte)
Indications: Intermediate or high-risk myelofibrosis, polycythemia vera
Class: Janus kinase (JAK) inhibitor
Half-life: 3 hours
Clinically important, potentially hazardous interactions with: boceprevir, clarithromycin, conivaptan, fluconazole, grapefruit juice, indinavir, itraconazole, ketoconazole, lopinavir, mibefradil, nefazodone, nelfinavir, posaconazole, ritonavir, ritonavir, saquinavir, strong CYP3A4 inhibitors, telaprevir, telithromycin, voriconazole
Important contra-indications noted in the prescribing guidelines for: nursing mothers; pediatric patients
Warning: WARNING: SERIOUS INFECTIONS, MORTALITY, MALIGNANCY, MAJOR ADVERSE CARDIOVASCULAR EVENTS (MACE), AND THROMBOSIS SEE FULL PRESCRIBING INFORMATION FOR COMPLETE BOXED WARNING.
SERIOUS INFECTIONS LEADING TO HOSPITALIZATION OR DEATH, INCLUDING TUBERCULOSIS AND BACTERIAL, INVASIVE FUNGAL, VIRAL, AND OTHER OPPORTUNISTIC INFECTIONS, HAVE OCCURRED IN PATIENTS RECEIVING JANUS KINASE INHIBITORS FOR INFLAMMATORY CONDITIONS.
HIGHER RATE OF ALL-CAUSE MORTALITY, INCLUDING SUDDEN CARDIOVASCULAR DEATH HAVE BEEN OBSERVED IN PATIENTS TREATED WITH JANUS KINASE INHIBITORS FOR INFLAMMATORY CONDITIONS.
LYMPHOMA AND OTHER MALIGNANCIES HAVE BEEN OBSERVED IN PATIENTS TREATED WITH JANUS KINASE INHIBITORS FOR INFLAMMATORY CONDITIONS.
HIGHER RATE OF MACE (INCLUDING CARDIOVASCULAR DEATH, MYOCARDIAL INFARCTION, AND STROKE) HAS BEEN OBSERVED IN PATIENTS TREATED WITH JANUS KINASE INHIBITORS FOR INFLAMMATORY CONDITIONS.
THROMBOSIS, INCLUDING DEEP VENOUS THROMBOSIS, PULMONARY EMBOLISM, AND ARTERIAL THROMBOSIS, SOME FATAL, HAVE OCCURRED IN PATIENTS TREATED WITH JANUS KINASE INHIBITORS FOR INFLAMMATORY CONDITIONS.

Skin
Bruise / bruising / contusion / ecchymosis (ecchymoses) (23%)
Hematoma / cutaneous hematoma (23%)
Herpes zoster (2%)
Petechiae (23%)
Purpura (23%)

Cardiovascular
Hypertension [2]

Central Nervous System
Balance disorder (18%)
Headache [3]
Vertigo / dizziness (18%) [2]

Endocrine/Metabolic
ALT increased (25%)
AST increased (17%)
Weight gain (7%)

Gastrointestinal/Hepatic
Diarrhea [4]
Hepatitis (reactivation) [2]

Genitourinary
Cystitis (includes interstitial cystitis / bladder pain syndrome) (9%)
Pyuria (9%)
Urinary tract infection (9%)
Urosepsis (9%)

Hematologic
Anemia (96%) [22]
Cytopenia [2]
Hemotoxicity [2]
Neutropenia (neutrophils decreased) (19%) [3]
Thrombocytopenia / platelets decreased (70%) [27]

Local
Injection-site hematoma (23%)

Neuromuscular/Skeletal
Asthenia / fatigue [3]

Ocular
Periorbital hematoma (23%)

Other
Adverse effects / adverse reactions [6]
Death [2]
Infection [8]

SACUBITRIL/VALSARTAN

Trade name: Entresto (Novartis)
Indications: To reduce risk of cardiovascular death and hospitalization for heart failure in chronic heart failure
Class: Angiotensin receptor neprilysin inhibitor (ARNI)
Half-life: <12 hours
Clinically important, potentially hazardous interactions with: ACE inhibitors, aliskiren, lithium, NSAIDs, potassium-sparing diuretics
Pregnancy category: Can cause fetal harm
Important contra-indications noted in the prescribing guidelines for: nursing mothers; pediatric patients
Note: Contra-indicated in patients with a history of angioedema related to previous therapy with angiotensin-converting enzyme inhibitor or angiotensin II receptor blocker. See also separate profile for valsartan.
Warning: FETAL TOXICITY

Skin
Angioedema (formerly named angioneurotic edema) (<2%) [2]
Peripheral edema [2]

Cardiovascular
Hypotension (18%) [8]
Orthostatic hypotension (2%)

Central Nervous System
Gait instability / postural instability (2%)
Vertigo / dizziness (6%) [2]

Endocrine/Metabolic
Hyperkalemia (12%) [6]
Hyponatremia [2]
Serum creatinine increased [2]

Gastrointestinal/Hepatic
Constipation [2]

Neuromuscular/Skeletal
Arthralgia [2]
Rhabdomyolysis [3]

Renal
Nephrotoxicity / kidney injury / acute kidney injury (AKI) / drug-induced kidney injury [3]
Renal failure (5%)
Renal function abnormal / renal dysfunction [2]

Respiratory
Cough (9%) [4]
Nasopharyngitis [2]

Other
Adverse effects / adverse reactions [3]

SAFINAMIDE

Trade name: Xadago (Newron)
Indications: Adjunctive treatment to levodopa/carbidopa in patients with Parkinson's disease experiencing 'off' episodes
Class: Monoamine oxidase B inhibitor
Half-life: 20–26 hours
Clinically important, potentially hazardous interactions with: cyclobenzaprine, dextromethorphan, dopaminergic antagonists, imatinib, irinotecan, isoniazid, lapatinib, linezolid, meperidine, methadone, methylphenidate, metoclopramide, mitoxantrone, other MAO inhibitors, propoxyphene, rosuvastatin, serotonergic drugs, St John's wort, sulfasalazine, sympathomimetics, topotecan, tramadol, tricyclic or tetracyclic antidepressants, viloxazine
Important contra-indications noted in the prescribing guidelines for: nursing mothers; pediatric patients

---

Skin
Peripheral edema [2]
Cardiovascular
Hypertension [4]
Orthostatic hypotension (2%)
Central Nervous System
Anxiety (2%)
Dyskinesia (17–21%) [8]
Fever (pyrexia) (includes hyperpyrexia) [3]
Gait instability / postural instability (4–6%) [2]
Headache [3]
Insomnia (<4%) [2]
Parkinsonism (exacerbation) [2]
Tremor [2]
Vertigo / dizziness [2]
Endocrine/Metabolic
ALT increased (3–7%)
AST increased (6–7%)
Weight loss [2]
Gastrointestinal/Hepatic
Abdominal pain [2]
Constipation [2]
Dyspepsia / functional dyspepsia (indigestion) (see also gastroparesis) (<2%)
Nausea (3–6%) [3]
Vomiting [2]
Neuromuscular/Skeletal
Asthenia / fatigue [2]
Back pain [3]
Ocular
Cataract [3]
Vision blurred [2]
Respiratory
Cough (2%) [2]
Nasopharyngitis [3]

SALMETEROL

Trade names: Advair (GSK), Serevent (GSK)
Indications: Asthma
Class: Beta-2 adrenergic agonist, Bronchodilator
Half-life: 3–4 hours
Clinically important, potentially hazardous interactions with: alpha blockers, aprepitant, atazanavir, beta blockers, betahistine, boceprevir, cobicistat/elvitegravir/emtricitabine/tenofovir alafenamide, cobicistat/elvitegravir/emtricitabine/tenofovir disoproxil, conivaptan, CYP3A4 inhibitors, darunavir, delavirdine, efavirenz, indinavir, iobenguane, lapatinib, loop diuretics, lopinavir, ombitasvir/paritaprevir/ritonavir, sympathomimetics, telaprevir, telithromycin, tipranavir, tricyclic antidepressants, voriconazole
Important contra-indications noted in the prescribing guidelines for: nursing mothers
Note: Advair is salmeterol and fluticasone.
Warning: ASTHMA-RELATED DEATH

Skin
Rash (<3%) [2]
Urticaria / hives (<3%)
Mucosal
Nasal congestion (4–9%)
Oropharyngeal pain [2]
Xerostomia (dry mouth) (<3%)
Cardiovascular
Hypertension (4%)
Central Nervous System
Fever (pyrexia) (includes hyperpyrexia) [2]
Headache (13–16%) [6]
Pain (<12%)
Tremor (<10%) [2]
Vertigo / dizziness (4%)
Gastrointestinal/Hepatic
Throat irritation/pain (7%)
Genitourinary
Urinary tract infection [2]
Neuromuscular/Skeletal
Back pain [4]
Myalgia/Myopathy (<3%)
Respiratory
Asthma [3]
COPD (exacerbation) [3]
Cough (5%) [3]
Influenza- ('flu)-like syndrome (5%)
Nasopharyngitis [5]
Pharyngitis (sore throat) (6%)
Pneumonia [5]
Rhinitis / rhinosinusitis (see also sinusitis) (4%)
Sinusitis (see also rhinitis / rhinosinusitis) (4–5%)
Upper respiratory tract infection (5%) [4]
Other
Adverse effects / adverse reactions [3]
Death [8]
Infection (2–12%)

SALSALATE

Trade name: Mono-Gesic (Schwarz)
Indications: Arthritis
Class: Non-steroidal anti-inflammatory (NSAID), Salicylate
Half-life: 7–8 hours
Clinically important, potentially hazardous interactions with: dichlorphenamide, methotrexate
Important contra-indications noted in the prescribing guidelines for: nursing mothers; pediatric patients
Note: NSAIDs may cause an increased risk of serious cardiovascular and gastrointestinal adverse events, which can be fatal. This risk may increase with duration of use.

Skin
Anaphylactoid reactions / anaphylaxis (includes anaphylactic shock) (<10%)
Rash (<10%)

SAPROPTERIN

Trade name: Kuvan (BioMarin)
Indications: Phenylketonuria
Class: Enzyme
Half-life: 6.7 hours
Clinically important, potentially hazardous interactions with: levodopa, methotrexate, pralatrexate, sildenafil, tadalafil, vardenafil
Important contra-indications noted in the prescribing guidelines for: the elderly; nursing mothers; pediatric patients

---

Skin
Rash (5%)
Mucosal
Nasal congestion (4%)
Rhinorrhea (11%)
Central Nervous System
Confusion (5%)
Headache (15%)
Gastrointestinal/Hepatic
Abdominal pain (5%)
Diarrhea (8%)
Vomiting (8%)
Respiratory
Cough (7%)
Pharyngolaryngeal pain (10%)
Upper respiratory tract infection (12%)
Other
Adverse effects / adverse reactions [2]

SAQUINAVIR

Trade name: Invirase (Roche)
Indications: Advanced HIV infection
Class: Antiretroviral, CYP3A4 inhibitor, HIV-1 protease inhibitor
Half-life: 12 hours
Clinically important, potentially hazardous interactions with: abiraterone, afatinib, alprazolam, amitriptyline, amprenavir, astemizole, atazanavir, atorvastatin, avanafil, brigatinib, cabazitaxel, cabozantinib, calcifediol, clindamycin, clozapine, copanlisib, crizotinib, darifenacin, darunavir, dasatinib, delavirdine, dihydroergotamine, dronedarone, efavirenz, elbasvir & grazoprevir, eluxadoline, eplerenone, ergot derivatives, erlotinib, everolimus, fentanyl, fesoterodine, flibanserin, fluticasone propionate, itraconazole, ixabepilone, ketoconazole, lapatinib, levomepromazine, lomitapide, lopinavir, maraviroc, methysergide, midazolam, midostaurin, mifepristone, naldemedine, nelfinavir, neratinib, olaparib, omeprazole, paclitaxel, palbociclib, pantoprazole, pazopanib, pentamidine, phenytoin, pimozide, ponatinib, quinine, ribociclib, rifampin, rilpivirine, ritonavir, rivaroxaban, romidepsin, rosuvastatin, ruxolitinib, sildenafil, simeprevir, simvastatin, solifenacin, sonidegib, St John's wort, sunitinib, tadalafil, telithromycin, temsirolimus, ticagrelor, tipranavir, tolvaptan, vardenafil, vemurafenib, viloxazine, vorapaxar, voriconazole

Important contra-indications noted in the prescribing guidelines for: nursing mothers
Note: Protease inhibitors cause dyslipidemia which includes elevated triglycerides and cholesterol and redistribution of body fat centrally to produce the so-called 'protease paunch', breast enlargement, facial atrophy, and 'buffalo hump'.

Skin
Acneiform eruption / acneiform dermatitis / acneiform rash (<2%)
Candidiasis / candidosis (<2%)
Dermatitis (<2%)
Diaphoresis (<2%)
Eczema / eczematous reaction / eczematous eruption (<2%)
Erythema (<2%)
Exanthems (<2%)
Folliculitis (<2%)
Herpes simplex (<2%)
Herpes zoster (<2%)
Photosensitivity (<2%)
Pigmentation (Skin) (includes hyperpigmentation) (<2%)
Seborrheic dermatitis (<2%)
Ulcerations (<2%)
Urticaria / hives (<2%)
Verrucae vulgaris / warts / verrucae (<2%)
Xerosis / xeroderma (<2%)

Hair
Hair changes (<2%)

Mucosal
Cheilitis (inflammation of the lips) (<2%)
Gingivitis (<2%)
Glossitis (inflammation of the tongue) (<2%)
Oral ulceration (2%)
Stomatitis (oral mucositis) (<2%)
Xerostomia (dry mouth) (<2%)

Cardiovascular
QT interval prolonged / QT prolongation [3]

Central Nervous System
Dysesthesia (<2%)
Dysgeusia (taste perversion) (<2%)
Hyperesthesia (<2%)
Paresthesias (3%)

Endocrine/Metabolic
Gynecomastia [2]

Gastrointestinal/Hepatic
Hepatotoxicity / liver injury / acute liver injury / drug-induced liver injury (DILI) [2]
Vertigo / dizziness [2]

Gastrointestinal/Hepatic
Nausea [2]

Respiratory
Nasopharyngitis [2]

SARECYCLINE

Trade name: Seysara (Allergan)
Indications: indicated for the treatment of inflammatory lesions of non-nodular moderate to severe acne vulgaris in patients 9 years of age and older
Class: Antibiotic, Antibiotic; tetracycline
Half-life: 21–22 hours
Clinically important, potentially hazardous interactions with: acitretin, isotretinoin
Pregnancy category: may cause fetal harm
Important contra-indications noted in the prescribing guidelines for: nursing mothers

---

Skin
Photosensitivity [2]

Central Nervous System
Headache [2]

SARILUMAB

Trade name: Kevzara (Sanofi)
Indications: Rheumatoid arthritis
Class: Covid-19 putative drug, Interleukin-6 inhibitor / anti-interleukin 6 receptor monoclonal antibody, Monoclonal antibody
Half-life: 8–10 days (concentration-dependent)
Clinically important, potentially hazardous interactions with: live vaccines
Pregnancy category: Based on animal data, may cause fetal harm
Important contra-indications noted in the prescribing guidelines for: the elderly; nursing mothers; pediatric patients
Warning: RISK OF SERIOUS INFECTIONS

Endocrine/Metabolic
ALT increased (5%) [4]
AST increased (38–43%)
Hypercholesterolemia [2]
Hypertriglyceridemia (includes triglycerides increased) (<3%)

Gastrointestinal/Hepatic
Hepatotoxicity / liver injury / acute liver injury / drug-induced liver injury (DILI) [3]

Genitourinary
Urinary tract infection (3%) [2]

Hematologic
Leukocytopenia (leukopenia) / leukocytes (white blood cells) decreased (<2%)
Neutropenia (neutrophils decreased) (7–10%) [15]

Local
Injection-site erythema (4–5%) [4]
Injection-site pruritus (2%)
Injection-site reaction (6–7%) [2]

Respiratory
Nasopharyngitis (>3%) [3]
Upper respiratory tract infection (3–4%) [3]

Other
Adverse effects / adverse reactions [3]
Infection [9]

SARSAPARILLA

Family: Smilacaceae
Scientific names: *Smilax aristolochiaefolia, Smilax febrifuga, Smilax glabra, Smilax japicanga, Smilax officinalis, Smilax ornata, Smilax regelii, Smilax rotundifolia*
Indications: Blood purifier, general tonic, gout, syphilis, gonorrhea, rheumatism, wounds, arthritis, fever, cough, scrofula, hypertension, digestive disorders, psoriasis, skin diseases, cancer
Class: Anti-inflammatory, Immunomodulator
Half-life: N/A
Clinically important, potentially hazardous interactions with: none known
Note: Sarsaparilla vine should not be confused with sasparilla and sassafras (the root and bark of which were once used to flavor root beer). Sarsaparilla is only used in root beer and other beverages for its foaming properties.

SAW PALMETTO

Family: Arecaceae; Palmae
Scientific names: *Sabal serrulata, Serenoa repens, Serenoa serrulata*
Indications: Benign prostatic hyperplasia, diuretic, sedative, prostate cancer (with other herbs), aphrodisiac, hair growth, colds, coughs, sore throat, asthma, chronic bronchitis, migraine
Class: 5-alpha reductase inhibitor, Anti-inflammatory, Hormone modulator
Half-life: N/A
Clinically important, potentially hazardous interactions with: none known

---

Central Nervous System
Headache [2]

Gastrointestinal/Hepatic
Abdominal pain [3]
Diarrhea [2]
Hepatotoxicity / liver injury / acute liver injury / drug-induced liver injury (DILI) [2]
Nausea [3]
Pancreatitis / acute pancreatitis [2]
Vomiting [2]

Neuromuscular/Skeletal
Asthenia / fatigue [2]

Respiratory
Rhinitis / rhinosinusitis (see also sinusitis) [2]

Other
Adverse effects / adverse reactions [10]

SAXAGLIPTIN

Trade names: Onglyza (Bristol-Myers Squibb), Qtern (AstraZeneca)
Indications: Type II diabetes mellitus
Class: Antidiabetic, Dipeptidyl peptidase-4 (DPP-4) (gliptin) inhibitor
Half-life: 2.5–3.1 hours
Clinically important, potentially hazardous interactions with: ACE inhibitors, alcohol, aprepitant, beta blockers, bexarotene, colchicine, conivaptan, corticosteroids, CYP3A4 inducers, darunavir, dasatinib, delavirdine, diazoxide, diuretics, efavirenz, estradiol, estrogens, hypoglycemic agents, indinavir, ketoconazole, lapatinib, MAO inhibitors, oxcarbazepine, P-glycoprotein inhibitors and inducers, pegvisomant, pioglitazone, rifapentine, somatropin, strong CYP3A4/5 inhibitors, telithromycin, terbinafine, testosterone, voriconazole
Important contra-indications noted in the prescribing guidelines for: nursing mothers; pediatric patients
Note: Qtern is saxagliptin and dapagliflozin.

Skin
Hypersensitivity (<2%)
Peripheral edema (2–3%)

Cardiovascular
Cardiac disorder / cardiac dysfunction [2]
Cardiac failure [3]
Myocardial infarction [2]

Central Nervous System
Headache (7%) [7]
Stroke / cerebrovascular accident [2]

Endocrine/Metabolic
Hypoglycemia [10]

Gastrointestinal/Hepatic
Abdominal pain (2%)
Diarrhea [5]
Gastroenteritis (2%)
Hepatotoxicity / liver injury / acute liver injury / drug-induced liver injury (DILI) [2]
Vomiting (2%)

Genitourinary
Urinary tract infection (7%) [7]

Respiratory
Nasopharyngitis [4]
Sinusitis (see also rhinitis / rhinosinusitis) (3%) [2]
Upper respiratory tract infection (8%) [8]

Other
Adverse effects / adverse reactions [7]
Death [2]
Infection [2]

SCOPOLAMINE

Synonym: hyoscine
Trade names: Kwells (Bayer), Scopoderm-TTS (Novartis), Transderm-Scop Patch (Novartis)
Indications: Nausea and vomiting, excess salivation
Class: Anticholinergic, Antiemetic, Muscarinic antagonist
Half-life: 8 hours
Clinically important, potentially hazardous interactions with: anticholinergics, arbutamine
Note: The UK Medicines and Healthcare products Regulatory Agency: Safety update (July 2023) Hyoscine hydrobromide patches (Scopoderm 1.5mg Patch or Scopoderm TTS Patch): risk of anticholinergic side effects, including hyperthermia There have been a small number of reports of serious and life-threatening anticholinergic side effects associated with hyoscine hydrobromide patches, particularly when used outside the licence. Healthcare professionals, patients, parents and carers should be aware of the signs and symptoms of serious side effects and the need to seek medical help if they occur.
Systemic adverse effects have been reported following ophthalmic administration.

Skin
Anaphylactoid reactions / anaphylaxis (includes anaphylactic shock) [2]
Dermatitis (transdermal patch and ophthalmic) [8]
Erythema multiforme [2]
Photosensitivity (<10%)
Rash [2]
Xerosis / xeroderma (>10%)

Mucosal
Xerostomia (dry mouth) (>60%) [9]

Cardiovascular
Bradycardia / sinus bradycardia [2]

Central Nervous System
Agitation [2]
Amnesia [4]
Hallucinations [5]
Hallucinations, visual [4]
Psychosis [5]

Genitourinary
Urinary retention [2]

Local
Injection-site irritation (>10%)

Ocular
Dilated pupils [3]
Mydriasis [2]
Vision blurred [2]

Other
Death [2]

SEBELIPASE ALFA

Trade name: Kanuma (Alexion)
Indications: Lysosomal acid lipase deficiency
Class: Enzyme replacement
Half-life: 5–7 minutes
Clinically important, potentially hazardous interactions with: none known
Pregnancy category: No available data
Important contra-indications noted in the prescribing guidelines for: nursing mothers

---

Skin
Hypersensitivity (20%)
Urticaria / hives (33%)

Mucosal
Oropharyngeal pain (17%)

Cardiovascular
Chest pain (<8%)
Tachycardia (<30%)

Central Nervous System
Anxiety (<8%)
Fever (pyrexia) (includes hyperpyrexia) (25–56%)
Headache (28%)

Gastrointestinal/Hepatic
Constipation (8%)
Diarrhea (67%)
Nausea (8%)
Vomiting (67%)

Hematologic
Anemia (44%)

Neuromuscular/Skeletal
Asthenia / fatigue (8%)
Hypotonia (<30%)

Respiratory
Cough (33%)
Nasopharyngitis (11–33%)
Rhinitis / rhinosinusitis (see also sinusitis) (56%)

Other
Sneezing (sternutation) (<30%)

SECOBARBITAL

Trade name: Seconal (Ranbaxy)
Indications: Insomnia
Class: Barbiturate
Half-life: 15–40 hours
Clinically important, potentially hazardous interactions with: alcohol, anticoagulants, antihistamines, brompheniramine, buclizine, chlorpheniramine, dicumarol, ethanolamine, imatinib, warfarin

---

Local
Injection-site pain (>10%)

SECRETIN

Trade name: Secretin-Ferring (Ferring)
Indications: Diagnosis of gastrinoma (Zollinger–Ellison syndrome)
Class: Hormone, polypeptide
Half-life: N/A
Clinically important, potentially hazardous interactions with: anticholinergics, fesoterodine, oxybutynin, tiotropium, trospium
Important contra-indications noted in the prescribing guidelines for: nursing mothers; pediatric patients
Note: SecreFlo is porcine-derived; ChiRhoStim is human-derived.

SECUKINUMAB

Trade name: Cosentyx (Novartis)
Indications: Moderate-to-severe plaque psoriasis, psoriatic arthritis, ankylosing spondylitis
Class: Antipsoriatic agent, Biologic, Interleukin-17 (IL-17) antagonist / interleukin-17 inhibitor, Monoclonal antibody
Half-life: 22–31 days
Clinically important, potentially hazardous interactions with: live vaccines
Important contra-indications noted in the prescribing guidelines for: nursing mothers; pediatric patients
Note: Use with caution in patients with inflammatory bowel disease.

Skin
Behçet's disease [5]
Candidiasis / candidosis [9]
Eczema / eczematous reaction / eczematous eruption [2]
Henoch-Schönlein purpura / IgA vasculitis / immunoglobulin A vasculitis [3]
Hidradenitis suppurativa (acne inversa) [3]
Lupus erythematosus (subacute cutaneous lupus erythematosus (SCLE)) [3]
Pompholyx / dyshidrotic eczema [3]
Pruritus (itching) [4]
Psoriasis (exacerbation) [2]
Pyoderma gangrenosum [4]
Vasculitis (angiitis) / cutaneous vasculitis (angiitis) [3]
Vitiligo [4]

Hair
Alopecia areata [4]

Mucosal
Behçet's disease / Behçet's syndrome [4]
Oral candidiasis [2]

Cardiovascular
Cardiac disorder / cardiac dysfunction [2]
Hypertension [3]

Central Nervous System
Headache [15]

Gastrointestinal/Hepatic
Colitis [3]
Crohn's disease [5]
Diarrhea (3–4%) [7]
Inflammatory bowel disease [3]

Hematologic
Neutropenia (neutrophils decreased) [6]

Local
Injection-site reaction [3]

Neuromuscular/Skeletal
Arthralgia [4]

Asthenia / fatigue [2]
Back pain [2]

Respiratory
Nasopharyngitis (11–12%) [23]
Upper respiratory tract infection (3%) [15]

Other
Adverse effects / adverse reactions [10]
Infection (29%) [15]
Malignancies [2]
Neoplasms [2]

SELEGILINE

Synonyms: deprenyl; L-deprenyl
Trade names: Eldepryl (Somerset), Emsam (Mylan Specialty), Zelapar (Valeant)
Indications: Parkinsonism
Class: Antidepressant, Monoamine oxidase B inhibitor, Neuroprotectant
Half-life: 9 minutes
Clinically important, potentially hazardous interactions with: amitriptyline, carbidopa, citalopram, doxepin, ephedra, ephedrine, escitalopram, fluoxetine, fluvoxamine, levodopa, meperidine, methadone, moclobemide, naratriptan, nefazodone, oral contraceptives, oxcarbazepine, ozanimod, paroxetine hydrochloride, propoxyphene, sertraline, tramadol, valbenazine, venlafaxine, viloxazine
Important contra-indications noted in the prescribing guidelines for: nursing mothers; pediatric patients
Warning: SUICIDALITY IN CHILDREN AND ADOLESCENTS

Mucosal
Xerostomia (dry mouth) (>10%) [2]

Cardiovascular
Hypertension [2]

Central Nervous System
Hallucinations [2]
Headache [2]
Serotonin syndrome [2]

Gastrointestinal/Hepatic
Nausea [2]

Local
Application-site reactions [5]

Other
Bruxism (teeth grinding) (<10%)

SELENIUM

Trade names: Bio-Active Selenium (Solaray), Head & Shoulders Shampoo (Procter & Gamble), SelenoMax (Source Naturals), Selsun Blue (Chattem), Selsun Shampoo (Chattem)
Indications: Anticancer (stomach, colorectal, lung, prostate), arthritis, asthma, heart disease, HIV inhibitor, treatment of dandruff, fungal infections (tinea versicolor), and seborrhea
Class: Antioxidant, Trace element
Half-life: 12–41 hours; selenomethionine: 252 days, selenite: 102 days
Clinically important, potentially hazardous interactions with: baloxavir marboxil, cholesterol-lowering drugs, cisplatin, clozapine, dimercaprol, eltrombopag, niacin, oral corticosteroids, simvastatin
Note: Selenium is an essential component of glutathione peroxidase. Inadequate concentrations of dietary selenium account, in part, for Keshan disease (a fatal cardiomyopathy). Paradise nuts (Lecythis ollaria) are a natural selenium source.

Skin
Carcinoma [5]
Cutaneous toxicity / skin toxicity [3]
Dermatitis [2]

Hair
Alopecia / hair loss [6]
Hair changes [2]

Nails
Brittle nails [5]
Nail pigmentation [2]

Central Nervous System
Amyotrophic lateral sclerosis [4]

Gastrointestinal/Hepatic
Nausea [3]
Vomiting [2]

Other
Adverse effects / adverse reactions [3]

SELEXIPAG

Trade name: Uptravi (Actelion)
Indications: Pulmonary arterial hypertension
Class: Prostacyclin receptor agonist
Half-life: <3 hours
Clinically important, potentially hazardous interactions with: gemfibrozil, strong CYP2C8 inhibitors
Pregnancy category: No data available
Important contra-indications noted in the prescribing guidelines for: nursing mothers

---

Skin
Flushing / rubefaction (12%)
Rash (11%)

Central Nervous System
Headache (65%) [8]

Endocrine/Metabolic
Appetite decreased (6%)

Gastrointestinal/Hepatic
Diarrhea (42%) [4]
Nausea (33%) [6]
Vomiting (18%)

Hematologic
Anemia (8%)

Neuromuscular/Skeletal
Arthralgia (11%)
Jaw pain (26%) [6]
Myalgia/Myopathy (16%) [2]
Pain in extremities (17%)

SELPERCATINIB

Trade name: Retevmo (Loxo Oncology Inc)
Indications: Non-small cell lung cancer, thyroid cancer.
Note: (2020) FDA approved under accelerated approval based on overall response rate and duration of response. Continued approval may be contingent upon verification and description of clinical benefit in confirmatory trial(s).
Class: Kinase inhibitor, RET (Rearranged during Transfection) kinase inhibitor
Half-life: 32 hours
Clinically important, potentially hazardous interactions with: acid-reducing agents (proton pump inhibitors, H2 receptor antagonists, locally-acting antacids), CYP2C8 and CYP3A substrates, CYP3A inducers, CYP3A inhibitors, itraconazole, midazolam, omeprazole, repaglinide, rifampin
Pregnancy category: Can cause fetal harm. Advise females of reproductive potential of the possible risk to the fetus and to use effective contraception.

Skin
Edema / fluid retention (33%)
Hypersensitivity (4%)
Rash (27%)

Mucosal
Xerostomia (dry mouth) (39%)

Cardiovascular
Hypertension (35%) [6]
QT interval prolonged / QT prolongation (17%) [2]

Central Nervous System
Headache (23%)

Endocrine/Metabolic
ALP increased (36%)
ALT increased (45%) [6]
AST increased (51%) [6]
Hyperbilirubinemia (23%) [2]
Hypercholesterolemia (31%)
Hyperglycemia (includes glucose increased) (44%)
Hypoalbuminemia / albumin decreased (42%) [2]
Hypocalcemia (41%)
Hypoglycemia (22%)
Hypomagnesemia (24%)
Hyponatremia (27%) [3]
Serum creatinine increased (37%)

Gastrointestinal/Hepatic
Abdominal pain (23%)
Constipation (25%)
Diarrhea (37%) [3]
Nausea (23%)
Vomiting (15%)

Hematologic
Hemorrhage (15%)
Leukocytopenia (leukopenia) / leukocytes (white blood cells) decreased (43%)
Thrombocytopenia / platelets decreased [3]

Neuromuscular/Skeletal
Asthenia / fatigue (35%)

Respiratory
Cough (18%)
Dyspnea / shortness of breath (16%)

Other
Adverse effects / adverse reactions [2]

SEMAGLUTIDE

Trade name: Ozempic (Novo Nordisk)
Indications: Antidiabetic. Treatment of type 2 diabetes mellitus.
Adjunct for the treatment of obesity and for weight loss management in defined populations and health conditions.
Class: Anti-obesity / weight loss pharmacotherapy, Antidiabetic, Glucagon-like peptide-1 (GLP-1) receptor agonist
Half-life: Approximately 1 week
Clinically important, potentially hazardous interactions with: insulin, insulin secretagogues
Pregnancy category: Discontinue semaglutide in women at least 2 months before a planned pregnancy due to the long washout period for this drug.
Note: Not indicated for use in type 1 diabetes mellitus or for the treatment of diabetic ketoacidosis. Semaglutide causes a delay of gastric emptying, and thereby has the potential to impact the absorption of concomitantly administered oral medications.
An oral formulation of semaglutide and sodium salcaprozate (an intestinal permeation enhancer) is available in the United States and Europe.
Warning: IN RODENTS, SEMAGLUTIDE CAUSES THYROID C-CELL TUMORS. IT IS UNKNOWN WHETHER SEMAGLUTIDE CAUSES THYROID C-CELL TUMORS, INCLUDING MEDULLARY THYROID CARCINOMA (MTC), IN HUMANS AS THE HUMAN RELEVANCE OF SEMAGLUTIDE-INDUCED RODENT THYROID C-CELL TUMORS HAS NOT BEEN DETERMINED. SEMAGLUTIDE IS CONTRAINDICATED IN PATIENTS WITH A PERSONAL OR FAMILY HISTORY OF MTC OR IN PATIENTS WITH MULTIPLE ENDOCRINE NEOPLASIA SYNDROME TYPE 2. COUNSEL PATIENTS REGARDING THE POTENTIAL RISK OF MTC AND SYMPTOMS OF THYROID TUMORS.

Skin
- Lupus erythematosus (subacute cutaneous lupus erythematosus (SCLE)) [2]

Cardiovascular
- Cardiovascular adverse effect (includes major adverse cardiovascular events (MACE)) [2]

Central Nervous System
- Suicidal ideation [5]

Gastrointestinal/Hepatic
- Abdominal pain (6%)
- Constipation (3%)
- Diarrhea (9%) [5]
- Dyspepsia / functional dyspepsia (indigestion) (see also gastroparesis) (3%)
- Eructation (belching) (3%)
- Flatulence (2%)
- Gastroesophageal reflux (2%)
- Gastrointestinal adverse reaction [10]
- Gastrointestinal disorder / discomfort [5]
- Gastroparesis (delayed gastric emptying) [4]
- Hepatic (liver) disorder / hepatobiliary disorder / hepatic (liver) dysfunction [2]
- Nausea (20%) [5]
- Pancreatitis / acute pancreatitis [5]
- Vomiting (9%)

Other
- Adverse effects / adverse reactions [5]

SENNA

Family: Caesalpiniaceae; Fabaceae
Scientific names: *Cassia acutifolia, Cassia angustifolia, Cassia obtusifloia, Cassia senna, Cassia tora, Senna alexandrina, Senna obtusifolia, Senna tora*
Indications: Laxative, cathartic, cholagogue, purgative
Class: Stimulant laxative
Half-life: N/A
Clinically important, potentially hazardous interactions with: squill
Note: Part used: Leaves and/or seed pods. Prolonged or excessive laxative use can lead to electrolyte and fluid disturbances, development of carthartic colon, and possible increased risk of colorectal cancer. Treatment should be limited to 8 to 10 days.

Skin
- AGEP [2]

Gastrointestinal/Hepatic
- Hepatotoxicity / liver injury / acute liver injury / drug-induced liver injury (DILI) [2]

Neuromuscular/Skeletal
- Arthralgia (from abuse) [2]
- Finger clubbing (from abuse) (reversible) [3]

Other
- Adverse effects / adverse reactions [4]

SERMORELIN

Trade name: Geref (Merck)
Class: Growth hormone-releasing hormone analog
Half-life: ~12 minutes
Clinically important, potentially hazardous interactions with: aspirin, drugs affecting pituitary secretion of somatotropin, glucocorticoids, indomethacin, insulin

SERTINDOLE

Trade name: Serdolect (Lundbeck)
Indications: Schizophrenia
Class: Antipsychotic
Half-life: 2–4 days
Clinically important, potentially hazardous interactions with: antiarrhythmics, antidepressants, antihistamines, astemizole, cimetidine, CYP3A inhibitors, macrolides, quinidine, quinolones, sotalol, terfenadine
Important contra-indications noted in the prescribing guidelines for: nursing mothers
Note: Contra-indicated in patients with a history of clinically significant cardiovascular disease, congestive heart failure, cardiac hypertrophy, arrhythmia, or bradycardia.
Not available in the USA.

Mucosal
- Nasal congestion [2]
- Xerostomia (dry mouth) [2]

Cardiovascular
- Arrhythmias [2]
- Cardiac disorder / cardiac dysfunction [3]
- QT interval prolonged / QT prolongation [21]

Central Nervous System
- Extrapyramidal symptoms [3]
- Headache [2]

Endocrine/Metabolic
- Weight gain [7]

Genitourinary
- Ejaculatory dysfunction [4]
- Sexual dysfunction [3]

Respiratory
- Rhinitis / rhinosinusitis (see also sinusitis) [4]

Other
- Adverse effects / adverse reactions [5]

SERTRALINE

Trade name: Zoloft (Pfizer)
Indications: Depression, panic disorders, obsessive compulsive disorders
Class: Antidepressant, Selective serotonin reuptake inhibitor (SSRI)
Half-life: 24–26 hours
Clinically important, potentially hazardous interactions with: amphetamines, astemizole, clarithromycin, clozapine, darunavir, dextroamphetamine, diethylpropion, droperidol, efavirenz, erythromycin, gilteritinib, isocarboxazid, linezolid, MAO inhibitors, mazindol, methamphetamine, metoclopramide, phendimetrazine, phenelzine, phentermine, phenylpropanolamine, pimozide, pseudoephedrine, selegiline, sibutramine, St John's wort, sumatriptan, sympathomimetics, tranylcypromine, trazodone, troleandomycin, zolmitriptan

---

Skin
- Angioedema (formerly named angioneurotic edema) [3]
- Diaphoresis (8%) [6]
- Flushing / rubefaction (2%)
- Rash (<10%)
- Stevens-Johnson syndrome and toxic epidermal necrolysis (SJS/TEN) [2]

Hair
- Alopecia / hair loss [3]

Mucosal
- Xerostomia (dry mouth) (16%) [7]

Cardiovascular
- Chest pain (<10%)
- Palpitation (<10%)
- QT interval prolonged / QT prolongation [3]
- Torsades de pointes [2]

Central Nervous System
- Akathisia [6]
- Anxiety (<10%)
- Coma [2]
- Hallucinations, visual [3]
- Headache (>10%)
- Hypoesthesia / hypesthesia (numbness) (5%)
- Insomnia (>10%)
- Mania [4]
- Pain (<10%)
- Paresthesias (<10%)
- Restless legs syndrome / Willis-Ekbom disease (includes restless arms syndrome variant) [3]
- Seizures [2]
- Serotonin syndrome [10]
- Somnolence (drowsiness) (>10%)

Tremor (<10%) [3]
Vertigo / dizziness (>10%) [3]
Yawning (<10%)

Endocrine/Metabolic
Galactorrhea [5]
Gynecomastia [2]
Hyponatremia [4]
Libido decreased (>10%)
SIADH [15]
Weight gain (<10%)

Gastrointestinal/Hepatic
Constipation (<10%)
Diarrhea (>10%) [3]
Hepatotoxicity / liver injury / acute liver injury / drug-induced liver injury (DILI) [6]
Nausea (10%) [3]
Pancreatitis / acute pancreatitis [3]
Vomiting (>10%)

Genitourinary
Impotence (<10%)
Priapism [5]
Sexual dysfunction (10%) [5]
Urinary retention [2]

Neuromuscular/Skeletal
Asthenia / fatigue (>10%)
Back pain (<10%)
Rhabdomyolysis [3]
Trismus [2]

Ocular
Abnormal vision (<10%)
Papilledema [2]

Otic
Tinnitus (<10%)

Respiratory
Eosinophilic pneumonia [6]
Rhinitis / rhinosinusitis (see also sinusitis) (<10%)

Other
Adverse effects / adverse reactions [5]
Allergic reactions [2]
Bruxism (teeth grinding) [3]
Death [5]

SEVELAMER

Trade names: Renagel (Genzyme), Renvela (Genzyme)
Indications: Hyperphosphatemia
Class: Phosphate binding agent
Half-life: N/A
Clinically important, potentially hazardous interactions with: ciprofloxacin, cyclosporine, gemifloxacin, levothyroxine, moxifloxacin, mycophenolate, ofloxacin, tacrolimus
Important contra-indications noted in the prescribing guidelines for: pediatric patients
Note: Contra-indicated in patients with bowel obstruction.

Endocrine/Metabolic
Acidosis (includes lactic acidosis) [8]

Gastrointestinal/Hepatic
Abdominal pain (9%)
Colitis [4]
Constipation (8%) [9]
Diarrhea [4]
Dyspepsia / functional dyspepsia (indigestion) (see also gastroparesis) (16%) [3]
Flatulence (8%)
Gastrointestinal ulceration [2]
Intestinal bleeding [2]
Nausea (20%) [4]
Vomiting (22%) [3]

Other
Adverse effects / adverse reactions [2]

SEVOFLURANE

Trade name: Ultane (AbbVie)
Indications: Induction and maintenance of general anesthesia
Class: Anesthetic; inhalation
Half-life: 15–23 hours
Clinically important, potentially hazardous interactions with: mivacurium

---

Mucosal
Sialorrhea (ptyalism; hypersalivation) (4%)

Cardiovascular
Arrhythmias [3]
Bradycardia / sinus bradycardia [2]
QT interval prolonged / QT prolongation [7]
Torsades de pointes [2]

Central Nervous System
Agitation [3]
Hyperthermia [4]
Malignant hyperthermia [8]
Seizures [8]
Shivering (6%)

Gastrointestinal/Hepatic
Hepatotoxicity / liver injury / acute liver injury / drug-induced liver injury (DILI) [4]
Nausea [2]
Vomiting [2]

Local
Application-site burning [2]
Application-site erythema [3]

Neuromuscular/Skeletal
Rhabdomyolysis [2]

Renal
Nephrogenic diabetes insipidus / arginine vasopressin resistance [5]

Respiratory
Alveolar hemorrhage (pulmonary) [2]
Cough (5%)
Laryngospasm (laryngeal dystonia / spasmodic dysphonia) [2]

SIBERIAN GINSENG

Family: Araliaceae
Scientific names: *Acanthopanax senticosus, Eleutherococcus senticosus*
Indications: Alzheimer's disease, anaphylaxis, arthritis, colds, depression, fatigue, flu, impotence, infertility, menopause, multiple sclerosis, osteoporosis, perimenopause, PMS, stress
Class: Immunomodulator
Half-life: N/A
Clinically important, potentially hazardous interactions with: antihypertensives
Note: Eleutherococcus may prevent biotransformation of some drugs to less toxic compounds.

SIBUTRAMINE

Trade name: Meridia (AbbVie)
Indications: Obesity
Class: Anti-obesity / weight loss pharmacotherapy, Norepinephrine antagonist, Serotonin antagonist
Half-life: 1.1 hours
Clinically important, potentially hazardous interactions with: amitriptyline, citalopram, desvenlafaxine, dextromethorphan, dihydroergotamine, duloxetine, ephedra, ergot, fluoxetine, fluvoxamine, isocarboxazid, linezolid, lithium, MAO inhibitors, meperidine, methysergide, milnacipran, naratriptan, nefazodone, paroxetine hydrochloride, phenelzine, rizatriptan, sertraline, sumatriptan, tapentadol, tranylcypromine, tryptophan, venlafaxine, verapamil, zolmitriptan, zuclopenthixol
Note: Due to an increased risk of heart attack and stroke in patients with cardiovascular disease, sibutramine should not be used in patients with a history of coronary artery disease, congestive heart failure, arrhythmias, or stroke. Sibutramine has been withdrawn in the USA and the European Union due to risk of serious cardiovascular events.

Skin
Diaphoresis (2%)
Edema / fluid retention (2%)
Rash (4%)

Mucosal
Xerostomia (dry mouth) (17%) [8]

Cardiovascular
Arrhythmias [2]
Cardiac arrest [2]
Cardiotoxicity [2]
Hypertension [4]
Myocardial infarction [3]
Palpitation [2]
QT interval prolonged / QT prolongation [5]
Tachycardia [4]

Central Nervous System
Amnesia [2]
Dysgeusia (taste perversion) (2%)
Headache [6]
Paresthesias (2%)
Serotonin syndrome [2]
Stroke / cerebrovascular accident [2]
Vertigo / dizziness [2]

Gastrointestinal/Hepatic
Constipation [2]

Neuromuscular/Skeletal
Asthenia / fatigue [2]
Myalgia/Myopathy (2%)

Respiratory
Influenza- ('flu)-like syndrome (<10%)

Other
Allergic reactions (2%)
Death [2]

SILDENAFIL

Trade names: Revatio (Pfizer), Viagra (Pfizer)
Indications: Erectile dysfunction, hypertension
Class: Covid-19 putative drug, Phosphodiesterase type 5 (PDE5) inhibitor
Half-life: 4 hours
Clinically important, potentially hazardous interactions with: alfuzosin, alpha blockers, amlodipine, amprenavir, amyl nitrite, antifungals, antihypertensives, atazanavir, boceprevir, bosentan, cimetidine, clarithromycin, cobicistat/elvitegravir/emtricitabine/tenofovir alafenamide, cobicistat/elvitegravir/emtricitabine/tenofovir disoproxil, conivaptan, CYP3A4 inhibitors and inducers, darunavir, dasatinib, deferasirox, delavirdine, disopyramide, erythromycin, etravirine, fosamprenavir, grapefruit juice, high-fat foods, HMG-CoA reductase inhibitors, indinavir, isosorbide, isosorbide dinitrate, isosorbide mononitrate, itraconazole, ketoconazole, lopinavir, macrolide antibiotics, nelfinavir, nicorandil, nitrates, nitroglycerin, ombitasvir/paritaprevir/ritonavir, ombitasvir/paritaprevir/ritonavir and dasabuvir, other phosphodiesterase 5 inhibitors, paclitaxel, PEG-interferon, riociguat, ritonavir, sapropterin, saquinavir, St John's wort, telaprevir, telithromycin, tipranavir, vericiguat
Important contra-indications noted in the prescribing guidelines for: nursing mothers; pediatric patients

---

Skin
Dermatitis (<2%)
Diaphoresis (<2%)
DRESS syndrome (Drug-induced hypersensitivity syndrome) [2]
Edema / fluid retention (<2%)
Erythema (6%)
Exfoliative dermatitis (<2%)
Facial edema (<2%)
Flushing / rubefaction (10–25%) [34]
Genital edema (<2%)
Herpes simplex (<2%)
Lichenoid eruption / lichenoid reaction [2]
Peripheral edema (<2%)
Photosensitivity (<2%)
Pruritus (itching) (<2%)
Rash (2%)
Ulcerations (<2%)
Urticaria / hives (<2%)

Mucosal
Epistaxis (nosebleed) (9–13%) [2]
Gingivitis (<2%)
Glossitis (inflammation of the tongue) (<2%)
Nasal congestion [7]
Rectal hemorrhage / rectal bleeding (<2%)
Stomatitis (oral mucositis) (<2%)
Xerostomia (dry mouth) (<2%)

Cardiovascular
Angina (<2%)
Atrial fibrillation [2]
Atrioventricular block (<2%)
Cardiac arrest (<2%) [2]
Cardiac failure (<2%)
Cardiomyopathy (<2%)
Chest pain (<2%) [2]
Congestive heart failure [2]
Hypotension (<2%) [5]
Myocardial infarction [4]
Myocardial ischemia (<2%)
Palpitation (<2%)
Postural hypotension (<2%)
Tachycardia (<2%)
Vasodilation [3]
Ventricular arrhythmia [2]

Central Nervous System
Abnormal dreams (<2%)
Amnesia [3]
Anorgasmia (<2%)
Chills (<2%)
Depression (<2%)
Fever (pyrexia) (includes hyperpyrexia) (6%)
Headache (16–46%) [41]
Hyperesthesia (<2%)
Insomnia (7%)
Migraine (<2%)
Neurotoxicity (<2%)
Pain (<2%)
Paresthesias (3%)
Seizures [3]
Somnolence (drowsiness) (<2%)
Stroke / cerebrovascular accident [2]
Subarachnoid hemorrhage [2]
Syncope / fainting (<2%)
Tremor (<2%)
Vertigo / dizziness (2%) [7]

Endocrine/Metabolic
Gynecomastia (<2%)
Hyperglycemia (includes glucose increased) (<2%)
Hypernatremia (<2%)
Hyperuricemia (<2%)

Gastrointestinal/Hepatic
Abdominal pain (<2%) [3]
Colitis (<2%)
Diarrhea (3–9%) [4]
Dyspepsia / functional dyspepsia (indigestion) (see also gastroparesis) (7–17%) [15]
Dysphagia (<2%)
Esophagitis (<2%)
Gastritis / pangastritis / gastric irritation (<2%)
Gastroenteritis (<2%)
Gastrointestinal disorder / discomfort [2]
Hepatotoxicity / liver injury / acute liver injury / drug-induced liver injury (DILI) [2]
Nausea [4]
Vomiting (<2%)

Genitourinary
Cystitis (includes interstitial cystitis / bladder pain syndrome) (<2%)
Ejaculatory dysfunction (<2%)
Enuresis (urinary incontinence) (<2%)
Nocturia (<2%)
Priapism [6]
Urinary frequency (<2%)
Urinary tract infection (3%)

Hematologic
Anemia (<2%)
Leukocytopenia (leukopenia) / leukocytes (white blood cells) decreased (<2%)

Neuromuscular/Skeletal
Arthralgia (<2%)
Asthenia / fatigue (<2%) [2]
Ataxia (<2%)
Back pain [3]
Bone pain / joint pain (<2%)
Gouty tophi (<2%)
Hypertonia (<2%)
Myalgia/Myopathy (7%) [4]
Tendinopathy/Tendon rupture (<2%)

Ocular
Abnormal vision [3]
Cataract (<2%)
Conjunctivitis (conjunctival inflammation) (<2%)
Dyschromatopsia (blue-green vision) (3–11%) [5]
Mydriasis (<2%)
Ocular hemorrhage (<2%)
Ocular pain (<2%)
Ocular pigmentation (<2%)
Optic neuropathy [18]
Photophobia (<2%)
Retinal vein occlusion [2]
Vision blurred [4]
Visual disturbances [5]
Xerophthalmia (dry eyes) (<2%)

Otic
Ear pain (<2%)
Hearing loss (hypoacusis) (<2%) [4]
Tinnitus (<2%) [2]

Respiratory
Asthma (<2%)
Bronchitis (<2%)
Cough (<2%)
Dyspnea / shortness of breath (7%) [4]
Hemoptysis [2]
Hypoxia [3]
Laryngitis (<2%)
Pharyngitis (sore throat) (<2%)
Pneumonia [2]
Respiratory failure [3]
Rhinitis / rhinosinusitis (see also sinusitis) (4%) [6]
Sinusitis (see also rhinitis / rhinosinusitis) (<2%)
Stridor [2]
Upper respiratory tract infection [2]

Other
Adverse effects / adverse reactions [7]
Allergic reactions (<2%)
Death [3]
Dipsia (thirst) / polydipsia (<2%)

SILODOSIN

Trade names: Rapaflo (Watson), Urief (Kissei)
Indications: Benign prostatic hyperplasia
Class: Adrenergic alpha-receptor antagonist
Half-life: 4.7–6 hours
Clinically important, potentially hazardous interactions with: alpha blockers, antihypertensives, atorvastatin, clarithromycin, conivaptan, cyclosporine, darunavir, delavirdine, diltiazem, erythromycin, indinavir, itraconazole, ketoconazole, lapatinib, ritonavir, stong CYP3A4 inhibitors, telithromycin, vasodilators, verapamil, voriconazole
Pregnancy category: Not indicated for use in women
Important contra-indications noted in the prescribing guidelines for: pediatric patients
Note: Contra-indicated in patients with severe hepatic or renal impairment.

Mucosal
Nasal congestion (2%) [3]
Rhinorrhea (<2%)

Cardiovascular
Orthostatic hypotension (3%) [9]
Postural hypotension [2]

Central Nervous System
Headache (2%) [3]
Insomnia (<2%)
Vertigo / dizziness (3%) [8]

Gastrointestinal/Hepatic
Abdominal pain (<2%)
Diarrhea (3%) [2]

Genitourinary
Ejaculatory dysfunction (25%) [29]
Retrograde ejaculation (28%) [5]

Neuromuscular/Skeletal
Asthenia / fatigue (<2%)

Ocular
Floppy iris syndrome [2]

Respiratory
Nasopharyngitis (2%)
Sinusitis (see also rhinitis / rhinosinusitis) (<2%)

Other
Adverse effects / adverse reactions [2]
Dipsia (thirst) / polydipsia (7%) [2]

SIMEPREVIR

Trade name: Olysio (Janssen)
Indications: Hepatitis C
Class: Direct-acting antiviral, Hepatitis C virus NS3/4A protease inhibitor
Half-life: 10–13 hours
Clinically important, potentially hazardous interactions with: atazanavir, carbamazepine, cisapride, clarithromycin, cobicistat/elvitegravir/emtricitabine/tenofovir disoproxil, darunavir, delavirdine, dexamethasone, efavirenz, erythromycin, etravirine, fluconazole, fosamprenavir, indinavir, itraconazole, ketoconazole, ledipasvir & sofosbuvir, lopinavir, milk thistle, nelfinavir, nevirapine, oxcarbazepine, phenobarbital, phenytoin, posaconazole, rifabutin, rifampin, rifapentine, ritonavir, saquinavir, St John's wort, telithromycin, tipranavir, voriconazole
Pregnancy category: simeprevir is pregnancy category C but must not be used in monotherapy
Important contra-indications noted in the prescribing guidelines for: nursing mothers; pediatric patients
Note: Must be used in combination with PEG-interferon and ribavirin (see separate entries).
Warning: RISK OF HEPATITIS B VIRUS REACTIVATION IN PATIENTS COINFECTED WITH HCV AND HBV

Skin
Photosensitivity (28%) [5]
Pruritus (itching) (22%) [8]
Rash (28%) [10]

Central Nervous System
Fever (pyrexia) (includes hyperpyrexia) [2]
Headache [13]
Insomnia [3]

Endocrine/Metabolic
Hyperbilirubinemia [9]

Gastrointestinal/Hepatic
Nausea (22%) [9]
Vomiting [2]

Hematologic
Anemia [11]
Neutropenia (neutrophils decreased) [3]

Neuromuscular/Skeletal
Asthenia / fatigue [10]
Myalgia/Myopathy (16%)

Respiratory
Dyspnea / shortness of breath (12%)
Influenza- ('flu)-like syndrome [3]

Other
Adverse effects / adverse reactions [7]

SIMVASTATIN

Trade names: Inegy (MSD), Simcor (AbbVie), Vytorin (MSD), Zocor (Merck)
Indications: Hypercholesterolemia
Class: HMG-CoA reductase inhibitor / statin
Half-life: 1.9 hours
Clinically important, potentially hazardous interactions with: alitretinoin, amiodarone, amlodipine, amprenavir, atazanavir, azithromycin, bempedoic acid, boceprevir, bosentan, carbamazepine, ciprofibrate, clarithromycin, clopidogrel, colchicine, conivaptan, coumarins, cyclosporine, danazol, darunavir, dasatinib, delavirdine, diltiazem, dronedarone, efavirenz, elbasvir & grazoprevir, erythromycin, fosamprenavir, fusidic acid, gemfibrozil, glecaprevir & pibrentasvir, grapefruit juice, HIV protease inhibitors, imatinib, imidazoles, indinavir, itraconazole, ketoconazole, letermovir, lomitapide, lonafarnib, lopinavir, miconazole, mifepristone, nefazodone, nelfinavir, ombitasvir/paritaprevir/ritonavir, ombitasvir/paritaprevir/ritonavir and dasabuvir, paclitaxel, pazopanib, posaconazole, rabeprazole, ranolazine, red rice yeast, rifampin, ritonavir, roxithromycin, saquinavir, selenium, St John's wort, tacrolimus, telaprevir, telithromycin, ticagrelor, tipranavir, triazoles, verapamil, viloxazine, voriconazole, warfarin
Important contra-indications noted in the prescribing guidelines for: nursing mothers; pediatric patients
Note: Simcor is simvastatin and niacin; Vytorin is simvastatin and ezetimibe.

Skin
Dermatomyositis [5]
Eczema / eczematous reaction / eczematous eruption (5%) [4]
Edema / fluid retention (3%) [2]
Eosinophilic fasciitis (Shulman syndrome / Shulman disease) [2]
Erythema multiforme [2]
Lichen planus pemphigoides [2]
Lichenoid eruption / lichenoid reaction [2]
Lupus erythematosus (subacute cutaneous lupus erythematosus (SCLE)) [5]
Peripheral edema [2]
Photosensitivity [7]
Pruritus (itching) [3]
Purpura [3]
Rash (<10%) [4]
Vasculitis (angiitis) / cutaneous vasculitis (angiitis) [2]

Mucosal
Stomatitis (oral mucositis) [2]

Cardiovascular
Atrial fibrillation (6%)

Central Nervous System
Cognitive impairment [3]
Headache (3–7%)
Memory loss/memory impaired [2]
Vertigo / dizziness (5%)

Endocrine/Metabolic
ALT increased [2]
Creatine phosphokinase (CPK) / creatine kinase increased (hyperCKemia) [3]
Diabetes mellitus [4]

Gastrointestinal/Hepatic
Abdominal pain (7%)
Constipation (2–7%)
Diarrhea [6]
Gastritis / pangastritis / gastric irritation (5%)
Hepatitis [4]
Hepatotoxicity / liver injury / acute liver injury / drug-induced liver injury (DILI) [8]
Nausea (5%)
Pancreatitis / acute pancreatitis [7]

Hematologic
Leukocytopenia (leukopenia) / leukocytes (white blood cells) decreased [2]

Neuromuscular/Skeletal
Asthenia / fatigue (9%) [3]
Compartment syndrome [2]
Myalgia/Myopathy (<10%) [37]
Necrotizing myopathy / immune-mediated necrotizing myopathy [2]
Rhabdomyolysis [94]
Tendinopathy/Tendon rupture [3]

Renal
Nephrotoxicity / kidney injury / acute kidney injury (AKI) / drug-induced kidney injury [2]
Renal failure [9]

Respiratory
Bronchitis (7%)
Cough [2]
Upper respiratory tract infection (9%)

Other
Adverse effects / adverse reactions [10]
Death [5]

SIPONIMOD

Synonym: Mayzent
Trade name: Mayzent (Novartis)
Indications: A sphingosine1-phosphate receptor modulator indicated for the treatment of relapsing forms of multiple sclerosis (MS), to include clinically isolated syndrome, relapsing-remitting disease, and active secondary progressive disease, in adults
Class: Sphingosine1-phosphate receptor modulator
Half-life: ~30 hours
Clinically important, potentially hazardous interactions with: CYP2C9 and CYP3A4 inducers, CYP2C9 and CYP3A4 inhibitors, vaccines
Pregnancy category: There are no adequate data on the developmental risk associated with the use of MAYZENT (SIPONIMOD) in pregnant women. Based on animal data and its mechanism of action, siponimod can cause fetal harm when administered to a pregnant woman. Women of childbearing potential should use effective contraception during and for 10 days after stopping siponimod.

Skin
Edema / fluid retention (>5%)
Herpes zoster (<5%)

Cardiovascular
Atrioventricular block (<5%)
Bradycardia / sinus bradycardia (>5%)
Hypertension (>10%) [2]

Central Nervous System
Fall (>10%)
Headache (>10%)
Seizures (2%)
Tremor (<5%)

Vertigo / dizziness (>5%)

Endocrine/Metabolic

Hypertransaminasemia (hepatic transaminitis) / elevated transaminases (>10%)

Gastrointestinal/Hepatic

Diarrhea (>5%)
Nausea (>5%)

Hematologic

Lymphopenia (lymphocytopenia) / lymphocytes decreased (<5%)

Neuromuscular/Skeletal

Asthenia / fatigue (<5%)
Pain in extremities (>5%)

Ocular

Macular edema (<5%)

Respiratory

Pulmonary function test decreased (<5%)

Other

Adverse effects / adverse reactions [2]

SIROLIMUS

Synonym: rapamycin
Trade name: Rapamune (Wyeth)
Indications: Prophylaxis of organ rejection in renal transplants, lymphangioleiomyomatosis
Class: Immunosuppressant, Macrolactam, Non-calcineurin inhibitor
Half-life: 62 hours
Clinically important, potentially hazardous interactions with: atazanavir, benazepril, boceprevir, captopril, ceritinib, cobicistat/elvitegravir/emtricitabine/tenofovir disoproxil, crizotinib, cyclosporine, darunavir, dasatinib, delavirdine, dronedarone, efavirenz, eluxadoline, enalapril, enzalutamide, fosinopril, Hemophilus B vaccine, indinavir, itraconazole, letermovir, lisinopril, lopinavir, micafungin, mifepristone, posaconazole, quinapril, ramipril, ribociclib, St John's wort, tacrolimus, telaprevir, telithromycin, tipranavir, venetoclax, viloxazine, voriconazole, zotarolimus
Important contra-indications noted in the prescribing guidelines for: the elderly; nursing mothers; pediatric patients
Warning: IMMUNOSUPPRESSION, USE IS NOT RECOMMENDED IN LIVER OR LUNG TRANSPLANT PATIENTS

Skin

Abscess (3–20%)
Acne vulgaris ('acne') [2]
Acneiform eruption / acneiform dermatitis / acneiform rash (20–31%) [10]
Angioedema (formerly named angioneurotic edema) [6]
Bruise / bruising / contusion / ecchymosis (ecchymoses) (3–20%)
Cellulitis and pseudocellulitis (3–20%)
Contact dermatitis [3]
Cutaneous toxicity / skin toxicity [3]
Dermatitis [3]
Diaphoresis (3–20%)
Edema / fluid retention (16–24%) [6]
Facial edema (3–20%) [2]
Folliculitis [3]
Fungal dermatitis (3–20%)
Hypertrophy (3–20%)
Lymphedema [2]
Maculopapular rash / morbilliform rash [2]
Peripheral edema (54–64%) [3]
Pruritus (itching) (3–20%) [2]
Purpura (3–20%)
Rash (10–20%) [5]
Ulcerations (3–20%)
Vasculitis (angiitis) / cutaneous vasculitis (angiitis) [2]

Hair

Hirsutism (3–20%)

Nails

Onychopathy [2]

Mucosal

Aphthous stomatitis / aphthous ulcer / aphtha (aphthae) (9%) [8]
Gingival hyperplasia / gingival hypertrophy / gingival enlargement / gingival overgrowth (3–20%) [2]
Gingivitis (3–20%)
Mucositis [2]
Oral candidiasis (3–20%)
Oral ulceration (3–20%) [10]
Stomatitis (oral mucositis) (3–20%) [12]

Cardiovascular

Thrombophlebitis (3–20%)

Central Nervous System

Chills (3–20%)
Depression (3–20%)
Fever (pyrexia) (includes hyperpyrexia) [2]
Hyperesthesia (3–20%)
Paresthesias (3–20%)
Tremor (21–31%) [2]

Endocrine/Metabolic

Dyslipidemia [5]
Hypercholesterolemia [5]
Hyperlipidemia / lipids elevated [3]
Hypertriglyceridemia (includes triglycerides increased) [5]
Menstrual irregularities [2]

Gastrointestinal/Hepatic

Diarrhea [5]
Hepatitis [3]
Hepatotoxicity / liver injury / acute liver injury / drug-induced liver injury (DILI) [3]
Pancreatitis / acute pancreatitis [2]

Hematologic

Anemia [5]
Hemolytic uremic syndrome [2]
Leukocytopenia (leukopenia) / leukocytes (white blood cells) decreased [2]
Neutropenia (neutrophils decreased) [3]
Thrombocytopenia / platelets decreased [4]
Thrombosis [3]

Local

Application-site pruritus [2]

Neuromuscular/Skeletal

Arthralgia (25–31%) [3]
Asthenia / fatigue [4]
Myalgia/Myopathy [2]

Ocular

Eyelid edema / palpebral edema / blepharedema (40%) [2]

Otic

Tinnitus (3–20%)

Renal

Nephrotoxicity / kidney injury / acute kidney injury (AKI) / drug-induced kidney injury [2]
Proteinuria [5]

Respiratory

Cough [2]
Influenza- ('flu)-like syndrome (3–20%)
Interstitial lung disease / interstitial pneumonitis / interstitial pneumonia (cryptogenic organizing pneumonia) / drug-induced interstitial lung disease [3]
Pneumonitis [7]
Pulmonary toxicity [3]
Upper respiratory tract infection (20–26%) [3]

Other

Adverse effects / adverse reactions [6]
Death [4]
Infection [5]

SITAGLIPTIN

Trade names: Janumet (Merck Sharpe & Dohme), Januvia (Merck Sharpe & Dohme)
Indications: Type II diabetes mellitus
Class: Antidiabetic, Dipeptidyl peptidase-4 (DPP-4) (gliptin) inhibitor
Half-life: 12 hours
Clinically important, potentially hazardous interactions with: alcohol, anabolic steroids, beta blockers, corticosteroids, diazoxide, digoxin, estrogens, loop diuretics, MAO inhibitors, progestogens, testosterone, thiazides
Important contra-indications noted in the prescribing guidelines for: the elderly; nursing mothers; pediatric patients
Note: Janumet is sitagliptin and metformin.

Skin

Angioedema (formerly named angioneurotic edema) [3]
Bullous pemphigoid / pemphigoid [3]
Edema / fluid retention [3]
Rash [2]

Central Nervous System

Headache [6]
Stroke / cerebrovascular accident [2]

Endocrine/Metabolic

Creatine phosphokinase (CPK) / creatine kinase increased (hyperCKemia) [2]
Hypoglycemia [14]
Weight gain [4]
Weight loss [2]

Gastrointestinal/Hepatic

Abdominal pain (2%)
Constipation [3]
Diarrhea [9]
Hepatotoxicity / liver injury / acute liver injury / drug-induced liver injury (DILI) [2]
Nausea [11]
Pancreatitis / acute pancreatitis [12]
Vomiting [6]

Neuromuscular/Skeletal

Arthralgia [2]
Bone pain / joint pain [2]
Rhabdomyolysis [4]

Renal

Renal failure [2]

Respiratory

Nasopharyngitis [5]
Upper respiratory tract infection [2]

Other

Adverse effects / adverse reactions [8]
Cancer [3]
Death [2]

SITAXENTAN

Synonym: sitaxsentan
Trade name: Thelin (Pfizer)
Indications: Pulmonary arterial hypertension
Class: Endothelin receptor (ETR) antagonist
Half-life: 10 hours
Clinically important, potentially hazardous interactions with: warfarin
Note: This drug has been withdrawn.

Skin
Peripheral edema (9%) [2]

Central Nervous System
Headache (15%) [2]
Vertigo / dizziness (>2%)

Gastrointestinal/Hepatic
Abdominal pain (>2%)
Hepatitis [2]
Hepatotoxicity / liver injury / acute liver injury / drug-induced liver injury (DILI) [5]

Neuromuscular/Skeletal
Myalgia/Myopathy (>2%)

Other
Death [2]

SODIUM OXYBATE

Synonym: GHB
Trade name: Xyrem (Jazz)
Indications: Cataplexy (in patients with narcolepsy)
Class: Anesthetic; general
Half-life: 0.3–1 hour
Clinically important, potentially hazardous interactions with: alcohol, amitriptyline, antipsychotics, benzodiazepines, clobazam, hydromorphone, hypnotics, levomepromazine, phenobarbital, risperidone, sedatives, tricyclic depressants, zuclopenthixol
Important contra-indications noted in the prescribing guidelines for: nursing mothers; pediatric patients
Note: Sodium oxybate is a class of drugs that are also known as: designer drugs, party drugs, club drugs, recreational drugs, rave drugs, fantasy drugs, date rape drugs or abuse drugs.
Warning: Central nervous system depressant with abuse potential. Should not be used with alcohol or other CNS depressants.

Skin
Diaphoresis [3]
Hyperhidrosis (3–6%)

Cardiovascular
Hypertension (6%)

Central Nervous System
Agitation [2]
Anxiety [2]
Cataplexy (9%)
Confusion (3–6%)
Depression (6%)
Disorientation (3–9%)
Headache (22%) [5]
Hypoesthesia / hypesthesia (numbness) (6%)
Impaired concentration (<9%)
Nightmares (3–6%)
Pain (3–6%)
Psychosis [3]
Seizures [10]
Sleep-related disorder (3–14%) [2]
Somnolence (drowsiness) (6%) [2]
Tremor [6]
Vertigo / dizziness (17%) [10]

Gastrointestinal/Hepatic
Abdominal pain (3–11%)
Dyspepsia / functional dyspepsia (indigestion) (see also gastroparesis) (3–9%)
Gastroenteritis (6%)
Nausea (21%) [10]
Vomiting (8%) [4]

Genitourinary
Enuresis (urinary incontinence) (7%) [4]

Neuromuscular/Skeletal
Asthenia / fatigue (3–6%) [2]
Back pain (6%)

Ocular
Vision blurred (6%)

Otic
Tinnitus (6%)

Respiratory
Nasopharyngitis (8%)
Pharyngolaryngeal pain (3–9%)
Upper respiratory tract infection (3–6%)

Other
Death [9]

SODIUM PICOSULFATE

Trade names: Pico-Salax (Ferring), Prepopik (Ferring)
Indications: Laxative for colon cleansing prior to colonoscopy
Class: Stimulant laxative
Half-life: ~7 hours
Clinically important, potentially hazardous interactions with: antibiotics, antipsychotics, carbamazepine, cardiac glycosides, chlorpromazine, corticosteroids, digoxin, diuretics, NSAIDs, oral iron, penicillamine, SSRIs, tetracycline, tricyclic antidepressants
Important contra-indications noted in the prescribing guidelines for: nursing mothers; pediatric patients
Note: Prepopik is a combination of sodium picosulfate and magnesium citrate. Contra-indicated in patients with severely reduced renal function, gastrointestinal obstruction or ileus, bowel perforation, toxic colitis or toxic megacolon, or gastric retention.

Central Nervous System
Headache [6]

Gastrointestinal/Hepatic
Abdominal pain [2]
Nausea (3%) [6]
Vomiting [4]

Other
Adverse effects / adverse reactions [3]

SOFOSBUVIR

Trade name: Sovaldi (Gilead)
Indications: Hepatitis C
Class: Direct-acting antiviral, Hepatitis C virus nucleotide analog NS5B polymerase inhibitor
Half-life: <27 hours
Clinically important, potentially hazardous interactions with: carbamazepine, oxcarbazepine, phenobarbital, phenytoin, rifabutin, rifampin, rifapentine, ritonavir, St John's wort, tipranavir
Pregnancy category: May cause fetal harm
Important contra-indications noted in the prescribing guidelines for: nursing mothers; pediatric patients
Note: Used in combination with daclatasvir, ledipasvir, ribavirin, velpatasvir or with PEG-interferon and ribavirin (see separate entries).

Skin
Pruritus (itching) (11–27%) [14]
Rash (8–18%) [10]

Cardiovascular
Bradyarrhythmia [2]
Bradycardia / sinus bradycardia [2]
Chest pain [2]

Central Nervous System
Chills (2–18%) [2]
Fever (pyrexia) (includes hyperpyrexia) (4–18%) [3]
Headache (24–44%) [56]
Insomnia (15–29%) [22]
Irritability (10–16%) [7]
Vertigo / dizziness [4]

Endocrine/Metabolic
Appetite decreased (6–18%)
Hyperbilirubinemia [3]

Gastrointestinal/Hepatic
Abdominal pain [2]
Diarrhea (9–17%) [8]
Dyspepsia / functional dyspepsia (indigestion) (see also gastroparesis) [2]
Hepatotoxicity / liver injury / acute liver injury / drug-induced liver injury (DILI) [2]
Nausea (13–34%) [43]
Vomiting [5]

Hematologic
Anemia (6–21%) [40]
Lymphopenia (lymphocytopenia) / lymphocytes decreased [2]
Neutropenia (neutrophils decreased) (<17%) [5]

Neuromuscular/Skeletal
Arthralgia [3]
Asthenia / fatigue (30–59%) [56]
Back pain [2]
Myalgia/Myopathy (6–16%) [5]

Renal
Renal failure [2]

Respiratory
Cough [4]
Dyspnea / shortness of breath [3]
Influenza- ('flu)-like syndrome (3–18%) [4]
Nasopharyngitis [2]
Upper respiratory tract infection [4]

Other
Adverse effects / adverse reactions [10]
Infection [2]

SOFOSBUVIR & VELPATASVIR

Trade name: Epclusa (Gilead)
Indications: Hepatitis C
Class: Direct-acting antiviral, Hepatitis C virus NS5A inhibitor (velpatasvir), Hepatitis C virus nucleotide analog NS5B polymerase inhibitor (sofosbuvir)
Half-life: <27 hours (sofosbuvir); 15 hours (velpatasvir)
Clinically important, potentially hazardous interactions with: amiodarone, carbamazepine, doravirine/lamiduvine/tenofovir disoproxil, efavirenz, omeprazole, oxcarbazepine, phenobarbital, phenytoin, rifabutin, rifampin, rifapentine, St John's wort, topotecan
Pregnancy category: Insufficient evidence to inform drug-associated risk; contra-indicated in pregnancy when given with ribavirin
Important contra-indications noted in the prescribing guidelines for: nursing mothers; pediatric patients
Note: See also separate entry for sofosbuvir.

Skin
Pruritus (itching) [2]
Rash (2%) [2]

Central Nervous System
Headache (22%) [17]
Insomnia (5%) [8]

Endocrine/Metabolic
Creatine phosphokinase (CPK) / creatine kinase increased (hyperCKemia) (<2%)

Gastrointestinal/Hepatic
Diarrhea [2]
Hepatotoxicity / liver injury / acute liver injury / drug-induced liver injury (DILI) (2–6%)
Nausea (9%) [12]

Hematologic
Anemia [3]
Lymphopenia (lymphocytopenia) / lymphocytes decreased [2]
Thrombocytopenia / platelets decreased [2]

Neuromuscular/Skeletal
Arthralgia [2]
Asthenia / fatigue (5–15%) [17]

Respiratory
Nasopharyngitis [5]

Other
Adverse effects / adverse reactions [2]

SOFOSBUVIR/ VELPATASVIR/ VOXILAPREVIR

Trade name: Vosevi (Gilead)
Indications: Chronic HCV infection
Class: Direct-acting antiviral, Hepatitis C virus NS3/4A protease inhibitor (voxilaprevir), Hepatitis C virus NS5A inhibitor (velpatasvir), Hepatitis C virus nucleotide analog NS5B polymerase inhibitor (sofosbuvir)
Half-life: <29 hours (sofosbuvir); 17 hours (velpatasvir); 33 hours (voxilaprevir)
Clinically important, potentially hazardous interactions with: amiodarone, atazanavir, carbamazepine, cyclosporine, efavirenz, lopinavir, oxcarbazepine, phenobarbital, phenytoin, pitavastatin, rifabutin, rifampin, rifapentine, ritonavir, rosuvastatin, St John's wort, tipranavir
Pregnancy category: Insufficient evidence to inform drug-associated risk
Important contra-indications noted in the prescribing guidelines for: nursing mothers; pediatric patients
Note: See also separate entries for sofosbuvir and sofosbuvir & velpatasvir.
Warning: RISK OF HEPATITIS B VIRUS REACTIVATION IN PATIENTS COINFECTED WITH HCV AND HBV

Skin
Rash (<2%)

Central Nervous System
Headache (21–23%) [9]
Insomnia (3–6%)

Endocrine/Metabolic
Hyperbilirubinemia (4–13%)
Hyperlipasemia (2–3%)

Gastrointestinal/Hepatic
Diarrhea (13–14%) [9]
Nausea (10–13%) [9]

Hematologic
Anemia [2]

Neuromuscular/Skeletal
Asthenia / fatigue (6–19%) [11]

SOLIFENACIN

Trade name: Vesicare (Astellas)
Indications: Overactive bladder
Class: Muscarinic antagonist
Half-life: 45–68 hours
Clinically important, potentially hazardous interactions with: atazanavir, carbamazepine, clarithromycin, indinavir, itraconazole, ketoconazole, nefazodone, nelfinavir, phenobarbital, phenytoin, rifabutin, rifampin, rifapentine, ritonavir, saquinavir, St John's wort, troleandomycin, voriconazole
Important contra-indications noted in the prescribing guidelines for: nursing mothers; pediatric patients

---

Mucosal
Xerostomia (dry mouth) (11–27%) [25]

Cardiovascular
QT interval prolonged / QT prolongation [3]

Central Nervous System
Vertigo / dizziness (2%) [3]

Gastrointestinal/Hepatic
Abdominal pain (2%)
Constipation [15]

Neuromuscular/Skeletal
Asthenia / fatigue (<2%)

Ocular
Vision blurred (4–5%) [7]
Xerophthalmia (dry eyes) (2%)

Other
Adverse effects / adverse reactions [5]

SOLRIAMFETOL

Synonym: Sunosi
Trade name: Sunosi (Jazz)
Indications: A dopamine and norepinephrine reuptake inhibitor indicated to improve wakefulness in adult patients with excessive daytime sleepiness associated with narcolepsy or obstructive sleep apnea
Class: Dopamine reuptake inhibitor, Norepinephrine reuptake inhibitor
Half-life: ~ 7 hours
Clinically important, potentially hazardous interactions with: dopaminergic drugs, drugs that increase blood pressure and/or heart rate, monoamine oxidase (mao) inhibitors
Pregnancy category: Available data from case reports are not sufficient to determine drug-associated risks of major birth defects, miscarriage, or adverse maternal or fetal outcomes.

Skin
Hyperhidrosis (≥2%)

Mucosal
Xerostomia (dry mouth) (≥2%) [4]

Cardiovascular
Chest discomfort (≥2%)
Chest pain (<2%)
Palpitation (≥2%)

Central Nervous System
Agitation (<2%)
Anxiety (≥2%) [4]
Attention disturbances (<2%)
Headache (≥5%) [5]
Insomnia (≥5%) [5]
Irritability (≥2%)
Jittery feelings (≥2%)
Restlessness (<2%)
Tremor (<2%)
Vertigo / dizziness (≥2%) [2]

Endocrine/Metabolic
Appetite decreased (≥5%) [4]
Weight loss (<2%)

Gastrointestinal/Hepatic
Abdominal pain (≥2%)
Constipation (≥2%)
Diarrhea (≥2%)
Nausea (≥5%) [5]
Vomiting (<2%)

Respiratory
Cough (<2%)
Dyspnea / shortness of breath (<2%)
Nasopharyngitis [3]

Other
Bruxism (teeth grinding) (<2%)
Dipsia (thirst) / polydipsia (<2%)

SOMATROPIN

Synonym: somatostatin
Trade names: Genotropin (Pfizer), Humatrope (Lilly), Norditropin (Novo Nordisk), Norditropin SimpleXx (Novo Nordisk), Nutropin (Genentech), NutropinAq (Ipsen), Saizen (Merck Serono), Scitropin A (Teva), Serostim (Merck Serono), Tev-Tropin (Teva), Zomacton (Ferring), Zorbtive (Merck Serono)
Indications: Growth failure, growth hormone deficiency, short stature (in Turner's syndrome), muscle wasting (in HIV positive patients)
Class: Growth hormone analog
Half-life: 0.4 hours (intravenous); 3 hours (subcutaneous); 5 hours (intramuscular)
Clinically important, potentially hazardous interactions with: acarbose, corticosteroids, estradiol, estrogens, exenatide, glucocorticoids, insulin aspart, insulin degludec, insulin detemir, insulin glargine, insulin glulisine, metformin, pioglitazone, saxagliptin, triamcinolone
Important contra-indications noted in the prescribing guidelines for: the elderly; nursing mothers
Note: Contra-indicated in patients with acute critical illiness; children with Prader-Willi syndrome who are severely obese or have severe respiratory impairment; active malignancy; active proliferative or severe non-proliferative diabetic retinopathy; or children with closed epiphyses.

Skin
Edema / fluid retention (11%)
Peripheral edema (18%)

Central Nervous System
Fever (pyrexia) (includes hyperpyrexia) [2]
Headache (7%) [2]
Pain (14%)
Paresthesias (14%)

Gastrointestinal/Hepatic
Abdominal pain [2]

Neuromuscular/Skeletal
Arthralgia (14%) [3]
Back pain (9%)
Myalgia/Myopathy (9%)
Pain in extremities [2]

Respiratory
Influenza- ('flu)-like syndrome (7%)
Rhinitis / rhinosinusitis (see also sinusitis) (11%)

Other
Adverse effects / adverse reactions [4]
Death [3]

SONIDEGIB

Trade name: Odomzo (Novartis)
Indications: Basal cell carcinoma
Class: Hedgehog (Hh) signaling pathway inhibitor
Half-life: 28 days
Clinically important, potentially hazardous interactions with: atazanavir, carbamazepine, diltiazem, efavirenz, fluconazole, itraconazole, ketoconazole, modafinil, nefazodone, phenobarbital, phenytoin, posaconazole, rifabutin, rifampin, saquinavir, St John's wort, telithromycin, voriconazole
Pregnancy category: Can cause fetal harm
Important contra-indications noted in the prescribing guidelines for: nursing mothers; pediatric patients
Note: Patients should not donate blood or blood products while receiving sonidegib and for at least 20 months after the last dose.
Warning: EMBRYO-FETAL TOXICITY

Skin
Pruritus (itching) (10%)

Hair
Alopecia / hair loss (53%) [8]

Central Nervous System
Anorexia [2]
Dysgeusia (taste perversion) (46%) [7]
Headache (15%)
Pain (14%)
Vertigo / dizziness [2]

Endocrine/Metabolic
ALT increased (19%)
Appetite decreased (30%) [2]
AST increased (19%)
Creatine phosphokinase (CPK) / creatine kinase increased (hyperCKemia) (61%) [10]
Hyperbilirubinemia [2]
Hyperglycemia (includes glucose increased) (51%)
Weight loss (30%) [4]

Gastrointestinal/Hepatic
Abdominal pain (18%)
Diarrhea (32%) [2]
Hepatotoxicity / liver injury / acute liver injury / drug-induced liver injury (DILI) [2]
Nausea (39%) [5]
Vomiting (11%) [3]

Hematologic
Anemia (32%)
Lymphopenia (lymphocytopenia) / lymphocytes decreased (28%)

Neuromuscular/Skeletal
Asthenia / fatigue (41%) [6]
Bone pain / joint pain (32%)
Muscle spasm (54%) [8]
Myalgia/Myopathy (19%) [6]

Other
Adverse effects / adverse reactions [2]

SORAFENIB

Trade name: Nexavar (Bayer)
Indications: Advanced renal cell carcinoma
Class: Angiogenesis inhibitor / antiangiogenic agent, Antineoplastic / anticancer agent (see also Immune checkpoint inhibitor), RET (Rearranged during Transfection) kinase inhibitor, Tyrosine kinase inhibitor, Vascular endothelial growth factor (VEGF) inhibitor / antagonist
Half-life: 25–48 hours
Clinically important, potentially hazardous interactions with: bevacizumab, carbamazepine, clozapine, conivaptan, coumarins, CYP3A4 inducers, darunavir, delavirdine, dexamethasone, digoxin, docetaxel, doxorubicin, efavirenz, indinavir, irinotecan, neomycin, oxcarbazepine, phenobarbital, phenytoin, rifabutin, rifampin, rifapentine, St John's wort, telithromycin, voriconazole, warfarin
Important contra-indications noted in the prescribing guidelines for: nursing mothers; pediatric patients
Note: In combination with carboplatin and paclitaxel, Nexavar is contra-indicated in patients with squamous cell lung cancer.

Skin
Acneiform eruption / acneiform dermatitis / acneiform rash (<10%) [7]
Actinic keratoses [4]
AGEP [4]
Cutaneous toxicity / skin toxicity [20]
Desquamation (19–40%) [10]
Eczema / eczematous reaction / eczematous eruption [2]
Edema / fluid retention [3]
Erythema (>10%) [4]
Erythema multiforme [11]
Exanthems [3]
Exfoliative dermatitis (<10%)
Facial erythema [3]
Flushing / rubefaction (<10%)
Folliculitis [3]
Hand–foot syndrome (palmar–plantar erythrodysesthesia) (21–30%) [133]
Hidradenitis suppurativa (acne inversa) [3]
Hyperkeratosis [4]
Hypersensitivity [2]
Keratoacanthoma (Grzybowski syndrome) [5]
Keratosis pilaris [2]
Milia [2]
Nevi (naevi) [3]
Nodulocystic lesions [2]
Palmar–plantar toxicity [2]
Pigmentation (Skin) (includes hyperpigmentation) [2]
Pruritus (itching) (14–19%) [10]
Psoriasis [3]
Radiation recall dermatitis [3]
Rash (19–40%) [56]
Recall reaction [2]
Seborrheic dermatitis [2]
Squamous cell carcinoma [8]
Stevens-Johnson syndrome and toxic epidermal necrolysis (SJS/TEN) [3]
Xerosis / xeroderma (10–11%) [6]

Hair
Alopecia / hair loss (14–27%) [31]
Hair pigmentation [2]

Nails
Splinter hemorrhage [4]
Subungual hematoma / subungual hemorrhage [2]

Mucosal
Burning Mouth Syndrome / glossodynia / glossalgia / glossopyrosis (also includes stomatodynia / oral dysesthesia / stomatopyrosis) (<10%)
Epistaxis (nosebleed) [2]
Mucositis (<10%) [14]
Stomatitis (oral mucositis) (<10%) [14]
Xerostomia (dry mouth) (<10%)

Cardiovascular
Cardiac failure [3]
Cardiotoxicity (3%) [7]
Congestive heart failure (<10%)
Hypertension (9–17%) [63]
Myocardial infarction (<10%)

Central Nervous System
Anorexia (16–29%) [18]
Depression (<10%)

Dysgeusia (taste perversion) [2]
Encephalopathy (includes hepatic encephalopathy) [3]
Fever (pyrexia) (includes hyperpyrexia) (<10%) [8]
Headache (10%) [5]
Neurotoxicity (2–40%) [4]
Pain (>10%) [4]

Endocrine/Metabolic
ALT increased [12]
Appetite decreased (<10%) [9]
AST increased [10]
Creatine phosphokinase (CPK) / creatine kinase increased (hyperCKemia) [2]
Hyperbilirubinemia [6]
Hyperlipasemia [2]
Hypoalbuminemia / albumin decreased (56%)
Hypocalcemia [2]
Hypokalemia [2]
Hyponatremia [5]
Hypophosphatemia (35–45%) [10]
Hypothyroidism [8]
Thyroid dysfunction [4]
Thyroiditis [4]
Weight loss (10–30%) [15]

Gastrointestinal/Hepatic
Abdominal pain (11–31%) [10]
Acute-on-chronic liver failure [2]
Ascites [3]
Constipation (14–15%) [4]
Diarrhea (43–55%) [77]
Dyspepsia / functional dyspepsia (indigestion) (see also gastroparesis) (<10%)
Dysphagia (<10%)
Gastrointestinal bleeding [5]
Hepatotoxicity / liver injury / acute liver injury / drug-induced liver injury (DILI) (11%) [27]
Nausea (23–24%) [15]
Pancreatitis / acute pancreatitis [8]
Pneumatosis intestinalis / pneumatosis cystoides intestinalis [2]
Vomiting (15–16%) [9]

Genitourinary
Erectile dysfunction (<10%)

Hematologic
Anemia (44%) [10]
Bleeding [3]
Cytopenia [2]
Hemorrhage (15–18%) [4]
Hemotoxicity [2]
Leukocytopenia (leukopenia) / leukocytes (white blood cells) decreased (>10%) [4]
Lymphopenia (lymphocytopenia) / lymphocytes decreased (23–47%) [5]
Myelosuppression / bone marrow suppression / myelotoxicity [2]
Neutropenia (neutrophils decreased) (<10%) [8]
Thrombocytopenia / platelets decreased (12–46%) [21]
Thrombosis [3]

Neuromuscular/Skeletal
Arthralgia (<10%)
Asthenia / fatigue (37–46%) [61]
Back pain [3]
Bone pain / joint pain (>10%) [3]
Myalgia/Myopathy (<10%) [2]

Renal
Nephrotoxicity / kidney injury / acute kidney injury (AKI) / drug-induced kidney injury [2]
Proteinuria [5]
Renal failure (<10%) [3]

Respiratory
Cough (13%) [2]
Dysphonia (includes voice disorders / voice changes) [6]
Dyspnea / shortness of breath (14%) [4]
Hoarseness (<10%) [2]
Influenza- ('flu)-like syndrome (<10%)
Pulmonary toxicity [2]

Other
Adverse effects / adverse reactions [19]
Death [9]
Infection [2]
Side effects (71%) [4]

SOTALOL

Trade name: Betapace (Bayer)
Indications: Ventricular arrhythmias
Class: Antiarrhythmic, Antiarrhythmic class II, Antiarrhythmic class III, Beta adrenergic blocker, Beta blocker
Half-life: 7–18 hours
Clinically important, potentially hazardous interactions with: abarelix, amiodarone, amisulpride, amitriptyline, arsenic, artemether/lumefantrine, asenapine, astemizole, atomoxetine, bepridil, ciprofloxacin, class I and class III antiarrhythmics, clonidine, degarelix, disopyramide, dronedarone, droperidol, enoxacin, gatifloxacin, guanethidine, haloperidol, insulin, isoprenaline, ivabradine, levomepromazine, lomefloxacin, loop diuretics, mizolastine, moxifloxacin, nilotinib, norfloxacin, ofloxacin, oral macrolides, phenothiazines, pimavanserin, pimozide, ponesimod, procainamide, quinidine, quinine, quinolones, ranolazine, reserpine, ribociclib, salbutamol, sertindole, sparfloxacin, sulpiride / levosulpiride, terbutaline, tetrabenazine, thiazides and related diruetics, tolterodine, tricyclic antidepressants, trifluoperazine, vandetanib, zuclopenthixol
Important contra-indications noted in the prescribing guidelines for: nursing mothers; pediatric patients
Note: Contra-indicated in patients with bronchial asthma, sinus bradycardia, second and third degree AV block, unless a functioning pacemaker is present, congenital or acquired long QT syndromes, cardiogenic shock, or uncontrolled congestive heart failure.

Skin
Edema / fluid retention (5%)
Pruritus (itching) (<10%)
Psoriasis [3]
Rash (3%)
Scleroderma [3]

Cardiovascular
Arrhythmias [2]
Atrioventricular block [2]
Bradycardia / sinus bradycardia [11]
Cardiac failure [2]
Cardiogenic shock [2]
Cardiotoxicity [3]
Hypotension [4]
QT interval prolonged / QT prolongation [20]
Torsades de pointes [25]

Central Nervous System
Depression [2]
Paresthesias (3%)

Neuromuscular/Skeletal
Asthenia / fatigue (6%) [2]

Other
Adverse effects / adverse reactions [2]

SOTORASIB

Trade name: Lumakras (Amgen)
Indications: Advanced or metastatic non-small cell lung cancer in patients with the *KRAS* p.G12C-mutation.
This indication is approved under accelerated approval based on overall response rate and duration of response. Continued approval for this indication may be contingent upon verification and description of clinical benefit in a confirmatory trial(s).

Class: Ras–GTPase inhibitor
Half-life: 5 hours
Clinically important, potentially hazardous interactions with: CYP3A4 inducers, CYP3A4 substrates, digoxin, famotidine, H2 receptor antagonists, itraconazole, metformin, omeprazole, P-gp substrates, proton pump inhibitors, rifampin
Pregnancy category: No available data for use in pregnant women.

Skin
Edema / fluid retention (15%)
Rash (12%)

Endocrine/Metabolic
ALP increased (33%)
ALT increased (38%) [2]
Appetite decreased (13%)
AST increased (39%) [2]
Hypoalbuminemia / albumin decreased (22%)
Hypocalcemia (35%)
Hyponatremia (28%)

Gastrointestinal/Hepatic
Abdominal pain (15%)
Constipation (16%)
Diarrhea (42%) [2]
Hepatotoxicity / liver injury / acute liver injury / drug-induced liver injury (DILI) (12% grade 3–4) (25%) [5]
Nausea (26%) [2]
Vomiting (17%)

Hematologic
Hemoglobin decreased (43%)
Lymphopenia (lymphocytopenia) / lymphocytes decreased (48%)
Prothrombin time (INR) increased (23%)

Neuromuscular/Skeletal
Arthralgia (12%)
Asthenia / fatigue (26%)
Musculoskeletal pain (35%)

Renal
Proteinuria (29%)

Respiratory
Dyspnea / shortness of breath (3% grade 3–4) (16%)
Pneumonia (12%)

SPARFLOXACIN

Trade name: Zagam (LGM Pharma)
Indications: Community-acquired pneumonia
Class: Antibiotic, Antibiotic; fluoroquinolone, Antimicrobial
Half-life: 16–30 hours
Clinically important, potentially hazardous interactions with: amiodarone, amisulpride, amitriptyline, amoxapine, arsenic, bepridil, bretylium, calcium, chlorpromazine, clomipramine, desipramine, disopyramide, doxepin, erythromycin, fluphenazine, imipramine, iron salts, magnesium, mesoridazine, nortriptyline, pentamidine, perphenazine, phenothiazines, pimozide, procainamide, prochlorperazine, promazine, promethazine, protriptyline, quinidine, sotalol, sucralfate, thioridazine, tricyclic antidepressants, trifluoperazine, trimipramine, zinc salts
Important contra-indications noted in the prescribing guidelines for: the elderly; nursing mothers; pediatric patients
Note: Fluoroquinolones are associated with an increased risk of tendinitis and tendon rupture in all ages. This risk is further increased in older patients usually over 60 years of age, in patients taking corticosteroid drugs, and in patients with kidney, heart or lung transplants.
Fluoroquinolones may exacerbate muscle weakness in persons with myasthenia gravis.

Skin
Photosensitivity (4%) [9]
Phototoxicity (8%) [5]
Pruritus (itching) (3%)

Nails
Photo-onycholysis [2]

Cardiovascular
QT interval prolonged / QT prolongation [3]
Torsades de pointes [3]

Genitourinary
Vulvovaginal candidiasis (3%)

SPECTINOMYCIN

Trade name: Trobicin (Pfizer)
Indications: Gonorrhea
Class: Antibiotic, Antimicrobial
Half-life: 1–3 hours
Clinically important, potentially hazardous interactions with: mivacurium

Skin
Anaphylactoid reactions / anaphylaxis (includes anaphylactic shock) [2]
Dermatitis [2]

Central Nervous System
Perioral paresthesias [3]
Vertigo / dizziness [3]

Local
Injection-site pain [3]

SPIRONOLACTONE

Trade names: Aldactazide (Pfizer), Aldactone (Pfizer)
Indications: Hyperaldosteronism, hirsutism, hypertension, edema for patients with congestive heart failure, cirrhosis of the liver or nephrotic syndrome
Class: Aldosterone antagonist / mineralocorticoid receptor antagonist (MRA), Diuretic
Half-life: 78–84 minutes
Clinically important, potentially hazardous interactions with: ACE inhibitors, alcohol, amiloride, barbiturates, benazepril, captopril, cyclosporine, enalapril, fosinopril, lisinopril, mitotane, moexipril, narcotics, NSAIDs, potassium chloride, potassium iodide, quinapril, ramipril, trandolapril, triamterene, zofenopril
Important contra-indications noted in the prescribing guidelines for: nursing mothers; pediatric patients
Note: Aldactazide is spironolactone and hydrochlorothiazide. Hydrochlorothiazide is a sulfonamide and can be absorbed systemically. Sulfonamides can produce severe, possibly fatal, reactions such as toxic epidermal necrolysis and Stevens-Johnson syndrome.
Warning: Spironolactone has been shown to be a tumorigen in chronic toxicity studies in rats

Skin
Bullous pemphigoid / pemphigoid [2]
Dermatitis [6]
Eczema / eczematous reaction / eczematous eruption [2]
Exanthems (<5%) [6]
Lichenoid eruption / lichenoid reaction [3]
Melasma [2]
Pigmentation (Skin) (includes hyperpigmentation) [3]
Pruritus (itching) [4]
Rash (<10%) [2]
Urticaria / hives [2]
Xerosis / xeroderma (40%) [2]

Hair
Alopecia / hair loss [2]

Endocrine/Metabolic
Amenorrhea [2]
Gynecomastia [31]
Hyperkalemia [9]

Renal
Renal function abnormal / renal dysfunction [2]

Other
Adverse effects / adverse reactions [6]

SQUILL

Family: Liliaceae
Scientific names: *Drimia indica, Drimia maritima, Scilla indica, Scilla maritima, Urginea indica, Urginea maritima, Urginea scilla*
Indications: Arrhythmias, asthma, edema, bronchitis, whooping cough, abortifacient. Also used as a rodenticide
Class: Diuretic
Half-life: N/A
Clinically important, potentially hazardous interactions with: ginger, ginseng, hawthorn (fruit, leaf, flower extract), licorice, mistletoe, senna
Note: Squill is unsafe for self-medication.

ST JOHN'S WORT

Family: Hypericaceae
Scientific names: *Hypericum perforatum, Kira (Lichtwer), Quanterra Emotional Balance (Warner Lambert)*
Indications: Depression, dysthymic disorder, fatigue, insomnia, loss of appetite, anxiety, obsessive-compulsive disorders, mood disturbances, migraine headaches, neuralgia, fibrositis, sciatica, palpitations, exhaustion, headache, muscle pain, vitiligo, diuretic, bruises, abrasions, first-degree burns, hemorrhoids
Class: Anxyolytic, CYP3A4 inducer
Half-life: 24–48 hours
Clinically important, potentially hazardous interactions with: acetaminophen, acitretin, afatinib, alfuzosin, alitretinoin, alprazolam, ambrisentan, aminophylline, amiodarone, amitriptyline, amlodipine, amprenavir, apixaban, aprepitant, artemether/lumefantrine, atazanavir, atorvastatin, berotralstat, bexarotene, bictegravir/emtricitabine/tenofovir alafenamide, boceprevir, bosentan, brigatinib, buspirone, cabazitaxel, cabozantinib, carbamazepine, ceritinib, cilostazol, ciprofloxacin, citalopram, cobimetinib, conivaptan, copanlisib, crizotinib, cyclosporine, cyproterone, dabigatran, daclatasvir, darunavir, dasatinib, delavirdine, demeclocycline, desipramine, digoxin, docetaxel, doravirine, doravirine/lamiduvine/tenofovir disoproxil, doxycycline, dronedarone, duloxetine, efavirenz, eliglustat, emtricitabine/rilpivirine/tenofovir alafenamide, enzalutamide, eplerenone, erlotinib, escitalopram, esomeprazole, estradiol, eszopiclone, ethosuximide, etoposide, etravirine, everolimus, fenfluramine, fesoterodine, fexofenadine, flibanserin, fluoxetine, fluvoxamine, fosamprenavir, fostemsavir, gefitinib, gemifloxacin, ginkgo biloba, glecaprevir & pibrentasvir, hydromorphone, ibrexafungerp, ibrutinib, idelalisib, imatinib, indinavir, irinotecan, isavuconazonium sulfate, isotretinoin, ivabradine, ivacaftor, ixabepilone, ixazomib, lacosamide, lapatinib, ledipasvir & sofosbuvir, lemborexant, levonorgestrel, loperamide, lopinavir, lorcaserin, lumacaftor/ivacaftor, lumateperone, maraviroc, metaxalone, methadone, midazolam, midostaurin, mifepristone, milnacipran, minocycline, naldemedine, naratriptan, nefazodone, nelfinavir, neratinib, nevirapine, nifedipine, nilotinib, nintedanib, ofloxacin, olaparib, ombitasvir/paritaprevir/ritonavir, ombitasvir/paritaprevir/ritonavir and dasabuvir, omeprazole, oral contraceptives, osimertinib, oxcarbazepine, palbociclib, paroxetine hydrochloride, pazopanib, perampanel, phenobarbitone, phenprocoumon, phenytoin, pimavanserin, ponatinib, quinolones, raltegravir, ramelteon, red rice yeast, regorafenib, reserpine, rilpivirine, riociguat, ritonavir, rivaroxaban, rizatriptan, romidepsin, safinamide, saquinavir, sertraline, sildenafil, simeprevir, simvastatin, sirolimus, sofosbuvir, sofosbuvir & velpatasvir, sofosbuvir/velpatasvir/voxilaprevir, solifenacin, sonidegib, sorafenib, SSRIs, sumatriptan, sunitinib, tacrolimus, tadalafil, tapentadol, telaprevir, telithromycin, temsirolimus, tenofovir alafenamide, tetracyclines, tezacaftor/ivacaftor, thalidomide, tiagabine, tibolone, tipranavir, tolvaptan, trabectedin, tricyclic antidepressants, ubrogepant, ulipristal, valbenazine, vandetanib,

venetoclax, venlafaxine, vigabatrin, vorapaxar, voriconazole, warfarin, ziprasidone, zolmitriptan
Note: St John's wort is a natural source of flavoring in Europe. Although not indigenous to Australia, and long considered a weed, St John's wort is now grown there as a cash crop and produces 20% of the world's supply.

Skin
Hyperhidrosis [2]
Photosensitivity [11]
Pruritus (itching) [2]
Rash [2]

Mucosal
Xerostomia (dry mouth) [5]

Cardiovascular
Hypertension [3]

Central Nervous System
Headache [5]
Insomnia [3]
Irritability [2]
Mania [2]
Neurotoxicity [2]
Psychosis [2]
Restlessness [4]
Serotonin syndrome [8]
Sleep disturbances [3]
Somnolence (drowsiness) [3]
Vertigo / dizziness [4]

Gastrointestinal/Hepatic
Abdominal pain [2]
Constipation [2]
Diarrhea [2]
Hepatotoxicity / liver injury / acute liver injury / drug-induced liver injury (DILI) [6]
Nausea [4]

Neuromuscular/Skeletal
Asthenia / fatigue [6]

Other
Adverse effects / adverse reactions [20]
Allergic reactions [2]

STANOZOLOL

Trade name: Winstrol (Ovation)
Indications: Hereditary angioedema
Class: Anabolic steroid
Half-life: N/A
Clinically important, potentially hazardous interactions with: anticoagulants, warfarin
Important contra-indications noted in the prescribing guidelines for: nursing mothers

---

Skin
Acneiform eruption / acneiform dermatitis / acneiform rash (>10%) [2]
Pigmentation (Skin) (includes hyperpigmentation) (<10%)

Hair
Hirsutism (in women) [3]

Cardiovascular
Cardiomyopathy [2]
Hypertension [2]
Myocardial infarction [2]
Myocardial ischemia [2]

Central Nervous System
Chills (<10%)

Endocrine/Metabolic
Gynecomastia (>10%)

Gastrointestinal/Hepatic
Hepatotoxicity / liver injury / acute liver injury / drug-induced liver injury (DILI) [3]

Genitourinary
Priapism (>10%)

Renal
Nephrotoxicity / kidney injury / acute kidney injury (AKI) / drug-induced kidney injury [3]

Other
Death [3]

STAR ANISE (CHINESE)

Family: Illiciaceae
Scientific name: *Illicium verum*
Indications: Bronchitis, colic, cough, flatulence, menstrual complaints, respiratory tract inflammation. Culinary spice, fragrance component in cosmetics
Class: Antimycobacterial (including antitubercular), Insecticide
Half-life: N/A
Clinically important, potentially hazardous interactions with: none known
Note: Star anise preparations are sometimes contaminated with highly poisonous Japanese star anise (*Illicium anisatum*). Star anise contains a compound used in the manufacture of Tamiflu.

Central Nervous System
Seizures [2]

STAVUDINE

Synonym: D4T
Trade name: Zerit (Bristol-Myers Squibb)
Indications: HIV infection
Class: Antiretroviral, Nucleoside analog reverse transcriptase inhibitor
Half-life: 1.44 hours
Clinically important, potentially hazardous interactions with: doxorubicin, ribavirin, zidovudine
Important contra-indications noted in the prescribing guidelines for: nursing mothers
Warning: LACTIC ACIDOSIS and HEPATOMEGALY with STEATOSIS; PANCREATITIS

Skin
Cutaneous toxicity / skin toxicity [2]
Diaphoresis (19%)
Lipoatrophy [7]
Lipodystrophy / acquired generalized lipodystrophy [9]
Rash (40%)
Stevens-Johnson syndrome and toxic epidermal necrolysis (SJS/TEN) [3]

Central Nervous System
Chills (50%)
Neurotoxicity [4]
Peripheral neuropathy (52%) [11]

Endocrine/Metabolic
Acidosis (includes lactic acidosis) [11]
Diabetes mellitus [2]
Fat distribution abnormality [4]
Gynecomastia [4]

Gastrointestinal/Hepatic
Diarrhea (50%)
Hepatotoxicity / liver injury / acute liver injury / drug-induced liver injury (DILI) [2]
Nausea (39%)
Pancreatitis / acute pancreatitis [6]
Vomiting (39%)

Neuromuscular/Skeletal
Myalgia/Myopathy (32%) [2]

Renal
Fanconi syndrome (proximal tubular dysfunction) [2]

Other
Adverse effects / adverse reactions [3]
Allergic reactions (9%)

STREPTOKINASE

Trade names: Kabikinase (Pfizer), Streptase (AstraZeneca)
Indications: Pulmonary embolism, acute myocardial infarction
Class: Fibrinolytic
Half-life: 83 minutes
Clinically important, potentially hazardous interactions with: bivalirudin, lepirudin

---

Skin
Anaphylactoid reactions / anaphylaxis (includes anaphylactic shock) [2]
Angioedema (formerly named angioneurotic edema) (>10%) [2]
Diaphoresis (<10%)
Exanthems (<5%) [2]
Pruritus (itching) (<10%)
Purpura [2]
Rash (<10%)
Serum sickness [4]
Serum sickness-like reaction [3]
Urticaria / hives (<5%)
Vasculitis (angiitis) / cutaneous vasculitis (angiitis) [7]

Neuromuscular/Skeletal
Rhabdomyolysis [2]

Ocular
Periorbital edema (>10%)

Other
Allergic reactions (4%) [4]

STREPTOMYCIN

Trade name: Streptomycin (Pfizer)
Indications: Tuberculosis
Class: Antibiotic, Antibiotic; aminoglycoside, Antimicrobial, Drug-resistant antituberculosis agent
Half-life: 2–5 hours
Clinically important, potentially hazardous interactions with: aldesleukin, aminoglycosides, atracurium, bacitracin, bumetanide, doxacurium, ethacrynic acid, furosemide, methoxyflurane, neostigmine, non-depolarizing muscle relaxants, pancuronium, polypeptide antibiotics, rocuronium, succinylcholine, teicoplanin, torsemide, vecuronium
Important contra-indications noted in the prescribing guidelines for: nursing mothers
Note: Aminoglycosides may cause neurotoxicity and/or nephrotoxicity.

Skin
Anaphylactoid reactions / anaphylaxis (includes anaphylactic shock) [3]
Dermatitis [2]

DRESS syndrome (Drug-induced hypersensitivity syndrome) [3]
Erythema multiforme [4]
Exanthems (>5%) [8]
Exfoliative dermatitis [11]
Lupus erythematosus (subacute cutaneous lupus erythematosus (SCLE)) [5]
Nicolau syndrome [2]
Photosensitivity [2]
Pruritus (itching) [2]
Purpura [3]
Stevens-Johnson syndrome and toxic epidermal necrolysis (SJS/TEN) [12]
Urticaria / hives [3]

Mucosal
Cheilitis (inflammation of the lips) (2%)
Glossitis (inflammation of the tongue) (2%)
Oral mucosal eruption [2]
Stomatitis (oral mucositis) [2]

Ocular
Optic neuropathy [2]

Otic
Ototoxicity [7]

Renal
Nephrotoxicity / kidney injury / acute kidney injury (AKI) / drug-induced kidney injury [2]

Other
Adverse effects / adverse reactions [2]
Allergic reactions [2]

STREPTOZOCIN

Trade name: Zanosar (Gensia)
Indications: Carcinoma of the pancreas, carcinoid tumor, Hodgkin's disease
Class: Alkylating agent, Antineoplastic / anticancer agent (see also Immune checkpoint inhibitor)
Half-life: 35 minutes
Clinically important, potentially hazardous interactions with: aldesleukin
Important contra-indications noted in the prescribing guidelines for: nursing mothers

---

Gastrointestinal/Hepatic
Abdominal pain [2]
Nausea [2]
Vomiting [2]

Hematologic
Neutropenia (neutrophils decreased) [2]

Local
Injection-site pain (<10%)

Neuromuscular/Skeletal
Asthenia / fatigue [2]

Renal
Nephrotoxicity / kidney injury / acute kidney injury (AKI) / drug-induced kidney injury [2]

STRONTIUM RANELATE

Trade name: Protelos (Servier)
Indications: Postmenopausal osteoporosis
Class: Bone formation stimulant, Bone resorption inhibitor
Half-life: 60 hours
Clinically important, potentially hazardous interactions with: antacids, calcium products, chlortetracycline, ciprofloxacin, demeclocycline, doxycycline, levofloxacin, lymecycline, minocycline, moxifloxacin, norfloxacin, ofloxacin, oxytetracycline, quinolone antibiotics, tetracycline, tigecycline
Important contra-indications noted in the prescribing guidelines for: nursing mothers; pediatric patients

---

Skin
Dermatitis (2%) [2]
DRESS syndrome (Drug-induced hypersensitivity syndrome) [12]
Eczema / eczematous reaction / eczematous eruption (2%)
Hypersensitivity [4]
Stevens-Johnson syndrome and toxic epidermal necrolysis (SJS/TEN) [4]

Hair
Alopecia / hair loss [2]

Cardiovascular
Venous thromboembolism (3%) [4]

Central Nervous System
Headache (3%) [5]
Memory loss/memory impaired (2%)

Gastrointestinal/Hepatic
Diarrhea (7%) [8]
Gastritis / pangastritis / gastric irritation [3]
Nausea (7%) [6]

Other
Adverse effects / adverse reactions [6]
Death [2]

SUCCIMER

Synonym: DMSA
Trade name: Chemet (Sanofi-Aventis)
Indications: Heavy metal poisoning
Class: Chelator
Half-life: 2 days
Clinically important, potentially hazardous interactions with: other chelating agents
Important contra-indications noted in the prescribing guidelines for: nursing mothers; pediatric patients

---

Skin
Candidiasis / candidosis (16%)
Exanthems (11%)
Pruritus (itching) (11%)
Rash (<11%) [2]

Mucosal
Mucocutaneous eruption (includes fixed eruption) (11%)

Central Nervous System
Chills (16%)
Dysgeusia (taste perversion) (metallic) (21%)
Fever (pyrexia) (includes hyperpyrexia) (16%)
Headache (16%)
Pain (3%)
Paresthesias (13%)

Gastrointestinal/Hepatic
Abdominal pain (16%)

Neuromuscular/Skeletal
Back pain (16%)

Respiratory
Influenza- ('flu)-like syndrome (16%)

SUCCINYLCHOLINE

Synonym: suxamethonium
Trade name: Anectine (Sabex)
Indications: Skeletal muscle relaxation during general anesthesia
Class: Cholinesterase inhibitor, Depolarizing muscle relaxant
Half-life: N/A
Clinically important, potentially hazardous interactions with: amikacin, aminoglycosides, donepezil, galantamine, gentamicin, hydromorphone, kanamycin, levomepromazine, neomycin, neostigmine, paromomycin, physostigmine, pipecuronium, pralidoxime, quinine, streptomycin, tapentadol, thalidomide, tobramycin, vancomycin, vecuronium
Important contra-indications noted in the prescribing guidelines for: the elderly; nursing mothers
Warning: RISK OF CARDIAC ARREST FROM HYPERKALEMIC RHABDOMYOLYSIS

Skin
Anaphylactoid reactions / anaphylaxis (includes anaphylactic shock) [13]

Mucosal
Sialorrhea (ptyalism; hypersalivation) (<10%)

Cardiovascular
Bradycardia / sinus bradycardia [3]

Central Nervous System
Malignant hyperthermia [7]
Myokymia / twitching / fasciculation [7]
Paralysis / paraplegia [3]

Endocrine/Metabolic
Hyperkalemia [8]

Neuromuscular/Skeletal
Myalgia/Myopathy [12]
Rhabdomyolysis [27]

Other
Death [3]

SUCRALFATE

Trade name: Carafate (Aptalis)
Indications: Duodenal ulcer
Class: Chelator
Half-life: N/A
Clinically important, potentially hazardous interactions with: anagrelide, chlortetracycline, ciprofloxacin, clorazepate, demeclocycline, doxycycline, gemifloxacin, ketoconazole, lansoprazole, levofloxacin, lomefloxacin, lymecycline, minocycline, moxifloxacin, norfloxacin, ofloxacin, oxtriphylline, oxytetracycline, paricalcitol, phenytoin, sparfloxacin, tetracycline, tigecycline, voriconazole
Important contra-indications noted in the prescribing guidelines for: the elderly; nursing mothers; pediatric patients
Note: Sucralfate use can lead to symptoms of aluminum toxicity.

Mucosal
Xerostomia (dry mouth) [2]

Gastrointestinal/Hepatic
Constipation (2%)

SUCRALOSE

Trade name: Splenda (McNeil)
Indications: Weight reduction
Class: Sweetening agent
Half-life: 2–5 hours
Clinically important, potentially hazardous interactions with: none known

Central Nervous System
Migraine [3]

SUFENTANIL

Trade name: Sufenta (Akorn)
Indications: Epidural and general anesthesia
Class: Anesthetic; general, Opiate agonist
Half-life: 152 minutes
Clinically important, potentially hazardous interactions with: cimetidine

Skin
Pruritus (itching) [10]

Cardiovascular
Bradycardia / sinus bradycardia [2]
Hypotension [2]

Gastrointestinal/Hepatic
Nausea [3]
Vomiting [4]

Respiratory
Cough [7]
Respiratory depression [2]

SUGAMMADEX

Trade name: Bridion (Organon)
Indications: Reversal of neuromuscular blockade induced by rocuronium bromide and vecuronium bromide in adults undergoing surgery
Class: Cyclodextrin, Selective relaxant binding agent
Half-life: ~2 hours
Clinically important, potentially hazardous interactions with: toremifene
Pregnancy category: No data available
Important contra-indications noted in the prescribing guidelines for: the elderly; nursing mothers; pediatric patients

Skin
Anaphylactoid reactions / anaphylaxis (includes anaphylactic shock) [16]
Erythema (<2%)
Hypersensitivity [7]
Pruritus (itching) (2–3%)

Mucosal
Oropharyngeal pain (3–5%)
Xerostomia (dry mouth) (<2%) [2]

Cardiovascular
Atrioventricular block [2]
Bradycardia / sinus bradycardia (<5%) [9]
Cardiac arrest [3]
Hypotension [3]
QT interval prolonged / QT prolongation (<6%) [2]
Tachycardia (2–5%)

Central Nervous System
Anxiety (<3%)
Chills (3–7%)
Depression (<2%)
Dysgeusia (taste perversion) [3]
Fever (pyrexia) (includes hyperpyrexia) (5–9%)
Headache (5–10%) [2]
Hypoesthesia / hypesthesia (numbness) (<3%)
Insomnia (2–5%)
Pain (36–52%)
Restlessness (<2%)
Somnolence (drowsiness) [2]
Vertigo / dizziness (3–6%)

Endocrine/Metabolic
Creatine phosphokinase (CPK) / creatine kinase increased (hyperCKemia) (<2%)
Hypocalcemia (<2%)

Gastrointestinal/Hepatic
Abdominal pain (4–6%)
Diarrhea [2]
Flatulence (<3%)
Nausea (23–26%) [3]
Vomiting (11–15%) [2]

Hematologic
Anemia (<2%)

Local
Injection-site pain (4–6%)

Neuromuscular/Skeletal
Bone pain / joint pain (<2%)
Myalgia/Myopathy (<2%)
Pain in extremities (<6%)

Respiratory
Bronchospasm [4]
Cough (<8%)

Other
Adverse effects / adverse reactions [2]
Allergic reactions [2]

SULFACETAMIDE

Trade names: Blephamide (Allergan), Klaron (Dermik), Ovace (Healthpoint), Plexion (Medicis), Rosula (Doak), Sulfacet Sodium (Dermik), Sulfacet-R (Dermik), Vasocidin (Novartis), Vasosulf (Novartis)
Indications: Infectious conjunctivitis, acne vulgaris, seborrheic dermatitis
Class: Antibiotic, Antibiotic; sulfonamide, Antimicrobial
Half-life: 7–13 hours
Clinically important, potentially hazardous interactions with: anticoagulants, cyclosporine, silver salts
Note: Sulfacetamide is a sulfonamide and can be absorbed systemically. Sulfonamides can produce severe, possibly fatal, reactions such as toxic epidermal necrolysis and Stevens-Johnson syndrome.

Skin
Exfoliative dermatitis (<10%)
Stevens-Johnson syndrome and toxic epidermal necrolysis (SJS/TEN) (<10%) [2]

SULFADIAZINE

Indications: Various infections caused by susceptible organisms
Class: Antibiotic, Antibiotic; sulfonamide, Antimicrobial
Half-life: 17 hours
Clinically important, potentially hazardous interactions with: anticoagulants, BCG vaccine, cyclosporine, methotrexate
Important contra-indications noted in the prescribing guidelines for: nursing mothers
Note: Sulfadiazine is a sulfonamide and can be absorbed systemically. Sulfonamides can produce severe, possibly fatal, reactions such as toxic epidermal necrolysis and Stevens-Johnson syndrome.

Skin
DRESS syndrome (Drug-induced hypersensitivity syndrome) [2]
Fixed eruption / fixed drug eruption (12%) [2]
Hypersensitivity [4]
Photosensitivity (>10%)
Pruritus (itching) (>10%)
Rash (>10%)
Stevens-Johnson syndrome and toxic epidermal necrolysis (SJS/TEN) (<10%) [4]

Genitourinary
Crystalluria [5]

Renal
Nephrolithiasis (kidney stones / renal calculi) [3]
Nephrotoxicity / kidney injury / acute kidney injury (AKI) / drug-induced kidney injury [2]
Renal failure [7]

SULFA-METHOXAZOLE

Trade names: Bactrim (Women First), Septra (Monarch)
Indications: Various infections caused by susceptible organisms
Class: Antibiotic, Antibiotic; sulfonamide, Antimicrobial, Folic acid antagonist
Half-life: 7–12 hours
Clinically important, potentially hazardous interactions with: anticoagulants, azathioprine, cyclosporine, methotrexate, pralatrexate, probenecid, warfarin
Note: Sulfamethoxazole is a sulfonamide and can be absorbed systemically. Sulfonamides can produce severe, possibly fatal, reactions such as toxic epidermal necrolysis and Stevens-Johnson syndrome.
Sulfamethoxazole is commonly used in conjunction with trimethoprim (see separate entry for co-trimoxazole).

Skin
AGEP [3]
Anaphylactoid reactions / anaphylaxis (includes anaphylactic shock) [4]
Angioedema (formerly named angioneurotic edema) (<5%)
Dermatitis [4]
DRESS syndrome (Drug-induced hypersensitivity syndrome) [4]

Erythema multiforme [15]
Erythema nodosum [2]
Exanthems (<5%) [30]
Exfoliative dermatitis [3]
Fixed eruption / fixed drug eruption [29]
Hypersensitivity [6]
Linear IgA bullous dermatosis [3]
Lupus erythematosus (subacute cutaneous lupus erythematosus (SCLE)) [3]
Photosensitivity (>10%) [3]
Pruritus (itching) (10%) [7]
Purpura [3]
Pustules / pustular eruption [6]
Radiation recall dermatitis [3]
Rash (>10%) [3]
Stevens-Johnson syndrome and toxic epidermal necrolysis (SJS/TEN) (<10%) [47]
Sweet's syndrome [3]
Urticaria / hives [9]
Vasculitis (angiitis) / cutaneous vasculitis (angiitis) [6]

Mucosal
Oral mucosal eruption [2]
Oral ulceration [2]

Hematologic
Thrombocytopenia / platelets decreased [2]

Neuromuscular/Skeletal
Rhabdomyolysis [4]

Renal
Nephrotoxicity / kidney injury / acute kidney injury (AKI) / drug-induced kidney injury [2]

Other
Allergic reactions [2]
Side effects (2%) [2]

SULFASALAZINE

Synonyms: salicylazosulfapyridine; salazopyrin; salazosulfapyridine
Trade name: Azulfidine (Pfizer)
Indications: Inflammatory bowel disease, ulcerative colitis, rheumatoid arthritis
Class: Aminosalicylate, Disease-modifying antirheumatic drug (DMARD), Sulfonamide
Half-life: 5–10 hours
Clinically important, potentially hazardous interactions with: cholestyramine, methotrexate, safinamide
Important contra-indications noted in the prescribing guidelines for: nursing mothers; pediatric patients
Note: Sulfasalazine is a sulfonamide and can be absorbed systemically. Sulfonamides can produce severe, possibly fatal, reactions such as toxic epidermal necrolysis and Stevens-Johnson syndrome.
Contra-indicated in patients with intestinal or urinary obstruction, or with porphyria.

Skin
AGEP [3]
Anaphylactoid reactions / anaphylaxis (includes anaphylactic shock) [4]
Angioedema (formerly named angioneurotic edema) [3]
Bullous pemphigoid / pemphigoid [3]
Cyanosis / acrocyanosis (<10%)
Dermatitis [2]
DRESS syndrome (Drug-induced hypersensitivity syndrome) [42]
Erythema multiforme [8]
Erythema nodosum [3]
Exanthems (2–23%) [23]
Exfoliative dermatitis [5]
Fixed eruption / fixed drug eruption [7]
Flushing / rubefaction [2]
Hypersensitivity (<5%) [23]
Lichen planus (includes hypertrophic lichen planus) [3]
Lupus erythematosus (subacute cutaneous lupus erythematosus (SCLE)) [34]
Photosensitivity (10%) [4]
Pigmentation (Skin) (includes hyperpigmentation) [3]
Pruritus (itching) (10%) [8]
Pseudolymphoma / cutaneous pseudolymphoma [2]
Pustules / pustular eruption [2]
Rash (>10%) [19]
Raynaud's phenomenon [3]
Stevens-Johnson syndrome and toxic epidermal necrolysis (SJS/TEN) [20]
Sweet's syndrome [2]
Urticaria / hives (<5%) [11]
Vasculitis (angiitis) / cutaneous vasculitis (angiitis) [4]

Hair
Alopecia / hair loss [6]

Mucosal
Mucocutaneous reactions (6%) [2]
Oral mucosal eruption [4]
Oral ulceration [3]
Stomatitis (oral mucositis) (<10%)

Central Nervous System
Anorexia (10%)
Aseptic meningitis [3]
Fever (pyrexia) (includes hyperpyrexia) [4]
Headache (10%) [7]
Vertigo / dizziness (<10%)

Gastrointestinal/Hepatic
Abdominal pain (<10%)
Dyspepsia / functional dyspepsia (indigestion) (see also gastroparesis) (10%) [3]
Hepatotoxicity / liver injury / acute liver injury / drug-induced liver injury (DILI) [14]
Nausea (10%) [7]
Neutropenic enterocolitis [2]
Pancreatitis / acute pancreatitis [6]
Vomiting (10%) [2]

Hematologic
Agranulocytosis / severe selective neutropenia [8]
Anemia (<10%)
Leukocytopenia (leukopenia) / leukocytes (white blood cells) decreased (<10%) [4]
Neutropenia (neutrophils decreased) [3]
Thrombocytopenia / platelets decreased (<10%)

Neuromuscular/Skeletal
Arthralgia [2]
Asthenia / fatigue [5]

Ocular
Conjunctival pigmentation [2]

Renal
Nephrotoxicity / kidney injury / acute kidney injury (AKI) / drug-induced kidney injury [4]
Renal failure [2]

Respiratory
Pulmonary toxicity [3]
Upper respiratory tract infection [3]

Other
Adverse effects / adverse reactions [9]
Death [5]
Side effects (5%)

SULFINPYRAZONE

Trade name: Anturane (Novartis)
Indications: Gouty arthritis
Class: Sulfonamide, Uricosuric
Half-life: 2–7 hours
Clinically important, potentially hazardous interactions with: anisindione, anticoagulants, ceftobiprole, dabigatran, dicumarol, enoxaparin, penicillin G, penicillin V, tinzaparin, warfarin
Pregnancy category: category C in first and second trimester; category D in third trimester
Note: Sulfinpyrazone is a sulfonamide and can be absorbed systemically. Sulfonamides can produce severe, possibly fatal, reactions such as toxic epidermal necrolysis and Stevens-Johnson syndrome.

Skin
Dermatitis (<10%)
Exanthems (<3%)
Rash (<10%)

Renal
Nephrotoxicity / kidney injury / acute kidney injury (AKI) / drug-induced kidney injury [15]

SULFISOXAZOLE

Trade name: Gantrisin (Roche)
Indications: Various infections caused by susceptible organisms
Class: Antibiotic, Antibiotic; sulfonamide, Antimicrobial
Half-life: 3–7 hours
Clinically important, potentially hazardous interactions with: anticoagulants, cyclosporine, methotrexate, warfarin
Note: Sulfisoxazole is a sulfonamide and can be absorbed systemically. Sulfonamides can produce severe, possibly fatal, reactions such as toxic epidermal necrolysis and Stevens-Johnson syndrome.

Skin
Anaphylactoid reactions / anaphylaxis (includes anaphylactic shock) [2]
Erythema multiforme [7]
Exanthems (<5%) [9]
Exfoliative dermatitis [2]
Fixed eruption / fixed drug eruption [6]
Lupus erythematosus (subacute cutaneous lupus erythematosus (SCLE)) [2]
Photosensitivity (>10%) [4]
Pruritus (itching) (<10%) [4]
Purpura [4]
Rash (>10%)
Stevens-Johnson syndrome and toxic epidermal necrolysis (SJS/TEN) (<10%) [8]
Urticaria / hives [4]
Vasculitis (angiitis) / cutaneous vasculitis (angiitis) [3]

Mucosal
Oral ulceration [2]

Other
Allergic reactions (3%)
Side effects (2%)

SULFITES

Family: N/A
Scientific names: *Ammonium bisulfite [AB], potassium bisulfite [PB], potassium metabisulfite [PM], sodium bisulfite [SB], sodium metabisulfite [SM], sodium sulfite [SS], sulfur dioxide [SD]*
Indications: Food additive, drug additive, sanitary agent
Class: Trace element
Half-life: N/A
Clinically important, potentially hazardous interactions with: aspirin, NSAIDs

---

Skin
- Anaphylactoid reactions / anaphylaxis (includes anaphylactic shock) [11]
- Angioedema (formerly named angioneurotic edema) [2]
- Dermatitis [15]
- Edema / fluid retention [2]
- Hypersensitivity [6]
- Rash [2]
- Sensitivity [4]
- Urticaria / hives [6]

Respiratory
- Pulmonary toxicity [2]
- Rhinitis / rhinosinusitis (see also sinusitis) [3]

Other
- Adverse effects / adverse reactions [5]
- Allergic reactions [6]
- Death [2]

SULINDAC

Trade name: Clinoril (Merck)
Indications: Arthritis
Class: Non-steroidal anti-inflammatory (NSAID)
Half-life: 7.8–16.4 hours
Clinically important, potentially hazardous interactions with: methotrexate, warfarin
Pregnancy category: category C in first and second trimesters; category D in third trimester
Important contra-indications noted in the prescribing guidelines for: nursing mothers; pediatric patients
Note: NSAIDs may cause an increased risk of serious cardiovascular and gastrointestinal adverse events, which can be fatal. This risk may increase with duration of use.

Skin
- Anaphylactoid reactions / anaphylaxis (includes anaphylactic shock) [4]
- Erythema multiforme [8]
- Exanthems (<5%) [9]
- Fixed eruption / fixed drug eruption [5]
- Photosensitivity [2]
- Pruritus (itching) (<10%) [5]
- Purpura [2]
- Rash (>10%)
- Stevens-Johnson syndrome and toxic epidermal necrolysis (SJS/TEN) [16]
- Urticaria / hives [4]

Mucosal
- Oral mucosal eruption (3%) [2]
- Stomatitis (oral mucositis) [2]
- Xerostomia (dry mouth) [2]

Gastrointestinal/Hepatic
- Hepatotoxicity / liver injury / acute liver injury / drug-induced liver injury (DILI) [4]
- Pancreatitis / acute pancreatitis [3]

SULPIRIDE / LEVOSULPIRIDE

Synonym: Levosulpiride
Trade name: Dolmatil (Sanofi-Aventis)
Indications: Acute and chronic schizophrenia
Class: Dopamine receptor antagonist
Half-life: 8 hours
Clinically important, potentially hazardous interactions with: alcohol, amiodarone, amphotericin B, cisapride, clonidine, digitalis, diltiazem, disopyramide, droperidol, erythromycin, glucocorticoids, halofantrine, haloperidol, hypokalemic diruretics, levodopa, lithium, pentamidine, pimozide, quinidine, sotalol, stimulant laxatives, tetracosactides, thioridazine
Important contra-indications noted in the prescribing guidelines for: the elderly; nursing mothers; pediatric patients
Note: Levosulpiride is the (S)-isomer.

Skin
- Jaundice (see also cholestasis / cholestatic jaundice) [2]
- Ulcerations [2]

Cardiovascular
- QT interval prolonged / QT prolongation [3]
- Torsades de pointes [3]
- Ventricular arrhythmia [2]

Central Nervous System
- Akathisia [2]
- Movement disorder(s) [3]
- Neuroleptic malignant syndrome [3]
- Parkinsonism [6]
- Rabbit syndrome (oral vertical dyskinesia) [2]
- Tardive syndrome / tardive dyskinesia [7]
- Tremor [3]

Endocrine/Metabolic
- Amenorrhea [5]
- Galactorrhea [5]
- Hyperprolactinemia [4]

Gastrointestinal/Hepatic
- Constipation [2]

Multi-Organ and/or Multi-Metabolic Adverse Reactions
- Pheochromocytoma crisis / paraganglioma crisis [2]

Neuromuscular/Skeletal
- Dystonia [3]

Other
- Death [2]

SUMATRIPTAN

Trade names: Alsuma (King), Imigran (GSK), Imitrex (GSK), Onzetra Xsail (Avanir), Sumavel DosePro (Endo), Zecuity (Teva)
Indications: Migraine attacks, cluster headaches
Class: 5-HT1 agonist, Serotonin receptor agonist, Triptan
Half-life: 2.5 hours
Clinically important, potentially hazardous interactions with: citalopram, dihydroergotamine, ergot-containing drugs, escitalopram, fluoxetine, fluvoxamine, isocarboxazid, MAO inhibitors, methysergide, naratriptan, nefazodone, paroxetine hydrochloride, phenelzine, rizatriptan, sertraline, sibutramine, SNRIs, SSRIs, St John's wort, tranylcypromine, venlafaxine, zolmitriptan
Important contra-indications noted in the prescribing guidelines for: the elderly; nursing mothers; pediatric patients
Note: Contra-indicated in patients with Wolff-Parkinson-White syndrome, peripheral vascular disease, ischemic bowel disease, uncontrolled hypertension, severe hepatic impairment or a history of coronary artery disease, coronary vasospasm, stroke, transient ischemic attack, or hemiplegic or basilar migraine; or with recent (within 24 hours) use of another 5-HT1 agonist (e.g. another triptan) or an ergotamine-containing medication, or current or recent (past 2 weeks) use of a monoamine oxidase-A inhibitor.

Skin
- Burning / skin burning sensation (<10%)
- Diaphoresis (2%)
- Flushing / rubefaction (7%) [4]
- Hot flashes / hot flushes (>10%)
- Hypersensitivity [2]

Mucosal
- Nasal discomfort [3]
- Rhinorrhea [2]
- Xerostomia (dry mouth) [2]

Cardiovascular
- Chest pain (<2%) [7]
- Hypertension [2]
- Myocardial infarction [5]

Central Nervous System
- Dysgeusia (taste perversion) [11]
- Headache [2]
- Neurotoxicity [3]
- Pain (<2%) [4]
- Paresthesias (3–5%) [11]
- Somnolence (drowsiness) [3]
- Stroke / cerebrovascular accident [2]
- Vertigo / dizziness (<2%) [10]
- Warm feeling (includes feeling hot) (2–3%)

Gastrointestinal/Hepatic
- Colitis [2]
- Nausea [13]

Local
- Application-site erythema [2]
- Injection-site edema [2]
- Injection-site reaction (10–58%) [2]

Neuromuscular/Skeletal
- Asthenia / fatigue (2–3%) [5]
- Jaw pain (<3%)
- Muscle spasm [2]
- Myalgia/Myopathy (2%) [2]
- Neck pain (<3%)

Respiratory
- Nasopharyngitis [2]
- Rhinitis / rhinosinusitis (see also sinusitis) [2]
- Upper respiratory tract infection [2]

Other
- Adverse effects / adverse reactions [10]

SUNITINIB

Trade name: Sutent (Pfizer)
Indications: Gastrointestinal stromal tumor, advanced renal cell carcinoma, advanced pancreatic neuroendocrine tumor
Class: Angiogenesis inhibitor / antiangiogenic agent, Antineoplastic / anticancer agent (see also Immune checkpoint inhibitor), RET (Rearranged during Transfection) kinase inhibitor, Tyrosine kinase inhibitor, Vascular endothelial growth factor (VEGF) inhibitor / antagonist
Half-life: 40–60 hours
Clinically important, potentially hazardous interactions with: atazanavir, bevacizumab, carbamazepine, clarithromycin, clozapine, dexamethasone, digoxin, efavirenz, grapefruit juice, indinavir, itraconazole, ketoconazole, nefazodone, nelfinavir, phenobarbital, phenytoin, rifabutin, rifampin, rifapentine, ritonavir, saquinavir, St John's wort, telithromycin, temsirolimus, voriconazole
Important contra-indications noted in the prescribing guidelines for: nursing mothers; pediatric patients
Note: [G] = treated for gastrointestinal tumor; [R] = treated for renal cell carcinoma; [P] treated for pancreatic neuroendocrine tumor.
Warning: HEPATOTOXICITY

Skin
Acral erythema [2]
Cutaneous toxicity / skin toxicity [24]
Edema / fluid retention [6]
Erythema [6]
Facial edema [3]
Hand–foot syndrome (palmar–plantar erythrodysesthesia) (12–14%) [78]
Lesions (includes skin lesions) [2]
Nevi (naevi) [2]
Peripheral edema [R] (17%)
Pigmentation (Skin) (includes hyperpigmentation) [15]
Pruritus (itching) [R] [3]
Pyoderma gangrenosum [10]
Rash (14–38%) [17]
Thrombocytopenic purpura [4]
Xerosis / xeroderma (17%) [3]

Hair
Alopecia / hair loss (5–12%) [6]
Hair pigmentation [G] [8]

Nails
Splinter hemorrhage [2]
Subungual hematoma / subungual hemorrhage [4]

Mucosal
Burning Mouth Syndrome / glossodynia / glossalgia / glossopyrosis (also includes stomatodynia / oral dysesthesia / stomatopyrosis) [R] [P] (15%)
Epistaxis (nosebleed) [2]
Mucosal inflammation [4]
Mucositis (29–53%) [19]
Stomatitis (oral mucositis) [21]
Xerostomia (dry mouth) [R] [P] [2]

Cardiovascular
Aortic dissection [3]
Cardiac failure [2]
Cardiomyopathy [2]
Cardiotoxicity [9]
Congestive heart failure [2]
Hypertension [64]
QT interval prolonged / QT prolongation [2]
Ventricular arrhythmia [2]

Central Nervous System
Anorexia [8]
Dysgeusia (taste perversion) (21–43%) [6]
Encephalopathy (includes hepatic encephalopathy) [8]
Fever (pyrexia) (includes hyperpyrexia) [R] (15–18%) [2]
Guillain-Barré syndrome / acute inflammatory demyelinating polyradiculoneuropathy / acute motor axonal neuropathy [3]
Headache (13–25%) [4]
Leukoencephalopathy / posterior reversible encephalopathy syndrome (PRES) [9]
Neurotoxicity [R] (10%)
Pain [R] (18%)
Vertigo / dizziness [R] (16%)

Endocrine/Metabolic
ALT increased [4]
Appetite decreased [2]
AST increased [2]
Hyperammonemia [8]
Hyperlipasemia [2]
Hypothyroidism [R] [31]
Serum creatinine increased [2]
Thyroid dysfunction [8]

Gastrointestinal/Hepatic
Abdominal pain (20–33%) [3]
Constipation [3]
Diarrhea [42]
Dyspepsia / functional dyspepsia (indigestion) (see also gastroparesis) [R] [P] [3]
Esophagitis [2]
Gastrointestinal bleeding [4]
Gastrointestinal disorder / discomfort [2]
Hepatotoxicity / liver injury / acute liver injury / drug-induced liver injury (DILI) [9]
Nausea [18]
Pneumatosis intestinalis / pneumatosis cystoides intestinalis [6]
Vomiting [16]

Hematologic
Anemia [22]
Bleeding [5]
Cytopenia [2]
Hemorrhage [2]
Hemotoxicity [3]
Leukocytopenia (leukopenia) / leukocytes (white blood cells) decreased [21]
Lymphopenia (lymphocytopenia) / lymphocytes decreased [10]
Myelosuppression / bone marrow suppression / myelotoxicity [6]
Neutropenia (neutrophils decreased) [50]
Thrombocytopenia / platelets decreased [47]
Thrombotic microangiopathy [3]

Neuromuscular/Skeletal
Arthralgia [R] (12–28%)
Asthenia / fatigue (22%) [76]
Back pain [R] (11–17%)
Myalgia/Myopathy [G] (14–17%) [2]
Osteonecrosis / avascular necrosis (includes steroid-induced osteonecrosis of the femoral head) [4]

Ocular
Epiphora [R] (6%)
Periorbital edema [R] (7%)

Renal
Nephrotoxicity / kidney injury / acute kidney injury (AKI) / drug-induced kidney injury [5]
Proteinuria [6]
Renal function abnormal / renal dysfunction [2]

Respiratory
Cough [R] (8–17%) [2]
Dyspnea / shortness of breath [5]
Pulmonary toxicity [3]
Radiation recall pneumonitis [2]

Other
Adverse effects / adverse reactions [17]
Death [9]
Side effects [3]

TACRINE

Trade name: Cognex (First Horizon)
Indications: Dementia of Alzheimer's disease
Class: Cholinesterase inhibitor
Half-life: 1.5–4 hours
Clinically important, potentially hazardous interactions with: fluvoxamine, galantamine, ibuprofen, norfloxacin, oxtriphylline

---

Skin
Exanthems (7%)
Flushing / rubefaction (3%)
Pruritus (itching) (7%)
Purpura (2%)
Rash (7%)
Urticaria / hives (7%)

Cardiovascular
Bradycardia / sinus bradycardia [2]

Central Nervous System
Parkinsonism [2]
Tremor (<10%)

Gastrointestinal/Hepatic
Hepatotoxicity / liver injury / acute liver injury / drug-induced liver injury (DILI) [12]

Neuromuscular/Skeletal
Myalgia/Myopathy (9%)

TACROLIMUS

Trade names: Envarsus XR (Veloxis), Prograf (Astellas), Protopic (Astellas)
Indications: Prophylaxis of organ rejection, atopic dermatitis (topical)
Class: Calcineurin inhibitor, Immunosuppressant, Macrolactam
Half-life: ~8.7 hours
Clinically important, potentially hazardous interactions with: abatacept, afatinib, alefacept, amiodarone, amprenavir, atazanavir, azacitidine, beta blockers, betamethasone, boceprevir, bosentan, cabazitaxel, caspofungin, ceritinib, cinacalcet, cobicistat/elvitegravir/emtricitabine/tenofovir disoproxil, crizotinib, cyclosporine, CYP3A4 inhibitors and inducers, dabigatran, dairy products, danazol, darunavir, dasatinib, delavirdine, denileukin, dexlansoprazole, diclofenac, docetaxel, dronedarone, efavirenz, elbasvir & grazoprevir, eluxadoline, enzalutamide, erythromycin, etoricoxib, fingolimod, gefitinib, grapefruit juice, Hemophilus B vaccine, HMG-CoA reductase inhibitors, ibuprofen, immunosuppressants, indinavir, irbesartan, itraconazole, ketoconazole, leflunomide, lenalidomide, letermovir, lopinavir, lovastatin, meloxicam, mifepristone, mycophenolate, nelfinavir, nifedipine, olmesartan, omeprazole, oxaliplatin, pazopanib, pemetrexed, posaconazole, potassium, potassium-sparing

diuretics, pralatrexate, ribociclib, rifabutin, rifampin, rifapentine, sevelamer, simvastatin, sirolimus, St John's wort, telaprevir, telithromycin, temsirolimus, tinidazole, tipranavir, tofacitinib, triamcinolone, vaccines, viloxazine, voriconazole
Important contra-indications noted in the prescribing guidelines for: the elderly; nursing mothers; pediatric patients
Note: Between 25% and 31% of patients who receive tacrolimus are reported to experience some form of neurotoxic adverse events.
Warning: MALIGNANCIES AND SERIOUS INFECTIONS

Skin
Anaphylactoid reactions / anaphylaxis (includes anaphylactic shock) [4]
Bruise / bruising / contusion / ecchymosis (ecchymoses) (>3%)
Burning / skin burning sensation (46%) [13]
Cutaneous toxicity / skin toxicity [3]
Dermatitis [2]
Diaphoresis (>3%)
Edema / fluid retention (>10%)
Erythema (12%) [3]
Exanthems (4%) [2]
Flushing / rubefaction [4]
Folliculitis (10%) [2]
Graft-versus-host reaction [2]
Herpes simplex (13%) [4]
Herpes zoster [3]
Kaposi's sarcoma [2]
Kaposi's varicelliform eruption [2]
Lymphoma [2]
Peripheral edema (26%)
Photosensitivity (>3%)
Pigmentation (Skin) (includes hyperpigmentation) [2]
Pruritus (itching) (25–36%) [13]
Pustules / pustular eruption (6%)
Rash (24%) [2]
Rosacea [5]
Thrombocytopenic purpura [2]

Hair
Alopecia / hair loss (>3%) [7]
Hypertrichosis [2]

Mucosal
Gingival hyperplasia / gingival hypertrophy / gingival enlargement / gingival overgrowth [6]
Oral candidiasis (>3%)
Oral pigmentation [2]
Oral ulceration [2]

Cardiovascular
Cardiomyopathy [3]
Hypertension (49%) [10]
QT interval prolonged / QT prolongation [2]

Central Nervous System
Akinetic mutism / mutism [3]
Bradykinesia [2]
Catatonia [2]
Central pontine myelinolysis [3]
Dysarthria [2]
Encephalopathy (includes hepatic encephalopathy) [11]
Fever (pyrexia) (includes hyperpyrexia) (>10%) [2]
Headache [10]
Insomnia [2]
Leukoencephalopathy / posterior reversible encephalopathy syndrome (PRES) [20]
Neurotoxicity [14]
Pain [3]
Paresthesias (40%) [5]
Parkinsonism [5]
Psychosis [3]
Reversible cerebral vasoconstriction syndrome (RCVS) [2]
Seizures (<10%) [6]
Tremor (>10%) [13]
Vertigo / dizziness [3]

Endocrine/Metabolic
Diabetes mellitus [8]
Diabetic ketoacidosis [9]
Dyslipidemia [3]
Gynecomastia [3]
Hyperglycemia (includes glucose increased) [12]
Hyperkalemia [6]
Hyperlipidemia / lipids elevated [2]
Hypomagnesemia (>10%) [2]
Hyponatremia [6]
Hypophosphatemia (>10%)
Serum creatinine increased [4]
SIADH [2]
Weight loss [2]

Gastrointestinal/Hepatic
Abdominal pain [3]
Constipation (>10%)
Diarrhea (>10%) [7]
Dyspepsia / functional dyspepsia (indigestion) (see also gastroparesis) (>10%)
Dysphagia (>3%)
Hepatotoxicity / liver injury / acute liver injury / drug-induced liver injury (DILI) [12]
Nausea (>10%) [3]
Pancreatitis / acute pancreatitis [4]
Vomiting (>10%)

Genitourinary
Urinary tract infection [3]

Hematologic
Anemia (>10%) [2]
Angiopathy [4]
Hemolytic anemia [3]
Hemolytic uremic syndrome [18]
Leukocytopenia (leukopenia) / leukocytes (white blood cells) decreased (>10%) [5]
Myelosuppression / bone marrow suppression / myelotoxicity [2]
Neutropenia (neutrophils decreased) [4]
Pure red cell aplasia [3]
Thrombocytopenia / platelets decreased [2]
Thrombotic microangiopathy [9]

Local
Application-site burning [7]
Application-site erythema [3]
Application-site infection [2]
Application-site irritation [2]
Application-site pain [2]
Application-site pruritus [9]

Neuromuscular/Skeletal
Arthralgia (>10%) [2]
Asthenia / fatigue (>10%) [4]
Back pain (>10%)
Bone pain / joint pain [2]
Myalgia/Myopathy (>3%)

Ocular
Diplopia (double vision) [2]
Ocular burning [3]
Optic neuropathy [4]
Vision blurred [2]
Vision loss [4]

Otic
Tinnitus [2]

Renal
Nephropathy [3]
Nephrotoxicity / kidney injury / acute kidney injury (AKI) / drug-induced kidney injury [51]
Renal failure [2]
Renal function abnormal / renal dysfunction [5]

Respiratory
Cough (>10%)
Dyspnea / shortness of breath (>10%)
Influenza [2]
Pneumonia [3]
Pulmonary toxicity [2]

Other
Adverse effects / adverse reactions [23]
Cancer [2]
Cytomegalovirus infection [2]
Death [2]
Infection (>10%) [17]
Multiorgan failure [2]
Neoplasms [2]

TADALAFIL

Trade names: Adcirca (Lilly), Cialis (Lilly)
Indications: Erectile dysfunction, pulmonary arterial hypertension
Class: Phosphodiesterase type 5 (PDE5) inhibitor
Half-life: 15–18 hours
Clinically important, potentially hazardous interactions with: alcohol, alfuzosin, alpha blockers, amlodipine, amyl nitrite, angiotensin II receptor blockers, antifungals, antihypertensives, atazanavir, bendroflumethiazide, boceprevir, bosentan, clarithromycin, cobicistat/elvitegravir/emtricitabine/tenofovir alafenamide, cobicistat/elvitegravir/emtricitabine/tenofovir disoproxil, conivaptan, CYP3A4 inhibitors or inducers, darunavir, dasatinib, delavirdine, disopyramide, doxazosin, efavirenz, enalapril, erythromycin, etravirine, fosamprenavir, grapefruit juice, indinavir, itraconazole, ketoconazole, lopinavir, macrolide antibiotics, metoprolol, nelfinavir, nicorandil, nitrates, nitroglycerin, nitroprusside, oxcarbazepine, phosphodiesterase 5 inhibitors, rifampin, rifapentine, riociguat, ritonavir, sapropterin, saquinavir, St John's wort, tamsulosin, telaprevir, telithromycin, voriconazole
Pregnancy category: Cialis is not indicated for use in women
Important contra-indications noted in the prescribing guidelines for: pediatric patients

---

Skin
Diaphoresis (<2%)
Facial edema (<2%)
Fixed eruption / fixed drug eruption [6]
Flushing / rubefaction (2–3%) [16]
Peripheral edema [2]
Pruritus (itching) (<2%)
Rash (<2%)

Mucosal
Epistaxis (nosebleed) (<2%) [2]
Nasal congestion [4]
Rectal hemorrhage / rectal bleeding (<2%)
Xerostomia (dry mouth) (<2%)

Cardiovascular
Angina (<2%)
Chest pain (<2%)
Hypotension (<2%)
Myocardial infarction (<2%)

Palpitation (<2%)
Postural hypotension (<2%)
Tachycardia (<2%)

Central Nervous System
Amnesia [3]
Headache (4–15%) [38]
Hyperesthesia (<2%)
Hypoesthesia / hypesthesia (numbness) (<2%)
Insomnia (<2%)
Pain (<3%)
Paresthesias (<2%)
Somnolence (drowsiness) (<2%)
Syncope / fainting (<2%)
Vertigo / dizziness (<2%) [8]

Endocrine/Metabolic
GGT increased (<2%)

Gastrointestinal/Hepatic
Diarrhea [2]
Dyspepsia / functional dyspepsia (indigestion) (see also gastroparesis) [8]
Dysphagia (<2%)
Esophagitis (<2%)
Gastritis / pangastritis / gastric irritation (<2%)
Gastroesophageal reflux (<2%)
Hepatotoxicity / liver injury / acute liver injury / drug-induced liver injury (DILI) [2]
Loose stools / soft feces (<2%)
Nausea (<2%) [3]
Vomiting (<2%)

Genitourinary
Erection (<2%)
Priapism (spontaneous) (<2%) [2]

Hematologic
Anemia [2]

Neuromuscular/Skeletal
Arthralgia (<2%)
Asthenia / fatigue (<2%)
Back pain (2–6%) [22]
Myalgia/Myopathy (<4%) [15]
Neck pain (<2%)

Ocular
Chorioretinopathy [2]
Conjunctival hyperemia / conjunctival injection (<2%)
Conjunctivitis (conjunctival inflammation) (<2%)
Dyschromatopsia (<2%)
Eyelid edema / palpebral edema / blepharedema (<2%)
Eyelid pain (<2%)
Lacrimation (<2%)
Optic neuropathy [7]
Vision blurred (<2%)

Otic
Hearing loss (hypoacusis) (<2%) [4]
Tinnitus (<2%)

Respiratory
Dyspnea / shortness of breath (<2%)
Nasopharyngitis [2]
Pharyngitis (sore throat) (<2%)

Other
Adverse effects / adverse reactions [6]

TAFAMIDIS MEGLUMINE

Trade name: Vyndaqel (FoldRx Pharmaceuticals)
Indications: Cardiomyopathy of wild type or hereditary transthyretin-mediated amyloidosis in adults. Transthyretin familial amyloid polyneuropathy (TTR-FAP)
Class: Transthyretin stabilizer
Half-life: 49 hours
Clinically important, potentially hazardous interactions with: breast cancer resistance protein inhibitors, imatinib, methotrexate, rosuvastatin
Pregnancy category: Based on findings from animal studies, tafamidis may cause fetal harm when administered to a pregnant woman.

Gastrointestinal/Hepatic
Diarrhea [4]

Genitourinary
Urinary tract infection [2]

Other
Adverse effects / adverse reactions [2]

TAFENOQUINE

Trade name: Krintafel (GSK)
Indications: indicated for the radical cure (prevention of relapse) of *Plasmodium vivax* malaria in patients aged 16 years and older who are receiving appropriate antimalarial therapy for acute *P. vivax* infection
Class: Antimalarial
Half-life: ~15 days
Clinically important, potentially hazardous interactions with: none known
Pregnancy category: May cause hemolytic anemia in a fetus who is G6PD deficient. Treatment during pregnancy is not recommended
Important contra-indications noted in the prescribing guidelines for: nursing mothers

---

Skin
Hypersensitivity (<3%)

Central Nervous System
Abnormal dreams (<3%)
Anxiety (<3%)
Headache (5%)
Insomnia (<3%)
Somnolence (drowsiness) (<3%)
Vertigo / dizziness (8%)

Endocrine/Metabolic
ALT increased (<3%)
Creatine phosphokinase (CPK) / creatine kinase increased (hyperCKemia) (<3%)

Gastrointestinal/Hepatic
Abdominal pain [2]
Diarrhea [2]
Nausea (6%) [4]
Vomiting (6%)

Hematologic
Hemoglobin decreased (5%)
Methemoglobinemia (<3%)

Ocular
Keratopathy (<3%)
Photophobia (<3%)

Other
Adverse effects / adverse reactions [3]

TALAZOPARIB

Trade name: Talzenna (Pfizer)
Indications: indicated for the treatment of adult patients with deleterious or suspected deleterious germline BRCA-mutated (gBRCAm) HER2-negative locally advanced or metastatic breast cancer
Class: Poly (ADP-ribose) polymerase (PARP) inhibitor
Half-life: 90 hours
Clinically important, potentially hazardous interactions with: amiodarone, carvedilol, clarithromycin, itraconazole, verapamil
Pregnancy category: can cause embryo-fetal harm
Important contra-indications noted in the prescribing guidelines for: nursing mothers

---

Hair
Alopecia / hair loss (25%)

Mucosal
Stomatitis (oral mucositis) (8%) [2]

Central Nervous System
Dysgeusia (taste perversion) (10%)
Headache (33%)
Vertigo / dizziness (17%) [2]

Endocrine/Metabolic
ALP increased (36%)
ALT increased (33%)
Appetite decreased (21%)
AST increased (37%)
Hypocalcemia (28%)

Gastrointestinal/Hepatic
Abdominal pain (19%)
Diarrhea (22%)
Nausea (49%) [3]
Vomiting (25%)

Hematologic
Anemia (53%) [7]
Hemoglobin decreased (90%)
Leukocytopenia (leukopenia) / leukocytes (white blood cells) decreased (84%) [2]
Lymphopenia (lymphocytopenia) / lymphocytes decreased (7%)
Neutropenia (neutrophils decreased) (35%) [4]
Thrombocytopenia / platelets decreased (27%) [4]

Neuromuscular/Skeletal
Asthenia / fatigue (62%) [5]

TAMOXIFEN

Trade name: Nolvadex (AstraZeneca)
Indications: Advanced breast cancer
Class: Selective estrogen receptor modulator (SERM)
Half-life: 5–7 days
Clinically important, potentially hazardous interactions with: anastrozole, bexarotene, cinacalcet, delavirdine, droperidol, duloxetine, gadobenate, ginseng, norfloxacin, norfloxacin, paroxetine hydrochloride, rifapentine, terbinafine, tipranavir
Important contra-indications noted in the prescribing guidelines for: nursing mothers; pediatric patients

---

Skin
Carcinosarcoma [2]

Cutaneous toxicity / skin toxicity [3]
Diaphoresis [4]
Edema / fluid retention (2–6%) [3]
Exanthems (3%) [3]
Flushing / rubefaction (>10%) [9]
Hot flashes / hot flushes [18]
Lupus erythematosus (subacute cutaneous lupus erythematosus (SCLE)) [2]
Pruritus ani et vulvae [2]
Radiation recall dermatitis [6]
Rash (<10%) [2]
Sarcoma [9]
Tumors [3]
Vasculitis (angiitis) / cutaneous vasculitis (angiitis) [6]
Xerosis / xeroderma (7%)

Hair
Alopecia / hair loss [7]
Hirsutism [2]

Mucosal
Stomatitis (oral mucositis) [2]
Xerostomia (dry mouth) (7%) [2]

Cardiovascular
Myocardial ischemia [2]
QT interval prolonged / QT prolongation [3]
Thromboembolism [6]
Thrombophlebitis [3]
Venous thromboembolism [6]

Central Nervous System
Depression [5]
Headache [3]
Insomnia [4]
Mood changes (includes mood disorder) [3]
Parkinsonism [2]
Stroke / cerebrovascular accident [4]
Vertigo / dizziness [3]

Endocrine/Metabolic
ALP increased [2]
Amenorrhea [8]
Galactorrhea (<10%)
Hypercholesterolemia [2]
Hypertriglyceridemia (includes triglycerides increased) [7]
Libido decreased [4]
Weight gain [4]

Gastrointestinal/Hepatic
Hepatic steatosis [2]
Hepatotoxicity / liver injury / acute liver injury / drug-induced liver injury (DILI) [12]
Nausea [5]
Pancreatitis / acute pancreatitis [4]
Vomiting [4]

Genitourinary
Dyspareunia [4]
Endometrial cancer [5]
Ovarian cyst [2]
Ovarian hyperstimulation syndrome [2]
Sexual dysfunction [2]
Vaginal bleeding [4]
Vaginal discharge [5]
Vaginal dryness [5]

Hematologic
Hemolytic uremic syndrome [2]
Thrombosis [9]

Neuromuscular/Skeletal
Asthenia / fatigue [5]
Bone pain / joint pain [4]
Fractures [3]
Leg cramps [2]
Myalgia/Myopathy [4]
Osteoporosis [2]

Ocular
Cataract [9]
Keratopathy [4]
Macular edema [2]
Maculopathy [5]
Ocular adverse effect [6]
Ocular toxicity [6]
Optic neuritis / papillitis [2]
Retinopathy [5]
Vision impaired [3]

Respiratory
Pulmonary embolism [7]

Other
Death [3]
Teratogenicity [2]

TAMSULOSIN

Trade names: Flomax (Boehringer Ingelheim), Jalyn (GSK)
Indications: Benign prostatic hypertrophy
Class: Adrenergic alpha-receptor antagonist
Half-life: 9–13 hours
Clinically important, potentially hazardous interactions with: alpha adrenergic blockers, cimetidine, conivaptan, darunavir, delavirdine, erythromycin, indinavir, ketoconazole, paroxetine hydrochloride, phosphodiesterase 5 inhibitors, tadalafil, telithromycin, terbinafine, vardenafil, voriconazole, warfarin
Pregnancy category: not indicated for use in women; Jalyn is pregnancy category X
Important contra-indications noted in the prescribing guidelines for: nursing mothers; pediatric patients
Note: Jalyn is tamsulosin and dutasteride.

Mucosal
Xerostomia (dry mouth) [5]

Cardiovascular
Atrial fibrillation [2]
Chest pain (4%)
Hypotension (6–19%) [4]
Orthostatic hypotension [3]
Postural hypotension [3]

Central Nervous System
Headache (19–21%) [9]
Insomnia (<2%)
Somnolence (drowsiness) (3–4%)
Vertigo / dizziness (15–17%) [19]

Endocrine/Metabolic
Libido decreased (<2%)

Gastrointestinal/Hepatic
Constipation [3]
Diarrhea (4–6%)
Dyspepsia / functional dyspepsia (indigestion) (see also gastroparesis) [2]
Nausea (3–4%)

Genitourinary
Ejaculatory dysfunction (8–18%) [9]
Enuresis (urinary incontinence) [2]
Erectile dysfunction [2]
Priapism [8]
Retrograde ejaculation [2]
Urinary retention [3]

Neuromuscular/Skeletal
Asthenia / fatigue (8–9%) [3]
Back pain (7–8%) [2]

Ocular
Floppy iris syndrome [35]
Vision blurred (<2%)

Respiratory
Cough (3–5%)
Pharyngitis (sore throat) (5–6%)
Rhinitis / rhinosinusitis (see also sinusitis) (13–18%) [2]
Sinusitis (see also rhinitis / rhinosinusitis) (2–4%)

Other
Adverse effects / adverse reactions [4]
Infection (9–11%)
Tooth disorder (<2%)

TAPENTADOL

Trade names: Nucynta (Janssen), Nucynta ER (Janssen), Palexia (Grunenthal)
Indications: Immediate release formulation: moderate to severe acute pain, extended release formulation: moderate to severe chronic pain and neuropathic pain associated with diabetic peripheral neuropathy when a continuous analgesic is needed for an extended period of time
Class: Analgesic; opioid
Half-life: 5 hours
Clinically important, potentially hazardous interactions with: alcohol, alvimopan, amphetamines, anesthetics, anitemetics, anticholinergics, buprenorphine, butorphanol, CNS depressants, desmopressin, droperidol, hypnotics, linezolid, MAO inhibitors, mirtazapine, nalbuphine, PEG-interferon, pegvisomant, pentazocine, phenothiazines, sedatives, sibutramine, SNRIs, SSRIs, St John's wort, succinylcholine, thiazide diuretics, tramadol, tranquilizers, trazodone, tricyclic antidepressants, triptans
Important contra-indications noted in the prescribing guidelines for: the elderly; nursing mothers; pediatric patients
Note: Contra-indicated in patients with impaired pulmonary function or paralytic ileus. Should not be used in patients currently using or within 14 days of using a monoamine oxidase inhibitor.
Warning: For extended release oral tablets: ABUSE POTENTIAL, LIFE-THREATENING RESPIRATORY DEPRESSION, ACCIDENTAL EXPOSURE, and INTERACTION WITH ALCOHOL

Mucosal
Xerostomia (dry mouth) [4]

Central Nervous System
Headache [5]
Neurotoxicity [2]
Somnolence (drowsiness) [9]
Vertigo / dizziness (4%) [10]

Gastrointestinal/Hepatic
Constipation [15]
Diarrhea [2]
Gastrointestinal disorder / discomfort [2]
Nausea (4%) [23]
Vomiting (3%) [15]

Neuromuscular/Skeletal
Asthenia / fatigue [3]

Other
Adverse effects / adverse reactions [5]

TASIMELTEON

Trade name: Hetlioz (Vanda)
Indications: Non-24-hour sleep-wake disorder
Class: Melatonin receptor agonist
Half-life: 2–3 hours
Clinically important, potentially hazardous interactions with: fluvoxamine, ketoconazole, rifampin, viloxazine
Important contra-indications noted in the prescribing guidelines for: the elderly; nursing mothers; pediatric patients

---

Central Nervous System
- Abnormal dreams (10%) [3]
- Headache (17%) [3]
- Nightmares (10%) [3]

Endocrine/Metabolic
- ALT increased (10%) [2]

Genitourinary
- Urinary tract infection (7%) [3]

Respiratory
- Upper respiratory tract infection (7%) [2]

TASONERMIN

Trade name: Beromun (Boehringer Ingelheim)
Indications: As an adjunct to surgery for subsequent removal of various tumors
Class: Immune stimulant, TNF alpha agonist
Half-life: 0.37 hours
Clinically important, potentially hazardous interactions with: anthracyclines, interferon gamma, melphalan

---

Skin
- Edema / fluid retention (10%)
- Hypersensitivity (<10%)
- Necrosis (skin necrosis) (<10%)

Nails
- Onycholysis (<10%)

Cardiovascular
- Arrhythmias (10%)
- Cardiac failure (<10%)
- Hypotension (<10%)
- Shock (<10%)

Central Nervous System
- Chills (10%)
- Fever (pyrexia) (includes hyperpyrexia) (10%)
- Headache (<10%)
- Neurotoxicity (<10%)

Gastrointestinal/Hepatic
- Diarrhea (<10%)
- Hepatotoxicity / liver injury / acute liver injury / drug-induced liver injury (DILI) (10%)
- Nausea (10%)
- Vomiting (10%)

Hematologic
- Sepsis (<10%)
- Thrombosis (<10%)

Neuromuscular/Skeletal
- Asthenia / fatigue (10%)
- Myalgia/Myopathy (<10%)
- Rhabdomyolysis (<10%)

Renal
- Proteinuria (10%)

Respiratory
- Acute respiratory distress syndrome (<10%)

TAZAROTENE

Trade names: Avage (Allergan), Fabior (GSK), Tazorac (Allergan), Zorac (Allergan)
Indications: Acne vulgaris, mild to moderate plaque psoriasis involving up to 10% body surface area
Half-life: 18 hours
Clinically important, potentially hazardous interactions with: none known
Important contra-indications noted in the prescribing guidelines for: the elderly; nursing mothers; pediatric patients

---

Skin
- Burning / skin burning sensation (10–20%) [5]
- Contact dermatitis (5–10%)
- Desquamation (5–10%)
- Erythema (10–20%) [5]
- Pruritus (itching) (10–25%) [12]
- Psoriasis (5–10%)
- Rash (5–10%)
- Scaling [2]
- Stinging (<3%) [2]
- Xerosis / xeroderma (<3%) [5]

Local
- Application-site reactions [2]

Other
- Adverse effects / adverse reactions [2]
- Side effects [2]

TEA TREE

Family: Myrtaceae
Scientific names: *Melaleuca alternifolia, Melaleuca cajeputi, Melaleuca dissitifolia, Melaleuca linafolia*
Indications: Gram-negative and Gram-positive bacteria, acne, vaginal infection, burns, onychomycosis, tinea pedis, bruises, insect bites, skin infections, mouthwash, genital herpes, antiperspirant, gingivitis, disinfectant, scabies
Class: Antiseptic
Half-life: N/A
Clinically important, potentially hazardous interactions with: colophony, turpentine
Note: Tea tree oil in bottles may undergo photooxidation, and degradation products are moderate to strong sensitizers.
The plant was discovered and named by Captain James Cook of the Royal Navy in 1770, who found groves of trees with sticky, aromatic leaves that, when boiled, made a spicy tea.

Skin
- Burning / skin burning sensation [2]
- Dermatitis [22]
- Hypersensitivity [3]
- Pruritus (itching) [2]

Endocrine/Metabolic
- Gynecomastia [3]

Other
- Adverse effects / adverse reactions [4]
- Allergic reactions [8]

TEGAFUR/GIMERACIL/ OTERACIL

Synonyms: TS-1; S-1
Trade name: Teysuno (Taiho Pharma)
Indications: Gastric, colorectal, head and neck cancers, non-small cell lung cancer, inoperable or recurrent breast cancer, pancreatic cancer
Class: Antineoplastic / anticancer agent (see also Immune checkpoint inhibitor)
Half-life: N/A
Clinically important, potentially hazardous interactions with: capecitabine, flucytosine, fluorouracil, other fluoropyrimidine-group antineoplastics, phenytoin, uracil/tegafur, warfarin
Pregnancy category: Contra-indicated in pregnancy
Important contra-indications noted in the prescribing guidelines for: the elderly; nursing mothers; pediatric patients
Note: Contra-indicated in patients with severe bone marrow depression, hepatic or renal impairment.
Not available in the USA.

Skin
- Dermatitis (<5%)
- Desquamation (<5%)
- Edema / fluid retention (<5%) [3]
- Erythema (<5%)
- Flushing / rubefaction (<5%)
- Hand–foot syndrome (palmar–plantar erythrodysesthesia) (<5%) [13]
- Herpes simplex (<5%)
- Jaundice (see also cholestasis / cholestatic jaundice) (<5%)
- Pigmentation (Skin) (includes hyperpigmentation) (21%) [10]
- Pruritus (itching) (<5%)
- Rash (12%) [6]
- Raynaud's phenomenon (<5%)
- Stevens-Johnson syndrome and toxic epidermal necrolysis (SJS/TEN) [3]
- Ulcerations (<5%)
- Xerosis / xeroderma (<5%) [2]

Hair
- Alopecia / hair loss (<5%) [4]

Nails
- Nail disorder (<5%)
- Paronychia (<5%) [2]

Mucosal
- Mucositis [7]
- Stomatitis (oral mucositis) (17%) [12]

Cardiovascular
- Hypertension (<5%) [2]
- Hypotension (<5%)

Central Nervous System
- Anorexia (34%) [29]
- Fever (pyrexia) (includes hyperpyrexia) (<5%) [2]
- Headache (<5%)
- Neurotoxicity [4]
- Paresthesias (<5%)
- Peripheral neuropathy [4]
- Vertigo / dizziness (<5%)
- Warm feeling (includes feeling hot) (<5%)

Endocrine/Metabolic
- ALT increased (12%) [6]
- Appetite decreased [6]
- AST increased (12%) [5]
- Hyperbilirubinemia [4]

Hypoalbuminemia / albumin decreased [2]
Hyponatremia [5]
Weight loss (<5%)

Gastrointestinal/Hepatic
Diarrhea (19%) [43]
Hepatotoxicity / liver injury / acute liver injury / drug-induced liver injury (DILI) [6]
Nausea (23%) [25]
Vomiting (8%) [14]

Genitourinary
Glycosuria (<5%)
Hematuria (<5%)

Hematologic
Anemia [31]
Bleeding (<5%)
Febrile neutropenia [13]
Hemotoxicity [5]
Leukocytopenia (leukopenia) / leukocytes (white blood cells) decreased (87%) [28]
Myelosuppression / bone marrow suppression / myelotoxicity [8]
Neutropenia (neutrophils decreased) (44%) [55]
Thrombocytopenia / platelets decreased (11%) [25]

Neuromuscular/Skeletal
Arthralgia (<5%)
Asthenia / fatigue (22%) [20]
Myalgia/Myopathy (<5%)

Ocular
Conjunctivitis (conjunctival inflammation) (<5%)
Keratitis (ocular keratitis) / corneal inflammation) (<5%)
Lacrimation (<5%) [3]
Ocular adverse effect [2]
Ocular pain (<5%)
Reduced visual acuity (<5%)

Renal
Nephrotoxicity / kidney injury / acute kidney injury (AKI) / drug-induced kidney injury [2]
Proteinuria (<5%)

Respiratory
Pharyngitis (sore throat) (<5%)
Pneumonitis [5]
Rhinitis / rhinosinusitis (see also sinusitis) (<5%)

Other
Adverse effects / adverse reactions [23]
Death [4]
Infection [2]

TEGASEROD

Trade name: Zelnorm (Novartis)
Indications: Irritable bowel syndrome
Class: 5-HT4 agonist, Serotonin type 4 receptor agonist
Half-life: 11±5 hours
Clinically important, potentially hazardous interactions with: none known
Important contra-indications noted in the prescribing guidelines for: nursing mothers; pediatric patients
Note: Contra-indicated in patients with severe renal impairment, moderate or severe hepatic impairment, a history of bowel obstruction, symptomatic gallbladder disease, suspected sphincter of Oddi dysfunction, or abdominal adhesions.

Cardiovascular
Cardiotoxicity [2]
Myocardial infarction [3]

Central Nervous System
Headache (15%) [8]
Insomnia (<2%)
Migraine (2%)
Vertigo / dizziness (<4%)

Gastrointestinal/Hepatic
Abdominal distension (3–4%)
Abdominal pain (5–12%) [6]
Diarrhea (4–9%) [2]
Flatulence (6%)
Nausea (5–8%)

Genitourinary
Dysmenorrhea (<2%)
Urinary tract infection (<2%)

Neuromuscular/Skeletal
Arthralgia (2%)
Back pain (2–5%)

Respiratory
Sinusitis (see also rhinitis / rhinosinusitis) (3%)
Upper respiratory tract infection (3–4%)

TEICOPLANIN

Trade name: Targocid (Sanofi-Aventis)
Indications: Staphylococcal infections
Class: Antibiotic, Antibiotic; glycopeptide, Antimicrobial
Half-life: 150 hours
Clinically important, potentially hazardous interactions with: amikacin, cephaloridine, colistin, gentamicin, kanamycin, neomycin, streptomycin, tobramycin, vancomycin
Pregnancy category: Not recommended in pregnancy
Important contra-indications noted in the prescribing guidelines for: nursing mothers

---

Skin
DRESS syndrome (Drug-induced hypersensitivity syndrome) [4]
Erythema (<10%)
Exanthems [2]
Hypersensitivity [4]
Pruritus (itching) (<10%)
Rash (<10%) [4]
Red man syndrome / flushing syndrome [3]
Urticaria / hives [2]

Central Nervous System
Fever (pyrexia) (includes hyperpyrexia) (<10%)

Gastrointestinal/Hepatic
Hepatotoxicity / liver injury / acute liver injury / drug-induced liver injury (DILI) (2%) [2]

Hematologic
Neutropenia (neutrophils decreased) [2]
Thrombocytopenia / platelets decreased [4]

Otic
Ototoxicity [2]

Renal
Nephrotoxicity / kidney injury / acute kidney injury (AKI) / drug-induced kidney injury [2]

Other
Adverse effects / adverse reactions [2]

TELAPREVIR

Trade name: Incivek (Vertex)
Indications: Hepatitis C (must only be used in combination with PEG-interferon alfa and ribavirin)
Class: CYP3A4 inhibitor, Direct-acting antiviral, Hepatitis C virus NS3/4A protease inhibitor
Half-life: 4–11 hours
Clinically important, potentially hazardous interactions with: alfuzosin, alprazolam, amiodarone, amlodipine, atazanavir, atorvastatin, bepridil, bosentan, budesonide, carbamazepine, cisapride, dabigatran, darunavir, desipramine, dexamethasone, digoxin, dihydroergotamine, diltiazem, efavirenz, ergotamine, escitalopram, estradiol, felodipine, flecainide, flibanserin, fluticasone propionate, fosamprenavir, itraconazole, ketoconazole, lidocaine, lomitapide, lovastatin, methylergonovine, methylprednisolone, midazolam, mifepristone, nicardipine, nisoldipine, olaparib, palbociclib, phenobarbital, phenytoin, pimozide, ponatinib, posaconazole, propafenone, quinidine, rifampin, ritonavir, ruxolitinib, salmeterol, sildenafil, simvastatin, sirolimus, St John's wort, tacrolimus, tadalafil, telithromycin, tenofovir disoproxil, trazodone, triazolam, vardenafil, venetoclax, verapamil, vorapaxar, voriconazole, warfarin, zolpidem
Important contra-indications noted in the prescribing guidelines for: the elderly; nursing mothers; pediatric patients
Note: Must be used in combination with PEG-interferon alfa and ribavirin (see separate entries).
Warning: SERIOUS SKIN REACTIONS

Skin
Cutaneous toxicity / skin toxicity [2]
Dermatitis [2]
DRESS syndrome (Drug-induced hypersensitivity syndrome) [7]
Exanthems [6]
Pruritus (itching) (including anal pruritus) (53%) [14]
Rash (56%) [38]
Stevens-Johnson syndrome and toxic epidermal necrolysis (SJS/TEN) [3]

Central Nervous System
Dysgeusia (taste perversion) (10%)

Gastrointestinal/Hepatic
Anorectal discomfort (11%)
Diarrhea (26%) [2]
Hemorrhoids (12%)
Hepatotoxicity / liver injury / acute liver injury / drug-induced liver injury (DILI) [5]
Nausea (39%) [4]
Vomiting (13%)

Hematologic
Anemia [36]
Neutropenia (neutrophils decreased) [6]
Thrombocytopenia / platelets decreased [6]

Neuromuscular/Skeletal
Asthenia / fatigue (56%) [4]

Renal
Nephrotoxicity / kidney injury / acute kidney injury (AKI) / drug-induced kidney injury [3]

Other
Adverse effects / adverse reactions [19]
Infection [4]

TELAVANCIN

Trade name: Vibativ (Astellas)
Indications: Complicated skin and skin structure infections (cSSSI)
Class: Antibiotic, Antibiotic; lipoglycopeptide, Antimicrobial
Half-life: 7–10 hours
Clinically important, potentially hazardous interactions with: alfuzosin, artemether/ lumefantrine, BCG vaccine, chloroquine, ciprofloxacin, dronedarone, gadobutrol, indacaterol, nilotinib, pimozide, QT prolonging agents, quetiapine, quinine, tetrabenazine, thioridazine, toremifene, typhoid vaccine, vandetanib, vemurafenib, ziprasidone
Important contra-indications noted in the prescribing guidelines for: nursing mothers; pediatric patients
Note: Contra-indicated in patients with known hypersensitivity to vancomycin.
Warning: FETAL RISK

Skin
Pruritus (itching) (6%) [3]
Rash (4%) [3]

Cardiovascular
Hypotension [2]
QT interval prolonged / QT prolongation [2]

Central Nervous System
Dysgeusia (taste perversion) (33%) [10]
Headache [5]
Insomnia [5]
Rigors (4%)
Vertigo / dizziness (6%)

Endocrine/Metabolic
Appetite decreased (3%)
Hypokalemia [5]
Serum creatinine increased [6]

Gastrointestinal/Hepatic
Abdominal pain (2%)
Constipation [4]
Diarrhea (7%) [3]
Nausea (27%) [13]
Vomiting (14%) [10]

Genitourinary
Hematuria [2]

Hematologic
Anemia [4]

Local
Infusion-related reactions [2]
Infusion-site erythema (3%)
Infusion-site pain (4%)

Renal
Foamy urine (13%) [4]
Nephrotoxicity / kidney injury / acute kidney injury (AKI) / drug-induced kidney injury [9]
Renal failure [4]
Renal function abnormal / renal dysfunction [2]

Other
Adverse effects / adverse reactions [6]

TELBIVUDINE

Trade names: Sebvio (Novartis), Tyzeka (Novartis)
Indications: Hepatitis B (chronic)
Class: Nucleoside analog reverse transcriptase inhibitor
Half-life: ~15 hours
Clinically important, potentially hazardous interactions with: interferon alfa, PEG-interferon
Important contra-indications noted in the prescribing guidelines for: the elderly; nursing mothers; pediatric patients

---

Skin
Pruritus (itching) (2%)
Rash (4%)

Cardiovascular
Arrhythmias [2]

Central Nervous System
Fever (pyrexia) (includes hyperpyrexia) (4%)
Headache (11%)
Insomnia (3%)
Neurotoxicity [2]
Peripheral neuropathy [2]
Vertigo / dizziness (4%)

Endocrine/Metabolic
Acidosis (includes lactic acidosis) [2]
ALT increased (3%)
Creatine phosphokinase (CPK) / creatine kinase increased (hyperCKemia) [5]

Gastrointestinal/Hepatic
Abdominal distension (3%)
Abdominal pain (12%)
Diarrhea [2]
Dyspepsia / functional dyspepsia (indigestion) (see also gastroparesis) (3%)
Hepatitis (exacerbation) (2%)

Hematologic
Neutropenia (neutrophils decreased) (2%)

Neuromuscular/Skeletal
Arthralgia (4%)
Asthenia / fatigue (>5%) [2]
Back pain (4%)
Myalgia/Myopathy (3%) [9]

Respiratory
Cough (7%)
Influenza- ('flu)-like syndrome (7%)
Pharyngolaryngeal pain (5%)
Upper respiratory tract infection (>5%)

TELITHROMYCIN

Trade name: Ketek (Sanofi-Aventis)
Indications: Community-acquired pneumonia, chronic bronchitis
Class: Antibiotic, Antibiotic; macrolide, Antimicrobial, CYP3A4 inhibitor
Half-life: 10–13 hours
Clinically important, potentially hazardous interactions with: abiraterone, alfentanil, alfuzosin, almotriptan, alosetron, antifungals, antineoplastics, aprepitant, artemether/ lumefantrine, atazanavir, atorvastatin, avanafil, BCG vaccine, benzodiazepines, bortezomib, brinzolamide, buspirone, cabazitaxel, cabozantinib, calcifediol, calcium channel blockers, carbamazepine, cardiac glycosides, ceritinib, chloroquine, ciclesonide, cilostazol, ciprofloxacin, cisapride, clopidogrel, clozapine, cobicistat/elvitegravir/emtricitabine/tenofovir alafenamide, cobicistat/elvitegravir/emtricitabine/ tenofovir disoproxil, colchicine, conivaptan, corticosteroids, crizotinib, cyclosporine, CYP3A4 inhibitors or inducers, CYP3A4 substrates, deferasirox, dienogest, digoxin, dihydroergotamine, disopyramide, dronedarone, dutasteride, eletriptan, eplerenone, ergot derivatives, ergotamine, eszopiclone, etravirine, everolimus, fentanyl, fesoterodine, flibanserin, fluticasone propionate, fosamprenavir, gadobutrol, guanfacine, halofantrine, hexobarbital, HMG-CoA reductase inhibitors, ibrutinib, indinavir, itraconazole, ivabradine, ixabepilone, ketoconazole, lapatinib, lomitapide, lopinavir, lovastatin, maraviroc, methylprednisolone, methysergide, metoprolol, midazolam, mifepristone, mometasone, nelfinavir, nilotinib, nisoldipine, olaparib, oral typhoid vaccines, osimertinib, oxycodone, paclitaxel, palbociclib, paricalcitol, pazopanib, phenobarbital, phenytoin, phosphodiesterase 5 inhibitors, pimecrolimus, pimozide, ponatinib, prasugrel, pravastatin, primidone, QT prolonging agents, quinidine, quinine, ranolazine, regorafenib, repaglinide, rifampin, rifamycin derivatives, rimonabant, ritonavir, rivaroxaban, romidepsin, ruxolitinib, salmeterol, saquinavir, saxagliptin, sildenafil, silodosin, simeprevir, simvastatin, sirolimus, sonidegib, sorafenib, SSRIs, St John's wort, sunitinib, tacrolimus, tadalafil, tamsulosin, telaprevir, temsirolimus, tetrabenazine, tezacaftor/ivacaftor, thioridazine, ticagrelor, tipranavir, tolvaptan, triazolam, ulipristal, vemurafenib, verapamil, vitamin K antagonists, vorapaxar, warfarin, ziprasidone
Important contra-indications noted in the prescribing guidelines for: nursing mothers; pediatric patients
Warning: CONTRA-INDICATION IN MYASTHENIA GRAVIS

Skin
Candidiasis / candidosis (<2%)
Hypersensitivity (<2%)
Jaundice (see also cholestasis / cholestatic jaundice) [2]
Rash (<2%)
Vasculitis (angiitis) / cutaneous vasculitis (angiitis) (<2%)

Mucosal
Glossitis (inflammation of the tongue) (<2%)
Oral candidiasis (<2%)
Stomatitis (oral mucositis) (<2%)
Xerostomia (dry mouth) (<2%)

Cardiovascular
QT interval prolonged / QT prolongation [2]

Central Nervous System
Anorexia (<2%)
Dysgeusia (taste perversion) (2%)
Fever (pyrexia) (includes hyperpyrexia) [2]
Headache (6%) [3]
Insomnia (<2%)
Somnolence (drowsiness) (<2%)
Tremor (<2%)
Vertigo / dizziness (2–6%) [2]

Endocrine/Metabolic
ALT increased (<2%)
AST increased (<2%)

Gastrointestinal/Hepatic
Abdominal distension (<2%)
Abdominal pain (<2%) [2]

Ascites [2]
Constipation (<2%)
Diarrhea (11%)
Dyspepsia / functional dyspepsia (indigestion) (see also gastroparesis) (<2%)
Flatulence (<2%)
Gastritis / pangastritis / gastric irritation (<2%)
Gastroenteritis (<2%)
Hepatitis (<2%)
Hepatotoxicity / liver injury / acute liver injury / drug-induced liver injury (DILI) [12]
Loose stools / soft feces (2%)
Nausea (7%)
Vomiting (3%)

Genitourinary
Vaginitis (includes vulvitis) (<2%)
Vulvovaginal candidiasis (<2%)

Hematologic
Thrombocythemia (thrombocytosis) / platelets increased (<2%)

Neuromuscular/Skeletal
Asthenia / fatigue (<2%)
Myasthenia gravis (exacerbation) [7]

Ocular
Accommodation disorder [3]
Diplopia (double vision) (<2%) [2]
Vision blurred (<2%)
Visual disturbances (<2%) [2]

Other
Adverse effects / adverse reactions [2]
Death [4]
Tooth pigmentation / discoloration (<2%)

TELMISARTAN

Trade name: Micardis (Boehringer Ingelheim)
Indications: Hypertension
Class: Angiotensin receptor antagonist (blocker), Antihypertensive
Half-life: 24 hours
Clinically important, potentially hazardous interactions with: ramipril
Pregnancy category: category C in first trimester; category D in second and third trimesters
Important contra-indications noted in the prescribing guidelines for: nursing mothers; pediatric patients
Warning: FETAL TOXICITY

Skin
Angioedema (formerly named angioneurotic edema) [5]
Peripheral edema [2]

Cardiovascular
Hypotension [2]

Central Nervous System
Headache [6]
Vertigo / dizziness [6]

Endocrine/Metabolic
Hyperkalemia [2]

Gastrointestinal/Hepatic
Enteropathy [3]

Neuromuscular/Skeletal
Asthenia / fatigue [4]

Respiratory
Cough [9]

TEMAZEPAM

Trade name: Restoril (Mallinckrodt)
Indications: Insomnia, anxiety
Class: Benzodiazepine
Half-life: 8–15 hours
Clinically important, potentially hazardous interactions with: amprenavir, chlorpheniramine, clarithromycin, efavirenz, esomeprazole, imatinib, mianserin, nelfinavir
Important contra-indications noted in the prescribing guidelines for: the elderly; nursing mothers; pediatric patients

---

Skin
Dermatitis (<10%)
Diaphoresis (>10%)
Rash (>10%)

Mucosal
Sialopenia (>10%)
Sialorrhea (ptyalism; hypersalivation) (<10%)
Xerostomia (dry mouth) (2%)

Other
Adverse effects / adverse reactions [2]

TEMOZOLOMIDE

Trade name: Temodar (MSD)
Indications: Anaplastic astrocytoma, newly diagnosed glioblastoma multiforme concomitantly with radiotherapy and then as maintenance treatment
Class: Alkylating agent, Antineoplastic / anticancer agent (see also Immune checkpoint inhibitor)
Half-life: 1.8 hours
Clinically important, potentially hazardous interactions with: clozapine, digoxin, valproic acid
Important contra-indications noted in the prescribing guidelines for: the elderly; nursing mothers; pediatric patients

---

Skin
Cutaneous toxicity / skin toxicity [3]
Peripheral edema (11%)
Pruritus (itching) (8%)
Rash (8%) [8]

Hair
Alopecia / hair loss [3]

Mucosal
Mucositis [2]

Cardiovascular
Thromboembolism [2]
Venous thromboembolism [2]

Central Nervous System
Anorexia [3]
Cerebral hemorrhage [2]
Fever (pyrexia) (includes hyperpyrexia) [2]
Headache [3]
Paresthesias (9%)

Endocrine/Metabolic
Mastodynia (6%)

Gastrointestinal/Hepatic
Constipation [2]
Diarrhea [8]
Gastrointestinal perforation / perforated colon / gastric perforation [2]
Hepatotoxicity / liver injury / acute liver injury / drug-induced liver injury (DILI) [6]
Nausea [11]
Vanishing bile duct syndrome / ductopenia [3]
Vomiting [4]

Hematologic
Anemia [3]
Aplastic anemia [11]
Febrile neutropenia [2]
Hemotoxicity [6]
Leukocytopenia (leukopenia) / leukocytes (white blood cells) decreased [6]
Lymphopenia (lymphocytopenia) / lymphocytes decreased [8]
Myelosuppression / bone marrow suppression / myelotoxicity [3]
Neutropenia (neutrophils decreased) [12]
Thrombocytopenia / platelets decreased [14]

Neuromuscular/Skeletal
Asthenia / fatigue [15]
Myalgia/Myopathy (5%)

Other
Adverse effects / adverse reactions [2]
Death [8]
Infection [5]

TEMSIROLIMUS

Trade name: Torisel (Wyeth)
Indications: Renal cell carcinoma, other cancers
Class: Analog of sirolimus, Antineoplastic / anticancer agent (see also Immune checkpoint inhibitor), mTOR inhibitor
Half-life: 17 hours
Clinically important, potentially hazardous interactions with: ACE inhibitors, atazanavir, BCG vaccine, benazepril, captopril, carbamazepine, clarithromycin, clozapine, conivaptan, cyclosporine, darunavir, dasatinib, denosumab, dexamethasone, digoxin, enalapril, fluconazole, fosinopril, grapefruit juice, hypoglycemic agents, indinavir, itraconazole, ketoconazole, leflunomide, lisinopril, live and inactive vaccines, macolide antibiotics, natalizumab, nefazodone, nelfinavir, P-glycoprotein inhibitors, phenobarbital, phenytoin, pimecrolimus, posaconazole, protease inhibitors, quinapril, ramipril, rifabutin, rifampin, rifapentine, ritonavir, saquinavir, St John's wort, sunitinib, tacrolimus, telithromycin, tipranavir, trastuzumab, voriconazole
Important contra-indications noted in the prescribing guidelines for: the elderly; nursing mothers; pediatric patients
Note: Contra-indicated in patients with bilirubin >1.5xULN.

Skin
Acneiform eruption / acneiform dermatitis / acneiform rash (10%) [4]
Cutaneous toxicity / skin toxicity [4]
Edema / fluid retention [2]
Exanthems [3]
Hypersensitivity (9%) [3]
Pruritus (itching) (19%) [3]
Rash (47%) [14]
Xerosis / xeroderma (11%)

Nails
Nail disorder (14%)
Paronychia [2]

Mucosal
Mucositis (30%) [12]
Stomatitis (oral mucositis) [19]

Cardiovascular
Chest pain (16%)
Hypertension (7%) [3]

Central Nervous System
Anorexia (30%) [4]
Chills (8%)
Depression (4%)
Dysgeusia (taste perversion) (20%) [2]
Fever (pyrexia) (includes hyperpyrexia) (24%)
Headache (15%)
Insomnia (12%) [2]
Neurotoxicity [2]
Pain (28%)

Endocrine/Metabolic
ALT increased [4]
AST increased [2]
Dehydration [2]
Hypercholesterolemia [4]
Hyperglycemia (includes glucose increased) [14]
Hyperlipidemia / lipids elevated [2]
Hypertriglyceridemia (includes triglycerides increased) [5]
Hypokalemia [3]
Hypophosphatemia [4]
Serum creatinine increased [2]

Gastrointestinal/Hepatic
Abdominal pain (21%)
Diarrhea [7]
Nausea [8]
Vomiting [3]

Genitourinary
Urinary tract infection (15%)

Hematologic
Anemia [10]
Febrile neutropenia [3]
Hemorrhage [2]
Hemotoxicity [3]
Immunosupression [2]
Leukocytopenia (leukopenia) / leukocytes (white blood cells) decreased [4]
Lymphopenia (lymphocytopenia) / lymphocytes decreased [5]
Neutropenia (neutrophils decreased) [5]
Thrombocytopenia / platelets decreased [17]

Neuromuscular/Skeletal
Arthralgia (18%)
Asthenia / fatigue (30%) [22]
Back pain (20%)
Myalgia/Myopathy (8%)

Ocular
Conjunctivitis (conjunctival inflammation) (7%)

Respiratory
Cough (26%) [3]
Dyspnea / shortness of breath [7]
Pharyngitis (sore throat) (12%)
Pneumonia [2]
Pneumonitis (36%) [11]
Rhinitis / rhinosinusitis (see also sinusitis) (10%)
Upper respiratory tract infection (7%)

Other
Adverse effects / adverse reactions [10]
Death [2]
Infection (20%) [5]

TENIPOSIDE

Trade name: Vumon (Bristol-Myers Squibb)
Indications: Acute lymphocytic leukemia, non-Hodgkin's lymphoma, small cell lung cancer
Class: Antineoplastic / anticancer agent (see also Immune checkpoint inhibitor), Topoisomerase 2 inhibitor
Half-life: 45 minutes
Clinically important, potentially hazardous interactions with: phenobarbital, phenytoin, propranolol
Important contra-indications noted in the prescribing guidelines for: nursing mothers

---

Skin
Anaphylactoid reactions / anaphylaxis (includes anaphylactic shock) [3]
Hypersensitivity (2–11%) [4]

Hair
Alopecia / hair loss (31%) [6]

Mucosal
Stomatitis (oral mucositis) (3%)

Cardiovascular
Hypertension [2]
Hypotension [3]

Gastrointestinal/Hepatic
Hepatotoxicity / liver injury / acute liver injury / drug-induced liver injury (DILI) (2%)

Renal
Nephrotoxicity / kidney injury / acute kidney injury (AKI) / drug-induced kidney injury (2%)

Other
Allergic reactions (5–15%) [2]
Death [3]

TENOFOVIR ALAFENAMIDE

Trade names: Descovy (Gilead), Vemlidy (Gilead)
Indications: Hepatitis B
Class: Antiviral, Hepatitis B virus necleoside analog reverse transcriptase inhibitor
Half-life: <1 hour
Clinically important, potentially hazardous interactions with: carbamazepine, oxcarbazepine, phenobarbital, phenytoin, rifabutin, rifampin, rifapentine, St John's wort
Pregnancy category: No available data to inform drug-associated risk
Important contra-indications noted in the prescribing guidelines for: nursing mothers; pediatric patients
Note: Descovy is tenofovir alafenamide and emtricitabine. See also separate profile for tenofovir alafenamide in combination with cobicistat, elvitegravir and emtricitabine.
Warning: LACTIC ACIDOSIS/SEVERE HEPATOMEGALY WITH STEATOSIS and POST TREATMENT SEVERE ACUTE EXACERBATION OF HEPATITIS B

Central Nervous System
Headache (9%) [5]

Endocrine/Metabolic
ALT increased (8%) [2]
AST increased (3%)
Creatine phosphokinase (CPK) / creatine kinase increased (hyperCKemia) (3%)
Hyperamylasemia (3%)
Hypercholesterolemia (4%)
Hypophosphatemia [2]

Gastrointestinal/Hepatic
Abdominal pain (7%)
Nausea (5%)

Genitourinary
Glycosuria (5%)

Neuromuscular/Skeletal
Asthenia / fatigue (6%)
Back pain (5%)

Respiratory
Cough (6%)
Nasopharyngitis [4]
Upper respiratory tract infection [4]

Other
Adverse effects / adverse reactions [3]

TENOFOVIR DISOPROXIL

Trade names: Atripla (Gilead), Complera (Gilead), Truvada (Gilead), Viread (Gilead)
Indications: HIV infection in combination with at least two other antiretroviral agents
Class: Antiretroviral, Covid-19 putative drug, Nucleoside analog reverse transcriptase inhibitor
Half-life: 12–18 hours
Clinically important, potentially hazardous interactions with: acyclovir, adefovir, atazanavir, cidofovir, cobicistat/elvitegravir/emtricitabine/tenofovir disoproxil, darunavir, didanosine, ganciclovir, high-fat foods, indinavir, ledipasvir & sofosbuvir, lopinavir, protease inhibitors, ritonavir, telaprevir, tipranavir, trospium, valacyclovir, valganciclovir
Important contra-indications noted in the prescribing guidelines for: nursing mothers; pediatric patients
Note: Atripla is tenofovir disoproxil, efavirenz and emtricitabine; Complera is tenofovir disoproxil, emtricitabine and rilpivirine; Truvada is tenofovir disoproxil and emtricitabine. See also separate profile for tenofovir disoproxil in combination with cobicistat, elvitegravir and emtricitabine.
Warning: LACTIC ACIDOSIS/SEVERE HEPATOMEGALY WITH STEATOSIS and POST TREATMENT EXACERBATION OF HEPATITIS

Skin
Diaphoresis (3%)
DRESS syndrome (Drug-induced hypersensitivity syndrome) [2]
Lichenoid eruption / lichenoid reaction [2]
Rash (5–18%) [5]
Stevens-Johnson syndrome and toxic epidermal necrolysis (SJS/TEN) [3]

Cardiovascular
Chest pain (3%)

Central Nervous System
Abnormal dreams [3]
Anorexia (3%)
Anxiety (6%) [2]
Depression (4–11%)
Fever (pyrexia) (includes hyperpyrexia) (2–8%)
Headache (5–14%) [11]
Insomnia (3–5%) [2]

Neurotoxicity (3%) [6]
Pain (7–13%)
Peripheral neuropathy (<3%)
Somnolence (drowsiness) [2]
Vertigo / dizziness (<3%) [4]

Endocrine/Metabolic
Acidosis (includes lactic acidosis) [3]
ALT increased [3]
Creatine phosphokinase (CPK) / creatine kinase increased (hyperCKemia) [3]
Hypokalemia [2]
Hypophosphatemia [4]
Weight loss (2%)

Gastrointestinal/Hepatic
Abdominal pain (4–7%) [2]
Diarrhea (11%) [7]
Dyspepsia / functional dyspepsia (indigestion) (see also gastroparesis) (3–4%)
Flatulence (3%)
Hepatic failure [2]
Hepatotoxicity / liver injury / acute liver injury / drug-induced liver injury (DILI) [3]
Nausea (8%) [10]
Pancreatitis / acute pancreatitis [5]
Vomiting (4–5%) [6]

Neuromuscular/Skeletal
Arthralgia (5%)
Asthenia / fatigue (6–7%) [6]
Back pain (3–9%)
Bone pain / joint pain [5]
Fractures [2]
Myalgia/Myopathy (3%) [2]
Osteomalacia [6]

Renal
Fanconi syndrome (proximal tubular dysfunction) [29]
Nephrotoxicity / kidney injury / acute kidney injury (AKI) / drug-induced kidney injury [42]
Proteinuria [4]
Renal failure [10]
Renal tubular acidosis [2]
Renal tubular necrosis [2]

Respiratory
Nasopharyngitis [3]
Pneumonia (2–5%)
Upper respiratory tract infection [2]

Other
Adverse effects / adverse reactions [11]

TENOXICAM

Trade name: Mobiflex (Roche)
Indications: Osteoarthritis, rheumatoid arthritis, ankylosing spondylitits and hyperuricemia
Class: Non-steroidal anti-inflammatory (NSAID)
Half-life: 72 hours
Clinically important, potentially hazardous interactions with: cyclosporine, lithium, methotrexate, mifepristone, NSAIDs, quinolones, salicylates
Note: NSAIDs may cause an increased risk of serious cardiovascular and gastrointestinal adverse events, which can be fatal. This risk may increase with duration of use.

Gastrointestinal/Hepatic
Hepatotoxicity / liver injury / acute liver injury / drug-induced liver injury (DILI) [4]

TERAZOSIN

Trade name: Hytrin (AbbVie)
Indications: Hypertension, benign prostatic hypertrophy
Class: Adrenergic alpha-receptor antagonist
Half-life: 12 hours
Clinically important, potentially hazardous interactions with: vardenafil

---

Skin
Edema / fluid retention (<10%)
Lichenoid eruption / lichenoid reaction [2]
Peripheral edema (6%)

Mucosal
Xerostomia (dry mouth) (<10%)

Cardiovascular
Postural hypotension [2]

Central Nervous System
Paresthesias (3%)
Vertigo / dizziness [3]

Genitourinary
Priapism [2]

Ocular
Floppy iris syndrome [2]

TERBINAFINE

Trade name: Lamisil (Novartis)
Indications: Fungal infections of the skin and nails
Class: Antifungal / antimycotic, Antimicrobial
Half-life: ~36 hours
Clinically important, potentially hazardous interactions with: amitriptyline, amphotericin B, atomoxetine, caffeine, carbamazepine, cimetidine, codeine, conivaptan, cyclosporine, CYP2D6 substrates, desipramine, estrogens, fesoterodine, fluconazole, nebivolol, progestogens, rifampin, rifapentine, saxagliptin, tamoxifen, tamsulosin, tetrabenazine, thioridazine, tramadol, tricyclic antidepressants
Important contra-indications noted in the prescribing guidelines for: nursing mothers; pediatric patients

---

Skin
AGEP [29]
Baboon syndrome / symmetrical drug-related intertriginous and flexural exanthema (SDRIFE) [2]
Dermatitis (<10%)
DRESS syndrome (Drug-induced hypersensitivity syndrome) [2]
Eczema / eczematous reaction / eczematous eruption [2]
Erythema multiforme [9]
Erythroderma [2]
Exanthems [5]
Fixed eruption / fixed drug eruption [3]
Hypersensitivity [3]
Lichenoid eruption / lichenoid reaction [3]
Lupus erythematosus (subacute cutaneous lupus erythematosus (SCLE)) [30]
Pityriasis rosea [3]
Pruritus (itching) (3%) [6]
Psoriasis [15]
Pustules / pustular eruption [3]
Rash (6%) [3]
Rowell syndrome / Rowell's syndrome [2]
Stevens-Johnson syndrome and toxic epidermal necrolysis (SJS/TEN) [7]
Urticaria / hives [7]

Hair
Alopecia / hair loss (<10%)

Nails
Onychocryptosis (ingrowing toe nail) [2]

Central Nervous System
Ageusia (taste loss) / taste disorder [17]
Dysgeusia (taste perversion) (3%) [8]
Headache (13%)

Gastrointestinal/Hepatic
Abdominal pain (2%)
Diarrhea (6%)
Dyspepsia / functional dyspepsia (indigestion) (see also gastroparesis) (4%)
Flatulence (2%)
Hepatotoxicity / liver injury / acute liver injury / drug-induced liver injury (DILI) [13]
Nausea (3%)

Other
Adverse effects / adverse reactions [4]
Allergic reactions (<10%)
Death [2]
Side effects (3%)

TERBUTALINE

Trade names: Brethine (aaiPharma), Bricanyl (AstraZeneca)
Indications: Bronchospasm
Class: Beta-2 adrenergic agonist, Bronchodilator, Tocolytic
Half-life: 11–16 hours
Clinically important, potentially hazardous interactions with: alpha blockers, atomoxetine, beta blockers, betahistine, cannabinoids, epinephrine, insulin aspart, insulin degludec, insulin detemir, insulin glargine, insulin glulisine, iobenguane, loop diuretics, MAO inhibitors, propranolol, sotalol, sympathomimetics, tricyclic antidepressants, yohimbine
Important contra-indications noted in the prescribing guidelines for: nursing mothers; pediatric patients
Warning: PROLONGED TOCOLYSIS

Skin
Diaphoresis (<10%)

Mucosal
Xerostomia (dry mouth) (<10%)

Cardiovascular
Arrhythmias [2]

Central Nervous System
Dysgeusia (taste perversion) (<10%)
Tremor [2]

Gastrointestinal/Hepatic
Nausea [2]

Other
Side effects [2]

TERFENADINE

Class: Histamine H1 receptor antagonist
Half-life: 16–22 hours
Clinically important, potentially hazardous interactions with: amisulpride, aprepitant, artemether/lumefantrine, astemizole, darunavir, dasatinib, delavirdine, devil's claw, erythromycin, grapefruit juice, itraconazole, nilotinib, quinine, roxithromycin, sertindole, troglitazone, troleandomycin
Note: This drug has been withdrawn.

Skin
Photosensitivity [3]
Psoriasis (exacerbation) [2]

Hair
Alopecia / hair loss [3]

Mucosal
Xerostomia (dry mouth) (<10%)

Cardiovascular
QT interval prolonged / QT prolongation [3]
Torsades de pointes [4]

TERIFLUNOMIDE

Trade name: Aubagio (Sanofi-Aventis)
Indications: Relapsing forms of multiple sclerosis
Class: Pyrimidine synthesis inhibitor
Half-life: N/A
Clinically important, potentially hazardous interactions with: alosetron, caffeine, duloxetine, ethinylestradiol, leflunomide, live vaccines, oral contraceptives, paclitaxel, pioglitazone, repaglinide, rosiglitazone, theophylline, tizanidine, warfarin
Important contra-indications noted in the prescribing guidelines for: the elderly; nursing mothers; pediatric patients
Warning: HEPATOTOXICITY and RISK OF TERATOGENICITY

Skin
Acneiform eruption / acneiform dermatitis / acneiform rash (<3%)
Burning / skin burning sensation (2–3%)
Herpes (oral) (2–4%)
Lichenoid eruption / lichenoid reaction [2]
Lupus erythematosus (subacute cutaneous lupus erythematosus (SCLE)) [2]
Pruritus (itching) (3–4%)
Psoriasiform eruption [2]

Hair
Alopecia / hair loss (10–13%) [17]

Nails
Nail loss [2]

Cardiovascular
Hypertension (4%) [3]
Palpitation (2–3%)

Central Nervous System
Anxiety (3–4%)
Carpal tunnel syndrome (<3%)
Headache (19–22%) [4]
Paresthesias (9–10%) [3]
Peripheral neuropathy (<2%) [2]

Endocrine/Metabolic
ALT increased (12–14%) [12]
AST increased (2–3%)
GGT increased (3–5%)
Hypophosphatemia (mild) (18%)
Weight loss (2–3%)

Gastrointestinal/Hepatic
Abdominal distension (<2%)
Abdominal pain (5–6%)
Diarrhea (15–18%) [11]
Gastroenteritis (2–4%)
Hepatotoxicity / liver injury / acute liver injury / drug-induced liver injury (DILI) [5]
Nausea (9–14%) [9]

Genitourinary
Cystitis (includes interstitial cystitis / bladder pain syndrome) (2–4%)

Hematologic
Immunosupression (10–15%)
Leukocytopenia (leukopenia) / leukocytes (white blood cells) decreased (<2%) [2]
Lymphopenia (lymphocytopenia) / lymphocytes decreased [3]
Neutropenia (neutrophils decreased) (2–4%) [5]

Neuromuscular/Skeletal
Asthenia / fatigue [2]
Back pain (<3%) [2]
Bone pain / joint pain (4–5%)
Myalgia/Myopathy (3–4%)

Ocular
Conjunctivitis (conjunctival inflammation) (<3%)
Vision blurred (3%)

Renal
Renal failure [2]

Respiratory
Bronchitis (5–8%)
Influenza (9–12%) [2]
Nasopharyngitis [2]
Sinusitis (see also rhinitis / rhinosinusitis) (4–6%)
Upper respiratory tract infection (9%)

Other
Adverse effects / adverse reactions [5]
Allergic reactions (2–3%)
Infection [5]
Side effects [2]
Toothache (odontalgia) (4%)

TERIPARATIDE

Trade name: Forteo (Lilly)
Indications: Osteoporosis in postmenopausal women and men at increased risk of fractures
Class: Parathyroid hormone analog
Half-life: 1 hour
Clinically important, potentially hazardous interactions with: alcohol, digoxin
Important contra-indications noted in the prescribing guidelines for: nursing mothers; pediatric patients
Warning: POTENTIAL RISK OF OSTEOSARCOMA

Skin
Diaphoresis (2%)
Herpes zoster (3%)
Rash (5%)

Cardiovascular
Angina (3%)
Hypertension (7%)

Central Nervous System
Anxiety (4%)
Depression (4%)
Dysgeusia (taste perversion) (<2%)
Headache (8%) [10]
Insomnia (4–5%)
Pain (21%)
Paresthesias (<2%)
Syncope / fainting (3%)
Vertigo / dizziness (4–8%) [7]

Endocrine/Metabolic
Hypercalcemia [6]

Gastrointestinal/Hepatic
Constipation (5%)
Diarrhea (5%)
Dyspepsia / functional dyspepsia (indigestion) (see also gastroparesis) (5%)
Gastritis / pangastritis / gastric irritation (2–7%)
Nausea (9–14%) [10]
Vomiting (3%) [3]

Local
Injection-site pain (<2%)

Neuromuscular/Skeletal
Arthralgia (10%) [3]
Asthenia / fatigue (9%)
Bone tumor [2]
Leg cramps (3%) [4]
Myalgia/Myopathy [2]
Neck pain (3%)
Pain in extremities [3]

Respiratory
Cough (6%)
Dyspnea / shortness of breath (4–6%)
Pharyngitis (sore throat) (6%)
Pneumonia (4–6%)
Rhinitis / rhinosinusitis (see also sinusitis) (10%)

Other
Adverse effects / adverse reactions [5]
Tooth disorder (2%)

TERLIPRESSIN

Synonym: Terlipressin acetate
Trade names: Glypressin (IS Pharma), Terlipressin (Ferring) (Bissendorf Peptide)
Indications: Esophageal variceal hemorrhage
Class: Vasopressin agonist
Half-life: 50–70 minutes
Clinically important, potentially hazardous interactions with: none known
Pregnancy category: Contra-indicated in pregnancy

Skin
Gangrene [2]
Necrosis (skin necrosis) [16]

Cardiovascular
Hypertension [2]
Myocardial infarction [3]
Peripheral ischemia [3]
QT interval prolonged / QT prolongation [2]
Torsades de pointes [2]

Central Nervous System
Seizures [3]

Endocrine/Metabolic
Hyponatremia [14]

Neuromuscular/Skeletal
Rhabdomyolysis [3]

Other
Adverse effects / adverse reactions [2]

TESTOSTERONE

Trade names: Androderm (Actavis), AndroGel (AbbVie), Delatestryl (Endo), Fortesta (Endo), Natesto (Endo), Testim (Auxilium)
Indications: Androgen replacement, hypogonadism, postpartum breast pain
Class: Androgen
Half-life: 10–100 minutes
Clinically important, potentially hazardous interactions with: acarbose, anisindione, anticoagulants, cyclosporine, dicumarol, metformin, saxagliptin, sitagliptin, warfarin
Pregnancy category: Contra-indicated in pregnancy

Important contra-indications noted in the prescribing guidelines for: nursing mothers; pediatric patients
Note: Contra-indicated in men with carcinoma of the breast or known or suspected carcinoma of the prostate.
Warning: SECONDARY EXPOSURE TO TESTOSTERONE

Skin
- Acneiform eruption / acneiform dermatitis / acneiform rash (>10%) [20]
- Carcinoma [2]
- Dermatitis (4%) [2]
- Edema / fluid retention (<10%)
- Flushing / rubefaction (<10%)
- Rash (2%)

Hair
- Alopecia / hair loss [3]
- Hirsutism (<10%) [12]

Cardiovascular
- Cardiotoxicity [2]
- Cardiovascular adverse effect (includes major adverse cardiovascular events (MACE)) [3]
- Myocardial infarction [3]

Endocrine/Metabolic
- Gynecomastia [2]
- Mastodynia (>10%)

Genitourinary
- Priapism (>10%) [10]

Hematologic
- Hematocrit (packed cell volume (PCV)) increased [2]
- Polycythemia / erythrocytosis [2]
- Thrombosis [4]

Local
- Application-site bullae (12%)
- Application-site burning (3%)
- Application-site erythema (7%)
- Application-site induration (3%)
- Application-site pruritus (37%)
- Application-site vesicles (6%)
- Injection-site pain [2]

Other
- Adverse effects / adverse reactions [3]

TETRABENAZINE

Trade names: Nitoman (aaiPharma), Xenazine (Alliance)
Indications: Hyperkinetic movement disorders: Huntington's chorea, hemiballismus, senile chorea, Tourette syndrome, and tardive dyskinesia
Class: Vesicular monoamine transporter 2 inhibitor
Half-life: 2–8 hours
Clinically important, potentially hazardous interactions with: alcohol, amantadine, amiodarone, amitriptyline, amoxapine, antiarrhythmics, antibiotics, antipsychotics, arsenic, chlorpromazine, cinacalcet, citalopram, cyclic antidepressants, dasatinib, degarelix, delavirdine, deutetrabenazine, dolasetron, haloperidol, lapatinib, levodopa, levofloxacin, levomepromazine, linezolid, lithium, lurasidone, MAO inhibitors, metoclopramide, moxifloxacin, olanzapine, paliperidone, paroxetine hydrochloride, pazopanib, procainamide, QT prolonging drugs, quinidine, reserpine, risperidone, sotalol, telavancin, telithromycin, terbinafine, thioridazine, tipranavir, voriconazole, vorinostat, ziprasidone, zuclopenthixol
Pregnancy category: Based on animal data, may cause fetal harm
Important contra-indications noted in the prescribing guidelines for: the elderly; nursing mothers; pediatric patients
Warning: DEPRESSION AND SUICIDALITY

Skin
- Bruise / bruising / contusion / ecchymosis (ecchymoses) (6%)

Central Nervous System
- Akathisia (19%) [9]
- Anxiety (15%) [7]
- Balance disorder (9%)
- Bradykinesia (9%)
- Compulsions / obsessive-compulsive symptoms / obsessive-compulsive disorder (4%)
- Confusion (2%)
- Depression (19%) [16]
- Dysarthria (4%)
- Extrapyramidal symptoms (15%)
- Gait instability / postural instability (4%)
- Headache (4%)
- Insomnia (11%) [5]
- Irritability (9%)
- Memory loss/memory impaired (2%)
- Nervousness (10%) [2]
- Neuroleptic malignant syndrome [5]
- Parkinsonism (9%) [21]
- Sedation (31%) [3]
- Somnolence (drowsiness) (31%) [14]
- Suicidal ideation [4]
- Tremor (3%)
- Vertigo / dizziness (4%)

Endocrine/Metabolic
- Appetite decreased (4%)
- Hyperprolactinemia [2]

Gastrointestinal/Hepatic
- Nausea (13%) [2]
- Vomiting (6%)

Genitourinary
- Dysuria (4%)

Neuromuscular/Skeletal
- Asthenia / fatigue (22%) [3]
- Dystonia (3%)

Respiratory
- Bronchitis (4%)
- Dyspnea / shortness of breath (4%)
- Upper respiratory tract infection (11%)

TETRACAINE & OXYMETAZOLINE

Trade name: Kovanaze (St Renatus)
Indications: Regional anesthesia in restorative dentistry
Class: Alpha adrenoceptor agonist (oxymetazoline), Anesthetic; local (tetracaine)
Half-life: <2 hours
Clinically important, potentially hazardous interactions with: beta blockers, MAO inhibitors, other intranasal products, tricyclic antidepressants
Pregnancy category: Insufficient evidence to inform drug-associated risk
Important contra-indications noted in the prescribing guidelines for: the elderly; nursing mothers; pediatric patients
Note: For intranasal use only. See separate entry for oxymetazoline as topical formulation.

Mucosal
- Epistaxis (nosebleed) (2%)
- Mucosal ulceration (2–3%)
- Nasal congestion (32%) [3]
- Nasal discomfort (26%)
- Nasal dryness (2%)
- Oropharyngeal pain (14%)
- Rhinorrhea (52%) [3]

Cardiovascular
- Blood pressure variations (3–5%)
- Bradycardia / sinus bradycardia (3%)
- Hypertension (3%)

Central Nervous System
- Dysgeusia (taste perversion) (8%)
- Headache (10%)
- Hypoesthesia / hypesthesia (numbness) (intranasal and pharyngeal) (10%)
- Sensory disturbances (2%)
- Vertigo / dizziness (3%)

Ocular
- Lacrimation (13%)

Other
- Sneezing (sternutation) (4%)

TETRACYCLINE

Trade names: Helidac (Prometheus), Sumycin (Par)
Indications: Various infections caused by susceptible organisms
Class: Antibiotic, Antibiotic; tetracycline, Antimicrobial
Half-life: 6–11 hours
Clinically important, potentially hazardous interactions with: ACE inhibitors, acitretin, aluminum, amoxicillin, ampicillin, antacids, atovaquone, atovaquone/proguanil, bacampicillin, betamethasone, bismuth, bromelain, calcium salts, carbenicillin, cholestyramine, cloxacillin, colestipol, corticosteroids, coumarins, dairy products, dicloxacillin, didanosine, digoxin, ergotamine, food, gliclazide, isotretinoin, kaolin, methicillin, methotrexate, methoxyflurane, methysergide, mezlocillin, nafcillin, oral iron, oral typhoid vaccine, oxacillin, penicillins, phenindione, piperacillin, quinapril, retinoids, rocuronium, sodium picosulfate, strontium ranelate, sucralfate, sulfonylureas, ticarcillin, tripotassium dicitratobismuthate, vitamin A, zinc

---

Skin
- Acneiform eruption / acneiform dermatitis / acneiform rash [2]
- Angioedema (formerly named angioneurotic edema) [2]
- Candidiasis / candidosis [2]
- Erythema multiforme [7]
- Exanthems [3]
- Exfoliative dermatitis [2]
- Fixed eruption / fixed drug eruption (15%) [43]
- Hypersensitivity [2]
- Jarisch–Herxheimer reaction [3]
- Lichenoid eruption / lichenoid reaction [3]
- Lupus erythematosus (subacute cutaneous lupus erythematosus (SCLE)) [6]

Photosensitivity (<10%) [12]
Phototoxicity [4]
Pigmentation (Skin) (includes hyperpigmentation) [4]
Psoriasis (exacerbation) [2]
Stevens-Johnson syndrome and toxic epidermal necrolysis (SJS/TEN) [15]
Urticaria / hives [5]

Nails

Onycholysis [5]
Photo-onycholysis [10]

Central Nervous System

Pseudotumor cerebri [6]

Gastrointestinal/Hepatic

Diarrhea [2]
Hepatotoxicity / liver injury / acute liver injury / drug-induced liver injury (DILI) [2]
Pancreatitis / acute pancreatitis [3]

Genitourinary

Vaginitis (includes vulvitis) [3]

Other

Adverse effects / adverse reactions [4]
Tooth pigmentation / discoloration (>10%) [14]

TETRAZEPAM

Indications: Alcohol withdrawal, anxiety disorders, convulsive disorders
Class: Anticonvulsant (see also antiepileptic (anti-seizure)), Anxiolytic, Benzodiazepine, Hypnotic, Skeletal muscle relaxant
Half-life: 18–26 hours
Clinically important, potentially hazardous interactions with: cisipride, clozapine
Important contra-indications noted in the prescribing guidelines for: nursing mothers

---

Skin

Contact dermatitis [4]
Dermatitis [4]
Erythema multiforme [2]
Exanthems [2]
Phototoxicity [2]
Stevens-Johnson syndrome and toxic epidermal necrolysis (SJS/TEN) [4]

Other

Adverse effects / adverse reactions [2]

TEZACAFTOR/ IVACAFTOR

Trade name: Symdeko (Vertex)
Indications: Cystic fibrosis in patients aged 12 years and older who are homozygous for the *F508del* mutation in the *CFTR* gene
Class: CFTR potentiator (ivacaftor), CFTR protein corrector (tezacaftor)
Half-life: 15 hours (tezacaftor); 14 hours (ivacaftor)
Clinically important, potentially hazardous interactions with: carbamazepine, clarithromycin, erythromycin, fluconazole, grapefruit juice, itraconazole, ketoconazole, phenobarbital, phenytoin, posaconazole, rifabutin, rifampin, seville oranges, St John's wort, strong cy3pa inducers, strong or moderate CYP3A inhibitors, telithromycin, voriconazole
Pregnancy category: Insufficient evidence to inform drug-associated risk
Important contra-indications noted in the prescribing guidelines for: nursing mothers; pediatric patients
Note: See also separate profile for ivacaftor.

Mucosal

Nasal congestion (4%)
Oropharyngeal pain [2]

Central Nervous System

Fever (pyrexia) (includes hyperpyrexia) [2]
Headache (15%) [3]
Vertigo / dizziness (4%)

Gastrointestinal/Hepatic

Nausea (9%)

Neuromuscular/Skeletal

Asthenia / fatigue [2]

Respiratory

Cough [3]
Hemoptysis [2]
Nasopharyngitis [2]

Other

Adverse effects / adverse reactions [2]

THALIDOMIDE

Trade name: Thalomid (Celgene)
Indications: Graft-versus-host reactions, recalcitrant aphthous stomatitis
Class: Covid-19 putative drug, Immunosuppressant, TNF modulator
Half-life: 5–7 hours
Clinically important, potentially hazardous interactions with: alcohol, amiodarone, antihistamines, antipsychotics, bortezomib, calcium channel blockers, carbamazepine, cimetidine, cisplatin, CNS depressants, digoxin, disulfiram, docetaxel, famotidine, griseofulvin, lithium, metronidazole, modafinil, opioids, paclitaxel, penicillins, phenytoin, rifabutin, rifampin, St John's wort, succinylcholine, vincristine
Important contra-indications noted in the prescribing guidelines for: nursing mothers; pediatric patients
Note: Thalidomide is a potent teratogen, an agent that causes congenital malformations and developmental abnormalities if introduced during gestation. Some of these teratogenic side effects of thalidomide include fetal limb growth retardation (arms, legs, hands, feet), ingrown genitalia, absence of lung, partial/total loss of hearing or sight, malformed digestive tract, heart, kidney, and stillborn infant.
Warning: FETAL RISK AND VENOUS THROMBOEMBOLIC EVENTS

Skin

Bullous dermatosis (5%)
Dermatitis [2]
Diaphoresis (13%)
Edema / fluid retention (57%) [11]
Erythema [2]
Erythema nodosum [2]
Erythroderma [2]
Exanthems [2]
Exfoliative dermatitis [4]
Facial erythema (<5%) [2]
Hypersensitivity [3]
Peripheral edema (3–8%) [4]
Pruritus (itching) (3–8%) [3]
Psoriasis [2]
Purpura [2]
Rash (11–50%) [29]
Stevens-Johnson syndrome and toxic epidermal necrolysis (SJS/TEN) [7]
Urticaria / hives (3%) [2]
Vasculitis (angiitis) / cutaneous vasculitis (angiitis) [2]
Xerosis / xeroderma (21%) [5]

Mucosal

Oral candidiasis (4–11%)
Xerostomia (dry mouth) (8%) [10]

Cardiovascular

Bradycardia / sinus bradycardia [5]
Cardiotoxicity [2]
Hypotension (16%)
Thromboembolism [2]
Venous thromboembolism [5]

Central Nervous System

Agitation (9–26%)
Fever (pyrexia) (includes hyperpyrexia) (19–23%) [2]
Headache [2]
Hyperesthesia [2]
Insomnia (9%)
Neurotoxicity (22%) [24]
Paresthesias (6–16%) [9]
Parkinsonism [2]
Peripheral neuropathy [32]
Somnolence (drowsiness) (36%) [17]
Tremor (4–26%) [6]
Vertigo / dizziness (4–20%) [18]

Endocrine/Metabolic

Amenorrhea [6]
Gynecomastia [2]
Weight gain (22%)
Weight loss (23%)

Gastrointestinal/Hepatic

Abdominal pain (3%)
Constipation [17]
Diarrhea (4–19%)
Flatulence (8%)
Hepatotoxicity / liver injury / acute liver injury / drug-induced liver injury (DILI) [4]
Pancreatitis / acute pancreatitis [2]

Genitourinary

Erectile dysfunction [2]
Impotence (38%)
Leukorrhea (17–35%)

Hematologic

Anemia (6–13%) [5]
Neutropenia (neutrophils decreased) (31%) [9]
Thrombocytopenia / platelets decreased [6]
Thrombosis [13]

Neuromuscular/Skeletal

Arthralgia (13%)
Asthenia / fatigue (79%) [18]
Myalgia/Myopathy (7%)

Respiratory

Dyspnea / shortness of breath (42%)
Pharyngitis (sore throat) (4–8%)
Pneumonia [2]
Rhinitis / rhinosinusitis (see also sinusitis) (4%)
Sinusitis (see also rhinitis / rhinosinusitis) (3–8%)

Other

Adverse effects / adverse reactions [10]
Death [2]
Infection (6–8%) [7]
Teratogenicity [6]
Toothache (odontalgia) (4%)

THIAMINE

Synonym: vitamin B_1
Indications: Thiamine deficiency
Class: Vitamin
Half-life: N/A
Clinically important, potentially hazardous interactions with: none known
Pregnancy category: the pregnancy category will be C if used in doses above the RDA

Skin
Anaphylactoid reactions / anaphylaxis (includes anaphylactic shock) [4]
Dermatitis [2]
Purpura [2]

THIOGUANINE

Indications: Leukemias, inflammatory bowel disease
Class: Antimetabolite, Antineoplastic / anticancer agent (see also Immune checkpoint inhibitor)
Half-life: 11 hours
Clinically important, potentially hazardous interactions with: aldesleukin, vaccines

---

Skin
Rash (<10%)
Hair
Alopecia / hair loss [2]
Mucosal
Stomatitis (oral mucositis) (<10%)
Endocrine/Metabolic
Hypertransaminasemia (hepatic transaminitis) / elevated transaminases [2]
Gastrointestinal/Hepatic
Hepatotoxicity / liver injury / acute liver injury / drug-induced liver injury (DILI) [3]
Nodular regenerative hyperplasia [2]

THIOPENTAL

Trade name: Thiopental (Baxter)
Indications: Induction of anesthesia
Class: Barbiturate
Half-life: 3–12 hours
Clinically important, potentially hazardous interactions with: droperidol, ethanol, ethanolamine

---

Skin
Anaphylactoid reactions / anaphylaxis (includes anaphylactic shock) [9]
Angioedema (formerly named angioneurotic edema) [4]
Bullous dermatosis [2]
Erythema multiforme [2]
Exanthems (3%) [3]
Fixed eruption / fixed drug eruption [3]
Purpura [2]
Stevens-Johnson syndrome and toxic epidermal necrolysis (SJS/TEN) [2]
Urticaria / hives [4]
Central Nervous System
Shivering (27%)
Endocrine/Metabolic
Porphyria [4]
Local
Injection-site pain (>10%)
Injection-site phlebitis (6%)

THIORIDAZINE

Trade name: Mellaril (Novartis)
Indications: Psychotic disorders
Class: Antipsychotic, Phenothiazine
Half-life: 21–25 hours
Clinically important, potentially hazardous interactions with: abiraterone, amisulpride, amitriptyline, amoxapine, antihistamines, arsenic, asenapine, chlorpheniramine, cinacalcet, citalopram, cobicistat/elvitegravir/emtricitabine/tenofovir alafenamide, cobicistat/elvitegravir/emtricitabine/tenofovir disoproxil, darifenacin, dasatinib, degarelix, delavirdine, dofetilide, dolasetron, duloxetine, epinephrine, lapatinib, levofloxacin, miconazole, mirabegron, moxifloxacin, naloxone, paroxetine hydrochloride, paroxetine mesylate, pazopanib, pimavanserin, pimozide, piperazine, quinolones, ranolazine, rolapitant, sparfloxacin, sulpiride / levosulpiride, telavancin, telithromycin, terbinafine, tetrabenazine, tipranavir, voriconazole, vorinostat, zaleplon, ziprasidone, zuclopenthixol
Note: This drug has been withdrawn.

Skin
Photosensitivity (<10%) [2]
Phototoxicity [2]
Pigmentation (Skin) (includes hyperpigmentation) (blue-gray) [3]
Rash (<10%) [3]
Cardiovascular
QT interval prolonged / QT prolongation [8]
Torsades de pointes [2]
Central Nervous System
Neuroleptic malignant syndrome [2]
Parkinsonism (>10%)
Tardive syndrome / tardive dyskinesia [2]
Tic disorder [2]
Endocrine/Metabolic
Mastodynia (<10%)
SIADH [2]
Genitourinary
Priapism [4]
Ocular
Retinopathy [3]
Other
Death [2]

THIOTEPA

Trade name: Thioplex (Amgen)
Indications: Breast, ovarian and bladder carcinomas
Class: Alkylating agent
Half-life: 109 minutes
Clinically important, potentially hazardous interactions with: aldesleukin

---

Skin
Angioedema (formerly named angioneurotic edema) [5]
Leukoderma [4]
Pigmentation (Skin) (includes hyperpigmentation) (<10%) [4]
Pruritus (itching) (<10%) [5]
Rash (<10%)
Toxic erythema of chemotherapy (TEC) [3]
Urticaria / hives (3%) [6]
Hair
Alopecia / hair loss (<10%) [2]
Central Nervous System
Neurotoxicity [2]
Endocrine/Metabolic
SIADH [2]
Hematologic
Febrile neutropenia [2]
Local
Injection-site pain (>10%)
Other
Allergic reactions (<10%)

TIAGABINE

Trade name: Gabitril (Cephalon)
Indications: Partial seizures
Class: Anticonvulsant (see also antiepileptic (anti-seizure)), Mood stabilizer
Half-life: 7–9 hours
Clinically important, potentially hazardous interactions with: alcohol, antipsychotics, carbamazepine, chloroquine, conivaptan, CYP3A4 inhibitors and inducers, dasatinib, deferasirox, droperidol, hydroxychloroquine, ketorolac, levomepromazine, MAO inhibitors, mefloquine, orlistat, phenobarbital, phenytoin, SSRIs, St John's wort, tricyclic antidepressants
Important contra-indications noted in the prescribing guidelines for: the elderly; nursing mothers; pediatric patients

---

Skin
Bruise / bruising / contusion / ecchymosis (ecchymoses) (<6%)
Pruritus (itching) (2%)
Rash (5%) [2]
Cardiovascular
Vasodilation (2%)
Central Nervous System
Confusion (5%)
Depression (<7%) [4]
Emotional lability (3%)
Gait instability / postural instability (3–5%)
Headache [8]
Hostility (2–5%)
Impaired concentration (6–14%) [2]
Insomnia (5–6%)
Nervousness (10–14%) [10]
Pain (2–7%)
Paresthesias (4%)
Seizures [4]
Somnolence (drowsiness) (18–21%) [9]
Speech disorder (4%)
Status epilepticus (non-convulsive) [17]
Syncope / fainting [2]
Tremor (9–21%) [7]
Vertigo / dizziness (27–31%) [22]
Endocrine/Metabolic
Appetite increased (2%)
Gastrointestinal/Hepatic
Abdominal pain (5–7%)
Diarrhea (2–10%)
Nausea (11%) [7]
Vomiting (7%)
Genitourinary
Urinary tract infection (<5%)

Neuromuscular/Skeletal
Asthenia / fatigue (18–23%) [16]
Ataxia (5–9%)
Dystonia [5]
Myalgia/Myopathy (2–5%)

Ocular
Amblyopia (4–9%)
Nystagmus (2%)

Respiratory
Cough (4%)
Influenza- ('flu)-like syndrome (6–9%)
Pharyngitis (sore throat) (7–8%)

Other
Adverse effects / adverse reactions [6]
Infection (10–19%) [3]

TIANEPTINE

Trade name: Stablon (Servier)
Indications: Depression
Class: Antidepressant, Serotonin agonist
Half-life: 2.5 hours
Clinically important, potentially hazardous interactions with: tramadol
Pregnancy category: Not recommended in pregnancy
Important contra-indications noted in the prescribing guidelines for: nursing mothers; pediatric patients
Note: Immediate postpartum period is a high-risk time for depression, especially in women who have had prior depressive episodes, so tianeptine may need to be reinstituted late in the third trimester or shortly after childbirth to prevent a recurrence during the postpartum period.
Not available in USA or UK.

Mucosal
Xerostomia (dry mouth) [2]

Central Nervous System
Vertigo / dizziness [2]

Gastrointestinal/Hepatic
Abdominal pain [2]
Constipation [4]
Hepatotoxicity / liver injury / acute liver injury / drug-induced liver injury (DILI) [5]
Nausea [3]

Other
Adverse effects / adverse reactions [2]

TIBOLONE

Trade name: Livial (Organon)
Indications: Estrogen deficiency, prevention of osteoporosis
Class: Androgen agonist, Derivative of norethynodel, Estrogen agonist, Progesterone agonist, Selective estrogen receptor modulator (SERM)
Half-life: 1–4 hours
Clinically important, potentially hazardous interactions with: cyp3q4 inducers, midazolam, St John's wort, warfarin
Important contra-indications noted in the prescribing guidelines for: nursing mothers

Hair
Hypertrichosis (<10%)

Central Nervous System
Stroke / cerebrovascular accident [3]

Endocrine/Metabolic
Mastodynia [2]
Weight gain (<10%)

Gastrointestinal/Hepatic
Abdominal pain (<10%)

Genitourinary
Candidal vaginitis (<10%)
Endometrial cancer [5]
Vaginal discharge (<10%)

Other
Breast cancer [8]

TICAGRELOR

Trade name: Brilinta (AstraZeneca)
Indications: Thrombotic cardiovascular events
Class: Antiplatelet (antithrombotic), Antiplatelet; cyclopentyl triazolo-pyrimidine (CPTP)
Half-life: 7 hours
Clinically important, potentially hazardous interactions with: atazanavir, carbamazepine, clarithromycin, dexamethasone, digoxin, efavirenz, indinavir, inotersen, itraconazole, ketoconazole, lovastatin, nefazodone, nelfinavir, phenobarbital, phenytoin, rifampin, ritonavir, saquinavir, simvastatin, telithromycin, venetoclax, voriconazole
Important contra-indications noted in the prescribing guidelines for: nursing mothers; pediatric patients
Note: Maintenance doses of aspirin above 100 mg reduce the effectiveness of ticagrelor and should be avoided. Contra-indicated in patients with a history of intracranial hemorrhage, or active pathological bleeding, and in patients with severe hepatic impairment.
Warning: BLEEDING RISK

Skin
Angioedema (formerly named angioneurotic edema) [4]
Hypersensitivity [2]

Cardiovascular
Asystole [3]
Atrial fibrillation (4%)
Bradycardia / sinus bradycardia [2]
Chest pain (3–4%)
Hypertension (4%)
Hypotension (3%)
Sinus node dysfunction (sick sinus syndrome) [2]
Ventricular arrhythmia [7]

Central Nervous System
Headache (7%)
Vertigo / dizziness (5%)

Gastrointestinal/Hepatic
Diarrhea (4%)
Nausea (4%)

Hematologic
Bleeding (12%) [21]

Neuromuscular/Skeletal
Asthenia / fatigue (3%)
Back pain (4%)
Rhabdomyolysis [4]

Respiratory
Cough (5%)
Dyspnea / shortness of breath (14%) [21]
Pneumonitis [2]

Other
Adverse effects / adverse reactions [2]
Death [2]

TICARCILLIN

Trade names: Ticar (GSK), Timentin (GSK)
Indications: Various infections caused by susceptible organisms
Class: Antibiotic, Antibiotic; beta-lactam, Antibiotic; penicillin, Antimicrobial
Half-life: 1.0–1.2 hours
Clinically important, potentially hazardous interactions with: anticoagulants, ceftobiprole, cyclosporine, demeclocycline, doxycycline, imipenem/cilastatin, methotrexate, minocycline, oral contraceptives, oxytetracycline, probenecid, tetracycline
Important contra-indications noted in the prescribing guidelines for: nursing mothers
Note: Timentin is ticarcillin and clavulanic acid.

Local
Injection-site pain [2]
Injection-site phlebitis [3]

TICLOPIDINE

Trade name: Ticlid (Roche)
Indications: To reduce risk of thrombotic stroke
Class: Antiplatelet; thienopyridine, CYP1A2 inhibitor
Half-life: 24 hours
Clinically important, potentially hazardous interactions with: alteplase, clobazam, dabigatran, fondaparinux, inotersen, lepirudin, oxtriphylline, phenytoin, tinzaparin

Skin
Diaphoresis (<2%)
Exanthems (<12%) [5]
Fixed eruption / fixed drug eruption [3]
Hematoma / cutaneous hematoma (2%)
Lupus erythematosus (subacute cutaneous lupus erythematosus (SCLE)) (positive ANA) [4]
Petechiae (2%)
Pruritus (itching) [3]
Purpura (<5%) [26]
Rash (5%) [5]
Thrombocytopenic purpura [2]
Urticaria / hives (<5%) [4]

Central Nervous System
Fever (pyrexia) (includes hyperpyrexia) [2]

Gastrointestinal/Hepatic
Hepatotoxicity / liver injury / acute liver injury / drug-induced liver injury (DILI) [3]

Hematologic
Agranulocytosis / severe selective neutropenia [4]
Neutropenia (neutrophils decreased) [3]

Other
Side effects (8%)

TIGECYCLINE

Trade name: Tygacil (Wyeth)
Indications: Complicated skin or intra-abdominal infections, community-acquired bacterial pneumonia
Class: Antibiotic, Antibiotic, Antibiotic; glycylcycline, Antibiotic; tetracycline, Antimicrobial
Half-life: 36 hours
Clinically important, potentially hazardous interactions with: acitretin, antacids, coumarins, dairy products, ergotamine, kaolin, methysergide, oral contraceptives, oral iron, phenindione, quinapril, retinoids, strontium ranelate, sucralfate, sulfonylureas, tripotassium dicitratobismuthate, typhoid vaccine, warfarin
Important contra-indications noted in the prescribing guidelines for: nursing mothers; pediatric patients
Warning: ALL-CAUSE MORTALITY

Skin
Abscess (2%)
Jaundice (see also cholestasis / cholestatic jaundice) (<2%) [2]
Pruritus (itching) (<2%)
Rash (3%)
Stevens-Johnson syndrome and toxic epidermal necrolysis (SJS/TEN) [2]
Wound complications (3%)

Mucosal
Xerostomia (dry mouth) (<2%)

Cardiovascular
Bradycardia / sinus bradycardia (<2%)
Phlebitis (3%)
Tachycardia (<2%)

Central Nervous System
Anorexia (<2%)
Chills (<2%)
Dysgeusia (taste perversion) (<2%)
Fever (pyrexia) (includes hyperpyrexia) [3]
Headache (6%) [4]
Vertigo / dizziness (3%)

Endocrine/Metabolic
ALP increased (3%) [2]
ALT increased [2]
AST increased [2]
Creatine phosphokinase (CPK) / creatine kinase increased (hyperCKemia) (<2%)
Hypocalcemia (<2%)
Hypoglycemia (<2%) [5]
Hyponatremia (2%)
Hypoproteinemia (5%)

Gastrointestinal/Hepatic
Abdominal pain (6%) [2]
Cholestasis / cholestatic jaundice [2]
Diarrhea (12%) [8]
Dyspepsia / functional dyspepsia (indigestion) (see also gastroparesis) (2%)
Hepatotoxicity / liver injury / acute liver injury / drug-induced liver injury (DILI) [4]
Nausea (26%) [35]
Pancreatitis / acute pancreatitis [18]
Vomiting (18%) [32]

Genitourinary
Leukorrhea (<2%)
Vaginitis (includes vulvitis) (<2%)
Vulvovaginal candidiasis (<2%)

Hematologic
Anemia (5%)
Coagulopathy / coagulation dysfunction / clotting factor deficiency (includes disseminated intravascular coagulation / DIC) [8]
Eosinophilia / eosinophils increased (<2%)
Hypofibrinogenemia [17]
Leukocytosis (elevated white blood cell (WBC) count) [2]
Prothrombin time (INR) increased (<2%) [2]
Thrombocytopenia / platelets decreased (<2%)

Local
Injection-site edema (<2%)
Injection-site inflammation (<2%)
Injection-site pain (<2%)
Injection-site phlebitis (<2%)
Injection-site reaction (<2%)

Neuromuscular/Skeletal
Asthenia / fatigue (3%)

Respiratory
Pneumonia (2%)

Other
Adverse effects / adverse reactions [9]
Allergic reactions (<2%)
Death [3]
Infection (7%) [2]

TILDRAKIZUMAB

Trade name: Ilumya (Merck Sharpe & Dohme)
Indications: Moderate-to-severe plaque psoriasis
Class: Interleukin-17 (IL-17) antagonist / interleukin-17 inhibitor, Interleukin-23 inhibitor, Monoclonal antibody
Half-life: 23 days
Clinically important, potentially hazardous interactions with: live vaccines
Pregnancy category: Insufficient data to inform drug-associated risk
Important contra-indications noted in the prescribing guidelines for: nursing mothers; pediatric patients

---

Central Nervous System
Headache [3]

Gastrointestinal/Hepatic
Diarrhea (2%)

Local
Injection-site reaction (3%)

Respiratory
Cough [2]
Nasopharyngitis [2]
Upper respiratory tract infection (14%) [4]

Other
Adverse effects / adverse reactions [4]

TILUDRONATE

Trade name: Skelid (Sanofi-Aventis)
Indications: Paget's disease of the bone
Class: Bisphosphonate
Half-life: 150 hours
Clinically important, potentially hazardous interactions with: indomethacin
Important contra-indications noted in the prescribing guidelines for: nursing mothers; pediatric patients

---

Skin
Edema / fluid retention (3%)
Peripheral edema (3%)
Rash (3%)

Cardiovascular
Chest pain (3%)

Central Nervous System
Headache (7%)
Pain (21%)
Paresthesias (4%)
Vertigo / dizziness (4%)

Endocrine/Metabolic
Hyperparathyroidism (3%)

Gastrointestinal/Hepatic
Diarrhea (9%)
Dyspepsia / functional dyspepsia (indigestion) (see also gastroparesis) (5%)
Flatulence (3%)
Nausea [2]
Vomiting (4%) [2]

Neuromuscular/Skeletal
Arthralgia (3%)
Back pain (8%)

Ocular
Cataract (3%)
Conjunctivitis (conjunctival inflammation) (3%)
Glaucoma (includes acute angle-closure glaucoma) (3%)

Renal
Nephrotoxicity / kidney injury / acute kidney injury (AKI) / drug-induced kidney injury [2]

Respiratory
Cough (3%)
Pharyngitis (sore throat) (3%)
Rhinitis / rhinosinusitis (see also sinusitis) (5%)
Sinusitis (see also rhinitis / rhinosinusitis) (5%)
Upper respiratory tract infection (5%)

Other
Infection (3%)
Tooth disorder (3%)

TIMOLOL

Trade names: Blocadren (Merck), Cosopt (Merck), Timolide (Merck), Timoptic (Merck) (ophthalmic)
Indications: Hypertension
Class: Adrenergic beta-receptor antagonist
Half-life: 2–2.7 hours
Clinically important, potentially hazardous interactions with: clonidine, cobicistat/elvitegravir/emtricitabine/tenofovir alafenamide, cobicistat/elvitegravir/emtricitabine/tenofovir disoproxil, epinephrine, ergot, prednisone, verapamil
Note: Cosopt is timolol and dorzolamide; Timolide is timolol and hydrochlorothiazide. Dorzolamide and hydrochlorothiazide are sulfonamides and can be absorbed systemically. Sulfonamides can produce severe, possibly fatal, reactions such as toxic epidermal necrolysis and Stevens-Johnson syndrome.
Cutaneous side-effects of beta-receptor blockers are clinically polymorphous. They apparently appear after several months of continuous therapy.

Skin
Dermatitis (eyedrops) [7]
Eczema / eczematous reaction / eczematous eruption [2]
Erythroderma [2]
Lichenoid eruption / lichenoid reaction [2]
Lupus erythematosus (subacute cutaneous lupus erythematosus (SCLE)) [2]
Pruritus (itching) (<5%)
Psoriasis [5]
Rash (<10%) [3]
Raynaud's phenomenon [3]

Hair
Alopecia / hair loss (<10%)

Mucosal
Xerostomia (dry mouth) (19%) [3]

Cardiovascular
Arrhythmias [3]
Bradycardia / sinus bradycardia [8]
Chest pain [4]
Hypotension [2]

Central Nervous System
Dysgeusia (taste perversion) [6]
Headache [5]
Syncope / fainting [3]
Vertigo / dizziness [2]

Gastrointestinal/Hepatic
Nausea [3]

Ocular
Blepharitis [2]
Choroidal detachment [3]
Conjunctival hyperemia / conjunctival injection [18]
Conjunctivitis (conjunctival inflammation) [3]
Eyelid dermatitis [3]
Foreign body sensation [4]
Keratitis (ocular keratitis) / corneal inflammation) [2]
Lacrimation [2]
Ocular adverse effect [5]
Ocular allergy [2]
Ocular burning [8]
Ocular hyperemia [6]
Ocular itching / ocular pruritus [15]
Ocular pain [5]
Ocular stinging [11]
Punctate keratitis [6]
Uveitis / anterior uveitis / posterior uveitis / panuveitis [2]
Vision blurred [11]

Respiratory
Asthma [2]
Dyspnea / shortness of breath [2]

Other
Adverse effects / adverse reactions [6]

TINIDAZOLE

Trade names: Fasigyn (Pfizer), Tindamax (Mission)
Indications: Amebiasis, giardiasis, trichomoniasis
Class: Antibiotic, Antibiotic; nitroimidazole, Antimicrobial
Half-life: 12–14 hours
Clinically important, potentially hazardous interactions with: alcohol, anticoagulants, cyclosporine, CYP3A4 inducers or inhibitors, fluorouracil, fosphenytoin, lithium, phenytoin, tacrolimus, typhoid vaccine, warfarin
Important contra-indications noted in the prescribing guidelines for: nursing mothers; pediatric patients
Warning: POTENTIAL RISK FOR CARCINOGENICITY

Skin
Fixed eruption / fixed drug eruption [5]

Central Nervous System
Anorexia (2–3%)
Dysgeusia (taste perversion) (4–6%) [2]
Headache [3]

Gastrointestinal/Hepatic
Abdominal pain [2]
Constipation (<2%)
Dyspepsia / functional dyspepsia (indigestion) (see also gastroparesis) (2%)
Nausea (3–5%)
Vomiting (<2%)

Neuromuscular/Skeletal
Asthenia / fatigue (2%)

TINZAPARIN

Trade name: Innohep (Leo Pharma)
Indications: Acute symptomatic deep vein thrombosis
Class: Anticoagulant (antithrombotic), Heparin, low molecular weight
Half-life: 3–4 hours
Clinically important, potentially hazardous interactions with: aliskiren, angiotensin II recepton antagonists, aspirin, butabarbital, clopidogrel, collagenase, dasatinib, dextran, diclofenac, dipyridamole, drotrecogin alfa, glyceryl trinitrate, ibritumomab, iloprost, ketorolac, NSAIDs, oral anticoagulants, pentosan, pentoxifylline, platelet inhibitors, prostacyclin analogues, salicylates, sulfinpyrazone, throbolytics, ticlopidine, tositumomab & iodine[131]
Important contra-indications noted in the prescribing guidelines for: the elderly; nursing mothers; pediatric patients
Warning: SPINAL / EPIDURAL HEMATOMAS

Skin
Bullous dermatosis (<10%)
Pruritus (itching) (<10%)

Mucosal
Epistaxis (nosebleed) (2%)

Cardiovascular
Chest pain (2%)

Central Nervous System
Fever (pyrexia) (includes hyperpyrexia) (2%)
Headache (2%)
Pain (2%)

Endocrine/Metabolic
ALT increased (13%)
AST increased (9%)

Genitourinary
Urinary tract infection (4%)

Hematologic
Bleeding [4]
Hemorrhage (2%)

Local
Injection-site hematoma (16%)

Neuromuscular/Skeletal
Back pain (2%)

Respiratory
Pulmonary embolism (2%)

TIOTROPIUM

Trade names: Spiriva (Boehringer Ingelheim), Stiolto Respimat (Boehringer Ingelheim)
Indications: Bronchospasm (associated with COPD)
Class: Anticholinergic, Muscarinic antagonist
Half-life: 5–6 days
Clinically important, potentially hazardous interactions with: acetylcholinesterase inhibitors, anticholinergics, antihistamines, botulinum toxin (A & B), cannabinoids, conivaptan, disopyramide, domperidone, haloperidol, ketoconazole, levodopa, MAO inhibitors, memantine, metoclopramide, nefopam, parasympathomimetics, PEG-interferon, phenothiazines, potassium chloride, pramlintide, secretin, sublingual nitrates, tricyclic antidepressants
Important contra-indications noted in the prescribing guidelines for: nursing mothers; pediatric patients
Note: Stiolto Respimat is tiotropium and olodaterol.

Skin
Candidiasis / candidosis (4%)
Edema / fluid retention (5%)
Herpes zoster (<3%)
Rash (4%)

Mucosal
Epistaxis (nosebleed) (4%)
Oral candidiasis [2]
Stomatitis (oral mucositis) (<3%)
Xerostomia (dry mouth) (10–16%) [22]

Cardiovascular
Angina (<3%)
Cardiotoxicity [2]
Chest pain (7%) [2]
Hypertension [2]

Central Nervous System
Depression (<3%)
Headache [6]
Paresthesias (<3%)
Vertigo / dizziness [2]

Endocrine/Metabolic
Hypercholesterolemia (<3%)
Hyperglycemia (includes glucose increased) (<3%)

Gastrointestinal/Hepatic
Abdominal pain (5%)
Constipation (4%) [2]
Diarrhea [3]
Dyspepsia / functional dyspepsia (indigestion) (see also gastroparesis) (6%)
Gastroesophageal reflux (<3%)
Vomiting (4%)

Genitourinary
Urinary tract infection (7%)

Neuromuscular/Skeletal
Arthralgia (>3%)
Back pain [4]
Bone pain / joint pain (<3%)
Leg pain (<3%)
Myalgia/Myopathy (4%)

Ocular
Cataract (<3%)

Respiratory
Asthma [4]
Bronchitis [4]
COPD (exacerbation) [5]

Cough (>3%) [8]
Dysphonia (includes voice disorders / voice changes) (<3%)
Dyspnea / shortness of breath [4]
Influenza [3]
Influenza- ('flu)-like syndrome (>3%)
Laryngitis (<3%)
Nasopharyngitis [11]
Pharyngitis (sore throat) (9%)
Pneumonia [3]
Rhinitis / rhinosinusitis (see also sinusitis) (6%) [3]
Sinusitis (see also rhinitis / rhinosinusitis) (11%)
Upper respiratory tract infection (41%) [4]

Other
Adverse effects / adverse reactions [13]
Allergic reactions (<3%)
Death [7]
Infection (4%)

TIPRANAVIR

Trade name: Aptivus (Boehringer Ingelheim)
Indications: Antiretroviral treatment of HIV-1
Class: HIV-1 protease inhibitor, Sulfonamide
Half-life: 4.8–6.0 hours
Clinically important, potentially hazardous interactions with: abacavir, alcohol, alfuzosin, alprazolam, amiodarone, antacids, antifungals, apixaban, artemether/lumefantrine, atazanavir, atomoxetine, atorvastatin, bepridil, bosentan, buprenorphine, calcium channel blockers, carbamazepine, cisapride, clarithromycin, codeine, conivaptan, copanlisib, corticosteroids, cyclosporine, CYP2D6 substrates, CYP3A4 inducers, dabigatran, darifenacin, deferasirox, delavirdine, didanosine, digoxin, dihydroergotamine, disulfiram, efavirenz, elbasvir & grazoprevir, eluxadoline, enfuvirtide, eplerenone, ergotamine, esomeprazole, estradiol, estrogens, etravirine, fesoterodine, flecainide, fluconazole, fosamprenavir, fusidic acid, garlic, HMG-CoA reductase inhibitors, lopinavir, lovastatin, meperidine, methadone, metoprolol, metronidazole, midazolam, midostaurin, nebivolol, nefazodone, neratinib, omeprazole, P-glycoprotein substrates, pantoprazole, phenobarbital, phenytoin, pimozide, propafenone, protease inhibitors, proton pump inhibitors, quetiapine, quinidine, quinine, raltegravir, ranolazine, rifabutin, rifampin, rilpivirine, rivaroxaban, rosuvastatin, salmeterol, saquinavir, sildenafil, simeprevir, simvastatin, sirolimus, sofosbuvir, sofosbuvir/velpatasvir/voxilaprevir, St John's wort, tacrolimus, tamoxifen, telithromycin, temsirolimus, tenofovir disoproxil, tetrabenazine, theophylline, thioridazine, tramadol, trazodone, triazolam, tricyclic antidepressants, valproic acid, vardenafil, viloxazine, vitamin E, zidovudine
Important contra-indications noted in the prescribing guidelines for: the elderly; nursing mothers; pediatric patients
Note: Tipranavir is a sulfonamide and can be absorbed systemically. Sulfonamides can produce severe, possibly fatal, reactions such as toxic epidermal necrolysis and Stevens-Johnson syndrome.
Tipranavir is co-administered with ritonavir. Contra-indicated in patients with moderate or severe (Child-Pugh Class B or C) hepatic impairment.
Warning: HEPATOTOXICITY and INTRACRANIAL HEMORRHAGE

Skin
Exanthems (<2%)
Herpes simplex (<2%)
Herpes zoster (<2%)
Hypersensitivity (<2%)
Lipoatrophy (<2%)
Lipodystrophy / acquired generalized lipodystrophy (<2%)
Lipohypertrophy (<2%)
Pruritus (itching) (<2%)
Rash (3%) [2]

Central Nervous System
Anorexia (<2%)
Depression (2%)
Fever (pyrexia) (includes hyperpyrexia) (14%)
Headache (5%)
Insomnia (2%)
Intracranial hemorrhage (<2%) [3]
Neurotoxicity (<2%)
Peripheral neuropathy (2%)
Sleep-related disorder (<2%)
Somnolence (drowsiness) (<2%)
Vertigo / dizziness (<2%)

Endocrine/Metabolic
ALT increased (2%) [2]
Appetite decreased (<2%)
Dehydration (2%)
Diabetes mellitus (<2%)
GGT increased (2%)
Hyperamylasemia (<2%)
Hypercholesterolemia (<2%)
Hyperglycemia (includes glucose increased) (<2%)
Hyperlipidemia / lipids elevated (3%)
Hypertriglyceridemia (includes triglycerides increased) (4%) [2]
Weight loss (3%)

Gastrointestinal/Hepatic
Abdominal distension (<2%)
Abdominal pain (6%)
Dyspepsia / functional dyspepsia (indigestion) (see also gastroparesis) (<2%)
Flatulence (<2%)
Gastroesophageal reflux (<2%)
Hepatic failure (<2%)
Hepatitis (<2%)
Hepatotoxicity / liver injury / acute liver injury / drug-induced liver injury (DILI) [4]
Nausea (9%)
Pancreatitis / acute pancreatitis (<2%)
Vomiting (6%)

Hematologic
Anemia (3%)
Neutropenia (neutrophils decreased) (2%)
Thrombocytopenia / platelets decreased (<2%)

Neuromuscular/Skeletal
Asthenia / fatigue (2%)
Cramps (<2%)
Myalgia/Myopathy (2%)

Respiratory
Dyspnea / shortness of breath (2%)
Influenza- ('flu)-like syndrome (<2%)

Other
Adverse effects / adverse reactions [3]

TIROFIBAN

Trade name: Aggrastat (Merck)
Indications: Acute coronary syndrome
Class: Antiplatelet (antithrombotic), Glycoprotein IIb/IIIa inhibitor
Half-life: 2 hours
Clinically important, potentially hazardous interactions with: aspirin, fondaparinux, heparin, iloprost, lepirudin, NSAIDs

---

Skin
Diaphoresis (2%)
Edema / fluid retention (2%)

Cardiovascular
Myocardial ischemia [2]

Hematologic
Thrombocytopenia / platelets decreased [25]
Thrombotic microangiopathy [2]

Respiratory
Alveolar hemorrhage (pulmonary) [4]

TIZANIDINE

Trade name: Zanaflex (Acorda)
Indications: Muscle spasticity, multiple sclerosis
Class: Adrenergic alpha2-receptor agonist
Half-life: 2.5 hours
Clinically important, potentially hazardous interactions with: acebutolol, alfuzosin, benazepril, captopril, cilazapril, ciprofloxacin, enalapril, fluvoxamine, fosinopril, irbesartan, lisinopril, norfloxacin, obeticholic acid, olmesartan, phenytoin, quinapril, ramipril, rofecoxib, teriflunomide, trandolapril, viloxazine
Important contra-indications noted in the prescribing guidelines for: the elderly; pediatric patients

---

Skin
Pallor [2]
Pruritus (itching) (<10%)
Rash (<10%)

Mucosal
Xerostomia (dry mouth) (49–88%) [14]

Cardiovascular
Bradycardia / sinus bradycardia (<10%) [5]
Hypotension (16–33%) [4]

Central Nervous System
Dyskinesia (3%)
Nervousness (3%)
Somnolence (drowsiness) (48–92%) [4]
Speech disorder (3%)
Tremor (<10%)
Vertigo / dizziness (41–45%) [3]

Gastrointestinal/Hepatic
Constipation (4%)
Hepatotoxicity / liver injury / acute liver injury / drug-induced liver injury (DILI) (6%) [4]
Vomiting (3%)

Genitourinary
Urinary frequency (3%)
Urinary tract infection (10%)

Neuromuscular/Skeletal
Asthenia / fatigue (41–78%) [5]

Ocular
Amblyopia (3%)

Respiratory
Influenza- ('flu)-like syndrome (3%)

Pharyngitis (sore throat) (3%)
Rhinitis / rhinosinusitis (see also sinusitis) (3%)

Other

Infection (6%)

TOBRAMYCIN

Trade names: TOBI (Chiron), TobraDex (Alcon)
Indications: Various serious infections caused by susceptible organisms, superficial ocular infections
Class: Antibiotic, Antibiotic; aminoglycoside, Antimicrobial
Half-life: 2–3 hours
Clinically important, potentially hazardous interactions with: adefovir, aldesleukin, aminoglycosides, atracurium, bumetanide, daptomycin, doxacurium, ethacrynic acid, furosemide, neuromuscular blockers, pancuronium, polypeptide antibiotics, rocuronium, succinylcholine, teicoplanin, torsemide, vecuronium
Pregnancy category: Category D for injection and inhalation; category B for ophthalmic use
Important contra-indications noted in the prescribing guidelines for: the elderly; nursing mothers; pediatric patients
Note: Aminoglycosides may cause neurotoxicity and/or nephrotoxicity.
TobraDex is tobramycin and dexamethasone.

Skin

Exanthems [4]
Hypersensitivity [3]
Rash [2]

Central Nervous System

Dysgeusia (taste perversion) [2]
Fever (pyrexia) (includes hyperpyrexia) [2]

Ocular

Conjunctivitis (conjunctival inflammation) [2]
Eyelid dermatitis [2]
Intraocular pressure increased [2]

Renal

Nephrotoxicity / kidney injury / acute kidney injury (AKI) / drug-induced kidney injury [6]

Respiratory

Cough [3]

TOCILIZUMAB

Trade names: Actemra (Roche), RoActemra (Roche)
Indications: Rheumatoid arthritis, juvenile idiopathic arthritis, Castleman's disease
Class: Biologic, Biologic disease-modifying antirheumatic drug (bDMARD), Covid-19 putative drug, Disease-modifying antirheumatic drug (DMARD), Interleukin-6 inhibitor / anti-interleukin 6 receptor monoclonal antibody, Monoclonal antibody
Half-life: 8–14 days
Clinically important, potentially hazardous interactions with: dolasetron, efavirenz, fesoterodine, fingolimod, infliximab, lurasidone, paricalcitol, pazopanib, typhoid vaccine, yellow fever vaccine
Pregnancy category: Based on animal data, may cause fetal harm
Important contra-indications noted in the prescribing guidelines for: nursing mothers; pediatric patients
Note: Tocilizumab-bavi (Tofidence) is biosimilar to Tocilizumab (Actemra). Approved 09/29/2023
Tocilizumab-Aazg (Tyenne) is biosimilar to Tocilizumab (Actemra). Approved 03/05/2024.
Warning: RISK OF SERIOUS INFECTIONS

Skin

Anaphylactoid reactions / anaphylaxis (includes anaphylactic shock) [5]
Cellulitis and pseudocellulitis [9]
Herpes zoster [8]
Hypersensitivity [6]
Peripheral edema (<2%)
Psoriasis [4]
Rash (2%) [9]
Urticaria / hives [2]

Mucosal

Aphthous stomatitis / aphthous ulcer / aphtha (aphthae) [2]
Mucosal ulceration [2]
Oral ulceration (2%) [2]
Stomatitis (oral mucositis) (<2%)

Cardiovascular

Cardiotoxicity [3]
Hypertension (6%) [4]

Central Nervous System

Headache (7%) [7]
Neurotoxicity [2]
Vertigo / dizziness (3%)

Endocrine/Metabolic

ALT increased (6%) [10]
AST increased [4]
Hypercholesterolemia [8]
Hyperlipidemia / lipids elevated [7]
Hypertransaminasemia (hepatic transaminitis) / elevated transaminases [5]
Hypertriglyceridemia (includes triglycerides increased) [3]
Hypothyroidism (<2%)
Weight gain (<2%)

Gastrointestinal/Hepatic

Abdominal pain (2%)
Diarrhea [2]
Gastroenteritis [6]
Gastrointestinal bleeding [3]
Gastrointestinal perforation / perforated colon / gastric perforation [10]
Gastrointestinal ulceration (<2%)
Hepatotoxicity / liver injury / acute liver injury / drug-induced liver injury (DILI) [17]
Nausea [4]
Pancreatitis / acute pancreatitis [2]

Genitourinary

Urinary tract infection [3]

Hematologic

Hemotoxicity [2]
Hypofibrinogenemia [2]
Leukocytopenia (leukopenia) / leukocytes (white blood cells) decreased (<2%) [7]
Lymphopenia (lymphocytopenia) / lymphocytes decreased [2]
Neutropenia (neutrophils decreased) [23]
Sepsis [2]

Local

Infusion-related reactions [3]
Infusion-site reactions [2]

Neuromuscular/Skeletal

Arthralgia [4]
Fractures [2]

Ocular

Conjunctivitis (conjunctival inflammation) (<2%)

Renal

Nephrolithiasis (kidney stones / renal calculi) (<2%)
Pyelonephritis [3]

Respiratory

Bronchitis (3%) [6]
Cough (<2%)
Dyspnea / shortness of breath (<2%)
Influenza [3]
Nasopharyngitis (7%) [7]
Pharyngitis (sore throat) [4]
Pneumonia [13]
Pneumothorax [2]
Pulmonary toxicity [5]
Upper respiratory tract infection (7%) [12]

Other

Adverse effects / adverse reactions [16]
Death [6]
Infection [42]
Malignancies [2]

TOFACITINIB

Trade name: Xeljanz (Pfizer)
Indications: Rheumatoid arthritis
Class: Disease-modifying antirheumatic drug (DMARD), Janus kinase (JAK) inhibitor
Half-life: ~3 hours
Clinically important, potentially hazardous interactions with: azathioprine, biologic disease-modifying antirheumatics, cyclosporine, CYP3A4 inhibitors, fluconazole, ketoconazole, live vaccines, potent immunosuppressives, rifampin, strong CYP inducers, strong CYP2C19 inhibitors, tacrolimus
Important contra-indications noted in the prescribing guidelines for: the elderly; nursing mothers; pediatric patients
Warning: ◆ INCREASED RISK OF SERIOUS BACTERIAL, FUNGAL, VIRAL, AND OPPORTUNISTIC INFECTIONS LEADING TO HOSPITALIZATION OR DEATH, INCLUDING TUBERCULOSIS (TB). INTERRUPT TREATMENT WITH TOFACITINIB ORAL SOLUTION IF SERIOUS INFECTION OCCURS UNTIL THE INFECTION IS CONTROLLED. TEST FOR LATENT TB BEFORE AND DURING THERAPY; TREAT LATENT TB PRIOR TO USE. MONITOR ALL PATIENTS FOR ACTIVE TB DURING TREATMENT, EVEN PATIENTS WITH INITIAL NEGATIVE LATENT TB TEST.
◆ HIGHER RATE OF ALL-CAUSE MORTALITY, INCLUDING SUDDEN CARDIOVASCULAR DEATH WITH TOFACITINIB VS. TNF BLOCKERS IN RHEUMATOID ARTHRITIS (RA) PATIENTS.
◆ MALIGNANCIES HAVE OCCURRED IN PATIENTS TREATED WITH TOFACITINIB. HIGHER RATE OF LYMPHOMAS AND LUNG CANCERS WITH TOFACITINIB VS. TNF BLOCKERS IN RA PATIENTS.
◆ HIGHER RATE OF MACE (DEFINED AS CARDIOVASCULAR DEATH, MYOCARDIAL INFARCTION, AND STROKE) WITH TOFACITINIB VS. TNF BLOCKERS IN RA PATIENTS.
◆ THROMBOSIS HAS OCCURRED IN PATIENTS TREATED WITH TOFACITINIB. INCREASED INCIDENCE OF PULMONARY

EMBOLISM, VENOUS AND ARTERIAL THROMBOSIS WITH XELJANZ VS. TNF BLOCKERS IN RA PATIENTS.

Skin
- Acneiform eruption / acneiform dermatitis / acneiform rash [3]
- Baboon syndrome / symmetrical drug-related intertriginous and flexural exanthema (SDRIFE) [2]
- Erythema (<2%)
- Herpes zoster [17]
- Peripheral edema (<2%)
- Pruritus (itching) (<2%)
- Psoriasis [2]
- Rash (<2%) [3]

Mucosal
- Nasal congestion (<2%)

Cardiovascular
- Cardiotoxicity [3]
- Hypertension (2%)

Central Nervous System
- Fever (pyrexia) (includes hyperpyrexia) (<2%)
- Headache (3–4%) [11]
- Insomnia (<2%)
- Paresthesias (<2%)

Endocrine/Metabolic
- ALT increased [3]
- AST increased [3]
- Creatine phosphokinase (CPK) / creatine kinase increased (hyperCKemia) [2]
- Dehydration (<2%)
- Dyslipidemia [2]
- Hypercholesterolemia [2]
- Hyperlipidemia / lipids elevated [3]

Gastrointestinal/Hepatic
- Abdominal pain (<2%) [2]
- Diarrhea (3–4%) [9]
- Dyspepsia / functional dyspepsia (indigestion) (see also gastroparesis) (<2%) [2]
- Gastritis / pangastritis / gastric irritation (<2%)
- Nausea (<2%) [4]
- Vomiting (<2%)

Genitourinary
- Urinary tract infection (2%) [5]

Hematologic
- Anemia (<2%)
- Neutropenia (neutrophils decreased) [3]

Neuromuscular/Skeletal
- Arthralgia (<2%)
- Bone pain / joint pain (<2%)
- Tendinitis (<2%)

Respiratory
- Bronchitis [4]
- Cough (<2%)
- Dyspnea / shortness of breath (<2%)
- Influenza [3]
- Nasopharyngitis (3–4%) [11]
- Tuberculosis [5]
- Upper respiratory tract infection (4–5%) [12]

Other
- Adverse effects / adverse reactions [13]
- Death [2]
- Infection (20–22%) [18]
- Malignant neoplasms [2]

TOLBUTAMIDE

Trade name: Orinase (Pfizer)
Indications: Non-insulin dependent diabetes Type II
Class: Antidiabetic, Hypoglycemic (antihyperglycemic) agent, Sulfonylurea
Half-life: 4–25 hours
Clinically important, potentially hazardous interactions with: aprepitant, leflunomide, phenylbutazones, prednisone, propranolol
Important contra-indications noted in the prescribing guidelines for: nursing mothers; pediatric patients
Note: Tolbutamide is a sulfonamide and can be absorbed systemically. Sulfonamides can produce severe, possibly fatal, reactions such as toxic epidermal necrolysis and Stevens-Johnson syndrome.

Skin
- Exanthems (<5%) [3]
- Flushing / rubefaction [3]
- Photosensitivity (<10%) [2]
- Purpura [2]
- Rash (<10%)
- Urticaria / hives (<10%)

Endocrine/Metabolic
- Hypoglycemia [6]

Other
- Side effects [3]

TOLMETIN

Trade name: Tolectin (Ortho-McNeil)
Indications: Rheumatoid arthritis, osteoarthritis, juvenile rheumatoid arthritis
Class: Non-steroidal anti-inflammatory (NSAID)
Half-life: 1–2 hours
Clinically important, potentially hazardous interactions with: ACE inhibitors, aspirin, furosemide, lithium, methotrexate, thiazide diuretics, warfarin
Important contra-indications noted in the prescribing guidelines for: nursing mothers; pediatric patients
Note: NSAIDs may cause an increased risk of serious cardiovascular and gastrointestinal adverse events, which can be fatal. This risk may increase with duration of use.

Skin
- Anaphylactoid reactions / anaphylaxis (includes anaphylactic shock) [7]
- Angioedema (formerly named angioneurotic edema) [2]
- Edema / fluid retention (3–9%)
- Exanthems (9%) [4]
- Pruritus (itching) (<10%) [3]
- Rash (>10%)
- Stevens-Johnson syndrome and toxic epidermal necrolysis (SJS/TEN) [3]
- Urticaria / hives (<5%) [5]

TOLTERODINE

Trade name: Detrol (Pharmacia & Upjohn)
Indications: Urinary incontinence
Class: Muscarinic antagonist
Half-life: 2–4 hours
Clinically important, potentially hazardous interactions with: itraconazole, ketoconazole, lopinavir, nelfinavir, sotalol, viloxazine, voriconazole, warfarin
Important contra-indications noted in the prescribing guidelines for: nursing mothers; pediatric patients

---

Skin
- Erythema (2%)
- Rash (2%)

Mucosal
- Xerostomia (dry mouth) (35%) [39]

Cardiovascular
- Chest pain (2%)

Central Nervous System
- Headache (7%) [5]
- Somnolence (drowsiness) (3%)
- Vertigo / dizziness (5%) [4]

Gastrointestinal/Hepatic
- Abdominal pain (5%) [2]
- Constipation (7%) [13]
- Diarrhea (4%)
- Dyspepsia / functional dyspepsia (indigestion) (see also gastroparesis) (4%)

Genitourinary
- Dysuria (2%)

Neuromuscular/Skeletal
- Arthralgia (2%)
- Asthenia / fatigue (4%)

Ocular
- Vision blurred [3]
- Xerophthalmia (dry eyes) (3%) [2]

Respiratory
- Influenza- ('flu)-like syndrome (3%)
- Upper respiratory tract infection (6%)

Other
- Adverse effects / adverse reactions [6]

TOLVAPTAN

Trade name: Samsca (Otsuka)
Indications: Chronic heart failure, hyponatremia, polycystic kidneys
Class: Vasopressin receptor antagonist
Half-life: 6–8 hours
Clinically important, potentially hazardous interactions with: aprepitant, barbiturates, benazepril, captopril, carbamazepine, clarithromycin, conivaptan, cyclosporine, darunavir, delavirdine, digoxin, efavirenz, enalapril, fosinopril, grapefruit juice, indinavir, irbesartan, itraconazole, ketoconazole, lapatinib, lisinopril, lovastatin, miconazole, nefazodone, nelfinavir, olmesartan, oxcarbazepine, P-gp inhibitors, phenytoin, quinapril, ramipril, rifabutin, rifampin, rifapentin, rifapentine, ritonavir, saquinavir, St John's wort, strong CYP3A inhibitors, telithromycin, voriconazole
Important contra-indications noted in the prescribing guidelines for: nursing mothers; pediatric patients
Note: March 2013. The U.S. Food and Drug Administration (FDA) has determined that

tolvaptan should not be used for longer than 30 days and should not be used in patients with underlying liver disease because it can cause liver injury, potentially requiring liver transplant or death.
Warning: INITIATE AND RE-INITIATE IN A HOSPITAL AND MONITOR SERUM SODIUM

Mucosal
Xerostomia (dry mouth) (13%) [14]
Cardiovascular
Intracardiac thrombus (<2%)
Ventricular fibrillation (<2%)
Central Nervous System
Anorexia (4%)
Fever (pyrexia) (includes hyperpyrexia) (4%)
Vertigo / dizziness [2]
Endocrine/Metabolic
ALT increased (4%) [2]
Appetite decreased (4%)
Dehydration [3]
Hyperglycemia (includes glucose increased) (6%)
Hypernatremia [6]
Hypertransaminasemia (hepatic transaminitis) / elevated transaminases [3]
Gastrointestinal/Hepatic
Abdominal distension [2]
Constipation (7%) [4]
Diarrhea [2]
Hepatotoxicity / liver injury / acute liver injury / drug-induced liver injury (DILI) [8]
Vomiting [2]
Genitourinary
Nocturia [2]
Pollakiuria (11%) [5]
Polyuria (includes polyuric syndrome) (11%) [8]
Hematologic
Hemorrhage (<2%)
Thrombosis (<2%)
Neuromuscular/Skeletal
Asthenia / fatigue (9%) [2]
Rhabdomyolysis (<2%)
Renal
Aquaresis [2]
Nephrotoxicity / kidney injury / acute kidney injury (AKI) / drug-induced kidney injury [2]
Respiratory
Pulmonary embolism (<2%)
Other
Adverse effects / adverse reactions [3]
Dipsia (thirst) / polydipsia (16%) [22]

TOPIRAMATE

Trade names: Qsymia (Vivus), Qudexy (Upsher-Smith), Topamax (Janssen), Trokendi XR (Supernus)
Indications: Partial onset seizures, migraine. Adjunct for the treatment of obesity and for weight loss management in defined populations and health conditions.

Class: Anti-obesity / weight loss pharmacotherapy, Anticonvulsant (see also antiepileptic (anti-seizure)), Mood stabilizer, Neuroprotectant
Half-life: 21 hours
Clinically important, potentially hazardous interactions with: eslicarbazepine, levonorgestrel, metformin, rufinamide, ulipristal, valproic acid
Important contra-indications noted in the prescribing guidelines for: nursing mothers; pediatric patients
Note: Qsymia, a combination of phentermine and topiramate, has been approved by the FDA for chronic weight management.

Skin
Anhidrosis [2]
Bromhidrosis (2%)
Diaphoresis (2%)
Edema / fluid retention (2%)
Fixed eruption / fixed drug eruption [2]
Flushing / rubefaction (>5%)
Hot flashes / hot flushes (<10%)
Hypohidrosis [2]
Palmar erythema [2]
Pruritus (itching) (2%) [3]
Rash (4%) [3]
Hair
Alopecia / hair loss [2]
Mucosal
Gingival hyperplasia / gingival hypertrophy / gingival enlargement / gingival overgrowth [2]
Gingivitis (2%)
Xerostomia (dry mouth) (3%) [7]
Cardiovascular
Tachycardia [4]
Central Nervous System
Anorexia (>5%) [4]
Anxiety [3]
Cognitive impairment (>5%) [17]
Confusion (>5%)
Depression [11]
Dysgeusia (taste perversion) (>5%) [11]
Encephalopathy (includes hepatic encephalopathy) [4]
Fever (pyrexia) (includes hyperpyrexia) (>5%)
Headache [2]
Hyperthermia [3]
Impaired concentration [4]
Insomnia [8]
Irritability [3]
Nervousness (>5%)
Neurotoxicity [6]
Palinopsia / visual perseveration [3]
Paresthesias (>5%) [38]
Peripheral neuropathy [2]
Psychosis [3]
Seizures [3]
Somnambulism (sleepwalking; noctambulism) [2]
Somnolence (drowsiness) (>5%) [7]
Stuttering (dysphemia) / stammering [3]
Suicidal ideation [2]
Tremor (>10%)
Vertigo / dizziness (>5%) [15]
Endocrine/Metabolic
Acidosis (includes lactic acidosis) [5]
Appetite decreased [5]
Gynecomastia (8%)
Hyperammonemia [3]
Mastodynia (3–9%)
Weight gain [2]
Weight loss (>5%) [17]
Gastrointestinal/Hepatic
Constipation [7]
Diarrhea [3]
Nausea [5]
Genitourinary
Erectile dysfunction [2]
Neuromuscular/Skeletal
Asthenia / fatigue (>5%) [10]
Ataxia [2]
Ocular
Ciliochoroidal effusion / uveal effusion (includes ciliary body effusion) [2]
Diplopia (double vision) [2]
Eyelid twitching / eyelid myokymia [2]
Glaucoma (includes acute angle-closure glaucoma) [21]
Hypopyon [2]
Myopia [14]
Uveitis / anterior uveitis / posterior uveitis / panuveitis [7]
Vision loss [3]
Renal
Nephrolithiasis (kidney stones / renal calculi) [5]
Respiratory
Influenza- ('flu)-like syndrome (<2%)
Other
Adverse effects / adverse reactions [11]
Death [2]
Infection (>5%)
Side effects [3]
Teratogenicity [8]

TOPOTECAN

Trade name: Hycamtin (GSK)
Indications: Metastatic ovarian carcinoma
Class: Antineoplastic / anticancer agent (see also Immune checkpoint inhibitor), Topoisomerase I inhibitor
Half-life: 3–6 hours
Clinically important, potentially hazardous interactions with: atorvastatin, darunavir, gefitinib, lapatinib, oxaliplatin, pantoprazole, safinamide, sofosbuvir & velpatasvir
Important contra-indications noted in the prescribing guidelines for: nursing mothers; pediatric patients
Warning: BONE MARROW SUPPRESSION

Hair
Alopecia / hair loss (59%) [7]
Mucosal
Mucositis [2]
Stomatitis (oral mucositis) (24%) [4]

Central Nervous System
Fever (pyrexia) (includes hyperpyrexia) [2]
Paresthesias (9%)

Gastrointestinal/Hepatic
Abdominal pain [2]
Diarrhea [5]
Hepatotoxicity / liver injury / acute liver injury / drug-induced liver injury (DILI) [3]
Nausea [3]
Vomiting [4]

Hematologic
Anemia [11]
Febrile neutropenia [5]
Granulocytopenia [2]
Myelosuppression / bone marrow suppression / myelotoxicity [3]
Neutropenia (neutrophils decreased) [16]
Thrombocytopenia / platelets decreased [15]

Neuromuscular/Skeletal
Asthenia / fatigue [9]

Renal
Nephrotoxicity / kidney injury / acute kidney injury (AKI) / drug-induced kidney injury [2]

Respiratory
Dyspnea / shortness of breath [3]

Other
Adverse effects / adverse reactions [2]
Death [5]
Infection [2]

TOREMIFENE

Trade name: Fareston (ProStrakan)
Indications: Metastatic breast cancer
Class: Selective estrogen receptor modulator (SERM)
Half-life: ~5 days
Clinically important, potentially hazardous interactions with: amoxapine, arsenic, dolasetron, efavirenz, pazopanib, sugammadex, telavancin
Important contra-indications noted in the prescribing guidelines for: nursing mothers; pediatric patients
Warning: QT PROLONGATION

Skin
Diaphoresis (20%) [6]
Edema / fluid retention (5%) [2]
Flushing / rubefaction [3]
Hot flashes / hot flushes (35%) [4]

Cardiovascular
Thromboembolism [3]
Venous thromboembolism [2]

Central Nervous System
Headache [2]
Vertigo / dizziness [2]

Endocrine/Metabolic
ALP increased [2]
Galactorrhea (<10%)

Gastrointestinal/Hepatic
Hepatotoxicity / liver injury / acute liver injury / drug-induced liver injury (DILI) [3]
Nausea [2]
Vomiting [2]

Genitourinary
Priapism (<10%)
Vaginal bleeding [2]
Vaginal discharge [2]

Ocular
Cataract [3]

TORSEMIDE

Synonym: Torasemide
Trade names: Demadex (Roche), Torem (Roche)
Indications: Essential hypertension, edema due to congestive heart failure, hepatic, pulmonary or renal edema
Class: Diuretic, loop
Half-life: 2–4 hours
Clinically important, potentially hazardous interactions with: ACE inhibitors, amikacin, aminoglycosides, aminophylline, anti-diabetics, antihypertensives, cephalosporins, cisplatin, gentamicin, indomethacin, kanamycin, neomycin, probenecid, salicylates, streptomycin, tobramycin
Important contra-indications noted in the prescribing guidelines for: nursing mothers; pediatric patients
Note: Torsemide is a sulfonamide and can be absorbed systemically. Sulfonamides can produce severe, possibly fatal, reactions such as toxic epidermal necrolysis and Stevens-Johnson syndrome.

Skin
Photosensitivity (<10%)
Pseudoporphyria [2]
Purpura [2]
Urticaria / hives (<10%)
Vasculitis (angiitis) / cutaneous vasculitis (angiitis) [2]

Central Nervous System
Headache (7%)
Vertigo / dizziness (3%)

Gastrointestinal/Hepatic
Constipation (2%)
Diarrhea (2%)
Dyspepsia / functional dyspepsia (indigestion) (see also gastroparesis) (2%)
Nausea (2%)

Neuromuscular/Skeletal
Arthralgia (2%)
Asthenia / fatigue (2%)
Myalgia/Myopathy (2%)

Respiratory
Cough (2%)
Pharyngolaryngeal pain (2%)
Rhinitis / rhinosinusitis (see also sinusitis) (3%)

TOSITUMOMAB & IODINE[131]

Trade names: Bexxar (Corixa) (GSK), Iodine[131] I-Tositumomab (MDS Nordion)
Indications: Non-Hodgkin's lymphoma
Class: Antineoplastic / anticancer agent (see also Immune checkpoint inhibitor), Biologic, Monoclonal antibody
Half-life: 8 days
Clinically important, potentially hazardous interactions with: abciximab, argatroban, cilostazol, citalopram, clopidogrel, dabigatran, eptifibatide, meloxicam, tinzaparin
Important contra-indications noted in the prescribing guidelines for: nursing mothers; pediatric patients
Warning: SERIOUS ALLERGIC REACTIONS / ANAPHYLAXIS, PROLONGED AND SEVERE CYTOPENIAS, AND RADIATION EXPOSURE

Skin
Diaphoresis (8%)
Peripheral edema (9%)
Pruritus (itching) (10%) [2]
Rash (17%) [2]

Cardiovascular
Chest pain (7%)
Hypotension (7%)
Vasodilation (5%)

Central Nervous System
Anorexia (14%)
Chills (18%) [2]
Fever (pyrexia) (includes hyperpyrexia) (37%) [2]
Headache (16%) [2]
Pain (19%)
Somnolence (drowsiness) (5%) [2]
Vertigo / dizziness (5%)

Endocrine/Metabolic
Hypothyroidism (7%) [2]
Weight loss (6%)

Gastrointestinal/Hepatic
Abdominal pain (15%)
Constipation (6%)
Diarrhea (12%)
Dyspepsia / functional dyspepsia (indigestion) (see also gastroparesis) (6%)
Nausea (36%) [3]
Vomiting (15%)

Hematologic
Anemia [2]
Cytopenia [2]
Hemotoxicity [5]
Neutropenia (neutrophils decreased) [5]
Thrombocytopenia / platelets decreased [3]

Neuromuscular/Skeletal
Arthralgia (10%) [2]
Asthenia / fatigue (46%) [2]
Back pain (8%)
Myalgia/Myopathy (13%) [5]
Neck pain (6%)

Respiratory
Cough (21%)
Dyspnea / shortness of breath (11%)
Pharyngitis (sore throat) (12%)
Pneumonia (6%) [2]
Rhinitis / rhinosinusitis (see also sinusitis) (10%)

Other
Infection (21%) [2]

TRABECTEDIN

Trade name: Yondelis (Janssen)
Indications: Advanced soft tissue sarcoma
Class: Antineoplastic / anticancer agent (see also Immune checkpoint inhibitor)
Half-life: 180 hours
Clinically important, potentially hazardous interactions with: alcohol, aprepitant, atorvastatin, clarithromycin, cyclosporine, fluconazole, ketoconazole, phenobarbital, rifampin, ritonavir, rosuvastatin, St John's wort, strong CYP3A inducers or inhibitors, verapamil
Pregnancy category: Can cause fetal harm
Important contra-indications noted in the prescribing guidelines for: nursing mothers; pediatric patients

Skin
Edema / fluid retention (<10%)

Flushing / rubefaction (<10%)
Necrosis (skin necrosis) [2]
Peripheral edema [2]

Hair
Alopecia / hair loss (<10%)

Mucosal
Mucositis [3]

Cardiovascular
Cardiomyopathy [2]
Hypotension (<10%)

Central Nervous System
Anorexia (>10%) [4]
Dysgeusia (taste perversion) (<10%)
Headache (>10%) [3]
Insomnia (<10%)
Neurotoxicity (<10%)
Paresthesias (<10%)
Vertigo / dizziness (<10%)

Endocrine/Metabolic
ALT increased [14]
Appetite decreased (<10%) [3]
AST increased [7]
GGT increased [2]
Hypertransaminasemia (hepatic transaminitis) / elevated transaminases [2]
Weight loss (<10%)

Gastrointestinal/Hepatic
Abdominal pain (<10%)
Constipation (<10%) [6]
Diarrhea (<10%) [5]
Dyspepsia / functional dyspepsia (indigestion) (see also gastroparesis) (<10%)
Hepatotoxicity / liver injury / acute liver injury / drug-induced liver injury (DILI) [13]
Nausea (<10%) [17]
Vomiting (<10%) [15]

Hematologic
Anemia (>10%) [8]
Febrile neutropenia [6]
Leukocytopenia (leukopenia) / leukocytes (white blood cells) decreased [4]
Myelosuppression / bone marrow suppression / myelotoxicity [4]
Neutropenia (neutrophils decreased) [20]
Sepsis [2]
Thrombocytopenia / platelets decreased [8]

Local
Injection-site reaction (<10%)

Neuromuscular/Skeletal
Arthralgia (<10%)
Asthenia / fatigue (>10%) [18]
Back pain (<10%)
Myalgia/Myopathy (<10%)
Rhabdomyolysis [10]

Respiratory
Cough (<10%)
Dyspnea / shortness of breath (<10%) [3]

Other
Adverse effects / adverse reactions [2]
Death [2]

TRAGACANTH GUM

Family: Fabaceae; Leguminosae
Scientific names: *Astragalus gossypinus, Astragalus gummifer*
Indications: Diarrhea. Ingredient in pharmaceuticals, foods, toothpaste, denture adhesives, emulsifier, binding agent, demulcent, stabilizer
Class: Food additive, Laxative
Half-life: N/A
Clinically important, potentially hazardous interactions with: none known
Note: See also Astragalus root.

TRAMADOL

Trade names: Rybix ODT (Victory Pharma), Ultracet (Ortho-McNeil), Ultram (Ortho-McNeil)
Indications: Pain
Class: Opiate agonist
Half-life: 6–7 hours
Clinically important, potentially hazardous interactions with: alcohol, amitriptyline, carbamazepine, cinacalcet, citalopram, delavirdine, desflurane, desipramine, desvenlafaxine, duloxetine, erythromycin, fluoxetine, fluvoxamine, ketoconazole, levomepromazine, linezolid, lorcaserin, MAO inhibitors, nefazodone, ondansetron, paroxetine hydrochloride, phenelzine, quinidine, risperidone, safinamide, selegiline, selegiline, tapentadol, terbinafine, tianeptine, tipranavir, tranylcypromine, venlafaxine, vilazodone, warfarin, zuclopenthixol
Important contra-indications noted in the prescribing guidelines for: the elderly; nursing mothers; pediatric patients
Note: The UK MHRA issued the following advice: Taking warfarin and tramadol together can cause harmful drug interactions, which can raise the International Normalised Ratio (INR), and result in severe bruising and bleeding, which in some patients could be fatal.

Skin
Anaphylactoid reactions / anaphylaxis (includes anaphylactic shock) [2]
Angioedema (formerly named angioneurotic edema) [2]
Contact dermatitis [2]
Diaphoresis (9%) [3]
Flushing / rubefaction [2]
Hypersensitivity [2]
Peripheral edema [2]
Pruritus (itching) (<10%) [4]
Rash (<5%) [2]
Urticaria / hives (<18%)

Mucosal
Xerostomia (dry mouth) (10%) [5]

Cardiovascular
Vasodilation (<5%)

Central Nervous System
Anorexia (<5%)
Anxiety (<5%)
Catatonia [2]
Confusion (<5%)
Euphoria / elation (<5%)
Fever (pyrexia) (includes hyperpyrexia) [2]
Hallucinations, auditory [2]
Hallucinations, visual [3]
Headache [8]
Insomnia [3]
Nervousness (<5%)
Restless legs syndrome / Willis-Ekbom disease (includes restless arms syndrome variant) [5]
Seizures [19]
Serotonin syndrome [18]
Sleep-related disorder (<5%)
Somnolence (drowsiness) [8]
Tic disorder [2]
Tremor (5–10%)
Vertigo / dizziness [19]

Endocrine/Metabolic
Adrenal insufficiency (hypoadrenalism) / Addisonian crisis (includes Addison's disease) [2]
Hypoglycemia [15]
Hyponatremia [4]

Gastrointestinal/Hepatic
Abdominal pain (<5%) [3]
Constipation [9]
Diarrhea [2]
Flatulence (<5%)
Nausea [27]
Vomiting [25]

Genitourinary
Urinary frequency (<5%)
Urinary retention (<5%)

Hematologic
Prothrombin time (INR) increased [6]

Neuromuscular/Skeletal
Asthenia / fatigue (<5%) [3]
Hypertonia (<5%)

Ocular
Mydriasis [2]
Visual disturbances (<5%)

Respiratory
Apnea [2]
Respiratory depression [2]

Other
Adverse effects / adverse reactions [8]
Death [2]
Hiccups / singultus [2]

TRAMETINIB

Trade name: Mekinist (Novartis)
Indications: Melanoma (unresectable or metastatic) in patients with BRAF V600E or V600K mutations
Class: MEK inhibitor (mitogen-activated protein kinase (MEK1 and MEK2) inhibitor)
Half-life: 4–5 days
Clinically important, potentially hazardous interactions with: none known
Important contra-indications noted in the prescribing guidelines for: nursing mothers; pediatric patients

---

Skin
Acneiform eruption / acneiform dermatitis / acneiform rash (19%) [8]
Actinic keratoses [2]
Cellulitis and pseudocellulitis (<10%)
Cutaneous toxicity / skin toxicity (87%) [5]
Dermatitis (19%) [2]
Edema / fluid retention (32%)
Erythema [2]
Exanthems [2]
Folliculitis (<10%)
Hand–foot syndrome (palmar–plantar erythrodysesthesia) [2]

Hyperkeratosis [3]
Keratosis pilaris [2]
Lymphedema (32%)
Panniculitis [4]
Papillomas [2]
Papulopustular eruption [2]
Peripheral edema (32%) [9]
Pruritus (itching) (10%) [4]
Pustules / pustular eruption (<10%)
Rash (57%) [19]
Squamous cell carcinoma [4]
Sweet's syndrome [3]
Xerosis / xeroderma (11%) [3]

Hair
Alopecia / hair loss [4]

Nails
Paronychia (10%)

Mucosal
Aphthous stomatitis / aphthous ulcer / aphtha (aphthae) (15%)
Epistaxis (nosebleed) (13%)
Gingival bleeding (13%)
Mucosal inflammation (15%)
Oral ulceration (15%)
Rectal hemorrhage / rectal bleeding (13%)
Stomatitis (oral mucositis) (15%) [2]
Xerostomia (dry mouth) (<10%)

Cardiovascular
Bradycardia / sinus bradycardia (<10%)
Cardiomyopathy (7%)
Cardiotoxicity [6]
Hypertension (15%) [7]

Central Nervous System
Chills [4]
Dysgeusia (taste perversion) (<10%)
Fever (pyrexia) (includes hyperpyrexia) [18]
Headache [5]
Vertigo / dizziness (<10%)

Endocrine/Metabolic
ALP increased (24%)
ALT increased (39%) [4]
Appetite decreased [2]
AST increased (60%) [6]
Hypoalbuminemia / albumin decreased (42%)

Gastrointestinal/Hepatic
Abdominal pain (13%)
Black stools / melena (13%)
Constipation [3]
Diarrhea (43%) [21]
Hepatotoxicity / liver injury / acute liver injury / drug-induced liver injury (DILI) [2]
Nausea [14]
Vomiting [9]

Genitourinary
Hematuria (13%)
Vaginal bleeding (13%)

Hematologic
Anemia (38%) [3]
Hemophagocytic lymphohistiocytosis / hemophagocytic syndrome [4]
Hemorrhage (13%)
Neutropenia (neutrophils decreased) [3]
Thrombocytopenia / platelets decreased [3]

Neuromuscular/Skeletal
Arthralgia [6]
Asthenia / fatigue [18]
Rhabdomyolysis (<10%) [2]

Ocular
Chorioretinopathy [3]
Conjunctival hemorrhage (13%)
Retinopathy [4]
Uveitis / anterior uveitis / posterior uveitis / panuveitis [4]
Vision blurred (<10%) [4]
Xerophthalmia (dry eyes) (<10%)

Respiratory
Cough [2]
Pneumonitis (2%)

Other
Adverse effects / adverse reactions [7]

TRANDOLAPRIL

Trade names: Mavik (AbbVie), Tarka (AbbVie)
Indications: Hypertension
Class: Angiotensin-converting enzyme (ACE) inhibitor, Antihypertensive, Vasodilator
Half-life: 6 hours
Clinically important, potentially hazardous interactions with: alcohol, aldesleukin, aliskiren, allopurinol, alpha blockers, amiloride, angiotensin II receptor antagonists, antacids, antidiabetics, antipsychotics, anxiolytics and hypnotics, baclofen, beta blockers, calcium channel blockers, clonidine, corticosteroids, cyclosporine, diazoxide, diuretics, estrogens, general anesthetics, gold & gold compounds, heparins, hydralazine, insulin, levodopa, lithium, MAO inhibitors, metformin, methyldopa, minoxidil, moxisylyte, moxonidine, nitrates, nitroprusside, NSAIDs, potassium salts, spironolactone, sulfonylureas, tizanidine, triamterene, trimethoprim
Pregnancy category: category C in first trimester; category D in second and third trimesters
Important contra-indications noted in the prescribing guidelines for: nursing mothers; pediatric patients
Note: Contra-indicated in patients with hereditary/idiopathic angioedema and in patients with a history of angioedema related to previous treatment with an ACE inhibitor. Tarka is trandolapril and verapamil.
Warning: FETAL TOXICITY

Skin
Angioedema (formerly named angioneurotic edema) [3]
Edema / fluid retention (>3%)

Mucosal
Xerostomia (dry mouth) (>3%)

Cardiovascular
Bradycardia / sinus bradycardia (5%)
Cardiogenic shock (4%)
Hypotension (11%)

Central Nervous System
Hyperesthesia (>3%)
Stroke / cerebrovascular accident (3%)
Syncope / fainting (6%)
Vertigo / dizziness (23%)

Endocrine/Metabolic
Creatine phosphokinase (CPK) / creatine kinase increased (hyperCKemia) (5%)
Hyperkalemia (5%)
Hypocalcemia (5%)

Gastrointestinal/Hepatic
Dyspepsia / functional dyspepsia (indigestion) (see also gastroparesis) (6%)
Gastritis / pangastritis / gastric irritation (4%)

Neuromuscular/Skeletal
Asthenia / fatigue (3%)
Myalgia/Myopathy (5%)

Respiratory
Cough (35%) [5]

TRANEXAMIC ACID

Trade name: Cyklokapron (Pharmacia)
Indications: Fibrinolysis
Class: Antifibrinolytic
Half-life: 2 hours
Clinically important, potentially hazardous interactions with: none known

---

Skin
Anaphylactoid reactions / anaphylaxis (includes anaphylactic shock) [2]
Fixed eruption / fixed drug eruption [2]

Central Nervous System
Headache [3]
Seizures [12]

Endocrine/Metabolic
Menstrual irregularities [3]

Gastrointestinal/Hepatic
Abdominal pain [2]

Renal
Nephrotoxicity / kidney injury / acute kidney injury (AKI) / drug-induced kidney injury [4]

Other
Adverse effects / adverse reactions [4]

TRANYLCYPROMINE

Trade name: Parnate (Concordia)
Indications: Depression
Class: Antidepressant, Monoamine oxidase (MAO) inhibitor
Half-life: 2.5 hours
Clinically important, potentially hazardous interactions with: amitriptyline, amoxapine, amphetamines, bupropion, citalopram, clomipramine, cyproheptadine, desipramine, dextroamphetamine, dextromethorphan, diethylpropion, dopamine, doxepin, entacapone, ephedrine, epinephrine, fluoxetine, fluvoxamine, imipramine, levodopa, mazindol, meperidine, methamphetamine, nefazodone, nortriptyline, opicapone, paroxetine hydrochloride, phendimetrazine, phentermine, phenylephrine, phenylpropanolamine, pizotifen, protriptyline, pseudoephedrine, rizatriptan, sertraline, sibutramine, sumatriptan, sympathomimetics, tramadol, tricyclic antidepressants, trimipramine, tryptophan, tyramine-containing foods, venlafaxine, viloxazine, zolmitriptan
Important contra-indications noted in the prescribing guidelines for: nursing mothers; pediatric patients
Note: Consuming tyramine-containing foods or drinks while you are taking tranylcypromine can raise your blood pressure to dangerous levels. These include the following: aged cheeses, avocados, banana skins, bologna and other processed luncheon meats, chicken livers, chocolate, figs, canned pickled herring, meat extracts, pepperoni, raisins, raspberries, soy sauce, vermouth, sherry and red wines.
Warning: SUICIDALITY AND ANTIDEPRESSANT DRUGS

Central Nervous System
Delirium [2]
Serotonin syndrome [3]

TRASTUZUMAB

Trade name: Herceptin (Genentech)
Indications: Metastatic breast cancer, stomach cancer
Class: Antineoplastic / anticancer agent (see also Immune checkpoint inhibitor), Biologic, HER2/neu receptor antagonist (HER2 receptor antagonist), Monoclonal antibody, Tyrosine kinase inhibitor
Half-life: 2–16 days (dose dependent)
Clinically important, potentially hazardous interactions with: abatacept, abciximab, alefacept, antineoplastics, azacitidine, betamethasone, cabazitaxel, denileukin, docetaxel, doxorubicin, fingolimod, gefitinib, immunosuppressants, leflunomide, lenalidomide, oxaliplatin, paclitaxel, pazopanib, pemetrexed, pralatrexate, temsirolimus
Important contra-indications noted in the prescribing guidelines for: nursing mothers; pediatric patients
Note: Trastuzumab-dkst (Ogivri) is biosimilar to Trastuzumab (Herceptin). Approved 12/01/2017 Trastuzumab-pkrb (Herzuma) is biosimilar to Trastuzumab (Herceptin). Approved 12/14/2018 Trastuzumab-dttb (Ontruzant) is biosimilar to Trastuzumab (Herceptin). Approved 01/18/2019 Trastuzumab-qyyp (Trazimera) is biosimilar to Trastuzumab (Herceptin). Approved 03/11/2019 Trastuzumab-anns (Kanjinti) is biosimilar to Trastuzumab (Herceptin). Approved 06/13/2019 Trastuzumab-strf (Hercessi) is biosimilar to Trastuzumab (Herceptin). Approved 04/25/2024.
Warning: CARDIOMYOPATHY, INFUSION REACTIONS, EMBRYO-FETAL TOXICITY, and PULMONARY TOXICITY

Skin
Acneiform eruption / acneiform dermatitis / acneiform rash (2%) [4]
Cutaneous toxicity / skin toxicity [3]
Dermatomyositis [3]
Edema / fluid retention (8%)
Erythema [2]
Hand–foot syndrome (palmar–plantar erythrodysesthesia) [11]
Herpes simplex (2%)
Hypersensitivity [3]
Peripheral edema (5–10%)
Photosensitivity [2]
Pruritus (itching) (2%)
Radiation recall dermatitis [3]
Rash (4–18%) [12]

Hair
Alopecia / hair loss [6]

Nails
Nail disorder (2%)

Mucosal
Epistaxis (nosebleed) (2%)
Mucositis [4]
Stomatitis (oral mucositis) [5]

Cardiovascular
Arrhythmias (3%)
Cardiac disorder / cardiac dysfunction [5]
Cardiac failure [5]
Cardiomyopathy [2]
Cardiotoxicity [32]
Congestive heart failure (2–7%) [8]
Hypertension (4%) [3]
Myocardial toxicity [3]
Palpitation (3%)
Tachycardia (5%)

Central Nervous System
Anorexia (14%) [6]
Chills (5–32%) [8]
Depression (6%)
Fever (pyrexia) (includes hyperpyrexia) (6–36%) [7]
Headache (10–26%) [3]
Insomnia (14%)
Neurotoxicity [4]
Pain (47%) [2]
Paresthesias (2–9%)
Peripheral neuropathy [9]
Vertigo / dizziness (4–13%)

Endocrine/Metabolic
ALT increased [7]
Appetite decreased [2]
AST increased [3]
Hyperbilirubinemia [2]
Hyperglycemia (includes glucose increased) [4]
Hypertransaminasemia (hepatic transaminitis) / elevated transaminases [2]

Gastrointestinal/Hepatic
Abdominal pain (2–22%)
Constipation (2%)
Diarrhea (7–25%) [35]
Dyspepsia / functional dyspepsia (indigestion) (see also gastroparesis) (2%)
Hepatotoxicity / liver injury / acute liver injury / drug-induced liver injury (DILI) [8]
Nausea (6–33%) [11]
Vomiting (4–23%) [5]

Genitourinary
Urinary tract infection (3–5%)

Hematologic
Anemia (4%) [9]
Febrile neutropenia [18]
Leukocytopenia (leukopenia) / leukocytes (white blood cells) decreased (3%) [13]
Neutropenia (neutrophils decreased) [38]
Thrombocytopenia / platelets decreased [8]

Local
Infusion-related reactions [5]
Injection-site reaction (21–40%) [7]

Neuromuscular/Skeletal
Arthralgia (6–8%) [5]
Asthenia / fatigue (5–47%) [24]
Back pain (5–22%)
Bone pain / joint pain (3–7%)
Muscle spasm (3%)
Myalgia/Myopathy (4%) [4]

Ocular
Corneal ulceration (see also corneal melting) [2]

Respiratory
Cough (5–26%)
Dyspnea / shortness of breath (3–22%) [2]
Influenza (4%)
Influenza- ('flu)-like syndrome (10%) [3]
Interstitial lung disease / interstitial pneumonitis / interstitial pneumonia (cryptogenic organizing pneumonia) / drug-induced interstitial lung disease [2]
Nasopharyngitis (8%)
Pharyngitis (sore throat) (12%)
Pharyngolaryngeal pain (2%)
Pneumonia [3]
Pneumonitis [2]
Pulmonary toxicity [4]
Rhinitis / rhinosinusitis (see also sinusitis) (2–14%)
Sinusitis (see also rhinitis / rhinosinusitis) (2–9%)
Upper respiratory tract infection (3%)

Other
Adverse effects / adverse reactions [9]
Allergic reactions (3%) [2]
Death [5]
Infection (20%) [3]

TRASTUZUMAB EMTANSINE / ADO-TRASTUZUMAB EMTANSINE

Synonym: T-DM1
Trade name: Kadcyla (Genentech)
Indications: HER2-positive, metastatic breast cancer in patients who previously received trastuzumab and a taxane, separately or in combination
Class: Antibody-drug conjugate (ADC), Biologic, HER2-targeted antibody-drug conjugate, Monoclonal antibody
Half-life: 4 days
Clinically important, potentially hazardous interactions with: none known
Important contra-indications noted in the prescribing guidelines for: nursing mothers; pediatric patients
Note: Formerly named Trastuzumab Emtansine.
Warning: HEPATOTOXICITY, CARDIAC TOXICITY, EMBRYO-FETAL TOXICITY

Skin
Hypersensitivity (2%)
Peripheral edema (7%)
Pruritus (itching) (6%)
Rash (12%)
Telangiectasia [7]

Mucosal
Epistaxis (nosebleed) (23%) [2]
Stomatitis (oral mucositis) (14%)
Xerostomia (dry mouth) (17%)

Cardiovascular
Cardiotoxicity [2]
Hypertension (5%)
Systolic dysfunction / ejection fraction reduced [2]

Central Nervous System
Chills (8%)
Dysgeusia (taste perversion) (8%)
Fever (pyrexia) (includes hyperpyrexia) (19%) [2]
Headache (28%) [4]
Insomnia (12%)
Peripheral neuropathy (21%) [4]
Vertigo / dizziness (10%)

Endocrine/Metabolic
ALP increased (5%)
ALT increased (82%) [4]
AST increased (98%) [7]
Hypokalemia (10%) [3]

Gastrointestinal/Hepatic
Abdominal pain (19%)
Constipation (27%) [3]
Diarrhea (24%) [6]

Dyspepsia / functional dyspepsia (indigestion) (see also gastroparesis) (9%)
Hepatotoxicity / liver injury / acute liver injury / drug-induced liver injury (DILI) [16]
Nausea (40%) [10]
Vomiting (19%)

Genitourinary
Urinary tract infection (9%)

Hematologic
Anemia (14%) [10]
Febrile neutropenia [3]
Hemorrhage (32%) [2]
Neutropenia (neutrophils decreased) (7%) [5]
Thrombocytopenia / platelets decreased (31%) [32]

Neuromuscular/Skeletal
Arthralgia (19%) [3]
Asthenia / fatigue (18–36%) [15]
Bone pain / joint pain (36%)
Myalgia/Myopathy (14%)

Ocular
Conjunctivitis (conjunctival inflammation) (4%)
Lacrimation (3%)
Vision blurred (5%)
Xerophthalmia (dry eyes) (4%)

Respiratory
Cough (18%)
Dyspnea / shortness of breath (12%)
Pneumonia [3]
Pulmonary hypertension [2]

Other
Adverse effects / adverse reactions [5]
Death [3]

TRAZODONE

Trade names: Desyrel (Bristol-Myers Squibb), Oleptro (Angelini)
Indications: Depression
Class: Antidepressant; tricyclic, Serotonin reuptake inhibitor
Half-life: 3–6 hours
Clinically important, potentially hazardous interactions with: amiodarone, amprenavir, atazanavir, boceprevir, citalopram, cobicistat/elvitegravir/emtricitabine/tenofovir alafenamide, cobicistat/elvitegravir/emtricitabine/tenofovir disoproxil, darunavir, delavirdine, fluoxetine, fluvoxamine, ginkgo biloba, indinavir, linezolid, lopinavir, MAO inhibitors, nefazodone, paroxetine hydrochloride, sertraline, tapentadol, telaprevir, tipranavir, venlafaxine
Important contra-indications noted in the prescribing guidelines for: nursing mothers; pediatric patients
Warning: SUICIDALITY IN CHILDREN AND ADOLESCENTS

Skin
Edema / fluid retention (<10%)
Exanthems [6]
Photosensitivity [2]
Psoriasis (exacerbation) [2]
Urticaria / hives [3]

Hair
Alopecia / hair loss [2]

Mucosal
Xerostomia (dry mouth) (>10%) [6]

Cardiovascular
Arrhythmias [2]
QT interval prolonged / QT prolongation [2]

Central Nervous System
Delirium [3]
Dysgeusia (taste perversion) (>10%)
Headache [3]
Parkinsonism [5]
Sedation (>5%)
Serotonin syndrome [7]
Somnolence (drowsiness) (>5%) [3]
Tremor (<10%)
Vertigo / dizziness (>5%) [4]

Gastrointestinal/Hepatic
Constipation (>5%)
Hepatotoxicity / liver injury / acute liver injury / drug-induced liver injury (DILI) [2]
Nausea [2]

Genitourinary
Priapism (12%) [25]
Sexual dysfunction [2]

Neuromuscular/Skeletal
Myalgia/Myopathy (<10%)

Ocular
Vision blurred (>5%)

TREPROSTINIL

Synonym: Treprostinil palmitil (an ester prodrug)
Trade names: Remodulin (United Therapeutics), Tyvaso (United Therapeutics)
Indications: Pulmonary arterial hypertension, patients requiring transition from epoprostenol
Class: Antihypertensive, Platelet aggregation inhibitor, Prostaglandin
Half-life: 2–4 hours
Clinically important, potentially hazardous interactions with: anticoagulants, antihypertensives, CYP2C8 inhibitors or inducers, diuretics, gemfibrozil, meloxicam, rifampin, rifapentine, vasodilators
Important contra-indications noted in the prescribing guidelines for: the elderly; nursing mothers; pediatric patients

---

Skin
Edema / fluid retention (9%)
Flushing / rubefaction [5]
Hot flashes / hot flushes [2]
Pruritus (itching) (8%)
Rash (14%)

Mucosal
Throat irritation [2]

Cardiovascular
Hypotension (4%) [2]
Vasodilation (11%)

Central Nervous System
Headache (27%) [13]
Pain (13%)
Vertigo / dizziness (9%) [2]

Gastrointestinal/Hepatic
Diarrhea (25%) [8]
Nausea (22%) [7]

Local
Application-site reactions (83%)
Injection-site bleeding (33%)
Injection-site pain (85%) [4]
Injection-site reaction (83%) [2]

Neuromuscular/Skeletal
Jaw pain (13%) [6]

Respiratory
Cough [5]

Other
Adverse effects / adverse reactions [3]

TRETINOIN

Synonyms: all-trans-retinoic acid; ATRA
Trade names: Aknemycin Plus (EM Industries), Renova (Ortho), Retin-A Micro (Ortho), Solage (Galderma), Vesanoid (Roche)
Indications: Acne vulgaris, skin aging, facial roughness, fine wrinkles, hyperpigmentation [T], acute promyelocytic leukemia [O]
Class: Antineoplastic / anticancer agent (see also Immune checkpoint inhibitor), Retinoid
Half-life: 0.5–2 hours
Clinically important, potentially hazardous interactions with: aldesleukin, bexarotene
Pregnancy category: category B (topical), category C (oral), category D in third trimester
Important contra-indications noted in the prescribing guidelines for: nursing mothers; pediatric patients
Note: Oral retinoids can cause birth defects, and women should avoid tretinoin when pregnant or trying to conceive. Avoid prolonged exposure to sunlight.
[T] = Topical; [O] = Oral.

Skin
Bullous dermatosis [2]
Burning / skin burning sensation [O][T] (10–40%) [20]
Cellulitis and pseudocellulitis [O] (<10%)
Crusting [2]
Dermatitis [7]
Desquamation (14%)
Diaphoresis (20%)
Differentiation syndrome [O] (25%) [19]
Edema / fluid retention (29%) [8]
Erythema [O][T] (<49%) [19]
Erythema nodosum [4]
Exfoliative dermatitis [O] (8%) [3]
Facial edema [O] (<10%)
Flaking [O] (23%)
Hyperkeratosis [O] (78%)
Hypomelanosis (5%) [2]
Pallor [O] (<10%)
Palmar–plantar desquamation [O] (<10%)
Peeling [4]
Photosensitivity [O][T] (10%) [3]
Pigmentation (Skin) (includes hyperpigmentation) (5%) [3]
Pruritus (itching) [O][T] (5–40%) [14]
Rash [O][T] (54%) [3]
Scaling (10–40%) [16]
Stinging (<26%) [8]
Sweet's syndrome [22]
Ulcerations (scrotal) [9]
Vasculitis (angiitis) / cutaneous vasculitis (angiitis) [2]
Xerosis / xeroderma [O] (49–100%) [19]

Hair
Alopecia areata [O] (14%)

Nails
Pyogenic granuloma [3]

Mucosal
Cheilitis (inflammation of the lips) [O] (10%)
Xerostomia (dry mouth) [O] (10%)

Cardiovascular
Phlebitis (11%)

Central Nervous System
Depression [O] (14%)
Fever (pyrexia) (includes hyperpyrexia) [O] [6]
Headache [3]
Intracranial pressure increased (intracranial hypertension) [3]
Pain [O] (37%)
Paresthesias [O] (17%)
Pseudotumor cerebri [O] [12]
Shivering [O] (63%)
Tremor [O] (<10%)

Gastrointestinal/Hepatic
Hepatotoxicity / liver injury / acute liver injury / drug-induced liver injury (DILI) [3]
Pancreatitis / acute pancreatitis [2]

Hematologic
Hemorrhage [2]

Local
Injection-site reaction (17%)

Neuromuscular/Skeletal
Arthralgia [O] (10%) [3]
Bone pain / joint pain [O] (77%) [3]
Myalgia/Myopathy (14%) [3]

Ocular
Diplopia (double vision) [2]
Ocular itching / ocular pruritus [O] (10%)
Ocular pigmentation [O] (<10%)
Xerophthalmia (dry eyes) [O] (<10%) [2]

Other
Death [O] [2]
Infection [O] (58%)

TRIAMCINOLONE

Trade names: Aristospan (Sabex), Azmacort (Kos), Kenalog (Apothecon), Nasacort (Aventis), Triacet (Teva)
Indications: Arthralgias, asthma, dermatoses, inflammatory ocular conditions, rhinitis
Class: Corticosteroid / Glucocorticoid, Corticosteroid, systemic, Corticosteroid, topical
Half-life: 17–25 days
Clinically important, potentially hazardous interactions with: ACE inhibitors, acetazolamide, adrenergic neurone blockers, aldesleukin, alpha blockers, aminoglutethimide, aminophylline, amphotericin B, angiotensin II receptor antagonists, antacids, antidiabetics, antifungals, aprepitant, aspirin, barbiturates, beta blockers, beta$_2$ sympathomimetics, calcium channel blockers, calcium salts, carbamazepine, cardiac glycosides, clonidine, denosumab, diazoxide, diuretics, erythromycin, estrogens, fluconazole, fosaprepitant, histamine, hydralazine, isoniazid, itraconazole, ketoconazole, leflunomide, leflunomide, live vaccines, loop diuretics, macrolide antibiotics, methyl salicylate, methyldopa, mifamurtide, mifepristone, minoxidil, mitotane, moxonidine, natalizumab, neuromuscular blocking agents, nitrates, nitroprusside, NSAIDs, oral contraceptives, pancuronium, phenindione, phenobarbital, phenytoin, pimecrolimus, primidone, quinolones, rifampin, rifamycin derivatives, salicylates, sipuleucel-T, sodium benzoate, sodium phenylbutyrate, somatropin, tacrolimus, thiazides, vaccines, vecuronium, warfarin
Important contra-indications noted in the prescribing guidelines for: nursing mothers

---

Skin
Anaphylactoid reactions / anaphylaxis (includes anaphylactic shock) [2]
Atrophy / Skin atrophy [4]
Bruise / bruising / contusion / ecchymosis (ecchymoses) [2]
Burning / skin burning sensation [2]
Dermatitis [3]
Erythema [5]
Moon face [2]
Nicolau syndrome [2]
Pigmentation (Skin) (includes hyperpigmentation) [7]
Scaling [2]
Urticaria / hives [2]

Nails
Nail pigmentation [2]
Subungual hematoma / subungual hemorrhage [2]

Central Nervous System
Headache [7]
Pain [4]

Endocrine/Metabolic
Cushing's syndrome [6]

Local
Injection-site lipoatrophy/lipohypertrophy [4]
Injection-site pain [2]

Neuromuscular/Skeletal
Osteoporosis [3]

Ocular
Cataract [30]
Chorioretinopathy [5]
Conjunctival ulceration [2]
Endophthalmitis [20]
Eyelid ptosis / blepharoptosis [3]
Glaucoma (includes acute angle-closure glaucoma) [11]
Intraocular hypertension [8]
Intraocular pressure increased [7]
Maculopathy [2]
Ocular hypertension [7]
Ocular pressure [22]
Retinal detachment [3]
Uveitis / anterior uveitis / posterior uveitis / panuveitis [3]
Vision impaired [3]

Other
Adverse effects / adverse reactions [4]
Allergic reactions [3]
Hoigne's syndrome [2]

TRIAMTERENE

Trade names: Dyazide (GSK), Dyrenium (Concordia)
Indications: Edema
Class: Diuretic, potassium-sparing
Half-life: 1–2 hours
Clinically important, potentially hazardous interactions with: ACE inhibitors, acemetacin, benazepril, captopril, cyclosporine, enalapril, fosinopril, indomethacin, lisinopril, metformin, moexipril, potassium iodide, potassium salts, quinapril, ramipril, spironolactone, trandolapril, zofenopril
Important contra-indications noted in the prescribing guidelines for: nursing mothers; pediatric patients
Note: Dyazide and Maxzide are triamterene and hydrochlorothiazide. Hydrochlorothiazide is a sulfonamide and can be absorbed systemically. Sulfonamides can produce severe, possibly fatal, reactions such as toxic epidermal necrolysis and Stevens-Johnson syndrome.

Skin
Edema / fluid retention (<10%)
Lupus erythematosus (subacute cutaneous lupus erythematosus (SCLE)) (with hydrochlorothiazide) [2]
Photosensitivity [2]
Rash (<10%)

TRIAZOLAM

Trade name: Halcion (Pfizer)
Indications: Insomnia
Class: Benzodiazepine
Half-life: 1.5–5.5 hours
Clinically important, potentially hazardous interactions with: amprenavir, atazanavir, boceprevir, clarithromycin, darunavir, delavirdine, efavirenz, erythromycin, fosamprenavir, indinavir, itraconazole, ketoconazole, lopinavir, nelfinavir, ombitasvir/paritaprevir/ritonavir, ombitasvir/paritaprevir/ritonavir and dasabuvir, paclitaxel, posaconazole, rifampin, ritonavir, telaprevir, telithromycin, tipranavir, viloxazine

---

Skin
Dermatitis (<10%)
Diaphoresis (>10%) [2]
Pruritus (itching) [2]
Rash (>10%)

Mucosal
Sialopenia (>10%)
Sialorrhea (ptyalism; hypersalivation) (<10%)
Xerostomia (dry mouth) (>10%) [4]

Central Nervous System
Amnesia [19]
Dysgeusia (taste perversion) [2]
Tremor (<10%)

Neuromuscular/Skeletal
Ataxia [2]

Ocular
Diplopia (double vision) [2]

TRICHLORMETHIAZIDE

Indications: Edema, hypertension
Class: Diuretic, thiazide
Half-life: N/A
Clinically important, potentially hazardous interactions with: digoxin, lithium
Important contra-indications noted in the prescribing guidelines for: nursing mothers; pediatric patients
Note: Trichlormethiazide is a sulfonamide and can be absorbed systemically. Sulfonamides can produce severe, possibly fatal, reactions such as toxic epidermal necrolysis and Stevens-Johnson syndrome.

TRIENTINE

Synonym: triethylenetetramine
Trade names: Cufence (Univar Solutions), Cuprior (Orphalan), Cuvrior (Orphalan), Syprine (Bausch Health US)
Indications: Wilson's disease
Class: Chelator
Half-life: 13.8 to 16.5 hours (trientine tetrahydrochloride)
Clinically important, potentially hazardous interactions with: ferrous sulfate, mineral supplements (e.g. iron, zinc, calcium, or magnesium)
Pregnancy category: Chelator-induced copper deficiency may have adverse effects on the fetus.
Important contra-indications noted in the prescribing guidelines for: the elderly; nursing mothers
Note: Trientine hydrochloride is the USAN for trientine dihydrochloride. Administer trientine formulations at least 1 hour apart from any other oral drug. Worsening of clinical symptoms, including neurological deterioration, may occur at the beginning of trientine therapy due to mobilization of excess stores of copper. Adjust the dosage or discontinue trientine if the patient's clinical condition worsens.

Skin
Rash (12%)

Hair
Alopecia / hair loss (8%)

Central Nervous System
Mood changes (includes mood disorder) (8%)

Gastrointestinal/Hepatic
Abdominal pain (19%)
Colitis [2]
Gastrointestinal adverse reaction (15%)

Hematologic
Sideroblastic anemia / acquired sideroblastic anemia [2]

TRIFAROTENE

Trade name: Aklief (Galderma)
Indications: Indicated for the topical treatment of acne vulgaris in patients 9 years of age and older
Class: Retinoic acid receptors (RAR) agonist, Retinoid
Half-life: 2–9 hours
Clinically important, potentially hazardous interactions with: none known
Pregnancy category: Available data from clinical trials in pregnant women have not identified a drug-associated risk of major birth defects, miscarriage or adverse maternal or fetal outcomes.
Note: For topical use only. Not for oral, ophthalmic or intravaginal use.

Skin
Sunburn (3%)

Local
Application-site irritation (8%)
Application-site pruritus (2%)

TRIFLUOPERAZINE

Indications: Psychoses, anxiety
Class: Antipsychotic, Neuroleptic, Phenothiazine
Half-life: 10–20 hours
Clinically important, potentially hazardous interactions with: ACE inhibitors, adrenergic neurone blockers, antihistamines, arsenic, beta blockers, chlorpheniramine, diazoxide, diuretics, dofetilide, hydralazine, kaolin, lithium, minoxidil, moxonidine, myelosuppressives, nitrates, nitroprusside, pentamidine, pimozide, piperazine, quinolones, sotalol, sparfloxacin
Important contra-indications noted in the prescribing guidelines for: the elderly; nursing mothers
Warning: INCREASED MORTALITY IN ELDERLY PATIENTS WITH DEMENTIA-RELATED PSYCHOSIS

Skin
Photosensitivity (<10%)
Rash (<10%)

Central Nervous System
Neuroleptic malignant syndrome [2]
Parkinsonism (>10%) [3]

Endocrine/Metabolic
Mastodynia (<10%)

TRIFLURIDINE & TIPIRACIL

Trade name: Lonsurf (Monarch)
Indications: Metastatic colorectal cancer in patients who have been previously treated with fluoropyrimidine-, oxaliplatin-and irinotecan-based chemotherapy, an anti-VEGF biological therapy, and if RAS wild-type, an anti-EGFR therapy
Class: Antineoplastic / anticancer agent (see also Immune checkpoint inhibitor), Thymidine phosphorylase inhibitor, Thymidine-based nucleoside analogue
Half-life: 2 hours
Clinically important, potentially hazardous interactions with: none known
Pregnancy category: Can cause fetal harm
Important contra-indications noted in the prescribing guidelines for: nursing mothers; pediatric patients
Note: See also separate entry for trifluridine.

Hair
Alopecia / hair loss (7%)

Mucosal
Stomatitis (oral mucositis) (8%)

Central Nervous System
Anorexia [3]
Dysgeusia (taste perversion) (7%)
Fever (pyrexia) (includes hyperpyrexia) (19%)

Endocrine/Metabolic
Appetite decreased (39%) [3]

Gastrointestinal/Hepatic
Abdominal pain (21%) [3]
Diarrhea (32%) [4]
Nausea (48%) [7]
Vomiting (28%) [3]

Genitourinary
Urinary tract infection (4%)

Hematologic
Anemia (77%) [21]
Febrile neutropenia [3]
Granulocytopenia [3]
Leukocytopenia (leukopenia) / leukocytes (white blood cells) decreased [13]
Neutropenia (neutrophils decreased) (67%) [26]
Thrombocytopenia / platelets decreased (42%) [5]

Neuromuscular/Skeletal
Asthenia / fatigue (52%) [9]

Respiratory
Nasopharyngitis (4%)
Pulmonary embolism (2%)

Other
Adverse effects / adverse reactions [4]
Death [2]
Infection (27%)

TRIHEXYPHENIDYL

Indications: Parkinsonism
Class: Muscarinic antagonist
Half-life: 3–4 hours
Clinically important, potentially hazardous interactions with: anticholinergics, arbutamine
Important contra-indications noted in the prescribing guidelines for: pediatric patients

---

Skin
Photosensitivity (<10%)
Xerosis / xeroderma (>10%)

Mucosal
Xerostomia (dry mouth) (30–50%)

Central Nervous System
Hallucinations [3]

TRILACICLIB

Trade name: Cosela (G1 Therapeutics)
Indications: Reduction of the incidence of chemotherapy-induced myelosuppression in adult patients when administered prior to a platinum/etoposide-containing regimen or topotecan-containing regimen for extensive-stage small cell lung cancer
Class: Cyclin-dependent kinase (CDK) 4/6 inhibitor, Kinase inhibitor
Half-life: ~14 hours
Clinically important, potentially hazardous interactions with: cisplatin, dalfampridine, dofetilide, metformin
Pregnancy category: Trilaciclib can cause fetal harm when administered to pregnant women. Advise female patients of reproductive potential to use effective contraception during treatment with trilaciclib and for at least 3 weeks after the final dose.
Important contra-indications noted in the prescribing guidelines for: nursing mothers

---

Skin
Peripheral edema (7%)
Rash (9%)

Central Nervous System
Headache (13%)

Endocrine/Metabolic
AST increased (17%)
Hyperglycemia (includes glucose increased) (6%)

Hypocalcemia (24%)
Hypokalemia (22%)
Hypophosphatemia (21%)

Gastrointestinal/Hepatic
Abdominal pain (7%)

Hematologic
Thrombosis (7%)

Local
Infusion-site reactions (8%)

Neuromuscular/Skeletal
Asthenia / fatigue (34%)

Respiratory
Pneumonia (10%)

TRIMETHOPRIM

Trade names: Bactrim (Women First), Septra (Monarch)
Indications: Various urinary tract infections caused by susceptible organisms, acute otitis media in children, acute and chronic bronchitis
Class: Antibiotic, Antimicrobial
Half-life: 8–10 hours
Clinically important, potentially hazardous interactions with: ACE inhibitors, amantadine, angiotensin II receptor antagonists, antidiabetics, azathioprine, benazepril, captopril, carvedilol, cilazapril, conivaptan, coumarins, cyclosporine, CYP2C8 substrates, CYP2C9 inhibitors, CYP3A4 inducers, dapsone, deferasirox, digoxin, dofetilide, enalapril, eplerenone, fosinopril, irbesartan, lamivudine, leucovorin, levoleucovorin, lisinopril, memantine, mercaptopurine, metformin, methotrexate, olmesartan, oral typhoid vaccine, PEG-interferon, phenytoin, pioglitazone, pralatrexate, procainamide, pyrimethamine, quinapril, ramipril, repaglinide, rifampin, sulfonylureas, trandolapril
Important contra-indications noted in the prescribing guidelines for: nursing mothers
Note: Although trimethoprim has been known to elicit occasional adverse reactions by itself, it is most commonly used in conjunction with sulfamethoxazole (co-trimoxazole - see separate entry).

Skin
DRESS syndrome (Drug-induced hypersensitivity syndrome) [2]
Fixed eruption / fixed drug eruption [6]
Pruritus (itching) (<10%)
Rash (3–7%)
Stevens-Johnson syndrome and toxic epidermal necrolysis (SJS/TEN) [6]

Central Nervous System
Aseptic meningitis [3]

Endocrine/Metabolic
Hyperkalemia [3]
Hyponatremia [3]

Gastrointestinal/Hepatic
Hepatotoxicity / liver injury / acute liver injury / drug-induced liver injury (DILI) [2]

Hematologic
Anemia [2]
Thrombocytopenia / platelets decreased [2]

Neuromuscular/Skeletal
Rhabdomyolysis [3]

TRIMIPRAMINE

Trade name: Surmontil (Odyssey)
Indications: Major depression
Class: Antidepressant; tricyclic
Half-life: 20–26 hours
Clinically important, potentially hazardous interactions with: amprenavir, arbutamine, bupropion, clonidine, epinephrine, formoterol, guanethidine, isocarboxazid, linezolid, MAO inhibitors, phenelzine, quinolones, sparfloxacin, tranylcypromine, venlafaxine
Important contra-indications noted in the prescribing guidelines for: pediatric patients
Warning: SUICIDALITY AND ANTIDEPRESSANT DRUGS

Skin
Diaphoresis (<10%)

Mucosal
Xerostomia (dry mouth) (>10%) [2]

Cardiovascular
QT interval prolonged / QT prolongation [2]

Central Nervous System
Dysgeusia (taste perversion) (>10%)
Parkinsonism (<10%)
Seizures [4]

TRIPELENNAMINE

Trade name: PBZ (Novartis)
Indications: Allergic rhinitis, urticaria
Class: Histamine H1 receptor antagonist
Half-life: N/A
Clinically important, potentially hazardous interactions with: alcohol, barbiturates, chloral hydrate, ethchlorvynol, paraldehyde, phenothiazines
Note: The intravenous use of a pentazocine/ tripelennamine combination (T's and Blues) was a major drug abuse problem in the 1970s.

Skin
Purpura [2]

Mucosal
Xerostomia (dry mouth) (<10%)

Central Nervous System
Seizures [2]

TRIPTORELIN

Trade names: Decapeptyl (Ipsen), Trelstar (Debiopharma)
Indications: Palliative treatment of advanced prostate carcinoma
Class: Gonadotropin-releasing hormone (GnRH) agonist
Half-life: ~3 hours
Clinically important, potentially hazardous interactions with: hyperprolactinemic drugs
Important contra-indications noted in the prescribing guidelines for: pediatric patients

---

Skin
Edema / fluid retention (<10%)
Hot flashes / hot flushes (59–73%) [6]
Hyperhidrosis (<10%)
Rash (2%)

Cardiovascular
Chest pain (2%)
Hypertension (<4%)

Central Nervous System
Anorexia (2%)
Headache (2–7%)
Insomnia (<2%)
Pain (2–3%)
Paresthesias (<10%)
Vertigo / dizziness (<3%)

Endocrine/Metabolic
ALP increased (2%)
Gynecomastia (2%)
Libido decreased (2%)
Mastodynia (2%)
Pituitary apoplexy [2]

Gastrointestinal/Hepatic
Constipation (2%)
Dyspepsia / functional dyspepsia (indigestion) (see also gastroparesis) (2%)
Nausea (<10%)
Vomiting (2%)

Genitourinary
Dysuria (5%)
Erectile dysfunction (10%)
Impotence (2–7%)
Testicular atrophy (8%)

Local
Injection-site erythema (<10%)
Injection-site inflammation (<10%)
Injection-site pain (4%)
Injection-site reaction (<10%)

Neuromuscular/Skeletal
Arthralgia (2%)
Asthenia / fatigue (2%)
Back pain (<10%)
Bone pain / joint pain (12–13%)
Leg cramps (2%)
Leg pain (2–5%)

Respiratory
Cough (2%)

Other
Adverse effects / adverse reactions [3]

TROGLITAZONE

Trade names: Prelay (Sankyo), Rezulin (Pfizer)
Indications: Management of Type II diabetes (noninsulin-dependent diabetes mellitus (NIDDM) also known as adult-onset diabetes)
Class: Antidiabetic, CYP3A4 inducer, Thiazolidinedione
Half-life: 16–34 hours
Clinically important, potentially hazardous interactions with: cholestyramine, digoxin, terfenadine
Important contra-indications noted in the prescribing guidelines for: nursing mothers; pediatric patients
Note: Troglitazone should not be used in Type I diabetes or for the treatment of diabetic keto-acidosis.
Not available in USA, UK or Japan.
Warning: HEPATOTOXICITY

Skin
Peripheral edema (5%)

Central Nervous System
Headache (11%)
Pain (10%)
Vertigo / dizziness (6%)

Endocrine/Metabolic
ALT increased (2%)

Gastrointestinal/Hepatic
Diarrhea (5%)
Hepatotoxicity / liver injury / acute liver injury / drug-induced liver injury (DILI) [5]
Nausea (6%)

Genitourinary
Urinary tract infection (5%)

Neuromuscular/Skeletal
Asthenia / fatigue (6%)
Back pain (6%)

Respiratory
Pharyngitis (sore throat) (5%)
Rhinitis / rhinosinusitis (see also sinusitis) (5%)

Other
Infection (18%)

TROLEANDOMYCIN

Trade name: TAO (Pfizer)
Indications: Various infections caused by susceptible organisms
Class: Antibiotic, Antibiotic; macrolide, Antimicrobial
Half-life: N/A
Clinically important, potentially hazardous interactions with: aprepitant, astemizole, carbamazepine, colchicine, copanlisib, crizotinib, cyclosporine, dihydroergotamine, dutasteride, eletriptan, ergot alkaloids, ergotamine, erlotinib, erythromycin, fluoxetine, fluvoxamine, methylergonovine, methylprednisolone, methysergide, midostaurin, neratinib, oral contraceptives, paroxetine hydrochloride, pimozide, prednisolone, rifampin, rilpivirine, sertraline, solifenacin, terfenadine, warfarin

---

Skin
Exanthems [2]
Pruritus (itching) [2]
Rash (<10%)
Urticaria / hives (<10%)

Gastrointestinal/Hepatic
Hepatotoxicity / liver injury / acute liver injury / drug-induced liver injury (DILI) [8]

TROSPIUM

Trade name: Sanctura (Allergan)
Indications: Overactive bladder
Class: Anticholinergic, Antispasmodic, Muscarinic antagonist
Half-life: 20 hours
Clinically important, potentially hazardous interactions with: anticholinergics, antihistamines, botulinum toxin (A & B), cannabinoids, clozapine, disopyramide, domperidone, haloperidol, ketoconazole, levodopa, maois, memantine, metformin, metoclopramide, morphine, nefopam, pancuronium, parasypathomimetics, phenothiazines, pramlintide, procainamide, secretin, tenofovir disoproxil, tricyclic antidepressants, vancomycin
Important contra-indications noted in the prescribing guidelines for: the elderly; nursing mothers; pediatric patients

---

Mucosal
Xerostomia (dry mouth) (20%) [16]

Central Nervous System
Dysgeusia (taste perversion) (<10%)
Headache (4%) [4]

Gastrointestinal/Hepatic
Abdominal pain (2%)
Constipation (10%) [6]

Neuromuscular/Skeletal
Asthenia / fatigue (2%)

Other
Adverse effects / adverse reactions [4]

TRYPTOPHAN

Other common trade names: 5-HT, 5-HTP, 5-hydroxytryptophan, 5-OHTrp, L-2-amino-3-(indole-3yl) propionic acid, L-trypt, L-tryptophan
Indications: Insomnia, depression, myofascial pain, premenstrual syndrome, aid to smoking cessation, bruxism
Class: Amino acid, Antidepressant
Half-life: N/A
Clinically important, potentially hazardous interactions with: citalopram, desipramine, duloxetine, fluoxetine, fluvoxamine, isocarboxazid, linezolid, milnacipran, paroxetine hydrochloride, phenelzine, sibutramine, tranylcypromine, vilazodone
Important contra-indications noted in the prescribing guidelines for: nursing mothers; pediatric patients
Note: Tryptophan is an essential amino acid. It is a precursor of serotonin and is also converted to nicotinic acid and nicotinamide.

Skin
Eosinophilia–myalgia syndrome [23]
Eosinophilic fasciitis (Shulman syndrome / Shulman disease) [13]
Scleroderma [8]

Neuromuscular/Skeletal
Myalgia/Myopathy [2]

Respiratory
Pulmonary hypertension [2]

TUCATINIB

Trade name: Tukysa (Seattle Genetics)
Indications: In combination with **trastuzumab** and **capecitabine**, for the treatment of unresectable or metastatic HER2-positive breast cancer.
Class: Kinase inhibitor, Tyrosine kinase inhibitor
Half-life: approx. 8.5 hours
Clinically important, potentially hazardous interactions with: CYP2C8 inducers, CYP2C8 inhibitors, CYP3A inducers, CYP3A substrates, CYP3A substrates, digoxin, gemfibrozil, itraconazole, metformin, midazolam, P-gp substrates, repaglinide, rifampin
Pregnancy category: Tucatinib can cause fetal harm when administered to a pregnant woman. Advise pregnant women and females of reproductive potential of the potential risk to the fetus.

Skin
Hand–foot syndrome (palmar–plantar erythrodysesthesia) (with trastuzumab and capecitabine) (63%)
Rash (with trastuzumab and capecitabine) (20%)

Mucosal
Epistaxis (nosebleed) (with trastuzumab and capecitabine) (12%)
Stomatitis (oral mucositis) (with trastuzumab and capecitabine) (32%)

Central Nervous System
Peripheral neuropathy (with trastuzumab and capecitabine) (13%)

Endocrine/Metabolic
ALP increased (with trastuzumab and capecitabine) (26%)
ALT increased (with trastuzumab and capecitabine) (46%)
Appetite decreased (with trastuzumab and capecitabine) (25%)
AST increased (with trastuzumab and capecitabine) (43%)
Hyperbilirubinemia (with trastuzumab and capecitabine) (47%)
Hypertransaminasemia (hepatic transaminitis) / elevated transaminases [2]
Hypokalemia (with trastuzumab and capecitabine) (36%)
Hypomagnesemia (with trastuzumab and capecitabine) (40%)
Hyponatremia (with trastuzumab and capecitabine) (28%)
Hypophosphatemia (with trastuzumab and capecitabine) (57%)
Serum creatinine increased (with trastuzumab and capecitabine) (14–33%)
Weight loss (with trastuzumab and capecitabine) (13%)

Gastrointestinal/Hepatic
Diarrhea (with trastuzumab and capecitabine) (81%) [2]
Hepatotoxicity / liver injury / acute liver injury / drug-induced liver injury (DILI) (with trastuzumab and capecitabine) (42%)
Nausea (with trastuzumab and capecitabine) (58%) [3]
Vomiting (with trastuzumab and capecitabine) (36%)

Hematologic
Anemia (with trastuzumab and capecitabine) (21%)
Hemoglobin decreased (with trastuzumab and capecitabine) (59%)

Neuromuscular/Skeletal
Arthralgia (with trastuzumab and capecitabine) (15%)
Asthenia / fatigue [2]

TURMERIC

Family: Zingiberaceae
Scientific names: *Curcuma aromatica, Curcuma domestica, Curcuma longa, Curcuma xanthorrhiza*
Indications: Arthritis, anticarcinogen, stimulant, carminative, amenorrhea, angina, asthma, colorectal cancer, delirium, diarrhea, dyspepsia, flatulence, hemorrhage, hepatitis, hypercholesterolemia, hypertension, jaundice, mania, menstrual disorders, ophthalmia, tendonitis. **Topical:** conjuctivitis, skin cancer, smallpox, chickenpox, leg ulcers. Food coloring in cheese, margarine, sweets, snack foods, cosmetics, essential oil in perfumes, culinary spice
Class: Anti-inflammatory, Anti-Tumor Necrosis Factor-alpha (TNF-α antagonist)
Half-life: N/A
Clinically important, potentially hazardous interactions with: none known

Note: Persons with symptoms of gallstones or obstruction of bile passages should avoid turmeric.

Skin
- Dermatitis [6]
- Rash [3]

Mucosal
- Stomatitis (oral mucositis) [2]

Central Nervous System
- Headache [2]

Gastrointestinal/Hepatic
- Abdominal pain [2]
- Diarrhea [6]
- Hepatotoxicity / liver injury / acute liver injury / drug-induced liver injury (DILI) [3]
- Nausea [2]

Other
- Adverse effects / adverse reactions [4]

TYPHOID VACCINE

Trade names: Typherix (GSK), Typhim Vi (Sanofi Pasteur), Vivotif (Berna Biotech)
Indications: Immunization against typhoid fever
Class: Vaccine
Half-life: N/A
Clinically important, potentially hazardous interactions with: alcohol, antibiotics, antimalarials, atovaquone/proguanil, azathioprine, belimumab, cefixime, ceftaroline fosamil, ceftobiprole, chloroquine, ciprofloxacin, corticosteroids, daptomycin, fingolimod, gemifloxacin, hydroxychloroquine, immunosuppressants, interferon gamma, leflunomide, mefloquine, mercaptopurine, sulfonamides, telavancin, tigecycline, tinidazole, tocilizumab, ustekinumab
Important contra-indications noted in the prescribing guidelines for: nursing mothers; pediatric patients
Note: Vivotif is a live oral vaccine.

Skin
- Anaphylactoid reactions / anaphylaxis (includes anaphylactic shock) [2]

Central Nervous System
- Fever (pyrexia) (includes hyperpyrexia) (<3%) [6]
- Headache (5–20%) [3]
- Myelitis / myeloradiculitis [2]

Gastrointestinal/Hepatic
- Abdominal pain (6%) [2]
- Diarrhea (<3%)
- Nausea (2–8%)
- Vomiting (2%)

Local
- Injection-site edema [3]
- Injection-site erythema (4–5%) [2]
- Injection-site induration (5–15%)
- Injection-site pain (27–41%) [6]

Neuromuscular/Skeletal
- Asthenia / fatigue (4–24%) [3]
- Myalgia/Myopathy (3–7%) [3]

Other
- Adverse effects / adverse reactions [4]
- Death [2]

UBROGEPANT

Trade name: Ubrelvy (Allergan)
Indications: Acute treatment of migraine with or without aura in adults
Class: Calcitonin gene-related peptide (CGRP) receptor antagonist
Half-life: ~5–7 hours
Clinically important, potentially hazardous interactions with: bcrp and/or P-gp only inhibitors, CYP3A4 inhibitors, CYP3A4 inducers, ciprofloxacin, clarithromycin, cyclosporine, fluconazole, fluvoxamine, grapefruit juice, itraconazole, ketoconazole, phenytoin, rifampin, St John's wort, verapamil
Pregnancy category: There are no adequate data on the developmental risk associated with use in pregnant women.
Note: Ubrogepant is not indicated for the preventive treatment of migraine. Avoid use in patients with end-stage renal disease.

Mucosal
- Xerostomia (dry mouth) (1–2%) [2]

Central Nervous System
- Somnolence (drowsiness) (2–3%)
- Vertigo / dizziness [2]

Endocrine/Metabolic
- ALT increased [2]

Gastrointestinal/Hepatic
- Nausea (2–4%) [4]

ULIPRISTAL

Trade names: ella (Watson), ellaOne (HRA Pharma)
Indications: Emergency contraception within 120 hours (5 days) of unprotected sexual intercourse or contraceptive failure
Class: Progestogen antagonist
Half-life: 32 hours
Clinically important, potentially hazardous interactions with: antacids, barbiturates, bosentan, carbamazepine, clarithromycin, conivaptan, CYP3A4 inducers, dabigatran, deferasirox, digoxin, efavirenz, felbamate, griseofulvin, H2-receptor antagonists, hypericum perforatum, itraconazole, ketoconazole, levonorgestrel, nefazodone, omeprazole, oxcarbazepine, pantoprazole, phenobarbital, phenytoin, progestogens, proton pump inhibitors, rifampin, rifapentine, ritonavir, St John's wort, telithromycin, topiramate
Important contra-indications noted in the prescribing guidelines for: the elderly; nursing mothers; pediatric patients

---

Skin
- Hot flashes / hot flushes [3]

Central Nervous System
- Headache (18–19%) [8]
- Mood changes (includes mood disorder) (<10%)
- Vertigo / dizziness (5%) [2]

Endocrine/Metabolic
- Mastodynia (<10%) [2]
- Menstrual irregularities [3]

Gastrointestinal/Hepatic
- Abdominal pain (8–15%) [5]
- Dyspepsia / functional dyspepsia (indigestion) (see also gastroparesis) (<10%)
- Nausea (12–13%) [7]
- Vomiting (<10%)

Genitourinary
- Dysmenorrhea (7–13%)
- Pelvic pain (<10%)

Neuromuscular/Skeletal
- Asthenia / fatigue (6%)
- Back pain (<10%)
- Myalgia/Myopathy (<10%)

Other
- Infection (<10%)

UMECLIDINIUM

Trade name: Incruse (GSK)
Indications: Chronic obstructive pulmonary disease (COPD)
Class: Anticholinergic, Muscarinic antagonist
Half-life: 11 hours
Clinically important, potentially hazardous interactions with: anticholinergics
Important contra-indications noted in the prescribing guidelines for: nursing mothers; pediatric patients

---

Mucosal
- Oropharyngeal pain [2]

Cardiovascular
- Angina [2]
- Arrhythmias [2]
- Extrasystoles [3]
- Hypertension [3]
- Supraventricular tachycardia [2]
- Tachycardia [2]

Central Nervous System
- Dysgeusia (taste perversion) [3]
- Headache [12]

Gastrointestinal/Hepatic
- Constipation [2]

Genitourinary
- Urinary tract infection [2]

Neuromuscular/Skeletal
- Arthralgia (2%) [2]
- Back pain [5]

Respiratory
- Bronchitis [2]
- COPD (exacerbation) [5]
- Cough (3%) [6]
- Dysphonia (includes voice disorders / voice changes) [4]
- Influenza [2]
- Nasopharyngitis (8%) [12]
- Pharyngitis (sore throat) [2]
- Pneumonia [4]
- Sinusitis (see also rhinitis / rhinosinusitis) [3]
- Upper respiratory tract infection [5]

Other
- Adverse effects / adverse reactions [4]

UPADACITINIB HEMIHYDRATE

Trade name: Rinvoq (AbbVie)
Other common trade names: ABT-494* (AbbVie)
Indications: Treatment of adults with moderately to severely active rheumatoid arthritis who have had an inadequate response or intolerance to methotrexate.
Class: Janus kinase (JAK) inhibitor
Half-life: 8–14 hours
Clinically important, potentially hazardous interactions with: coadministration of upadacitinib with strong CYP3A4 inducers (e.g. rifampin) is not recommended, rifampin, upadacitinib should be used with caution in patients receiving chronic treatment with strong CYP3A4 inhibitors (e.g. ketoconazole).
Pregnancy category: Based on animal studies, upadacitinib may cause embryo-fetal harm when administered to pregnant women. Advise female patients of reproductive potential to use effective contraception during treatment with upadacitinib and for 4 weeks after the final dose.
Important contra-indications noted in the prescribing guidelines for: nursing mothers
Note: Use of in combination with other Janus kinase (JAK) inhibitors, biologic disease-modifying antirheumatic drugs (DMARDs), or with potent immunosuppressants such as azathioprine and cyclosporine, is not recommended. Advise patients not to breastfeed. Upadacitinib is not recommended in patients with severe hepatic impairment.
Warning: ♦ INCREASED RISK OF SERIOUS BACTERIAL, FUNGAL, VIRAL, AND OPPORTUNISTIC INFECTIONS LEADING TO HOSPITALIZATION OR DEATH, INCLUDING TUBERCULOSIS (TB). INTERRUPT TREATMENT WITH UPADACITINIB IF SERIOUS INFECTION OCCURS UNTIL THE INFECTION IS CONTROLLED. TEST FOR LATENT TB BEFORE AND DURING THERAPY; TREAT LATENT TB PRIOR TO USE. MONITOR ALL PATIENTS FOR ACTIVE TB DURING TREATMENT, EVEN PATIENTS WITH INITIAL NEGATIVE, LATENT TB TEST.
♦ HIGHER RATE OF ALL-CAUSE MORTALITY, INCLUDING SUDDEN CARDIOVASCULAR DEATH WITH ANOTHER JANUS KINASE (JAK) INHIBITOR VS. TUMOR NECROSIS FACTOR (TNF) BLOCKERS IN RHEUMATOID ARTHRITIS (RA) PATIENTS.
♦ MALIGNANCIES HAVE OCCURRED IN PATIENTS TREATED WITH UPADACITINIB. HIGHER RATE OF LYMPHOMAS AND LUNG CANCERS WITH ANOTHER JAK INHIBITOR VS. TNF BLOCKERS IN RA PATIENTS.
♦ HIGHER RATE OF MACE (DEFINED AS CARDIOVASCULAR DEATH, MYOCARDIAL INFARCTION, AND STROKE) WITH ANOTHER JAK INHIBITOR VS. TNF BLOCKERS IN RA PATIENTS.
♦ THROMBOSIS HAS OCCURRED IN PATIENTS TREATED WITH UPADACITINIB. INCREASED INCIDENCE OF PULMONARY EMBOLISM, VENOUS AND ARTERIAL THROMBOSIS WITH ANOTHER JAK INHIBITOR VS. TNF BLOCKERS.

Skin
Acne (unspecified) [4]
Herpes zoster [4]

Cardiovascular
Arterial thromboembolism (2 cases)
Venous thromboembolism (9 cases)

Central Nervous System
Headache [3]

Endocrine/Metabolic
Creatine phosphokinase (CPK) / creatine kinase increased (hyperCKemia) (2%) [3]
Hypercholesterolemia [2]

Gastrointestinal/Hepatic
Gastrointestinal perforation / perforated colon / gastric perforation (5 cases)
Nausea (4%)

Genitourinary
Urinary tract infection [2]

Hematologic
Anemia [2]
Lymphopenia (lymphocytopenia) / lymphocytes decreased (1–2%)
Neutropenia (neutrophils decreased) (1–2%)

Respiratory
Cough (2%)
Nasopharyngitis [4]
Tuberculosis (<1%; 3 cases)
Upper respiratory tract infection (14%) [4]

Other
Adverse effects / adverse reactions [4]
Infection [5]

URACIL/TEGAFUR

Trade name: Uftoral (Bristol-Myers Squibb)
Indications: Metastatic colorectal cancer
Class: Antimetabolite, Folic acid antagonist
Half-life: 6.5 hours
Clinically important, potentially hazardous interactions with: allopurinol, cimetidine, clozapine, metronidazole, phenytoin, tegafur/gimeracil/oteracil, warfarin
Important contra-indications noted in the prescribing guidelines for: nursing mothers; pediatric patients
Note: Tegafur is a prodrug of fluorouracil (see separate entry).

Skin
Acral erythema [2]
Hand–foot syndrome (palmar–plantar erythrodysesthesia) [6]
Keratoderma [2]
Photosensitivity [3]

Nails
Nail pigmentation [2]

Mucosal
Mucositis [4]
Stomatitis (oral mucositis) [6]

Central Nervous System
Anosmia (smell loss) / smell disorder [2]
Pain [2]

Endocrine/Metabolic
ALT increased [2]

Gastrointestinal/Hepatic
Abdominal pain [2]
Diarrhea [2]
Hepatotoxicity / liver injury / acute liver injury / drug-induced liver injury (DILI) [3]
Nausea [2]

Neuromuscular/Skeletal
Asthenia / fatigue [9]

Other
Side effects [2]

URAPIDIL

Trade name: Eupressyl (Nycomed)
Indications: Hypertension
Class: Adrenergic alpha-receptor antagonist, Serotonin agonist
Half-life: 4.7 hours (oral); 2.7 hours (intravenous)
Clinically important, potentially hazardous interactions with: none known
Note: Not approved by the FDA. Approved on a national level in several countries in Europe, South America, Japan and other Asian regions.

Cardiovascular
Bradycardia / sinus bradycardia [2]
Tachycardia [2]

Central Nervous System
Headache [8]
Intracranial pressure increased (intracranial hypertension) [2]
Somnolence (drowsiness) [2]
Vertigo / dizziness [8]

Neuromuscular/Skeletal
Asthenia / fatigue [4]

UROKINASE

Trade name: Abbokinase (AbbVie)
Indications: Acute myocardial infarction, coronary artery thrombosis, pulmonary embolism
Class: Fibrinolytic, Plasminogen activator
Half-life: 10–20 minutes
Clinically important, potentially hazardous interactions with: aspirin, bivalirudin, ibuprofen, indomethacin

---

Skin
Anaphylactoid reactions / anaphylaxis (includes anaphylactic shock) (>10%)
Angioedema (formerly named angioneurotic edema) (>10%)

Ocular
Periorbital edema (>10%)

URSODIOL

Synonyms: ursodeoxycholic acid; UDCA
Trade names: Actigall (Watson), Destolit (Norgine), Urdox (Wockhardt), Urso 250 (Aptalis), Urso Forte (Aptalis), Ursogal (Galen)
Indications: The dissolution of radiolucent (i.e. non-radio opaque) cholesterol gallstones in patients with a functioning gallbladder, primary biliary cirrhosis, biliary calculus, cholelithiasis
Class: Cholesterol antagonist, Urolithic
Half-life: 100 hours
Clinically important, potentially hazardous interactions with: aluminum based antacids, aluminum hydroxide, charcoal, cholestyramine, clofibrate, colestimide, colestipol, cyclosporine, dapsone, estradiol, estrogens, nitrendipine, oral contraceptives, P4503A substrates

Important contra-indications noted in the prescribing guidelines for: the elderly; nursing mothers; pediatric patients

---

Skin
- Lichenoid eruption / lichenoid reaction [3]
- Pruritus (itching) [3]
- Rash (3%)

Hair
- Alopecia / hair loss (<5%)

Cardiovascular
- Chest pain (3%)

Central Nervous System
- Headache (18–25%)
- Insomnia (2%)
- Vertigo / dizziness (17%)

Endocrine/Metabolic
- Weight gain [2]

Gastrointestinal/Hepatic
- Abdominal pain (43%)
- Cholecystitis (calculous / acalculous) (5%)
- Constipation (26%)
- Diarrhea (27%) [4]
- Dyspepsia / functional dyspepsia (indigestion) (see also gastroparesis) (16%) [2]
- Flatulence (7%)
- Gastrointestinal disorder / discomfort [2]
- Nausea (14%) [4]
- Vomiting (9–14%) [3]

Genitourinary
- Dysmenorrhea (5%)
- Urinary tract infection (6%)

Hematologic
- Leukocytopenia (leukopenia) / leukocytes (white blood cells) decreased (3%)

Neuromuscular/Skeletal
- Arthralgia (7%)
- Asthenia / fatigue (3–7%)
- Back pain (7–12%)
- Bone pain / joint pain (6%)
- Myalgia/Myopathy (5%)

Respiratory
- Bronchitis (6%)
- Cough (7%)
- Influenza- ('flu)-like syndrome (6%)
- Pharyngitis (sore throat) (8%)
- Rhinitis / rhinosinusitis (see also sinusitis) (5%)
- Sinusitis (see also rhinitis / rhinosinusitis) (5–11%)
- Upper respiratory tract infection (12–15%)

Other
- Adverse effects / adverse reactions [3]
- Allergic reactions (5%)
- Infection (viral) (9–19%)

USTEKINUMAB

Trade name: Stelara (Centocor)
Indications: Plaque psoriasis (moderate to severe), active psoriatic arthritis, active Crohn's disease (moderate to severe)
Class: Antipsoriatic agent, Biologic, Interleukin-12/23 antagonist, Interleukin-17 (IL-17) antagonist / interleukin-17 inhibitor, Monoclonal antibody
Half-life: 15–32 days
Clinically important, potentially hazardous interactions with: live vaccines, typhoid vaccine, yellow fever vaccine
Important contra-indications noted in the prescribing guidelines for: nursing mothers; pediatric patients
Note: Ustekinumab-aekn (Selarsdi) is biosimilar to Ustekinumab (Stelara). Approved 04/16/2024 Ustekinumab-auub (Wezlana) is biosimilar to Ustekinumab (Stelara). Approved 10/31/2023.

Skin
- Bullous pemphigoid / pemphigoid [5]
- Cellulitis and pseudocellulitis (<10%)
- Eosinophilic cellulitis / Wells' syndrome [2]
- Herpes zoster [2]
- Pruritus (itching) (<10%)
- Psoriasis [3]
- Pustules / pustular eruption [2]

Mucosal
- Nasal congestion (<10%)

Cardiovascular
- Cardiotoxicity [3]

Central Nervous System
- Depression (<10%)
- Headache (<10%) [9]
- Leukoencephalopathy / posterior reversible encephalopathy syndrome (PRES) [5]
- Vertigo / dizziness (<10%)

Gastrointestinal/Hepatic
- Diarrhea (<10%)
- Hepatotoxicity / liver injury / acute liver injury / drug-induced liver injury (DILI) [3]

Local
- Injection-site reaction [7]

Neuromuscular/Skeletal
- Arthralgia [3]
- Asthenia / fatigue (<10%) [3]
- Back pain (<10%)
- Myalgia/Myopathy (<10%)
- Psoriatic arthralgia / psoriatic arthritis [2]

Respiratory
- Nasopharyngitis (10%) [12]
- Pharyngolaryngeal pain (<10%)
- Tuberculosis [2]
- Upper respiratory tract infection (10%) [9]

Other
- Adverse effects / adverse reactions [17]
- Infection [15]
- Malignancies [2]

VALACYCLOVIR

Trade name: Valtrex (GSK)
Indications: Genital herpes, herpes simplex, herpes zoster
Class: Antiviral, Guanine nucleoside analog
Half-life: 3 hours
Clinically important, potentially hazardous interactions with: cobicistat/elvitegravir/emtricitabine/tenofovir alafenamide, cobicistat/elvitegravir/emtricitabine/tenofovir disoproxil, immunosuppressants, meperidine, tenofovir disoproxil
Important contra-indications noted in the prescribing guidelines for: the elderly; pediatric patients

---

Central Nervous System
- Hallucinations [3]
- Headache [5]
- Neurotoxicity [6]

Gastrointestinal/Hepatic
- Abdominal pain [2]
- Nausea [4]
- Vomiting [3]

Renal
- Nephrotoxicity / kidney injury / acute kidney injury (AKI) / drug-induced kidney injury [6]

VALBENAZINE

Trade name: Ingrezza (Neurocrine Biosciences)
Indications: Tardive dyskinesia
Class: Vesicular monoamine transporter 2 inhibitor
Half-life: 15–22 hours
Clinically important, potentially hazardous interactions with: carbamazepine, clarithromycin, digoxin, fluoxetine, isocarboxazid, itraconazole, ketoconazole, MAO inhibitors, paroxetine hydrochloride, phenelzine, phenytoin, quinidine, rifampin, selegiline, St John's wort, strong CYP2D6 inducers, strong CYP3A4 inducers or inhibitors
Pregnancy category: May cause fetal harm
Important contra-indications noted in the prescribing guidelines for: nursing mothers; pediatric patients
Note: Valbenazine tosylate.

Mucosal
- Xerostomia (dry mouth) (<5%) [2]

Central Nervous System
- Akathisia (<3%)
- Depression [2]
- Gait instability / postural instability (<4%)
- Headache (3%) [6]
- Impaired concentration (<5%)
- Restlessness (<3%)
- Sedation (<11%)
- Somnolence (drowsiness) (<11%) [6]
- Suicidal ideation [2]
- Vertigo / dizziness (<4%) [2]

Endocrine/Metabolic
- Appetite decreased [2]

Gastrointestinal/Hepatic
- Constipation (<5%) [2]
- Diarrhea [2]
- Nausea (2%) [3]
- Vomiting (3%)

Genitourinary
- Urinary retention (<5%)
- Urinary tract infection [3]

Neuromuscular/Skeletal
- Arthralgia (2%)
- Asthenia / fatigue (<11%) [6]

Ocular
- Vision blurred (<5%)

VALDECOXIB

Trade name: Bextra (Pfizer)
Indications: Osteoarthritis, adult rheumatoid arthritis, dysmenorrhea
Class: COX-2 inhibitor, Non-steroidal anti-inflammatory (NSAID), Sulfonamide
Half-life: 8–11 hours
Clinically important, potentially hazardous interactions with: aspirin, dextromethorphan, lithium, warfarin
Note: Valdecoxib is a sulfonamide and can be absorbed systemically. Sulfonamides can produce severe, possibly fatal, reactions such as toxic epidermal necrolysis and Stevens-Johnson

syndrome. NSAIDs may cause an increased risk of serious cardiovascular and gastrointestinal adverse events, which can be fatal. This risk may increase with duration of use.
This drug has been withdrawn.
Warning: CARDIOVASCULAR AND GASTROINTESTINAL RISKS

Skin
Acneiform eruption / acneiform dermatitis / acneiform rash (<2%)
Bruise / bruising / contusion / ecchymosis (ecchymoses) (<2%)
Cellulitis and pseudocellulitis (<2%)
Dermatitis (<2%)
Diaphoresis (<2%)
Eczema / eczematous reaction / eczematous eruption (<2%)
Edema / fluid retention (<2%)
Exanthems (<2%)
Facial edema (<2%)
Hematoma / cutaneous hematoma (<2%)
Hot flashes / hot flushes (<2%)
Lipomatosis (<2%)
Peripheral edema (2–3%)
Photosensitivity (<2%)
Pruritus (itching) (<2%)
Psoriasis (<2%)
Rash (<2%)
Stevens-Johnson syndrome and toxic epidermal necrolysis (SJS/TEN) [4]
Ulcerations (<2%)
Urticaria / hives (<2%) [2]
Xerosis / xeroderma (<2%)

Hair
Alopecia / hair loss (<2%)

Mucosal
Stomatitis (oral mucositis) (<2%)
Xerostomia (dry mouth) (<2%)

Cardiovascular
Myocardial infarction [4]
Myocardial toxicity [2]
Thrombophlebitis (<2%)

Central Nervous System
Chills (<2%)
Depression (<2%)
Dysgeusia (taste perversion) (<2%)
Hyperesthesia (<2%)
Myokymia / twitching / fasciculation (<2%)
Paresthesias (<2%)
Stroke / cerebrovascular accident [3]
Tremor (<2%)

Neuromuscular/Skeletal
Arthralgia (<2%)
Back pain (2–3%)
Myalgia/Myopathy (2%)
Tendinopathy/Tendon rupture (<2%)

Ocular
Periorbital edema (<2%)

Otic
Tinnitus (2–10%)

Renal
Nephrotoxicity / kidney injury / acute kidney injury (AKI) / drug-induced kidney injury [2]

Respiratory
Cough (<2%)
Influenza- ('flu)-like syndrome (2%)
Upper respiratory tract infection (6–7%)

Other
Allergic reactions (<2%)

VALERIAN

Family: Valerianaceae
Scientific names: *Valeriana edulis, Valeriana jatamansii, Valeriana officinalis, Valeriana sitchensis, Valeriana wallichii*
Indications: Depression, tremors, epilepsy, attention deficit hyperactivity disorder, rheumatism, nervous asthma, gastric spasms, colic, menstrual cramps, hot flashes. Flavoring in foods and beverages
Class: Anxiolytic
Half-life: N/A
Clinically important, potentially hazardous interactions with: amitriptyline, escitalopram, eszopiclone

Central Nervous System
Somnolence (drowsiness) [2]
Tremor [2]

Gastrointestinal/Hepatic
Hepatotoxicity / liver injury / acute liver injury / drug-induced liver injury (DILI) [2]

Other
Adverse effects / adverse reactions [2]

VALGANCICLOVIR

Trade name: Valcyte (Roche)
Indications: Cytomegalovirus retinitis (CMV) in patients with AIDS, prevention of CMV disease in high-risk transplant patients
Class: Antiviral, Guanine nucleoside analog
Half-life: 4 hours (in severe renal impairment up to 68%)
Clinically important, potentially hazardous interactions with: abacavir, cobicistat/elvitegravir/emtricitabine/tenofovir alafenamide, cobicistat/elvitegravir/emtricitabine/tenofovir disoproxil, emtricitabine, tenofovir disoproxil
Pregnancy category: May cause fetal toxicity based on findings in animal studies
Important contra-indications noted in the prescribing guidelines for: nursing mothers
Note: Valganciclovir is rapidly converted to ganciclovir in the body.
Warning: HEMATOLOGIC TOXICITY, IMPAIRMENT OF FERTILITY, FETAL TOXICITY, MUTAGENESIS AND CARCINOGENESIS

Mucosal
Oral candidiasis [2]

Central Nervous System
Fever (pyrexia) (includes hyperpyrexia) [3]
Headache [2]
Neurotoxicity [2]
Paresthesias (8%)

Hematologic
Neutropenia (neutrophils decreased) [10]

Other
Allergic reactions (<5%)
Infection (<5%)

VALPROIC ACID

Synonyms: valproate sodium; divalproex; divalproate
Trade names: Depacon (AbbVie), Depakene (AbbVie), Depakote (AbbVie)
Indications: Seizures, migraine
Class: Anticonvulsant (see also antiepileptic (anti-seizure)), Antipsychotic, Mood stabilizer
Half-life: 6–16 hours
Clinically important, potentially hazardous interactions with: amitriptyline, aspirin, ceftobiprole, cholestyramine, clobazam, clozapine, doripenem, eslicarbazepine, ethosuximide, imipenem/cilastatin/relebactam, indinavir, ivermectin, lesinurad, levomepromazine, lumateperone, meropenem, meropenem & vaborbactam, olanzapine, oxcarbazepine, paliperidone, risperidone, rufinamide, temozolomide, tipranavir, topiramate, topiramate, vorinostat, zidovudine, zinc, zuclopenthixol
Note: Gestational exposure to valproate is associated with an unacceptably high risk of major congenital malformations, neurodevelopmental disorders, and other adverse outcomes. Prescription of valproate to reproductive-age women is therefore strongly discouraged in many parts of the world. From January 2024, the United Kingdom began regulating that no one under the age of 55 will be newly prescribed sodium valproate unless two specialists agree that no other effective or tolerable treatment is available, or unless there are 'compelling reasons that reproductive risks do not apply' (Medicines and Healthcare Products Regulatory Agency. Date of Issue: 28 November 2023; Reference No: NatPSA/2023/013/MHRA).
Divalproate (divalproex) is an equimolar combination of valproic acid and sodium valproate.
Warning: LIFE-THREATENING ADVERSE REACTIONS

Skin
Bruise / bruising / contusion / ecchymosis (ecchymoses) (<5%) [4]
DRESS syndrome (Drug-induced hypersensitivity syndrome) [17]
Edema / fluid retention [3]
Erythema multiforme [3]
Erythroderma [3]
Exanthems (5%) [3]
Facial edema (>5%)
Furunculosis (<5%)
Hypersensitivity [5]
Lupus erythematosus (subacute cutaneous lupus erythematosus (SCLE)) [6]
Peripheral edema (<5%)
Petechiae (<5%)
Pruritus (itching) (>5%)
Pseudolymphoma / cutaneous pseudolymphoma [2]
Purpura [2]
Rash (>5%) [7]
Stevens-Johnson syndrome and toxic epidermal necrolysis (SJS/TEN) [19]
Vasculitis (angiitis) / cutaneous vasculitis (angiitis) [3]

Hair
Alopecia / hair loss (7%) [23]
Curly hair [6]
Hirsutism [2]

Nails
- Nail pigmentation [2]

Mucosal
- Gingival hyperplasia / gingival hypertrophy / gingival enlargement / gingival overgrowth [8]
- Glossitis (inflammation of the tongue) (<5%)
- Stomatitis (oral mucositis) (<5%)
- Xerostomia (dry mouth) (<5%) [2]

Central Nervous System
- Akathisia [2]
- Brain atrophy / cerebral atrophy / cerebellar atrophy [2]
- Cerebral edema / brain edema [2]
- Cognitive impairment [2]
- Coma [3]
- Confusion [2]
- Delirium [2]
- Dysgeusia (taste perversion) (<5%)
- Encephalopathy (includes hepatic encephalopathy) [36]
- Gait instability / postural instability [2]
- Headache [2]
- Movement disorder(s) [3]
- Neurotoxicity [4]
- Paresthesias (<5%)
- Parkinsonism [16]
- Sedation [3]
- Seizures [10]
- Sleep apnea [3]
- Somnolence (drowsiness) [11]
- Tremor [16]
- Vertigo / dizziness [7]

Endocrine/Metabolic
- Acute intermittent porphyria [2]
- Appetite increased [2]
- AST increased [2]
- Carnitine deficiency [2]
- GGT increased [2]
- Hyperammonemia [32]
- Hyponatremia [2]
- Metabolic syndrome (includes metabolic disorder) [4]
- Porphyria [2]
- SIADH [6]
- Weight gain [23]

Gastrointestinal/Hepatic
- Constipation [2]
- Dyspepsia / functional dyspepsia (indigestion) (see also gastroparesis) [2]
- Hepatic steatosis [2]
- Hepatotoxicity / liver injury / acute liver injury / drug-induced liver injury (DILI) [22]
- Nausea [5]
- Pancreatitis / acute pancreatitis [34]
- Vomiting [3]

Genitourinary
- Enuresis (urinary incontinence) [7]
- Vaginitis (includes vulvitis) (<5%)

Hematologic
- Coagulopathy / coagulation dysfunction / clotting factor deficiency (includes disseminated intravascular coagulation / DIC) [6]
- Eosinophilia / eosinophils increased [2]
- Hemotoxicity [3]
- Hypofibrinogenemia [2]
- Myelosuppression / bone marrow suppression / myelotoxicity [4]
- Neutropenia (neutrophils decreased) [4]
- Pancytopenia (includes bicytopenia) [8]
- Pure red cell aplasia [2]
- Thrombocytopenia / platelets decreased [7]

Neuromuscular/Skeletal
- Asthenia / fatigue [4]
- Myoclonus (see also hypnic jerk) [3]
- Osteoporosis [3]
- Rhabdomyolysis [3]

Ocular
- Cataract [2]
- Ocular adverse effect [2]

Otic
- Hearing loss (hypoacusis) [3]

Renal
- Fanconi syndrome (proximal tubular dysfunction) [4]

Respiratory
- Pleural effusion [4]
- Pneumonitis [2]

Other
- Adverse effects / adverse reactions [9]
- Allergic reactions (<5%)
- Congenital malformations [7]
- Death [9]
- Teratogenicity [31]

VALSARTAN

Trade names: Byvalson (Forest), Diovan (Novartis), Diovan HCT (Novartis), Exforge (Novartis), Valturna (Novartis)
Indications: Hypertension
Class: Angiotensin receptor antagonist (blocker), Antihypertensive
Half-life: 9 hours
Clinically important, potentially hazardous interactions with: none known
Important contra-indications noted in the prescribing guidelines for: nursing mothers; pediatric patients
Note: Byvalson is valsartan and nebivolol; Exforge is valsartan and amlodipine; Valturna is valsartan and aliskiren; Diovan HCT is valsartan and hydrochlorothiazide. Hydrochlorothiazide is a sulfonamide and can be absorbed systemically. Sulfonamides can produce severe, possibly fatal, reactions such as toxic epidermal necrolysis and Stevens-Johnson syndrome.
See also separate profile for Sacubitril/Valsartan.
Warning: FETAL TOXICITY

Skin
- Angioedema (formerly named angioneurotic edema) (>2%) [10]
- Edema / fluid retention [6]
- Peripheral edema [4]
- Photosensitivity [3]
- Pruritus (itching) (>2%)
- Pseudolymphoma / cutaneous pseudolymphoma [2]
- Rash (>2%)

Mucosal
- Aphthous stomatitis / aphthous ulcer / aphtha (aphthae) (<10%)
- Xerostomia (dry mouth) (>10%)

Cardiovascular
- Hypotension [2]

Central Nervous System
- Dysgeusia (taste perversion) (>10%)
- Headache [7]
- Paresthesias (>2%)
- Vertigo / dizziness [10]

Endocrine/Metabolic
- Hyperkalemia [3]

Gastrointestinal/Hepatic
- Enteropathy [2]

Neuromuscular/Skeletal
- Arthralgia (<10%)
- Myalgia/Myopathy (10–29%)

Respiratory
- Cough [2]
- Nasopharyngitis [3]
- Upper respiratory tract infection [3]

Other
- Adverse effects / adverse reactions [6]
- Allergic reactions (>2%)

VANCOMYCIN

Trade name: Vancocin (Lilly)
Indications: Various infections caused by susceptible organisms
Class: Antibiotic, Antibiotic; glycopeptide, Antimicrobial
Half-life: 5–11 hours
Clinically important, potentially hazardous interactions with: meloxicam, metformin, pentamidine, rocuronium, succinylcholine, teicoplanin, trospium

---

Skin
- Abscess [2]
- AGEP [10]
- Anaphylactoid reactions / anaphylaxis (includes anaphylactic shock) [14]
- Angioedema (formerly named angioneurotic edema) [3]
- Bullous dermatosis [5]
- Cellulitis and pseudocellulitis [3]
- DRESS syndrome (Drug-induced hypersensitivity syndrome) [33]
- Erythema multiforme [5]
- Exanthems [16]
- Exfoliative dermatitis [4]
- Fixed eruption / fixed drug eruption [2]
- Flushing / rubefaction (<10%)
- Hypersensitivity [8]
- Leukocytoclastic vasculitis (angiitis) [8]
- Linear IgA bullous dermatosis [64]
- Lupus erythematosus (subacute cutaneous lupus erythematosus (SCLE)) [2]
- Maculopapular rash / morbilliform rash [7]
- Pruritus (itching) [12]
- Purpura [2]
- Rash [22]
- Red man syndrome / flushing syndrome (<14%) [58]
- Red neck syndrome [2]
- Stevens-Johnson syndrome and toxic epidermal necrolysis (SJS/TEN) [18]
- Urticaria / hives [8]
- Vasculitis (angiitis) / cutaneous vasculitis (angiitis) [2]

Cardiovascular
- Cardiac arrest [3]
- Extravasation [2]
- Hypotension [3]
- Phlebitis (14–23%) [6]

Central Nervous System
- Chills (>10%) [2]
- Dysgeusia (taste perversion) (>10%)
- Fever (pyrexia) (includes hyperpyrexia) [9]
- Headache [5]
- Vertigo / dizziness [2]

Endocrine/Metabolic
- ALT increased [2]

AST increased [3]
Hypokalemia [2]

Gastrointestinal/Hepatic
Constipation [3]
Diarrhea [7]
Gastrointestinal disorder / discomfort [2]
Hepatotoxicity / liver injury / acute liver injury / drug-induced liver injury (DILI) [2]
Nausea [12]
Vomiting [6]

Hematologic
Agranulocytosis / severe selective neutropenia [2]
Anemia [2]
Eosinophilia / eosinophils increased [4]
Leukocytopenia (leukopenia) / leukocytes (white blood cells) decreased [2]
Leukocytosis (elevated white blood cell (WBC) count) [2]
Neutropenia (neutrophils decreased) [14]
Thrombocytopenia / platelets decreased [25]

Local
Infusion-related reactions [2]
Injection-site extravasation [2]

Ocular
Retinal vasculitis (includes hemorrhagic occlusive retinal vasculitis (HORV)) [9]

Otic
Ototoxicity [5]
Tinnitus [2]

Renal
Nephritis / interstitial nephritis / tubulointerstitial nephritis [4]
Nephrotoxicity / kidney injury / acute kidney injury (AKI) / drug-induced kidney injury [40]
Renal failure [4]

Other
Adverse effects / adverse reactions [7]
Allergic reactions (<5%) [5]
Death [7]

VANDETANIB

Trade name: Caprelsa (AstraZeneca)
Indications: Medullary thyroid cancer
Class: Angiogenesis inhibitor / antiangiogenic agent, Epidermal growth factor receptor (EGFR) inhibitor / antagonist, RET (Rearranged during Transfection) kinase inhibitor, Tyrosine kinase inhibitor
Half-life: 19 days
Clinically important, potentially hazardous interactions with: amiodarone, amoxapine, antiarrhythmics, arsenic, carbamazepine, chloroquine, clarithromycin, CYP3A4 inducers, dexamethasone, disopyramide, dofetilide, dolasetron, efavirenz, granisetron, haloperidol, methadone, moxifloxacin, pazopanib, phenobarbital, phenytoin, pimozide, procainamide, QT prolonging agents, rifabutin, rifampin, rifapentine, sotalol, St John's wort, telavancin
Important contra-indications noted in the prescribing guidelines for: nursing mothers; pediatric patients
Note: Contra-indicated in patients with congenital long QT syndrome.
Warning: QT PROLONGATION, TORSADES DE POINTES, AND SUDDEN DEATH

Skin
Acneiform eruption / acneiform dermatitis / acneiform rash (35%) [4]
Cutaneous toxicity / skin toxicity [9]
Folliculitis [5]
Hand–foot syndrome (palmar–plantar erythrodysesthesia) [4]
Photosensitivity (13%) [8]
Phototoxicity [4]
Pigmentation (Skin) (includes hyperpigmentation) [6]
Pruritus (itching) (11%) [2]
Rash (53%) [35]
Stevens-Johnson syndrome and toxic epidermal necrolysis (SJS/TEN) [4]
Xerosis / xeroderma (15%) [3]

Hair
Hair changes [2]

Nails
Paronychia [5]
Photo-onycholysis [2]
Splinter hemorrhage [2]

Mucosal
Mucositis [2]
Stomatitis (oral mucositis) [2]

Cardiovascular
Hypertension (33%) [25]
QT interval prolonged / QT prolongation (14%) [26]

Central Nervous System
Anorexia [3]
Depression (10%)
Headache (26%) [4]
Insomnia (13%)
Neurotoxicity [2]

Endocrine/Metabolic
ALT increased (51%) [3]
Appetite decreased (21%) [3]
Hypocalcemia (11%) [2]
Hypothyroidism [2]
Thyroid dysfunction [2]
Weight loss (10%) [2]

Gastrointestinal/Hepatic
Abdominal pain (21%)
Constipation [2]
Diarrhea (57%) [46]
Dyspepsia / functional dyspepsia (indigestion) (see also gastroparesis) (11%)
Hepatotoxicity / liver injury / acute liver injury / drug-induced liver injury (DILI) [4]
Nausea (33%) [14]
Vomiting (15%) [6]

Hematologic
Anemia [3]
Hemorrhage [2]
Hemotoxicity [2]
Myelosuppression / bone marrow suppression / myelotoxicity [2]
Neutropenia (neutrophils decreased) [5]

Neuromuscular/Skeletal
Asthenia / fatigue (15–24%) [18]

Ocular
Keratopathy [2]

Renal
Proteinuria (10%) [2]

Respiratory
Cough (11%)
Dyspnea / shortness of breath [3]
Nasopharyngitis (11%)

Other
Adverse effects / adverse reactions [6]
Death [3]

VARDENAFIL

Trade name: Levitra (Bayer)
Indications: Erectile dysfunction
Class: Phosphodiesterase type 5 (PDE5) inhibitor
Half-life: 4–5 hours
Clinically important, potentially hazardous interactions with: alfuzosin, alpha blockers, amyl nitrite, antifungals, antihypertensives, atazanavir, boceprevir, bosentan, cobicistat/elvitegravir/emtricitabine/tenofovir alafenamide, cobicistat/elvitegravir/emtricitabine/tenofovir disoproxil, conivaptan, CYP3A4 inhibitors, darunavir, dasatinib, disopyramide, doxazosin, erythromycin, etravirine, fosamprenavir, grapefruit juice, high-fat foods, indinavir, itraconazole, ketoconazole, lopinavir, macrolide antibiotics, nelfinavir, nicorandil, nifedipine, nitrates, nitroglycerin, nitroprusside, phosphodiesterase 5 inhibitors, protease inhibitors, riociguat, ritonavir, sapropterin, saquinavir, tamsulosin, telaprevir, terazosin, tipranavir, viloxazine
Pregnancy category: not indicated for use in women
Important contra-indications noted in the prescribing guidelines for: pediatric patients

---

Skin
Anaphylactoid reactions / anaphylaxis (includes anaphylactic shock) (<2%)
Angioedema (formerly named angioneurotic edema) (<2%)
Diaphoresis (<2%)
Erythema (<2%)
Facial edema (<2%)
Flushing / rubefaction (11%) [14]
Photosensitivity (<2%)
Pruritus (itching) (<2%)
Rash (<2%)

Mucosal
Nasal congestion [4]
Xerostomia (dry mouth) (<2%)

Cardiovascular
Angina (<2%)
Chest pain (<2%)
Hypotension (<2%)
Myocardial infarction (<2%)
Palpitation (<2%)
QT interval prolonged / QT prolongation [2]
Tachycardia (<2%)
Ventricular arrhythmia (<2%)

Central Nervous System
Amnesia (<2%)
Dysesthesia (<2%)
Headache (7–15%) [16]
Pain (<2%)
Paresthesias (<2%)
Seizures (<2%)
Sleep-related disorder (<2%)
Somnolence (drowsiness) (<2%)
Syncope / fainting (<2%)
Vertigo / dizziness (2%) [3]

Endocrine/Metabolic
ALT increased (<2%)
Creatine phosphokinase (CPK) / creatine kinase increased (hyperCKemia) (<2%)

Gastrointestinal/Hepatic
Abdominal pain (<2%)
Diarrhea (<2%)
Dyspepsia / functional dyspepsia (indigestion) (see also gastroparesis) [3]
Gastritis / pangastritis / gastric irritation (<2%)
Gastroesophageal reflux (<2%)
Nausea (<2%)
Vomiting (<2%)

Genitourinary
Erection (<2%)
Priapism (<2%)

Neuromuscular/Skeletal
Arthralgia (<2%)
Back pain (<2%)
Cramps (<2%)
Myalgia/Myopathy (<2%)

Ocular
Conjunctivitis (conjunctival inflammation) (<2%)
Dyschromatopsia (<2%)
Intraocular pressure increased (<2%)
Ocular hyperemia (<2%)
Ocular pain (<2%)
Photophobia (<2%)
Visual disturbances (<2%)

Otic
Hearing loss (hypoacusis) [2]
Tinnitus (<2%)

Respiratory
Dyspnea / shortness of breath (<2%)
Influenza- ('flu)-like syndrome (3%)
Rhinitis / rhinosinusitis (see also sinusitis) (9%) [10]
Sinusitis (see also rhinitis / rhinosinusitis) (3%)

Other
Allergic reactions (<2%)

VARENICLINE

Trade names: Champix (Pfizer), Chantix (Pfizer)
Indications: Smoking deterrent
Class: Nicotinic antagonist
Half-life: 24 hours
Clinically important, potentially hazardous interactions with: none known
Important contra-indications noted in the prescribing guidelines for: nursing mothers; pediatric patients
Warning: SERIOUS NEUROPSYCHIATRIC EVENTS

Skin
AGEP [4]
Rash (<3%)

Mucosal
Stomatitis (oral mucositis) [2]
Xerostomia (dry mouth) (4–6%)

Cardiovascular
Cardiotoxicity [5]

Central Nervous System
Abnormal dreams (9–13%) [19]
Aggression (includes anger) [3]
Anorexia (<2%)
Anxiety [6]
Depression [11]
Dysgeusia (taste perversion) (5–8%)
Hallucinations [2]
Hallucinations, visual [2]
Headache (15–19%) [14]
Insomnia (18–19%) [17]
Irritability [3]
Mania [5]
Mood changes (includes mood disorder) [4]
Neuropsychiatric / neuropsychological adverse effect [2]
Nightmares (<2%)
Psychosis [7]
Sleep disturbances [8]
Sleep-related disorder (2–5%) [3]
Somnolence (drowsiness) (3%) [2]
Suicidal ideation [7]

Endocrine/Metabolic
Appetite decreased (<2%)
Appetite increased (3–4%) [2]

Gastrointestinal/Hepatic
Abdominal pain (5–7%) [4]
Constipation (5–8%) [5]
Dyspepsia / functional dyspepsia (indigestion) (see also gastroparesis) (5%) [4]
Flatulence (6–9%)
Hepatotoxicity / liver injury / acute liver injury / drug-induced liver injury (DILI) [2]
Nausea (16–30%) [33]
Vomiting (<5%) [4]

Neuromuscular/Skeletal
Asthenia / fatigue (<7%) [6]

Respiratory
Dyspnea / shortness of breath (<2%)
Nasopharyngitis [2]
Upper respiratory tract infection (5–7%)

Other
Adverse effects / adverse reactions [10]
Death [3]
Sneezing (sternutation) [2]

VECURONIUM

Indications: Adjunct to general anesthesia
Class: Non-depolarizing neuromuscular blocker
Half-life: 65–75 minutes
Clinically important, potentially hazardous interactions with: aminoglycosides, betamethasone, cyclosporine, gentamicin, halothane, inhalational anesthetics, kanamycin, magnesium salts, neomycin, quinidine, streptomycin, succinylcholine, tazobactam, tobramycin, triamcinolone

---

Skin
Anaphylactoid reactions / anaphylaxis (includes anaphylactic shock) [11]

Cardiovascular
Bradycardia / sinus bradycardia [8]

Local
Injection-site pain [4]

VEDOLIZUMAB

Trade name: Entyvio (Takeda)
Indications: Ulcerative colitis, Crohn's disease
Class: Biologic, Integrin receptor antagonist, Monoclonal antibody
Half-life: 25 days
Clinically important, potentially hazardous interactions with: live vaccines, natalizumab, TNF blockers
Important contra-indications noted in the prescribing guidelines for: nursing mothers; pediatric patients

---

Skin
Pruritus (itching) (3%)
Rash (3%) [3]

Mucosal
Oropharyngeal pain (3%)

Central Nervous System
Fever (pyrexia) (includes hyperpyrexia) (9%) [5]
Headache (12%) [11]

Gastrointestinal/Hepatic
Abdominal pain [7]
Cholestatic liver injury / cholestatic hepatitis [2]
Colitis [6]
Crohn's disease (exacerbation) [2]
Nausea (9%) [9]
Pancreatitis / acute pancreatitis [4]
Vomiting [4]

Hematologic
Anemia [4]

Local
Infusion-related reactions (4%) [4]

Neuromuscular/Skeletal
Arthralgia (12%) [9]
Asthenia / fatigue (6%) [6]
Back pain (4%) [3]
Pain in extremities (3%)

Renal
Nephritis / interstitial nephritis / tubulointerstitial nephritis [6]

Respiratory
Bronchitis (4%)
Cough (5%) [3]
Influenza (4%)
Interstitial lung disease / interstitial pneumonitis / interstitial pneumonia (cryptogenic organizing pneumonia) / drug-induced interstitial lung disease [2]
Nasopharyngitis (13%) [11]
Sinusitis (see also rhinitis / rhinosinusitis) (3%)
Upper respiratory tract infection (7%) [7]

Other
Adverse effects / adverse reactions [15]
Cancer [2]
Infection [9]
Malignancies [2]

VEMURAFENIB

Trade name: Zelboraf (Roche)
Indications: Melanoma (metastatic or unresectable)
Class: BRAF inhibitor, Kinase inhibitor
Half-life: 57 hours
Clinically important, potentially hazardous interactions with: amoxapine, arsenic, atazanavir, carbamazepine, clarithromycin, CYP substrates, dolasetron, efavirenz, indinavir, itraconazole, ketoconazole, nefazodone, nelfinavir, pazopanib, phenobarbital, phenytoin, rifabutin, rifampin, rifapentine, ritonavir, saquinavir, telavancin, telithromycin, voriconazole, warfarin
Important contra-indications noted in the prescribing guidelines for: nursing mothers; pediatric patients

---

Skin
Acneiform eruption / acneiform dermatitis / acneiform rash [6]

Actinic keratoses [4]
Basal cell carcinoma [2]
Cutaneous toxicity / skin toxicity [12]
DRESS syndrome (Drug-induced hypersensitivity syndrome) [8]
Eccrine squamous syringometaplasia [2]
Erythema (14%) [2]
Exanthems [9]
Fibromatosis [includes palmar fibromatosis (Dupuytren's contracture / Dupuytren's disease), plantar fibromatosis (Ledderhose disease) and penile fibromatosis (Peyronie disease)] [3]
Granulomas [2]
Hand–foot syndrome (palmar–plantar erythrodysesthesia) [8]
Hyperkeratosis (24%) [18]
Keratoacanthoma (Grzybowski syndrome) [28]
Keratoses [4]
Keratosis pilaris [10]
Lymphoma [2]
Melanoma [3]
Milia [2]
Nevi (naevi) [6]
Panniculitis [10]
Papillomas (21%) [2]
Papular lesions (5%)
Peripheral edema (17%)
Photosensitivity (33%) [30]
Pruritus (itching) (23%) [10]
Radiation recall dermatitis [2]
Rash (37%) [27]
Squamous cell carcinoma (24%) [36]
Stevens-Johnson syndrome and toxic epidermal necrolysis (SJS/TEN) [10]
Sunburn (10%)
Transient acantholytic dermatosis (Grover's disease) [4]
Vasculitis (angiitis) / cutaneous vasculitis (angiitis) [2]
Verrucae vulgaris / warts / verrucae [2]
Verrucous lesions [3]
Vitiligo [2]
Xerosis / xeroderma [5]

Hair
Alopecia / hair loss (45%) [19]
Hair changes [2]

Nails
Paronychia [3]
Pyogenic granuloma [2]

Mucosal
Gingival hyperplasia / gingival hypertrophy / gingival enlargement / gingival overgrowth [2]

Cardiovascular
QT interval prolonged / QT prolongation [4]

Central Nervous System
Bell's palsy (facial palsy) [2]
Dysgeusia (taste perversion) (14%)
Fever (pyrexia) (includes hyperpyrexia) (19%) [6]
Headache (23%) [3]
Paralysis / paraplegia [2]

Endocrine/Metabolic
ALT increased [6]
Appetite decreased (18%) [2]
AST increased [5]
GGT increased [2]

Gastrointestinal/Hepatic
Constipation (12%)
Diarrhea (28%) [9]
Hepatotoxicity / liver injury / acute liver injury / drug-induced liver injury (DILI) [4]
Nausea (35%) [10]
Pancreatitis / acute pancreatitis [2]
Vomiting (18%) [4]

Neuromuscular/Skeletal
Arthralgia (53%) [23]
Asthenia / fatigue (38%) [20]
Back pain (8%)
Bone pain / joint pain (8%)
Myalgia/Myopathy (8–13%) [2]
Pain in extremities (18%)

Ocular
Chorioretinopathy [2]
Ocular adverse effect [2]
Uveitis / anterior uveitis / posterior uveitis / panuveitis [9]
Vision blurred [2]

Respiratory
Cough (8%)

Other
Adverse effects / adverse reactions [12]
Neoplasms [2]
Vogt-Koyanagi-Harada syndrome [4]

VENETOCLAX

Trade name: Venclexta (AbbVie)
Indications: Chronic lymphocytic leukemia in patients with 17p deletion, as detected by an FDA approved test, who have received at least one prior therapy
Class: BCL-2 inhibitor
Half-life: 26 hours
Clinically important, potentially hazardous interactions with: amiodarone, azithromycin, bosentan, captopril, carbamazepine, carvedilol, ciprofloxacin, clarithromycin, conivaptan, cyclosporine, digoxin, diltiazem, dronedarone, efavirenz, erythromycin, etravirine, everolimus, felodipine, fluconazole, grapefruit juice, indinavir, itraconazole, ketoconazole, live vaccines, lopinavir, modafinil, nafcillin, phenytoin, posaconazole, quercetin, quinidine, ranolazine, rifampin, ritonavir, sirolimus, St John's wort, stong or moderate P-gp inhibitors or substrates, strong or moderate CYP3A inducers or inhibitors, telaprevir, ticagrelor, verapamil, voriconazole
Pregnancy category: May cause fetal harm
Important contra-indications noted in the prescribing guidelines for: nursing mothers; pediatric patients
Note: Concomitant use of strong CYP3A inhibitors during initiation and ramp-up phase is contra-indicated.

Skin
Peripheral edema (11%)

Central Nervous System
Fever (pyrexia) (includes hyperpyrexia) (16%) [4]
Headache (15%) [2]

Endocrine/Metabolic
Hyperkalemia (20%)
Hyperphosphatemia (15%)
Hyperuricemia (6%)
Hypocalcemia (9%)
Hypokalemia (12%)

Gastrointestinal/Hepatic
Constipation (14%)
Diarrhea (35%) [13]
Nausea (33%) [15]
Vomiting (15%) [5]

Hematologic
Anemia (29%) [13]
Febrile neutropenia [7]
Leukocytopenia (leukopenia) / leukocytes (white blood cells) decreased [5]
Neutropenia (neutrophils decreased) (45%) [19]
Thrombocytopenia / platelets decreased (22%) [15]

Neuromuscular/Skeletal
Asthenia / fatigue (21%) [9]
Back pain (10%)

Renal
Tumor lysis syndrome (TLS) [13]

Respiratory
Cough (13%)
Pneumonia (8%) [4]
Upper respiratory tract infection (22%) [6]

Other
Adverse effects / adverse reactions [3]
Death [5]
Infection [2]

VENLAFAXINE

Trade names: Effexor (Wyeth), Effexor XL (Wyeth)
Indications: Major depressive disorder
Class: Antidepressant, Serotonin-norepinephrine reuptake inhibitor
Half-life: 3–7 hours
Clinically important, potentially hazardous interactions with: 5HT1 agonists, artemether/lumefantrine, aspirin, atomoxetine, clozapine, desvenlafaxine, dexibuprofen, diclofenac, duloxetine, entacapone, haloperidol, indinavir, isocarboxazid, ketoconazole, linezolid, lithium, MAO inhibitors, meloxicam, metoclopramide, metoprolol, mirtazapine, moclobemide, naratriptan, NSAIDs, phenelzine, selegiline, sibutramine, SNRIs, SSRIs, St John's wort, sumatriptan, tramadol, tranylcypromine, trazodone, trimipramine, triptans, viloxazine, voriconazole, warfarin
Important contra-indications noted in the prescribing guidelines for: the elderly; nursing mothers; pediatric patients
Warning: SUICIDALITY AND ANTIDEPRESSANT DRUGS

Skin
Angioedema (formerly named angioneurotic edema) [2]
Bruise / bruising / contusion / ecchymosis (ecchymoses) [2]
Diaphoresis [7]
Hyperhidrosis [2]
Pruritus (itching) (<10%)
Rash (3%)

Hair
Alopecia / hair loss [2]

Mucosal
Xerostomia (dry mouth) (22%) [10]

Cardiovascular
Cardiac failure [2]
Cardiomyopathy [3]
Hypertension [7]
Myocardial infarction [2]
Orthostatic hypotension [2]
Preeclampsia [2]

QT interval prolonged / QT prolongation [6]
Tachycardia [2]

Central Nervous System
Akathisia [2]
Delirium [2]
Dysgeusia (taste perversion) (2%)
Hallucinations, visual [3]
Headache [8]
Insomnia [5]
Mania [10]
Paresthesias (3%)
Psychosis [3]
Restless legs syndrome / Willis-Ekbom disease (includes restless arms syndrome variant) [3]
Seizures [8]
Serotonin syndrome [24]
Somnolence (drowsiness) [9]
Tremor (<10%) [3]
Vertigo / dizziness [10]
Yawning [2]

Endocrine/Metabolic
Appetite decreased [2]
Galactorrhea [5]
Hyponatremia [4]
Libido increased [2]
Mastodynia [2]
SIADH [6]
Weight gain [2]

Gastrointestinal/Hepatic
Constipation [6]
Hepatotoxicity / liver injury / acute liver injury / drug-induced liver injury (DILI) [8]
Nausea [16]
Vomiting [3]

Genitourinary
Ejaculatory dysfunction [2]
Enuresis (urinary incontinence) [2]
Sexual dysfunction [8]
Urinary retention [2]

Hematologic
Thrombocytopenia / platelets decreased [2]

Neuromuscular/Skeletal
Asthenia / fatigue [5]
Dystonia [2]
Rhabdomyolysis [3]

Ocular
Glaucoma (includes acute angle-closure glaucoma) [2]

Respiratory
Pneumonitis [3]

Other
Adverse effects / adverse reactions [3]
Bruxism (teeth grinding) [7]

VERAPAMIL

Trade names: Calan (Pfizer), Covera-HS (Pfizer), Isoptin (AbbVie), Tarka (AbbVie), Verelan (Schwarz)
Indications: Angina, arrhythmias, hypertension
Class: Antiarrhythmic class IV, Calcium channel blocker, CYP3A4 inhibitor
Half-life: 2–8 hours
Clinically important, potentially hazardous interactions with: acebutolol, afatinib, aliskiren, amiodarone, amitriptyline, amprenavir, aspirin, atazanavir, atenolol, atorvastatin, avanafil, betaxolol, betrixaban, bisoprolol, carbamazepine, carteolol, celiprolol, clonidine, cobicistat/elvitegravir/emtricitabine/tenofovir alafenamide, cobicistat/elvitegravir/emtricitabine/tenofovir disoproxil, colchicine, dabigatran, dantrolene, darifenacin, deflazacort, delavirdine, digoxin, dofetilide, dronedarone, dutasteride, epirubicin, eplerenone, erythromycin, esmolol, everolimus, fingolimod, flibanserin, indacaterol, ivabradine, lemborexant, lovastatin, lumateperone, metoprolol, mifepristone, nadolol, naldemedine, naloxegol, neratinib, nevirapine, olaparib, oxprenolol, oxtriphylline, palbociclib, penbutolol, pindolol, ponesimod, posaconazole, propranolol, quinidine, ranolazine, sibutramine, silodosin, simvastatin, talazoparib, telaprevir, telithromycin, timolol, trabectedin, ubrogepant, venetoclax, voclosporin
Important contra-indications noted in the prescribing guidelines for: nursing mothers; pediatric patients
Note: Tarka is verapamil and trandolapril.

Skin
Angioedema (formerly named angioneurotic edema) [3]
Diaphoresis [2]
Edema / fluid retention (2%)
Erythema multiforme [4]
Erythromelalgia / erythermalgia [2]
Exanthems [8]
Exfoliative dermatitis [2]
Flushing / rubefaction (<7%) [4]
Hyperkeratosis (palms) [2]
Lupus erythematosus (subacute cutaneous lupus erythematosus (SCLE)) [2]
Peripheral edema (<10%)
Photosensitivity [4]
Pruritus (itching) [6]
Rash [2]
Stevens-Johnson syndrome and toxic epidermal necrolysis (SJS/TEN) [5]
Urticaria / hives [5]
Vasculitis (angiitis) / cutaneous vasculitis (angiitis) [2]

Hair
Alopecia / hair loss [5]

Mucosal
Gingival hyperplasia / gingival hypertrophy / gingival enlargement / gingival overgrowth (19%) [10]

Cardiovascular
Atrial fibrillation [2]
Atrioventricular block [2]
Bradycardia / sinus bradycardia [11]
Congestive heart failure [2]
Hypotension [3]
QT interval prolonged / QT prolongation [2]
Torsades de pointes [2]

Central Nervous System
Parkinsonism [2]
Seizures [3]

Endocrine/Metabolic
Gynecomastia [8]

Gastrointestinal/Hepatic
Hepatotoxicity / liver injury / acute liver injury / drug-induced liver injury (DILI) [2]

Neuromuscular/Skeletal
Rhabdomyolysis [2]

Other
Death [2]
Side effects [2]

VERNAKALANT

Trade name: Kynapid (Cardiome)
Indications: Atrial fibrillation
Class: Antiarrhythmic class III, Potassium channel antagonist, Sodium channel antagonist
Half-life: 2–3 hours
Clinically important, potentially hazardous interactions with: none known
Important contra-indications noted in the prescribing guidelines for: nursing mothers; pediatric patients

---

Cardiovascular
Bradycardia / sinus bradycardia [3]
Hypotension [3]

Central Nervous System
Dysgeusia (taste perversion) [6]
Paresthesias [3]

Gastrointestinal/Hepatic
Nausea [2]

Other
Sneezing (sternutation) [3]

VIBEGRON

Trade name: Gemtesa (Urovant)
Indications: Treatment of an overactive bladder

Class: Beta-3 adrenergic agonist
Half-life: approximately 31 hours
Clinically important, potentially hazardous interactions with: digoxin
Pregnancy category: No available data to evaluate drug-associated risk of major birth defects, miscarriage, or adverse maternal or fetal outcomes.
Note: Clinical trials of vibegron were conducted in patients with an overactive bladder, the majority of whom were Caucasian (78%) and female (85%) with a mean age of 60 years (range 18 to 93 years).

Skin
Hot flashes / hot flushes (<2%)

Mucosal
Xerostomia (dry mouth) (<2%) [3]

Cardiovascular
Hypertension [2]

Central Nervous System
Headache (4%) [2]

Gastrointestinal/Hepatic
Constipation (<2%) [2]
Diarrhea (2%)
Nausea (2%)

Genitourinary
Residual urine volume increased / post-void residual (PVR) urine (<2%)
Urinary retention (<2%)
Urinary tract infection (7%) [2]

Respiratory
Bronchitis (3%)
Nasopharyngitis (3%) [2]
Upper respiratory tract infection (2%)

VIDARABINE

Synonyms: adenine arabinoside; ara-A
Trade name: Vira-A Ophthalmic (Pfizer)
Indications: Herpetic keratoconjunctivitis
Class: Antiviral; nucleoside analog
Half-life: 3.3 hours
Clinically important, potentially hazardous interactions with: allopurinol, insulin
Important contra-indications noted in the prescribing guidelines for: nursing mothers; pediatric patients

---

Central Nervous System
Neurotoxicity [9]
Pain [2]
Tremor [4]

Other
Death [2]

VIGABATRIN

Trade names: Sabril (Lundbeck), Vigafyde (Pyros)
Indications: Epilepsy, infantile spasms (West's syndrome)
Class: Anticonvulsant (see also antiepileptic (anti-seizure)), Antiepileptic (anti-seizure)
Half-life: 7.5 hours
Clinically important, potentially hazardous interactions with: antipsychotics, chloroquine, hydroxychloroquine, MAO inhibitors, mefloquine, orlistat, phenytoin, rufinamide, SSRIs, St John's wort, tricyclic antidepressants
Important contra-indications noted in the prescribing guidelines for: nursing mothers; pediatric patients
Warning: VISION LOSS

Skin
Peripheral edema (5–7%)
Rash (6%) [2]

Cardiovascular
Chest pain (<5%)

Central Nervous System
Abnormal dreams (<5%)
Anxiety (4%)
Confusion (4–14%)
Depression (8%) [4]
Dysarthria (2%)
Encephalopathy (includes hepatic encephalopathy) [4]
Fever (pyrexia) (includes hyperpyrexia) (4–7%)
Gait instability / postural instability (6–12%)
Headache (18%)
Hypoesthesia / hypesthesia (numbness) (4–5%)
Hyporeflexia (4–5%)
Impaired concentration (9%)
Incoordination (7%)
Insomnia (7%)
Irritability (7%)
Memory loss/memory impaired (7%)
Nervousness (2–5%)
Peripheral neuropathy (4%)
Psychosis [2]
Sedation (4%)
Seizures (11%) [4]
Somnolence (drowsiness) (17%) [3]
Status epilepticus (2–5%)
Tremor (7%)
Vertigo / dizziness (15%)

Endocrine/Metabolic
Appetite increased (<5%)
Weight gain (10%) [4]

Gastrointestinal/Hepatic
Abdominal distension (2%)
Abdominal pain (2–3%)
Constipation (5–8%)
Diarrhea (7%)
Dyspepsia / functional dyspepsia (indigestion) (see also gastroparesis) (4–5%)
Nausea (7%)
Vomiting (6%)

Genitourinary
Dysmenorrhea (5–9%)
Erectile dysfunction (5%)
Urinary tract infection (4–5%)

Hematologic
Anemia (6%)

Neuromuscular/Skeletal
Arthralgia (5–10%)
Asthenia / fatigue (16%) [2]
Back pain (4–7%)
Muscle spasm (3%)
Myalgia/Myopathy (3–5%)
Pain in extremities (2–6%)

Ocular
Diplopia (double vision) (6%)
Nystagmus (7%)
Ocular pain (5%)
Optic atrophy [2]
Retinopathy [12]
Vision blurred (6%)
Vision impaired [20]

Otic
Tinnitus (2%)

Respiratory
Bronchitis (5%)
Cough (2–14%)
Influenza (5–7%)
Nasopharyngitis (10%)
Pharyngolaryngeal pain (7–14%)
Upper respiratory tract infection (10%)

Other
Adverse effects / adverse reactions [4]
Dipsia (thirst) / polydipsia (2%)
Toothache (odontalgia) (2–5%)

VILAZODONE

Trade name: Viibryd (Merck KGaA)
Indications: Major depressive disorder
Class: Antidepressant, Serotonin-norepinephrine reuptake inhibitor
Half-life: 25 hours
Clinically important, potentially hazardous interactions with: anticoagulants, aspirin, buspirone, CNS-active agents, CYP3A4 inhibitors or inducers, efavirenz, erythromycin, ketoconazole, MAO inhibitors, NSAIDs, SNRIs, SSRIs, tramadol, triptans, tryptophan, warfarin
Important contra-indications noted in the prescribing guidelines for: nursing mothers; pediatric patients
Warning: SUICIDALITY AND ANTIDEPRESSANT DRUGS

Mucosal
Xerostomia (dry mouth) (8%) [2]

Cardiovascular
Palpitation (2%)

Central Nervous System
Abnormal dreams (4%)
Headache [4]
Insomnia (6%) [5]
Paresthesias (3%)
Restlessness (3%)
Somnolence (drowsiness) (3%) [3]
Tremor (2%)
Vertigo / dizziness (9%) [2]

Endocrine/Metabolic
Appetite increased (2%)
Libido decreased (4–5%)

Gastrointestinal/Hepatic
Diarrhea (28%) [15]
Dyspepsia / functional dyspepsia (indigestion) (see also gastroparesis) (3%)
Flatulence (3%)
Gastroenteritis (3%)
Nausea (23%) [15]
Vomiting (5%) [5]

Genitourinary
Ejaculatory dysfunction (2%)
Erectile dysfunction (2%)
Sexual dysfunction (3%) [2]

Neuromuscular/Skeletal
Arthralgia (3%)
Asthenia / fatigue (4%)

Other
Adverse effects / adverse reactions [3]

VILDAGLIPTIN

Trade name: Galvus (Novartis)
Indications: Type II diabetes mellitus
Class: Antidiabetic, Dipeptidyl peptidase-4 (DPP-4) (gliptin) inhibitor
Half-life: 2–3 hours
Clinically important, potentially hazardous interactions with: corticosteroids, sympathomimetics, thiazides, thyroid products
Important contra-indications noted in the prescribing guidelines for: nursing mothers; pediatric patients

---

Skin
Angioedema (formerly named angioneurotic edema) [2]
Bullous pemphigoid / pemphigoid [6]
Peripheral edema [3]

Central Nervous System
Headache [6]
Vertigo / dizziness [2]

Endocrine/Metabolic
Hypoglycemia [8]

Gastrointestinal/Hepatic
Hepatotoxicity / liver injury / acute liver injury / drug-induced liver injury (DILI) [2]
Pancreatitis / acute pancreatitis [4]

Respiratory
Nasopharyngitis [3]

Other
Adverse effects / adverse reactions [18]

VILOXAZINE

Trade name: Qelbree (Supernus)
Indications: Treatment of Attention Deficit Hyperactivity Disorder (ADHD) in pediatric patients 6 to 17 years of age
Class: Norepinephrine reuptake inhibitor
Half-life: ~7 hours
Clinically important, potentially hazardous interactions with: alfentanil, alosetron, atomoxetine, avanafil, clozapine, conivaptan, CYP1A2 substrates, CYP2D6 substrates, CYP3A4 substrates, darunavir, desipramine, dextromethorphan, duloxetine, everolimus, ibrutinib, isocarboxazid, lomitapide, lovastatin, lurasidone, metoprolol, midazolam, monoamine oxidase inhibitors, naloxegol, nebivolol, nisoldipine, nortriptyline, perphenazine, phenelzine, pirfenidone, ramelteon, rasagiline, risperidone, safinamide, saquinavir, selegiline, simvastatin, sirolimus, tacrolimus, tasimelteon, theophylline, tipranavir, tizanidine, tolterodine, tranylcypromine, triazolam, vardenafil, venlafaxine
Pregnancy category: May cause maternal harm; discontinue when pregnancy is recognized.
Warning: IN CLINICAL TRIALS, HIGHER RATES OF SUICIDAL THOUGHTS AND BEHAVIOR WERE REPORTED IN PEDIATRIC PATIENTS TREATED WITH VILOXAZINE THAN IN PATIENTS TREATED WITH PLACEBO. CLOSELY MONITOR FOR WORSENING AND EMERGENCE OF SUICIDAL THOUGHTS AND BEHAVIORS.

Cardiovascular
Heart rate alteration (pediatric patients) (22%)

Central Nervous System
Fever (pyrexia) (includes hyperpyrexia) (2%)
Headache (11%) [3]
Insomnia (4%) [2]
Irritability (pediatric ADHD patients) (3%)
Somnolence (drowsiness) (pediatric ADHD patients) (16%)

Endocrine/Metabolic
Appetite decreased (pediatric ADHD patients) (7%) [2]

Gastrointestinal/Hepatic
Abdominal pain (pediatric ADHD patients) (5%)
Nausea (pediatric ADHD patients) (5%) [2]
Vomiting (pediatric ADHD patients) (4%)

Neuromuscular/Skeletal
Asthenia / fatigue (6%) [2]

Respiratory
Upper respiratory tract infection (pediatric ADHD patients) (7%)

Other
Adverse effects / adverse reactions [2]

VINBLASTINE

Trade names: Velban (Lilly), Velbe (Lilly), Velsar (Lilly)
Indications: Lymphomas, melanoma, carcinomas
Class: Antimitotic, Vinca alkaloid
Half-life: initial: 3.7 minutes; terminal: 24.8 hours
Clinically important, potentially hazardous interactions with: aldesleukin, aprepitant, erythromycin, fluconazole, itraconazole, ketoconazole, lopinavir, miconazole, posaconazole
Important contra-indications noted in the prescribing guidelines for: nursing mothers

---

Skin
Acral necrosis [2]
Dermatitis (<10%)
Photosensitivity (<10%) [2]
Pigmentation (Skin) (includes hyperpigmentation) [3]
Radiation recall dermatitis [2]
Rash (<10%)
Raynaud's phenomenon (<10%) [17]

Hair
Alopecia / hair loss (>10%)

Mucosal
Mucositis [2]
Oral lesions (<5%)
Stomatitis (oral mucositis) (>10%)

Central Nervous System
Dysgeusia (taste perversion) (metallic taste) (>10%)
Paresthesias (<10%)
Peripheral neuropathy [2]

Endocrine/Metabolic
SIADH [4]

Gastrointestinal/Hepatic
Diarrhea [2]

Hematologic
Hemolytic uremic syndrome [2]
Neutropenia (neutrophils decreased) [3]

Local
Injection-site necrosis [2]

Neuromuscular/Skeletal
Myalgia/Myopathy (<10%)

Otic
Tinnitus [2]

Renal
Nephrotoxicity / kidney injury / acute kidney injury (AKI) / drug-induced kidney injury [2]

Other
Adverse effects / adverse reactions [2]

VINCRISTINE

Synonym: oncovin
Trade name: Vincasar (Teva)
Indications: Leukemias, lymphomas, neuroblastoma, Wilm's tumor
Class: Antimitotic, Vinca alkaloid
Half-life: 24 hours
Clinically important, potentially hazardous interactions with: aldesleukin, aprepitant, bromelain, fluconazole, gadobenate, influenza vaccine, itraconazole, ketoconazole, lopinavir, miconazole, nifedipine, posaconazole, thalidomide
Important contra-indications noted in the prescribing guidelines for: nursing mothers

---

Skin
Erythroderma [2]
Exanthems [3]
Hand–foot syndrome (palmar–plantar erythrodysesthesia) [2]
Rash (<10%)
Raynaud's phenomenon [2]

Hair
Alopecia / hair loss (20–70%) [9]

Nails
Beau's lines (transverse nail bands) [3]
Leukonychia striata (Mees' lines) [6]
Nail pigmentation [2]

Mucosal
Oral lesions (<10%) [2]
Oral ulceration (<10%)

Cardiovascular
Hypertension [2]
Phlebitis (<10%)

Central Nervous System
Anorexia [2]
Cranial neuropathy (includes types of palsy) [3]
Dysgeusia (taste perversion) (<10%)
Neurotoxicity [18]
Paresthesias (<10%)
Peripheral neuropathy [26]
Seizures [7]

Endocrine/Metabolic
Hyponatremia [2]
SIADH [10]

Gastrointestinal/Hepatic
Abdominal pain [2]
Constipation [2]
Ileus / adynamic ileus / paralytic ileus [2]
Intestinal pseudo-obstruction (Ogilvie syndrome) [3]

Hematologic
Anemia [2]
Febrile neutropenia [5]
Hemolytic uremic syndrome [4]
Hemotoxicity [2]
Leukocytopenia (leukopenia) / leukocytes (white blood cells) decreased [3]
Neutropenia (neutrophils decreased) [10]
Thrombocytopenia / platelets decreased [10]

Local
Injection-site cellulitis (>10%)
Injection-site necrosis (>10%)

Neuromuscular/Skeletal
Asthenia / fatigue [2]
Myalgia/Myopathy (<10%)

Ocular
Eyelid ptosis / blepharoptosis [5]
Optic neuropathy [3]

Respiratory
Pneumonia [2]

Other
Adverse effects / adverse reactions [7]
Death [6]
Infection [3]
Vocal cord / vocal fold paralysis (vocal cord / vocal fold palsy) [6]

VINORELBINE

Trade name: Navelbine (Kyowa Kirin)
Indications: Non-small cell lung cancer
Class: Antimitotic, Vinca alkaloid
Half-life: 28–44 hours
Clinically important, potentially hazardous interactions with: aldesleukin, itraconazole
Important contra-indications noted in the prescribing guidelines for: nursing mothers; pediatric patients
Warning: MYELOSUPPRESSION

Skin
Acneiform eruption / acneiform dermatitis / acneiform rash [3]

Hand–foot syndrome (palmar–plantar erythrodysesthesia) [9]
Rash (<5%) [2]
Recall reaction [2]

Hair
Alopecia / hair loss (12%) [5]

Mucosal
Mucositis [2]
Stomatitis (oral mucositis) (>10%) [6]

Cardiovascular
Extravasation [2]
Hypertension [2]
Phlebitis (7%)

Central Nervous System
Anorexia [7]
Dysgeusia (taste perversion) (metallic taste) (>10%)
Hyperesthesia (<10%)
Neurotoxicity [4]
Paresthesias (<10%)
Peripheral neuropathy [2]

Endocrine/Metabolic
ALT increased [2]
AST increased [2]
SIADH [3]

Gastrointestinal/Hepatic
Constipation [5]
Diarrhea [14]
Esophagitis [2]
Hepatotoxicity / liver injury / acute liver injury / drug-induced liver injury (DILI) [2]
Nausea [12]
Vomiting [8]

Hematologic
Anemia [8]
Febrile neutropenia [6]
Leukocytopenia (leukopenia) / leukocytes (white blood cells) decreased [12]
Myelosuppression / bone marrow suppression / myelotoxicity [2]
Neutropenia (neutrophils decreased) [31]
Thrombocytopenia / platelets decreased [4]

Local
Injection-site irritation (<10%)
Injection-site necrosis (<10%)
Injection-site phlebitis (12%) [2]

Neuromuscular/Skeletal
Asthenia / fatigue [14]
Bone pain / joint pain [3]
Myalgia/Myopathy (<5%)

Other
Adverse effects / adverse reactions [2]
Death [2]
Infection [4]

VITAMIN A

Trade name: Aquasol A (aaiPharma)
Indications: Vitamin A deficiency
Class: Vitamin
Half-life: N/A
Clinically important, potentially hazardous interactions with: acitretin, alitretinoin, bexarotene, cholestyramine, fish oil supplements, isotretinoin, minocycline, orlistat, prednisone, tetracycline, warfarin
Pregnancy category: the pregnancy category will be X if used in doses above the RDA

Skin
Dermatitis [7]
Pruritus (itching) [2]
Xerosis / xeroderma (<10%)

Hair
Alopecia / hair loss [11]

Mucosal
Oral mucosal eruption [2]

VITAMIN E

Synonym: alpha tocopherol
Trade name: Aquasol E (aaiPharma)
Indications: Vitamin E deficiency
Class: Vitamin
Half-life: N/A
Clinically important, potentially hazardous interactions with: amprenavir, cholestyramine, orlistat, tipranavir, warfarin
Pregnancy category: the pregnancy category will be C if used in doses above the RDA

Skin
Dermatitis [13]
Erythema multiforme [3]
Sclerosing lipogranuloma [2]

Genitourinary
Prostate cancer (increased risk) [4]

VOCLOSPORIN

Trade name: Lupkynis (Aurinia Pharmaceuticals)
Indications: Treatment of adult patients with active lupus nephritis (in combination with immunosuppressive therapy)
Class: Calcineurin inhibitor
Half-life: Approximately 30 hours
Clinically important, potentially hazardous interactions with: clarithromycin, CYP3A4 inducers, CYP3A4 inhibitors, diltiazem, fluconazole, itraconazole, ketoconazole, P-gp substrates, verapamil
Pregnancy category: May cause fetal harm. Advise patient not to breastfeed.
Important contra-indications noted in the prescribing guidelines for: nursing mothers
Warning: INCREASED RISK FOR DEVELOPING MALIGNANCIES AND SERIOUS INFECTIONS WITH VOCLOSPORIN OR OTHER IMMUNOSUPPRESSANTS THAT MAY LEAD TO HOSPITALIZATION OR DEATH

Hair
Alopecia / hair loss (in combination with mycophenolate mofetil and a tapered dose of a corticosteroid) (6%)

Mucosal
Oral ulceration (in combination with mycophenolate mofetil and a tapered dose of a corticosteroid) (4%)

Cardiovascular
Hypertension (in combination with mycophenolate mofetil and a tapered dose of a corticosteroid) (19%)

Central Nervous System
Headache (in combination with mycophenolate mofetil and a tapered dose of a corticosteroid) (15%)
Tremor (in combination with mycophenolate mofetil and a tapered dose of a corticosteroid) (3%)

Endocrine/Metabolic
Appetite decreased (in combination with mycophenolate mofetil and a tapered dose of a corticosteroid) (3%)

Gastrointestinal/Hepatic
Abdominal pain (in combination with mycophenolate mofetil and a tapered dose of a corticosteroid) (7%)
Diarrhea (in combination with mycophenolate mofetil and a tapered dose of a corticosteroid) (19%)
Dyspepsia / functional dyspepsia (indigestion) (see also gastroparesis) (in combination with mycophenolate mofetil and a tapered dose of a corticosteroid) (6%)

Genitourinary
Urinary tract infection (in combination with mycophenolate mofetil and a tapered dose of a corticosteroid) (10%)

Hematologic
Anemia (in combination with mycophenolate mofetil and a tapered dose of a corticosteroid) (12%)

Neuromuscular/Skeletal
Asthenia / fatigue (in combination with mycophenolate mofetil and a tapered dose of a corticosteroid) (4%)

Renal
Glomerular filtration rate decreased (in combination with mycophenolate mofetil and a tapered dose of a corticosteroid) (26%)
Nephrotoxicity / kidney injury / acute kidney injury (AKI) / drug-induced kidney injury (in combination with mycophenolate mofetil and a tapered dose of a corticosteroid) (3%)
Renal function abnormal / renal dysfunction (in combination with mycophenolate mofetil and a tapered dose of a corticosteroid) (6%)

Respiratory
Cough (in combination with mycophenolate mofetil and a tapered dose of a corticosteroid) (11%)

Other
Adverse effects / adverse reactions [2]

VORAPAXAR

Trade name: Zontivity (Merck)
Indications: Reduction of thrombotic cardiovascular events in patients with a history of myocardial infarction or with peripheral arterial disease
Class: Protease-activated receptor-1 (PAR-1) antagonist
Half-life: 3–4 days
Clinically important, potentially hazardous interactions with: boceprevir, carbamazepine, clarithromycin, conivaptan, indinavir, itraconazole, ketoconazole, nefazodone, nelfinavir, phenytoin, posaconazole, rifampin, ritonavir, saquinavir, St John's wort, strong CYP3A inhibitors or inducers, telaprevir, telithromycin
Important contra-indications noted in the prescribing guidelines for: nursing mothers; pediatric patients
Note: Contra-indicated in patients with a history of stroke, transient ischemic attack, or intracranial hemorrhage, or with active pathological bleeding.
Warning: BLEEDING RISK

Skin
Exanthems (2%)
Rash (2%)
Cardiovascular
Cardiotoxicity [2]
Central Nervous System
Depression (2%)
Intracranial hemorrhage [5]
Hematologic
Anemia (5%)
Bleeding (25%) [10]
Ocular
Diplopia (double vision) (<2%)
Retinopathy (<2%)
Other
Adverse effects / adverse reactions [3]

VORICONAZOLE

Trade name: Vfend (Pfizer)
Indications: Invasive aspergillosis
Class: Antifungal / antimycotic, Antifungal; triazole, Antimicrobial, CYP3A4 inhibitor
Half-life: 6–24 hours (dose dependent)
Clinically important, potentially hazardous interactions with: abiraterone, alfentanil, alfuzosin, almotriptan, alosetron, amphotericin B, antineoplastics, apixaban, aprepitant, artemether/lumefantrine, astemizole, atazanavir, atorvastatin, barbiturates, benzodiazepines, boceprevir, bortezomib, bosentan, brigatinib, brinzolamide, buspirone, busulfan, cabazitaxel, cabozantinib, calcifediol, calcium channel blockers, carbamazepine, carvedilol, chloramphenicol, chloroquine, ciclesonide, cilostazol, cinacalcet, ciprofloxacin, cisapride, clopidogrel, cobicistat/elvitegravir/emtricitabine/tenofovir alafenamide, cobicistat/elvitegravir/emtricitabine/tenofovir disoproxil, colchicine, conivaptan, copanlisib, coumarins, crizotinib, cyclosporine, CYP2C19 inhibitors and inducers, CYP2C9 inhibitors and substrates, CYP3A4 substrates, darunavir, diazepam, diclofenac, didanosine, dienogest, docetaxel, dofetilide, dronedarone, dutasteride, efavirenz, eletriptan, eplerenone, ergot alkaloids, ergotamine, erlotinib, esomeprazole, estrogens, eszopiclone, etravirine, everolimus, fentanyl, fesoterodine, food, gadobutrol, gefitinib, grapefruit juice, guanfacine, halofantrine, HMG-CoA reductase inhibitors, ibrutinib, ibuprofen, imatinib, irinotecan, ixabepilone, lapatinib, letermovir, lomitapide, lopinavir, losartan, lumateperone, macrolide antibiotics, maraviroc, meloxicam, methadone, methylergonovine, methylprednisolone, methysergide, midazolam, midostaurin, mifepristone, mometasone, neratinib, nilotinib, nisoldipine, olaparib, ombitasvir/paritaprevir/ritonavir, omeprazole, oxycodone, palbociclib, pantoprazole, paricalcitol, pazopanib, PEG-interferon, phenobarbital, phenytoin, phosphodiesterase 5 inhibitors, pimecrolimus, pimozide, ponatinib, prasugrel, progestins, progestogens, protease inhibitors, proton pump inhibitors, QT prolonging agents, quetiapine, quinidine, quinine, ramelteon, ranolazine, reboxetine, regorafenib, repaglinide, ribociclib, rifabutin, rifampin, rifapentine, rilpivirine, ritonavir, rivaroxaban, romidepsin, ruxolitinib, salmeterol, saquinavir, saxagliptin, silodosin, simeprevir, simvastatin, sirolimus, solifenacin, sonidegib, sorafenib, St John's wort, sucralfate, sulfonylureas, sunitinib, tacrolimus, tadalafil, tamsulosin, telaprevir, temsirolimus, tetrabenazine, tezacaftor/ivacaftor, thioridazine, ticagrelor, tolterodine, tolvaptan, vemurafenib, venetoclax, venlafaxine, vitamin K antagonists, ziprasidone, zolpidem
Important contra-indications noted in the prescribing guidelines for: nursing mothers; pediatric patients

Skin
Actinic keratoses [2]
Anaphylactoid reactions / anaphylaxis (includes anaphylactic shock) (<2%)
Angioedema (formerly named angioneurotic edema) (<2%)
Bruise / bruising / contusion / ecchymosis (ecchymoses) (<2%)
Cellulitis and pseudocellulitis (<2%)
Contact dermatitis (<2%)
Cyanosis / acrocyanosis (<2%)
Dermatitis (<2%)
Diaphoresis (<2%) [2]
Eczema / eczematous reaction / eczematous eruption (<2%)
Edema / fluid retention (<2%)
Erythema [5]
Erythema multiforme (<2%)
Exfoliative dermatitis (<2%)
Facial edema (<2%)
Fixed eruption / fixed drug eruption (<2%)
Furunculosis (<2%)
Graft-versus-host reaction (<2%)
Granulomas (<2%)
Herpes simplex (<2%)
Lentigo (lentigines; lentigos (pl)) [3]
Lupus erythematosus (subacute cutaneous lupus erythematosus (SCLE)) (<2%) [5]
Lymphadenopathy (<2%)
Melanoma (<2%)
Melanosis / melanocytosis (<2%)
Peripheral edema (<2%)
Petechiae (<2%)
Photosensitivity (8%) [18]
Phototoxicity [13]
Pigmentation (Skin) (includes hyperpigmentation) (<2%)
Pruritus (itching) (8%) [2]
Pseudoporphyria [8]
Psoriasis (<2%)
Purpura (<2%)
Rash (5%) [8]
Squamous cell carcinoma (<2%) [11]
Stevens-Johnson syndrome and toxic epidermal necrolysis (SJS/TEN) (<2%) [6]
Urticaria / hives (<2%)
Xerosis / xeroderma (<2%) [2]
Hair
Alopecia / hair loss (<2%) [4]
Nails
Nail changes [3]
Mucosal
Cheilitis (inflammation of the lips) (<2%) [4]
Gingival bleeding (<2%)
Gingival hyperplasia / gingival hypertrophy / gingival enlargement / gingival overgrowth (<2%)
Gingivitis (<2%)
Glossitis (inflammation of the tongue) (<2%)
Rectal hemorrhage / rectal bleeding (<2%)
Stomatitis (oral mucositis) (<2%)
Tongue edema (<2%)
Xerostomia (dry mouth) (<2%)
Cardiovascular
Arrhythmias (<2%)
Atrial fibrillation (<2%)
Atrioventricular block (<2%)
Bradycardia / sinus bradycardia (<2%)
Bundle branch block (<2%)
Cardiac arrest (<2%)
Cardiomyopathy (<2%)
Chest pain (<2%)
Congestive heart failure (<2%)
Extrasystoles (<2%)
Hypertension (<2%)
Hypotension (<2%)
Myocardial infarction (<2%)
Palpitation (<2%)
Phlebitis (<2%)
Postural hypotension (<2%)
QT interval prolonged / QT prolongation (<2%) [13]
Supraventricular tachycardia (<2%)
Tachycardia (2%) [2]
Thrombophlebitis (<2%)
Torsades de pointes [8]
Vasodilation (<2%)
Ventricular arrhythmia (<2%)
Ventricular fibrillation (<2%)
Ventricular tachycardia (<2%)
Central Nervous System
Abnormal dreams (<2%)
Ageusia (taste loss) / taste disorder (<2%)
Agitation (<2%)
Akathisia (<2%)
Amnesia (<2%)
Anorexia (<2%)
Anxiety (<2%)
Cerebral edema / brain edema (<2%)
Cerebral hemorrhage (<2%)
Cerebral ischemia (<2%)
Chills (4%)
Coma (<2%)
Confusion (<2%) [2]
Delirium (<2%) [2]
Dementia (<2%)
Depersonalization (<2%)
Depression (<2%)
Dysgeusia (taste perversion) (<2%)
Encephalitis (<2%)
Encephalopathy (includes hepatic encephalopathy) (<2%) [3]
Euphoria / elation (<2%)
Extrapyramidal symptoms (<2%)
Fever (pyrexia) (includes hyperpyrexia) (6%)
Guillain-Barré syndrome / acute inflammatory demyelinating polyradiculoneuropathy / acute motor axonal neuropathy (<2%)
Hallucinations (2%) [9]
Hallucinations, visual [9]
Headache (3%) [3]
Hypoesthesia / hypesthesia (numbness) (<2%)
Insomnia (<2%) [2]
Intracranial pressure increased (intracranial hypertension) (<2%)
Neurotoxicity [7]
Paresthesias (<2%)
Peripheral neuropathy [4]
Psychosis (<2%) [3]
Seizures (<2%)
Somnolence (drowsiness) (<2%)
Status epilepticus (<2%)
Stroke / cerebrovascular accident (<2%)
Suicidal ideation (<2%)
Syncope / fainting (<2%)

Tremor (<2%)
Vertigo / dizziness (<2%)

Endocrine/Metabolic
ALP increased (4%)
ALT increased [2]
AST increased [2]
Creatine phosphokinase (CPK) / creatine kinase increased (hyperCKemia) (<2%)
Diabetes insipidus (<2%)
GGT increased (<2%)
Hypercalcemia (<2%)
Hypercholesterolemia (<2%)
Hyperglycemia (includes glucose increased) (<2%)
Hyperkalemia (<2%) [2]
Hypermagnesemia (<2%)
Hypernatremia (<2%)
Hyperthyroidism (includes 'thyroid storm') (<2%)
Hyperuricemia (<2%)
Hypervolemia (fluid overload) (<2%)
Hypocalcemia (<2%)
Hypoglycemia (<2%)
Hypokalemia (2%) [4]
Hypomagnesemia (<2%)
Hyponatremia (<2%)
Hypophosphatemia (<2%)
Hypothyroidism (<2%)
Libido decreased (<2%)

Gastrointestinal/Hepatic
Abdominal pain (<2%)
Ascites (<2%)
Black stools / melena (<2%)
Cholecystitis (calculous / acalculous) (<2%)
Cholelithiasis (gallstones in the gall bladder or the bile duct) (<2%)
Constipation (<2%)
Diarrhea (<2%) [2]
Duodenitis (<2%)
Dyspepsia / functional dyspepsia (indigestion) (see also gastroparesis) (<2%)
Dysphagia (<2%)
Esophagitis (<2%)
Flatulence (<2%)
Gastroenteritis (<2%)
Gastrointestinal bleeding (<2%)
Gastrointestinal perforation / perforated colon / gastric perforation (<2%)
Gastrointestinal ulceration (<2%)
Hematemesis (<2%)
Hepatic failure (<2%)
Hepatotoxicity / liver injury / acute liver injury / drug-induced liver injury (DILI) [24]
Nausea (5%) [3]
Pancreatitis / acute pancreatitis (<2%) [2]
Peritonitis (<2%)
Pseudomembranous colitis (<2%)
Vomiting (4%) [2]

Genitourinary
Anuria (<2%)
Cystitis (includes interstitial cystitis / bladder pain syndrome) (<2%)
Dysmenorrhea (<2%)
Dysuria (<2%)
Enuresis (urinary incontinence) (<2%)
Epididymitis (<2%)
Glycosuria (<2%)
Hematuria (<2%)
Impotence (<2%)
Oliguria (<2%)
Urinary retention (<2%)
Urinary tract infection (<2%)
Uterine bleeding (<2%)
Vaginal bleeding (<2%)

Hematologic
Agranulocytosis / severe selective neutropenia (<2%)
Anemia (<2%)
Eosinophilia / eosinophils increased (<2%)
Hemolytic anemia (<2%)
Leukocytopenia (leukopenia) / leukocytes (white blood cells) decreased (<2%)
Myelosuppression / bone marrow suppression / myelotoxicity (<2%)
Pancytopenia (includes bicytopenia) (<2%)
Prothrombin time (INR) increased (<2%)
Sepsis (<2%)
Thrombocytopenia / platelets decreased (<2%)

Local
Injection-site infection (<2%)
Injection-site inflammation (<2%)
Injection-site pain (<2%)

Neuromuscular/Skeletal
Arthralgia (<2%) [2]
Asthenia / fatigue (<2%) [2]
Ataxia (<2%)
Back pain (<2%)
Bone pain / joint pain (<2%)
Hypertonia (<2%)
Leg cramps (<2%)
Myalgia/Myopathy (<2%) [4]
Myasthenia gravis [2]
Osteomalacia (<2%)
Osteoporosis (<2%)
Periostitis / periostitis deformans [32]
Rhabdomyolysis [2]
Skeletal fluorosis [2]

Ocular
Abnormal vision (19%)
Accommodation disorder (<2%)
Blepharitis (<2%)
Conjunctivitis (conjunctival inflammation) (<2%)
Corneal opacity (<2%)
Diplopia (double vision) (<2%)
Keratitis (ocular keratitis) / corneal inflammation) (<2%)
Keratoconjunctivitis (<2%)
Mydriasis (<2%)
Night blindness (<2%)
Nystagmus (<2%)
Ocular adverse effect [3]
Ocular hemorrhage (<2%)
Ocular pain (<2%)
Oculogyric crisis / oculogyric dystonic reaction (<2%)
Optic atrophy (<2%)
Optic neuritis / papillitis (<2%)
Papilledema (<2%)
Photophobia (2%) [2]
Retinitis (<2%)
Scleritis (<2%)
Uveitis / anterior uveitis / posterior uveitis / panuveitis (<2%)
Visual disturbances (19%) [18]
Xerophthalmia (dry eyes) (<2%)

Otic
Ear pain (<2%)
Hearing loss (hypoacusis) (<2%)
Tinnitus (<2%)

Renal
Nephrotoxicity / kidney injury / acute kidney injury (AKI) / drug-induced kidney injury (<2%) [5]
Renal tubular necrosis (<2%)

Respiratory
Cough (<2%)
Dysphonia (includes voice disorders / voice changes) (<2%)
Dyspnea / shortness of breath (<2%)
Hemoptysis (<2%)
Hypoxia (<2%)
Influenza- ('flu)-like syndrome (<2%)
Pharyngitis (sore throat) (<2%)
Pleural effusion (<2%)
Pneumonia (<2%)
Pneumonitis [2]
Pulmonary embolism (<2%)
Respiratory distress (<2%)
Rhinitis / rhinosinusitis (see also sinusitis) (<2%)
Sinusitis (see also rhinitis / rhinosinusitis) (<2%)
Upper respiratory tract infection (<2%)

Other
Adverse effects / adverse reactions (20%) [12]
Infection (<2%)
Malignancies [2]
Multiorgan failure (<2%)
Periodontal infection (<2%)

VORINOSTAT

Trade name: Zolinza (Merck)
Indications: Cutaneous T-cell lymphoma
Class: Antineoplastic / anticancer agent (see also Immune checkpoint inhibitor), Histone deacetylase (HDAC) inhibitor
Half-life: ~2 hours
Clinically important, potentially hazardous interactions with: alfuzosin, artemether/lumefantrine, chloroquine, ciprofloxacin, coumarins, dronedarone, gadobutrol, nilotinib, pimozide, QT prolonging agents, quinine, tetrabenazine, thioridazine, valproic acid, vitamin K antagonists, ziprasidone
Important contra-indications noted in the prescribing guidelines for: nursing mothers; pediatric patients

---

Skin
Exanthems [2]
Peripheral edema (13%)
Pruritus (itching) (12%)

Hair
Alopecia / hair loss (19%) [2]

Mucosal
Mucositis [2]
Stomatitis (oral mucositis) [2]
Xerostomia (dry mouth) (16%)

Cardiovascular
QT interval prolonged / QT prolongation [3]

Central Nervous System
Anorexia [5]
Chills (16%)
Dysgeusia (taste perversion) (28%)
Fever (pyrexia) (includes hyperpyrexia) (10%)
Headache (12%)
Vertigo / dizziness (15%)

Endocrine/Metabolic
Creatine phosphokinase (CPK) / creatine kinase increased (hyperCKemia) [2]
Dehydration [2]
Hyperglycemia (includes glucose increased) [3]

Weight loss [4]

Gastrointestinal/Hepatic

Abdominal pain [2]
Constipation [2]
Diarrhea [7]
Nausea [10]
Vomiting [4]

Hematologic

Anemia (14%) [7]
Febrile neutropenia [2]
Hemotoxicity [2]
Leukocytopenia (leukopenia) / leukocytes (white blood cells) decreased [3]
Lymphopenia (lymphocytopenia) / lymphocytes decreased [6]
Neutropenia (neutrophils decreased) [10]
Thrombocytopenia / platelets decreased [16]

Neuromuscular/Skeletal

Asthenia / fatigue (52%) [11]

Renal

Renal failure [2]

Respiratory

Cough (11%)
Upper respiratory tract infection (10%)

Other

Adverse effects / adverse reactions [2]

VORTIOXETINE

Trade name: Trintellix (formerly Brintellix) (Takeda)
Indications: Major depressive disorder
Class: Antidepressant, Serotonin receptor agonist, Serotonin receptor antagonist, Serotonin reuptake inhibitor
Half-life: ~66 hours
Clinically important, potentially hazardous interactions with: bupropion, carbamazepine, fluoxetine, MAO inhibitors, paroxetine hydrochloride, phenytoin, quinidine, rifampin
Important contra-indications noted in the prescribing guidelines for: nursing mothers; pediatric patients
Warning: SUICIDAL THOUGHTS AND BEHAVIORS

Skin

Hyperhidrosis [6]
Pruritus (itching) (<3%) [2]

Mucosal

Xerostomia (dry mouth) (6–8%) [18]

Central Nervous System

Abnormal dreams (<3%) [2]
Agitation [2]
Anxiety [2]
Headache [26]
Hypomania [2]
Insomnia [7]
Somnolence (drowsiness) [4]
Vertigo / dizziness (6–9%) [19]

Endocrine/Metabolic

Weight gain [2]

Gastrointestinal/Hepatic

Constipation (3–6%) [13]
Diarrhea (7–10%) [16]
Flatulence (<3%)
Nausea (21–32%) [41]
Vomiting (3–6%) [17]

Genitourinary

Sexual dysfunction (<5%) [10]

Neuromuscular/Skeletal

Asthenia / fatigue [7]

Respiratory

Nasopharyngitis [7]
Upper respiratory tract infection [2]

Other

Adverse effects / adverse reactions [3]

VOXELOTOR

Trade name: Oxbryta (Global Blood Therapeutics)
Indications: Sickle cell disease in adults and pediatric patients 12 years of age and older
Class: Hemoglobin modulator, Hemoglobin S (HbS) polymerization inhibitor
Half-life: 35.5 hours
Clinically important, potentially hazardous interactions with: fluconazole, midazolam, strong CYP3A4 inhibitors, strong or moderate CYP3A4 inducers, CYP3A4 substrates
Note: Women with sickle cell disease have an increased risk of adverse pregnancy outcomes for the mother and the fetus. Voxelotor should only be used during pregnancy if the benefit of the drug outweighs the potential risk.
September 2024: The sickle cell treatment voxelotor (Oxbryta) has been withdrawn from all markets by the manufacturer Pfizer after a "higher than anticipated" number of deaths were reported and clinical evidence showed that the drug's benefits no longer outweighed the risks.

Skin

Hypersensitivity (<10%)
Rash (grade 3 / 4 cases) (14%)

Central Nervous System

Fever (pyrexia) (includes hyperpyrexia) (12%)
Headache (26%)

Gastrointestinal/Hepatic

Abdominal pain (19%)
Diarrhea (grade 3 / 1 case) (20%)
Nausea (grade 3 / 1 case) (17%)

Neuromuscular/Skeletal

Asthenia / fatigue (14%)

WARFARIN

Trade name: Coumadin (Bristol-Myers Squibb)
Indications: Thromboembolic disease, pulmonary embolism
Class: Anticoagulant (antithrombotic), Coumarin
Half-life: 1.5–2.5 days (highly variable)
Clinically important, potentially hazardous interactions with: acemetacin, amiodarone, amobarbital, amprenavir, antithyroid agents, aprepitant, aprobarbital, aspirin, atazanavir, atorvastatin, azathioprine, azithromycin, barbiturates, beclomethasone, betamethasone, bezafibrate, bismuth, bivalirudin, boceprevir, bosentan, butabarbital, capecitabine, cefixime, celecoxib, ceritinib, chondroitin, cimetidine, ciprofloxacin, clarithromycin, clofibrate, clopidogrel, clorazepate, co-trimoxazole, cobicistat/elvitegravir/emtricitabine/tenofovir alafenamide, cobicistat/elvitegravir/emtricitabine/tenofovir disoproxil, colesevelam, cyclosporine, danazol, daptomycin, darunavir, dasiglucagon, delavirdine, desvenlafaxine, dexamethasone, dexibuprofen, dexlansoprazole, diclofenac, dicloxacillin, dirithromycin, disulfiram, dronedarone, duloxetine, econazole, efavirenz, enzalutamide, ergotamine, erlotinib, erythromycin, eslicarbazepine, etoricoxib, exenatide, fenofibrate, fluconazole, flunisolide, fluoxymesterone, fosamprenavir, gefitinib, gemfibrozil, glucagon, grapefruit juice, heparin, imatinib, influenza vaccine, inotersen, itraconazole, ketoconazole, leflunomide, lepirudin, letermovir, levofloxacin, levothyroxine, liothyronine, liraglutide, lomitapide, lopinavir, menadione, mephobarbital, methimazole, methyl salicylate, methylprednisolone, methyltestosterone, metronidazole, miconazole, mifepristone, moricizine, moxifloxacin, nafcillin, nalidixic acid, nandrolone, nilutamide, norfloxacin, obeticholic acid, ofloxacin, omeprazole, oritavancin, orlistat, pantoprazole, PEG-interferon, penicillin G, penicillin V, penicillins, pentobarbital, phenobarbital, phenylbutazones, phytonadione, piperacillin, piroxicam, prasugrel, primidone, propoxyphene, propranolol, propylthiouracil, quinidine, quinine, rabeprazole, resveratrol, rifampin, rifapentine, rofecoxib, romidepsin, ropinirole, rosuvastatin, roxithromycin, salicylates, secobarbital, simvastatin, sitaxentan, sorafenib, St John's wort, stanozolol, sulfamethoxazole, sulfinpyrazone, sulfisoxazole, sulfonamides, sulindac, tamsulosin, tegafur/gimeracil/oteracil, telaprevir, telithromycin, teriflunomide, testosterone, tibolone, tigecycline, tinidazole, tolmetin, tolterodine, tramadol, triamcinolone, troleandomycin, uracil/tegafur, valdecoxib, vemurafenib, venlafaxine, vilazodone, vitamin A, vitamin E, zafirlukast, zileuton
Pregnancy category: category D for women with mechanical heart valves
Note: June 2024. Tramadol and warfarin drug interaction. The UK MHRA issued the following advice: Taking warfarin and tramadol together can cause harmful drug interactions, which can raise the International Normalised Ratio (INR), and result in severe bruising and bleeding, which in some patients could be fatal.
Alternative remedies, including herbals, may potentially increase the risk of bleeding or potentiate the effects of warfarin therapy. Some of these include the following: angelica root, arnica flower, anise, asafetida, bogbean, borage seed oil, bromelain, dan-shen, devil's claw, fenugreek, feverfew, garlic, ginger, ginkgo biloba, ginseng, horse chestnut, lovage root, meadowsweet, onion, parsley, passionflower herb, poplar, quassia, red clover, rue, turmeric and willow bark.
Warning: BLEEDING RISK

Skin

Blue toe syndrome / purple toe syndrome [5]
Bruise / bruising / contusion / ecchymosis (ecchymoses) [2]
Calcinosis cutis / calcification (includes calciphylaxis) [9]
Dermatitis [2]
Exanthems [7]
Gangrene [6]
Hematoma / cutaneous hematoma [3]
Hypersensitivity [3]
Leukocytoclastic vasculitis (angiitis) [3]
Necrosis (skin necrosis) (>10%) [118]
Pruritus (itching) [2]

Purplish erythema (feet and toes) [8]
Purpura [3]
Rash [2]
Stevens-Johnson syndrome and toxic epidermal necrolysis (SJS/TEN) [3]
Urticaria / hives [3]
Vasculitis (angiitis) / cutaneous vasculitis (angiitis) [7]

Hair
Alopecia / hair loss (>10%) [8]

Mucosal
Tongue hematoma / lingual hematoma [4]

Cardiovascular
Myocardial infarction [2]

Central Nervous System
Headache [2]
Intracranial hemorrhage [2]
Vertigo / dizziness [2]

Gastrointestinal/Hepatic
Black stools / melena [2]
Gastrointestinal bleeding [7]
Hematemesis [2]
Hepatotoxicity / liver injury / acute liver injury / drug-induced liver injury (DILI) [3]

Genitourinary
Priapism [4]

Hematologic
Anticoagulation [3]
Bleeding [19]
Hemorrhage [9]
Prothrombin time (INR) increased [11]
Thrombosis [2]

Neuromuscular/Skeletal
Rhabdomyolysis [2]
Spinal epidural hematoma [3]

Renal
Nephropathy [5]
Nephrotoxicity / kidney injury / acute kidney injury (AKI) / drug-induced kidney injury [4]

Other
Adverse effects / adverse reactions [9]
Death [4]

WILLOW BARK

Family: Salicaceae
Scientific names: *Salix alba, Salix fragilis, Salix purpurea*
Indications: Colds, infections, headaches, pain, muscle and joint aches, influenza, gouty arthritis, ankylosing spondylitis, rheumatoid arthritis, osteoarthritis
Class: Anti-inflammatory
Half-life: N/A
Clinically important, potentially hazardous interactions with: NSAIDs, salicylates

XIPAMIDE

Trade name: Diurexan (Meda)
Indications: Hypertension
Class: Antihypertensive
Half-life: N/A
Clinically important, potentially hazardous interactions with: ACTH, amphotericin, carbenoxolone, corticosteroids, laxatives, lithium

---

Cardiovascular
Ventricular fibrillation [2]

XYLOMETAZOLINE

Trade name: Otrivine (Novartis)
Indications: Nasal congestion, perennial and allergic rhinitis, sinusitis
Class: Alpha adrenoceptor agonist
Half-life: N/A
Clinically important, potentially hazardous interactions with: none known
Important contra-indications noted in the prescribing guidelines for: nursing mothers

---

Mucosal
Epistaxis (nosebleed) [2]
Mucosal bleeding [2]

YARROW

Family: Compositae
Scientific name: *Achillea millefolium*
Indications: Fevers, common cold, essential hypertension, digestive complaints, loss of appetite, amenorrhea, dysentery, diarrhea, cerebral and coronary thromboses, menstrual pain, bleeding piles, toothache, muscle spasms, gastrointestinal disorders. **Topical:** slow-healing wounds, skin inflammations, cosmetics
Class: Anti-inflammatory
Half-life: N/A
Clinically important, potentially hazardous interactions with: anticoagulants, antiepileptics, hypertensives, hypotensives

---

Skin
Dermatitis [4]

YELLOW FEVER VACCINE

Trade names: Stamaril (Sanofi Pasteur), YF-VAX (Sanofi Pasteur)
Indications: Immunization against yellow fever
Class: Vaccine
Half-life: N/A
Clinically important, potentially hazardous interactions with: azathioprine, belimumab, corticosteroids, fingolimod, hydroxychloroquine, immunosuppressants, interferon-gamma, leflunomide, mercaptopurine, prednisone, tocilizumab, ustekinumab
Important contra-indications noted in the prescribing guidelines for: the elderly; nursing mothers; pediatric patients
Note: Contra-indicated in patients with hypersensitivity to egg or chick embryo protein.

Skin
Anaphylactoid reactions / anaphylaxis (includes anaphylactic shock) [8]
Hypersensitivity [2]
Rash (3%)
Urticaria / hives [2]

Central Nervous System
Encephalopathy (includes hepatic encephalopathy) [4]
Fever (pyrexia) (includes hyperpyrexia) (low-grade) (<5%) [3]
Headache (<30%) [2]
Myelitis / myeloradiculitis [2]
Neurotoxicity [11]

Gastrointestinal/Hepatic
Diarrhea (<10%) [2]
Hepatitis [2]
Nausea (<10%)
Vomiting (<10%) [2]

Local
Infusion-site erythema (<5%)
Infusion-site pain (<5%)

Neuromuscular/Skeletal
Asthenia / fatigue (10–30%) [2]
Myalgia/Myopathy (10–30%) [2]

Respiratory
Influenza [2]

Other
Adverse effects / adverse reactions [15]
Death [13]
Multiorgan failure [3]
Viscerotropic disease / multiple organ system dysfunction [20]

YOHIMBINE

Family: Rubiaceae
Scientific name: *Pausinystalia yohimbe*
Indications: Impotence, alpha2-adrenergic blocker, orthostatic hypertension
Class: Rauwolfia alkaloid
Half-life: 36 minutes
Clinically important, potentially hazardous interactions with: amitriptyline, benazepril, captopril, clevidipine, lisinopril, terbutaline, tricyclic antidepressants

---

Skin
Flushing / rubefaction [2]

Mucosal
Sialorrhea (ptyalism; hypersalivation) [2]

Cardiovascular
Hypertension [5]
Tachycardia [4]

Central Nervous System
Agitation [2]
Anxiety [6]
Headache [3]

Gastrointestinal/Hepatic
Hepatotoxicity / liver injury / acute liver injury / drug-induced liver injury (DILI) [4]

Genitourinary
Urinary frequency [2]

ZAFIRLUKAST

Trade name: Accolate (AstraZeneca)
Indications: Asthma
Class: Leukotriene receptor antagonist
Half-life: 10 hours
Clinically important, potentially hazardous interactions with: aminophylline, aspirin, carvedilol, CYP2C9 substrates, CYP3A4 substrates, erythromycin, high protein foods, interferon alfa, primidone, vitamin K antagonists, warfarin
Important contra-indications noted in the prescribing guidelines for: nursing mothers; pediatric patients
Note: Contra-indicated in patients with hepatic impairment including hepatic cirrhosis.

Skin
Churg-Strauss syndrome [6]

Central Nervous System
Fever (pyrexia) (includes hyperpyrexia) (2%)

Headache (13%)
Pain (generalized) (2%)
Vertigo / dizziness (2%)

Gastrointestinal/Hepatic
Abdominal pain (2%)
Diarrhea (3%)
Nausea (3%)
Vomiting (2%)

Neuromuscular/Skeletal
Asthenia / fatigue (2%)
Back pain (2%)
Myalgia/Myopathy (2%)

Respiratory
Cough [2]

Other
Infection (4%)

ZALEPLON

Trade name: Sonata (Wyeth)
Indications: Insomnia
Class: Hypnotic, non-benzodiazepine
Half-life: 1 hour
Clinically important, potentially hazardous interactions with: alcohol, cimetidine, erythromycin, imipramine, ketoconazole, promethazine, rifampin, rifapentine, thioridazine
Important contra-indications noted in the prescribing guidelines for: nursing mothers; pediatric patients

---

Cardiovascular
Tachycardia [2]

Central Nervous System
Amnesia (2–4%)
Anorexia (<2%)
Confusion [2]
Depersonalization (<2%)
Hallucinations [3]
Headache (30–42%) [3]
Hypoesthesia / hypesthesia (numbness) (<2%)
Paresthesias (3%)
Parosmia (<2%)
Slurred speech [2]
Somnambulism (sleepwalking; noctambulism) [2]
Somnolence (drowsiness) (5–6%) [4]
Tremor (2%)
Vertigo / dizziness (7–9%) [4]

Gastrointestinal/Hepatic
Abdominal pain (6%)
Nausea (6–8%)
Vomiting [2]

Genitourinary
Dysmenorrhea (3–4%)

Neuromuscular/Skeletal
Asthenia / fatigue (5–7%)
Ataxia [2]

Ocular
Ocular pain (3–4%)

Otic
Hyperacusis (<2%)

Other
Adverse effects / adverse reactions [2]
Viscerotropic disease / multiple organ system dysfunction [2]

ZANUBRUTINIB

Trade name: Brukinsa (BeiGene)
Indications: Adult patients with mantle cell lymphoma who have received at least one prior therapy
Class: Bruton's tyrosine kinase (BTK) inhibitor, Kinase inhibitor, Tyrosine kinase inhibitor
Half-life: ~2–4 hours
Clinically important, potentially hazardous interactions with: CYP3A inhibitors and CYP3A inducers
Pregnancy category: Can cause fetal harm. Advise women of the potential risk to a fetus and to avoid pregnancy.

Skin
Bruise / bruising / contusion / ecchymosis (ecchymoses) (14%) [2]
Rash (36%) [2]

Cardiovascular
Atrial fibrillation [2]
Hypertension (3% ≥ grade 3) (12%) [3]

Endocrine/Metabolic
ALT increased (1% grade 3 or 4) (28%)
Hyperbilirubinemia (1% grade 3 or 4) (24%)
Hyperuricemia (3% grade 3 or 4) (29%)
Hypokalemia (2% ≥ grade 3) (14%)

Gastrointestinal/Hepatic
Constipation (13%) [2]
Diarrhea (< 1%) (23%) [3]

Genitourinary
Urinary tract infection (< 1% ≥ grade 3) (11%)

Hematologic
Anemia (8% ≥ grade 3) (14%)
Hemoglobin decreased (6% grade 3 or 4) (27%)
Hemorrhage (3% ≥ grade 3) (11%) [2]
Leukocytopenia (leukopenia) / leukocytes (white blood cells) decreased (5% ≥ grade 3) (25%)
Lymphocytosis / lymphocytes increased (16% grade 3 or 4) (asymptomatic lymphocytosis is a known effect of BTK inhibition) (41%)
Neutropenia (neutrophils decreased) (15% ≥ grade 3) (38%) [4]
Thrombocytopenia / platelets decreased (7% grade 3 or 4) (27%) [2]

Neuromuscular/Skeletal
Musculoskeletal pain (3% ≥ grade 3) (14%)

Respiratory
Cough (12%)
Pneumonia (10% ≥ grade 3) (2 cases fatal) (15%) [3]
Upper respiratory tract infection (39%) [3]

Other
Death (8 cases (7%))

ZICONOTIDE

Trade name: Prialt (Jazz)
Indications: Analgesic, severe chronic pain
Class: Neuronal calcium channel blocker, Neuroprotectant
Half-life: 4.6 hours
Clinically important, potentially hazardous interactions with: CNS depressants
Important contra-indications noted in the prescribing guidelines for: the elderly; nursing mothers; pediatric patients
Note: Ziconotide is a synthetic analog of a substance isolated from the venom of carnivorous oceanic snails that sting their prey with a cocktail of neurotoxins injected through a harpoon-like tube. Ziconotide is 100 to 1,000 times more powerful than morphine.
Warning: NEUROPSYCHIATRIC ADVERSE REACTIONS

Skin
Bruise / bruising / contusion / ecchymosis (ecchymoses) (~2%)
Cellulitis and pseudocellulitis (~2%)
Diaphoresis (5%)
Edema / fluid retention (~2%)
Pruritus (itching) (7%)
Xerosis / xeroderma (~2%)

Mucosal
Xerostomia (dry mouth) (~2%)

Cardiovascular
Atrial fibrillation (~2%)
Chest pain (~2%)
Hypertension (~2%)
Hypotension (~2%)
Tachycardia (~2%)

Central Nervous System
Amnesia (8%)
Anorexia (6%)
Anxiety (8%)
Chills (~2%)
Confusion (15%) [8]
Depression (~2%) [2]
Dysarthria (7%)
Dysesthesia (7%)
Dysgeusia (taste perversion) (5%)
Fever (pyrexia) (includes hyperpyrexia) (5%)
Gait instability / postural instability [3]
Hallucinations [4]
Hallucinations, auditory [2]
Headache (13%)
Hyperesthesia (~2%)
Insomnia (6%)
Myokymia / twitching / fasciculation (~2%)
Pain (11%)
Paresthesias (7%)
Rigors (7%)
Seizures (<2%)
Somnolence (drowsiness) (17%) [4]
Suicidal ideation (<2%)
Tremor (7%)
Vertigo / dizziness (47%) [10]

Endocrine/Metabolic
Creatine phosphokinase (CPK) / creatine kinase increased (hyperCKemia) [2]

Gastrointestinal/Hepatic
Abdominal pain (~2%)
Diarrhea (18%)
Nausea (40%) [5]
Vomiting (16%) [3]

Genitourinary
Urinary retention (9%) [4]

Neuromuscular/Skeletal
Arthralgia (~2%)
Asthenia / fatigue (18%)
Ataxia (14%)
Back pain (~2%)
Muscle spasm (6%)
Myalgia/Myopathy (~2%)
Rhabdomyolysis (<2%)

Ocular
Diplopia (double vision) (~2%)
Nystagmus (8%) [3]
Periorbital edema (~2%)
Photophobia (~2%)
Vision blurred (12%) [2]
Visual disturbances (10%)

Otic
Tinnitus (~2%)

Respiratory
Influenza- ('flu)-like syndrome (~2%)
Sinusitis (see also rhinitis / rhinosinusitis) (5%)

Other
Adverse effects / adverse reactions [3]
Infection (~2%)

ZIDOVUDINE

Synonyms: azidothymidine; AZT
Trade names: Combivir (ViiV), Retrovir (ViiV), Trizivir (ViiV)
Indications: HIV infection
Class: Antiretroviral, Nucleoside analog reverse transcriptase inhibitor
Half-life: 0.5–3 hours
Clinically important, potentially hazardous interactions with: atovaquone, bone marrow suppressives, clarithromycin, darunavir, diclofenac, doxorubicin, fluconazole, ganciclovir, indinavir, interferon alfa, interferon beta, lopinavir, meloxicam, methadone, NSAIDs, PEG-interferon, phenytoin, probenecid, pyrimethamine, ribavirin, rifampin, rifapentine, stavudine, tipranavir, valproic acid
Important contra-indications noted in the prescribing guidelines for: the elderly; nursing mothers
Note: Combivir is zidovudine and lamivudine; Trizivir is zidovudine, abacavir and lamivudine.
Warning: HEMATOLOGICAL TOXICITY, MYOPATHY, LACTIC ACIDOSIS AND SEVERE HEPATOMEGALY, and EXACERBATIONS OF HEPATITIS B

Skin
Acneiform eruption / acneiform dermatitis / acneiform rash (<5%)
Bromhidrosis (<5%)
Diaphoresis (5–19%)
Edema of lip (<5%)
Erythema multiforme [2]
Exanthems (<5%) [6]
Lipoatrophy [2]
Lipodystrophy / acquired generalized lipodystrophy [2]
Pigmentation (Skin) (includes hyperpigmentation) [10]
Pruritus (itching) [4]
Rash (17%) [8]
Stevens-Johnson syndrome and toxic epidermal necrolysis (SJS/TEN) [6]
Urticaria / hives (<5%) [2]
Vasculitis (angiitis) / cutaneous vasculitis (angiitis) [2]

Hair
Alopecia / hair loss [2]
Hypertrichosis (eyelashes) [2]

Nails
Nail pigmentation [27]

Mucosal
Oral lichenoid eruption [2]
Oral pigmentation [8]
Oral ulceration (<5%)
Tongue edema (<5%)
Tongue pigmentation [4]

Central Nervous System
Dysgeusia (taste perversion) (5–19%) [2]
Headache [3]
Paresthesias (<8%)

Endocrine/Metabolic
Acidosis (includes lactic acidosis) [6]

Gastrointestinal/Hepatic
Abdominal pain [3]
Diarrhea [2]
Hepatotoxicity / liver injury / acute liver injury / drug-induced liver injury (DILI) [2]
Nausea [3]
Pancreatitis / acute pancreatitis [3]
Vomiting [2]

Hematologic
Anemia [15]
Neutropenia (neutrophils decreased) [3]

Neuromuscular/Skeletal
Asthenia / fatigue [3]
Myalgia/Myopathy [5]

Other
Adverse effects / adverse reactions [9]
Teratogenicity [2]

ZILEUTON

Trade name: Zyflo (AbbVie)
Indications: Asthma
Class: Leukotriene receptor antagonist
Half-life: 2.5 hours
Clinically important, potentially hazardous interactions with: anisindione, anticoagulants, astemizole, dicumarol, methylergonovine, pimozide, propranolol, warfarin
Important contra-indications noted in the prescribing guidelines for: nursing mothers; pediatric patients

---

Neuromuscular/Skeletal
Myalgia/Myopathy (3%)

ZINC

Trade name: Cold-Eeze (The Quigley Corp)
Indications: Supplement to intravenous solutions given for total parenteral nutrition (TPN)
Class: Food supplement, Trace element
Half-life: N/A
Clinically important, potentially hazardous interactions with: baloxavir marboxil, chlorothiazide, chlortetracycline, chlorthalidone, ciprofloxacin, cisplatin, deferoxamine, demeclocycline, doxycycline, eltrombopag, ethambutol, ferrous sulfate, gatifloxacin, gemifloxacin, hydrochlorothiazide, indapamide, levofloxacin, lymecycline, metolozone, minocycline, moxifloxacin, norfloxacin, ofloxacin, oxytetracycline, propofol, tetracycline, valproic acid
Note: Zinc is found in meats, seafood, dairy products, legumes, nuts, whole grains. Zinc oxide and zinc sulfate are used to fortify wheat products.

Skin
Churg-Strauss syndrome [2]
Dermatitis [4]

Mucosal
Oral mucosal irritation [2]

Central Nervous System
Anosmia (smell loss) / smell disorder [3]
Dysgeusia (taste perversion) [5]

Endocrine/Metabolic
Hypocupremia [2]

Hematologic
Pancytopenia (includes bicytopenia) [2]
Sideroblastic anemia / acquired sideroblastic anemia [2]

ZIPRASIDONE

Trade name: Geodon (Pfizer)
Indications: Schizophrenia, bipolar I disorder
Class: Antipsychotic, Antipsychotic, atypical
Half-life: 7 hours
Clinically important, potentially hazardous interactions with: acetylcholinesterase inhibitors, alcohol, alfuzosin, amitriptyline, amoxapine, amphetamines, antifungals, arsenic, artemether/lumefantrine, asenapine, astemizole, carbamazepine, chloroquine, ciprofloxacin, citalopram, CNS depressants, conivaptan, dasatinib, degarelix, dolasetron, dopamine agonists, dopamine agonists, dronedarone, food, gadobutrol, ketoconazole, lapatinib, levodopa, levofloxacin, lithium, methylphenidate, metoclopramide, moxifloxacin, nilotinib, pazopanib, pimavanserin, pimozide, QT prolonging agents, quinagolide, quinine, ranolazine, St John's wort, telavancin, telithromycin, tetrabenazine, thioridazine, voriconazole, vorinostat
Important contra-indications noted in the prescribing guidelines for: the elderly; nursing mothers; pediatric patients
Note: Ziprasidone should be avoided in patients with congenital long QT syndrome or a history of cardiac arrhythmias.
Warning: INCREASED MORTALITY IN ELDERLY PATIENTS WITH DEMENTIA-RELATED PSYCHOSIS

Skin
Angioedema (formerly named angioneurotic edema) [2]
Diaphoresis (2%)
DRESS syndrome (Drug-induced hypersensitivity syndrome) [2]
Fungal dermatitis (2%)
Furunculosis (2%)
Lupus erythematosus (subacute cutaneous lupus erythematosus (SCLE)) [2]
Rash (4%)
Urticaria / hives (5%)

Mucosal
Rectal hemorrhage / rectal bleeding (2%)
Sialorrhea (ptyalism; hypersalivation) (4%)
Tongue edema (3%)
Xerostomia (dry mouth) (<5%)

Cardiovascular
Bradycardia / sinus bradycardia (2%)
Chest pain (3%)
Hypertension (2–3%)
Postural hypotension (5%)
QT interval prolonged / QT prolongation [22]
Tachycardia (2%) [2]
Torsades de pointes [6]

Central Nervous System
Agitation (2%) [3]
Akathisia (2–10%) [5]
Anorexia (2%)
Anxiety (2–5%) [2]
Depression [2]
Dyskinesia (<10%) [2]
Extrapyramidal symptoms (2–31%) [6]
Headache (3–18%) [3]
Hyperesthesia (<2%)
Hypokinesia (<5%)
Insomnia (3%) [5]
Mania [2]
Myokymia / twitching / fasciculation (<10%)
Neuroleptic malignant syndrome [10]
Paralysis / paraplegia (<10%)
Paresthesias (<2%)
Sedation [4]
Somnolence (drowsiness) (8–31%) [12]
Speech disorder (2%)
Tardive syndrome / tardive dyskinesia [5]
Tremor (<10%) [2]
Vertigo / dizziness (3–16%) [2]

Endocrine/Metabolic
Diabetes mellitus [2]
Galactorrhea [3]
Weight gain [7]

Gastrointestinal/Hepatic
Abdominal pain (<2%)
Constipation (2–9%)
Diarrhea (3–5%)
Dyspepsia / functional dyspepsia (indigestion) (see also gastroparesis) (<8%)
Dysphagia (2%)
Nausea (4–12%) [4]
Vomiting (3–5%)

Genitourinary
Dysmenorrhea (2%)
Priapism [4]

Local
Infusion-site pain (7–9%)

Neuromuscular/Skeletal
Asthenia / fatigue (2–6%) [4]
Dystonia (<10%) [6]
Hypertonia (<10%)
Myalgia/Myopathy (2%)
Rhabdomyolysis [2]

Ocular
Abnormal vision (3–6%)
Oculogyric crisis / oculogyric dystonic reaction [3]

Respiratory
Cough (increased) (3%)
Dyspnea / shortness of breath (2%)
Pharyngitis (sore throat) (3%)
Respiratory tract infection (8%)
Rhinitis / rhinosinusitis (see also sinusitis) (<4%)
Upper respiratory tract infection (8%)

Other
Adverse effects / adverse reactions [8]
Death [2]

ZOFENOPRIL

Trade names: Bifril (Menarini), Zantipres (Menarini), Zofenil (Menarini), Zofepril (Menarini), Zofil (Menarini), Zopranol (Menarini)
Indications: Hypertension, myocardial infarction
Class: Angiotensin-converting enzyme (ACE) inhibitor, Antihypertensive
Half-life: 5.5 hours
Clinically important, potentially hazardous interactions with: allopurinol, amiloride, cimetidine, corticosteroids, cyclosporine, insulin, lithium, potassium sparing diuretics, potassium supplements, procainamide, spironolactone, triamterene
Pregnancy category: not recommended in pregnancy
Important contra-indications noted in the prescribing guidelines for: pediatric patients

---

Cardiovascular
Hypotension [5]

Central Nervous System
Headache [2]
Vertigo / dizziness [2]

Genitourinary
Polyuria (includes polyuric syndrome) [2]

Neuromuscular/Skeletal
Asthenia / fatigue (3%)

Respiratory
Cough [5]

Other
Adverse effects / adverse reactions [3]

ZOLEDRONATE

Synonym: zoledronic acid
Trade names: Aclasta (Novartis), Reclast (Novartis), Zometa (Novartis)
Indications: Hypercalcemia of malignancy, Paget's disease, osteoporosis
Class: Bisphosphonate
Half-life: 7 days
Clinically important, potentially hazardous interactions with: aminoglycosides, bisphosphonates, loop diuretics, nephrotoxics
Important contra-indications noted in the prescribing guidelines for: the elderly; nursing mothers; pediatric patients

---

Skin
Baboon syndrome / symmetrical drug-related intertriginous and flexural exanthema (SDRIFE) [2]
Candidiasis / candidosis (12%)
Dermatitis (11%)
Dermatomyositis [3]
Edema / fluid retention [3]
Peripheral edema (5–21%)
Rash [3]

Hair
Alopecia / hair loss (12%)

Mucosal
Mucositis (5–10%)
Stomatitis (oral mucositis) (8%)

Cardiovascular
Atrial fibrillation [3]
Chest pain (5–10%)
Hypotension (11%)

Central Nervous System
Agitation (13%)
Anorexia (9–22%)
Anxiety (11–14%)
Chills [2]
Confusion (7–13%)
Depression (14%)
Fever (pyrexia) (includes hyperpyrexia) (32–44%) [20]
Headache (5–19%) [4]
Hypoesthesia / hypesthesia (numbness) (12%)
Insomnia (15–16%)
Paresthesias (15%)
Rigors (11%)
Seizures [2]
Somnolence (drowsiness) (5–10%)
Vertigo / dizziness (18%)

Endocrine/Metabolic
Appetite decreased (13%)
Creatine phosphokinase (CPK) / creatine kinase increased (hyperCKemia) [2]
Dehydration (5–14%)
Hyperparathyroidism [2]
Hypocalcemia (5–10%) [29]
Hypokalemia (12%)
Hypomagnesemia (11%)
Hypophosphatemia (13%) [6]
Weight loss (16%)

Gastrointestinal/Hepatic
Abdominal pain (14–16%)
Constipation (27–31%) [3]
Diarrhea (17–24%) [2]
Dyspepsia / functional dyspepsia (indigestion) (see also gastroparesis) (10%)
Dysphagia (5–10%)
Hepatotoxicity / liver injury / acute liver injury / drug-induced liver injury (DILI) [7]
Nausea (29–46%) [12]
Vomiting (14–32%) [2]

Genitourinary
Urinary tract infection (12–14%)

Hematologic
Acute-phase reaction [7]
Anemia (22–33%) [8]
Granulocytopenia (5–10%)
Neutropenia (neutrophils decreased) (12%)
Pancytopenia (includes bicytopenia) (5–10%)
Sepsis [2]
Thrombocytopenia / platelets decreased (5–10%)

Neuromuscular/Skeletal
Arthralgia (5–10%) [9]
Asthenia / fatigue (5–39%) [11]
Back pain (15%)
Bone pain / joint pain (12–55%) [15]
Fractures [4]
Myalgia/Myopathy (23%) [7]
Osteonecrosis / avascular necrosis (includes steroid-induced osteonecrosis of the femoral head) [56]
Pain in extremities (14%)

Ocular
Ocular adverse effect [2]
Ocular inflammation [3]
Scleritis [2]
Uveitis / anterior uveitis / posterior uveitis / panuveitis [14]

Renal
Fanconi syndrome (proximal tubular dysfunction) [2]

Nephrotoxicity / kidney injury / acute kidney injury (AKI) / drug-induced kidney injury [15]
Renal failure [4]
Renal function abnormal / renal dysfunction [2]

Respiratory
Cough (12–22%)
Dyspnea / shortness of breath (22–27%)
Influenza- ('flu)-like syndrome [9]
Pharyngolaryngeal pain (8%)
Upper respiratory tract infection (10%)

Other
Adverse effects / adverse reactions [7]
Infection (5–10%)
Neoplasms (malignant / aggrevated) (20%)
Systemic inflammatory response syndrome (SIRS) [2]

ZOLMITRIPTAN

Trade name: Zomig (AstraZeneca)
Indications: Migraine attacks
Class: 5-HT1 agonist, Serotonin receptor agonist, Triptan
Half-life: 3 hours
Clinically important, potentially hazardous interactions with: cimetidine, ciprofloxacin, dihydroergotamine, ergot-containing drugs, fluoxetine, fluvoxamine, isocarboxazid, levofloxacin, MAO inhibitors, methysergide, moclobemide, moxifloxacin, naratriptan, norfloxacin, ofloxacin, oral contraceptives, phenelzine, propranolol, rizatriptan, sertraline, sibutramine, SNRIs, SSRIs, St John's wort, sumatriptan, tranylcypromine
Important contra-indications noted in the prescribing guidelines for: nursing mothers; pediatric patients

---

Skin
Diaphoresis (2–3%)
Hot flashes / hot flushes (>10%)

Mucosal
Xerostomia (dry mouth) (3–5%)

Cardiovascular
Chest pain (2–4%)
Myocardial infarction [4]

Central Nervous System
Dysgeusia (taste perversion) [4]
Headache [2]
Neurotoxicity [2]
Paresthesias (5–9%) [6]
Somnolence (drowsiness) (5–8%)
Vertigo / dizziness (2–10%) [3]
Warm feeling (includes feeling hot) (5–7%)

Gastrointestinal/Hepatic
Dyspepsia / functional dyspepsia (indigestion) (see also gastroparesis) (<3%)
Dysphagia (<2%)
Nausea (4–9%) [2]

Neuromuscular/Skeletal
Jaw pain (4–10%)
Myalgia/Myopathy (2%) [2]
Neck pain (4–10%)

Renal
Nephrotoxicity / kidney injury / acute kidney injury (AKI) / drug-induced kidney injury [2]

Other
Adverse effects / adverse reactions [6]

ZOLPIDEM

Trade name: Ambien (Sanofi-Aventis)
Indications: Insomnia
Class: Hypnotic, non-benzodiazepine
Half-life: 2.6 hours
Clinically important, potentially hazardous interactions with: alcohol, antihistamines, azatadine, azelastine, brompheniramine, buclizine, chlorpheniramine, chlorpromazine, cimetidine, clemastine, cobicistat/elvitegravir/emtricitabine/tenofovir alafenamide, cobicistat/elvitegravir/emtricitabine/tenofovir disoproxil, dexchlorpheniramine, erythromycin, imipramine, ketoconazole, meclizine, pizotifen, ramelteon, rifampin, rifapentine, ritonavir, telaprevir, voriconazole
Important contra-indications noted in the prescribing guidelines for: nursing mothers; pediatric patients

---

Skin
Rash (2%)

Mucosal
Xerostomia (dry mouth) (3%) [3]

Cardiovascular
Palpitation (2%)
Tachycardia [2]
Torsades de pointes [2]

Central Nervous System
Amnesia [16]
Anxiety [2]
Compulsions / obsessive-compulsive symptoms / obsessive-compulsive disorder [2]
Confusion [3]
Delirium [5]
Depression (2%)
Dysgeusia (taste perversion) [4]
Euphoria / elation [2]
Gait instability / postural instability [3]
Hallucinations [13]
Hallucinations, visual [9]
Headache (7%) [11]
Mania [2]
Nightmares [2]
Seizures [7]
Sleep-related disorder [20]
Sleep-related eating disorder (SRED) [4]
Slurred speech [2]
Somnambulism (sleepwalking; noctambulism) [17]
Somnolence (drowsiness) (2–8%) [11]
Vertigo / dizziness (<5%) [12]

Gastrointestinal/Hepatic
Abdominal pain (2%)
Constipation (2%)
Diarrhea (<3%)
Hepatotoxicity / liver injury / acute liver injury / drug-induced liver injury (DILI) [2]
Nausea [5]
Vomiting [2]

Neuromuscular/Skeletal
Asthenia / fatigue (3%) [4]
Ataxia [3]
Back pain (3%)
Fractures [2]
Myalgia/Myopathy (7%)

Respiratory
Influenza- ('flu)-like syndrome (2%)
Pharyngitis (sore throat) (3%)
Sinusitis (see also rhinitis / rhinosinusitis) (4%)

Other
Adverse effects / adverse reactions [8]
Allergic reactions (4%)

ZONISAMIDE

Trade name: Zonegran (Concordia)
Indications: Epilepsy
Class: Anticonvulsant (see also antiepileptic (anti-seizure)), Antiepileptic; sulfonamide
Half-life: 63 hours
Clinically important, potentially hazardous interactions with: caffeine, metformin
Important contra-indications noted in the prescribing guidelines for: nursing mothers; pediatric patients
Note: Zonisamide is a sulfonamide and can be absorbed systemically. Sulfonamides can produce severe, possibly fatal, reactions such as toxic epidermal necrolysis and Stevens-Johnson syndrome.

Skin
Bruise / bruising / contusion / ecchymosis (ecchymoses) (2%)
DRESS syndrome (Drug-induced hypersensitivity syndrome) [5]
Hypersensitivity [4]
Oligohydrosis (reduced sweating) [8]
Purpura (2%)
Rash (3%) [6]
Stevens-Johnson syndrome and toxic epidermal necrolysis (SJS/TEN) [9]

Mucosal
Xerostomia (dry mouth) (2%)

Central Nervous System
Agitation (9%) [4]
Anorexia (13%) [10]
Anxiety (3%)
Cognitive impairment (6%) [4]
Confusion (6%)
Depression (6%) [4]
Dysgeusia (taste perversion) (2%)
Fever (pyrexia) (includes hyperpyrexia) [2]
Headache (10%) [8]
Insomnia (6%)
Irritability (9%) [4]
Mania [2]
Nervousness (2%)
Neuroleptic malignant syndrome [2]
Paresthesias (4%)
Psychosis [3]
Restless legs syndrome / Willis-Ekbom disease (includes restless arms syndrome variant) [3]
Schizophrenia (2%)
Somnolence (drowsiness) (17%) [22]
Speech disorder (2–5%)
Suicidal ideation [2]
Vertigo / dizziness (13%) [19]

Endocrine/Metabolic
Appetite decreased [8]
Weight loss (3%) [20]

Gastrointestinal/Hepatic
Abdominal pain (6%)
Constipation (2%)
Diarrhea (5%)
Dyspepsia / functional dyspepsia (indigestion) (see also gastroparesis) (3%)
Nausea (9%) [2]

Vanishing bile duct syndrome / ductopenia [2]
Vomiting [2]

Neuromuscular/Skeletal
Asthenia / fatigue (7–8%) [9]
Ataxia (6%) [3]

Ocular
Ciliochoroidal effusion / uveal effusion (includes ciliary body effusion) [2]
Diplopia (double vision) (6%) [2]
Nystagmus (4%)

Renal
Nephrolithiasis (kidney stones / renal calculi) [4]
Nephrotoxicity / kidney injury / acute kidney injury (AKI) / drug-induced kidney injury [2]

Respiratory
Influenza- ('flu)-like syndrome (4%)
Pneumonitis [2]
Rhinitis / rhinosinusitis (see also sinusitis) (2%)

Other
Adverse effects / adverse reactions [12]
Side effects [4]
Teratogenicity [2]

ZOTAROLIMUS

Trade names: Endeavor (Medtronic), ZoMaxx Drug-Eluting Coronary Stent (AbbVie)
Indications: Ischemic heart disease, restenosis
Class: Angiogenesis inhibitor / antiangiogenic agent, Macrolide immunosuppressant (derivative of sirolimus), mTOR inhibitor
Half-life: 33–36 hours
Clinically important, potentially hazardous interactions with: ketoconazole, sirolimus
Important contra-indications noted in the prescribing guidelines for: nursing mothers; pediatric patients

---

Skin
Rash (<6%)
Xerosis / xeroderma (<13%)

Cardiovascular
Cardiotoxicity [4]
Myocardial infarction [3]
Subacute thrombosis [2]

Central Nervous System
Headache (4–13%)
Pain (13–63%)

Gastrointestinal/Hepatic
Abdominal pain (<6%)
Diarrhea (<6%)

Genitourinary
Hematuria (<13%)

Local
Application-site reactions (13–63%)
Injection-site reaction (13–38%)

ZUCLOPENTHIXOL

Trade name: Clopixol (Lundbeck)
Indications: Psychoses, especially schizophrenia
Class: Antipsychotic
Half-life: 24 hours
Clinically important, potentially hazardous interactions with: ACE inhibitors, alcohol, alpha blockers, amantadine, amiodarone, angiotensin II receptor antagonists, antiarrythmics, anticholinergics, antihistamines, antipsychotics, anxiolytics and hypnotics, apomorphine, arsenic, artemether/lumefantrine, atomoxetine, atropine sulfate, barbiturates, bromocriptine, cabergoline, calcium channel blockers, carbamazepine, cisapride, clozapine, CNS depressants, corticosteroids, digoxin, disopyramide, dofetilide, doxazosin, efavirenz, erythromycin, ethosuximide, general anesthetics, guanethidine, histamine, hydralazine, levodopa, lithium, memantine, methadone, methyldopa, metoclopramide, moxifloxacin, opioid analgesics, oxcarbazepine, pergolide, phenytoin, piperazine, pramipexole, primidone, quinidine, ritonavir, ropinirole, rotigotine, sibutramine, sodium oxybate, sotalol, synpathomimetics, tetrabenazine, thiazide diuretics, thioridazine, tramadol, tricyclic antidepressants, valproic acid
Important contra-indications noted in the prescribing guidelines for: the elderly; pediatric patients

---

Skin
Hyperhidrosis (3%)
Pruritus (itching) (2%)
Seborrhea (2%)

Mucosal
Salivary hypersecretion (8%)
Xerostomia (dry mouth) (15%)

Central Nervous System
Anxiety (17%)
Depression (8%)
Extrapyramidal symptoms [2]
Headache (5%)
Hypokinesia (8%)
Insomnia (16%)
Neuroleptic malignant syndrome [4]
Somnolence (drowsiness) (32%)
Tremor (19%)
Vertigo / dizziness (11%)

Endocrine/Metabolic
Libido decreased (3%)

Gastrointestinal/Hepatic
Nausea (2%)
Vomiting (3%)

Genitourinary
Priapism [4]

Neuromuscular/Skeletal
Hypertonia (19%)

Ocular
Abnormal vision (4%)
Accommodation disorder (6%)

Other
Death [2]
Side effects [2]

ZUCLOPENTHIXOL DECANOATE

Trade name: Clopixol Depot (Lundbeck)
Indications: Schizophrenia
Class: Antipsychotic
Half-life: 19 days
Clinically important, potentially hazardous interactions with: guanethidine, levodopa, piperazine
Important contra-indications noted in the prescribing guidelines for: nursing mothers; pediatric patients

---

Central Nervous System
Neuroleptic malignant syndrome [3]

Genitourinary
Priapism [3]

Descriptions of Important Reactions

Acanthosis nigricans

Acanthosis nigricans (AN) is a process characterized by a soft, velvety, brown or grayish-black thickening of the skin that is symmetrically distributed over the axillae, neck, inguinal areas and other body folds.

While most cases of AN are seen in obese and prepubertal children, it can occur as a marker for various endocrinopathies as well as in female patients with elevated testosterone levels, irregular menses, and hirsutism. It is frequently a concomitant of an underlying malignant condition, principally an adenocarcinoma of the intestinal tract.

Acneiform eruption / acneiform dermatitis / acneiform rash

Acneiform eruptions are inflammatory follicular reactions that resemble acne vulgaris and that are manifested clinically as papules or pustules. They are monomorphic reactions, have a monomorphic appearance, and are found primarily on the upper parts of the body. Unlike acne vulgaris, there are rarely comedones present. Consider a drug-induced acneiform eruption if:

- The onset is sudden
- There is a worsening of existing acne lesions
- The extent is considerable from the outset
- The appearance is monomorphic
- The localization is unusual for acne as, for example, when the distal extremities are involved
- The patient's age is unusual for regular acne
- There is an exposure to a potentially responsible drug.

Acute febrile neutrophilic dermatosis (Sweet's / Sweet syndrome)

Acute febrile neutrophilic dermatosis is a disorder that appears more frequently in females and has several characteristic features. The lesions – tender, erythematous or purple, annular plaques or nodules – appear suddenly and are most prominent on the face, neck and upper extremities. Pain and fever often accompany the eruption. While the cause is unknown, about 15% of the patients have some type of myeloproliferative disorder, primarily leukemias.

Acute generalized exanthematous pustulosis (AGEP)

Arising on the face or intertriginous areas, acute generalized exanthematous pustulosis (AGEP) is characterized by a rapidly evolving, widespread, scarlatiniform eruption covered with hundreds of small superficial pustules.

Often accompanied by a high fever, AGEP usually occurs within 24 hours of the drug exposure.

Ageusia (taste loss) / taste disorder

Ageusia is the loss of taste functions of the tongue, essentially the inability to detect sweet, sour, bitter, or salty substances, and umami (the taste of monosodium glutamate).

Alopecia / hair loss

Many drugs have been reported to occasion hair loss. More commonly appearing as a diffuse alopecia, it affects women more frequently than men and is limited in most instances to the scalp. Axillary and pubic hairs are rarely affected except with anticoagulants.

The hair loss from cytostatic agents, which is dose-dependent and begins about 2 weeks after the onset of therapy, is a result of the interruption of the anagen (growing) cycle of hair. With other drugs the hair loss does not begin until 2–5 months after the medication has been begun. With cholesterol-lowering drugs, diffuse alopecia is a result of interference with normal keratinization.

The scalp is normal and the drug-induced alopecia is almost always reversible within 1–3 months after the therapy has been discontinued. The regrown hair is frequently depigmented and occasionally more curly.

Angioedema

Angioedema is a term applied to a variant of urticaria in which the subcutaneous tissues, rather than the dermis, are mainly involved. Also known as Quincke's edema, giant urticaria, and angioneurotic edema, this acute, evanescent, skin-colored, circumscribed edema usually affects the most distensible tissues: the lips, eyelids, earlobes, and genitalia. It can also affect the mucous membranes of the tongue, mouth, and larynx.

Symptoms of angioedema, frequently unilateral, asymmetrical and nonpruritic, last for an hour or two but can persist for 2–5 days.

Anosmia (smell loss) / smell disorder

Anosmia, or odor blindness, is the total absence of the sense of smell. It can be either temporary or permanent.

Aphthous stomatitis / aphthous ulcer / aphtha (aphthae)

Aphthous stomatitis – also known as canker sores – is a frequent disease of the oral mucous membranes. Arising as tiny, discrete or grouped, papules or vesicles, these painful lesions develop into small (2–5 mm in diameter), round, shallow ulcerations having a grayish, yellow base surrounded by a thin red border.

Located predominantly over the labial and buccal mucosae, these aphthae heal without scarring in 10–14 days. Recurrences are common.

Baboon syndrome / symmetrical drug-related intertriginous and flexural exanthema (SDRIFE)

Baboon syndrome or symmetric drug-related intertriginous and flexural exanthema (SDRIFE) is an unusual presentation of a drug eruption with a characteristic intertriginous distribution pattern.

Originally described as a type of systemic contact dermatitis characterized by pruritic exanthems involving the buttocks and major flexures (groins and axillae), some investigators believe that this entity is a form of recall phenomenon. In children, it is important in the differential diagnosis of viral exanthems.

Black tongue / black hairy tongue (lingua villosa nigra)

Black hairy tongue (BHT) represents a benign hyperplasia of the filiform papillae of the anterior two-thirds of the tongue. These papillary elongations, usually associated with black, brown, or yellow pigmentation attributed to the overgrowth of pigment-producing bacteria, may be as long as 2 cm.

Occurring only in adults, BHT has been associated with the administration of oral antibiotics, poor dental hygiene, and excessive smoking.

Bullous dermatosis

Bullous and vesicular drug eruptions are diseases in which blisters and vesicles occur as a complication of the administration of drugs. Blisters are a well-known manifestation of cutaneous reactions to drugs.

In many types of drug reactions, bullae and vesicles may be found in addition to other manifestations. Bullae are usually noted in: erythema multiforme, Stevens-Johnson syndrome/toxic epidermal necrolysis, fixed eruptions when very intense, urticaria, vasculitis, porphyria cutanea tarda, and phototoxic reactions (from furosemide and nalidixic acid). Tense, thick-walled bullae can be seen in bromoderma and iododerma as well as in barbiturate overdosage.

DRESS syndrome

DRESS syndrome is an acronym for Drug Rash with Eosinophilia and Systemic Symptoms. This syndrome also includes 'drug-induced

DOI: 10.1201/9781003715672-1499

pseudolymphoma', 'drug-induced hypersensitivity syndrome' (DIHS), and 'anticonvulsant hypersensitivity syndrome'. The characteristic features are fever, rash, and lymphadenopathy, which are accompanied by multiorgan-system abnormalities. Fatal outcomes are most often associated with liver failure.

The symptoms of DRESS syndrome usually begin 1–8 weeks after exposure to the offending drug.

Erythema multiforme

Erythema multiforme is a relatively common, acute, self-limited, inflammatory reaction pattern that is often associated with a preceding herpes simplex or mycoplasma infection. Other causes are associated with connective tissue disease, physical agents, X-ray therapy, pregnancy and internal malignancies, to mention a few. In 50% of the cases, no cause can be found. In a recent prospective study of erythema multiforme, only 10% were drug related.

The eruption rapidly occurs over a period of 12–24 hours. In about half the cases there are prodromal symptoms of an upper respiratory infection accompanied by fever, malaise, and varying degrees of muscular and joint pains.

Clinically, bluish-red, well-demarcated, macular, papular, or urticarial lesions, as well as the classical 'iris' or 'target lesions', sometimes with central vesicles, bullae, or purpura, are distributed preferentially over the distal extremities, especially over the dorsa of the hands and extensor aspects of the forearms. Lesions tend to spread peripherally and may involve the palms and trunk as well as the mucous membranes of the mouth and genitalia. Central healing and overlapping lesions often lead to arciform, annular and gyrate patterns. Lesions appear over the course of a week or 10 days and resolve over the next two weeks.

Erythema nodosum

Erythema nodosum is a cutaneous reaction pattern characterized by erythematous, tender or painful subcutaneous nodules frequently distributed over the anterior aspect of the lower legs, and occasionally elsewhere. More common in young women, erythema nodosum is often associated with increased estrogen levels as occurs during pregnancy and with the ingestion of oral contraceptives. It is also an occasional manifestation of streptococcal infection, sarcoidosis, secondary syphilis, tuberculosis, certain deep fungal infections, Hodgkin's disease, inflammatory bowel disease, leukemia, and radiation therapy and is often preceded by fever, fatigue, arthralgia, vomiting, and diarrhea.

The incidence of erythema nodosum due to drugs is low and it is impossible to distinguish clinically between erythema nodosum due to drugs and that caused by other factors.

Exanthems

Exanthems, often resembling viral rashes, represent the most frequent type of cutaneous drug eruption. Described as maculopapular or morbilliform eruptions, these flat, barely raised, erythematous patches, from one to several millimeters in diameter, are usually bilateral and symmetrical. They usually begin on the head and neck or upper torso and progress downward to the limbs. They may present or develop into confluent areas and may be accompanied by pruritus and a mild fever.

The exanthems caused by drugs can be classified as:

- Morbilliform eruptions: fingernail-sized erythematous patches
- Scarlatiniform eruptions: punctate, pinpoint, or pinhead-sized lesions in erythematous areas that have a tendency to coalesce. Circumoral pallor and the subsequent appearance of scaling may also be noted.

Maculopapular drug eruptions usually fade with desquamation and, occasionally, postinflammatory hyperpigmentation, in about 2 weeks. They invariably recur on rechallenge.

Exanthems often have a sudden onset during the first 2 weeks of administration, except in cases of semisynthetic penicillin administration, when the exanthems frequently develop after the first 2 weeks following the initial dose.

Exfoliative dermatitis

Exfoliative dermatitis is a rare but serious reaction pattern that is characterized by erythema, pruritus and scaling over the entire body (erythroderma).

Drug-induced exfoliative dermatitis usually begins a few weeks or longer following the administration of a culpable drug. Beginning as erythematous, edematous patches, often on the face, it spreads to involve the entire integument. The skin becomes swollen and scarlet and may ooze a straw-colored fluid; this is followed in a few days by desquamation. High fever, severe malaise and chills, along with enlargement of lymph nodes, often coexist with the cutaneous changes.

One of the most dangerous of all reaction patterns, exfoliative dermatitis can be accompanied by any or all of the following: hypothermia, fluid and electrolyte loss, cardiac failure, and gastrointestinal hemorrhage. Death may supervene if the drug is continued after the onset of the eruption.

Secondary infection often complicates the course of the disease. Once the active dermatitis has receded, hyperpigmentation as well as loss of hair and nails may ensue.

Fixed eruption

A fixed eruption is an unusual hypersensitivity reaction characterized by one or more well-demarcated erythematous plaques that recur at the same cutaneous (or mucosal) site or sites each time exposure to the offending agent occurs. The sizes of the lesions vary from a few millimeters to as much as 20 centimeters in diameter. Almost any drug that is ingested, injected, inhaled, or inserted into the body can trigger this skin reaction.

The eruption typically begins as a sharply marginated, solitary edematous papule or plaque – occasionally surmounted by a large bulla – which usually develops 30 minutes to 8 hours following the administration of a drug. If the offending agent is not promptly eliminated, the inflammation intensifies, producing a dusky red, violaceous or brown patch that may crust, desquamate, or blister within 7–10 days. The lesions are rarely pruritic. Favored sites are the hands, feet, face, and genitalia (especially the glans penis).

The reason for the specific localization of the skin lesions in a fixed drug eruption is unknown. The offending drug cannot be detected at the skin site. Certain drugs cause a fixed eruption at specific sites, for example, tetracycline and ampicillin often elicit a fixed eruption on the penis, whereas aspirin usually causes skin lesions on the face, limbs and trunk.

Gingival hyperplasia / gingival hypertrophy / gingival enlargement / gingival overgrowth

Gingival hyperplasia, a frequent, undesirable, non-allergic drug reaction, begins as a diffuse swelling of the interdental papillae.

Particularly prevalent with phenytoin therapy, gingival hyperplasia begins about 3 months after the onset of therapy and occurs in 30–70% of patients receiving it. The severity of the reaction is dose-dependent and children and young adults are more frequently affected. The most severe cases are noted in young women.

In many cases, gingival hyperplasia is accompanied by painful and bleeding gums. There is often superimposed secondary bacterial gingivitis. This can be so extensive that the teeth of the maxilla and mandible are completely overgrown.

Hand-foot syndrome (palmar-plantar erythrodysesthesia)

Hand-foot syndrome (also known as acral erythema, palmar-plantar erythrodysesthesia, palmoplantar erythrodysesthesia, palmar-plantar erythema, and Bergdorf's reaction) is a syndrome that is characterized by well-demarcated painful erythema, edema, numbness, and desquamation over the palms and soles that may develop following treatment with a variety of chemotherapeutic agents including bleomycin, cisplatin, cyclophosphamide, hydroxyurea, idarubicin, methotrexate, sorafenib, sunitinib, and others. Tenderness involving the skin overlying the fingers and toes, followed by bulla formation and subsequent desquamation, often supervenes.

This side effect results when a small amount of the culpable drug leaks out of the blood vessels, damaging tissues. This reaction predominates over the palms and soles, where eccrine glands are more numerous, and also as a result of the increased friction and heat that extremities are exposed to through daily activities.

Lichenoid eruption / lichenoid reaction

Lichenoid eruptions are so called because of their resemblance to lichen planus, a papulosquamous disorder that characteristically presents as multiple, discrete, violaceous, flat-topped papules, often polygonal in shape and which are extremely pruritic.

Not infrequently, lichenoid lesions appear weeks or months following exposure to the responsible drug. As a rule, the symptoms begin to recede a few weeks following the discontinuation of the drug.

Lupus erythematosus (subacute cutaneous lupus erythematosus (SCLE)

A reaction, clinically and pathologically resembling idiopathic systemic lupus erythematosus (SLE), has been reported in association with a large variety of drugs. There is some evidence that drug-induced SLE, invariably accompanied by a positive ANA reaction with 90% having antihistone antibodies, may have a genetically determined basis. These symptoms of SLE, a relatively benign form of lupus, recede within days or weeks following the discontinuation of the responsible drug. Skin lesions occur in about 20% of cases. Drugs cause fewer than 8% of all cases of SLE.

Onycholysis

Onycholysis, the painless separation of the nail plate from the nail bed, is one of the most frequent nail disorders. The unattached portion, which is white and opaque, usually begins at the free margin and proceeds proximally, causing part or most of the nail plate to become separated. The attached, healthy portion of the nail, by contrast, is pink and translucent.

Paresthesias

Paresthesias are abnormal neurological sensations such as burning, prickling, numbness, pruritus, formication, or tingling, often described as 'pins and needles' or of a limb being 'asleep'. It is a symptom of partial damage to a peripheral nerve, as occurs from a head or spinal injury, lack of blood supply to a nerve, or in many cases medications. Paresthesias can affect various parts of the body; hands, fingers, and feet are frequent sites but all areas are possibilities.

Pemphigus vulgaris

Pemphigus vulgaris (PV) is a rare, serious, acute or chronic, blistering disease involving the skin and mucous membranes. Characterized by thin-walled, easily ruptured, flaccid bullae that are seen to arise on normal or erythematous skin and over mucous membranes, the lesions of PV appear initially in the mouth (in about 60% of the cases) and then spread, after weeks or months, to involve the axillae and groin, scalp, face, and neck. The lesions may become generalized. Because of their fragile roofs, the bullae rupture, leaving painful erosions, and crusts may develop principally over the scalp.

Peyronie's disease

First described in 1743 by the French surgeon, François de la Peyronie, Peyronie's disease is a rare, benign connective tissue disorder involving the growth of fibrous plaques in the soft tissue of the penis. Beginning as a localized inflammation, it often develops into a hardened scar. Affecting as many as 1% of men, it may cause deformity, pain, cord-like lesions, or abnormal curvature of the penis when erect.

Photosensitivity

A photosensitive reaction is a chemically induced change in the skin that makes an individual unusually sensitive to electromagnetic radiation (light). On absorbing light of a specific wavelength, an oral, injected or topical drug may be chemically altered to produce a reaction ranging from macules and papules, vesicles and bullae, edema, urticaria, or an acute eczematous reaction. Any eruption that is prominent on the face, the dorsa of the hands, the 'V' of the neck, and the presternal area should suggest an adverse reaction to light. The distribution is the key to the diagnosis. Initially the eruption, which consists of erythema, edema, blisters, weeping and desquamation, involves the forehead, rims of the ears, the nose, the malar eminences and cheeks, the sides and back of the neck, the extensor surfaces of the forearms and the dorsa of the hands. These reactions frequently spare the shaded areas: those under the chin, under the nose, behind the ears, and inside the fold of the upper eyelids. There is usually a sharp cut-off at the site of jewelry and at clothing margins. All light-exposed areas need not be affected equally.

There are two main types of photosensitive reactions: the phototoxic and the photoallergic reaction. Phototoxic reactions, the most frequent type of drug-induced photosensitivity, resemble an exaggerated sunburn and occur within 5–20 hours after the skin has been exposed to a photosensitizing substance and light of the proper wavelength and intensity. It is not a form of allergy – prior sensitization is not required – and, theoretically, could occur in anyone given enough drug and light. Phototoxic reactions are dose-dependent both for drug and sunlight. Patients with phototoxicity reactions are frequently sensitive to ultraviolet A (UVA radiation), the so-called 'tanning rays' at 320–400 nm. Phototoxic reactions may cause onycholysis, as the nailbed is particularly susceptible because of its lack of melanin protection. Patients with a true photoallergy (the interaction of drug, light and the immune system), a less frequent form of drug-induced photosensitivity, are often sensitive to UVB radiation, the so-called 'burning rays' at 290–320 nm. Photoallergic reactions, unlike phototoxic responses, represent an immunologic change and require a latent period of from 24 to 48 hours during which sensitization occurs. They are not dose-related. If the photosensitizer acts internally, it is a photodrug reaction; if it acts externally, it is photocontact dermatitis.

Pigmentation

Drug-induced pigmentation on the skin, hair, nails, and mucous membranes is a result of either melanin synthesis, increased lipofuscin synthesis, or post-inflammatory pigmentation. Color changes, which can be localized or widespread, can also be a result of a deposition of bile pigments (jaundice), exogenous metal compounds, and direct deposition of elements such as carotene or quinacrine.

Post-inflammatory pigmentation can follow a variety of drug-induced inflammatory cutaneous reactions; fixed eruptions are known to leave a residual pigmentation that can persist for months.

Pityriasis rosea

Pityriasis rosea, often mistaken for ringworm, is a unique disorder that usually begins as a single, large, round or oval pinkish patch known as the 'mother' or 'herald' patch. The most common sites for this solitary lesion are the chest, the back, or the abdomen. This is followed in about 2 weeks by a blossoming of small, flat, round or oval, scaly patches of similar color, each with a central collarette scale, usually distributed in a Christmas tree pattern over the trunk and, to a lesser degree, the extremities. This eruption seldom itches and usually limits itself to areas from the neck to the knees. The etiology of idiopathic pityriasis rosea is unknown.

In drug-induced pityriasis rosea, the 'herald patch' is usually absent, and the eruption will often not follow the classic pattern.

Pruritus

Generalized itching, without any visible signs, is one of the rarer adverse reactions to drugs. More frequently than not, drug-induced itching – moderate or severe – is fairly generalized. For most drugs it is not known in what way they elicit pruritus; some drugs can cause itching directly or indirectly through cholestasis. Pruritus may develop by different pathogenetic mechanisms: allergic, pseudoallergic (histamine release), neurogenic, by vasodilatation, cholestatic effect, and others.

Pseudolymphoma

Pseudolymphoma is not a specific disease. It is an inflammatory response to various stimuli – known or unknown – that results in a lymphomatous–appearing, but benign, accumulation of inflammatory cells. It may resemble true lymphoma clinically and histologically. Localized, nodular pseudolymphomas typically mimic B-cell lymphoma.

Pseudoporphyria

Pseudoporphyria is an infrequent, reversible, photoinduced, cutaneous bullous disorder with clinical, histologic and immunofluorescent similarities to porphyria cutanea tarda but without the accompanying biochemical porphyrin abnormalities. It is commonly seen as localized bullae and skin fragility on sun-exposed skin, often on the dorsum of the hands and fingers.

While pseudoporphyria has been linked with numerous causes, including chronic renal failure, dialysis, and ultraviolet radiation, several medications, primarily naproxen and other nonsteroidal inflammatory drugs, have been reported to trigger this reaction pattern. Blue/gray eye color appears to be an independent risk factor for the development of pseudoporphyria.

Psoriasis

Many drugs, as a result of their pharmacological action, have been implicated in the precipitation or exacerbation of psoriasis or psoriasiform eruptions. Psoriasis is a frequent, chronic, papulosquamous disorder of unknown etiology with characteristic histopathological features and many biochemical, physiological, and immunological abnormalities. The effect and extent of drug-induced psoriatic eruptions are dose-dependent.

Purpura

Purpura, a result of hemorrhage into the skin, can be divided into thrombocytopenic purpura and non-thrombocytopenic purpura (vascular purpura). Both thrombocytopenic and vascular purpura may be due to drugs, and most of the drugs producing purpura may do so by giving rise to vascular damage and thrombocytopenia. In both types of purpura, allergic or toxic (nonallergic) mechanisms may be involved. Some drugs combine with platelets to form an antigen, stimulating formation of antibody to the platelet-drug combination. Thus, the drug appears to act as a hapten; subsequent antigen-antibody reaction causes platelet destruction leading to thrombocytopenia. The purpuric lesions are usually more marked over the lower portions of the body, notably the legs and dorsal aspects of the feet in ambulatory patients.

Other drug-induced cutaneous reactions – erythema multiforme, erythema nodosum, fixed eruption, necrotizing vasculitis, and others – can have a prominent purpuric component.

Raynaud's phenomenon

Raynaud's phenomenon is the paroxysmal, cold-induced constriction of small arteries and arterioles of the fingers and, less often, the toes. Although estimates vary, recent surveys show that Raynaud's phenomenon may affect 5–10 percent of the general population in the United States. Occurring more frequently in women, Raynaud's phenomenon is characterized by blanching, pallor, and cyanosis. In severe cases, secondary changes may occur: thinning and ridging of the nails, telangiectasias of the nail folds, and, in the later stages, sclerosis and atrophy of the digits.

Rhabdomyolysis

Rhabdomyolysis is the breakdown of muscle fibers, the result of skeletal muscle injury, that leads to the release of potentially toxic intracellular contents into the plasma. The causes are diverse: muscle trauma from vigorous exercise, electrolyte imbalance, extensive thermal burns, crush injuries, infections, various toxins and drugs, and a host of other factors. Rhabdomyolysis can result from direct muscle injury by myotoxic drugs such as cocaine, heroin and alcohol. About 10–40% of patients with rhabdomyolysis develop acute renal failure. The classic triad of symptoms of rhabdomyolysis is muscle pain, weakness and dark urine. Most frequently, the involved muscle groups are those of the back and lower calves. The primary diagnostic indicator of this syndrome is significantly elevated serum creatine phosphokinase.

Stevens-Johnson syndrome and toxic epidermal necrolysis (SJS/TEN)

Previously classified clinically and in the Litt database as two separate adverse drug reactions, Stevens-Johnson syndrome (SJS) and toxic epidermal necrolysis (TEN) (also known as Lyell's syndrome) are now considered to be at either end of a spectrum of severe epidermolytic and potentially fatal adverse cutaneous drug reactions, differing only by their extent of skin detachment. SJS and TEN are characterized by mucocutaneous tenderness and typically hemorrhagic erosions, erythema and more or less severe epidermal detachment presenting as blisters and areas of denuded skin. Other symptoms, which may precede the cutaneous manifestations, include fever, myalgia, malaise, headache, arthralgia and ocular involvement.

Drugs are usually identified as the main cause of SJS/TEN, but *Mycoplasma pneumoniae* and *Herpes simplex* virus infections have also been associated with SJS/TEN. Genetic susceptibility to SJS and TEN is likely as exemplified by the strong association observed in Han Chinese between a genetic marker, the human leukocyte antigen HLA-B*1502, and SJS induced by carbamazepine. Diagnosis relies mainly on clinical signs together with the histological analysis of a skin biopsy showing typical full-thickness epidermal necrolysis due to extensive keratinocyte apoptosis.

Tinnitus

Tinnitus (from the Latin word to tinkle or ring like a bell) is the perception of sound – ringing, buzzing, hissing, humming, whistling, whining, roaring, or ticking, clicking, banging, beeping, pulsating – in the human ear, when none exists. It has also been described as a 'whooshing' sound, like wind or waves, 'crickets' or 'tree frogs' or 'locusts.' To some it's a chirping, clanging, sizzling, rumbling, or a dreadful shrieking noise. And it can be like rushing water, breaking glass or chain saws running. Nearly 40 million Americans suffer from this disorder.

Urticaria / hives

Urticaria induced by drugs is, after exanthems, the second most frequent type of drug reaction. Urticaria, or hives, is a vascular reaction of the skin characterized by pruritic, erythematous wheals. These welts – or wheals – caused by localized edema, can vary in size from one millimeter in diameter to large palm-sized swellings, favor the covered areas (trunk, buttocks, chest), and are, more often than not, generalized. Urticaria usually develops within 36 hours following the administration of the responsible drug. Individual lesions rarely persist for more than 24 hours.

Urticaria may be the only symptom of drug sensitivity, or it may be a concomitant or followed by the manifestations of serum sickness. Urticaria may be accompanied by angioedema of the lips or eyelids. It may, on rare occasions, progress to anaphylactoid reactions or to anaphylaxis.

Vasculitis (angiitis) / cutaneous vasculitis (angiitis)

Drug-induced cutaneous necrotizing vasculitis, a clinicopathologic process characterized by inflammation and necrosis of blood vessels, often presents with a variety of small, palpable purpuric lesions most frequently distributed over the lower extremities: urticaria-like lesions, small ulcerations, and occasional hemorrhagic vesicles and pustules. The basic process involves an immunologically mediated response to antigens that result in vessel wall damage.

Beginning as small macules and papules, they ultimately eventuate into purpuric lesions and, in the more severe cases, into hemorrhagic blisters and frank ulcerations. A polymorphonuclear infiltrate and fibrinoid changes in the small dermal vessels characterize the vasculitic reaction.

Vertigo / dizziness

Vertigo, a specific type of dizziness, is a feeling of unsteadiness. It is the sensation of spinning or swaying while actually remaining stationary with respect to the surroundings. It is a result of either motion sickness, a viral infection of the organs of balance, low blood sugar, or medications. It is a symptom of multiple sclerosis, carbon monoxide poisoning, and Ménière's disease.

Vertigo is one of the most frequently reported health problems in adults. According to the National Institutes of Health, about 40% of people in the United States experience vertigo at least once during their lifetime. Prevalence is higher in women and increases with age.

Xerostomia (dry mouth)

Xerostomia is a dryness of the oral cavity that makes speaking, chewing and swallowing difficult. Some people also experience changes in taste and salivary gland enlargement. Lack of saliva may predispose one to oral infection, such as candidiasis, and increase the risk of dental caries. Resulting from a partial or complete absence of saliva production, xerostomia can be caused by many drugs.

Drugs that cause important reactions

Acanthosis nigricans
Amprenavir
Azathioprine
Diethylstilbestrol
Estrogens
Fusidic Acid
Heroin
Insulin
Mechlorethamine
Methsuximide
Methyltestosterone
Niacin
Niacinamide
Oral Contraceptives
Palifermin
Prednisolone
Prednisone
Somatropin
Thioridazine
Tryptophan

Acneiform eruption / acneiform dermatitis / acneiform rash
Abrocitinib
Acamprosate
Acyclovir
Adalimumab
Adapalene
Afatinib
Alosetron
Alprazolam
Aminolevulinic Acid
Androstenedione
Aprepitant
Aripiprazole
Atorvastatin
Azathioprine
Basiliximab
Bedaquiline
Belatacept
Betamethasone
Bevacizumab
Bexarotene
Bosutinib
Brimonidine
Budesonide
Bupropion
Buserelin
Buspirone
Cabergoline
Capecitabine
Carbamazepine
Ceritinib
Cetirizine
Cetuximab
Chasteberry
Chloral Hydrate
Chlorotrianisene
Cidofovir
Ciprofloxacin
Cisplatin
Clindamycin/Tretinoin
Clobetasol
Clofazimine
Clomipramine
Cobimetinib
Cocoa
Crofelemer
Cyanocobalamin
Cyclophosphamide
Cyclosporine
Dabrafenib
Daclizumab
Dacomitinib
Dactinomycin
Danazol
Dantrolene
Dapsone
Dasatinib
Deflazacort
Demeclocycline
Dexamethasone
Dexlansoprazole
Diazepam
Diltiazem
Disulfiram
Docetaxel
Doxycycline
Duloxetine
Durvalumab
Efalizumab
Eflornithine
Encorafenib
Epoetin Alfa
Erlotinib
Erythromycin
Escitalopram
Esmolol
Esomeprazole
Estazolam
Estramustine
Estrogens
Eszopiclone
Etanercept
Ethionamide
Everolimus
Famotidine
Felbamate
Fenoprofen
Finasteride
Fluconazole
Fluorides
Fluorouracil
Fluoxetine
Fluoxymesterone
Fluvoxamine
Folic Acid
Follitropin Alfa/Beta
Fosphenytoin
Gabapentin
Ganciclovir
Gefitinib
Gemcitabine
Gestrinone
Glatiramer
Gold & Gold Compounds
Goserelin
Granulocyte Colony-Stimulating Factor (G-CSF)
Grepafloxacin
Halothane
Heroin
Histrelin
Hyaluronic Acid
Hydroquinone
Imatinib
Infliximab
Interferon Alfa
Interferon Beta
Ipilimumab
Irinotecan
Isoniazid
Isotretinoin
Ivacaftor
Ixazomib
Lamotrigine
Lansoprazole
Lapatinib
Leflunomide
Lenalidomide
Letrozole
Leucovorin
Levonorgestrel
Lisdexamfetamine
Lithium
Lopinavir
Maprotiline
MDMA
Medroxyprogesterone
Mephenytoin
Mesalamine
Methotrexate
Methoxsalen
Methyltestosterone
Minoxidil
Mobocertinib
Mobocertinib
Mometasone
Mycophenolate
Nabumetone
Nadolol
Nafarelin
Naltrexone
Nandrolone
Naratriptan
Necitumumab
Nefazodone
Nicotine
Nilotinib
Nimodipine
Nisoldipine
Nitrofurantoin
Nivolumab
Nizatidine
Olsalazine
Oral Contraceptives
Osimertinib
Oxcarbazepine
Paclitaxel
Panitumumab
Panobinostat
Pantoprazole
Paroxetine Hydrochloride
Pentostatin
Phenobarbital
Phenylbutazone
Phenytoin
Pimecrolimus
Ponatinib
Potassium Iodide
Prednisolone
Prednisone
Pretomanid
Progestins
Propafenone
Propranolol
Propylthiouracil
Psoralens
Pyrazinamide
Pyridoxine
Quinidine
Quinine
Ramipril
Riboflavin
Rifampin
Rifapentine
Risperidone
Ritonavir
Rufinamide
Ruxolitinib
Saquinavir
Selumetinib
Sertraline
Sibutramine
Simvastatin
Sirolimus
Smallpox Vaccine
Sodium Oxybate
Sorafenib
Sparfloxacin
Stanozolol
Sunitinib
Tacrine
Temsirolimus
Teriflunomide
Testosterone
Tetracycline
Tiagabine
Tibolone
Tizanidine
Tofacitinib
Topiramate
Trametinib
Trastuzumab
Tretinoin
Trioxsalen
Triptorelin
Ulipristal
Valdecoxib
Vandetanib
Vedolizumab
Vemurafenib
Venlafaxine
Verapamil
Vinblastine
Vinorelbine
Vorinostat
Zalcitabine
Zaleplon
Zidovudine
Zolpidem
Zonisamide

DOI: 10.1201/9781003715672-1500

Acute febrile neutrophilic dermatosis (Sweet's / Sweet syndrome)
Abacavir
Aceclofenac
Acetaminophen
Adalimumab
Aldesleukin
Allopurinol
Amoxapine
Amoxicillin
Azacitidine
Azathioprine
BCG Vaccine
Bendamustine
Bortezomib
Capsicum
Cedazuridine & Decitabine
Celecoxib
Chloroquine
Ciprofloxacin
Citalopram
Clindamycin
Clindamycin/Tretinoin
Clofazimine
Clopidogrel
Clozapine
Co-Trimoxazole
Codeine
Covid-19 Vaccine, mRNA
Cytarabine
Dabigatran
Dabrafenib
Dapagliflozin
Dasatinib
Diazepam
Doxycycline
Dupilumab
Enasidenib
Erlotinib
Esomeprazole
Fluconazole
Furosemide
Gemcitabine
Gilterinib
Glucagon
Granulocyte Colony-Stimulating Factor (G-CSF)
Haloperidol
Hydralazine
Hydroxychloroquine
Ibrutinib
Imatinib
Infliximab
Influenza Vaccine
Ipilimumab
Isotretinoin
Ixazomib
Lamotrigine
Lenalidomide
Letrozole
Levofloxacin
Levomepromazine
Mercaptopurine
Midostaurin
Minocycline
Mirtazapine
Mitoxantrone
Nilotinib
Niraparib
Nitrofurantoin
Nivolumab
Norfloxacin
Ofloxacin
Omeprazole
Oral Contraceptives
Palbociclib
Pandemic Influenza Vaccine (H1N1)
PEG-Interferon
Pembrolizumab
Pemetrexed
Perphenazine
Phenylbutazone
Piperacillin
Pneumococcal Vaccine
Promethazine
Propylthiouracil
Quinupristin/Dalfopristin
Ribavirin
Risankizumab
Sulfamethoxazole
Sulfasalazine
Ticagrelor
Tocilizumab
Topotecan
Trametinib
Tretinoin
Verapamil
Vorinostat

Acute generalized exanthematous pustulosis (AGEP)
Acarbose
Acetaminophen
Acetazolamide
Aldesleukin
Allopurinol
Amoxapine
Amoxicillin
Amphotericin B
Ampicillin
Apalutamide
Apixaban
Aspirin
Atezolizumab
Atovaquone/Proguanil
Azathioprine
Azithromycin
Bacampicillin
Bendamustine
Benznidazole
Bupropion
Carbamazepine
Carbimazole
Cariprazine
Cefaclor
Cefazolin
Cefditoren
Cefepime
Cefotaxime
Ceftazidime
Ceftriaxone
Cefuroxime
Celecoxib
Cephalexin
Cephradine
Cetirizine
Cetuximab
Chloramphenicol
Chloroquine
Chlorzoxazone
Ciprofloxacin
Clindamycin
Clindamycin/Tretinoin
Clopidogrel
Cloxacillin
Clozapine
Co-Trimoxazole
Codeine
Cytarabine
Dalteparin
Dapsone
Daptomycin
Denosumab
Dexamethasone
Dextromethorphan
Dihydrocodeine
Diltiazem
Diphenhydramine
Docetaxel
Doripenem
Doxycycline
Dupilumab
Enzalutamide
Epoetin Alfa
Erlotinib
Ertapenem
Erythromycin
Etanercept
Etodolac
Exemestane
Famotidine
Fenofibrate
Fexofenadine
Finasteride
Flucloxacillin
Fluconazole
Fosfomycin
Furosemide
Gadobutrol
Galantamine
Gefitinib
Gemcitabine
Ginkgo Biloba
Haloperidol
Hyaluronic Acid
Hydrochlorothiazide
Hydroxychloroquine
Hydroxyzine
Ibuprofen
Icodextrin
Imatinib
Imipenem/Cilastatin
Immune Globulin IV
Infliximab
Influenza Vaccine
Iodixanol
Iohexol
Iomeprol
Ioversol
Isoniazid
Isotretinoin
Itraconazole
Ketoconazole
Lamivudine
Lamotrigine
Lansoprazole
Levetiracetam
Levofloxacin
Lincomycin
Lindane
Lopinavir
Meloxicam
Meropenem
Metamizole
Metformin
Methimazole
Methoxsalen
Methylphenidate
Methylprednisolone
Metronidazole
Mexiletine
Midodrine
Mifepristone
Minocycline
Minoxidil
Morphine
Moxifloxacin
Naltrexone
Nifedipine
Nimesulide
Nivolumab
Nystatin
Olanzapine
Omeprazole
Oxacillin
Paclitaxel
Pemetrexed
Phenobarbital
Phenytoin
Piperacillin
Piperacillin/Tazobactam
Piroxicam
Prednisolone
Pristinamycin
Progestins
Propafenone
Propoxyphene
Pseudoephedrine
Pyrazinamide
Pyrimethamine
Quetiapine
Quinidine
Ranibizumab
Ranitidine
Ranolazine
Rifabutin
Rifampin
Ritodrine
Rivaroxaban
Senna
Sertraline
Simvastatin
Sorafenib
Streptomycin
Sulfamethoxazole
Sulfasalazine
Teicoplanin
Telavancin
Terazosin
Terbinafine
Tetrazepam
Thalidomide
Thallium
Ticlopidine
Tigecycline
Tocilizumab
Tosufloxacin
Valdecoxib
Valproic Acid
Vancomycin
Varenicline
Vemurafenib
Zidovudine

Ageusia / taste loss / taste disorder
Acarbose
Aspirin
Atorvastatin
Azelastine
Betaxolol

Cabozantinib
Candesartan
Captopril
Carbamazepine
Cetirizine
Chlorhexidine
Clindamycin
Clopidogrel
Cocaine
Cyclobenzaprine
Doxorubicin
Enalapril
Eslicarbazepine
Etidronate
Feverfew
Fluoxetine
Fluvoxamine
Fosinopril
Grepafloxacin
Hydroxychloroquine
Indomethacin
Interferon Alfa
Isotretinoin
Lenalidomide
Losartan
Maribavir
Methimazole
Nefazodone
Nitroglycerin
Paroxetine Hydrochloride
Penicillamine
Phenylbutazone
Phenytoin
Propofol
Propylthiouracil
Ramipril
Rifabutin
Rifaximin
Rimantadine
Ritonavir
Rivastigmine
Sonidegib
Sulindac
Sunitinib
Terbinafine
Tiagabine
Tiopronin
Topiramate
Valrubicin
Venlafaxine
Vismodegib
Voriconazole
Zalcitabine

Alopecia / hair loss

Abemaciclib
Acetohexamide
Acitretin
Acyclovir
Adalimumab
Afatinib
Aflibercept
Albendazole
Aldesleukin
Alectinib
Alitretinoin
Allopurinol
Alpelisib
Altretamine
Amantadine
Amiloride
Aminolevulinic Acid
Aminosalicylate Sodium
Amiodarone
Amitriptyline
Amlodipine
Amoxapine
Anagrelide
Anastrozole
Androstenedione
Anidulafungin
Aprepitant
Arsenic
Aspirin
Astemizole
Atenolol
Atorvastatin
Atovaquone/Proguanil
Atropine Sulfate
Avapritinib
Axitinib
Azathioprine
Belatacept
Belinostat
Bendamustine
Benznidazole
Betamethasone
Betaxolol
Bevacizumab
Bexarotene
Bezafibrate
Bicalutamide
Bismuth
Bleomycin
Botulinum Toxin (A & B)
Brentuximab Vedotin
Brinzolamide
Bromocriptine
Budesonide
Bupropion
Buspirone
Busulfan
Cabazitaxel
Cabergoline
Cabozantinib
Calcipotriol
Capecitabine
Captopril
Carbamazepine
Carboplatin
Carmustine
Carvedilol
Celecoxib
Certolizumab
Cetirizine
Cetuximab
Cevimeline
Chlorambucil
Chloramphenicol
Chlordiazepoxide
Chlorpropamide
Cidofovir
Cimetidine
Cisplatin
Citalopram
Clarithromycin
Clofibrate
Clomiphene
Clomipramine
Clonazepam
Clonidine
Cobimetinib
Colchicine
Crizotinib
Cyclophosphamide
Cyclosporine
Cytarabine
Dabrafenib
Dacarbazine
Daclatasvir
Daclizumab
Dacomitinib
Dactinomycin
Dalteparin
Danazol
Dasatinib
Daunorubicin
Decitabine
Deferasirox
Deflazacort
Degarelix
Delavirdine
Desipramine
Dexamethasone
Diazoxide
Diclofenac
Dicumarol
Didanosine
Diethylpropion
Diflunisal
Diltiazem
Dimethyl Fumarate
Docetaxel
Donepezil
Doxazosin
Doxepin
Doxorubicin
Duloxetine
Dupilumab
Eculizumab
Efavirenz
Eflornithine
Eltrombopag
Enalapril
Encorafenib
Enoxaparin
Entecavir
Epinephrine
Epirubicin
Epoetin Alfa
Erdafitinib
Eribulin
Erlotinib
Erythromycin
Escitalopram
Eslicarbazepine
Estramustine
Estrogens
Eszopiclone
Etanercept
Ethambutol
Ethionamide
Etoposide
Everolimus
Evolocumab
Exemestane
Febuxostat
Fenofibrate
Fenoprofen
Fingolimod
Flecainide
Fluconazole
Fludarabine
Fluorouracil
Fluoxetine
Fluoxymesterone
Flurbiprofen
Fluvoxamine
Foscarnet
Fulvestrant
Gabapentin
Gadodiamide
Ganciclovir
Gefitinib
Gemcitabine
Gentamicin
Givosiran
Glasdegib
Glatiramer
Gold & Gold Compounds
Goserelin
Granisetron
Granulocyte Colony-Stimulating Factor (G-CSF)
Grepafloxacin
Haloperidol
Halothane
Heparin
Hepatitis B Vaccine
Human Papillomavirus Vaccine (Bivalent)
Hyaluronic Acid
Hydroxychloroquine
Hydroxyurea
Hyoscyamine
Ibandronate
Ibritumomab
Ibuprofen
Idarubicin
Ifosfamide
Imatinib
Imipramine
Imiquimod
Immune Globulin IV
Indinavir
Indomethacin
Infigratinib
Infliximab
Interferon Alfa
Interferon Beta
Ipilimumab
Ipratropium
Irinotecan
Isavuconazonium Sulfate
Isoniazid
Isotretinoin
Itraconazole
Ixabepilone
Ixazomib
Ketoconazole
Ketoprofen
Ketorolac
Labetalol
Lamivudine
Lamotrigine
Lanreotide
Lansoprazole
Lapatinib
Leflunomide
Lenvatinib
Letrozole
Leucovorin
Leuprolide
Levamisole
Levobetaxolol
Levobunolol
Levodopa
Levothyroxine
Liothyronine
Lisinopril
Lithium
Lomustine
Loperamide

Lopinavir
Loratadine
Losartan
Lovastatin
Lutetium Lu177 Dotatate
Maprotiline
Mebendazole
Mechlorethamine
Meclofenamate
Medroxyprogesterone
Mefloquine
Meloxicam
Melphalan
Memantine
Mepolizumab
Mercaptopurine
Mesalamine
Metformin
Methimazole
Methotrexate
Methyltestosterone
Methysergide
Metoprolol
Mexiletine
Minocycline
Minoxidil
Mirtazapine
Mitomycin
Mitotane
Mitoxantrone
Mizoribine
Mobocertinib
Moexipril
Mycophenolate
Nabumetone
Nadolol
Nalidixic Acid
Naltrexone
Naproxen
Naratriptan
Nefazodone
Neratinib
Nifedipine
Nilotinib
Nimodipine
Nintedanib
Nisoldipine
Nitisinone
Nitrofurantoin
Nivolumab
Nortriptyline
Octreotide
Olanzapine
Olaparib
Olaratumab
Omacetaxine
Omalizumab
Ombitasvir/Paritaprevir/Ritonavir
Omeprazole
Oral Contraceptives
Osilodrostat
Oxaliplatin
Oxerutins
Paclitaxel
Palbociclib
Panitumumab
Panobinostat
Pantoprazole
Paricalcitol
Paroxetine Hydrochloride
Pasireotide
Pazopanib
PEG-Interferon
Pegvisomant
Pembrolizumab
Pemetrexed
Pemigatinib
Penicillamine
Pentosan
Pentostatin
Peplomycin
Pergolide
Pertuzumab
Pexidartinib hydrochloride
Phentermine
Phenytoin
Piroxicam
Pramipexole
Praziquantel
Prazosin
Prednisolone
Prednisone
Procarbazine
Propafenone
Propranolol
Propylthiouracil
Protriptyline
Pyridostigmine
Quetiapine
Quinacrine
Quinapril
Quinidine
Rabeprazole
Raltitrexed
Ramipril
Regorafenib
Ribavirin
Ribociclib
Riluzole
Ripretinib
Risperidone
Ritonavir
Rituximab
Rivaroxaban
Rivastigmine
Rofecoxib
Ropinirole
Rucaparib
Ruxolitinib
Selenium
Sertraline
Setmelanotide
Sodium Oxybate
Sonidegib
Sorafenib
Sotalol
Sparfloxacin
Spinosad
Spironolactone
St John's Wort
Strontium Ranelate
Sulfasalazine
Sulfisoxazole
Sulindac
Sunitinib
Tacrine
Tacrolimus
Talazoparib
Tamoxifen
Tegafur/Gimeracil/Oteracil
Temozolomide
Temsirolimus
Teniposide
Tepotinib
Terbinafine
Terfenadine
Teriflunomide
Testosterone
Thalidomide
Thallium
Thioguanine
Thiotepa
Tiagabine
Timolol
Tinzaparin
Tiopronin
Tizanidine
Tocainide
Tolcapone
Topiramate
Topotecan
Trabectedin
Trametinib
Trastuzumab
Trastuzumab Emtansine / Ado-Trastuzumab Emtansine
Trazodone
Trientine
Trifluridine & Tipiracil
Trimethadione
Trimipramine
Triptorelin
Ursodiol
Valdecoxib
Valproic Acid
Vandetanib
Vasopressin
Vemurafenib
Venlafaxine
Verapamil
Vinblastine
Vincristine
Vinorelbine
Vismodegib
Vitamin A
Voclosporin
Voriconazole
Vorinostat
Warfarin
Zaleplon
Zidovudine
Ziprasidone
Zoledronate
Zonisamide
Zoster Vaccine

Angioedema

Acetaminophen
Acetylcysteine
Acitretin
Acyclovir
Adalimumab
Albendazole
Aldesleukin
Alefacept
Alemtuzumab
Alendronate
Aliskiren
Allopurinol
Alogliptin
Alprazolam
Alteplase
Aminoglutethimide
Aminosalicylate Sodium
Amiodarone
Amitriptyline
Amlodipine
Amodiaquine
Amoxicillin
Ampicillin
Ampicillin/Sulbactam
Anidulafungin
Anthrax Vaccine
Ascorbic Acid
Asenapine
Asparaginase
Aspartame
Aspirin
Atorvastatin
Atracurium
Avacopan
Azatadine
Azathioprine
Azithromycin
Aztreonam
Benazepril
Benznidazole
Bevacizumab
Bezafibrate
Bismuth
Bleomycin
Brivaracetam
Brompheniramine
Budesonide
Bupropion
Butabarbital
Canagliflozin
Candesartan
Captopril
Carbamazepine
Carisoprodol
Carvedilol
Cefaclor
Cefadroxil
Cefixime
Cefoxitin
Cefprozil
Ceftazidime
Ceftriaxone
Cefuroxime
Celecoxib
Cephalexin
Certolizumab
Cetirizine
Chloral Hydrate
Chlorambucil
Chloramphenicol
Chlordiazepoxide
Chloroquine
Chlorpheniramine
Chlorpromazine
Chlorpropamide
Chlorthalidone
Chlorzoxazone
Cilazapril
Cimetidine
Cinoxacin
Ciprofloxacin
Cisplatin
Clarithromycin
Clemastine
Clonazepam
Clonidine
Clopidogrel
Cloxacillin
Clozapine
Co-Trimoxazole
Cocaine
Codeine
Cromolyn
Cyanocobalamin
Cyclamate

Cyclobenzaprine
Cyclophosphamide
Cyclosporine
Cyproheptadine
Dacarbazine
Danazol
Darunavir
Daunorubicin
Deferoxamine
Deflazacort
Delavirdine
Desipramine
Dexchlorpheniramine
Diazepam
Diclofenac
Dicumarol
Diethylstilbestrol
Diflunisal
Dihydrocodeine
Diltiazem
Dimenhydrinate
Diphenhydramine
Dipyridamole
Disulfiram
Dofetilide
Doxazosin
Doxorubicin
Doxycycline
Dronedarone
Droperidol
Dulaglutide
Dupilumab
Dutasteride
Echinacea
Efalizumab
Enalapril
Enoxaparin
Epoetin Alfa
Erythromycin
Esomeprazole
Estramustine
Estrogens
Etanercept
Ethambutol
Etidronate
Etodolac
Etomidate
Etoricoxib
Everolimus
Exenatide
Ezetimibe
Famotidine
Febuxostat
Felodipine
Fenoprofen
Fentanyl
Feverfew
Fluconazole
Fluorouracil
Fluoxetine
Fluphenazine
Flurbiprofen
Fluvoxamine
Fosinopril
Fulvestrant
Glatiramer
Glucagon
Gold & Gold Compounds
Griseofulvin
Haloperidol
Halothane
Henna
Heparin
Hepatitis B Vaccine
Heroin
Histrelin
Hyaluronic Acid
Hydralazine
Hydrochlorothiazide
Hydrocortisone
Hydromorphone
Hydroxychloroquine
Hydroxyzine
Ibritumomab
Ibuprofen
Icatibant
Iloperidone
Imidapril
Imiglucerase
Imipenem/Cilastatin
Imipramine
Imiquimod
Indapamide
Indomethacin
Infliximab
Insulin
Interferon Alfa
Iodixanol
Iothalamate
Irbesartan
Isoniazid
Isotretinoin
Itraconazole
Ivacaftor
Ivermectin
Ixekizumab
Ketoconazole
Ketoprofen
Ketorolac
Labetalol
Lacosamide
Lamivudine
Lamotrigine
Ledipasvir & Sofosbuvir
Lepirudin
Levamisole
Levetiracetam
Levofloxacin
Levothyroxine
Lidocaine
Linezolid
Lisinopril
Lithium
Lixisenatide
Loratadine
Losartan
Lurasidone
MDMA
Mebendazole
Mebeverine
Mechlorethamine
Meclizine
Meclofenamate
Mefenamic Acid
Meloxicam
Melphalan
Meperidine
Mephenytoin
Mephobarbital
Mepivacaine
Meprobamate
Mesna
Metformin
Methohexital
Methotrexate
Methylphenidate
Metoclopramide
Metoprolol
Metronidazole
Miconazole
Midazolam
Miltefosine
Minocycline
Mirtazapine
Mitotane
Moexipril
Monosodium Glutamate
Montelukast
Nabumetone
Nalidixic Acid
Naloxone
Naproxen
Neomycin
Nevirapine
Nicardipine
Nifedipine
Nimesulide
Nitrofurantoin
Ofloxacin
Olanzapine
Olmesartan
Omalizumab
Ombitasvir/Paritaprevir/ Ritonavir and Dasabuvir
Omeprazole
Oral Contraceptives
Oritavancin
Oxaliplatin
Oxaprozin
Oxcarbazepine
Paclitaxel
Paliperidone
Pamidronate
Panitumumab
Pantoprazole
Paroxetine Hydrochloride
PEG-Interferon
Pegaptanib
Pegaspargase
Penicillin G
Penicillin V
Pentagastrin
Pentobarbital
Pentoxifylline
Perflutren
Perindopril
Phenelzine
Phenobarbital
Phenolphthalein
Phenylbutazone
Phenytoin
Pioglitazone
Piperacillin
Piperacillin/Tazobactam
Piroxicam
Pitavastatin
Potassium Iodide
Prasugrel
Praziquantel
Prazosin
Prilocaine
Primaquine
Pristinamycin
Procainamide
Procarbazine
Progestins
Promethazine
Propafenone
Propofol
Propranolol
Propylthiouracil
Protamine Sulfate
Pseudoephedrine
Pyrimethamine
Quinapril
Quinestrol
Quinidine
Quinine
Ramipril
Ranitidine
Riboflavin
Rifampin
Risperidone
Rituximab
Rivaroxaban
Rofecoxib
Ropinirole
Rosuvastatin
Sacubitril/Valsartan
Saxagliptin
Secobarbital
Sertraline
Simvastatin
Sirolimus
Sitagliptin
Solifenacin
Sorafenib
Sparfloxacin
Streptokinase
Streptomycin
Sulfadoxine
Sulfamethoxazole
Sulfasalazine
Sulfisoxazole
Sulfites
Sulindac
Sumatriptan
Tacrolimus
Tartrazine
Telithromycin
Telmisartan
Tenecteplase
Terbinafine
Terfenadine
Teriflunomide
Tetracycline
Thiamine
Thiopental
Thioridazine
Thiotepa
Ticagrelor
Ticlopidine
Tinidazole
Tiopronin
Tiotropium
Tocilizumab
Tolmetin
Tositumomab & Iodine[131]
Tosufloxacin
Tramadol
Trandolapril
Trastuzumab
Trazodone
Trifluoperazine
Trimeprazine
Trimetrexate
Tripelennamine
Triprolidine
Triptorelin
Troleandomycin
Trospium
Trovafloxacin

Urokinase
Valsartan
Vancomycin
Vardenafil
Vedolizumab
Venlafaxine
Verapamil
Vildagliptin
Vinblastine
Vincristine
Voriconazole
Vorinostat
Warfarin
Yellow Fever Vaccine
Zalcitabine
Zidovudine
Ziprasidone
Zofenopril

Anosmia (smell loss) / smell disorders

Amikacin
Aspirin
Cocaine
Dorzolamide
Doxycycline
Enalapril
Fluticasone Propionate
Interferon Alfa
Levodopa
Methazolamide
Methoxsalen
Midodrine
Nifedipine
Propofol
Pyrazinamide
Terbinafine
Uracil/Tegafur
Varenicline
Zinc

Aphthous stomatitis / aphthous ulcer / aphtha (aphthae)

Afatinib
Aldesleukin
Amodiaquine
Amoxicillin
Anagrelide
Artesunate
Asparaginase
Aspirin
Azathioprine
Azelastine
Azithromycin
Aztreonam
Belatacept
Benznidazole
Bupropion
Candesartan
Captopril
Cefaclor
Certolizumab
Cetuximab
Cisplatin
Co-Trimoxazole
Cyclophosphamide
Cyclosporine
Delavirdine
Diclofenac
Docetaxel
Doxepin
Doxorubicin
Epirubicin
Erlotinib
Everolimus
Exemestane
Fenoprofen
Fluorides
Fluorouracil
Fluoxetine
Gold & Gold Compounds
Hepatitis B Vaccine
Hydroxyurea
Imatinib
Imiquimod
Indinavir
Interferon Alfa
Ipilimumab
Ketorolac
Labetalol
Ledipasvir & Sofosbuvir
Lenvatinib
Losartan
Methotrexate
Mycophenolate
Naproxen
Nicorandil
Nivolumab
Olanzapine
Omacetaxine
Orlistat
Paclitaxel
Pantoprazole
Paroxetine Hydrochloride
Pemetrexed
Penicillamine
Piroxicam
Prednisone
Pyrimethamine
Rifabutin
Risdiplam
Rofecoxib
Sertraline
Siltuximab
Sirolimus
Sorafenib
Sulfadoxine
Sulfamethoxazole
Sulfasalazine
Sulfisoxazole
Tegafur/Gimeracil/Oteracil
Temsirolimus
Tocilizumab
Tosufloxacin
Trametinib
Valsartan
Vedolizumab
Zalcitabine

Baboon syndrome / symmetrical drug-related intertriginous and flexural exanthema (SDRIFE)

Acetaminophen
Afatinib
Allopurinol
Aminophylline
Amoxicillin
Ampicillin
Ampicillin/Sulbactam
Aspirin
Betamethasone
Cefadroxil
Cefuroxime
Celecoxib
Cephalexin
Cetuximab
Cimetidine
Ciprofloxacin
Cisplatin
Clarithromycin
Clindamycin
Cloxacillin
Clozapine
Co-Trimaxazole
Codeine
Covid-19 Vaccine, mRNA
Disulfiram
Docetaxel
Doxycycline
Erythromycin
Etoricoxib
Everolimus
Fluconazole
Fluorouracil
Gefitinib
Gemcitabine
Golimumab
Heparin
Hydrochlorothiazide
Hydroxyurea
Hydroxyzine
Immune Globulin IV
Infliximab
Iomeprol
Iopromide
Itraconazole
Ketoconazole
Lactulose
Lenalidomide
Levocetirizine
Levofloxacin
Mefenamic Acid
Meropenem
Mesalamine
Metronidazole
Mitomycin
Naproxen
Nystatin
Omeprazole
Oral Contraceptives
Osimertinib
Oxycodone
Pamidronate
Pantoprazole
Penicillin V
Piperacillin/Tazobactam
Pirfenidone
Prednisolone
Pristinamycin
Pseudoephedrine
Ranitidine
Remdesivir
Risperidone
Rivastigmine
Roxithromycin
Secnidazole
Tacrolimus
Tamoxifen
Telmisartan
Terbinafine
Tofacitinib
Valacyclovir
Valsartan
Vancomycin
Varenicline
Verurafenib
Zoledronate

Black tongue / black hairy tongue (lingua villosa nigra)

Amoxicillin
Benztropine
Ceftriaxone
Chloramphenicol
Clarithromycin
Clonazepam
Co-Trimoxazole
Cocaine
Doxycycline
Erlotinib
Erythromycin
Fluoxetine
Griseofulvin
Lansoprazole
Linezolid
Methyldopa
Minocycline
Moxifloxacin
Nicotine
Nortriptyline
Olanzapine
Oxytetracycline
PEG-Interferon
Piperacillin/Tazobactam
Ribavirin
Streptomycin
Sulfamethoxazole
Tetracycline
Thiothixene

Bullous dermatosis

Acetazolamide
Acitretin
Afatinib
Aldesleukin
Alemtuzumab
Amifostine
Aminocaproic Acid
Aminophylline
Aminosalicylate Sodium
Amitriptyline
Ampicillin
Anthrax Vaccine
Argatroban
Arsenic
Aspirin
Atropine Sulfate
Bergamot
Bleomycin
Bumetanide
Buspirone
Busulfan
Butabarbital
Butalbital
Capsicum
Captopril
Carbamazepine
Celecoxib
Cetirizine
Cevimeline
Chloral Hydrate
Chloramphenicol
Chlorpromazine
Chlorpropamide
Ciprofloxacin
Clonazepam
Clopidogrel
Co-Trimoxazole
Cocaine
Codeine
Colchicine
Cyanocobalamin
Cyclamate
Cyclosporine
Cytarabine

Dalteparin
Dapsone
Desoximetasone
Dextromethorphan
Diazepam
Diclofenac
Dicumarol
Diethylstilbestrol
Diflunisal
Digoxin
Disulfiram
Entacapone
Ephedrine
Erlotinib
Estrogens
Ethambutol
Ethchlorvynol
Felbamate
Fluconazole
Fluorouracil
Fluoxetine
Fluvoxamine
Fondaparinux
Fosphenytoin
Frovatriptan
Furosemide
Ganciclovir
Garlic
Gemcitabine
Glyburide
Gold & Gold Compounds
Griseofulvin
Henna
Hydralazine
Hydrochlorothiazide
Hydroxychloroquine
Ibuprofen
Ibutilide
Imipramine
Imiquimod
Indomethacin
Infliximab
Influenza Vaccine
Insulin
Interferon Alfa
Isoniazid
Ivermectin
Ketoprofen
Lamotrigine
Leflunomide
Lindane
Lisinopril
Lithium
Lomefloxacin
Mechlorethamine
Meloxicam
Mephenytoin
Meprobamate
Methicillin
Methotrexate
Methoxsalen
Miconazole
Minoxidil
Mitomycin
Mometasone
Moxifloxacin
Mycophenolate
Nabumetone
Nalidixic Acid
Naproxen
Nifedipine
Norfloxacin
Omeprazole
Oral Contraceptives
Oxacillin
Penicillamine
Pentamidine
Pentobarbital
Pentostatin
Phenobarbital
Phenolphthalein
Phenytoin
Piroxicam
Prednicarbate
Promethazine
Propranolol
Propyphenazone
Pyridoxine
Pyrimethamine
Quinethazone
Reserpine
Rifampin
Risperidone
Ritonavir
Rituximab
Rivastigmine
Rofecoxib
Rue
Senna
Sertraline
Smallpox Vaccine
Sparfloxacin
Streptomycin
Sulfadoxine
Sulfamethoxazole
Sulfisoxazole
Sunitinib
Temazepam
Tetracycline
Thalidomide
Thiopental
Tinzaparin
Tolbutamide
Tranexamic Acid
Tretinoin
Trioxsalen
Urokinase
Ustekinumab
Valproic Acid
Vancomycin
Vasopressin
Vinblastine
Warfarin
Zalcitabine
Zidovudine
Zolpidem

DRESS syndrome

Abacavir
Acenocoumarol
Acetaminophen
Afatinib
Allopurinol
Amikacin
Aminosalicylate Sodium
Amitriptyline
Amlodipine
Amoxicillin
Ampicillin
Anakinra
Apalutamide
Apixaban
Aspirin
Atenolol
Atorvastatin
Azithromycin
Benznidazole
Binimetinib
Boceprevir
Bortezomib
Bosentan
Bupropion
Caffeine
Canakinumab
Captopril
Carbamazepine
Cefadroxil
Cefepime
Cefixime
Cefotaxime
Ceftaroline Fosamil
Ceftazidime
Ceftriaxone
Celecoxib
Cenobamate
Chlorambucil
Cidofovir
Cilostazol
Ciprofloxacin
Clindamycin
Clomipramine
Clonazepam
Clopidogrel
Clozapine
Co-Trimoxazole
Cobimetinib
Codeine
Covid-19 Vaccine, mRNA
Cyclobenzaprine
Cycloserine
Daclatasvir
Dapsone
Daptomycin
Darunavir
Dextromethorphan
Diazoxide
Diclofenac
Doxycycline
Efalizumab
Efavirenz
Emtricitabine
Encorafenib
Enoxaparin
Erlotinib
Esomeprazole
Ethambutol
Ethosuximide
Febuxostat
Felbamate
Fenofibrate
Fluconazolw
Fluoxetine
Gabapentin
Ganciclovir
Ginseng
Heparin
Hydroxychloroquine
Ibuprofen
Imatinib
Ipilimumab
Isoniazid
Lamotrigine
Leflunomide
Lenalidomide
Leucovorin
Levetiracetam
Levofloxacin
Linezolid
Lithium
Meropenem
Mesalamine
Metamizole
Metformin
Methimazole
Methotrexate
Metronidazole
Minocycline
Mitoxantrone
Modafinil
Moxifloxacin
Naproxen
Nelfinavir
Nevirapine
Nitrazepam
Nitrofurantoin
Nivolumab
Olanzapine
Oxacillin
Oxazepam
Oxcarbazepine
Pandemic Influenza Vaccine (H1N1)
PEG-Interferon
Penicillin V
Perampanel
Perindopril
Phenobarbital
Phenylbutazone
Phenytoin
Piperacillin
Piperacillin/Tazobactam
Piroxicam
Primidone
Promethazine
Propylthiouracil
Pyrazinamide
Pyrimethamine
Quetiapine
Quinine
Raltegravir
Ramipril
Ribavirin
Ribociclib
Rifampin
Ritonavir
Rivaroxaban
Sildenafil
Sorafenib
Spironolactone
Streptomycin
Strontium Ranelate
Sulfadiazine
Sulfamethoxazole
Sulfasalazine
Teicoplanin
Telaprevir
Temozolomide
Tenofovir Disoproxil
Tenoxicam
Terbinafine
Teriflunomide
Thiamine
Tocilizumab
Torsemide
Trimethoprim
Valproic Acid
Vancomycin
Vemurafenib
Voxelotor
Warfarin
Ziprasidone
Zonisamide

Erythema multiforme

- Acamprosate
- Acarbose
- Acebutolol
- Acetaminophen
- Acetazolamide
- Adalimumab
- Aldesleukin
- Alectinib
- Alendronate
- Allopurinol
- Amifostine
- Aminosalicylate Sodium
- Amiodarone
- Amlodipine
- Amoxicillin
- Amphotericin B
- Ampicillin
- Anastrozole
- Anthrax Vaccine
- Arsenic
- Aspirin
- Atovaquone/Proguanil
- Atropine Sulfate
- Avelumab
- Azathioprine
- Aztreonam
- Benznidazole
- Bezafibrate
- Bortezomib
- Bosutinib
- Bumetanide
- Bupropion
- Busulfan
- Butabarbital
- Butalbital
- Candesartan
- Capsicum
- Carbamazepine
- Carisoprodol
- Cefaclor
- Cefadroxil
- Cefamandole
- Cefixime
- Cefotaxime
- Cefpodoxime
- Cefprozil
- Ceftazidime
- Ceftriaxone
- Cefuroxime
- Celecoxib
- Cephalexin
- Cephalothin
- Chloral Hydrate
- Chlorambucil
- Chloramphenicol
- Chlordiazepoxide
- Chloroquine
- Chlorpromazine
- Chlorpropamide
- Chlorzoxazone
- Cimetidine
- Ciprofloxacin
- Cisplatin
- Clindamycin
- Clofibrate
- Clonazepam
- Clozapine
- Co-Trimoxazole
- Codeine
- Collagen (Bovine)
- Covid-19 Vaccine, mRNA
- Crizotinib
- Cyclobenzaprine
- Cyclophosphamide
- Daclatasvir
- Danazol
- Dapsone
- Deflazacort
- Delavirdine
- Desoximetasone
- Dexamethasone
- Diclofenac
- Dicloxacillin
- Didanosine
- Diflunisal
- Dihydrocodeine
- Diltiazem
- Dimenhydrinate
- Docetaxel
- Dorzolamide
- Doxycycline
- Dupilumab
- Durvalumab
- Elotuzumab
- Enalapril
- Enoxacin
- Enoxaparin
- Erythromycin
- Estrogens
- Ethambutol
- Ethosuximide
- Etodolac
- Etoposide
- Etoricoxib
- Everolimus
- Famotidine
- Fenbufen
- Fenoprofen
- Flucloxacillin
- Fluconazole
- Fluorouracil
- Fluoxetine
- Flurbiprofen
- Fosphenytoin
- Furazolidone
- Furosemide
- Gadoversetamide
- Gemfibrozil
- Glucagon
- Glyburide
- Gold & Gold Compounds
- Golimumab
- Griseofulvin
- Henna
- Hepatitis B Vaccine
- Human Papillomavirus (HPV) Vaccine
- Hyaluronic Acid
- Hydrochlorothiazide
- Hydroxychloroquine
- Hydroxyurea
- Hydroxyzine
- Ibuprofen
- Icodextrin
- Imatinib
- Imipenem/Cilastatin
- Imiquimod
- Immune Globulin IV
- Indapamide
- Indomethacin
- Infliximab
- Interferon Beta
- Iomeprol
- Ipilimumab
- Isoniazid
- Isotretinoin
- Ixazomib
- Ketoprofen
- Lamotrigine
- Lansoprazole
- Ledipasvir & Sofosbuvir
- Leflunomide
- Lenalidomide
- Levamisole
- Levetiracetam
- Levofloxacin
- Lidocaine
- Lithium
- Loracarbef
- Loratadine
- Lorazepam
- Maprotiline
- Mechlorethamine
- Meclofenamate
- Mefenamic Acid
- Meloxicam
- Mephenytoin
- Meprobamate
- Metamizole
- Methenamine
- Methicillin
- Methotrexate
- Methyldopa
- Minocycline
- Minoxidil
- Misoprostol
- Mitomycin
- Mitotane
- Nabumetone
- Nalidixic Acid
- Naproxen
- Neomycin
- Nifedipine
- Nilotinib
- Nimesulide
- Nitrofurantoin
- Nitroglycerin
- Nivolumab
- Nystatin
- Ombitasvir/Paritaprevir/Ritonavir
- Omeprazole
- Oral Contraceptives
- Oritavancin
- Oxaprozin
- Oxazepam
- Oxybutynin
- Paclitaxel
- Palbociclib
- Pancreatin
- Pandemic Influenza Vaccine (H1N1)
- Pantoprazole
- Paramethadione
- Pembrolizumab
- Pemetrexed
- Penicillamine
- Pentobarbital
- Permethrin
- Phenobarbital
- Phenolphthalein
- Phensuximide
- Phenylbutazone
- Phenytoin
- Piroxicam
- Pneumococcal Vaccine
- Pravastatin
- Prednicarbate
- Prednisolone
- Primidone
- Probenecid
- Progestins
- Promethazine
- Propranolol
- Pseudoephedrine
- Pyrazinamide
- Pyrimethamine
- Quetiapine
- Quinidine
- Quinine
- Ramipril
- Regorafenib
- Ribavirin
- Ribociclib
- Rifampin
- Risedronate
- Risperidone
- Ritodrine
- Rivaroxaban
- Roxatidine
- Saquinavir
- Scopolamine
- Secukinumab
- Senna
- Sertraline
- Simvastatin
- Smallpox Vaccine
- Sofosbuvir
- Sorafenib
- Spironolactone
- Streptomycin
- Sulfacetamide
- Sulfadiazine
- Sulfadoxine
- Sulfamethoxazole
- Sulfasalazine
- Sulfisoxazole
- Sulindac
- Sunitinib
- Tamsulosin
- Tea Tree
- Telithromycin
- Telmisartan
- Terbinafine
- Tetracycline
- Tetrazepam
- Thalidomide
- Thiabendazole
- Thiopental
- Thioridazine
- Ticlopidine
- Tiopronin
- Tobramycin
- Tocainide
- Tolbutamide
- Tolcapone
- Tolmetin
- Trazodone
- Trihexyphenidyl
- Trimethadione
- Valproic Acid
- Vancomycin
- Vandetanib
- Vemurafenib
- Venlafaxine
- Verapamil
- Vinblastine
- Vitamin A
- Vitamin E
- Voriconazole
- Zalcitabine
- Zidovudine

Erythema nodosum
Abatacept
Acetaminophen
Acyclovir
Aldesleukin
Amiodarone
Anastrozole
Arsenic
Aspartame
Aspirin
Azathioprine
Benznidazole
Busulfan
Carbamazepine
Carbimazole
Certolizumab
Chlordiazepoxide
Chlorpropamide
Ciprofloxacin
Clomiphene
Co-Trimoxazole
Codeine
Colchicine
Dapsone
Dasatinib
Denosumab
Diclofenac
Disopyramide
Dupilumab
Echinacea
Estrogens
Etanercept
Fluoxetine
Furosemide
Glucagon
Gold & Gold Compounds
Granulocyte Colony-Stimulating Factor (G-CSF)
Hepatitis B Vaccine
Human Papillomavirus (HPV) Vaccine
Hydralazine
Hydroxychloroquine
Ibuprofen
Imatinib
Indomethacin
Interferon Alfa
Isotretinoin
Ixazomib
Levofloxacin
Lidocaine
Meclofenamate
Medroxyprogesterone
Meprobamate
Metamizole
Methimazole
Methyldopa
Minocycline
Montelukast
Naproxen
Nifedipine
Nitrofurantoin
Nivolumab
Omeprazole
Oral Contraceptives
Paroxetine Hydrochloride
Penicillamine
Ponatinib
Propylthiouracil
Quinacrine
Smallpox Vaccine
Streptomycin
Sulfamethoxazole
Sulfasalazine
Sulfisoxazole
Terbinafine
Thalidomide
Ticlopidine
Tretinoin
Trimethoprim
Verapamil
Zileuton
Zoledronate

Exanthems
Abacavir
Acamprosate
Acebutolol
Acenocoumarol
Acetaminophen
Acetazolamide
Acetohexamide
Acitretin
Acyclovir
Aldesleukin
Allopurinol
Alprazolam
Amantadine
Amcinonide
Amikacin
Amiloride
Aminocaproic Acid
Aminoglutethimide
Aminophylline
Aminosalicylate Sodium
Amiodarone
Amlodipine
Amoxapine
Amoxicillin
Amphotericin B
Ampicillin
Amprenavir
Anastrozole
Anidulafungin
Anistreplase
Anthrax Vaccine
Apalutamide
Aprotinin
Arsenic
Aspartame
Aspirin
Astemizole
Atazanavir
Atovaquone
Atovaquone/Proguanil
Azacitidine
Azathioprine
Azelastine
Azithromycin
Aztreonam
Bacampicillin
Baclofen
Benactyzine
Benazepril
Bendamustine
Bendroflumethiazide
Benznidazole
Betamethasone
Bevacizumab
Bexarotene
Bicalutamide
Bismuth
Bleomycin
Bortezomib
Bosentan
Bosutinib
Brompheniramine
Budesonide
Bupropion
Buserelin
Busulfan
Butabarbital
Butalbital
Candesartan
Captopril
Carbamazepine
Carboplatin
Carisoprodol
Carmustine
Carvedilol
Cefaclor
Cefadroxil
Cefamandole
Cefazolin
Cefdinir
Cefepime
Cefoperazone
Cefotaxime
Cefoxitin
Cefpodoxime
Ceftazidime
Ceftriaxone
Cefuroxime
Celecoxib
Cephalexin
Cephalothin
Cephapirin
Cephradine
Ceritinib
Cetirizine
Cetuximab
Cevimeline
Chloral Hydrate
Chlorambucil
Chloramphenicol
Chlordiazepoxide
Chlormezanone
Chloroquine
Chlorothiazide
Chlorpromazine
Chlorpropamide
Cimetidine
Ciprofloxacin
Cisplatin
Citalopram
Cladribine
Clarithromycin
Clemastine
Clindamycin
Clofibrate
Clomiphene
Clonazepam
Clopidogrel
Clorazepate
Cloxacillin
Clozapine
Co-Trimoxazole
Cobimetinib
Codeine
Colchicine
Colestipol
Cyanocobalamin
Cyclamate
Cyclophosphamide
Cycloserine
Cyclosporine
Cyclothiazide
Cyproheptadine
Cytarabine
Dabigatran
Dabrafenib
Dacarbazine
Daclizumab
Dalteparin
Danazol
Dantrolene
Dapsone
Daunorubicin
Deferasirox
Delavirdine
Denosumab
Desipramine
Dexamethasone
Diazepam
Diclofenac
Dicloxacillin
Dicumarol
Dicyclomine
Diethylpropion
Diethylstilbestrol
Diflunisal
Digoxin
Diltiazem
Dimenhydrinate
Diphenhydramine
Dipyridamole
Disopyramide
Disulfiram
Docetaxel
Docusate
Doxazosin
Doxepin
Doxorubicin
Doxycycline
Dronedarone
Durvalumab
Efavirenz
Eletriptan
Elotuzumab
Emtricitabine
Enalapril
Enoxacin
Enoxaparin
Entecavir
Ephedrine
Epoetin Alfa
Eprosartan
Erlotinib
Erythromycin
Esomeprazole
Estramustine
Estrogens
Etanercept
Ethacrynic Acid
Ethambutol
Ethionamide
Ethosuximide
Etodolac
Etoposide
Etoricoxib
Etravirine
Everolimus
Exemestane
Felodipine
Fenofibrate
Fenoprofen
Flecainide
Fluconazole
Flucytosine
Fludarabine
Fluorouracil
Fluoxetine
Flurazepam

Flurbiprofen
Flutamide
Folic Acid
Foscarnet
Fosfomycin
Furazolidone
Furosemide
Gabapentin
Galantamine
Ganciclovir
Gatifloxacin
Gefitinib
Gemcitabine
Gemfibrozil
Gemifloxacin
Gentamicin
Ginkgo Biloba
Glimepiride
Glipizide
Glucagon
Glyburide
Gold & Gold Compounds
Granulocyte Colony-Stimulating Factor (G-CSF)
Grepafloxacin
Griseofulvin
Halothane
Heparin
Heroin
Hydralazine
Hydrochlorothiazide
Hydromorphone
Hydroxychloroquine
Hydroxyurea
Hydroxyzine
Ibrutinib
Ibuprofen
Icodextrin
Idarubicin
Imatinib
Imipenem/Cilastatin
Imipramine
Imiquimod
Indapamide
Indinavir
Indomethacin
Infliximab
Insulin
Interferon Alfa
Iobenguane
Ipilimumab
Irbesartan
Irinotecan
Isocarboxazid
Isoniazid
Isosorbide Dinitrate
Isotretinoin
Isradipine
Itraconazole
Ivermectin
Ixazomib
Ketoconazole
Ketoprofen
Ketorolac
Labetalol
Lamivudine
Lamotrigine
Lapatinib
Lenalidomide
Lenvatinib
Letrozole
Levamisole
Levetiracetam
Levodopa
Levofloxacin
Lidocaine
Lincomycin
Linezolid
Lisinopril
Lithium
Loracarbef
Lovastatin
Maprotiline
Measles, Mumps & Rubella (MMR) Virus Vaccine
Mebendazole
Mechlorethamine
Meclofenamate
Mefenamic Acid
Mefloquine
Meloxicam
Melphalan
Memantine
Mephenytoin
Meprobamate
Mercaptopurine
Meropenem
Mesalamine
Mesna
Metamizole
Methazolamide
Methenamine
Methicillin
Methimazole
Methohexital
Methotrexate
Methoxsalen
Methsuximide
Methyldopa
Methylphenidate
Metoclopramide
Metoprolol
Metronidazole
Mexiletine
Miconazole
Minocycline
Minoxidil
Misoprostol
Mitomycin
Mitotane
Moexipril
Moricizine
Morphine
Nabumetone
Nadolol
Nafarelin
Nafcillin
Nalidixic Acid
Naltrexone
Naproxen
Naratriptan
Nefazodone
Nelfinavir
Neomycin
Nevirapine
Niacin
Nifedipine
Nilotinib
Nimesulide
Nimodipine
Nisoldipine
Nitisinone
Nitrofurantoin
Nivolumab
Norfloxacin
Nystatin
Octreotide
Ofloxacin
Olanzapine
Olmesartan
Olsalazine
Omega-3 Fatty Acids
Omeprazole
Oral Contraceptives
Oxacillin
Oxaliplatin
Oxaprozin
Oxcarbazepine
Paclitaxel
Paliperidone
Pamidronate
Panobinostat
Pantoprazole
Paromomycin
Paroxetine Hydrochloride
PEG-Interferon
Pembrolizumab
Pemoline
Penbutolol
Penicillamine
Penicillin V
Pentagastrin
Pentamidine
Pentazocine
Pentobarbital
Pentostatin
Perflutren
Perphenazine
Phenazopyridine
Phenobarbital
Phenolphthalein
Phenylbutazone
Phenytoin
Phytonadione
Piperacillin
Piperacillin/Tazobactam
Piroxicam
Potassium Iodide
Prazosin
Prednisolone
Primaquine
Primidone
Pristinamycin
Procainamide
Procarbazine
Prochlorperazine
Promazine
Promethazine
Propafenone
Propofol
Propolis
Propoxyphene
Propranolol
Propylthiouracil
Protamine Sulfate
Pseudoephedrine
Pyrazinamide
Pyrimethamine
Quinacrine
Quinapril
Quinethazone
Quinidine
Quinine
Quinupristin/Dalfopristin
Ramipril
Ranitidine
Rapacuronium
Regorafenib
Repaglinide
Ribavirin
Rifampin
Ritodrine
Ritonavir
Rituximab
Rivaroxaban
Rivastigmine
Rofecoxib
Ropinirole
Rucaparib
Saccharin
Saquinavir
Scopolamine
Sertraline
Simvastatin
Smallpox Vaccine
Sorafenib
Sparfloxacin
Spironolactone
Streptokinase
Streptomycin
Streptozocin
Succimer
Sucralfate
Sulfadiazine
Sulfadoxins
Sulfamethoxazole
Sulfasalazine
Sulfinpyrazone
Sulfisoxazole
Sulindac
Tacrine
Tacrolimus
Tamoxifen
Teicoplanin
Telaprevir
Telmisartan
Temozolomide
Temsirolimus
Terazosin
Terbinafine
Terfenadine
Testosterone
Tetracycline
Tetrazepam
Thalidomide
Thiabendazole
Thiamine
Thimerosal
Thioguanine
Thiopental
Thioridazine
Thiothixene
Tiagabine
Ticarcillin
Ticlopidine
Tinzaparin
Tiopronin
Tipranavir
Tizanidine
Tobramycin
Tocainide
Tolazamide
Tolazoline
Tolbutamide
Tolmetin
Topiramate
Tramadol
Trametinib
Trazodone
Triamcinolone
Trimeprazine
Trimethadione

Trimetrexate
Troleandomycin
Uracil/Tegafur
Valdecoxib
Valproic Acid
Valsartan
Vancomycin
Vardenafil
Varenicline
Vemurafenib
Venlafaxine
Verapamil
Vincristine
Vitamin A
Vorapaxar
Vorinostat
Warfarin
Zalcitabine
Zidovudine
Ziprasidone
Zoledronate
Zonisamide

Exfoliative dermatitis

Acamprosate
Acetaminophen
Acitretin
Afatinib
Aldesleukin
Alitretinoin
Allopurinol
Aminoglutethimide
Aminolevulinic Acid
Aminophylline
Aminosalicylate Sodium
Amiodarone
Amobarbital
Amoxicillin
Amphotericin B
Ampicillin
Arsenic
Aspirin
Avelumab
Azathioprine
Aztreonam
Benzyl Alcohol
Bexarotene
Bismuth
Bosutinib
Bumetanide
Butabarbital
Butalbital
Capecitabine
Captopril
Carbamazepine
Carvedilol
Cefoxitin
Cefpodoxime
Celecoxib
Chlorambucil
Chloroquine
Chlorpropamide
Cimetidine
Ciprofloxacin
Cisplatin
Clofazimine
Clofibrate
Clonazepam
Co-Trimoxazole
Codeine
Cytarabine
Dapsone
Dasatinib
Daunorubicin
Demeclocycline
Desipramine
Dexamethasone
Diazepam
Diclofenac
Dicloxacillin
Diethylstilbestrol
Diflunisal
Diltiazem
Doxorubicin
Efavirenz
Eletriptan
Enalapril
Enoxacin
Ephedrine
Esmolol
Esomeprazole
Estrogens
Ethambutol
Ethosuximide
Fenoprofen
Flecainide
Fluconazole
Flurbiprofen
Fluvoxamine
Fosphenytoin
Furosemide
Gefitinib
Gemcitabine
Gemfibrozil
Gentamicin
Gold & Gold Compounds
Granulocyte Colony-Stimulating Factor (G-CSF)
Grepafloxacin
Griseofulvin
Hydroxychloroquine
Ibuprofen
Icodextrin
Idelalisib
Imatinib
Imipramine
Indomethacin
Irinotecan
Isavuconazonium Sulfate
Isoniazid
Isotretinoin
Ixabepilone
Ixazomib
Ketoconazole
Ketoprofen
Ketorolac
Lansoprazole
Lapatinib
Leflunomide
Lenalidomide
Lidocaine
Lisinopril
Lithium
Lomefloxacin
Meclofenamate
Mefenamic Acid
Mefloquine
Mephenytoin
Mephobarbital
Methicillin
Methotrexate
Methsuximide
Methylphenidate
Mexiletine
Mezlocillin
Minocycline
Mitomycin
Nalidixic Acid
Nevirapine
Nifedipine
Nilotinib
Nisoldipine
Nitisinone
Nitrofurantoin
Nitroglycerin
Nivolumab
Omacetaxine
Ombitasvir/Paritaprevir/Ritonavir
Omeprazole
Oxaprozin
Oxcarbazepine
Oxytetracycline
Panitumumab
Paramethadione
Pazopanib
Pembrolizumab
Pentobarbital
Pentostatin
Phenobarbital
Phenolphthalein
Phenylbutazone
Phenytoin
Piroxicam
Procarbazine
Propranolol
Propylthiouracil
Pseudoephedrine
Pyrazinamide
Pyrimethamine
Quinacrine
Quinapril
Quinidine
Quinine
Raltitrexed
Rifampin
Risperidone
Rivastigmine
Romidepsin
Secobarbital
Senna
Sildenafil
Smallpox Vaccine
Sorafenib
Sparfloxacin
Streptomycin
Strontium Ranelate
Sulfacetamide
Sulfadoxine
Sulfamethoxazole
Sulfasalazine
Sulfisoxazole
Sulindac
Sunitinib
Tacrolimus
Teicoplanin
Terfenadine
Tetracycline
Thalidomide
Tiagabine
Ticlopidine
Tizanidine
Tobramycin
Tocainide
Trazodone
Tretinoin
Trimethadione
Trimethoprim
Trovafloxacin
Umbralisib
Vancomycin
Venlafaxine
Verapamil
Vitamin A
Voriconazole
Vorinostat
Yohimbine
Zalcitabine
Ziprasidone

Fixed eruption

Aceclofenac
Acetaminophen
Acyclovir
Adalimumab
Albendazole
Alendronate
Allopurinol
Aminosalicylate Sodium
Amitriptyline
Amlexanox
Amodiaquine
Amoxicillin
Amphotericin B
Ampicillin
Arsenic
Aspirin
Atenolol
Atorvastatin
Atropine Sulfate
Azathioprine
Azithromycin
Bacampicillin
BCG Vaccine
Bisacodyl
Bismuth
Bisoprolol
Bleomycin
Bucillamine
Butabarbital
Butalbital
Carbamazepine
Carisoprodol
Cefaclor
Cefazolin
Cefixime
Cefotaxime
Ceftazidime
Ceftriaxone
Celecoxib
Cephalexin
Cetirizine
Chloral Hydrate
Chloramphenicol
Chlordiazepoxide
Chlorhexidine
Chlormezanone
Chloroquine
Chlorothiazide
Chlorpromazine
Chlorpropamide
Chlorthalidone
Cimetidine
Ciprofloxacin
Clarithromycin
Clindamycin
Clioquinol
Clopidogrel
Co-Trimoxazole
Cocaine
Codeine
Colchicine
Cyproterone
Dacarbazine

Danazol
Dapsone
Demeclocycline
Dextromethorphan
Diazepam
Diclofenac
Diflunisal
Dimenhydrinate
Diphenhydramine
Disulfiram
Docetaxel
Doxorubicin
Doxycycline
Ephedrine
Erdosteine
Erythromycin
Esomeprazole
Estrogens
Etanercept
Ethchlorvynol
Etodolac
Etoricoxib
Finasteride
Flavoxate
Flecainide
Fluconazole
Flurbiprofen
Foscarnet
Furosemide
Ganciclovir
Ginkgo Biloba
Glipizide
Griseofulvin
Guanethidine
Heparin
Heroin
Hydralazine
Hydrochlorothiazide
Hydroxychloroquine
Hydroxyurea
Hydroxyzine
Ibuprofen
Imipramine
Indapamide
Indomethacin
Infliximab
Influenza Vaccine
Iohexol
Iopromide
Isotretinoin
Itraconazole
Ivermectin
Ketoconazole
Lamotrigine
Leuprolide
Levamisole
Levocetirizine
Levofloxacin
Licorice
Lidocaine
Loperamide
Loratadine
Lorazepam
Meclofenamate
Mefenamic Acid
Melatonin
Meloxicam
Meprobamate
Mesna
Metamizole
Metformin
Methenamine
Methimazole
Methyldopa
Methylphenidate
Metronidazole
Miconazole
Minocycline
Modafinil
Nabumetone
Naproxen
Neomycin
Niacin
Nifedipine
Nimesulide
Nitrofurantoin
Norfloxacin
Nystatin
Ofloxacin
Olanzapine
Olopatadine
Omeprazole
Ondansetron
Oral Contraceptives
Orphenadrine
Oxazepam
Oxcarbazepine
Oxybutynin
Oxytetracycline
Paclitaxel
Papaverine
Paroxetine Hydrochloride
PEG-Interferon
Pentobarbital
Phenobarbital
Phenolphthalein
Phenylbutazone
Phenylephrine
Phenylpropanolamine
Phenytoin
Piperacillin/Tazobactam
Piroxicam
Procarbazine
Prochlorperazine
Promethazine
Propofol
Propolis
Propranolol
Pseudoephedrine
Pyrazinamide
Pyridoxine
Pyrimethamine
Quinacrine
Quinidine
Quinine
Ranitidine
Ribavirin
Rifampin
Rofecoxib
Ropinirole
Roxithromycin
Rupatadine
Saccharin
Saquinavir
Scopolamine
Sorafenib
Streptomycin
Sulfadiazine
Sulfadoxine
Sulfamethoxazole
Sulfasalazine
Sulfisoxazole
Sulindac
Sunitinib
Tadalafil
Tartrazine
Temazepam
Terbinafine
Terfenadine
Tetracycline
Thiabendazole
Thiopental
Ticagrelor
Ticlopidine
Tinidazole
Tolbutamide
Topiramate
Topotecan
Tosufloxacin
Tranexamic Acid
Triamcinolone
Trifluoperazine
Trimethoprim
Tripelennamine
Triprolidine
Ursodiol
Valproic Acid
Vancomycin
Voriconazole
Zolmitriptan

Gingival hyperplasia / gingival hypertrophy / gingival enlargement / gingival overgrowth

Amlodipine
Basiliximab
Carbamazepine
Cevimeline
Clarithromycin
Clobazam
Co-Trimoxazole
Cycloserine
Cyclosporine
Diltiazem
Erythromycin
Eslicarbazepine
Everolimus
Felodipine
Fosphenytoin
Isradipine
Ketoconazole
Lamotrigine
Levetiracetam
Levonorgestrel
Lithium
Marihuana
Metoprolol
Mycophenolate
Nicardipine
Nifedipine
Nisoldipine
Oral Contraceptives
Palifermin
Penicillamine
Phenobarbital
Phenytoin
Primidone
Propranolol
Sertraline
Sirolimus
Tacrolimus
Tartrazine
Tiagabine
Topiramate
Valproic Acid
Vemurafenib
Verapamil
Vigabatrin
Voriconazole
Zonisamide

Hand-foot syndrome (palmar–plantar erythrodysesthesia)

Afatinib
Aflibercept
Avapritinib
Avelumab
Axitinib
Bevacizumab
Bleomycin
Bosutinib
Brentuximab Vedotin
Cabazitaxel
Cabozantinib
Capecitabine
Carboplatin
Cetuximab
Cisplatin
Clofarabine
Co-Trimoxazole
Cobimetinib
Cyclophosphamide
Cytarabine
Dabrafenib
Dacomitinib
Dasatinib
Daunorubicin
Docetaxel
Dolutegravir
Doxorubicin
Encorafenib
Epirubicin
Erdafitinib
Erlotinib
Etoposide
Everolimus
Fluorouracil
Gefitinib
Gemcitabine
Hydroxyurea
Ibandronate
Idarubicin
Imatinib
Infigratinib
Infliximab
Interferon Alfa
Ipilimumab
Irinotecan
Ixabepilone
Ketoconazole
Lapatinib
Lenvatinib
Letrozole
Leucovorin
Mercaptopurine
Mesalamine
Methotrexate
Mitomycin
Mobocertinib
Neratinib
Nilotinib
Nintedanib
Olaparib
Oxaliplatin
Paclitaxel
Palifermin
Panitumumab
Pazopanib
PEG-Interferon
Pemigatinib
Phenytoin
Regorafenib
Ripretinib

Rucaparib
Selumetinib
Sorafenib
Sunitinib
Tegafur/Gimeracil/Oteracil
Temozolomide
Temsirolimus
Tivozanib
Trabectedin
Trametinib
Trastuzumab
Tucatinib
Turmeric
Uracil/Tegafur
Valproic Acid
Vandetanib
Varenicline
Vemurafenib
Vincristine
Vinorelbine
Vorinostat

Lichenoid eruption / lichenoid reaction

Acebutolol
Acyclovir
Adalimumab
Alendronate
Allopurinol
Aminosalicylate Sodium
Amlodipine
Amoxicillin
Anakinra
Apalutamide
Apixaban
Aspirin
Atenolol
Atorvastatin
Avelumab
Azathioprine
BCG Vaccine
Captopril
Carbamazepine
Carvedilol
Ceftriaxone
Certolizumab
Chloral Hydrate
Chloroquine
Chlorothiazide
Chlorpromazine
Chlorpropamide
Cinnarizine
Clonazepam
Clopidogrel
Co-Trimoxazole
Colchicine
Crizotinib
Crizotinib
Cycloserine
Cyclosporine
Dactinomycin
Demeclocycline
Diazoxide
Diflunisal
Diltiazem
Dorzolamide
Durvalumab
Efavirenz
Enalapril
Esomeprazole
Etanercept
Ethambutol
Fluoxymesterone
Fluvastatin
Furosemide
Glimepiride
Glyburide
Gold & Gold Compounds
Griseofulvin
Henna
Hepatitis B Vaccine
Hydrochlorothiazide
Hydroxychloroquine
Hydroxyurea
Imatinib
Immune Globulin IV
Infliximab
Influenza Vaccine
Ipilimumab
Irbesartan
Isoniazid
Isotretinoin
Labetalol
Lansoprazole
Leflunomide
Levamisole
Lisinopril
Lovastatin
Mercaptopurine
Metformin
Methamphetamine
Methyldopa
Methyltestosterone
Metoprolol
Nadolol
Naproxen
Nebivolol
Nelfinavir
Nifedipine
Nilotinib
Nivolumab
Obinutuzumab
Olanzapine
Omeprazole
Oral Contraceptives
Orlistat
Osimertinib
Pantoprazole
PEG-Interferon
Pembrolizumab
Penicillamine
Peppermint
Phenytoin
Pindolol
Pirfenidone
Piroxicam
Pravastatin
Propranolol
Propylthiouracil
Pyrimethamine
Quinacrine
Quinidine
Quinine
Ranitidine
Relugolix
Ribavirin
Rifampin
Risperidone
Roxatidine
Salsalate
Sildenafil
Simeprevir
Simvastatin
Sofosbuvir
Solifenacin
Sotalol
Sparfloxacin
Spironolactone
Streptomycin
Sulfamethoxazole
Temazepam
Tenofovir Disoproxil
Terazosin
Terbinafine
Teriflunomide
Testosterone
Tetracycline
Thimerosal
Thioridazine
Timolol
Tiopronin
Tiotropium
Tolazamide
Tolbutamide
Torsemide
Trichlormethiazide
Tripelennamine
Triprolidine
Ursodiol
Venlafaxine
Zoster Vaccine

Lupus erythematosus (subacute cutaneous lupus erythematosus (SCLE)

Acebutolol
Acetazolamide
Adalimumab
Albuterol
Aldesleukin
Allopurinol
Aminoglutethimide
Aminosalicylate Sodium
Amiodarone
Amitriptyline
Amlodipine
Anastrozole
Anthrax Vaccine
Atenolol
Atorvastatin
Belatacept
Betaxolol
Bevacizumab
Bortezomib
Bupropion
Butabarbital
Butalbital
Capecitabine
Captopril
Carbamazepine
Carbimazole
Cefepime
Cefuroxime
Celecoxib
Celiprolol
Cenobamate
Chlorambucil
Chlordiazepoxide
Chlorothiazide
Chlorpromazine
Chlorpropamide
Chlorthalidone
Cilazapril
Cimetidine
Cinnarizine
Citalopram
Clobazam
Clofibrate
Clonidine
Clozapine
Co-Trimoxazole
Covid-19 Vaccine, mRNA
Cyclophosphamide
Cyclosporine
Cysteamine
Danazol
Dapsone
Dasatinib
Denosumab
Diethylstilbestrol
Diltiazem
Disopyramide
Docetaxel
Domperidone
Doxazosin
Doxorubicin
Doxycycline
Durvalumab
Efalizumab
Emtricitabine
Enalapril
Erlotinib
Esomeprazole
Estrogens
Etanercept
Ethambutol
Ethionamide
Ethosuximide
Fenofibrate
Fluorouracil
Fluoxymesterone
Fluphenazine
Flutamide
Fluvastatin
Fosphenytoin
Furosemide
Gemcitabine
Gold & Gold Compounds
Golimumab
Granulocyte Colony-Stimulating Factor (G-CSF)
Griseofulvin
Hepatitis B Vaccine
Human Papillomavirus (HPV) Vaccine
Hydralazine
Hydrochlorothiazide
Hydroxyurea
Ibandronate
Ibuprofen
Imipramine
Imiquimod
Immune Globulin IV
Immune Globulin SC
Infliximab
Interferon Alfa
Interferon Beta
Ipilimumab
Isoniazid
Labetalol
Lamotrigine
Lansoprazole
Leflunomide
Letrozole
Leuprolide
Levetiracetam
Levodopa
Lidocaine
Lisinopril
Lithium
Lovastatin
Mephenytoin
Meprobamate
Mercaptopurine

Mesalamine
Methimazole
Methoxsalen
Methsuximide
Methyldopa
Methyltestosterone
Methysergide
Metoprolol
Mexiletine
Minocycline
Minoxidil
Mitotane
Nafcillin
Nalidixic Acid
Naproxen
Nifedipine
Nitrofurantoin
Nivolumab
Olsalazine
Omeprazole
Oral Contraceptives
Osimertinib
Oxcarbazepine
Paclitaxel
Pantoprazole
PEG-Interferon
Pembrolizumab
Penicillamine
Pentobarbital
Perphenazine
Phenelzine
Phenobarbital
Phenolphthalein
Phenylbutazone
Phenytoin
Pindolol
Piroxicam
Potassium Iodide
Pravastatin
Prazosin
Prednicarbate
Primidone
Procainamide
Promethazine
Propafenone
Propranolol
Propylthiouracil
Psoralens
Quinidine
Quinine
Ranitidine
Reserpine
Ribavirin
Ribociclib
Rifabutin
Rifampin
Rilpivirine
Rituximab
Secukinumab
Semaglutide
Sertraline
Simvastatin
Smallpox Vaccine
Somatropin
Spironolactone
Streptomycin
Sulfadiazine
Sulfamethoxazole
Sulfasalazine
Sulfisoxazole
Tamoxifen
Tenofovir Disoproxil
Terbinafine
Terfenadine
Teriflunomide
Testosterone
Tetracycline
Thioridazine
Ticlopidine
Timolol
Tiopronin
Tiotropium
Tocainide
Triamterene
Trichlormethiazide
Trientine
Trimethadione
Trimethoprim
Trioxsalen
Uracil/Tegafur
Ustekinumab
Valproic Acid
Vancomycin
Verapamil
Vitamin E
Voriconazole
Yohimbine
Zafirlukast
Zinc
Ziprasidone
Zonisamide

Onycholysis

Acitretin
Adalimumab
Allopurinol
Bleomycin
Capecitabine
Captopril
Clofazimine
Dabrafenib
Docetaxel
Doxorubicin
Erdafitinib
Estrogens
Etoposide
Gold & Gold Compounds
Hydroxyurea
Ibuprofen
Irinotecan
Isotretinoin
Ketoprofen
Methotrexate
Mitoxantrone
Mycophenolate
Nintedanib
Nitrofurantoin
Nivolumab
Oral Contraceptives
Paclitaxel
Pemetrexed
Propranolol
Roxithromycin
Tasonermin
Tetracycline
Valproic Acid
Vemurafenib

Paresthesias

Acamprosate
Acetazolamide
Acitretin
Acyclovir
Adalimumab
Adenosine
Afamelanotide
Agalsidase
Alitretinoin
Allopurinol
Almotriptan
Alprazolam
Altretamine
Amifampridine
Amikacin
Amiloride
Amiodarone
Amlodipine
Amoxapine
Amphotericin B
Amprenavir
Anagrelide
Apraclonidine
Arbutamine
Arformoterol
Aripiprazole
Arsenic
Artemether/Lumefantrine
Articaine
Aspirin
Astemizole
Atorvastatin
Avacopan
Avanafil
Azatadine
Azithromycin
Baclofen
Basiliximab
Bedaquiline
Benazepril
Benznidazole
Benzthiazide
Bepridil
Betaxolol
Bicalutamide
Blinatumomab
Bortezomib
Bremelanotide
Brivaracetam
Bromocriptine
Brompheniramine
Bupivacaine
Bupropion
Buspirone
Cabergoline
Cabozantinib
Caffeine
Calcitonin
Candesartan
Capecitabine
Captopril
Carbamazepine
Carboplatin
Carfilzomib
Carisoprodol
Carteolol
Carvedilol
Caspofungin
Ceftazidime
Ceftibuten
Ceftizoxime
Ceftolozane & Tazobactam
Celecoxib
Cephapirin
Ceritinib
Cetirizine
Cevimeline
Chloramphenicol
Chlorothiazide
Chlorpheniramine
Chlorthalidone
Cidofovir
Cilostazol
Cinacalcet
Cinoxacin
Ciprofloxacin
Cisplatin
Citalopram
Clemastine
Clonazepam
Clopidogrel
Clozapine
Coagulation Factor IX (Recombinant)
Colistin
Copanlisib
Crisaborole
Cyclamate
Cyclobenzaprine
Cyclophosphamide
Cyclosporine
Cyproheptadine
Dalfampridine
Daptomycin
Dasatinib
Delafloxacin
Delavirdine
Demeclocycline
Denileukin
Desvenlafaxine
Dexamethasone
Dexchlorpheniramine
Dichlorphenamide
Diclofenac
Difelikefalin
Diflunisal
Dihydroergotamine
Diltiazem
Dimenhydrinate
Diphenhydramine
Dipyridamole
Dirithromycin
Disopyramide
Dobutamine
Docetaxel
Dofetilide
Dolutegravir
Donepezil
Doxycycline
Duloxetine
Efavirenz
Eflornithine
Eletriptan
Eltrombopag
Emtricitabine
Enalapril
Enoxacin
Entecavir
Entrectinib
Enzalutamide
Epirubicin
Epoetin Alfa
Epoprostenol
Eprosartan
Ergotamine
Ertapenem
Escitalopram
Esmolol
Esomeprazole
Estazolam
Eszopiclone
Etanercept
Etelcalcetide
Ethoxzolamide
Etravirine

Evolocumab
Exemestane
Ezetimibe
Ezogabine
Famciclovir
Famotidine
Febuxostat
Felbamate
Felodipine
Fentanyl
Ferric Gluconate
Ferumoxsil
Ferumoxytol
Fexinidazole
Fingolimod
Flecainide
Fluconazole
Flucytosine
Fludarabine
Flumazenil
Fluorouracil
Fluoxetine
Flurbiprofen
Flutamide
Fosamprenavir
Foscarnet
Fosfomycin
Fosinopril
Fosphenytoin
Frovatriptan
Fulvestrant
Gabapentin
Gadobenate
Gadobutrol
Gadodiamide
Gadofosveset
Gadopentetate
Gadoteridol
Gadoversetamide
Gadoxetate
Galantamine
Ganciclovir
Gatifloxacin
Gemcitabine
Gemfibrozil
Gentamicin
Glatiramer
Glipizide
Glucarpidase
Glyburide
Grepafloxacin
Griseofulvin
Guanadrel
Guanethidine
Guanfacine
Halofantrine
Histrelin
Human Papillomavirus Vaccine (Bivalent)
Hydrocodone
Hydroflumethiazide
Ibuprofen
Imatinib
Imipenem/Cilastatin
Indapamide
Indinavir
Indomethacin
Infliximab
Inotersen
Insulin
Interferon Alfa
Interferon Beta
Iodixanol
Iohexol
Iopromide
Ioversol
Ipilimumab
Ipratropium
Irbesartan
Isavuconazonium Sulfate
Isoniazid
Isradipine
Ixazomib
Ketoconazole
Ketoprofen
Ketorolac
Labetalol
Lamivudine
Lamotrigine
Lansoprazole
Laronidase
Lasmiditan
Leflunomide
Leucovorin
Leuprolide
Levalbuterol
Levamisole
Levetiracetam
Levobupivacaine
Levofloxacin
Levomilnacipran
Lidocaine
Lisinopril
Lomefloxacin
Loratadine
Lorcainide
Losartan
Lovastatin
Lubiprostone
Maraviroc
MDMA
Meclizine
Meclofenamate
Medroxyprogesterone
Mefloquine
Meloxicam
Menadione
Methazolamide
Methimazole
Methyclothiazide
Methyldopa
Metoclopramide
Metolazone
Metronidazole
Mexiletine
Midodrine
Miglustat
Milnacipran
Miltefosine
Minocycline
Mirtazapine
Mitapivat
Mitomycin
Modafinil
Monosodium Glutamate
Moricizine
Moxifloxacin
Nabumetone
Nadolol
Nafarelin
Naproxen
Naratriptan
Nebivolol
Nefazodone
Nelarabine
Nelfinavir
Nesiritide
Nevirapine
Niacin
Niacinamide
Nicardipine
Nifedipine
Nilotinib
Nilutamide
Nisoldipine
Nitrofurantoin
Nivolumab
Nizatidine
Nusinersen
Ofloxacin
Omacetaxine
Omalizumab
Omeprazole
Ondansetron
Oseltamivir
Oxaliplatin
Oxilan
Oxprenolol
Oxycodone
Oxymetazoline
Oxytetracycline
Paclitaxel
Palifermin
Pandemic Influenza Vaccine (H1N1)
Pantoprazole
Paricalcitol
Paroxetine Hydrochloride
Pegaspargase
Pegvisomant
Pembrolizumab
Pentamidine
Pentostatin
Pentoxifylline
Perampanel
Perflutren
Pergolide
Perindopril
Phentermine
Phenytoin
Pindolol
Piperacillin
Pirbuterol
Piroxicam
Pizotifen
Plasma (Human) Blood Product
Posaconazole
Pramipexole
Pravastatin
Prazosin
Prednicarbate
Pregabalin
Prilocaine
Procarbazine
Promethazine
Propafenone
Propylthiouracil
Pyridoxine
Quetiapine
Quinapril
Quinupristin/Dalfopristin
Rabeprazole
Ramipril
Ranolazine
Rasagiline
Rasburicase
Reboxetine
Repaglinide
Rifabutin
Rifampin
Riluzole
Rimantadine
Risedronate
Risperidone
Ritonavir
Rivaroxaban
Rivastigmine
Rizatriptan
Rofecoxib
Romiplostim
Ropinirole
Ropivacaine
Rosuvastatin
Rotigotine
Saquinavir
Sertraline
Sibutramine
Sildenafil
Siltuximab
Sincalide
Sipuleucel-T
Sirolimus
Smallpox Vaccine
Sodium Oxybate
Somatropin
Sonidegib
Sotalol
Sparfloxacin
St John's Wort
Stavudine
Streptomycin
Succimer
Sufentanil
Sugammadex
Sulfasalazine
Sulindac
Sumatriptan
Tacrine
Tacrolimus
Tadalafil
Taliglucerase
Tartrazine
Tecovirimat
Tegafur/Gimeracil/Oteracil
Telaprevir
Telbivudine
Telithromycin
Telmisartan
Temozolomide
Terazosin
Terfenadine
Teriflunomide
Teriparatide
Tesamorelin
Testosterone
Tetrabenazine
Tetracycline
Thalidomide
Thallium
Thiamine
Thyrotropin Alfa
Tiagabine
Tibolone
Tiludronate
Timolol
Tinidazole
Tiotropium
Tizanidine
Tobramycin
Tocainide
Tofacitinib

Tolcapone
Tolterodine
Topiramate
Topotecan
Torsemide
Trabectedin
Tramadol
Trandolapril
Trastuzumab
Travoprost
Trazodone
Tretinoin
Triazolam
Trihexyphenidyl
Trimeprazine
Tripelennamine
Triprolidine
Triptorelin
Trovafloxacin
Unoprostone
Valacyclovir
Valdecoxib
Valganciclovir
Valproic Acid
Valsartan
Vardenafil
Venlafaxine
Verapamil
Vernakalant
Vilazodone
Vinblastine
Vincristine
Vinorelbine
Voriconazole
Zaleplon
Ziconotide
Zidovudine
Zileuton
Ziprasidone
Zoledronate
Zolmitriptan
Zolpidem
Zonisamide
Zuclopenthixol

Pemphigus vulgaris

Aldesleukin
Amoxicillin
Bucillamine
Cefaclor
Cilazapril
Cocaine
Imiquimod
Ingenol Mebutate
Interferon Beta
Nifedipine
Penicillamine
Psoralens
Quinapril
Rifampin
Tiopronin
Typhoid Vaccine

Peyronie's disease

Acebutolol
Betaxolol
Carvedilol
Labetalol
Methotrexate
Metoprolol
Nadolol
Papaverine
Pindolol
Propranolol
Ropinirole
Timolol

Photosensitivity

Acamprosate
Aceclofenac
Acetohexamide
Acetylcysteine
Acitretin
Acyclovir
Aldesleukin
Alectinib
Allopurinol
Almotriptan
Aloe Vera (Gel, Juice, Leaf)
Alprazolam
Amantadine
Amiloride
Aminolevulinic Acid
Aminosalicylate Sodium
Amiodarone
Amitriptyline
Amlodipine
Amoxapine
Anagrelide
Apremilast
Arsenic
Astemizole
Atorvastatin
Atropine Sulfate
Azatadine
Azathioprine
Azilsartan
Azithromycin
Benazepril
Bendroflumethiazide
Benztropine
Bergamot
Bezafibrate
Bicalutamide
Brigatinib
Brompheniramine
Bumetanide
Bupropion
Butabarbital
Butalbital
Calcipotriol
Canagliflozin
Candesartan
Capecitabine
Captopril
Carbamazepine
Carisoprodol
Carvedilol
Cefazolin
Ceftazidime
Celecoxib
Ceritinib
Cetirizine
Cevimeline
Chlorambucil
Chlordiazepoxide
Chlorhexidine
Chloroquine
Chlorothiazide
Chlorpheniramine
Chlorpromazine
Chlorpropamide
Chlortetracycline
Chlorthalidone
Ciprofloxacin
Clemastine
Clofazimine
Clofibrate
Clomipramine
Clopidogrel
Clorazepate
Clozapine
Co-Trimoxazole
Cobimetinib
Colchicine
Crizotinib
Cyclamate
Cyproheptadine
Dabrafenib
Dacarbazine
Daclatasvir
Danazol
Dapsone
Dasatinib
Demeclocycline
Desipramine
Desoximetasone
Dexamethasone
Dexchlorpheniramine
Diazoxide
Diclofenac
Diflunisal
Diltiazem
Dimenhydrinate
Diphenhydramine
Disopyramide
Docetaxel
Dong Quai
Doxepin
Doxycycline
Dronedarone
Duloxetine
Eculizumab
Efavirenz
Enalapril
Enoxacin
Epoetin Alfa
Erlotinib
Esomeprazole
Estrogens
Eszopiclone
Ethambutol
Ethionamide
Etodolac
Febuxostat
Felbamate
Fenofibrate
Flucytosine
Fluorouracil
Fluoxetine
Flurbiprofen
Flutamide
Fluvoxamine
Fosinopril
Furazolidone
Furosemide
Ganciclovir
Gatifloxacin
Gemifloxacin
Gentamicin
Ginseng
Glimepiride
Glipizide
Glyburide
Glycopyrrolate
Gold & Gold Compounds
Goldenseal
Grepafloxacin
Griseofulvin
Haloperidol
Heroin
Hydralazine
Hydrochlorothiazide
Hydroflumethiazide
Hydroxychloroquine
Hydroxyurea
Hydroxyzine
Hyoscyamine
Ibuprofen
Imatinib
Imipramine
Indapamide
Indomethacin
Interferon Alfa
Interferon Beta
Irbesartan
Irinotecan
Isocarboxazid
Isoniazid
Isotretinoin
Itraconazole
Kanamycin
Ketoconazole
Ketoprofen
Ketorolac
Lamotrigine
Levofloxacin
Lisinopril
Lomefloxacin
Loncastuximab tesirine
Loratadine
Losartan
Loxapine
Maprotiline
Meclizine
Meclofenamate
Melatonin
Meloxicam
Meprobamate
Mercaptopurine
Mesalamine
Mesoridazine
Metformin
Methenamine
Methotrexate
Methoxsalen
Methyclothiazide
Methyldopa
Methylphenidate
Metolazone
Midostaurin
Minocycline
Mitomycin
Moexipril
Molindone
Moxifloxacin
Nabumetone
Nalidixic Acid
Naproxen
Naratriptan
Nefazodone
Nifedipine
Nimesulide
Nivolumab
Norfloxacin
Nortriptyline
Ofloxacin
Olanzapine
Olmesartan
Omalizumab
Ombitasvir/Paritaprevir/Ritonavir
Oral Contraceptives
Oxaprozin
Oxerutins

Oxytetracycline
Paclitaxel
Pantoprazole
Paroxetine Hydrochloride
PEG-Interferon
Pentobarbital
Pentosan
Pentostatin
Phenelzine
Phenobarbital
Phenytoin
Pilocarpine
Pimozide
Pirfenidone
Piroxicam
Polythiazide
Porfimer
Pravastatin
Procainamide
Prochlorperazine
Procyclidine
Promazine
Promethazine
Propranolol
Propylthiouracil
Protriptyline
Psoralens
Pyrazinamide
Pyridoxine
Pyrimethamine
Quetiapine
Quinacrine
Quinapril
Quinethazone
Quinidine
Quinine
Rabeprazole
Ramipril
Ranitidine
Regorafenib
Ribavirin
Ribociclib
Risperidone
Ritonavir
Ropinirole
Rosemary
Rucaparib
Rue
Saccharin
Saquinavir
Sarecycline
Scopolamine
Sertraline
Sildenafil
Simeprevir
Simvastatin
Sitagliptin
Smallpox Vaccine
Sofosbuvir
Sotalol
Sparfloxacin
St John's Wort
Streptomycin
Sulfadiazine
Sulfadoxine
Sulfamethoxazole
Sulfasalazine
Sulfisoxazole
Sulindac
Sumatriptan
Tacrolimus
Tartrazine
Tegafur/Gimeracil/Oteracil
Telmisartan
Tenofovir Disoproxil
Terfenadine
Tetracycline
Thimerosal
Thioguanine
Thioridazine
Thiothixene
Tiagabine
Tiopronin
Tiotropium
Tocilizumab
Tolazamide
Tolbutamide
Tolmetin
Topiramate
Torsemide
Trametinib
Tranylcypromine
Trastuzumab
Trazodone
Tretinoin
Triamterene
Triazolam
Trichlormethiazide
Trifluoperazine
Trihexyphenidyl
Trimeprazine
Trimethadione
Trimipramine
Trioxsalen
Tripelennamine
Triprolidine
Trovafloxacin
Uracil/Tegafur
Valdecoxib
Valproic Acid
Valsartan
Vandetanib
Vardenafil
Vemurafenib
Venlafaxine
Verapamil
Verteporfin
Vinblastine
Voriconazole
Xipamide
Yarrow
Zalcitabine
Zaleplon
Ziprasidone
Zolmitriptan
Zolpidem

Pigmentation

Abemaciclib
Acitretin
Adapalene
Afamelanotide
Alitretinoin
Amantadine
Amifostine
Aminolevulinic Acid
Amiodarone
Amitriptyline
Amlodipine
Amoxicillin
Apomorphine
Arformoterol
Arsenic
Azathioprine
Benznidazole
Bergamot
Betaxolol
Bevacizumab
Bimatoprost
Bismuth
Bleomycin
Bortezomib
Bremelanotide
Busulfan
Calcipotriol
Capecitabine
Captopril
Carboplatin
Carmustine
Ceftriaxone
Chloroquine
Chlorpromazine
Cidofovir
Ciprofloxacin
Cisplatin
Citalopram
Clobetasol
Clofazimine
Clomipramine
Clonidine
Co-Trimoxazole
Colistin
Collagen (Bovine)
Cyclophosphamide
Dactinomycin
Dapsone
Dasatinib
Daunorubicin
Deferasirox
Degarelix
Desipramine
Dexamethasone
Diazepam
Dicumarol
Diltiazem
Docetaxel
Donepezil
Doxorubicin
Doxycycline
Eletriptan
Elotuzumab
Eltrombopag
Emtricitabine
Emtricitabine
Enoxacin
Epirubicin
Esmolol
Estradiol
Estramustine
Estrogens
Eszopiclone
Etoposide
Ezogabine
Fluconazole
Fluorouracil
Fluoxetine
Fluphenazine
Fluvoxamine
Foscarnet
Ganciclovir
Gefitinib
Gold & Gold Compounds
Goserelin
Griseofulvin
Halobetasol
Haloperidol
Henna
Heroin
Human Papillomavirus (HPV) Vaccine
Hyaluronic Acid
Hydrochlorothiazide
Hydroquinone
Hydroxychloroquine
Hydroxyurea
Idarubicin
Ifosfamide
Imatinib
Imipramine
Imiquimod
Indapamide
Insulin
Interferon Alfa
Ipilimumab
Irinotecan
Isotretinoin
Ixabepilone
Ixazomib
Ketoconazole
Ketoprofen
Labetalol
Lamivudine
Lapatinib
Latanoprost
Leflunomide
Lenalidomide
Leuprolide
Levetiracetam
Levobupivacaine
Levofloxacin
Levonorgestrel
Levothyroxine
Lidocaine
Lithium
Loncastuximab tesirine
Loxapine
Lycopene
Mechlorethamine
Mephenytoin
Mercaptopurine
Mesoridazine
Methamphetamine
Methotrexate
Methoxsalen
Methyldopa
Minocycline
Minoxidil
Mirtazapine
Mitomycin
Mitotane
Molindone
Niacin
Nicotine
Nisoldipine
Nivolumab
Olanzapine
Omacetaxine
Omeprazole
Oral Contraceptives
Orphenadrine
Paclitaxel
Panitumumab
Paromomycin
Paroxetine Hydrochloride
Pazopanib
PEG-Interferon
Pembrolizumab
Pemetrexed
Pentazocine
Pentostatin
Perphenazine
Phenazopyridine
Phenobarbital

Phenolphthalein
Phenytoin
Pimozide
Polidocanol
Porfimer
Prilocaine
Procarbazine
Prochlorperazine
Promazine
Psoralens
Pyrimethamine
Quinacrine
Quinidine
Quinine
Rabeprazole
Ribavirin
Rifabutin
Rifapentine
Risperidone
Ropinirole
Ruxolitinib
Saquinavir
Sertraline
Setmelanotide
Siltuximab
Smallpox Vaccine
Sorafenib
Sparfloxacin
Spironolactone
Stanozolol
Sulfadiazine
Sulfasalazine
Sunitinib
Tacrolimus
Tegafur/Gimeracil/Oteracil
Telmisartan
Terbinafine
Tetracycline
Thioridazine
Thiotepa
Thiothixene
Tiagabine
Tigecycline
Tolcapone
Topiramate
Tretinoin
Triamcinolone
Trifluoperazine
Trioxsalen
Uracil/Tegafur
Vandetanib
Vinblastine
Vincristine
Vinorelbine
Vitamin A
Voriconazole
Warfarin
Zidovudine
Zinc

Pityriasis rosea

Acetaminophen
Acyclovir
Allopurinol
Ampicillin
Arsenic
Asenapine
Aspirin
Atenolol
BCG Vaccine
Bismuth
Captopril
Clonidine
Clozapine
Codeine
Covid-19 Vaccine, mRNA
Domperidone
Dupilumab
Everolimus
Gold & Gold Compounds
Hydrochlorothiazide
Imatinib
Isotretinoin
Ketotifen
Lamotrigine
Lisinopril
Meprobamate
Metronidazole
Mitomycin
Naproxen
Nimesulide
Nortriptyline
Omeprazole
Ondansetron
Pneumococcal Vaccine
Terbinafine
Tiopronin
Tripelennamine

Pruritus (itching)

Abacavir
Abametapir
Abatacept
Abciximab
Acamprosate
Acebutolol
Acetaminophen
Acetohexamide
Acetylcysteine
Acitretin
Acyclovir
Adalimumab
Adapalene
Adefovir
Afatinib
Albendazole
Albuterol
Aldesleukin
Alefacept
Alemtuzumab
Alendronate
Alfentanil
Alglucerase
Alitretinoin
Allopurinol
Almotriptan
Alogliptin
Alpelisib
Alpha-Lipoic Acid
Alprazolam
Altretamine
Alvimopan
Amantadine
Amcinonide
Amikacin
Amiloride
Aminoglutethimide
Aminolevulinic Acid
Aminophylline
Aminosalicylate Sodium
Amiodarone
Amitriptyline
Amlodipine
Amodiaquine
Amoxapine
Amoxicillin
Amphotericin B
Ampicillin
Anagrelide
Anastrozole
Anidulafungin
Anthrax Vaccine
Anti-Thymocyte Immunoglobulin (Rabbit)
Apalutamide
Apraclonidine
Aprepitant
Arsenic
Artemether/Lumefantrine
Artemisia
Artesunate
Asciminib
Asparaginase
Aspartame
Aspirin
Astemizole
Atazanavir
Atenolol
Atezolizumab
Atomoxetine
Atorvastatin
Atovaquone
Atovaquone/Proguanil
Atracurium
Avelumab
Axitinib
Azacitidine
Azathioprine
Azithromycin
Aztreonam
Bacampicillin
Bacitracin
Baclofen
Basiliximab
Becaplermin
Bedaquiline
Belinostat
Belumosudil
Benazepril
Bendamustine
Bendroflumethiazide
Benzalkonium
Benznidazole
Benzyl Alcohol
Betamethasone
Betaxolol
Bevacizumab
Bexarotene
Bezafibrate
Bicalutamide
Bismuth
Black Cohosh
Bleomycin
Boceprevir
Bortezomib
Bosentan
Bosutinib
Boswellia
Botulinum Toxin (A & B)
Brentuximab Vedotin
Brimonidine
Budesonide
Bumetanide
Bupivacaine
Buprenorphine
Bupropion
Buspirone
Butorphanol
Butterbur
Cabergoline
Calcipotriol
Calcium Hydroxylapatite
Canagliflozin
Capecitabine
Capsicum
Captopril
Carbamazepine
Carbetocin
Carboplatin
Carisoprodol
Carmustine
Carvedilol
Caspofungin
Cefaclor
Cefadroxil
Cefamandole
Cefazolin
Cefdinir
Cefditoren
Cefepime
Cefiderocol
Cefixime
Cefmetazole
Cefonicid
Cefoperazone
Cefotaxime
Cefotetan
Cefoxitin
Cefpodoxime
Ceftaroline Fosamil
Ceftazidime
Ceftibuten
Ceftizoxime
Ceftobiprole
Ceftolozane & Tazobactam
Ceftriaxone
Cefuroxime
Celecoxib
Cemiplimab
Cenobamate
Cephalexin
Cephalothin
Cephapirin
Cephradine
Certolizumab
Cetirizine
Cetuximab
Cevimeline
Chasteberry
Chloral Hydrate
Chlorambucil
Chloramphenicol
Chlordiazepoxide
Chlormezanone
Chloroquine
Chlorothiazide
Chlorpheniramine
Chlorpromazine
Chlorpropamide
Cholestyramine
Ciclopirox
Cidofovir
Cimetidine
Cinoxacin
Ciprofloxacin
Cisplatin
Citalopram
Cladribine
Clarithromycin
Clindamycin
Clindamycin/Tretinoin
Clobetasol
Clofarabine
Clofazimine

Clofibrate
Clomiphene
Clomipramine
Clonidine
Clopidogrel
Clotrimazole
Cloxacillin
Clozapine
Co-Trimoxazole
Coagulation Factor IX (Recombinant)
Cobicistat/Elvitegravir/ Emtricitabine/Tenofovir Alafenamide
Cobimetinib
Codeine
Colchicine
Collagen (Bovine)
Comfrey
Conivaptan
Crisaborole
Cromolyn
Cyanocobalamin
Cyclamate
Cyclobenzaprine
Cyclophosphamide
Cyclosporine
Cytarabine
Dabrafenib
Dacarbazine
Daclatasvir
Daclizumab
Dacomitinib
Dactinomycin
Dalbavancin
Dalteparin
Danaparoid
Danazol
Dapsone
Daptomycin
Darbepoetin Alfa
Darifenacin
Darunavir
Dasatinib
Daunorubicin
Decitabine
Deferasirox
Deferoxamine
Defibrotide
Delafloxacin
Delavirdine
Demeclocycline
Denileukin
Denosumab
Desipramine
Desonide
Dexamethasone
Dexlansoprazole
Diatrizoate
Diazepam
Diclofenac
Dicloxacillin
Dicumarol
Dicyclomine
Didanosine
Diethylpropion
Diethylstilbestrol
Difelikefalin
Diflunisal
Digoxin
Dihydrocodeine
Dihydrotachysterol
Diltiazem
Dimethyl Fumarate
Diphenhydramine
Diphenoxylate
Dipyridamole
Dirithromycin
Disopyramide
Dobutamine
Docetaxel
Dolasetron
Dolutegravir
Donepezil
Doripenem
Dostarlimab
Doxapram
Doxazosin
Doxepin
Doxercalciferol
Doxorubicin
Doxycycline
Dronedarone
Droperidol
Duloxetine
Durvalumab
Ecallantide
Echinacea
Econazole
Eculizumab
Efavirenz
Eflornithine
Elbasvir & Grazoprevir
Eletriptan
Emtricitabine
Enalapril
Encorafenib
Enfuvirtide
Enoxacin
Enoxaparin
Entecavir
Enzalutamide
Epinephrine
Epirubicin
Epoetin Alfa
Epoprostenol
Eprosartan
Ergocalciferol
Erlotinib
Ertapenem
Escitalopram
Esomeprazole
Estazolam
Estramustine
Estrogens
Eszopiclone
Etanercept
Etelcalcetide
Ethambutol
Etidronate
Etodolac
Everolimus
Evolocumab
Exemestane
Ezetimibe
Factor VIII - von Willebrand Factor
Famciclovir
Famotidine
Febuxostat
Felbamate
Felodipine
Fenofibrate
Fenoprofen
Fentanyl
Ferric Gluconate
Ferumoxytol
Fexinidazole
Fidaxomicin
Finasteride
Fingolimod
Flecainide
Fluconazole
Fludarabine
Fluocinonide
Fluorides
Fluorouracil
Fluoxetine
Fluphenazine
Flurbiprofen
Fluticasone Propionate
Folic Acid
Formoterol
Fosamprenavir
Foscarnet
Fosfomycin
Fosinopril
Fosphenytoin
Fostemsavir
Frovatriptan
Fulvestrant
Furazolidone
Furosemide
Gabapentin
Gadobenate
Gadobutrol
Gadodiamide
Gadofosveset
Gadopentetate
Gadoteridol
Gadoversetamide
Gadoxetate
Ganciclovir
Gatifloxacin
Gefitinib
Gemcitabine
Gemfibrozil
Gemifloxacin
Gemtuzumab
Gentamicin
Ginseng
Glatiramer
Glecaprevir & Pibrentasvir
Gliclazide
Glimepiride
Glipizide
Glucosamine
Glyburide
Gold & Gold Compounds
Goserelin
Granulocyte Colony-Stimulating Factor (G-CSF)
Grepafloxacin
Griseofulvin
Guanabenz
Guanfacine
Guselkumab
Halcinonide
Halobetasol
Halofantrine
Halometasone
Haloperidol
Henna
Heparin
Heroin
Histrelin
Human Papillomavirus Vaccine (Bivalent)
Hyaluronic Acid
Hydralazine
Hydrochlorothiazide
Hydrocodone
Hydrocortisone
Hydromorphone
Hydroquinone
Hydroxychloroquine
Hydroxyurea
Ibandronate
Ibritumomab
Ibuprofen
Icatibant
Icodextrin
Idursulfase
Imatinib
Imidapril
Imiglucerase
Imipenem/Cilastatin
Imipramine
Imiquimod
Immune Globulin IV
Immune Globulin SC
Indapamide
Indinavir
Indomethacin
Infliximab
Ingenol Mebutate
Insulin
Insulin Glulisine
Interferon Alfa
Iobenguane
Iodixanol
Iohexol
Iomeprol
Iopromide
Ioversol
Ipilimumab
Ipratropium
Irbesartan
Irinotecan
Isavuconazonium Sulfate
Isocarboxazid
Isoniazid
Isosorbide Mononitrate
Isotretinoin
Isradipine
Itraconazole
Ivermectin
Ixabepilone
Ixazomib
Ixekizumab
Japanese Encephalitis Vaccine
Kanamycin
Ketamine
Ketoconazole
Ketoprofen
Ketorolac
Ketotifen
Labetalol
Lacosamide
Lamivudine
Lamotrigine
Lansoprazole
Lapatinib
Latanoprost
Ledipasvir & Sofosbuvir
Leflunomide
Lenalidomide
Lepirudin
Letrozole
Leucovorin
Leuprolide
Levamisole

Levetiracetam
Levobunolol
Levobupivacaine
Levofloxacin
Levomilnacipran
Levothyroxine
Lidocaine
Linagliptin
Lincomycin
Lindane
Linezolid
Linseed
Liraglutide
Lisinopril
Lithium
Lomefloxacin
Lonafarnib
Loncastuximab tesirine
Loracarbef
Loratadine
Losartan
Lovastatin
Loxapine
Lurasidone
Mafenide
Maralixibat
Maraviroc
Mebendazole
Mechlorethamine
Meclofenamate
Medroxyprogesterone
Mefenamic Acid
Mefloquine
Meloxicam
Melphalan
Memantine
Meperidine
Mephenytoin
Mepivacaine
Mepolizumab
Meprobamate
Meropenem
Mesalamine
Mesna
Metformin
Methadone
Methenamine
Methimazole
Methotrexate
Methoxsalen
Methyl salicylate
Methyldopa
Methylprednisolone
Metolazone
Metoprolol
Metronidazole
Mexiletine
Micafungin
Miconazole
Midazolam
Midodrine
Midostaurin
Mifepristone
Milnacipran
Miltefosine
Minocycline
Minoxidil
Mirabegron
Mistletoe
Mitomycin
Mitotane
Mobocertinib
Modafinil
Moexipril
Molindone
Mometasone
Moricizine
Morphine
Moxidectin
Moxifloxacin
Mupirocin
Muromonab-CD3
Mycophenolate
Myrrh
Nabumetone
Nadolol
Nafarelin
Nalbuphine
Nalidixic Acid
Nalmefene
Naloxone
Naltrexone
Naproxen
Naratriptan
Natalizumab
Necitumumab
Nefazodone
Nelfinavir
Neostigmine
Nesiritide
Nevirapine
Niacin
Niacinamide
Nicotine
Nifedipine
Nilotinib
Nilutamide
Nimesulide
Nimodipine
Nintedanib
Nisoldipine
Nitazoxanide
Nitisinone
Nitrofurantoin
Nitrofurazone
Nitroglycerin
Nivolumab
Nizatidine
Norfloxacin
Nystatin
Obeticholic Acid
Octreotide
Ofatumumab
Ofloxacin
Olanzapine
Olaparib
Oliceridine
Olsalazine
Omacetaxine
Omadacycline
Omalizumab
Ombitasvir/Paritaprevir/Ritonavir
Ombitasvir/Paritaprevir/Ritonavir and Dasabuvir
Omega-3 Fatty Acids
Omeprazole
Ondansetron
Oral Contraceptives
Oritavancin
Osimertinib
Oxacillin
Oxaliplatin
Oxaprozin
Oxerutins
Oxilan
Oxybutynin
Oxycodone
Oxymorphone
Oxytetracycline
Paclitaxel
Pacritinib
Pafolacianine
Palifermin
Paliperidone
Palonosetron
Panitumumab
Pantoprazole
Papaverine
Paricalcitol
Paromomycin
Paroxetine Hydrochloride
Paroxetine Mesylate
Pasireotide
Pazopanib
PEG-Interferon
Pegaspargase
Pembrolizumab
Pemetrexed
Penicillamine
Penicillin V
Pentagastrin
Pentamidine
Pentazocine
Pentosan
Pentostatin
Pentoxifylline
Perflutren
Perindopril
Permethrin
Pertuzumab
Pexidartinib hydrochloride
Phenelzine
Phenobarbital
Phenolphthalein
Phenytoin
Pimecrolimus
Pindolol
Pirfenidone
Piroxicam
Plasma (Human) Blood Product
Pneumococcal Vaccine
Podophyllotoxin
Polypodium Leucotomos
Pomalidomide
Posaconazole
Pralatrexate
Pramipexole
Pravastatin
Praziquantel
Prazosin
Prednicarbate
Prednisolone
Prednisone
Pregabalin
Pretomanid
Prilocaine
Primaquine
Pristinamycin
Probenecid
Procainamide
Procarbazine
Prochlorperazine
Propafenone
Propofol
Propranolol
Propylthiouracil
Protriptyline
Psoralens
Pyrazinamide
Pyrimethamine
Quazepam
Quinacrine
Quinapril
Quinethazone
Quinidine
Quinine
Quinupristin/Dalfopristin
Rabeprazole
Raltegravir
Raltitrexed
Ramipril
Ranitidine
Rasburicase
Regorafenib
Remifentanil
Repaglinide
Retapamulin
Ribavirin
Ribociclib
Rifampin
Rifapentine
Rifaximin
Ripretinib
Risedronate
Risperidone
Ritonavir
Rituximab
Rivaroxaban
Rivastigmine
Rizatriptan
Rofecoxib
Romidepsin
Ropinirole
Ropivacaine
Rosuvastatin
Rotigotine
Rucaparib
Rufinamide
Saccharin
Sacubitril/Valsartan
Salmeterol
Saquinavir
Satralizumab
Saxagliptin
Scopolamine
Secukinumab
Selumetinib
Sertaconazole
Sertraline
Sevelamer
Sevoflurane
Sibutramine
Sildenafil
Siltuximab
Simeprevir
Simvastatin
Sirolimus
Smallpox Vaccine
Sodium Iodide I-131
Sodium Oxybate
Sofosbuvir
Sofosbuvir & Velpatasvir
Sonidegib
Sorafenib
Sotalol
Sparfloxacin
Spectinomycin
Spinosad
Spironolactone
St John's Wort

Streptokinase
Streptomycin
Streptozocin
Succimer
Succinylcholine
Sucralfate
Sufentanil
Sugammadex
Sulfadiazine
Sulfadoxine
Sulfamethoxazole
Sulfasalazine
Sulfisoxazole
Sulfites
Sulindac
Sumatriptan
Sunitinib
Tacrine
Tacrolimus
Tadalafil
Taliglucerase
Talimogene Laherparepvec
Tamoxifen
Tartrazine
Tazarotene
Tea Tree
Tecovirimat
Tedizolid
Tegafur/Gimeracil/Oteracil
Tegaserod
Teicoplanin
Telaprevir
Telavancin
Telbivudine
Telithromycin
Telmisartan
Temozolomide
Temsirolimus
Tepotinib
Terazosin
Terbinafine
Terbutaline
Terconazole
Teriflunomide
Tesamorelin
Testosterone
Tetracycline
Thalidomide
Thiabendazole
Thiamine
Thioguanine
Thiopental
Thiotepa
Thyrotropin Alfa
Tiagabine
Ticlopidine
Tigecycline
Tiludronate
Timolol
Tinidazole
Tinzaparin
Tiopronin
Tipranavir
Tizanidine
Tobramycin
Tocainide
Tocilizumab
Tofacitinib
Tolazamide
Tolbutamide
Tolcapone
Tolmetin
Tolterodine
Tolvaptan
Topiramate
Tositumomab & Iodine131
Tosufloxacin
Tramadol
Trametinib
Trandolapril
Tranexamic Acid
Trastuzumab
Trastuzumab Emtansine / Ado-Trastuzumab Emtansine
Travoprost
Trazodone
Treprostinil
Tretinoin
Triamcinolone
Triazolam
Triclabendazole
Trimeprazine
Trimethadione
Trimethoprim
Trimetrexate
Trioxsalen
Triprolidine
Triptorelin
Troleandomycin
Trovafloxacin
Typhoid Vaccine
Ulipristal
Unoprostone
Ursodiol
Ustekinumab
Valdecoxib
Valganciclovir
Valproic Acid
Valrubicin
Valsartan
Vancomycin
Vandetanib
Vardenafil
Varenicline
Varicella Vaccine
Vedolizumab
Vemurafenib
Venlafaxine
Verapamil
Vernakalant
Vestronidase
Vincristine
Vitamin A
Voriconazole
Vorinostat
Vortioxetine
Warfarin
Zalcitabine
Zaleplon
Ziconotide
Zidovudine
Zileuton
Zolmitriptan
Zolpidem
Zonisamide
Zuclopenthixol

Pseudolymphoma

Adalimumab
Aldesleukin
Allopurinol
Alprazolam
Amitriptyline
Amlodipine
Aspirin
Atenolol
Black Cohosh
Bromocriptine
Captopril
Carbamazepine
Cefixime
Cefuroxime
Chlorpromazine
Cimetidine
Clarithromycin
Clonazepam
Clonidine
Co-Trimoxazole
Cyclosporine
Dapsone
Desipramine
Diclofenac
Diflunisal
Diltiazem
Doxepin
Estrogens
Etanercept
Ethosuximide
Ethotoin
Fluorouracil
Fluoxetine
Fosinopril
Furosemide
Gemcitabine
Gemfibrozil
Glatiramer
Gold & Gold Compounds
Hepatitis A Vaccine
Hepatitis B Vaccine
Human Papillomavirus (HPV) Vaccine
Hydrochlorothiazide
Ibuprofen
Imatinib
Indomethacin
Infliximab
Interferon Alfa
Ketoprofen
Lamotrigine
Leucovorin
Lisinopril
Lithium
Lorazepam
Losartan
Lovastatin
Methotrexate
Methylphenidate
Metoprolol
Mexiletine
Nabumetone
Naproxen
Nitrofurantoin
Nizatidine
Oxaliplatin
Oxaprozin
Perphenazine
Phenobarbital
Phenytoin
Procainamide
Ranitidine
Sulfamethoxazole
Sulfasalazine
Sulindac
Tamoxifen
Terfenadine
Thioridazine
Valproic Acid
Valsartan
Zoledronate

Pseudoporphyria

Acitretin
Amiodarone
Ampicillin
Ampicillin/Sulbactam
Aspirin
Bumetanide
Carisoprodol
Cefepime
Celecoxib
Chlorthalidone
Ciprofloxacin
Cyclosporine
Diclofenac
Diflunisal
Fluorouracil
Flutamide
Furosemide
Hydrochlorothiazide
Ibuprofen
Imatinib
Indomethacin
Isotretinoin
Ketoprofen
Mefenamic Acid
Meloxicam
Metformin
Nabumetone
Nalidixic Acid
Naproxen
Olanzapine
Oral Contraceptives
Oxaprozin
Piroxicam
Psoralens
Pyridoxine
Quinidine
Rofecoxib
Tetracycline
Torsemide
Triamterene
Voriconazole

Psoriasis

Abatacept
Acebutolol
Aceclofenac
Acetazolamide
Acitretin
Adalimumab
Aldesleukin
Aminoglutethimide
Amiodarone
Amoxicillin
Ampicillin
Anakinra
Apremilast
Arsenic
Aspirin
Atenolol
Atezolizumab
Avelumab
Baricitinib
BCG Vaccine
Betamethasone
Bisoprolol
Bupropion
Calcipotriol
Candesartan
Captopril
Carbamazepine
Carvedilol
Certolizumab
Cetuximab

Chlorambucil
Chloroquine
Chlorthalidone
Cimetidine
Clarithromycin
Clonidine
Clopidogrel
Co-Trimoxazole
Cyclosporine
Dabrafenib
Daclizumab
Diclofenac
Digoxin
Diltiazem
Dipyridamole
Docetaxel
Donepezil
Doxorubicin
Doxycycline
Dupilumab
Durvalumab
Efalizumab
Eletriptan
Enalapril
Esmolol
Etanercept
Fexofenadine
Flecainide
Fluorouracil
Fluoxetine
Fluoxymesterone
Foscarnet
Gemfibrozil
Glyburide
Gold & Gold Compounds
Golimumab
Granulocyte Colony-Stimulating Factor (G-CSF)
Henna
Human Papillomavirus (HPV) Vaccine
Hydroxychloroquine
Hydroxyurea
Ibuprofen
Imatinib
Imiquimod
Indomethacin
Infliximab
Interferon Alfa
Interferon Beta
Interferon Gamma
Ipilimumab
Ketoprofen
L-Methylfolate
Labetalol
Lapatinib
Lenalidomide
Letrozole
Levamisole
Levetiracetam
Levobetaxolol
Lisinopril
Lithium
Losartan
MDMA
Meclofenamate
Mefloquine
Meloxicam
Mepolizumab
Mesalamine
Methicillin
Methotrexate
Methyltestosterone
Metipranolol
Metoprolol
Modafinil
Morphine
Mycophenolate
Nadolol
Nilotinib
Nivolumab
Olanzapine
Ombitasvir/Paritaprevir/Ritonavir
Omeprazole
Oral Contraceptives
Oxprenolol
Paroxetine Hydrochloride
PEG-Interferon
Pembrolizumab
Penicillamine
Pentostatin
Perindopril
Phenylbutazone
Pindolol
Ponatinib
Potassium Iodide
Prednisolone
Primaquine
Propafenone
Propranolol
Quinacrine
Quinidine
Rabeprazole
Ramipril
Ranitidine
Ribavirin
Risperidone
Ritonavir
Rituximab
Rivastigmine
Rofecoxib
Ropinirole
Saquinavir
Secukinumab
Sertraline
Siltuximab
Sitagliptin
Sorafenib
Sotalol
Sulfamethoxazole
Sulfasalazine
Tacrine
Tazarotene
Telmisartan
Terbinafine
Terfenadine
Teriflunomide
Testosterone
Tetracycline
Thalidomide
Thioguanine
Tiagabine
Timolol
Tocilizumab
Tofacitinib
Trazodone
Urapidil
Ustekinumab
Valdecoxib
Vedolizumab
Venlafaxine
Voriconazole

Purpura

Acenocoumarol
Acetaminophen
Acetazolamide
Acitretin
Aldesleukin
Alemtuzumab
Allopurinol
Alteplase
Aminocaproic Acid
Aminoglutethimide
Aminolevulinic Acid
Aminosalicylate Sodium
Amiodarone
Amitriptyline
Amlodipine
Amphotericin B
Ampicillin
Anastrozole
Anti-Thymocyte Globulin (Equine)
Arsenic
Artemether/Lumefantrine
Aspartame
Aspirin
Azathioprine
Azilsartan
Aztreonam
Bendamustine
Beta-Carotene
Betaxolol
Bevacizumab
Bortezomib
Botulinum Toxin (A & B)
Buspirone
Busulfan
Butabarbital
Butalbital
Capecitabine
Captopril
Carbamazepine
Carbenicillin
Carteolol
Carvedilol
Cefaclor
Cefoxitin
Celecoxib
Cephalothin
Cetirizine
Chloral Hydrate
Chlorambucil
Chloramphenicol
Chlordiazepoxide
Chlorothiazide
Chlorpromazine
Chlorpropamide
Chlorthalidone
Cilostazol
Cinacalcet
Ciprofloxacin
Citalopram
Cladribine
Clarithromycin
Clidinium
Clofibrate
Clomiphene
Clomipramine
Clonazepam
Clopidogrel
Clozapine
Co-Trimoxazole
Cocaine
Creatine
Cycloserine
Cyclosporine
Cytarabine
Dabigatran
Danazol
Dapsone
Delavirdine
Desipramine
Diazepam
Diclofenac
Dicumarol
Diethylpropion
Diethylstilbestrol
Digoxin
Diltiazem
Diphenhydramine
Dipyridamole
Disopyramide
Disulfiram
Donepezil
Doxazosin
Doxepin
Doxorubicin
Doxycycline
Drotrecogin Alfa
Duloxetine
Enalapril
Enoxacin
Enoxaparin
Entacapone
Ephedrine
Eprosartan
Erlotinib
Escitalopram
Estazolam
Estramustine
Estrogens
Ethacrynic Acid
Ethambutol
Ethchlorvynol
Ethionamide
Ethosuximide
Ethotoin
Famotidine
Febuxostat
Felodipine
Fenoprofen
Fentanyl
Flucloxacillin
Fluconazole
Fluoxetine
Fluvoxamine
Fondaparinux
Frovatriptan
Furosemide
Gabapentin
Galantamine
Gefitinib
Gentamicin
Glatiramer
Glyburide
Gold & Gold Compounds
Grapefruit Juice
Griseofulvin
Guanfacine
Heparin
Hepatitis B Vaccine
Heroin
Histrelin
Horse Chestnut (Bark, Flower, Leaf, Seed)
Hyaluronic Acid
Hydralazine
Hydrochlorothiazide
Hydrocortisone
Hydroxychloroquine

Hydroxyurea
Hydroxyzine
Ibritumomab
Ibuprofen
Imatinib
Imipramine
Indomethacin
Influenza Vaccine
Insulin
Interferon Alfa
Iohexol
Ipodate
Isoniazid
Isotretinoin
Itraconazole
Ketoconazole
Ketoprofen
Ketorolac
Labetalol
Lamotrigine
Leflunomide
Lenalidomide
Leuprolide
Levamisole
Levobupivacaine
Levodopa
Levofloxacin
Lidocaine
Lincomycin
Lindane
Linezolid
Lisinopril
Lithium
Lomefloxacin
Loratadine
Lovastatin
Maprotiline
Measles, Mumps & Rubella (MMR) Virus Vaccine
Mecasermin
Mechlorethamine
Meclofenamate
Mefloquine
Meloxicam
Mephenytoin
Meprobamate
Metformin
Methimazole
Methoxsalen
Methyldopa
Methylphenidate
Metoclopramide
Metolazone
Miconazole
Minocycline
Mirabegron
Mitomycin
Mitoxantrone
Montelukast
Nalidixic Acid
Naproxen
Naratriptan
Natalizumab
Nifedipine
Nimesulide
Nitrofurantoin
Nitroglycerin
Octreotide
Olanzapine
Omacetaxine
Oral Contraceptives
Oxaliplatin
Oxcarbazepine
Oxytetracycline
Paroxetine Hydrochloride
Pegaspargase
Penicillamine
Pentagastrin
Pentobarbital
Pentosan
Pentostatin
Perindopril
Phenobarbital
Phensuximide
Phenytoin
Piperacillin
Pirbuterol
Piroxicam
Plicamycin
Pravastatin
Prednisone
Prilocaine
Procainamide
Prochlorperazine
Promethazine
Propafenone
Propranolol
Propylthiouracil
Pyrimethamine
Quinidine
Quinine
Ramipril
Ranitidine
Rapacuronium
Rifampin
Rifapentine
Risperidone
Rituximab
Rivastigmine
Ropinirole
Rotigotine
Ruxolitinib
Sertraline
Simvastatin
Sirolimus
Smallpox Vaccine
Streptokinase
Streptomycin
Sulfadoxine
Sulfamethoxazole
Sulfasalazine
Sulfisoxazole
Sulindac
Tacrine
Tacrolimus
Tadalafil
Tamoxifen
Tartrazine
Tecovirimat
Teicoplanin
Tetracycline
Thalidomide
Thiamine
Thiopental
Ticlopidine
Tinzaparin
Tizanidine
Tolbutamide
Tolmetin
Topiramate
Topotecan
Torsemide
Tosufloxacin
Trichlormethiazide
Trimethadione
Tripelennamine
Valacyclovir
Valproic Acid
Vancomycin
Varicella Vaccine
Vasopressin
Verapamil
Voriconazole
Warfarin
Zolpidem
Zonisamide

Raynaud's phenomenon

Acebutolol
Amphotericin B
Aripiprazole
Arsenic
Atenolol
Bisoprolol
Bleomycin
Bromocriptine
Carboplatin
Carteolol
Cisplatin
Clonidine
Cocaine
Cyclosporine
Dextroamphetamine
Dopamine
Doxorubicin
Estrogens
Ethosuximide
Fluoxetine
Gemcitabine
Gemfibrozil
Hepatitis B Vaccine
Human Papillomavirus (HPV) Vaccine
Hydroxyurea
Iloprost
Interferon Alfa
Interferon Beta
Isotretinoin
Labetalol
Lamotrigine
Leflunomide
Methotrexate
Methylphenidate
Metoprolol
Minocycline
Nadolol
Octreotide
Phentermine
Pindolol
Propofol
Propranolol
Quinine
Ribavirin
Rofecoxib
Sotalol
Spironolactone
Sulfasalazine
Sulindac
Sumatriptan
Tegafur/Gimeracil/Oteracil
Tegaserod
Telmisartan
Tenofovir Disoproxil
Teriflunomide
Thiothixene
Timolol
Uracil/Tegafur
Vinblastine
Vincristine
Yohimbine
Zolmitriptan

Rhabdomyolysis

Abacavir
Abiraterone
Acetaminophen
Aldesleukin
Allopurinol
Alprazolam
Aminocaproic Acid
Aminophylline
Amiodarone
Amisulpride
Amitriptyline
Amlodipine
Amobarbital
Amoxicillin
Amphotericin B
Aprobarbital
Aripiprazole
Aspirin
Atorvastatin
Atropine Sulfate
Azacitidine
Azathioprine
Azithromycin
Baclofen
Benztropine
Bezafibrate
Buprenorphine
Bupropion
Butabarbital
Butalbital
Cabozantinib
Caffeine
Carbamazepine
Carbimazole
Chlorpromazine
Chlorthalidone
Cholestyramine
Ciprofibrate
Ciprofloxacin
Cisplatin
Citalopram
Clarithromycin
Clofibrate
Clopidogrel
Clozapine
Co-Trimoxazole
Cobicistat/Elvitegravir/Emtricitabine/Tenofovir Disoproxil
Cocaine
Colchicine
Colistin
Covid-19 Vaccine, mRNA
Creatine
Cyclosporine
Cytarabine
Dabrafenib
Dacarbazine
Danazol
Daptomycin
Dasatinib
Deferasirox
Delavirdine
Desipramine
Dexketoprofen
Dextroamphetamine
Diatrizoate
Diazepam
Diclofenac
Didanosine
Digoxin

Diltiazem
Diphenhydramine
Distigmine
Dolutegravir
Domperidone
Doxepin
Droperidol
Enflurane
Enoxacin
Epinephrine
Erlotinib
Erythromycin
Esomeprazole
Etoposide
Fenbufen
Fenofibrate
Fluconazole
Fluorouracil
Fluoxetine
Fluphenazine
Fluprednisolone
Fluvastatin
Fusidic Acid
Gabapentin
Gatifloxacin
Gemcitabine
Gemfibrozil
Granulocyte Colony-Stimulating Factor (G-CSF)
Grapefruit Juice
Haloperidol
Halothane
Heroin
Hydroxychloroquine
Ibuprofen
Imatinib
Indapamide
Infliximab
Influenza Vaccine
Interferon Alfa
Interferon Beta
Ipilimumab
Isoflurane
Isoniazid
Isotretinoin
Itraconazole
Ketoconazole
Labetalol
Lacosamide
Lamivudine
Lamotrigine
Leflunomide
Lenalidomide
Leuprolide
Levetiracetam
Levodopa
Levofloxacin
Levomepromazine
Licorice
Lindane
Linezolid
Lithium
Lorazepam
Lovastatin
Loxapine
Lurasidone
Maraviroc
MDMA
Meloxicam
Melphalan
Mephobarbital
Meprobamate
Metformin
Methadone
Methamphetamine
Methohexital
Metoprolol
Minocycline
Mirtazapine
Mizoribine
Molindone
Morphine
Moxifloxacin
Myrrh
Naltrexone
Naproxen
Nefazodone
Nelarabine
Nelfinavir
Nitrazepam
Nivolumab
Norfloxacin
Ofloxacin
Olanzapine
Omeprazole
Osimertinib
Paclitaxel
Palbociclib
Paliperidone
Pancuronium
Pantoprazole
PEG-Interferon
Pembrolizumab
Pemetrexed
Pemoline
Pentamidine
Pentobarbital
Perphenazine
Phendimetrazine
Phenelzine
Phenobarbital
Phenylpropanolamine
Phenytoin
Pioglitazone
Pravastatin
Pregabalin
Primidone
Propofol
Protamine Sulfate
Protriptyline
Pyrazinamide
Quetiapine
Quinacrine
Quinine
Rabeprazole
Raltegravir
Ranolazine
Red Rice Yeast
Ribavirin
Ribociclib
Rifampin
Rifaximin
Risperidone
Ritodrine
Ritonavir
Rosuvastatin
Sacubitril/Valsartan
Saw Palmetto
Secobarbital
Sertraline
Sevoflurane
Sildenafil
Simeprevir
Simvastatin
Sirolimus
Sitagliptin
Sofosbuvir & Velpatasvir
Sonidegib
Sotalol
St John's Wort
Stanozolol
Streptokinase
Streptomycin
Succinylcholine
Sulfamethoxazole
Sulfasalazine
Sulpiride /Levosulpiride
Sunitinib
Tacrolimus
Tasonermin
Tenecteplase
Tenofovir Disoproxil
Terbinafine
Terbutaline
Teriflunomide
Terlipressin
Thiopental
Ticagrelor
Tolcapone
Tolvaptan
Trabectedin
Trametinib
Trandolapril
Tranylcypromine
Trientine
Trifluoperazine
Trimethoprim
Trospium
Valproic Acid
Vasopressin
Venlafaxine
Verapamil
Vinblastine
Voriconazole
Warfarin
Ziconotide
Ziprasidone

Stevens-Johnson syndrome and toxic epidermal necrolysis (SJS/TEN)

Abacavir
Aceclofenac
Acetaminophen
Acetazolamide
Acyclovir
Adalimumab
Adefovir
Afatinib
Albendazole
Albuterol
Aldesleukin
Alfuzosin
Allopurinol
Alogliptin
Alprostadil
Amifostine
Aminophylline
Aminosalicylate Sodium
Amiodarone
Amitriptyline
Amlodipine
Amobarbital
Amoxapine
Amoxicillin
Ampicillin
Amprenavir
Anthrax Vaccine
Apalutamide
Aripiprazole
Arsenic
Asparaginase
Aspirin
Astemizole
Atorvastatin
Atovaquone
Atovaquone/Proguanil
Atropine Sulfate
Azathioprine
Azithromycin
Aztreonam
BCG Vaccine
Bendamustine
Benznidazole
Benzydamine
Bezafibrate
Bleomycin
Bortezomib
Bosutinib
Botulinum Toxin (A&B)
Bromfenac
Bucillamine
Bupropion
Busulfan
Butabarbital
Butalbital
Cabergoline
Capecitabine
Captopril
Carbamazepine
Carbenicillin
Carboplatin
Carvedilol
Caspofungin
Cefaclor
Cefadroxil
Cefamandole
Cefazolin
Cefdinir
Cefepime
Cefixime
Cefmetazole
Cefonicid
Cefoperazone
Cefotaxime
Cefotetan
Cefoxitin
Cefpodoxime
Cefprozil
Ceftazidime
Ceftazidime & Avibactam
Ceftibuten
Ceftizoxime
Ceftriaxone
Cefuroxime
Celecoxib
Cephalexin
Cephalothin
Cephapirin
Cephradine
Cetuximab
Chlorambucil
Chloramphenicol
Chlordiazepoxide
Chlormezanone
Chloroquine
Chlorpromazine
Chlorpropamide
Chlorthalidone
Cilostazol
Cimetidine
Cinnarizine
Ciprofloxacin

Cisplatin
Cladribine
Clarithromycin
Clindamycin
Clobazam
Clofibrate
Clomiphene
Clopidogrel
Cloxacillin
Clozapine
Co-Trimoxazole
Cobimetinib
Cocaine
Codeine
Colchicine
Cyclophosphamide
Cycloserine
Cyclosporine
Cytarabine
Danazol
Dapsone
Darunavir
Deflazacort
Delavirdine
Demeclocycline
Denileukin
Dexamethasone
Dextroamphetamine
Diatrizoate
Diclofenac
Dicloxacillin
Didanosine
Diflunisal
Diltiazem
Dimenhydrinate
Diphenhydramine
Dipyridamol
Disulfiram
Docetaxel
Dorzolamide
Doxycycline
Dronedarone
Duloxetine
Efavirenz
Enalapril
Enoxacin
Ephedrine
Erythromycin
Eslicarbazepine
Ethambutol
Ethosuximide
Etidronate
Etodolac
Etoposide
Etoricoxib
Famotidine
Febuxostat
Felbamate
Fenbufen
Fenofibrate
Fenoprofen
Fexofenadine
Flucloxacillin
Fluconazole
Fludarabine
Fluoxetine
Fluphenazine
Flurazepam
Flurbiprofen
Fluvoxamine
Foscarnet
Furosemide
Gabapentin
Galantamine
Gefitinib
Gemcitabine
Gemeprost
Gentamicin
Ginkgo Biloba
Ginseng
Glipizide
Gold & Gold Compounds
Grepafloxacin
Griseofulvin
Heparin
Heroin
Human Papillomavirus (HPV) Vaccine
Hydralazine
Hydrochlorothiazide
Hydroxychloroquine
Ibandronate
Ibuprofen
Idelalisib
Imatinib
Imipenem/Cilastatin
Imiquimod
Immune Globulin IV
Indapamide
Indinavir
Indomethacin
Infliximab
Iohexol
Ipilimumab
Isoniazid
Isotretinoin
Itraconazole
Ivermectin
Ixazomib
Ketoprofen
Ketorolac
Lacosamide
Lamivudine
Lamotrigine
Lansoprazole
Latanoprost
Leflunomide
Lenalidomide
Letrozole
Levamisole
Levetiracetam
Levofloxacin
Lidocaine
Lincomycin
Linezolid
Lomefloxacin
Lomustine
Loracarbef
Lorazepam
Lovastatin
Lymecycline
Maprotiline
Mebendazole
Mechlorethamine
Meclofenamate
Medroxyprogesterone
Mefenamic Acid
Mefloquine
Meloxicam
Meperidine
Mephenytoin
Mephobarbital
Meprobamate
Mercaptopurine
Meropenem
Mesna
Metamizole
Methamphetamine
Methazolamide
Methimazole
Methotrexate
Methsuximide
Methyldopa
Methylprednisolone
Metolazone
Metronidazole
Mexiletine
Miltefosine
Minocycline
Minoxidil
Mirtazapine
Mizoribine
Modafinil
Moxifloxacin
Mupirocin
Nabumetone
Nalidixic Acid
Naproxen
Neomycin
Nevirapine
Nifedipine
Nimesulide
Nitrofurantoin
Nivolumab
Norfloxacin
Nystatin
Ofloxacin
Omeprazole
Ondansetron
Oral Contraceptives
Oseltamivir
Osimertinib
Oxacillin
Oxaprozin
Oxazepam
Oxcarbazepine
Paclitaxel
Palbociclib
Panitumumab
Pantoprazole
Papaverine
PEG-Interferon
Pembrolizumab
Pemetrexed
Penicillamine
Penicillin G
Penicillin V
Pentamidine
Pentazocine
Pentobarbital
Peplomycin
Pertuzumab
Phenobarbital
Phenolphthalein
Phenylbutazone
Phenytoin
Piperacillin
Piperacillin/Tazobactam
Piroxicam
Plicamycin
Prednisolone
Primidone
Pristinamycin
Procarbazine
Prochlorperazine
Promethazine
Propranolol
Propylthiouracil
Pyrazinamide
Pyridoxine
Pyrimethamine
Quinidine
Quinine
Raltegravir
Ramipril
Ranitidine
Regorafenib
Reserpine
Ribavirin
Ribociclib
Rifampin
Rifaximin
Risedronate
Ritodrine
Rituximab
Rofecoxib
Secobarbital
Selpercatinib
Sertraline
Sibutramine
Sitagliptin
Smallpox Vaccine
Sofosbuvir
Sorafenib
Stavudine
Streptomycin
Streptozocin
Strontium Ranelate
Sulfacetamide
Sulfadiazine
Sulfadoxine
Sulfamethoxazole
Sulfasalazine
Sulfisoxazole
Sulindac
Sunitinib
Tamoxifen
Tegafur/Gimeracil/Oteracil
Teicoplanin
Telaprevir
Temozolomide
Tenofovir Disoproxil
Terbinafine
Terconazole
Teriflunomide
Tetracycline
Tetrazepam
Thalidomide
Thiabendazole
Thiopental
Thioridazine
Ticlopidine
Tigecycline
Tiludronate
Timolol
Tocainide
Tolbutamide
Tolmetin
Torsemide
Trastuzumab
Trimethadione
Trimethoprim
Trovafloxacin
Valdecoxib
Valproic Acid
Vancomycin
Vandetanib
Varicella Vaccine
Vemurafenib
Venlafaxine
Verapamil
Vinorelbine

Vitamin A
Voriconazole
Warfarin
Zidovudine
Zoledronate
Zonisamide

Tinnitus

Acamprosate
Acetaminophen
Acetazolamide
Acitretin
Adalimumab
Almotriptan
Amikacin
Amitriptyline
Anagrelide
Aprepitant
Arsenic
Artemether/Lumefantrine
Artesunate
Aspirin
Atorvastatin
Avanafil
Azithromycin
Baclofen
Bedaquiline
Betaxolol
Bismuth
Bleomycin
Bortezomib
Botulinum Toxin (A & B)
Bupropion
Carbimazole
Carboplatin
Carvedilol
Cefpodoxime
Chlorambucil
Chloramphenicol
Chloroquine
Chlorpromazine
Cilostazol
Ciprofloxacin
Cisplatin
Citalopram
Clarithromycin
Clindamycin
Clomipramine
Colistin
Cyclobenzaprine
Cycloserine
Cyclosporine
Dasatinib
Daunorubicin
Deferoxamine
Degarelix
Delafloxacin
Desvenlafaxine
Devil's Claw
Dexamethasone
Dexlansoprazole
Doxepin
Doxycycline
Dronabinol
Duloxetine
Eletriptan
Elotuzumab
Eprosartan
Erlotinib
Erythromycin
Escitalopram
Eslicarbazepine
Esomeprazole
Eszopiclone
Etanercept
Ethambutol
Etoposide
Febuxostat
Frovatriptan
Gadodiamide
Gadoteridol
Gadoversetamide
Gentamicin
Glatiramer
Halofantrine
Hepatitis B Vaccine
Hydroxychloroquine
Ibuprofen
Imipramine
Indomethacin
Interferon Alfa
Isavuconazonium Sulfate
Isoniazid
Kanamycin
Ketorolac
Lapatinib
Lenalidomide
Levobetaxolol
Levofloxacin
Lidocaine
Lofexidine
Mefloquine
Meloxicam
Mesalamine
Methyl salicylate
Metronidazole
Minocycline
Moexipril
Moxifloxacin
Muromonab-CD3
Nabumetone
Nadolol
Naproxen
Nitroprusside
Omacetaxine
Pamidronate
Paromomycin
PEG-Interferon
Perflutren
Phenelzine
Piroxicam
Propylthiouracil
Quinine
Rabeprazole
Ranitidine
Ranolazine
Ribavirin
Rifaximin
Rivastigmine
Ropivacaine
Rotigotine
Ruxolitinib
Salsalate
Sarecycline
Sertraline
Sildenafil
Sirolimus
Sodium Oxybate
Sorafenib
St John's Wort
Sumatriptan
Tacrolimus
Tadalafil
Teicoplanin
Tetracycline
Tiagabine
Tobramycin
Tramadol
Triptorelin
Valdecoxib
Valproic Acid
Vancomycin
Vardenafil
Venlafaxine
Vigabatrin
Vinblastine
Vincristine
Voriconazole
Zaleplon
Ziconotide
Ziprasidone
Zolpidem
Zonisamide

Urticaria

Abatacept
Acamprosate
Acarbose
Acebutolol
Aceclofenac
Acetaminophen
Acetohexamide
Acetylcysteine
Acyclovir
Adalimumab
Albendazole
Albiglutide
Albuterol
Alclometasone
Aldesleukin
Alefacept
Alemtuzumab
Alendronate
Alfentanil
Alglucerase
Alglucosidase Alfa
Alirocumab
Allopurinol
Alpha-Lipoic Acid
Alprostadil
Alteplase
Amcinonide
Aminolevulinic Acid
Aminophylline
Aminosalicylate Sodium
Amiodarone
Amlodipine
Amobarbital
Amodiaquine
Amoxapine
Amoxicillin
Amphotericin B
Ampicillin
Anagrelide
Anakinra
Anidulafungin
Anistreplase
Anthrax Vaccine
Anti-Thymocyte Globulin (Equine)
Aprepitant
Arsenic
Artemether/Lumefantrine
Artesunate
Artichoke
Asciminib
Asparaginase
Asparaginase *Erwinia chrysanthemi*
Aspartame
Aspirin
Astemizole
Atenolol
Atorvastatin
Atovaquone/Proguanil
Atracurium
Atropine Sulfate
Avelumab
Azacitidine
Azathioprine
Azithromycin
Aztreonam
Bacitracin
BCG Vaccine
Benazepril
Benralizumab
Benznidazole
Bepotastine
Betamethasone
Bezafibrate
Bictegravir/Emtricitabine/Tenofovir Alafenamide
Bismuth
Bosutinib
Brinzolamide
Brodalumab
Bumetanide
Bupropion
Buspirone
Busulfan
Butorphanol
Caffeine
Calcipotriol
Calcitonin
Canagliflozin
Capsicum
Captopril
Caraway
Carbamazepine
Carbenicillin
Carboplatin
Carisoprodol
Caspofungin
Cefaclor
Cefadroxil
Cefamandole
Cefazolin
Cefdinir
Cefditoren
Cefepime
Cefixime
Cefmetazole
Cefonicid
Cefoperazone
Cefotaxime
Cefotetan
Cefpodoxime
Cefprozil
Ceftaroline Fosamil
Ceftazidime
Ceftibuten
Ceftizoxime
Ceftolozane & Tazobactam
Ceftriaxone
Cefuroxime
Celecoxib
Cephalexin
Cephalothin
Cephapirin
Cephradine
Certolizumab
Cetirizine
Chasteberry
Chloral Hydrate

Chlorambucil
Chloramphenicol
Chlordiazepoxide
Chlorhexidine
Chloroquine
Chlorothiazide
Chlorpromazine
Chlorpropamide
Chlorthalidone
Chlorzoxazone
Cidofovir
Cilostazol
Cimetidine
Cinoxacin
Ciprofloxacin
Cisplatin
Clarithromycin
Clemastine
Clindamycin
Clioquinol
Clofibrate
Clomiphene
Clomipramine
Clonidine
Clopidogrel
Clorazepate
Cloxacillin
Clozapine
Co-Trimoxazole
Coagulation Factor IX (Recombinant)
Cocaine
Codeine
Colchicine
Colestipol
Crisaborole
Cromolyn
Cyanocobalamin
Cyclamate
Cyclobenzaprine
Cyclophosphamide
Cycloserine
Cyclosporine
Cysteamine
Cytarabine
Dacarbazine
Daclizumab
Dalbavancin
Dapagliflozin
Dapsone
Darunavir
Dasatinib
Daunorubicin
Decitabine
Deferasirox
Deferoxamine
Deflazacort
Degarelix
Delafloxacin
Delavirdine
Desipramine
Desloratadine
Dexamethasone
Dexlansoprazole
Dextroamphetamine
Diazepam
Diclofenac
Dicloxacillin
Dicumarol
Diethylstilbestrol
Diflunisal
Digoxin
Dihydrocodeine
Diltiazem
Dimenhydrinate
Dimethyl Fumarate
Dinutuximab
Diphenoxylate
Dipyridamole
Dirithromycin
Disulfiram
Docetaxel
Donepezil
Doxacurium
Doxazosin
Doxorubicin
Doxycycline
Dupilumab
Echinacea
Efalizumab
Efavirenz
Eletriptan
Emtricitabine
Enalapril
Enoxacin
Enoxaparin
Ephedrine
Ertapenem
Erythromycin
Esomeprazole
Estazolam
Estrogens
Eszopiclone
Etanercept
Etelcalcetide
Ethambutol
Ethionamide
Ethosuximide
Etodolac
Etoricoxib
Evolocumab
Exenatide
Famotidine
Febuxostat
Felbamate
Felodipine
Fenofibrate
Fenoprofen
Fentanyl
Ferric carboxymaltose (injection)
Ferumoxytol
Fexofenadine
Finasteride
Flecainide
Flucloxacillin
Flumazenil
Fluorides
Fluoxetine
Flurbiprofen
Fluvoxamine
Folic Acid
Foscarnet
Fosinopril
Fulvestrant
Furazolidone
Furosemide
Gadobenate
Gadodiamide
Gadopentetate
Gadoteridol
Gadoversetamide
Ganciclovir
Garlic
Gefitinib
Gemfibrozil
Gemifloxacin
Gentamicin
Glatiramer
Glimepiride
Glipizide
Glucagon
Glyburide
Gold & Gold Compounds
Granulocyte Colony-Stimulating Factor (G-CSF)
Grapefruit Juice
Grepafloxacin
Griseofulvin
Halothane
Henna
Heparin
Hepatitis B Vaccine
Heroin
Histrelin
Hops
Human Papillomavirus Vaccine (Bivalent)
Hydrochlorothiazide
Hydrocodone
Hydrocortisone
Hydromorphone
Hydroxychloroquine
Hydroxyzine
Ibritumomab
Ibuprofen
Idarubicin
Idursulfase
Imatinib
Imiglucerase
Imipenem/Cilastatin
Imipramine
Immune Globulin IV
Indapamide
Indinavir
Indomethacin
Infliximab
Insulin
Insulin Glulisine
Interferon Alfa
Interferon Beta
Iodixanol
Iohexol
Iomeprol
Iopromide
Ioversol
Ipilimumab
Ipratropium
Irbesartan
Isavuconazonium Sulfate
Isoniazid
Isotretinoin
Isradipine
Itraconazole
Ivacaftor
Ivermectin
Ixazomib
Ixekizumab
Japanese Encephalitis Vaccine
Kava
Ketamine
Ketoconazole
Ketoprofen
Ketorolac
Labetalol
Lamivudine
Lamotrigine
Lanreotide
Lansoprazole
Leflunomide
Lenalidomide
Lepirudin
Lesinurad
Leucovorin
Leuprolide
Levamisole
Levetiracetam
Levocetirizine
Levofloxacin
Levomilnacipran
Levonorgestrel
Levothyroxine
Lidocaine
Linaclotide
Linagliptin
Lincomycin
Lindane
Linezolid
Liothyronine
Liraglutide
Lisinopril
Lithium
Lixisenatide
Lomefloxacin
Loracarbef
Loratadine
Losartan
Lubiprostone
Maprotiline
Measles, Mumps & Rubella (MMR) Virus Vaccine
Mebeverine
Mechlorethamine
Meclofenamate
Medroxyprogesterone
Mefenamic Acid
Mefloquine
Meloxicam
Melphalan
Memantine
Meningococcal Group B Vaccine
Meperidine
Mephenytoin
Meprobamate
Mercaptopurine
Meropenem
Mesna
Metamizole
Metformin
Methadone
Methamphetamine
Methazolamide
Methimazole
Methohexital
Methotrexate
Methoxsalen
Methsuximide
Methyldopa
Methylphenidate
Methylprednisolone
Metoclopramide
Metolazone
Metronidazole
Mexiletine
Micafungin
Miconazole
Midazolam
Milk Thistle
Miltefosine
Minocycline
Mirabegron

Mistletoe
Mitomycin
Mitotane
Mivacurium
Moexipril
Monosodium Glutamate
Montelukast
Moricizine
Moxidectin
Moxifloxacin
Mycophenolate
Nabumetone
Nafarelin
Nalbuphine
Nalidixic Acid
Naloxone
Naproxen
Naratriptan
Nefazodone
Nelfinavir
Neomycin
Neostigmine
Nevirapine
Niacin
Nicardipine
Nifedipine
Nifurtimox
Nilotinib
Nimesulide
Nisoldipine
Nitrofurantoin
Nitroglycerin
Nivolumab
Nizatidine
Norfloxacin
Obeticholic Acid
Octreotide
Ofatumumab
Ofloxacin
Olanzapine
Olsalazine
Omadacycline
Omalizumab
Ombitasvir/Paritaprevir/Ritonavir
Omeprazole
Ondansetron
Oral Contraceptives
Oritavancin
Osimertinib
Oxacillin
Oxaliplatin
Oxaprozin
Oxerutins
Oxilan
Oxprenolol
Oxycodone
Oxymorphone
Paclitaxel
Paliperidone
Pantoprazole
Pantothenic Acid
Paroxetine Hydrochloride
PEG-Interferon
Pegaptanib
Pegaspargase
Pembrolizumab
Pemetrexed
Penicillamine
Penicillin G
Penicillin V
Pentamidine
Pentosan
Pentostatin
Perflutren
Permethrin
Perphenazine
Phenobarbital
Phenolphthalein
Phenylbutazone
Phenytoin
Phytonadione
Pilocarpine
Pipecuronium
Piperacillin
Piperacillin/Tazobactam
Piroxicam
Pitavastatin
Pizotifen
Plasma (Human) Blood Product
Pneumococcal Vaccine
Polidocanol
Pomalidomide
Porfimer
Potassium Iodide
Praziquantel
Prazosin
Prednicarbate
Prednisolone
Prednisone
Prilocaine
Primaquine
Primidone
Pristinamycin
Probenecid
Procainamide
Procarbazine
Progestins
Promethazine
Propafenone
Propofol
Propoxyphene
Propranolol
Propylthiouracil
Propyphenazone
Protamine Sulfate
Psoralens
Quinacrine
Quinapril
Quinestrol
Quinidine
Quinine
Quinupristin/Dalfopristin
Rabeprazole
Ramipril
Ranitidine
Rapacuronium
Remifentanil
Ribavirin
Riboflavin
Rifampin
Rifapentine
Rifaximin
Risankizumab
Risedronate
Risperidone
Ritonavir
Rituximab
Rivaroxaban
Rivastigmine
Rofecoxib
Ropinirole
Roxithromycin
Rupatadine
Saccharin
Salmeterol
Salsalate
Saquinavir
Sebelipase Alfa
Secretin
Secukinumab
Sertraline
Sildenafil
Simvastatin
Smallpox Vaccine
Sodium Oxybate
Solifenacin
Sorafenib
Sparfloxacin
Spectinomycin
Spironolactone
Streptokinase
Streptomycin
Sufentanil
Sulfadiazine
Sulfamethoxazole
Sulfasalazine
Sulfisoxazole
Sulfites
Sulindac
Sulpiride / Levosulpride
Sumatriptan
Tacrine
Tacrolimus
Tartrazine
Tedizolid
Tegafur/Gimeracil/Oteracil
Teicoplanin
Telithromycin
Telmisartan
Tenecteplase
Teniposide
Tenofovir Disoproxil
Terbinafine
Terfenadine
Teriflunomide
Tesamorelin
Tetracycline
Thalidomide
Thiabendazole
Thimerosal
Thiopental
Thiotepa
Thyrotropin Alfa
Tiagabine
Ticlopidine
Tigecycline
Tinidazole
Tinzaparin
Tirofiban
Tizanidine
Tocilizumab
Tolazamide
Tolbutamide
Tolcapone
Tolmetin
Topiramate
Torsemide
Tosufloxacin
Tramadol
Trazodone
Triamcinolone
Triclabendazole
Trimethadione
Trimethoprim
Tripelennamine
Troleandomycin
Trovafloxacin
Turmeric
Urofollitropin
Valdecoxib
Valsartan
Vancomycin
Vardenafil
Varicella Vaccine
Vasopressin
Vedolizumab
Velaglucerase Alfa
Venlafaxine
Verapamil
Viltolarsen
Voriconazole
Warfarin
Yarrow
Yellow Fever Vaccine
Zalcitabine
Zaleplon
Zanamivir
Zidovudine
Ziprasidone
Zolmitriptan
Zolpidem
Zonisamide

Vasculitis

Abatacept
Acebutolol
Aceclofenac
Acenocoumarol
Acetaminophen
Acyclovir
Adalimumab
Aldesleukin
Alemtuzumab
Allopurinol
Aminosalicylate Sodium
Amiodarone
Amitriptyline
Amlodipine
Amoxapine
Amoxicillin
Amphotericin B
Ampicillin
Anastrozole
Anistreplase
Anthrax Vaccine
Asparaginase
Aspartame
Aspirin
Atenolol
Atorvastatin
Azacitidine
Azatadine
Azathioprine
Azithromycin
BCG Vaccine
Bendamustine
Bevacizumab
Bexarotene
Blinatumomab
Bortezomib
Bromocriptine
Busulfan
Captopril
Carbamazepine
Carbimazole
Carvedilol
Caspofungin
Celecoxib
Certolizumab
Cetuximab
Cevimeline

Chloramphenicol
Chlordiazepoxide
Chlorothiazide
Chlorpromazine
Chlorpropamide
Chlorthalidone
Chlorzoxazone
Cimetidine
Cinacalcet
Ciprofloxacin
Citalopram
Cladribine
Clarithromycin
Clindamycin
Clorazepate
Clozapine
Co-Trimoxazole
Cocaine
Colchicine
Cromolyn
Cyclophosphamide
Cyclosporine
Cyproheptadine
Cytarabine
Daclizumab
Dapagliflozin
Deferasirox
Delavirdine
Diazepam
Diclofenac
Didanosine
Diflunisal
Digoxin
Diltiazem
Diphenhydramine
Disulfiram
Doxycycline
Dronedarone
Dupilumab
Efavirenz
Enalapril
Ephedrine
Epirubicin
Erlotinib
Erythromycin
Estrogens
Etanercept
Ethacrynic Acid
Etodolac
Etoposide
Everolimus
Exemestane
Ezetimibe
Famciclovir
Famotidine
Fenbufen
Flucloxacillin
Fluorouracil
Fluoxetine
Flurbiprofen
Fluticasone Propionate
Furosemide
Gabapentin
Gefitinib
Gemcitabine
Gemfibrozil
Gentamicin
Glatiramer
Glimepiride
Glucagon
Glyburide
Gold & Gold Compounds
Golimumab
Granulocyte Colony-Stimulating Factor (G-CSF)
Griseofulvin
Guanethidine
Heparin
Hepatitis B Vaccine
Heroin
Hydralazine
Hydrochlorothiazide
Hydroxychloroquine
Hydroxyurea
Ibrutinib
Ibuprofen
Icodextrin
Imatinib
Imipenem/Cilastatin
Imipramine
Imiquimod
Immune Globulin IV
Indapamide
Indinavir
Indomethacin
Infliximab
Influenza Vaccine
Insulin
Insulin Aspart
Interferon Alfa
Interferon Beta
Ipilimumab
Isoniazid
Isotretinoin
Itraconazole
Ixazomib
Ketoconazole
Ketorolac
Leflunomide
Leuprolide
Levamisole
Levetiracetam
Levofloxacin
Lisinopril
Lithium
Maprotiline
MDMA
Meclofenamate
Mefenamic Acid
Mefloquine
Meloxicam
Melphalan
Meningococcal Group B Vaccine
Meprobamate
Mercaptopurine
Mesalamine
Metformin
Methimazole
Methocarbamol
Methotrexate
Methoxsalen
Methyldopa
Methylphenidate
Metolazone
Minocycline
Mitotane
Nabumetone
Naproxen
Nelfinavir
Nicotine
Nifedipine
Nimesulide
Nivolumab
Nizatidine
Ofloxacin
Olanzapine
Olaparib
Omeprazole
Osimertinib
Oxacillin
Oxaliplatin
Pantoprazole
Paroxetine Hydrochloride
PEG-Interferon
Pembrolizumab
Pemetrexed
Penicillamine
Penicillin V
Pergolide
Phenobarbital
Phenylbutazone
Phenytoin
Phytonadione
Piroxicam
Potassium Iodide
Pramipexole
Pregabalin
Procainamide
Propylthiouracil
Psoralens
Pyridoxine
Quinapril
Quinidine
Quinine
Ramipril
Ranitidine
Ribavirin
Rifampin
Risedronate
Ritodrine
Rituximab
Rivastigmine
Rofecoxib
Secukinumab
Simvastatin
Sirolimus
Sofosbuvir
Sorafenib
Sotalol
Spironolactone
Streptokinase
Streptomycin
Sulfadiazine
Sulfamethoxazole
Sulfasalazine
Sulfisoxazole
Sulfites
Sulindac
Tacrolimus
Tamoxifen
Tartrazine
Telithromycin
Telmisartan
Terbinafine
Terbutaline
Tetracycline
Thalidomide
Thiamine
Thioridazine
Ticlopidine
Tinidazole
Tocainide
Tocilizumab
Torsemide
Trastuzumab Emtansine / Ado-Trastuzumab Emtansine
Trazodone
Tretinoin
Trichlormethiazide
Trimethadione
Trioxsalen
Triptorelin
Ustekinumab
Valproic Acid
Vancomycin
Vemurafenib
Verapamil
Vinorelbine
Warfarin
Zafirlukast
Zidovudine

Vertigo

Abacavir
Abaloparatide
Abarelix
Abatacept
Abemaciclib
Abiraterone
Abrocitinib
Acamprosate
Acebutolol
Aceclofenac
Acetaminophen
Acetohexamide
Acitretin
Adalimumab
Adenosine
Aducanumab
Afamelanotide
Afatinib
Aflibercept
Agalsidase
Albendazole
Albiglutide
Aldesleukin
Alectinib
Alefacept
Alemtuzumab
Alfuzosin
Alirocumab
Aliskiren
Allopurinol
Almotriptan
Alogliptin
Alosetron
Alpha-Lipoic Acid
Alprazolam
Alprostadil
Amantadine
Amifampridine
Amiloride
Amiodarone
Amisulpride
Amitriptyline
Amlodipine
Amodiaquine
Amoxapine
Amoxicillin
Anagrelide
Anidulafungin
Anti-Thymocyte Immunoglobulin (Rabbit)
Antihemophilic Factor
Apalutamide
Apixaban
Apomorphine
Apremilast
Aprepitant
Arformoterol
Aripiprazole
Armodafinil

Arsenic
Artemether/Lumefantrine
Artemisia
Artesunate
Articaine
Asciminib
Asenapine
Atazanavir
Atenolol
Atomoxetine
Atorvastatin
Atovaquone/Proguanil
Avacopan
Avanafil
Avapritinib
Avelumab
Axitinib
Azacitidine
Azathioprine
Azilsartan
Azithromycin
Baclofen
Basiliximab
Bedaquiline
Belatacept
Belinostat
Belzutifan
Bempedoic acid
Benazepril
Bendamustine
Benralizumab
Benznidazole
Benzphetamine
Bepridil
Betaxolol
Bezafibrate
Bictegravir/Emtricitabine/ Tenofovir Alafenamide
Binimetinib
Biperiden
Bismuth
Bisoprolol
Black Cohosh
Bleomycin
Blinatumomab
Bortezomib
Bosentan
Bosutinib
Botulinum Toxin (A & B)
Bremelanotide
Brentuximab Vedotin
Brexanolone
Brexpiprazole
Brinzolamide
Brivaracetam
Brodalumab
Bromocriptine
Bupivacaine
Buprenorphine
Bupropion
Burosumab
Butorphanol
C1-Esterase Inhibitor
Cabazitaxel
Cabergoline
Cabozantinib
Canagliflozin
Canakinumab
Candesartan
Cannabidiol
Capecitabine
Carbamazepine
Carbetocin
Carboplatin
Carfilzomib
Cariprazine
Carisoprodol
Carvedilol
Casimersen
Caspofungin
Cedazuridine & Decitabine
Cefditoren
Cefepime
Cefpodoxime
Ceftaroline Fosamil
Ceftazidime & Avibactam
Ceftolozane & Tazobactam
Ceftriaxone
Cefuroxime
Celecoxib
Celiprolol
Cenobamate
Certolizumab
Cevimeline
Chasteberry
Chloroquine
Chlorpromazine
Chlorthalidone
Chlorzoxazone
Cholera Vaccine
Choline Fenofibrate
Cilazapril
Cilostazol
Cinacalcet
Cinnarizine
Ciprofloxacin
Cisplatin
Citalopram
Clevidipine
Clobazam
Clofarabine
Clofazimine
Clomipramine
Clonidine
Clozapine
Co-Trimoxazole
Coagulation Factor IX (Recombinant)
Cobicistat/Elvitegravir/ Emtricitabine/Tenofovir Disoproxil
Codeine
Colesevelam
Crizotinib
Crofelemer
Cyclobenzaprine
Cycloserine
Cyclosporine
Cysteamine
Cytarabine
Dabigatran
Dabrafenib
Daclatasvir
Daclizumab
Dalbavancin
Dalfampridine
Dantrolene
Dapagliflozin
Dapsone
Daptomycin
Darbepoetin Alfa
Daridorexant
Darifenacin
Dasatinib
Daunorubicin
Decitabine
Deferasirox
Deflazacort
Degarelix
Delafloxacin
Denileukin
Denosumab
Desloratadine
Desmopressin
Desvenlafaxine
Deutetrabenazine
Dexamethasone
Dexketoprofen
Dexmedetomidine
Dextroamphetamine
Dextromethorphan
Diatrizoate
Diazepam
Diazoxide
Diclofenac
Dicyclomine
Diethylpropion
Difelikefalin
Dihydrocodeine
Dihydroergotamine
Diltiazem
Diphenhydramine
Dipyridamole
Disopyramide
Disulfiram
Docetaxel
Dofetilide
Dolasetron
Dolutegravir
Donepezil
Doravirine
Doravirine/Lamiduvine/ Tenofovir Disoproxil
Doxazosin
Doxepin
Doxercalciferol
Doxorubicin
Doxycycline
Dronabinol
Dronedarone
Droxidopa
Duloxetine
Dutasteride
Echinacea
Eculizumab
Edaravone
Edrophonium
Efavirenz
Eflornithine
Elagolix Sodium
Eletriptan
Eliglustat
Elotuzumab
Eluxadoline
Empagliflozin
Emtricitabine
Enalapril
Encorafenib
Entacapone
Entecavir
Entrectinib
Enzalutamide
Epinephrine
Eplerenone
Epoetin Alfa
Eprosartan
Eravacycline
Eribulin
Escitalopram
Eslicarbazepine
Esomeprazole
Estramustine
Eszopiclone
Etanercept
Etravirine
Everolimus
Evolocumab
Exenatide
Ezetimibe
Ezogabine
Factor VIII - von Willebrand Factor
Famotidine
Febuxostat
Fedratinib hydrochloride
Felbamate
Fentanyl
Ferric carboxymaltose (injection)
Ferric Gluconate
Ferumoxytol
Fesoterodine
Fexinidazole
Finasteride
Fingolimod
Flecainide
Flibanserin
Flumazenil
Fluorouracil
Fluoxetine
Fluphenazine
Flurbiprofen
Fluticasone Furoate
Fluticasone Propionate
Fluvoxamine
Follitropin Alfa/Beta
Fomepizole
Fomivirsen
Formoterol
Fosfomycin
Fosphenytoin
Fostamatinib
Fostemsavir
Frovatriptan
Fulvestrant
Furazolidone
Gabapentin
Gadobenate
Gadobutrol
Gadodiamide
Gadofosveset
Gadopentetate
Gadoteridol
Gadoversetamide
Gadoxetate
Galantamine
Gatifloxacin
Gefitinib
Gemifloxacin
Gentamicin
Gilteritinib
Glasdegib
Glatiramer
Gliclazide
Glimepiride
Glipizide
Glycopyrrolate
Golimumab
Golodirsen
Goserelin
Granisetron

Granulocyte Colony-Stimulating Factor (G-CSF)
Guanabenz
Guanadrel
Guanethidine
Guanfacine
Halofantrine
Haloperidol
Hawthorn (Fruit, Leaf, Flower Extract)
Human Papillomavirus (HPV) Vaccine
Human Papillomavirus Vaccine (Bivalent)
Hydrochlorothiazide
Hydrocodone
Hydromorphone
Hydroxychloroquine
Ibalizumab
Ibandronate
Ibrexafungerp
Ibritumomab
Ibrutinib
Icatibant
Icodextrin
Idebenone
Iloperidone
Iloprost
Imatinib
Imidapril
Imiglucerase
Imipramine
Imiquimod
Immune Globulin IV
Indapamide
Indinavir
Indoramin
Infliximab
Influenza Vaccine
Insulin
Insulin Detemir
Interferon Alfa
Interferon Beta
Iobenguane
Iodixanol
Iohexol
Iomeprol
Iopromide
Ioversol
Ipilimumab
Irinotecan
Isavuconazonium Sulfate
Isocarboxazid
Isosorbide Mononitrate
Isradipine
Istradefylline
Itraconazole
Ivabradine
Ivacaftor
Ivermectin
Ixabepilone
Japanese Encephalitis Vaccine
Kanamycin
Kava
Ketamine
Ketoconazole
Ketorolac
Lacosamide
Lamivudine
Lamotrigine
Lansoprazole
Lapatinib
Larotrectinib
Lasmiditan
Latanoprost
Ledipasvir & Sofosbuvir
Leflunomide
Lenalidomide
Lenvatinib
Lesinurad
Letrozole
Levetiracetam
Levodopa
Levofloxacin
Levomepromazine
Levomilnacipran
Levonorgestrel
Lidocaine
Linagliptin
Linezolid
Liothyronine
Liraglutide
Lisdexamfetamine
Lisinopril
Lithium
Lixisenatide
Lofexidine
Lomitapide
Lopinavir
Loratadine
Lorazepam
Lorcainide
Lorcaserin
Lorlatinib
Losartan
Lovastatin
Loxapine
Lubiprostone
Lumateperone
Lumiracoxib
Lurasidone
Lutetium Lu177 Dotatate
Macitentan
Maraviroc
Marihuana
Mazindol
MDMA
Mebendazole
Mefloquine
Melatonin
Meloxicam
Melphalan flufenamide
Memantine
Meperidine
Mepolizumab
Meptazinol
Mesalamine
Metamizole
Metaxalone
Metformin
Methocarbamol
Methotrexate
Methoxyflurane
Methylnaltrexone
Methylphenidate
Methylprednisolone
Metronidazole
Mexiletine
Micafungin
Midazolam
Midostaurin
Mifepristone
Miglustat
Milnacipran
Miltefosine
Minocycline
Minoxidil
Mirabegron
Mirtazapine
Mitapivat
Mivacurium
Mizoribine
Moclobemide
Modafinil
Moexipril
Montelukast
Morphine
Moxidectin
Moxifloxacin
Moxonidine
Mupirocin
Muromonab-CD3
Mycophenolate
Nabilone
Nabumetone
Nadolo
Nalbuphine
Nalmefene
Naloxegol
Naloxone
Naltrexone
Naproxen
Naratriptan
Nateglinide
Nebivolol
Nefazodone
Nelarabine
Nelfinavir
Nesiritide
Netupitant & Palonosetron
Niacin
Nicorandil
Nifedipine
Nifurtimox
Nilotinib
Nilutamide
Nintedanib
Niraparib
Nisoldipine
Nitazoxanide
Nivolumab
Nizatidine
Norfloxacin
Nortriptyline
Obeticholic Acid
Octreotide
Ofloxacin
Olanzapine
Oliceridine
Olmesartan
Olodaterol
Omacetaxine
Omadacycline
Omalizumab
Ombitasvir/Paritaprevir/Ritonavir
Ombitasvir/Paritaprevir/Ritonavir and Dasabuvir
Omeprazole
Ondansetron
Opicapone
Oral Contraceptives
Oritavancin
Orlistat
Osilodrostat
Oxaliplatin
Oxcarbazepine
Oxerutins
Oxilan
Oxprenolol
Oxybutynin
Oxycodone
Oxymorphone
Paclitaxel
Pacritinib
Palbociclib
Paliperidone
Palonosetron
Pancrelipase
Pandemic Influenza Vaccine (H1N1)
Panitumumab
Panobinostat
Pantoprazole
Paricalcitol
Paroxetine Hydrochloride
Paroxetine Mesylate
Pasireotide
Patisiran
PEG-Interferon
Pegaptanib
Pegaspargase
Peginesatide
Pegloticase
Pegvisomant
Pembrolizumab
Pemetrexed
Pentamidine
Pentazocine
Perampanel
Perflutren
Pergolide
Perindopril
Pertuzumab
Phendimetrazine
Phenelzine
Phenobarbital
Phenoxybenzamine
Phentermine
Pilocarpine
Pioglitazone
Piperacillin
Piracetam
Pirfenidone
Piroxicam
Pizotifen
Plazomicin
Pomalidomide
Ponatinib
Ponesimod
Posaconazole
Pramipexole
Pramlintide
Pranlukast
Prasugrel
Pravastatin
Praziquantel
Prazosin
Prednicarbate
Prednisolone
Pregabalin
Prenylamine
Pretomanid
Promazine
Promethazine
Propafenone
Propoxyphene
Propranolol
Prucalopride
Pseudoephedrine
Pyrimethamine
Quetiapine

Quinagolide
Quinapril
Quinidine
Quinine
Rabeprazole
Radium-223 Dichloride
Raltegravir
Ramelteon
Ramipril
Ranolazine
Rasagiline
Reboxetine
Regadenoson
Remifentanil
Remimazolam
Repaglinide
Reslizumab
Revefenacin
Ribavirin
Rifabutin
Rifampin
Rifapentine
Rifaximin
Rilpivirine
Riluzole
Rimantadine
Rimonabant
Riociguat
Risedronate
Risperidone
Ritonavir
Rituximab
Rivaroxaban
Rivastigmine
Rizatriptan
Rofecoxib
Roflumilast
Rolapitant
Romiplostim
Ropinirole
Ropivacaine
Rosuvastatin
Rotigotine
Roxatidine
Rucaparib
Rufinamide
Rupatadine
Ruxolitinib
Sacubitril/Valsartan
Safinamide
Salmeterol
Sarecycline
Saw Palmetto
Saxagliptin
Scopolamine
Secnidazole
Selegiline
Selenium
Selexipag
Selinexor
Sertraline
Setmelanotide
Sibutramine
Sildenafil
Silodosin
Simvastatin
Sincalide
Siponimod
Sipuleucel-T
Sitaxentan
Sodium Oxybate
Sofosbuvir
Solifenacin
Solriamfetol
Sonidegib
Sorafenib
Sotorasib
Spectinomycin
St John's Wort
Streptomycin
Strontium Ranelate
Sucralfate
Sufentanil
Sugammadex
Sulfadoxine
Sulfasalazine
Sumatriptan
Sunitinib
Suvorexant
Tacrine
Tacrolimus
Tadalafil
Tafenoquine
Talazoparib
Taliglucerase
Talimogene Laherparepvec
Tamoxifen
Tamsulosin
Tapentadol
Tedizolid
Tegafur/Gimeracil/Oteracil
Tegaserod
Teicoplanin
Telavancin
Telbivudine
Telithromycin
Telmisartan
Telotristat Ethyl
Temozolomide
Tenapanor hydrochloride
Tenapanor hydrochloride
Tenofovir Disoproxil
Tepotinib
Terazosin
Terbutaline
Teriparatide
Tetrabenazine
Tetracaine & Oxymetazoline
Tezacaftor/Ivacaftor
Thalidomide
Thiabendazole
Thioridazine
Thyrotropin Alfa
Tiagabine
Tianeptine
Ticagrelor
Tigecycline
Tildrakizumab
Tiludronate
Timolol
Tinidazole
Tiotropium
Tipranavir
Tizanidine
Tocainide
Tocilizumab
Tofacitinib
Tolcapone
Tolterodine
Tolvaptan
Topiramate
Toremifene
Torsemide
Tositumomab & Iodine131
Tosufloxacin
Trabectedin
Tramadol
Trametinib
Trandolapril
Tranylcypromine
Trastuzumab
Trastuzumab Emtansine / Ado-Trastuzumab Emtansine
Trazodone
Treprostinil
Triclabendazole
Trimipramine
Triptorelin
Troglitazone
Trospium
Trovafloxacin
Typhoid Vaccine
Ubrogepant
Ulipristal
Unoprostone
Urapidil
Ursodiol
Ustekinumab
Valbenazine
Valerian
Valproic Acid
Valrubicin
Valsartan
Vancomycin
Vardenafil
Varenicline
Varicella Vaccine
Velaglucerase Alfa
Venlafaxine
Verapamil
Verteporfin
Vigabatrin
Vilazodone
Vildagliptin
Vismodegib
Voriconazole
Vorinostat
Vortioxetine
Vosoritide
Warfarin
Zafirlukast
Zaleplon
Zanamivir
Ziconotide
Zidovudine
Ziprasidone
Zofenopril
Zoledronate
Zolmitriptan
Zolpidem
Zonisamide
Zoster Vaccine
Zuclopenthixol

Xerostomia

Abemaciclib
Acamprosate
Acebutolol
Acetaminophen
Acetazolamide
Acitretin
Aclidinium
Afatinib
Aflibercept
Albendazole
Albuterol
Aldesleukin
Almotriptan
Alprazolam
Alprostadil
Amantadine
Amifostine
Amiloride
Amisulpride
Amitriptyline
Amlodipine
Amoxapine
Amoxicillin
Apraclonidine
Aprepitant
Arbutamine
Aripiprazole
Armodafinil
Arsenic
Asenapine
Astemizole
Atomoxetine
Atropine Sulfate
Azatadine
Azelastine
Baclofen
Balsalazide
Bendamustine
Bendroflumethiazide
Benzphetamine
Benztropine
Bepridil
Betaxolol
Bexarotene
Bicalutamide
Bisacodyl
Bismuth
Bisoprolol
Botulinum Toxin (A & B)
Brexanolone
Brexpiprazole
Brimonidine
Brinzolamide
Bromelain
Bromocriptine
Brompheniramine
Bumetanide
Buprenorphine
Bupropion
Buspirone
Butorphanol
Cabergoline
Caffeine
Canagliflozin
Cannabidiol
Captopril
Cariprazine
Carisoprodol
Carvedilol
Cefditoren
Cefiderocol
Cefixime
Ceftibuten
Celecoxib
Cenobamate
Cetirizine
Cetuximab
Cevimeline
Chasteberry
Chlordiazepoxide
Chlormezanone
Chlorpheniramine
Chlorpromazine
Ciprofloxacin
Cisplatin
Citalopram
Clarithromycin
Clemastine

Clindamycin
Clomipramine
Clonazepam
Clonidine
Clorazepate
Clozapine
Codeine
Conivaptan
Crofelemer
Cromolyn
Cyclobenzaprine
Cyproheptadine
Daclatasvir
Dacomitinib
Dapagliflozin
Daridorexant
Darifenacin
Dasatinib
Daunorubicin
Degarelix
Delavirdine
Desipramine
Desloratadine
Desvenlafaxine
Deutetrabenazine
Dexamethasone
Dexchlorpheniramine
Dexketoprofen
Dexlansoprazole
Dexmedetomidine
Dexmethylphenidate
Dextroamphetamine
Dextromethorphan
Diazepam
Diclofenac
Dicyclomine
Didanosine
Diethylpropion
Diflunisal
Dihydrocodeine
Dihydroergotamine
Diltiazem
Dimenhydrinate
Diphenhydramine
Diphenoxylate
Dirithromycin
Disopyramide
Domperidone
Donepezil
Doxazosin
Doxepin
Dronabinol
Duloxetine
Dutasteride
Efavirenz
Eletriptan
Eltrombopag
Enalapril
Enfuvirtide
Enoxacin
Entacapone
Ephedra
Ephedrine
Epinephrine
Eprosartan
Erdafitinib
Eribulin
Escitalopram
Eslicarbazepine
Esmolol
Estazolam
Eszopiclone
Etravirine
Everolimus
Exemestane
Ezogabine
Famotidine
Felbamate
Felodipine
Fenoprofen
Fentanyl
Fesoterodine
Flavoxate
Flecainide
Flibanserin
Fluconazole
Flumazenil
Fluorides
Fluoxetine
Fluphenazine
Flurazepam
Flurbiprofen
Fluvoxamine
Formoterol
Fosfomycin
Fosinopril
Fosphenytoin
Frovatriptan
Furosemide
Gabapentin
Gadobenate
Gadodiamide
Gadopentetate
Gadoteridol
Gadoversetamide
Gadoxetate
Ganciclovir
Gemifloxacin
Glatiramer
Glycopyrrolate
Goserelin
Granisetron
Grepafloxacin
Griseofulvin
Guanabenz
Guanadrel
Guanethidine
Guanfacine
Haloperidol
Hydrocodone
Hydromorphone
Hydroxyzine
Hyoscyamine
Ibuprofen
Iloperidone
Imatinib
Imipramine
Indapamide
Indinavir
Infigratinib
Inotersen
Insulin
Interferon Alfa
Ioversol
Ipilimumab
Ipratropium
Isocarboxazid
Isoetharine
Isoproterenol
Isotretinoin
Isradipine
Itraconazole
Ketoprofen
Ketorolac
Ketotifen
Lamivudine
Lamotrigine
Lansoprazole
Leflunomide
Lenalidomide
Lenvatinib
Letrozole
Levocetirizine
Levodopa
Levofloxacin
Levomilnacipran
Liraglutide
Lisdexamfetamine
Lisinopril
Lithium
Lofexidine
Lomefloxacin
Loperamide
Loratadine
Lorazepam
Lorcaserin
Losartan
Lovastatin
Loxapine
Lubiprostone
Lumateperone
Maprotiline
Marihuana
Mazindol
MDMA
Meclizine
Meloxicam
Meperidine
Mesalamine
Metamizole
Methadone
Methamphetamine
Methantheline
Methazolamide
Methyldopa
Methylphenidat
Metoclopramide
Metolazone
Metronidazole
Mexiletine
Midodrine
Mifepristone
Miglustat
Milnacipran
Minocycline
Mirabegron
Mirtazapine
Mitapivat
Mizolastine
Modafinil
Moexipril
Molindone
Moricizine
Morphine
Moxifloxacin
Moxisylyte
Moxonidine
Mupirocin
Nabilone
Nabumetone
Nadolol
Nalbuphine
Nalmefene
Naloxone
Naltrexone
Naproxen
Nedocromil
Nefazodone
Neostigmine
Neratinib
Nevirapine
Nicardipine
Nicotine
Nifedipine
Nilotinib
Nilutamide
Niraparib
Nisoldipine
Nitrofurantoin
Nitroglycerin
Nivolumab
Nizatidine
Norfloxacin
Nortriptyline
Ofloxacin
Olanzapine
Olaparib
Olodaterol
Omacetaxine
Omeprazole
Ondansetron
Opicapone
Orlistat
Oxaliplatin
Oxazepam
Oxcarbazepine
Oxprenolol
Oxybutynin
Oxycodone
Oxymorphone
Oxytocin
Paliperidone
Palonosetron
Panobinostat
Pantoprazole
Papaverine
Paricalcitol
Paromomycin
Paroxetine Hydrochloride
PEG-Interferon
Pembrolizumab
Pemetrexed
Pemigatinib
Pentamidine
Pentazocine
Pentoxifylline
Perflutren
Pergolide
Perindopril
Pexidartinib hydrochloride
Phendimetrazine
Phenelzine
Phenobarbital
Phenoxybenzamine
Phentermine
Pilocarpine
Pimozide
Pirfenidone
Piroxicam
Pitolisant hydrochloride
Pizotifen
Posaconazole
Pralsetinib
Pramipexole
Prazepam
Prazosin
Pregabalin
Prochlorperazine
Procyclidine
Promethazine
Propafenone
Propantheline

Propofol
Propoxyphene
Propranolol
Protriptyline
Pseudoephedrine
Pyridostigmine
Pyrimethamine
Quazepam
Quetiapine
Quinapril
Rabeprazole
Raltitrexed
Ramipril
Ranolazine
Rasagiline
Reboxetine
Regadenoson
Regorafenib
Remifentanil
Reserpine
Rifaximin
Riluzole
Rimantadine
Risperidone
Ritonavir
Rivaroxaban
Rivastigmine
Rizatriptan
Rofecoxib
Rolapitant
Ropinirole
Rotigotine
Rucaparib
Rupatadine
Salmeterol
Saquinavir
Scopolamine
Selegiline
Selpercatinib
Sertindole
Sertraline
Setmelanotide
Sevoflurane
Sibutramine
Sildenafil
Sodium Oxybate
Solifenacin
Solriamfetol
Sorafenib
Sotalol
Sparfloxacin
Spironolactone
St John's Wort
Sucralfate
Sugammadex
Sulfamethoxazole
Sulfasalazine
Sulindac
Sulpiride / Levosulpiride
Sumatriptan
Sunitinib
Suvorexant
Tacrine
Tadalafil
Tamoxifen
Tamsulosin
Tapentadol
Tasimelteon
Tecovirimat
Tedizolid
Telithromycin
Telmisartan
Temazepam
Terazosin
Terbutaline
Terfenadine
Thalidomide
Thiabendazole
Thioguanine
Thioridazine
Thiothixene
Tiagabine
Tianeptine
Tigecycline
Tiludronate
Timolol
Tinidazole
Tiotropium
Tizanidine
Tocainide
Tolcapone
Tolterodine
Tolvaptan
Topiramate
Toremifene
Tosufloxacin
Tramadol
Trametinib
Trandolapril
Tranylcypromine
Trastuzumab Emtansine / Ado-Trastuzumab Emtansine
Trazodone
Tretinoin
Triamcinolone
Triamterene
Triazolam
Trihexyphenidyl
Trimeprazine
Trimipramine
Tripelennamine
Triprolidine
Trospium
Trovafloxacin
Tryptophan
Ubrogepant
Ulipristal
Umeclidinium
Unoprostone
Valbenazine
Valdecoxib
Valproic Acid
Valsartan
Vardenafil
Varenicline
Vemurafenib
Venlafaxine
Verapamil
Vibegron
Vilazodone
Viloxazine
Vitamin A
Voriconazole
Vorinostat
Vortioxetine
Zalcitabine
Zaleplon
Ziconotide
Zidovudine
Ziprasidone
Zolmitriptan
Zolpidem
Zonisamide
Zuclopenthixol

Main Classes of Drugs

5-HT1 agonists
- Almotriptan
- Eletriptan
- Frovatriptan
- Naratriptan
- Rizatriptan
- Sumatriptan
- Zolmitriptan

5-HT3 antagonists
- Alosetron
- Dolasetron
- Granisetron
- Ondansetron
- Palonosetron

Adrenergic alpha-receptor agonists
- Clonidine
- Dexmedetomidine
- Dopamine
- Ephedrine
- Guanabenz
- Guanadrel
- Guanethidine
- Guanfacine
- Methyldopa
- Midodrine
- Mirtazapine
- Phenylephrine
- Phenylpropanolamine
- Polythiazide
- Pseudoephedrine

Adrenergic alpha-receptor antagonists
- Alfuzosin
- Doxazosin
- Phenoxybenzamine
- Phentolamine
- Prazosin
- Silodosin
- Tamsulosin
- Terazosin
- Urapidil

Adrenergic alpha2-receptor agonists
- Apraclonidine
- Brimonidine
- Lofexidine
- Tizanidine

Adrenergic beta-receptor agonists
- Arbutamine
- Dobutamine
- Isoetharine
- Isoproterenol
- Isoxsuprine
- Metoprolol

Adrenergic beta-receptor antagonists (beta blockers)
- Acebutolol
- Atenolol
- Betaxolol
- Bisoprolol
- Carteolol
- Carvedilol
- Celiprolol
- Esmolol
- Labetalol
- Levobetaxolol
- Levobunolol
- Metipranolol
- Nadolol
- Nebivolol
- Penbutolol
- Pindolol
- Propranolol
- Sotalol
- Timolol

Alkylating agents
- Altretamine
- Bendamustine
- Busulfan
- Carboplatin
- Carmustine
- Chlorambucil
- Cisplatin
- Cyclophosphamide
- Dacarbazine
- Estramustine
- Ifosfamide
- Lomustine
- Loncastuximab tesirine
- Mechlorethamine
- Melphalan
- Melphalan flufenamide
- Mitomycin
- Oxaliplatin
- Procarbazine
- Streptozocin
- Temozolomide
- Thiotepa

Amphetamines
- Benzphetamine
- Dextroamphetamine
- Diethylpropion
- MDMA
- Methamphetamine
- Methylphenidate
- Pemoline
- Phendimetrazine
- Phentermine
- Prenylamine

Analeptics
- Doxapram
- Modafinil

Analgesics

narcotic
- Dextromethorphan

non-narcotic
- Acetaminophen

non-opioid
- Ketorolac

opioid
- Alfentanil
- Dihydrocodeine
- Fentanyl
- Meptazinol
- Tapentadol

urinary
- Pentosan
- Phenazopyridine

Anesthetics
- Alfentanil
- Edrophonium
- Fentanyl
- Ketamine

general
- Chloral Hydrate
- Propofol
- Sodium Oxybate
- Sufentanil

inhalation
- Desflurane
- Enflurane
- Halothane
- Isoflurane
- Methoxyflurane
- Sevoflurane

local
- Articaine
- Bupivacaine
- Cocaine
- Levobupivacaine
- Lidocaine
- Mepivacaine
- Ropivacaine
- Tetracaine & Oxymetazoline

Angiotensin Converting Enzyme (ACE) inhibitors
- Benazepril
- Captopril
- Cilazapril
- Enalapril
- Fosinopril
- Imidapril
- Lisinopril
- Moexipril
- Perindopril
- Quinapril
- Ramipril
- Trandolapril
- Zofenopril

Angiotensin receptor antagonists (blockers)
- Azilsartan
- Candesartan
- Eprosartan
- Irbesartan
- Losartan
- Olmesartan
- Telmisartan
- Valsartan

Anti-Tumor Necrosis Factor-alpha (TNF-α antagonists, TNF inhibitors)
- Adalimumab
- Certolizumab
- Etanercept
- Golimumab
- Green Tea
- Infliximab
- Turmeric

Antiarrhythmics

class Ia
- Disopyramide
- Procainamide
- Quinidine

class Ib
- Lidocaine
- Mexiletine
- Phenytoin

class Ic
- Flecainide
- Moricizine
- Propafenone

class II
- Acebutolol
- Atenolol
- Esmolol
- Labetalol
- Metoprolol
- Nadolol
- Propranolol
- Sotalol

class III
- Amiodarone
- Bretylium
- Dofetilide
- Dronedarone
- Ibutilide
- Sotalol
- Vernakalant

class IV
- Adenosine
- Amlodipine
- Bepridil
- Digoxin
- Diltiazem
- Verapamil

Antibiotics

aminoglycoside
- Amikacin
- Gentamicin
- Kanamycin
- Neomycin
- Paromomycin
- Plazomicin
- Streptomycin
- Tobramycin

anthracycline
- Bleomycin
- Dactinomycin
- Daunorubicin
- Doxorubicin
- Epirubicin
- Idarubicin
- Mitomycin
- Mitoxantrone
- Peplomycin
- Valrubicin

beta-lactam
- Amoxicillin
- Ampicillin
- Ampicillin/Sulbactam
- Aztreonam
- Becampicillin
- Carbenicillin

DOI: 10.1201/9781003715672-1501

Cefiderocol
Ceftazidime & Avibactam
Ceftolozane & Tazobactam
Cloxacillin
Dicloxacillin
Flucloxacillin
Methicillin
Mezlocillin
Nafcillin
Oxacillin
Penicillin G
Penicillin V
Piperacillin
Ticarcillin

carbapenem
Doripenem
Ertapenem
Imipenem/Cilastatin
Imipenem/Cilastatin/ Relebactam
Meropenem
Meropenem & Vaborbactam

fluouroquinolone
Besifloxacin
Ciprofloxacin
Dealfloxacin
Enoxacin
Finafloxacin
Gatifloxacin
Gemifloxacin
Levofloxacin
Lomefloxacin
Moxifloxacin
Norfloxacin
Ofloxacin
Sparfloxacin
Tosufloxacin

glycopeptide
Daptomycin
Teicoplanin
Vancomycin

lincosamide
Clindamycin
Clindamycin/Tretinoin
Lincomycin

macrolide
Azithromycin
Clarithromycin
Dirithromycin
Erythromycin
Fidaxomicin
Roxithromycin
Telithromycin
Troleandomycin

nitrofuran
Furazolidone
Nitrofurazone

oxazolidinone
Linezolid
Tedizolid

penicillin
Amoxicillin
Ampicillin
Ampicillin/Sulbactam
Bacampicillin
Carbenicillin
Cloxacillin
Dicloxacillin
Flucloxacillin
Methicillin
Mezlocillin
Nafcillin
Oxacillin
Penicillin G
Penicillin V
Piperacillin
Ticarcillin

quinolone
Cinoxacin
Ciprofloxacin
Grepafloxacin
Levofloxacin
Nalidixic Acid
Ofloxacin
Ozenoxacin
Trovafloxacin

rifamycin
Rifabutin
Rifampin
Rifapentine
Rifaximin

streptogramin
Pristinamycin
Quinupristin/Dalfopristin

sulphonamide
Co-Trimoxazole
Sulfacetamide
Sulfadiazine
Sulfadoxine
Sulfamethoxazole
Sulfisoxazole

tetracycline
Chlortetracycline
Demeclocycline
Doxycycline
Eravacycline
Lymecycline
Minocycline
Omadacycline
Oxytetracycline
Sarecycline
Tetracycline
Tigecycline

topical
Mupirocin
Retapamulin

miscellaneous
Aminosalicylate Sodium
Bacitracin
Benznidazole
Capreomycin
Ceftriaxone
Chloramphenicol
Cycloserine
Dapsone
Ethionamide
Fosfomycin
Isoniazid
Methenamine
Nitrofurantoin
Plicamycin
Pyrazinamide
Quinacrine
Spectinomycin
Trimethoprim

Anticonvulsants
Brivaracetam
Carbamazepine
Cenobamate
Clobazam
Eslicarbazepine
Ezogabine
Felbamate
Gabapentin
Lacosamide
Lamotrigine
Levetiracetam
Mephenytoin
Oxcarbazepine
Perampanel
Phenacemide
Phenobarbital
Phensuximide
Phenytoin
Pregabalin
Primidone
Rufinamide
Tetrazepam
Tiagabine
Topiramate
Valproic Acid
Vigabatrin 934
Zonisamide 693

Antidepressants
Bupropion
Citalopram
Desvenlafaxine
Duloxetine
Escitalopram
Fluoxetine
Fluvoxamine
Isocarboxazid
Levomilnacipran
Milnacipran
Moclobemide
Nefazodone
Paroxetine Hydrochloride
Phenelzine
Reboxetine
Selegiline
Sertraline
Tianeptine
Tranylcypromine
Tryptophan
Venlafaxine
Vilazodone
Vortioxetine

tetracyclic
Maprotiline
Mianserin
Mirtazapine

tricyclic
Amitriptyline
Amoxapine
Clomipramine
Desipramine
Doxepin
Imipramine
Nortriptyline
Protriptyline
Trazodone
Trimipramine

Antiemetics
Amisulpride
Aprepitant
Artichoke
Chlorpromazine
Dexamethasone
Dimenhydrinate
Diphenhydramine
Domperidone
Dronabinol
Droperidol
Granisetron
Haloperidol
Marihuana
Meclizine
Metoclopramide
Nabilone
Ondansetron
Palonosetron
Peppermint
Perphenazine
Prochlorperazine
Rolapitant
Scopolamine
Trimethobenzamide

Antiepileptic
Brivaracetam
Cenobamate
Clobazam
Eslicarbazepine
Lacosamide
Lamotrigine
Perampanel
Rufinamide
Vigabatrin

hydantoin
Ethotoin
Fosphenytoin
Mephenytoin
Phenytoin

oxazolidinedione
Paramethadione z
Trimethadione

succinimide
Ethosuximide
Methsuximide

Antifungals

antimycotic
Amphotericin B
Caspofungin
Ciclopirox
Clioquinol
Clotrimazole
Econazole
Efinaconazole
Fluconazole
Griseofulvin
Ibrexafungerp
Isavuconazonium Sulfate
Itraconazole
Ketoconazole
Luliconazole
Micafungin
Nystatin
Posaconazole
Rosemary
Sertaconazole
Tavabarole
Terbinafine
Terconazole
Thiabendazole
Voriconazole

imidazole
Clotrimazole
Econazole
Ketoconazole
Luliconazole
Miconazole
Sertaconazole
Thiabendazole

oxaborole
Tavaborole
triazole
Efinaconazole
Fluconazole
Isavuconazonium Sulfate
Itraconazole
Posaconazole
Terconazole
Voriconazole

Antiinflammatories
- Aloe Vera (Gel, Juice, Leaf)
- Amlexanox
- Amodiaquine
- Bloodroot
- Boswellia
- Bromelain
- Butterbur
- Caraway
- Clofazimine
- Colchicine
- Devil's Claw
- Eucalyptus
- Evening Primrose
- Fish Oils
- Fluprednisolone
- Henna
- Horsetail
- Juniper
- Licorice
- Linseed
- Meadowsweet
- Myrrh
- Omega-3 Fatty Acids
- Polypodium Leucotomos
- Roflumilast
- Sarsaparilla
- Saw Palmetto
- Turmeric
- Willow Bark
- Yarrow

Antimalarials
- Amodiaquine
- Artemether/Lumefantrine
- Artemisia
- Artesunate
- Atovaquone
- Atovaquone/Proguanil
- Chloroquine
- Halofantrine
- Hydroxychloroquine
- Mefloquine
- Primaquine
- Pyrimethamine
- Quinacrine
- Quinidine
- Quinine
- Sulfadoxine
- Tafenoquine

Antimycobacterials
- Aminosalicylate Sodium
- Bedaquiline
- Clofazimine
- Dapsone
- Ethambutol
- Ethionamide
- Flucytosine
- Isoniazid
- Para-Aminosalicylic Acid
- Potassium Iodide
- Pretomanid
- Pyrazinamide
- Rifampin
- Rifapentin
- Star Anise (Chinese)

echinocandin
- Anidulafungin
- Caspofungin
- Micafungin

Antineoplastics
- Anastrozole
- Arsenic
- Asparaginase
- Asparaginase *Erwinia chrysanthemi*
- Atezolizumab
- Avelumab
- Azacitidine
- Bexarotene
- Cabazitaxel
- Capecitabine
- Carboplatin
- Cemiplimab
- Cetuximab
- Cisplatin
- Cladribine
- Cytarabine
- Dacarbazine
- Dasatinib
- Decitabine
- Denileukin
- Docetaxel
- Durvalumab
- Eribulin
- Erlotinib
- Everolimus
- Floxuridine
- Fludarabine
- Fluorouracil
- Gefitinib
- Gemcitabine
- Gemtuzumab
- Hydroxyurea
- Ibritumomab
- Imatinib
- Irinotecan
- Ixabepilone
- Lapatinib
- Levamisole
- Mercaptopurine
- Mitotane
- Mitoxantrone
- Nelarabine
- Nilotinib
- Nilutamide
- Nivolumab
- Oxaliplatin
- Paclitaxel
- Panitumumab
- Pazopanib
- Pembrolizumab
- Pentostatin
- Porfimer
- Sorafenib
- Streptozocin
- Sunitinib
- Tegafur/Gimeracil/Oteracil
- Temozolomide
- Temsirolimus
- Teniposide
- Testolactone
- Thioguanine
- Topotecan
- Tositumomab & Iodine131
- Trabectedin
- Trastuzumab
- Tretinoin
- Trlfluridine & Tipiracil
- Vorinostat

Antiplatelets

antithrombotic
- Abciximab
- Aspirin
- Cangrelor
- Cilostazol
- Clopidogrel
- Dipyridamole
- Eptifibatide
- Ticagrelor
- Tirofiban

CPTP
- Cangrelor
- Ticagrelor

thienopyridine
- Clopidogrel
- Prasugrel
- Ticlopidine

Antiprotozoals
- Atovaquone
- Chloroquine
- Clioquinol
- Fexinidazole
- Hydroxychloroquine
- Mefloquine
- Metronidazle
- Nifurtimox
- Nitazoxanide
- Pentamidine
- Primaquine
- Pyrimethamine
- Quinidine
- Quinine

Antipsychotics
- Amisulpride
- Aripiprazole
- Asenapine
- Brexpiprazole
- Carbamazepine
- Cariprazine
- Chlorpromazine
- Clozapine
- Droperidol
- Fluphenazine
- Haloperidol
- Iloperidone
- Levomepromazine
- Lithium
- Loxapine
- Lumateperone
- Lurasidone
- Mesoridazine
- Molindone
- Olanzapine
- Paliperidone
- Perphenazine
- Pimavanserin
- Pimozide
- Prochlorperazine
- Promazine
- Quetiapine
- Risperidone
- Sertindole
- Thioridazine
- Thiothixene
- Trifluoperazine
- Trimeprazine
- Valproic Acid
- Ziprasidone
- Zuclopenthixol
- Zuclopenthixol Acetate
- Zuclopenthixol Decanoate
- Zuclopenthixol Dihydrochloride

Antiretrovirals
- Adefovir
- Amprenavir
- Atazanavir
- Bictegravir/Emtricitabine/Tenofovir Alafenamide
- Cobicistat/Elvitegravir/Emtricitabine/Tenofovir Alafenamide
- Cobicistat/Elvitegravir/Emtricitabine/Tenofovir Disoproxil
- Darunavir
- Delavirdine
- Didanosine
- Dolutegravir
- Efavirenz
- Emtricitabine
- Enfuvirtide
- Fosamprenavir
- Fostemsavir
- Hydroxyurea
- Ibalizumab
- Indinavir
- Lamivudine
- Lopinavir
- Maraviroc
- Nelfinavir
- Nevirapine
- Raltegravir
- Rilpivirine
- Ritonavir
- Saquinavir
- Stavudine
- Tenofovir Disoproxil
- Zalcitabine
- Zidovudine

Antiviral
- Acyclovir
- Amantadine
- Cytarabine
- Entecavir
- Famciclovir
- Foscarnet
- Fostemsavir
- Ganciclovir
- Imiquimod
- Letermovir
- Oseltamivir
- Penciclovir
- Peramivir
- Podophyllotoxin
- Remdesivir
- Rimantadine
- Tenofovir Alafenamide
- Trifluridine
- Valacyclovir
- Valganciclovir
- Zanamivir

nucleoside analog
- Ribavirin
- Vidarabine

nucleotide analog
- Cidofovir
- Remdesivir

topical
- Acyclovir
- Docosanol

Anxiolytics
- Buspirone
- Chlormezanone
- Kava
- Lavender
- Meprobamate
- Tetrazepam
- Valerian

Barbiturates
Amobarbital
Aprobarbital
Butabarbital
Butalbital
Mephobarbital
Methohexital
Pentobarbital
Phenobarbital
Primidone
Secobarbital
Thiopental

Benzodiazepines
Alprazolam
Chlordiazepoxide
Clobazam
Clonazepam
Clorazepate
Diazepam
Estazolam
Flurazepam
Lorazepam
Midazolam
Nitrazepam
Oxazepam
Prazepam
Quazepam
Remimazolam
Temazepam
Tetrazepam
Triazolam

Bisphosphonates
Alendronate
Etidronate
Ibandronate
Pamidronate
Risedronate
Tiludronate
Zoledronate

Calcium channel blockers
Amlodipine
Bepridil
Clevidipine
Diltiazem
Felodipine
Isradipine
Nicardipine
Nifedipine
Nimodipine
Nisoldipine
Prenylamine
Verapamil

Carbonic anhydrase inhibitors
Acetazolamide
Brinzolamide
Dichlorphenamide
Dorzolamide
Ethoxzolamide
Methazolamide

CB1 Cannabinoid receptor antagonists
Rimonabant

Central muscle relaxants
Carisoprodol
Chlormezanone
Chlorzoxazone
Cyclobenzaprine
Meprobamate
Metaxalone
Methocarbamol
Orphenadrine

Cephalosporins
1st generation
Cefadroxil
Cefazolin
Cephalexin
Cephalothin
Cephapirin
Cephradine
2nd generation
Cefaclor
Cefamandole
Cefmetazole
Cefonicid
Cefotetan
Cefoxirin
Cefuroxime
Loracarbef
3rd generation
Cefdinir
Cefditoren
Cefixime
Cefoperazone
Cefotaxime
Cefpodoxime
Ceftazidime
Ceftazidime & Avibactam
Ceftibuten
Ceftizoxone
Ceftriaxone
4th generation
Cefepime
Cefiderosol
5th generation
Ceftaroline Fosamil
Ceftobiprole
Ceftolozane & Tazobactam

Cholinesterase inhibitors
Donepezil
Edrophonium
Galantamine
Neostigmine
Physostigmine
Rivastigmine
Succinylcholine
Tacrine

CNS stimulants
Cocaine
Dexmethylphenidate
Dextroamphetamine
Lisdexamfetamine
Modafinil

Corticosteroids
Alclometasone
Amcinonide
Beclomethasone
Betamethasone
Budesonide
Ciclesonide
Clobetasol
Cortisone
Deflazacort
Desonide
Desoximetasone
Dexamethasone
Difluprednate
Fludrocortisone
Flumetasone
Flunisolide
Fluocinolone
Flucinonide
Fluprednisolone
Fluticasone Furoate
Fluticasone Propionate
Halcinonide
Halbetasol
Halometasone
Hydrocortisone
Loteprednol
Methylprednisolone
Mometasone
Prednicarbate
Prednisolone
Prednisone
Tixocortol
Triamcinolone
antagonist
Mifepristone
Misoprostol

COX-2 inhibitors
Celecoxib
Etodolac
Etoricoxib
Meloxicam
Nimesulide
Rofecoxib
Valdecoxib

CYP3A4 inhibitors
Amiodarone
Aprepitant
Boceprevir
Chloramphenicol
Cimetidine
Ciprofloxacin
Clarithromycin
Conivaptan
Delavirdine
Diltiazem
Erythromycin
Fluconazole
Fluvoxamine
Grapefruit Juice
Indinavir
Itraconazole
Ketoconazole
Mifepristone
Nefazodone
Nelfinavir
Norfloxacin
Ombitasvir/Paritaprevir/Ritonavir
Ombitasvir/Paritaprevir/Ritonavir & Dasabuvir
Ritonavir
Saquinavir
Telaprevir
Telithromycin
Verapamil
Voriconazole

Dermal fillers
Azficel-T
Calcium Hydroxylapatite
Hyaluronic Acid

Dipeptidyl peptidase-4 (DPP4) inhibitors
Alogliptin
Linagliptin
Saxagliptin
Sitagliptin
Vildagliptin

Disease-modifying antirheumatics (DMARD)
Abatacept
Adalimumab
Anakinra
Azathioprine
Bucillamine
Certolizumab
Chloroquine
Cyclosporine
Etanercept
Gold & Gold Compounds
Golimumab
Hydroxychloroquine
Infliximab
Leflunomide
Methotrexate
Minocycline
Penicillamine
Rituximab
Sulfasalazine
Tocilizumab
Tofacitinib

Diuretics
Acetazolamide
Blue Cohosh
Boswellia
Brinzolamide
Caffeine
Chicory
Cranberry
Dorzolamide
Eplerenone
Eucalyptus
Horse Chestnut (Bark, Flower, Leaf, Seed)
Horsetail
Isosorbide
Meadowsweet
Methazolamide
Spironolactone
Squill
loop
Bumetanide
Ethacrynic Acid
Furosemide
Torsemide
potassium-sparing
Amiloride
Triamterene
thiazide
Bendroflumethiazide
Benzthiazide
Chlorothiazide
Chlorthalidone
Cyclothiazide
Hydrochlorothiazide
Hydroflumethiazide
Indapamide
Methyclothiazide
Metolazone
Polythiazide
Quinethazone
Trichlormethiazide

Dopamine receptor agonists
Apomorphine
Bromocriptine
Cabergoline
Dopexamine
Fenoldopam
Pergolide
Pramipexole
Quinagolide
Ropinirole
Rotigotine

Dopamine receptor antagonists
- Amisulpride
- Domperidone
- Metoclopramide
- Sulpiride

Endothelin receptor (ETR) antagonists
- Ambrisentan
- Bosentan
- Macitentan
- Sitaxentan

Epidermal growth factor receptor (EGFR) inhibitors/ antagonists
- Afatinib
- Cetuximab
- Dacomitinib
- Erlotinib
- Gefitinib
- Lapatinib
- Mobocertinib
- Necitumumab
- Neratinib
- Osimertinib
- Panitumumab
- Vandetanib

Eugeroics
- Armodafinil

Fibrinolytics
- Alteplase
- Anistreplase
- Reteplase
- Streptokinase
- Tenecteplase
- Urokinase

Gonadotropin-releasing hormone (GnRH) agonists
- Buserelin
- Goserelin
- Histrelin
- Leuprolide
- Nafarelin
- Triptorelin

antagonist
- Abarelix
- Cetrorelix
- Degarelix
- Elagolix Sodium
- Ganirelix
- Relugolix

Histamines

H1 receptor antagonist
- Alcaftadine
- Astemizole
- Azatadine
- Azelastine
- Bepotastine
- Brompheniramine
- Buclizine
- Carbinoxamine
- Cetirizine
- Chlorpheniramine
- Cinnarizine
- Clemastine
- Cyproheptadine
- Desloratadine
- Dexchlorpheniramine
- Diphenhydramine
- Epinastine
- Fexofenadine
- Hydroxyzine
- Ketotifen
- Levocetirizine
- Loratadine
- Meclizine
- Mizolastine
- Olopatadine
- Phenindamine
- Promethazine
- Pyrilamine
- Rupatadine
- Terfenadine
- Trimeprazine
- Tripelennamine
- Tripolidine

H2 receptor antagonist
- Cimetidine
- Famotidine
- Nizatidine
- Ranitidine
- Roxatidine

Histone deacetylase (HDAC) inhibitors
- Belinostat
- Panobinostat
- Romidepsin
- Vorinostat

HMG-CoA reductase inhibitors (statins)
- Atorvastatin
- Fluvastatin
- Lovastatin
- Pitavastatin
- Pravastatin
- Red Rice Yeast
- Rosuvastatin
- Simvastatin

Hormones
- Drospirenone/Estetrol
- Estradiol
- Levonorgestrel
- Melatonin
- Oral Contraceptives
- Sincalide

Polypeptide
- Glucagon
- Insulin
- Insulin Aspart
- Mecasermin
- Nesiritide
- Pentagastrin
- Secretin

Immune checkpoint inhibitors (incl. Programmed death-ligand (PD-L1) inhibitors)
- Atezolizumab
- Avelumab
- Durvalumab

Programmed death receptor-1 (PD-1) inhibitor
- Cemiplimab
- Dostarlimab
- Ipilimumab
- Nivolumab
- Pembrolizumab

Immunomodulators
- Aldesleukin
- Aristolochia
- Arnica
- Bifidobacteria
- Brewer's Yeast
- Cladribine
- Cordyceps
- Dong Quai
- Echinacea
- Efalizumab
- Garlic
- Ginseng
- Glatiramer
- Goldenseal
- Imiquimod
- Immune Globulin IV
- Immune Globulin SC
- Interferon Alfa
- Interferon Beta
- Interferon Gamma
- Lactobacillus
- Lemon Balm
- Lenalidomide
- Levamisole
- Milk Thistle
- Mistletoe
- Natalizumab
- Palivizumab
- PEG-Interferon
- Pimecrolimus
- Pomalidomide
- Propolis
- Resveratrol
- Sarsaparilla
- Siberian Ginseng
- Sinecatechins

Immunosuppressants
- Alefacept
- Alemtuzumab
- Anti-Thymocyte Globulin (Equine)
- Anti-Thymocyte Immunoglobulin (Rabbit)
- Azathioprine
- Belatacept
- Belimumab
- Cyclosporine
- Daclizumab
- Everolimus
- Fingolimod
- Mizoribine
- Muromonab-CD3
- Mycophenolate
- Phellodendron
- Pirfenidone
- Rituximab
- Sirolimus
- Tacrolimus
- Thalidomide

Mast cell stabilizers
- Cromolyn
- Lodoxamide
- Nedocromil
- Pemirolast

Monoamine oxidase (MAO) inhibitors
- Isocarboxazid
- Phenelzine
- Tranylcypromine

mTOR inhibitors
- Everolimus
- Temsirolimus
- Zotarolimus

Muscarinic antagonists
- Aclidinium
- Amitriptyline
- Amoxapine
- Atropine Sulfate
- Benactyzine
- Benztropine
- Biperiden
- Chlorpheniramine
- Chlorpromazine
- Cinnarizine
- Clidinium
- Clomipramine
- Darifenacin
- Dicyclomine
- Diphenhydramine
- Disopyramide
- Doxepin
- Fesoterodine
- Flavoxate
- Glycopyrrolate
- Hydroxyzine
- Hyoscyamine
- Imipramine
- Ipratropium
- Maprotiline
- Mepenzolate
- Olanzapine
- Orphenadrine
- Oxybutynin
- Phenelzine
- Prochlorperazine
- Procyclidine
- Propantheline
- Scopolamine
- Solifenacin
- Tiotropium
- Tolterodine
- Trihexyphenidyl
- Trospium
- Umeclidinium

Muscarinic cholinergic agonists
- Bethanechol
- Carbachol
- Cevimeline
- Methantheline
- Pilocarpine

Non-depolarizing neuromuscular blockers
- Atracurium
- Cisatracurium
- Doxacurium
- Pancuronium
- Pipecuronium
- Rapacuronium
- Rocuronium
- Vecuronium

Non-nucleoside reverse transcriptase inhibitors
- Delavirdine
- Doravirine
- Efavirenz
- Emtricitabine/Rilpivirine/ Tenofovir Alafenamide
- Etravirine
- Nevirapine
- Rilpivirine

Non-steroidal antiinflammatories (NSAIDs)
- Aceclofenac
- Acemetacin
- Aspirin
- Benzydamine

Bromfenac
Celecoxib
Dexibuprofen
Dexketoprofen
Diclofenac
Diflunisal
Etodolac
Etoricoxib
Fenbufen
Flurbiprofen
Ibuprofen
Indomethacin
Ketoprofen
Ketorolac
Meclofenamate
Mefenamic Acid
Meloxicam
Metamizole
Methyl salicylate
Nabumetone
Naproxen
Nepafenac
Nimesulide
Oxaprozin
Phenylbutazone
Piroxicam
Pranoprofen
Rofecoxib
Salsalate
Sulindac
Tenoxicam
Tolmetin
Valdecoxib

Nucleoside analog reverse transcriptase inhibitors
Abacavir
Bictegravir/Emtricitabine/Tenofovir Alafenamide
Cobicistat/Elvitegravir/Emtricitabine/Tenofovir Alafenamide
Cobicistat/Elvitegravir/Emtricitabine/Tenofovir Disoproxil
Didanosine
Emtricitabine
Emtricitabine/Rilpivirine/Tenofovir Alafenamide
Lamivudine
Stavudine
Telbivudine
Tenofovir Disoproxil
Zalcitabine
Zidovudine

Oligonucleotides
Defibrotide

Opiate agonists
Codeine
Heroin
Hydrocodone
Hydromorphone
Loperamide
Meperidine
Methadone
Morphine
Nalbuphine
Oxycodone
Oxymorphone
Pentazocine
Propoxyphene
Sufentanil
Tramadol

Phosphodiesterase inhibitors
Apremilast
Cilostazol
Inamrinone
Milrinone
Roflumilast
type 5
Avanafil
Sldenafil
Tadalafil
Vardenafil

Prostaglandins
Alprostadil
Dinoprostone
Iloprost
Treprostinil
Unoprostone

Prostaglandin analogs
Bimatoprost
Gemeprost
Latanoprost
Tafluprost
Travoprost

Proton pump inhibitors (PPI)
Dexlansoprazole
Esomeprazole
Lansoprazole
Omeprazole
Pantoprazole
Rabeprazole

Retinoids
Acitretin
Adapalene
Alitretinoin
Bexarotene
Clindamycin/Tretinoin
Isotretinoin
Tretinoin
Trifarotene

Selective estrogen receptor modulators (SERM)
Chlorotrianisene
Clomiphene
Ospemifene
Raloxifene
Tamoxifen
Tibolone
Toremifene

Selective serotonin reuptake inhibitors (SSRI)
Citalopram
Escitalopram
Fluoxetine
Fluvoxamine
Paroxetine Hydrochloride
Paroxetine Mesylate
Sertraline

Serotonin antagonist
Buspirone
Sibutramine
serotonin receptor agonist
Almotriptan
Eletriptan
Frovatriptan
Lorcaserin
Rizatriptan
Sumatriptan
Vortioxetine
Zolmitriptan
serotonin receptor antagonist
Naratriptan
Vortioxetine
serotonin reuptake inhibitor
Duloxetine
Trazodone
Vortioxetine
serotonin type 3 receptor antagonist
Alosetron
Dolasetron
Granisetron
Netupitant & Palonosetron
Ondansetron
Palonosetron
serotonin type 4 receptor agonist
Prucalopride
Tegaserod
serotonin-norepinephrine reuptake inhibitor
Desvenlafaxine
Levomilnacipran
Venlafaxine
Vilazodone

Statins *(see HMG-CoA reductase inhibitors)*

Sulfonylureas
Acetohexamide
Chlorpropamide
Gliclazide
Glimepiride
Glipizide
Glyburide
Tolazamide
Tolazoline
Tolbutamide

Topoisomerase I inhibitors
Irinotecan
Topotecan

Topoisomerase 2 inhibitors
Etoposide
Teniposide

Trace elements
Arsenic
Selenium
Sulfites
Zinc

Tyrosine kinase inhibitors
Afatinib
Asciminib
Avapritinib
Axitinib
Bosutinib
Brigatinib
Cabozantinib
Crizotinib
Dacomitinib
Dasatinib
Erdafitinib
Erlotinib
Gefitinib
Imatinib
Lapatinib
Leflunomide
Lenvatinib
Mobocertinib
Neratinib
Nilotinib
Nintedanib
Osimertinib
Pazopanib
Ponatinib
Pralsetinib
Regorafenib
Ripretinib
Sorafenib
Sunitinib
Tivozanib
Trastuzumab
Tucatinib
Vandetanib
Zanubrutinib

Vaccines
Anthrax Vaccine
BCG Vaccine
Cholera Vaccine
Covid-19 Vaccine, mRNA
Diphtheria Antitoxin
Hemophilus B Vaccine
Hepatitis A Vaccine
Hepatitis B Vaccine
Human Papillomavirus (HPV) Vaccine
Human Papillomavirus Vaccine (Bivalent)
Inactivated Polio Vaccine
Influenza Vaccine
Japanese Encephalitis Vaccine
Measles, Mumps & Rubella (MMR) Virus Vaccine
Meningococcal Group B Vaccine
Meningococcal Groups C & Y & Haemophilus B Tetanus Toxoid Conjugate Vaccine
Pandemic Influenza Vaccine (H1N1)
Pneumococcal Vaccine
Sipuleucel-T
Smallpox Vaccine
Typhoid Vaccine
Varicella Vaccine
Yellow Fever Vaccine
Zoster Vaccine

Vasodilators
Ambrisentan
Amyl Nitrite
Astragalus Root
Benazepril
Bosentan
Captopril
Cilazapril
Diazoxide
Enalapril
Fosinopril
Hydralazine
Iloprost
Isosorbide Dinitrate
Isosorbide Mononitrate
Minoxidil
Nesiritide
Nitroglycerin
Nitroprusside
Prenylamine
Quinapril
Ramipril
Trandolapril
peripheral
Cilostazol
Cinnarizine
Epoprostenol
Papaverine
Pentoxifylline
Peppermint

Vitamins
- Ascorbic Acid
- Beta-Carotene
- Cyanocobalamin
- Ergocalciferol
- Folic Acid
- Niacin
- Niacinamide
- Pantothenic Acid
- Phytonadione
- Pyridoxine
- Riboflavin
- Thiamine
- Vitamin A
- Vitamin E

Vitamin D receptor agonists
- Dihydrotachysterol
- Doxercalciferol
- Paricalcitol

Xanthine alkaloids
- **Aminophylline**
- Caffeine
- Green Tea
- Pentoxifylline

CLASS REACTIONS*

ADRENERGIC BETA-RECEPTOR ANTAGONISTS (BETA BLOCKERS)

	A	B	Ca	Cr	Ce	N	P	S	T	=
SKIN										
Dermatitis	[1]		[3]			[1]	[2]		[7]	✓
Diaphoresis		•	[1]	•	[1]					
Eczema / eczematous reaction / eczematous eruption				[1]			[2]		[2]	
Edema / fluid retention		[1]		[2] (5–6%)				(5%)	•	
Lichenoid eruption / lichenoid reaction	[1]			[1]		[1]	[3]	[1]	[2]	✓
Peripheral edema		(<10%)	•	(<7%)		•				
Pruritus (itching)	(<5%)			[2]			[1]	(<10%)	[1] (<5%)	✓
Psoriasis	[7]	[1]		•			[21]	[3]	[5]	✓
Purpura			•	•			[1]			
Rash	[1]	(<10%)	[2]	•		•	[3] (<10%)	•	[3] (<10%)	✓
Raynaud's phenomenon	[2]	(<10%)	•				[3] (59%)	•	[3]	✓
Stevens-Johnson syndrome				[1]			[3]		[1]	
HAIR										
Alopecia / hair loss	[1]			•			[6]	•	[1] (<10%)	
MUCOSAL										
Xerostomia (dry mouth)		•		[1]			[1]	•	[3] (19%)	✓

A Atenolol; **B** Bisoprolol; **Ca** Carteolol; **Cr** Carvedilol; **Ce** Celiprolol; **N** Nebivolol; **P** Propranolol; **S** Sotalol; **T** Timolol

These tables concentrate on skin, hair, nails and mucosal reactions.

* The following conventions are followed in these tables:

- • reaction noted (package inserts)
- [3] number of published reports of a reaction
- (8%) highest incidence that has ever been noted or reported
- ? 20 reports or over or an incidence of 20% or over recorded for this reaction for a minority of drugs in the class
- ✓ at least half the drugs in the class selection have this reaction noted or reported
- ✓✓ all drugs in the class selection have this reaction noted or reported
- Note: reactions noted or reported for only one drug in a class selection have been excluded

DOI: 10.1201/9781003715672-1502

ANGIOTENSIN CONVERTING ENZYME (ACE) INHIBITORS

	B	Ca	Ci	E	F	I	L	M	P	Q	R	T	Z	=
SKIN														
Anaphylaxis		[1]		[1]			•	•	[1]		•			
Angioedema (formerly named angioneurotic edema)	[8]	[45] (15%)	[2]	[76]	[3]	[1]	[44] (70%)	[1]	[6]	[10]	[14]	[3]	[1]	✓✓
Bullous dermatosis		[1]					[1]							
Bullous pemphigoid / pemphigoid		[2]		[2]			[1]							
Dermatitis		[3]			[1]						[1]			
Diaphoresis	[1]			[1]	•		•	•	•	[3]	[2]			✓
DRESS syndrome (Drug-induced hypersensitivity syndrome)		[2]							[1]		[1]			
Edema / fluid retention			[1]	[1]	•				•	[4]	[1]	•		✓
Erythema		[1]		[1]			•		•		[1]			
Erythema multiforme				•							•			
Erythroderma		[2]		[1]	[1]									
Exanthems	[1]	[19] (10%)		[9]			[4]	•		[1]	[1]			✓
Exfoliative dermatitis		[4]		•			[2]			•				
Facial edema							[1]		•	[1]				
Flushing / rubefaction	[1]	[2]		[4]			[2]	[1]		•	[2]	•		✓
Jaundice (see also cholestasis / cholestatic jaundice)		[1]									[1]			
Kaposi's sarcoma		[2]	[1]				[2]			[1]				
Lichen planus pemphigoides		[2]									[3]			
Lichenoid eruption / lichenoid reaction		[12]		[2]			[2]							
Linear IgA	[1]	[5]												
Lupus erythematosus (subacute cutaneous lupus erythematosus (SCLE))		[8]	[1]	[2]			[1]							
Mycosis fungoides		[2]		[1]										
Palmoplantar pustulosis		[1]							[1]					
Pemphigus	[1]	[24]		[11]	[1]			•		[1]	[1]	•		✓
Pemphigus foliaceus	[1]	[2]	[1]	[2]	[1]		[2]	[1]	[1]	[1]	[1]	[1]		✓
Pemphigus vulgaris			[2]							[1]				
Peripheral edema	[3]			[2]			[1]	[1]	[4]	[3]				
Photosensitivity	•	[3]		[2]	•		•	•		[2]	[2]			✓
Pityriasis rosea		[6]					[2]							

B Benazepril; **Ca** Captopril; **Ci** Cilazapril; **E** Enalapril; **F** Fosinopril; **I** Imidapril; **L** Lisinopril; **M** Moexipril; **P** Perindopril; **Q** Quinapril; **R** Ramipril; **T** Trandolapril; **Z** Zofenopril

	B	Ca	Ci	E	F	I	L	M	P	Q	R	T	Z	=
Pruritus (itching)	[1]	[8] (10%)		[3]	[1]	[1]	•	•	(<10%)	[7]	[3]	•		✓
Pseudolymphoma / cutaneous pseudolymphoma		[2]			[1]		[1]							
Psoriasis		[8]		[3]			[1]		•		[1]			
Purpura		[1]		[1]			[2]		•		[1]			
Rash	[1]	[12]	[1]	[5]	[1]		[5]	•	[1] (<10%)	[5]	[4]	•	•	✓
Stevens-Johnson syndrome		[4]		[1] (5%)							[2]			
Urticaria / hives	[1]	[9] (7%)		[5]	•		[2]	•		•	•			✓
Vasculitis (angiitis) / cutaneous vasculitis (angiitis)		[7]		[2]			[1]			•	[1]			
Xerosis / xeroderma		[1]							•					
HAIR														
Alopecia / hair loss		[4]		[1]			[1]	•		•	(<10%)			
NAILS														
Nail dystrophy		[2]		[1]										
MUCOSAL														
Burning Mouth Syndrome / glossodynia / glossalgia / glossopyrosis		[2]		[2]			[1]							
Gingival bleeding				[1]							[1]			
Glossitis (inflammation of the tongue)		[3]		•										
Oral burn		[1]		[1]										
Oral ulceration		[4]		[2]										
Sialorrhea (ptyalism; hypersalivation)		[1]									•			
Tongue edema				[4]		[1]	[3]		[2]					
Xerostomia (dry mouth)		[1]		•	•		•	•	•	•	•	•		✓

B Benazepril; **Ca** Captopril; **Ci** Cilazapril; **E** Enalapril; **F** Fosinopril; **I** Imidapril; **L** Lisinopril; **M** Moexipril; **P** Perindopril; **Q** Quinapril; **R** Ramipril; **T** Trandolapril; **Z** Zofenopril

ANTIARRHYTHMICS

	A	Am	Aml	At	D	Di	Dr	F	I	L	M	P	Pr	Q	V	=
SKIN																
Acneiform eruption / acneiform dermatitis / acneiform rash						[2]						[8]	[2]	[2]	[1]	
Anaphylaxis		[3]		[2]			[2]			[7]		[1]	[1]			
Angioedema (formerly named angioneurotic edema)		[2]	[6] (6%)			[3]	[1]			[3]	[1]	[2]	[2]	•	[3]	✓
Bullous dermatosis					[1]				[1]			[1]	[1]			
Cutaneous toxicity / skin toxicity		[5]	[2]		[5]	[2]	[1]	[1]		[3]	[1]	[1]			[1]	✓
Dermatitis			(<10%)	[1]		[1]	[1] (<10%)			[27]			[2]	[4]		?
Diaphoresis	•	[2]	•		[1]	[2]		•	[1]	[1]					[2]	✓
Eczema / eczematous reaction / eczematous eruption			[2]			[1]	[1] (<10%)			[3]	[2]		[2]			
Edema / fluid retention		(<10%)	[22] (11%)			[4] (<10%)		•		[2]					[1]	?
Erythema						[2]	(5%)			[3]			[1]			
Erythema multiforme		[1]	[2]			[11] (31%)				[2]		[11]	[1]	[1]	[4]	✓
Erythema nodosum		[2]								[1]					[1]	
Exanthems		[5]	[2]		[2]	[17] (31%)	[1]	[1]		[2]	[1]	[22] (71%)	[4]	[6] (17%)	[8]	✓
Exfoliative dermatitis		[1]				[6]		•		[2]		[15]	[1]	[5]	[2]	✓
Fixed eruption / fixed drug eruption				[1]				[1]		[2]		[5]	[1]	[2]		
Flushing / rubefaction	[1] (18–44%)	(<10%)	[5] (<10%)			[6] (<10%)		•					[2]	[2]	[4] (<7%)	✓
Hypersensitivity		[1]	[1]			[2]	[1]			[9]		[47] (23%)		[1]		?
Leukocytoclastic vasculitis (angiitis)		[1]			[1]		[1]						[1]		[1]	
Lichenoid eruption / lichenoid reaction			[1]	[1]		[1]					[4]	[1]	[3]	[6]		
Lupus erythematosus (subacute cutaneous lupus erythematosus (SCLE))		[5] (5%)	[1]	[2]		[5]				[1]	[1]	[19]	[2]	[35]	[2]	✓
Necrosis (skin necrosis)		[1]		[3]									[3]			

A Adenosine; **Am** Amiodarone; **Aml** Amlodipine; **At** Atenolol; **D** Digoxin; **Di** Diltiazem; **Dr** Dronedarone; **F** Flecainide; **I** Ibutilide; **L** Lidocaine; **M** Metoprolol; **P** Phenytoin; **Pr** Propranolol; **Q** Quinidine; **V** Verapamil

	A	Am	Aml	At	D	Di	Dr	F	I	L	M	P	Pr	Q	V	=
Photosensitivity		[42] (10–75%)	[1]			[12]	[1]					[1]	[1]	[21]	[4]	✓
Phototoxicity		[4]				[2]	[2]						[1]	[1]		
Pigmentation (Skin) (includes hyperpigmentation)		[70] (<10%)	[2]			[12]				[1]		[4]		[3]		?
Pruritus (itching)		[2] (<5%)	[3]	(<5%)	[1]	[6]	[1] (<10%)	•		[3]	[1] (<5%)	[5]	[1]	[3]	[6]	✓
Pseudoporphyria		[1]												[1]		
Psoriasis		[2]		[7]	[2]	[3] (31%)		[2]			[8]		[21]	[5]		✓
Purpura		[1]	[2]		[1]	[3]				[1]		[4]	[1]	[13]	[1]	✓
Rash		[1]	(<10%)	[1]	[1]	[4]	[8] (<10%)	•		•	[3] (<5%)	[13] (17%)	[3] (<10%)	(<10%)	[2]	✓
Stevens-Johnson syndrome		[2]	[2]			[6]	[1]			[1]		[106] (68%)	[3]	[2]	[5]	✓
Urticaria / hives		[1]	[1]	[2]	[1]	[5]		•		[5]		[5]	[3]	[1]	[5]	✓
Vasculitis (angiitis) / cutaneous vasculitis (angiitis)		[6]	[2]	[1]	[1]	[6]	[1]					[11]		[5]	[2]	✓
HAIR																
Alopecia / hair loss		[5]	•	[1]		[2]		•			[1]	[3]	[6]	[1]	[5]	✓
MUCOSAL																
Oral ulceration						[1]				[1]		[1]	[1]		[1]	
Xerostomia (dry mouth)			[1]			[2]		•					[1]		•	

A Adenosine; **Am** Amiodarone; **Aml** Amlodipine; **At** Atenolol; **D** Digoxin; **Di** Diltiazem; **Dr** Dronedarone; **F** Flecainide; **I** Ibutilide; **L** Lidocaine; **M** Metoprolol; **P** Phenytoin; **Pr** Propranolol; **Q** Quinidine; **V** Verapamil

ANTIBIOTICS, FLUOROQUINOLONES

	C	E	Ga	Ge	L	M	N	O	S	=
SKIN										
Acneiform eruption / acneiform dermatitis / acneiform rash	[3]								•	
AGEP	[4]				[2]	[2]				
Anaphylaxis	[15]				[6]	[5]		[4]	•	✓
Angioedema (formerly named angioneurotic edema)	[8]				[1]			[3]	•	
Bruise / bruising / contusion / ecchymosis (ecchymoses)			•						•	
Bullous dermatosis	[1]					[2]	[1]		•	
Candidiasis / candidosis	[2]			•	•	•		[1]		✓
Cellulitis and pseudocellulitis	[1]								•	
Cutaneous adverse reaction	[1]				[1]					
Cutaneous toxicity / skin toxicity	[3]				[1]					
Dermatitis				•			[1]	[1]	•	
Desquamation					[1]	[1]				
Diaphoresis	[5]	•	•		[1]	•	•		•	✓
DRESS syndrome (Drug-induced hypersensitivity syndrome)	[2]				[4]	[4]				
Edema / fluid retention	•	•	•		[1]			•	•	✓
Erythema					[2]		[2]	[1]		
Erythema multiforme	[5]	•			[1]					
Erythema nodosum	[1]				[1]					
Exanthems	[4]	[1]	•	[1]	[2]		[2]	[3]	•	✓
Exfoliative dermatitis	•	•							•	
Facial edema	[2]		•	•					•	
Fixed eruption / fixed drug eruption	[14]				[2]		[3]	[5]		
Flushing / rubefaction	[1]			•		[1]				
Hot flashes / hot flushes	[1]			•						
Hypersensitivity	[5]				[5]	[5]		[2]		
Leukocytoclastic vasculitis (angiitis)	[2]				[1]					
Linear IgA	[2]						[1]			
Lupus syndrome / drug-induced lupus (DIL)	[1]				[1]					
Peripheral edema	[1]		•			[1]			•	

C Ciprofloxacin; **E** Enoxacin; **Ga** Gatifloxacin; **Ge** Gemifloxacin; **L** Levofloxacin; **M** Moxifloxacin; **N** Norfloxacin; **O** Ofloxacin; **S** Sparfloxacin

	C	E	Ga	Ge	L	M	N	O	S	=
Petechiae	[1]								•	
Photosensitivity	[20]	[5]	[2]	[2]	[3]	[5]	[1]	[8]	[9]	✓✓
Phototoxicity	[5]	[5]	[1]		[5]		[4]	[3]	[5] (8%)	✓
Pigmentation (Skin) (includes hyperpigmentation)	[1]	[1]			[1]				[1]	
Pruritus (itching)	[11]	[1] (8%)	•	•	[3]	[3]	[1]	[5]	•	✓✓
Purpura	[4]	•			[3]					
Pustules / pustular eruption							[1]		•	
Radiation recall dermatitis	[1]		[1]		[2]					
Rash	[14] (<10%)	•	•	[7] (2–7%)	[2]	[4]	•	[5] (<10%)	•	✓✓
SDRIFE	[1]				[1]					
Stevens-Johnson syndrome	[20]	•			[6] (5%)	[2]	[4]	[8]		✓
Sweet syndrome	[2]				[1]		[1]	[1]		
Thrombocytopenic purpura	[1]					[2]				
Toxic pustuloderma							[1]	[1]		
Urticaria / hives	[10]	[1]		•	[1]	[3]	[1]	[3]	•	✓
Vasculitis (angiitis) / cutaneous vasculitis (angiitis)	[11]				[3]			[4]		
Xerosis / xeroderma	[1]				[1]	•		[1]	•	✓
NAILS										
Photo-onycholysis						[1]	[2]	[3]	[2]	
MUCOSAL										
Gingivitis			•						•	
Glossitis (inflammation of the tongue)			•			•				
Oral candidiasis	[1]		•						•	
Oral ulceration			•						•	
Stomatitis (oral mucositis)	[4]	•	•			[1]			•	✓
Xerostomia (dry mouth)	[3]	•		•	[1]	[1]	•	•	•	✓

C Ciprofloxacin; **E** Enoxacin; **Ga** Gatifloxacin; **Ge** Gemifloxacin; **L** Levofloxacin; **M** Moxifloxacin; **N** Norfloxacin; **O** Ofloxacin; **S** Sparfloxacin

ANTIBIOTICS, MACROLIDE

	A	C	D	E	F	R	Te	Tr	=
SKIN									
AGEP	[3]			[3]					
Anaphylaxis	[2]	[2]		[2]			[1]		✓
Angioedema (formerly named angioneurotic edema)	[1]	[1]		[1]			[1]	[1]	✓
Candidiasis / candidosis	•						•		
Churg-Strauss syndrome	[2]					[1]			
Cutaneous toxicity / skin toxicity	[1]	[1]							
Dermatitis	[1]			[4]					
Erythema	[2]					[1]			
Erythema multiforme				[1]			•		
Exanthems	[3]	[3]		[4] (<5%)				[2]	✓
Fixed eruption / fixed drug eruption	[5]	[3]		[6]		[1]			✓
Hypersensitivity	[3]	[3]		[3] (<10%)	[1]	[1]	[1]		✓
Jarisch–Herxheimer reaction	[2]			[1]					
Jaundice (see also cholestasis / cholestatic jaundice)	[1]						[2]		
Pruritus (itching)	[5]	[1]	•		•		•	[2]	✓
Pustules / pustular eruption	[1]			[1]					
Rash	[7] (2–10%)	[2]	•	[3]	•	[2]	•	(<10%)	✓✓
SDRIFE		[3]		[2]		[1]			
Stevens-Johnson syndrome	[9] (5%)	[4]		[13] (10%)					?
Urticaria / hives	[2]	[1]	•	[4]		[2]	•	[1] (<10%)	✓
Vasculitis (angiitis) / cutaneous vasculitis (angiitis)	[1]	[3]		[1]			•		✓
HAIR									
Alopecia / hair loss		[1]		[1]					
MUCOSAL									
Black tongue / black hairy tongue (lingua villosa nigra)		[1]		[1]					
Gingival hyperplasia / gingival hypertrophy / gingival enlargement / gingival overgrowth		[1]		[1]					
Glossitis (inflammation of the tongue)		[1]					•		
Oral candidiasis				(<10%)			•		
Oral ulceration			•	[1]					
Stomatitis (oral mucositis)		[2]					•		
Xerostomia (dry mouth)		[1]	•				•		

A Azithromycin; **C** Clarithromycin; **D** Dirithromycin; **E** Erythromycin; **F** Fidaxomicin; **R** Roxithromycin; **Te** Telithromycin; **Tr** Troleandomycin

ANTICONVULSANTS

	C	Cl	E	G	L	La	Le	O	P	Ph	Phy	Pre	Pri	T	V	=
SKIN																
Acne keloid	[1]										[2]					
Acneiform eruption / acneiform dermatitis / acneiform rash	[1]			•		[1]		•		[1]	[8]			•		
AGEP	[7]					[1]	[1]			[1]	[5]				[1]	
Anaphylaxis						[1]	[2]				[1]					
Angioedema (formerly named angioneurotic edema)	[5]				[2]	[1] (<10%)	[1]	[2]		•	[2]					
Bruise / bruising / contusion / ecchymosis (ecchymoses)						•	•	•							[4] (<5%)	
Bullae	[1]	[1]								[1]						
Bullous dermatosis	[4]					[1]				[5]	[1]				[1]	
Bullous pemphigoid / pemphigoid				[2]			[1]									
Cutaneous adverse reaction	[8]					[1]		[1]			[5]					
Cutaneous toxicity / skin toxicity	[2]	[1]		[1]							[1]					
Dermatitis	[7]									[1]				•		
Diaphoresis	(<10%)					•		•		[1]				•	[1]	
DRESS syndrome (Drug-induced hypersensitivity syndrome)	[82] (77%)	[1]		[2]		[38] (11%)	[11]	[8]	[1]	[24] (6%)	[47] (68%)		[1]		[17]	✓
Eczema / eczematous reaction / eczematous eruption	[2]					•								•		
Edema / fluid retention				[5]			[1]	•		[1]		[10]		•	[3]	
Epidermolysis bullosa	[1]										[1]					
Erythema	[1]		•			[2] (~10%)	[2]									
Erythema multiforme	[17]					[4]	[2]			[7]	[11]		[2]		[3]	
Erythroderma	[12]						[1]			[2] (16%)	[9] (6%)				[3]	
Exanthems	[36] (17%)			[2]		[19] (20%)	[1]	[4]		[13] (70%)	[22] (71%)		[1] (<5%)	[1]	[3] (14%)	✓
Exfoliative dermatitis	[24]							[1]		[6]	[15]					?
Facial edema	[2]			•		•								[1]	•	
Facial skin hyperpigmentation																

C Carbamazepine; **Cl** Clobazam; **E** Eslicarbazepine; **G** Gabapentin; **L** Lacosamide; **La** Lamotrigine; **Le** Levetiracetam; **O** Oxcarbazepine; **P** Perampanel; **Ph** Phenobarbital; **Phy** Phenytoin; **Pre** Pregabalin; **Pri** Primidone; **T** Topiramate; **V** Valproic Acid

	C	Cl	E	G	L	La	Le	O	P	Ph	Phy	Pre	Pri	T	V	=
Fibromatosis [includes palmar fibromatosis (Dupuytren's contracture / Dupuytren's disease), plantar fibromatosis (Ledderhose disease) and penile fibromatosis (Peyronie disease)]										[2]			[1]			
Fixed eruption / fixed drug eruption	[10]					[1]		[1]		[9]	[5]			[2]	[1]	✓
Flushing / rubefaction						•								[1] (27%)		?
Granuloma annulare							[1]							[1]		
Hand–foot syndrome (palmar–plantar erythrodysesthesia)											[1]				[1]	
Hematoma / cutaneous hematoma					[1] (15%)				[1] (6%)							
Hot flashes / hot flushes				[1]		(<10%)		•						(<10%)		
Hyperhidrosis			•			[1]		•				[1]				
Hypersensitivity	[72]		•	[1]		[30] (<10%)	[2]	[6]		[12]	[47] (23%)	[2]	[2]		[5]	✓
Leukocytoclastic vasculitis (angiitis)				[1]			[1]			[1]						
Lichen planus	[2]										[1]					
Lichenoid eruption / lichenoid reaction	[8]										[1]					
Linear IgA	[1]										[8]					
Lupus erythematosus (subacute cutaneous lupus erythematosus (SCLE))	[35]	[1]				[5]	[1]	[2]		[2]	[19]		[7]		[6]	✓
Lupus syndrome / drug-induced lupus (DIL)						[2]					[1]					
Lymphadenopathy	[2]					[1]		[1]								
Lymphoma	[2]										[6]					
Lymphoproliferative disease / lymphoproliferative disorder	[5]										[1]					
Mycosis fungoides	[3]						[1]	[1]			[7]					
Pemphigus	[3]									[1]	[2]					
Peripheral edema	[1]		•	[14] (8%)					•	[1]	[1]	[16] (18%)			[1] (<5%)	✓
Petechiae	[1]					•									[1] (<5%)	
Photosensitivity	[9]					[2]				[1]	[1]			•	[1]	

C Carbamazepine; **Cl** Clobazam; **E** Eslicarbazepine; **G** Gabapentin; **L** Lacosamide; **La** Lamotrigine; **Le** Levetiracetam; **O** Oxcarbazepine; **P** Perampanel; **Ph** Phenobarbital; **Phy** Phenytoin; **Pre** Pregabalin; **Pri** Primidone; **T** Topiramate; **V** Valproic Acid

	C	Cl	E	G	L	La	Le	O	P	Ph	Phy	Pre	Pri	T	V	=
Pigmentation (Skin) (includes hyperpigmentation)							[1]			[1]	[4]			•		
Pruritus (itching)	[7]			[1]	[1]	[3]	[1]			[1]	[5]	[1]		[3]	[1]	✓
Pseudolymphoma / cutaneous pseudolymphoma	[17]					[1]				[1]	[31]				[2]	?
Psoriasis	[1]						[1]									
Purpura	[8]			[1]		[1]		•		[2]	[4]			•	[2]	✓
Pustules / pustular eruption	[5]									[1]	[3]					
Rash	[32] (12%)	[3]	[4]	[2]	[6]	[57] (12–22%)	[6]	[12] (9%)	[2]	[4]	[13] (17%)	[1]	[2]	[3] (6%)	[7]	✓✓
Scleroderma											[1]				[1]	
Stevens-Johnson syndrome	[155] (68%)	[3]	[1]	[2]	[3]	[89] (30%)	[5]	[15]		[40] (29%)	[106] (68%)		[5]		[19]	✓
Thrombocytopenic purpura	[1]				[1]											
Toxicoderma	[1]									[1]						
Urticaria / hives	[14] (7%)					[1]	[2]			[1]	[5]		[1]	[1]		
Vasculitis (angiitis) / cutaneous vasculitis (angiitis)	[7]			[1]			[1]			[1]	[11]	[1]			[3]	✓
Xerosis / xeroderma						•								[1]		
HAIR																
Alopecia / hair loss	[7] (~6%)		•	[2]		[2]					[3]			[2]	[23] (<10%)	
Alopecia areata						[1]				[1]						
Curly hair									[1]						[6]	
Hirsutism	[1] (25%)					•					[8] (13%)				[2] (60%)	?
Poliosis										[1]					[1]	
NAILS																
Nail changes											[2]			•		
Nail hypoplasia	[1]									[2]	[3]					
Nail pigmentation											[1]				[2]	
Onychomadesis	[2]														[1]	
MUCOSAL																
Epistaxis			•					•								

C Carbamazepine; **Cl** Clobazam; **E** Eslicarbazepine; **G** Gabapentin; **L** Lacosamide; **La** Lamotrigine; **Le** Levetiracetam; **O** Oxcarbazepine; **P** Perampanel; **Ph** Phenobarbital; **Phy** Phenytoin; **Pre** Pregabalin; **Pri** Primidone; **T** Topiramate; **V** Valproic Acid

	C	Cl	E	G	L	La	Le	O	P	Ph	Phy	Pre	Pri	T	V	=
Gingival hyperplasia / gingival hypertrophy / gingival enlargement / gingival overgrowth	[1]	[1]	•			•	[1]			[4] (16%)	[61] (16–94%)		[1]	[2]	[8] (42%)	✓
Gingivitis				•		•	•							•		
Mucocutaneous eruption	[4]										[2]					
Mucocutaneous lymph node syndrome	[2]										[1]					
Oral ulceration	[2]					[1]		[1]			[1]					
Sialorrhea (ptyalism; hypersalivation)		[1]				•								[1] (4–5%)		
Sjögren's syndrome (see also sicca syndrome)						[1]				[1]	[1]				[1]	
Stomatitis (oral mucositis)			•			•								•	(<5%)	
Xerostomia (dry mouth)			•	[1] (5%)		(6%)		•		[1]		[11] (17%)		[7] (16%)	[2] (<5%)	✓

C Carbamazepine; **Cl** Clobazam; **E** Eslicarbazepine; **G** Gabapentin; **L** Lacosamide; **La** Lamotrigine; **Le** Levetiracetam; **O** Oxcarbazepine; **P** Perampanel; **Ph** Phenobarbital; **Phy** Phenytoin; **Pre** Pregabalin; **Pri** Primidone; **T** Topiramate; **V** Valproic Acid

ANTIDEPRESSANTS, TRICYCLIC

	A	Am	C	De	Do	I	N	P	T	Tr	=
SKIN											
Angioedema (formerly named angioneurotic edema)	[1]			[1]		[1]			[1]		
Bullous dermatosis	[1]					[1]					
Cyanosis / acrocyanosis			[1]		[1]						
Dermatitis	[1]		[1]		[9]			[1]			
Diaphoresis	[1] (<10%)		[2] (43%)	[2] (<10%)	(<10%)	[8] (25%)	(<10%)	(<10%)	[1]	[1] (<10%)	✓
DRESS syndrome (Drug-induced hypersensitivity syndrome)	[2]		[1]								
Edema / fluid retention	[1]	(<10%)	•			[1]			(<10%)		✓
Erythroderma	[1]				[1]						
Exanthems		[2]		[5] (6%)	[1]	[6] (6%)			[6]		✓
Exfoliative dermatitis				[1]		[4]			[1]		
Fixed eruption / fixed drug eruption	[1]					[1]					
Flushing / rubefaction			(8%)	[1]	[1]	[1]					
Hypersensitivity	[1]		[2]								
Lichen planus	[1]					[1]					
Lupus erythematosus (subacute cutaneous lupus erythematosus (SCLE))	[1]					[1]					
Photosensitivity	[3]	•	[3]	[1]	[1]	[3]	[2]	[1]	[2]	•	✓✓
Pigmentation (Skin) (includes hyperpigmentation)	[4]		[1]	[3]		[13]					
Pruritus (itching)	[3]	[1]	[1] (6%)	[4]	[1]	[6]		[1] (<5%)	•		✓
Pseudolymphoma / cutaneous pseudolymphoma	[2]			[2]	[2]						
Purpura	[2]		•	[2]	[1]	[3]					✓
Rash		(<10%)	(8%)	[1]	[1]				[1]		✓
Stevens-Johnson syndrome	[1] (5%)	[2]									
Urticaria / hives		•	[1]	[3]		[6]			[3]		✓
Vasculitis (angiitis) / cutaneous vasculitis (angiitis)	[1]	[1]				[1]			[1]		
HAIR											
Alopecia / hair loss	[1]	•	•	[1]	•	[2]	•	•	[2]	•	✓✓

A Amitriptyline; **Am** Amoxapine; **C** Clomipramine; **De** Desipramine; **Do** Doxepin; **I** Imipramine; **N** Nortriptyline; **P** Protriptyline; **T** Trazodone; **Tr** Trimipramine

	A	Am	C	De	Do	I	N	P	T	Tr	=
Alopecia areata			[1]			[1]					
MUCOSAL											
Glossitis (inflammation of the tongue)					[1]	[2]					
Mucosal membrane desquamation				[1]		[1]					
Stomatitis (oral mucositis)	[1]				[1]	[2]					
Xerostomia (dry mouth)	[17] (79%)	[1] (14%)	[6] (84%)	[5]	[6] (5%)	[16] (21%)	[9]	•	[6]	[2]	✓✓

A Amitriptyline; **Am** Amoxapine; **C** Clomipramine; **De** Desipramine; **Do** Doxepin; **I** Imipramine; **N** Nortriptyline; **P** Protriptyline; **T** Trazodone; **Tr** Trimipramine

ANTIFUNGAL, IMIDAZOLE

	C	E	K	M	T	=
SKIN						
Angioedema (formerly named angioneurotic edema)			[3]	[1]		
Burning / skin burning sensation	[2]	•	[1]			✓
Contact dermatitis	[1]	[2]		[2]		✓
Dermatitis	[9]		[3]	[11]	[3]	✓
Erythema	[1]	•				
Exanthems			[7] (10%)	[5] (87%)	[4]	✓
Fixed eruption / fixed drug eruption			[2]	[1]	[2]	✓
Hypersensitivity		[1]	[3]		•	✓
Pruritus (itching)	[2]	[1]	[5] (10%)	[3] (36%)	[1]	✓✓
Purpura			[2]	[1]		
Rash		•	[3]	(9%)	(<10%)	✓
Urticaria / hives			[2]	[1]	[1] (<5%)	✓

C Clotrimazole; **E** Econazole; **K** Ketoconazole; **M** Miconazole; **T** Thiabendazole

ANTIMALARIALS

	Amo	A/L	Arm	Ars	At	A/P	C	Ha	Hy	Pr	Py	Qu	Qud	Qun	T	=
SKIN																
Acneiform eruption / acneiform dermatitis / acneiform rash													[2]	[2]		
AGEP						[1]	[1]		[28] (25%)		[1]		[2]			?
Anaphylaxis								[1]	[1]		•					
Angioedema (formerly named angioneurotic edema)	[1]						[1]		•	[1]	[2]		•	•		
Bullous dermatosis									[2]		[2]					
Cutaneous toxicity / skin toxicity							[2]		[1]							
Dermatitis		[1]					[2]		[1]		•		[4]	[6]		
DRESS syndrome (Drug-induced hypersensitivity syndrome)									[5]		[2]			[1]		
Erythema annulare centrifugum							[2]		[3]							
Erythema multiforme						[2]	•		[3]		[4]		[1]	[2]		
Erythema nodosum									[1]			[1]				
Erythroderma							[3]		[5]							
Exanthems					[1]	[1]	[3] (<5%)		[4] (<5%)	[1] (5%)	[3]	[3] (80%)	[6] (17%)	[3] (<5%)		✓
Exfoliative dermatitis							[4]		[3]		[2]	[3] (8%)	[5]	[2]		
Fixed eruption / fixed drug eruption	[1]						•		[1]		[3]	[3]	[2]	[12]		
Flushing / rubefaction													[2]	•		
Hypersensitivity		[1]									[1]		[1]	[1]	•	
Lichen planus									[1]				[7]	[3]		
Lichenoid eruption / lichenoid reaction							[6]		[4]		[2]	[6] (12%)	[6]	[3]		
Livedo reticularis / livedo racemosa													[6]	[3]		
Lupus erythematosus (subacute cutaneous lupus erythematosus (SCLE))													[35]	[1]		?
Lymphoproliferative disease / lympho-proliferative disorder									[1]		[1]		[1]			
Ochronosis												[2]		[1]		
Pemphigus							[1]		[1]							

Amo Amodiaquine; **A/L** Artemether/Lumefantrine; **Arm** Artemisia; **Ars** Artesunate; **At** Atovaquone; **A/P** Atovaquone/Proguanil; **C** Chloroquine; **Ha** Halofantrine; **Hy** Hydroxychloroquine; **Pr** Primaquine; **Py** Pyrimethamine; **Qu** Quinacrine; **Qud** Quinidine; **Qun** Quinine; **T** Tafenoquine

	Amo	A/L	Arm	Ars	At	A/P	C	Ha	Hy	Pr	Py	Qu	Qud	Qun	T	=
Photosensitivity							[8]		[6]		[3]	[1]	[21]	[19]		?
Phototoxicity						[1]	[1]		[3]				[1]			
Pigmentation (Skin) (includes hyperpigmentation)							[15]		[24] (<10%)		[5]	[9]	[3]	[6]		?
Pruritus (itching)	[4]	[2]	[2]	[4]	[2] (11%)	(<10%)	[36] (47%)	[3]	[13] (47%)	•	[2]	•	[3]	[1]		✓
Psoriasis							[19]		[17] (28%)	[1]		[1]	[5]			?
Purpura		[1]							[1]		[1]		[13]	[13]		
Pustules / pustular eruption		[1]					[1]		[1]		[1]		[1]			
Rash		[6] (11%)	[2]		[4] (23%)		[1]	[2]	[5] (<10%)		•	[1]	(<10%)	[1]		✓
Stevens-Johnson syndrome					[2]	[1]	[9]		[4]		[33] (<10%)		[2]	[5]		?
Sweet syndrome							[1]		[2]							
Thrombocytopenic purpura									[2]					[8]		
Urticaria / hives	[1]	[2]		[1]		[1]	[5]		[2]	[1]		[1]	[1]	[2]		✓
Vasculitis (angiitis) / cutaneous vasculitis (angiitis)									[1]				[5]	[5]		
HAIR																
Alopecia / hair loss						[1]			[2]			[2] (80%)	[1]			?
Hair pigmentation							[10]		[8] (<10%)							
NAILS																
Discoloration / nails (dyschromia)							[1]		[1]							
Nail pigmentation							[2]		[3]			[2]				
MUCOSAL																
Aphthous stomatitis / aphthous ulcer / aphtha (aphthae)	[1]			[1]							[1]					
Gingival pigmentation							[1]		[1]							
Oral edema				[1]							[1]					
Oral mucosal eruption													[2]	[1]		
Oral pigmentation							[14]		[7]			[4]	[1]			
Oral ulceration						[3] (6%)	[1]									
Stomatitis (oral mucositis)							•	•	[2]							

Amo Amodiaquine; **A/L** Artemether/Lumefantrine; **Arm** Artemisia; **Ars** Artesunate; **At** Atovaquone; **A/P** Atovaquone/Proguanil; **C** Chloroquine; **Ha** Halofantrine; **Hy** Hydroxychloroquine; **Pr** Primaquine; **Py** Pyrimethamine; **Qu** Quinacrine; **Qud** Quinidine; **Qun** Quinine; **T** Tafenoquine

ANTINEOPLASTICS

	At	Az	Ca	Cr	Cs	Cy	Da	Do	E	F	G	I	N	O	Pa	Pe	=
SKIN																	
Acneiform eruption / acneiform dermatitis / acneiform rash			[3] (10%)		[7] (38%)		[2] (<10%)	[1] (13%)	[30] (73–80%)	[3] (38%)	[3] (20%)	[3]	[1]		[6] (83%)		✓
Acral erythema			[1]		[1]	[16] (35%)		[1]		[4]					[4]		?
Actinic keratoses	[1]		[3]	[1]	[1]	[1]				[4]					[1]		
AGEP	[1]					[1]		[2]	[3]		[4]	[7]	[1]		[1]		✓
Anaphylaxis	[4]	(<5%)		[5]	[10]	[3]		[3]	[1] (30%)	[2]				[11]	[3]		✓
Angioedema (formerly named angioneurotic edema)					[4]					[1]				[1]	[1]		
Bullous dermatosis						[1]			[1]	[1]	[2]						
Bullous pemphigoid / pemphigoid	[1]	[1]							[1]				[13]			[21]	?
Cellulitis and pseudocellulitis		(8%)				[1] (7%)					[13]						
Cutaneous adverse reaction		[1]										[1] (71%)					?
Cutaneous toxicity / skin toxicity		[2]	[4] (33%)	[6] (15%)	[8] (49%)	[5] (41%)	[8] (36%)	[10] (56%)	[10] (84%)	[5] (16%)	[7] (80%)	[9] (30–44%)	[7] (7–17%)	[3] (80%)	[10] (15%)	[7] (10%)	✓
Dermatitis	[1]		[10] (37%)		[1]		[1] (<10%)	[1]	[5] (33%)	[4]	[6] (24%)		[3]	[1]	[2] (13%)	[6] (33%)	✓
Dermatomyositis	[1]		[1]					[1]			[2]	[1]	[7]		[1]	[5]	✓
Desquamation						[2]		[1]	[1]						[1] (7%)		
Diaphoresis		(11%)	•		[1]					[1]		(13%)		[2] (5%)		[1]	
DRESS syndrome (Drug-induced hypersensitivity syndrome)									[2]			[5]	[3]				
Eczema / eczematous reaction / eczematous eruption							(<10%)		[1]	[2]	[1]		[2]			[2]	
Edema / fluid retention		(14%)	[3] (18%)	[1] (30%)	[3] (29%)	[1]	[8] (38%)	[26] (100%)	[1]	[2] (29%)	[4] (13%)	[40] (80%)	[4] (17%)	[2] (13–15%)	[2] (21%)	[2]	✓

At Atezolizumab; **Az** Azacitidine; **Ca** Capecitabine; **Cr** Carboplatin; **Cs** Cisplatin; **Cy** Cytarabine; **Da** Dasatinib; **Do** Docetaxel; **E** Erlotinib; **F** Fluorouracil; **G** Gemcitabine; **I** Imatinib; **N** Nivolumab; **O** Oxaliplatin; **Pa** Paclitaxel; **Pe** Pembrolizumab

	At	Az	Ca	Cr	Cs	Cy	Da	Do	E	F	G	I	N	O	Pa	Pe	=
Eosinophilic fasciitis (Shulman syndrome / Shulman disease)													[6]			[5]	
Erosions										[1]						[1]	
Erythema		[1] (7–17%)		[2]	[3]	[7] (22%)	[2]	[4]	(18%)	[4] (10%)	[1]	[5] (<10%)	[5]	[4]	[6]	[3]	✓
Erythema multiforme					[1] (17%)			[1]		[3] (17%)		[2]	[2] (<10%)		[1]	[3]	
Erythema nodosum							•					[1]	[1]				
Erythroderma						[1]						[4]					
Exanthems		[1]		[3]	[4]	[7] (60%)		[3]	[3] (8%)	[3] (<10%)	[2]	[9]	[3]	[1]	[2]	[4]	✓
Exfoliative dermatitis			[1] (31–37%)		[1]	[1]	[1]				[1]	[4]	(<10%)			•	✓
Facial edema				[1]	[1]				[1]		[1]	[3] (<10%)					
Fissures									[1]	[1] (21%)							?
Fixed eruption / fixed drug eruption								[1]							[2]		
Flagellate dermatitis				[1]	[2]			[1]							[1]		
Flagellate erythema/ pigmentation					[1]			[3]									
Flushing / rubefaction				[3]	[5]		[1] (<10%)	[2] (6%)						[3] (47%)	[3] (28%)		?
Follicular pustular eruption									[1]							[1]	
Folliculitis									[9] (11%)	[2]		[1]		[1]	[2]		
Graft-versus-host reaction							[1]					[1]					
Granuloma annulare													[2]			[2]	
Granulomas			[1]													[1]	
Hand–foot syndrome (palmar–plantar erythro-dysesthesia)			[185] (89%)	[5] (14%)	[10] (14%)	[22]	[1]	[49] (33%)	[3] (30–60%)	[54] (63%)	[22] (44%)	[3]		[14] (63%)	[21] (40%)		✓
Hematoma / cutaneous hematoma		(9%)												[1]	[1]	[1]	

At Atezolizumab; **Az** Azacitidine; **Ca** Capecitabine; **Cr** Carboplatin; **Cs** Cisplatin; **Cy** Cytarabine; **Da** Dasatinib; **Do** Docetaxel; **E** Erlotinib; **F** Fluorouracil; **G** Gemcitabine; **I** Imatinib; **N** Nivolumab; **O** Oxaliplatin; **Pa** Paclitaxel; **Pe** Pembrolizumab

	At	Az	Ca	Cr	Cs	Cy	Da	Do	E	F	G	I	N	O	Pa	Pe	=
Henoch-Schönlein purpura / IgA vasculitis / immunoglobulin A vasculitis						[1]							[2]				
Herpes		[1]					(<10%)										
Herpes simplex		(9%)								[1]							
Hyperhidrosis							[1] (<10%)					[1]					
Hypersensitivity		(<5%)	[1]	[27] (30%)	[5] (20%)	[2]	•	[15] (28%)			[3]		[3]	[31] (20%)	[26] (52–54%)		✓
Hypomelanosis					[1]							[5]					
Jaundice (see also cholestasis / cholestatic jaundice)			[3] (35%)		[1]								[1]	[1]			?
Keratoacanthoma (Grzybowski syndrome)							[1]						[3]			[2]	
Keratoderma			[1]							[1]							
Lesions (includes skin lesions)								[1]	[1]			[1]				[1]	
Leukocytoclastic vasculitis (angiitis)											[1]	[1]		[1]			
Lichen planus	[1]											[7]	[4]			[7]	
Lichen planus pemphigoides	[1]												[4]			[7]	
Lichen sclerosus													[4]			[1]	
Lichenoid dermatitis	[2]												[4]			[4]	
Lichenoid eruption / lichenoid reaction												[15]	[6]			[7]	?
Linear IgA	[1]										[1]		[1]				
Lipodystrophy / acquired generalized lipodystrophy													[5]			[6]	
Lupus erythematosus (subacute cutaneous lupus erythematosus (SCLE))			[4]				[1]	[1]	[1]	[6]	[1]		[5]		[5]	[3]	✓
Lymphadenopathy													[3]			[1]	
Lymphedema					[1]						[1]						
Maculopapular rash / morbilliform rash									[1]			[1]				[2]	

At Atezolizumab; **Az** Azacitidine; **Ca** Capecitabine; **Cr** Carboplatin; **Cs** Cisplatin; **Cy** Cytarabine; **Da** Dasatinib; **Do** Docetaxel; **E** Erlotinib; **F** Fluorouracil; **G** Gemcitabine; **I** Imatinib; **N** Nivolumab; **O** Oxaliplatin; **Pa** Paclitaxel; **Pe** Pembrolizumab

	At	Az	Ca	Cr	Cs	Cy	Da	Do	E	F	G	I	N	O	Pa	Pe	=
Morphea / localized scleroderma													[4]			[4]	
Necrosis (skin necrosis)					[2]				[1]	[1]	[3]						
Neutrophilic dermatosis						[1]									[1]		
Neutrophilic eccrine hidradenitis						[11]						[3]					
Nevi (naevi)	[1]								[1]								
Panniculitis							[4]					[3]				[2]	
Papulopustular eruption			[1]						[9] (29%)						[1]		?
Peeling					[1] (5%)			[1] (5%)									
Pemphigus												[2]	[1]			[1]	
Peripheral edema	[2] (18%)	[1] (19%)			[2] (12%)		[3] (44%)	[9] (32%)		[2]	[4]	[5] (75%)		(11%)		[1] (17%)	✓
Petechiae		[1] (11–24%)				[1]					(16%)	[1] (<10%)					?
Photosensitivity			[2]				[1]	[6] (11%)	[1]	[3]		[3] (<10%)	[1]		[4]		✓
Pigmentation (Skin) (includes hyper-pigmentation)			[13] (18%)	[2]	[5] (52%)		[1]	[2]		[11] (11–17%)		[14] (60%)	[1]		[3] (5%)	[1]	✓
Porokeratosis					[1]								[1]				
Prurigo nodularis				[1]											[1]		
Pruritus (itching)	[6] (20%)	[1] (12%)	[2] (33%)	[2]	[8] (43%)	(<10%)	[5] (18%)	[1]	[10] (33%)	[5] (43%)	[2] (13%)	[3] (10%)	[30] (47%)	[6] (50%)	[6] (10%)	[21] (33%)	✓ ✓
Pseudolymphoma / cutaneous pseudo-lymphoma										[1]	[1]	[3]		[1]			
Pseudoporphyria										[1]		[6]					
Psoriasiform dermatitis													[2]			[3]	
Psoriasiform eruption	[1]											[1]					
Psoriasis	[6]							[3]		[1]		[3]	[10] (<10%)			[9]	
Purpura			•			[1]			[3]			[1]		[1]			
Pustules / pustular eruption													[1]		[2]		
Pyoderma gangrenosum		[2] (<5%)										[2]				[1]	

At Atezolizumab; **Az** Azacitidine; **Ca** Capecitabine; **Cr** Carboplatin; **Cs** Cisplatin; **Cy** Cytarabine; **Da** Dasatinib; **Do** Docetaxel; **E** Erlotinib; **F** Fluorouracil; **G** Gemcitabine; **I** Imatinib; **N** Nivolumab; **O** Oxaliplatin; **Pa** Paclitaxel; **Pe** Pembrolizumab

	At	Az	Ca	Cr	Cs	Cy	Da	Do	E	F	G	I	N	O	Pa	Pe	=
Radiation recall dermatitis			[6]	[2]	[1]	[1]		[18]	[1]	[3]	[17] (74%)			[3]	[11]	[4]	✓
Rash	[7] (18%)	[4] (10–14%)	[14] (65%)	[10] (43%)	[22] (76–91%)	[4] (61%)	[12] (34%)	[13] (22–44%)	[119] (80%)	[8] (42%)	[35] (100%)	[27] (69%)	[47] (55%)	[11] (21%)	[19] (83%)	[26] (50%)	✓ ✓
Raynaud's phenomenon				[1]	[14]						[3]						
Recall reaction					[2]			[3]		[3]	[1]				[2]		
Rosacea									[2]			[1]					
Sarcoidosis / sarcoid-like reaction (cutaneous sarcoidosis)	[2]												[10]			[12]	
Scleroderma			[1]	[2]				[9]		[1]	[2]		[5]		[9]	[8]	✓
Sclerosis											[1]				[1]		
SDRIFE					[1]			[1]		[1]	[1]						
Seborrheic dermatitis							[1]		[1]	[3]							
Seborrheic keratoses			[1]			[2]		[1]			[2]						
Squamous cell carcinoma										[1]		[2]					
Squamous syringometaplasia						[1]		[1]									
Stevens-Johnson syndrome			[3]	[2]	[3]	[2]		[4]			[4]	[15]	[11]		[3]	[19]	✓
Sweet syndrome		[10]			[1]	[1]	[1]		[1]		[2]	[4]	[1]			[1]	✓
Telangiectasia									[1]			[1]					
Thrombocytopenic purpura	[1]				[2]			[2]			[8]		[2]	[2]			
Thrombotic thrombocytopenic purpura													[4]			[1]	
Toxic erythema						[1] (55%)					[1]						?
Toxic erythema of chemotherapy (TEC)			[1]			[2]		[2]			[2]				[1]		
Transient acantholytic dermatosis (Grover's disease)													[2]			[2]	
Ulcerations						[1]	[1]	[1]		[2]			[1]				
Urticaria / hives		(6%)		[4]	[7] (8–11%)	[1]	[1] (<10%)	[1]				[3]	[2]	[3] (26%)	[4]	[1]	✓

At Atezolizumab; **Az** Azacitidine; **Ca** Capecitabine; **Cr** Carboplatin; **Cs** Cisplatin; **Cy** Cytarabine; **Da** Dasatinib; **Do** Docetaxel; **E** Erlotinib; **F** Fluorouracil; **G** Gemcitabine; **I** Imatinib; **N** Nivolumab; **O** Oxaliplatin; **Pa** Paclitaxel; **Pe** Pembrolizumab

	At	Az	Ca	Cr	Cs	Cy	Da	Do	E	F	G	I	N	O	Pa	Pe	=
Vasculitis (angiitis) / cutaneous vasculitis (angiitis)		[1]				[3]			[1]	[1]	[3]	[2]	[3]	[1]		[5]	✓
Vitiligo			[2]										[15] (5–11%)			[14] (25%)	?
Xerosis / xeroderma		(5%)	[2] (29%)		[2] (14%)		[1] (<10%)	[2]	[13] (56%)	[3] (40%)	[1]	[2] (<10%)		[1] (6%)			✓
HAIR																	
Alopecia / hair loss			[10] (55%)	[19] (59%)	[26] (100%)	[5] (100%)	[3] (<10%)	[34] (100%)	[10] (14%)	[19] (100%)	[15] (15%)	[2] (10–15%)	[1]	[4] (3–38%)	[52] (100%)	[2]	✓
Alopecia areata				[2]									[3]		[1]	[3]	
Lichen planopilaris													[3]			[2]	
NAILS																	
Beau's lines					[1]			[3] (45%)		[1]					[1] (29%)		?
Hyponychial dermatitis			[1]					[1]									
Leukonychia striata (Mees' lines)				[1]		[3] (33%)		[2]		[1]					[2]		?
Melanonychia			[1]		[1]			[2]							[1]		
Nail changes			[1] (53%)					[18] (58–89%)	[3] (25%)	[1]					[6]		?
Nail disorder			[1] (10%)				[1]	[2] (11–41%)		[1]		[1]			[1]		?
Nail dystrophy								[1]				[2]					
Nail loss			[1] (45%)					[3] (45%)					[1]				?
Nail pigmentation				[1] (7%)	[1] (16–31%)			[7] (10–50%)		[3] (50–67%)		[2]			[4] (52%)		?
Nail toxicity			[1] (40%)												[1] (40%)	[1]	?
Onychodystrophy	[1]									[1]							
Onycholysis			[3]					[15]					[2]		[11] (13%)		
Onychomadesis			[3] (24%)									[1] (29%)			[2]		?
Paronychia			[2] (27%)		[2] (21%)			[5]	[14] (23%)	[3] (25%)	[1] (16%)		[1]	[1]	[1]		✓
Pyogenic granuloma			[2]					[2]	[1]	[1]					[2]		

At Atezolizumab; **Az** Azacitidine; **Ca** Capecitabine; **Cr** Carboplatin; **Cs** Cisplatin; **Cy** Cytarabine; **Da** Dasatinib; **Do** Docetaxel; **E** Erlotinib; **F** Fluorouracil; **G** Gemcitabine; **I** Imatinib; **N** Nivolumab; **O** Oxaliplatin; **Pa** Paclitaxel; **Pe** Pembrolizumab

	At	Az	Ca	Cr	Cs	Cy	Da	Do	E	F	G	I	N	O	Pa	Pe	=
Subungual hematoma / subungual hemorrhage								[2]							[1] (9%)		
Subungual hyperkeratosis			[1]					[2]		[1]					[1]		
MUCOSAL																	
Aphthous stomatitis / aphthous ulcer / aphtha (aphthae)					[1] (8–32%)			[2] (30–33%)	[1]	[1] (8–67%)		[1]	[1]		[1] (19%)		?
Cheilitis (inflammation of the lips)			[1] (14%)		[1] (14%)					[1] (14%)		[1]					
Epistaxis				[2]	[3] (83%)			[1] (83%)		[2] (11%)				(<16%)	[2]		?
Gingival bleeding		(10%)			[1] (20%)			[1] (33%)									?
Gingivitis						[1]		[1]						•		[1]	
Mucocutaneous eruption							[1]					[1]					
Mucosal inflammation			[2] (13%)		[2] (55%)	[1]		[2] (55%)	[1] (18%)	[2] (14%)					[3] (69%)		?
Mucositis	[1]	[1] (24%)	[17] (58%)	[5] (17%)	[16] (80%)	[3] (32%)	[1] (16%)	[15] (20-30%)	[10] (21%)	[18] (79%)	[7] (36%)	[2] (15%)		[6] (22%)	[16] (17–35%)	[2]	✓
Mucous membrane pemphigoid													[1]			[3]	
Oral lesions				[1]	[2]	[5] (66%)									[1]		?
Oral lichenoid eruption												[3]	[1]				
Oral pigmentation			[2]									[4]					
Oral ulceration			[1] (18%)		[1]	•			[1]	[2]		[3] (15%)		[1] (18%)			
Oropharyngeal pain		[1]						[1]				[1]					
Rectal hemorrhage / rectal bleeding			[1]				[1]										
Sjögren's syndrome (see also sicca syndrome)	[2]												[2]			[3] (6%)	
Stomatitis (oral mucositis)		[1] (8%)	[19] (41%)	[2]	[18] (86%)	[2]	[1]	[26] (19–53%)	[12] (26%)	[31] (86%)	[14] (17%)		[2] (<10%)	[6] (47%)	[11] (62%)	[4] (9%)	✓
Tongue pigmentation										[2]			[1]				
Xerostomia (dry mouth)					[1] (12%)		[1] (33%)					[1] (44%)	[3]	(5%)		[2] (10%)	?

At Atezolizumab; **Az** Azacitidine; **Ca** Capecitabine; **Cr** Carboplatin; **Cs** Cisplatin; **Cy** Cytarabine; **Da** Dasatinib; **Do** Docetaxel; **E** Erlotinib; **F** Fluorouracil; **G** Gemcitabine; **I** Imatinib; **N** Nivolumab; **O** Oxaliplatin; **Pa** Paclitaxel; **Pe** Pembrolizumab

ANTIPSYCHOTICS

	Am	Ar	Ca	Ch	Cl	D	H	Le	Li	O	Q	R	V	Zi	Zu	=
SKIN																
Acneiform eruption / acneiform dermatitis / acneiform rash		[1]	[1]						[21] (11%)			•				?
AGEP			[7]		[1]		[1]			[2]	[1]		[1]			
Anaphylaxis				[1]		[3]				[1]						
Angioedema (formerly named angioneurotic edema)			[5]	[1]	[2]	[2]	[1]		[2]	[2]		[9]		[2]		✓
Bruise / bruising / contusion / ecchymosis (ecchymoses)										•			[4] (<5%)	•		
Bullous dermatosis			[4]	[1]					[1]			•	[1]			
Candidiasis / candidosis										•	•					
Cutaneous toxicity / skin toxicity	[1]		[2]		[5]				[2]							
Dermatitis			[7]	[1]	•		•		[4]	[1]						
Diaphoresis			(<10%)		[4] (31%)		[2]			•	(<10%)	•	[1]	[1]		✓
DRESS syndrome (Drug-induced hypersensitivity syndrome)			[82] (77%)		[1]				[2]	[1]	[3]		[17]	[2]		?
Eczema / eczematous reaction / eczematous eruption			[2]		•				[1]	•		[1]		•		
Edema / fluid retention					•				[3]	[3]	[2]	[3]	[3]			
Erythema			[1]		[1]				[2]							
Erythema multiforme			[17]	•	•				[1]		[1]	[1]	[3]			
Erythroderma			[12]										[3]			
Exanthems			[36] (17%)	[8] (13%)	[2]				[11]	•			[3] (14%)	•		?
Exfoliative dermatitis			[24]						[3]			•		•		?
Facial edema			[2]	[1]						•	•		•	•		
Fixed eruption / fixed drug eruption			[10]	•						[1]			[1]			
Flushing / rubefaction				[1]								[1]				
Furunculosis												•	(<5%)	•		
Hyperhidrosis		[1]			[2]						•				•	
Hypersensitivity			[72]							[2]			[5]			?
Lesions (includes skin lesions)									[1]			[1]				

Am Amisulpride; **Ar** Aripiprazole; **Ca** Carbamazepine; **Ch** Chlorpromazine; **Cl** Clozapine; **D** Droperidol; **H** Haloperidol; **Le** Levomepromazine; **Li** Lithium; **O** Olanzapine; **Q** Quetiapine; **R** Risperidone; **V** Valproic Acid; **Zi** Ziprasidone; **Zu** Zuclopenthixol

	Am	Ar	Ca	Ch	Cl	D	H	Le	Li	O	Q	R	V	Zi	Zu	=
Lichen planus			[2]						[1]							
Lichenoid eruption / lichenoid reaction			[8]	[1]						[1]		•				
Linear IgA			[1]						[4]							
Lupus erythematosus (subacute cutaneous lupus erythematosus (SCLE))			[35]	[12]	[4]				[5]				[6]	[2]		?
Lymphadenopathy			[2]											•		
Morphea / localized scleroderma									[1]				[1]			
Mycosis fungoides			[3]						[1]							
Pemphigus			[3]				[1]									
Peripheral edema			[1]							[5] (<10%)	[6]	[4] (16%)	[1] (<5%)	•		
Petechiae			[1]		•								[1] (<5%)			
Photosensitivity			[9]	[23] (<10%)	[1]		[3]			•	•	[2] (<10%)	[1]	•		✓
Pigmentation (Skin) (includes hyperpigmentation)				[16]			•		•	[1]		•				
Pruritus (itching)			[7]	[2] (<10%)	•	[1] (6%)	•		[9]	•		•	[1]		•	✓
Pseudolymphoma / cutaneous pseudolymphoma			[17]	[1]					[1]				[2]			
Psoriasis			[1]						[59]	[3]		•				?
Purpura			[8]	[6]	•				[2]	(<10%)		•	[2]			
Pustules / pustular eruption			[5]	[1]					[2]	[1]						
Rash		[2] (7%)	[32] (12%)	(<10%)	[2]		•		[1] (<10%)	[2]	•	[2]	[7]	•		✓
SDRIFE					[2]							[1]				
Seborrhea										•		•			•	
Seborrheic dermatitis				[4]			[2]		[3]							
Stevens-Johnson syndrome		[2]	[155] (68%)	[2]	[1]								[19]			?
Sweet syndrome					[3]		[1]	[1]								
Thrombocytopenic purpura			[1]								[3]					
Toxicoderma			[1]						[1]							
Ulcerations									[5]	•		•				
Urticaria / hives			[14] (7%)	[4]	[1]				[3]	•		[2]		[1] (5%)		

Am Amisulpride; **Ar** Aripiprazole; **Ca** Carbamazepine; **Ch** Chlorpromazine; **Cl** Clozapine; **D** Droperidol; **H** Haloperidol; **Le** Levomepromazine; **Li** Lithium; **O** Olanzapine; **Q** Quetiapine; **R** Risperidone; **V** Valproic Acid; **Zi** Ziprasidone; **Zu** Zuclopenthixol

	Am	Ar	Ca	Ch	Cl	D	H	Le	Li	O	Q	R	V	Zi	Zu	=
Vasculitis (angiitis) / cutaneous vasculitis (angiitis)			[7]	[3]	[1]				[4]	[1]			[3]			
Verrucae vulgaris / warts / verrucae									[1]			•				
Vesiculobullous eruption										•				•		
Xerosis / xeroderma									[1]	•	•	•				
HAIR																
Alopecia / hair loss			[7] (~6%)				[1]		[18] (12%)	[3]	[1]	[2]	[23] (<10%)	•		✓
Alopecia areata					[1]		[2]		[3]							
Hirsutism			[1] (25%)							•			[2] (60%)			?
Poliosis							[1]						[1]			
NAILS																
Nail pigmentation				[4]									[2]			
Onychomadesis			[2]						[1]				[1]			
Photo-onycholysis		[1]		[2]						[1]						
MUCOSAL																
Burning Mouth Syndrome / glossodynia / glossalgia / glossopyrosis					•				[1]							
Epistaxis										(<10%)		[1]		•		
Gingival bleeding												[1]		•		
Gingival hyperplasia / gingival hypertrophy / gingival enlargement / gingival overgrowth			[1]						[1]				[8] (42%)			?
Gingivitis										•	[1]	•		[1]		
Glossitis (inflammation of the tongue)								[1]		•	•		(<5%)			
Oral ulceration			[2]						[4]	•	•					
Sialorrhea (ptyalism; hypersalivation)		[5] (4–11%)			[86] (92%)		[1]		[4]	[4]	[3]	[12] (13%)		•		✓
Stomatitis (oral mucositis)									[2]	•	•	[1]	(<5%)			
Tongue edema										•	•	•		•		
Tongue pigmentation										•		•				
Xerostomia (dry mouth)	[1]	[7] (15%)		[1] (<10%)	[3] (6%)		[4] (21%)		[6]	[13] (19%)	[22] (31%)	[7] (18%)	[2] (<5%)	[1] (<5%)	(15%)	✓

Am Amisulpride; **Ar** Aripiprazole; **Ca** Carbamazepine; **Ch** Chlorpromazine; **Cl** Clozapine; **D** Droperidol; **H** Haloperidol; **Le** Levomepromazine; **Li** Lithium; **O** Olanzapine; **Q** Quetiapine; **R** Risperidone; **V** Valproic Acid; **Zi** Ziprasidone; **Zu** Zuclopenthixol

ANTIRETROVIRALS

	Am	At	B	C/A	C/D	Da	De	Do	E	H	I	L	N	R	T	Z	=
SKIN																	
Acneiform eruption / acneiform dermatitis / acneiform rash												(<10%)		•		[1] (<5%)	
AGEP												[1]				[1]	
Angioedema (formerly named angioneurotic edema)						•	•									[1]	
Bromhidrosis											•					[1] (<5%)	
Bruise / bruising / contusion / ecchymosis (ecchymoses)							•							•		[1]	
Bullous dermatosis														•		[1]	
Cutaneous toxicity / skin toxicity		[1] (21%)						[1]	[2] (39%)	[1] (5%)	[1]	[1] (6%)		[2]		[1]	✓
Dermatitis							•			[3]	•	[1]	•	[1]			
Diaphoresis							•		[1]		•		•	(<10%)	•	[1] (5–19%)	
DRESS syndrome (Drug-induced hypersensitivity syndrome)						[1]			[2]				[1]	[1]	[2]		
Eczema / eczematous reaction / eczematous eruption									•					•			
Edema of lip							•									[1] (<5%)	
Erythema							•		[1] (11%)								
Erythema multiforme							•			•						[2]	
Exanthems	[1]	[1]					(7%)		[3] (27%)	[1] (<10%)	[1]		[1]	[2]		[6] (<5%)	✓
Flushing / rubefaction									•		•			(13%)			
Folliculitis							•		•		•			•			
Hand–foot syndrome (palmar–plantar erythrodysesthesia)								[1]		[1]							
Hypersensitivity		[1]				[2]	[1]	[5]	[5]			[1]	[1]	(8%)	[1]		✓
Jaundice (see also cholestasis / cholestatic jaundice)		[11] (13%)									[1]	[1]		[3] (13%)		[1]	

Am Amprenavir; **At** Atazanavir; **B** Bictegravir/Emtricitabine/Tenofovir Alafenamide; **C/A** Cobicistat/Elvitegravir/Emtricitabine/Tenofovir Alafenamide; **C/D** Cobicistat/Elvitegravir/Emtricitabine/Tenofovir Disoproxil; **Da** Darunavir; **De** Delavirdine; **Do** Dolutegravir; **E** Efavirenz; **H** Hydroxyurea; **I** Indinavir; **L** Lopinavir; **N** Nelfinavir; **R** Ritonavir; **T** Tenofovir Disoproxil; **Z** Zidovudine

	Am	At	B	C/A	C/D	Da	De	Do	E	H	I	L	N	R	T	Z	=
Lesions (includes skin lesions)		[1]												[1]			
Lichenoid eruption / lichenoid reaction									[1]	[3]			[1]		[2]		
Lipoatrophy											[1]					[2]	
Lipodystrophy / acquired generalized lipodystrophy						[1]			[2]		[8] (14%)	(<10%)	[1]	[4]	•	[2]	✓
Lupus erythematosus (subacute cutaneous lupus erythematosus (SCLE))										[3]					[1]		
Peripheral edema							•		•	[1]				(6%)			
Photosensitivity									[5]	[1]				•	[1]		
Pigmentation (Skin) (includes hyperpigmentation)										[19] (59%)						[10]	?
Pruritus (itching)		[1]		[1]		•	•	[1]	(11%)	[3]	[2] (86%)		•	(12%)		[4]	✓
Psoriasis										[1]				•			
Purpura							•			[2]							
Rash	[6] (20–27%)	[7] (3–20%)	•		[3] (22%)	[9] (11%)	[5] (18–50%)	[3]	[16] (31%)		[2] (67%)	[5] (69%)	[4] (<10%)	[12] (69%)	[5] (5–18%)	[8] (69%)	✓
Raynaud's phenomenon										[1]					[1]		
Seborrhea							•				•			•			
Stevens-Johnson syndrome	[1]					[1]	[1]		[5] (8%)		[2]				[3]	[6]	
Urticaria / hives			[1]			•	•		[1]		•		[1]	(8%)	[1]	[2] (<5%)	✓
Vasculitis (angiitis) / cutaneous vasculitis (angiitis)							•		[1]	[6]	[1]		[1]			[2]	
Xerosis / xeroderma							•			[7] (<10%)	[2] (12%)			•			
HAIR																	
Alopecia / hair loss							•		•	[8] (<10%)	[5] (12%)	[3]		[2]		[2]	
Alopecia areata		[1]									[1]	[1]		[1]		[1]	
NAILS																	
Leukonychia striata (Mees' lines)										[1]						[1]	
Melanonychia										[9] (17%)						[1]	

Am Amprenavir; **At** Atazanavir; **B** Bictegravir/Emtricitabine/Tenofovir Alafenamide; **C/A** Cobicistat/Elvitegravir/Emtricitabine/Tenofovir Alafenamide; **C/D** Cobicistat/Elvitegravir/Emtricitabine/Tenofovir Disoproxil; **Da** Darunavir; **De** Delavirdine; **Do** Dolutegravir; **E** Efavirenz; **H** Hydroxyurea; **I** Indinavir; **L** Lopinavir; **N** Nelfinavir; **R** Ritonavir; **T** Tenofovir Disoproxil; **Z** Zidovudine

	Am	At	B	C/A	C/D	Da	De	Do	E	H	I	L	N	R	T	Z	=
Nail changes							•			[4]							
Nail pigmentation										[19] (5%)		[1]		[1]		[27] (42%)	?
Onychocryptosis (ingrowing toe nail)											[2]			[1]			
Paronychia											[5]					[1]	
MUCOSAL																	
Aphthous stomatitis / aphthous ulcer / aphtha (aphthae)							•			[1]	•						
Burning Mouth Syndrome / glossodynia / glossalgia / glossopyrosis									[1]							[1]	
Cheilitis (inflammation of the lips)											[4] (52%)			[1]			?
Gingivitis							•				•			•			
Oral pigmentation										[2]						[8]	
Oral ulceration							•			[8]			•	•		[1] (<5%)	
Oropharyngeal pain												[1]		(16%)		[1]	
Sialolithiasis		[1]												[1]			
Sialorrhea (ptyalism; hypersalivation)							•					[1]		[1]		[1]	
Stomatitis (oral mucositis)							•			[4]							
Tongue edema							•									[1] (<5%)	
Tongue pigmentation										[3] (<29%)						[4]	?
Xerostomia (dry mouth)							•		•		•			•		[1]	

Am Amprenavir; **At** Atazanavir; **B** Bictegravir/Emtricitabine/Tenofovir Alafenamide; **C/A** Cobicistat/Elvitegravir/Emtricitabine/Tenofovir Alafenamide; **C/D** Cobicistat/Elvitegravir/Emtricitabine/Tenofovir Disoproxil; **Da** Darunavir; **De** Delavirdine; **Do** Dolutegravir; **E** Efavirenz; **H** Hydroxyurea; **I** Indinavir; **L** Lopinavir; **N** Nelfinavir; **R** Ritonavir; **T** Tenofovir Disoproxil; **Z** Zidovudine

BENZODIAZEPINES

	A	Ch	Clb	Cln	Clr	D	L	M	O	Q	T	=
SKIN												
Acneiform eruption / acneiform dermatitis / acneiform rash	[1]					[1]						
Anaphylaxis						[1]		[1]				
Angioedema (formerly named angioneurotic edema)	[1]	[3]		[1]		[1]		[1]				
Bullous dermatosis				[2]		[1]						
Cutaneous toxicity / skin toxicity		[1]	[1]									
Dermatitis	[5]	(<10%)		(<10%)	(<10%)	[3] (<10%)	(<10%)		(<10%)	(<10%)	[1] (<10%)	✓
Diaphoresis	(16%)	•		[1]	•	•	•		•	•	[2]	✓
DRESS syndrome (Drug-induced hypersensitivity syndrome)			[1]	[1]					[1]			
Edema / fluid retention	(5%)	(<10%)						[2]				
Erythema multiforme		[5]		[1]			[1]		[1]			
Exanthems	[1]	[3]		[1]	[1]	[6]						✓
Exfoliative dermatitis				[1]		[2]						
Fixed eruption / fixed drug eruption		[7]				[2]	[1]		[1]			
Flushing / rubefaction						[1]		[1]				
Lupus erythematosus (subacute cutaneous lupus erythematosus (SCLE))		[3]	[1]									
Peripheral edema						[1]		•				
Photosensitivity	[4]	[6]			[1]						[1]	
Pruritus (itching)	[2] (<10%)	[1]				[1]		[3]		[1]	[2]	✓
Pseudolymphoma / cutaneous pseudolymphoma	[1]			[2]			[2]					
Purpura		[5]		[1]		[4]						
Rash	[4] (11%)	[1]	[3]	•	•	[2]	•	•	•	[1]	[1]	✓✓
Stevens-Johnson syndrome		[1]	[3]				[1]		[1]			
Urticaria / hives		[4]			[1]	[1]		[2]				

A Alprazolam; **Ch** Chlordiazepoxide; **Clb** Clobazam; **Cln** Clonazepam; **Clr** Clorazepate; **D** Diazepam; **L** Lorazepam; **M** Midazolam; **O** Oxazepam; **Q** Quazepam; **T** Triazolam

	A	Ch	Clb	Cln	Clr	D	L	M	O	Q	T	=
Vasculitis (angiitis) / cutaneous vasculitis (angiitis)		[2]			[1]	[1]						
HAIR												
Alopecia / hair loss		[3]		[2]								
MUCOSAL												
Burning Mouth Syndrome / glossodynia / glossalgia / glossopyrosis				[1]							•	
Nasal discomfort						[3] (6%)		[1] (12%)				
Sialopenia	(33%)	•		•	•		•		•	•	[1]	✓
Sialorrhea (ptyalism; hypersalivation)	•	(<10%)	[1]	(<10%)	(<10%)		[1]	•	(<10%)	(<10%)	(<10%)	✓
Xerostomia (dry mouth)	[6] (15%)	•		[1]	•	[1]	•		•	[1] (<5%)	[4]	✓

A Alprazolam; **Ch** Chlordiazepoxide; **Clb** Clobazam; **Cln** Clonazepam; **Clr** Clorazepate; **D** Diazepam; **L** Lorazepam; **M** Midazolam; **O** Oxazepam; **Q** Quazepam; **T** Triazolam

BISPHOSPHONATES

	A	E	I	P	R	T	Z	=
SKIN								
Angioedema (formerly named angioneurotic edema)	[2]	•		•				
Candidiasis / candidosis				(6%)			(12%)	
Eczema / eczematous reaction / eczematous eruption	[1] (13%)				[1]			
Edema / fluid retention				•		•	[3]	
Erythema	[1]						[1]	
Erythema multiforme	[2]				[1]			
Exanthems				[1]			[1]	
Flushing / rubefaction				[1]		•		
Hypersensitivity	[3] (19%)	•		•	[1]			✓
Lesions (includes skin lesions)			[1]			[1]		
Peripheral edema	[1]				(8%)	•	(5–21%)	✓
Pruritus (itching)	[1]	[1]	[1] (4–5%)		•	•		✓
Rash	[5]	•	[1]	[1]	[1] (8%)	•	[3] (6%)	✓✓
SDRIFE				[1]			[2]	
Stevens-Johnson syndrome		[1]	[1]		[1]	•	[1]	✓
Urticaria / hives	[1]				[1]			
HAIR								
Alopecia / hair loss			[1]				[1] (12%)	
MUCOSAL								
Stomatitis (oral mucositis)	[1]			•			(8%)	✓

A Alendronate; **E** Etidronate; **I** Ibandronate; **P** Pamidronate; **R** Risedronate; **T** Tiludronate; **Z** Zoledronate

CALCIUM CHANNEL BLOCKERS

	A	B	C	D	F	Nic	Nif	Nim	V	=
SKIN										
Acneiform eruption / acneiform dermatitis / acneiform rash				[2]				•	[1]	
AGEP				[21]			[3]			?
Anaphylaxis						[1]	[1]			
Angioedema (formerly named angioneurotic edema)	[6] (6%)			[3]	[1]	[1]	[2]		[3]	✓
Bruise / bruising / contusion / ecchymosis (ecchymoses)				•					[1]	
Cutaneous toxicity / skin toxicity	[2]			[2]					[1]	
Dermatitis	(<10%)			[1]			[1]			
Diaphoresis	•	•		[2]	[1]		[2]	•	[2]	✓
Eczema / eczematous reaction / eczematous eruption	[2]			[1]						
Edema / fluid retention	[22] (11%)	(<10%)		[4] (<10%)	[1]	•	[3]	•	[1]	✓
Erythema				[2]	•		[2]			
Erythema multiforme	[2]			[11] (31%)			[5]		[4]	?
Erythema nodosum							[2]		[1]	
Erythromelalgia / erythermalgia				[1]		[4]	[6]		[2]	
Exanthems	[2]			[17] (31%)	[2]		[9]	[2]	[8]	✓
Exfoliative dermatitis				[6]			[5]		[2]	
Facial edema	[1]				•		•			
Flushing / rubefaction	[5] (<10%)		[1]	[6] (<10%)	[10] (44%)	[2] (6%)	[9] (44%)	•	[4] (<7%)	✓
Hyperkeratosis				[1]					[2]	
Hypersensitivity	[1]			[2]						
Lichenoid eruption / lichenoid reaction	[1]			[1]			[3]			
Linear IgA	[1]								[1]	
Lupus erythematosus (subacute cutaneous lupus erythematosus (SCLE))	[1]			[5]			[3]		[2]	
Peripheral edema	[47] (34%)	•		[1] (5–8%)	[6] (22%)	[2] (7%)	[12] (6%)		[1] (<10%)	✓
Petechiae	[1]			•						

A Amlodipine; **B** Bepridil; **C** Clevidipine; **D** Diltiazem; **F** Felodipine; **Nic** Nicardipine; **Nif** Nifedipine; **Nim** Nimodipine; **V** Verapamil

	A	B	C	D	F	Nic	Nif	Nim	V	=
Photosensitivity	[1]			[12]			[5]		[4]	
Pigmentation (Skin) (includes hyperpigmentation)	[2]			[12]						
Pruritus (itching)	[3]			[6]	•		[3]	•	[6]	✓
Pseudolymphoma / cutaneous pseudolymphoma	[1]			[1]						
Purpura	[2]			[3]	[1]		[3]		[1]	✓
Rash	(<10%)	[1]		[4]	•	[3]	[2]	•	[2]	✓
Stevens-Johnson syndrome	[2]			[6]			[5]		[5]	
Telangiectasia	[6]				[2]		[2]			
Urticaria / hives	[1]			[5]	[1]	[3]	[7]		[5]	✓
Vasculitis (angiitis) / cutaneous vasculitis (angiitis)	[2]			[6]			[4]		[2]	
HAIR										
Alopecia / hair loss	•			[2]			[4]	[1]	[5]	✓
Hair pigmentation							[1]		[1]	
NAILS										
Nail dystrophy				[1]			[1]		[1]	
MUCOSAL										
Gingival hyperplasia / gingival hypertrophy / gingival enlargement / gingival overgrowth	[44] (31%)			[10] (21%)	[6]	[2]	[76] (75%)		[10] (19%)	✓
Oral ulceration				[1]					[1]	
Xerostomia (dry mouth)	[1]	[2] (<10%)		[2]	[1]	•	•		•	✓

A Amlodipine; **B** Bepridil; **C** Clevidipine; **D** Diltiazem; **F** Felodipine; **Nic** Nicardipine; **Nif** Nifedipine; **Nim** Nimodipine; **V** Verapamil

CEPHALOSPORINS

	Cef	Cnir	Cpm	Ctn	Ctxm	Cxim	Czim	Cple	Caxn	Coxm	Cxin	=
SKIN												
AGEP	[2]		[1]		[1]		[1]		[9]	[2]	[5]	✓
Anaphylaxis	[7] (13 cases)			[4]	[1]	•	[3]		[15]	[9]	[4]	✓
Angioedema (formerly named angioneurotic edema)							•		[3]	•	[2]	
Candidiasis / candidosis		•	•	•		[1]	•		[3] (5%)			✓
Dermatitis	[1]								[2]		[1]	
DRESS syndrome (Drug-induced hypersensitivity syndrome)			[1]		[5]		[2]		[4]			
Erythema								(9%)		[1]		
Erythema multiforme					[2]	[1]	[1]		[1]	•	[3]	✓
Exanthems	[3]	•	•	•	[3]	[1]	[1]		[7] (6%)	[2] (6%)	[3]	✓
Fixed eruption / fixed drug eruption	[1]				[1]		[1]		[3]		[1]	✓
Flushing / rubefaction						•			[2]			
Hypersensitivity	[3]		[2]	•	[2]		[1]	[1]	[4]	[4]		✓
Jarisch–Herxheimer reaction									[1]	[1]		
Lupus erythematosus (subacute cutaneous lupus erythematosus (SCLE))			[2]							[1]		
Pemphigus	[1]								[1]	[1]	[2]	
Pemphigus erythematodes (pemphigus erythematosus) (Senear-Usher syndrome)							[2]			[1]		
Photosensitivity	[1]						[1]					
Pruritus (itching)	[3]	•	[3]	•	[3]	•	[3]	[1] (9%)	[2]	•	[3]	✓✓
Pustules / pustular eruption	[3]									[1]	[2]	
Rash	[1]	•	[12] (51%)	[2]	[3]	[3]	[5]	[1]	[5]	[1]	•	✓✓
SDRIFE										[2]	[1]	
Serum sickness-like reaction	[2]	•		[2]		•			[2]	[2]	[1]	✓
Stevens-Johnson syndrome	[2]	•	[2]	•	[3]	•	[1]		[3]	[2]	[7]	✓
Thrombocytopenic purpura										[1]	[1]	
Urticaria / hives	•	•	[1]	[2]	•	•	•		[4]	[2]	[2]	✓
MUCOSAL												
Oral candidiasis	•		•						[1]	[1]		

Cef Cefazolin; **Cnir** Cefdinir; **Cpm** Cefepime; **Ctn** Cefoperazone; **Ctxm** Cefotaxime; **Cxim** Cefpodoxime; **Czim** Ceftazidime; **Cple** Ceftobiprole; **Caxn** Ceftriaxone; **Coxm** Cefuroxime; **Cxin** Cephalexin

CORTICOSTEROID TOPICAL

	A	Des	Dex	F	H	M	T	=
SKIN								
Acneiform eruption / acneiform dermatitis / acneiform rash			[6] (15%)			[1]		
Anaphylaxis			[3]		[18]		[2]	
Atrophy / Skin atrophy				[1]	[1]	[2]	[4]	✓
Bruise / bruising / contusion / ecchymosis (ecchymoses)			[1] (16%)	[1]	[1]		[2]	✓
Burning / skin burning sensation			[1]	[2]	[1]	[4]	[2]	✓
Churg-Strauss syndrome				[1]			[1]	
Cushingoid features			[1]	[1]				
Dermatitis	[3]	[4]	[5]		[11]		[3]	✓
Eczema / eczematous reaction / eczematous eruption					[4] (5%)		[1]	
Embolia cutis medicamentosa (Nicolau syndrome) / livedoid dermatitis			[1]				[2]	
Erythema			[1]			[2]	[5]	
Exanthems			[4] (16%)				[1]	
Hypersensitivity			[6] (52–54%)		[6]		[1]	?
Perioral dermatitis				[2]		[1]		
Peripheral edema			[9] (83%)	[1]				?
Photoallergic reaction	[1]				[1]			
Pigmentation (Skin) (includes hyperpigmentation)			[2] (16%)				[7]	
Pruritus (itching)		[1]	[7]	[3] (6%)	[2]	[2]	[1]	✓
Rash		[1]	[11] (67%)	(8%)	[2]			✓
Telangiectasia					[1]	[2]	[1] (41%)	?
Urticaria / hives	[1]		[1]		[5]		[2]	✓
Xerosis / xeroderma			[2] (16%)			[1]		
MUCOSAL								
Epistaxis				[1] (9%)		[2]		
Oral candidiasis			[2]	[12] (<31%)		[3]		?
Oropharyngeal pain				[4] (3–22%)		[1]		?
Xerostomia (dry mouth)			[1]				[1]	

A Alclometasone; **Des** Desonide; **Dex** Dexamethasone; **F** Fluticasone Propionate; **H** Hydrocortisone; **M** Mometasone; **T** Triamcinolone

DIPEPTIDYL PEPTIDASE-4 (DPP-4) INHIBITORS

	Alog	Lina	Saxa	Sita	Vild	=
SKIN						
Anaphylaxis	[1]			[1]		
Angioedema (formerly named angioneurotic edema)	[1]		[1]	[3]	[2]	✓
Bullous pemphigoid / pemphigoid	[2]	[1]		[3]	[6]	✓
Edema / fluid retention			[1]	[3]		
Hypersensitivity	[2]	[1]	[1]			✓
Lymphoma				[1]	[1]	
Peripheral edema	[1]	[1] (10%)	•		[3] (5%)	✓
Pruritus (itching)	[2]	[1]	[1]			✓
Rash	[1]		[1]	[2]	[1]	✓
Stevens-Johnson syndrome	[1]			[1]		
MUCOSAL						
Stomatitis (oral mucositis)	[1]				[1]	

Alog Alogliptin; **Lina** Linagliptin; **Saxa** Saxagliptin; **Sita** Sitagliptin; **Vild** Vildagliptin

DISEASE-MODIFYING ANTIRHEUMATIC DRUG (DMARDS)

	Ad	Az	H	I	L	M	R	Toc	Tof	=
SKIN										
Abscess	[1]			[4]		[2]			[1]	
Acneiform eruption / acneiform dermatitis / acneiform rash	[3]	[2]		[6]	(<10%)	[1] (67%)			[3] (20%)	✓
AGEP		[2]	[28] (25%)	[2]				[1]		?
Amicrobial pustulosis of the folds	[1]			[1]						
Anaphylaxis	[2]	[1]	[1]	[11]	•	[9] (<10%)	[8]	[5]		✓
Angioedema (formerly named angioneurotic edema)	[4]	[2]	•	[2] (11%)		[1]	[4] (11%)	[1]		✓
Basal cell carcinoma		[2]		[1]		[1]				
Bruise / bruising / contusion / ecchymosis (ecchymoses)			[1]	[1]		[2]				
Bullous dermatosis			[2]	[1]	[3]	[4]	[1]			✓
Candidiasis / candidosis	[1]			[4] (5%)		[1]		[1]		
Carcinoma	[2]	[3]				[2]				
Cellulitis and pseudocellulitis	[2] (<5%)			[5]		[1]	[1]	[9]		✓
Cutaneous toxicity / skin toxicity	[1]	[3] (6%)	[1]	[2] (75%)		[10] (10%)	[3] (12%)	[1]		✓
Dermatitis	[1]	[4]	[1]	[4]	(<10%)	[2]	[2]			✓
Dermatomyositis	[5]		[1]		[1]					
Diaphoresis					(<10%)		[2] (15%)			
DRESS syndrome (Drug-induced hypersensitivity syndrome)			[5]		[6]	[1]		[1]		✓
Eczema / eczematous reaction / eczematous eruption	[2]			[5] (19–30%)	[1]					?
Edema / fluid retention				[3]		[2]	[1]			
Eosinophilic cellulitis / Wells' syndrome	[2]			[1]						
Erythema	[1]	[1]		[1]		[1] (7%)	[2] (16%)		•	✓
Erythema annulare centrifugum			[3]				[1]	[1]		
Erythema multiforme	[4]	[2]	[3]	[4]	[1]	[4]				✓
Erythema nodosum		[5]	[1]							
Erythroderma			[5]			[2]		[1]		
Exanthems		[10] (5%)	[4] (<5%)	[4]		[5] (15%)	[1]			✓
Exfoliative dermatitis		[1]	[3]		[1]	[1]				✓
Facial edema				[1]		[1]	[1]	[1]		✓

Ad Adalimumab; **Az** Azathioprine; **H** Hydroxychloroquine; **I** Infliximab; **L** Leflunomide; **M** Methotrexate; **R** Rituximab; **Toc** Tocilizumab; **Tof** Tofacitinib

	Ad	Az	H	I	L	M	R	Toc	Tof	=
Fixed eruption / fixed drug eruption	[1]	[2]	[1]	[1]						
Flushing / rubefaction				[2] (39%)			(5%)			?
Folliculitis				[2]		[2]		[1]	[1] (13%)	
Furunculosis	[1]					[1]				
Granulomas	[1]			[1]						
Granulomatous reaction	[6]			[1]						
Hand–foot syndrome (palmar–plantar erythrodysesthesia)				[2] (31%)		[3]				?
Henoch-Schönlein purpura / IgA vasculitis / immunoglobulin A vasculitis	[3]			[5]			[1]			
Herpes	[1]			[2]						
Herpes simplex	[1]	[3] (35%)		[4] (10%)		[2]	[2]			✓
Herpes zoster	[10]	[8] (27%)		[11]	[1]	[7]	[7]	[8]	[17] (14%)	✓
Hidradenitis suppurativa (acne inversa)	[6]			[2]	[1]		[1]	[1]	[1]	✓
Hypersensitivity	[3]	[29]		[11] (11%)	[1]	[5]	[6] (9–11%)	[6]		✓
Ichthyosis				[1]		[1]				
Kaposi's sarcoma	[1]	[14]		[1]	[1]		[3]			✓
Keratoacanthoma (Grzybowski syndrome)		[1]		[1]						
Leprosy (Hansen disease)	[1]			[1]						
Lesions (includes skin lesions)	[2]		[1]	[2]						
Leukocytoclastic vasculitis (angiitis)	[1]			[6]		[1]	[1]			
Lichen planus			[1]	[4]	[1]					
Lichenoid eruption / lichenoid reaction	[5]	[1]	[4]	[4]	[2]					✓
Lupus erythematosus (subacute cutaneous lupus erythematosus (SCLE))	[18]			[35] (59%)	[9]		[1]			?
Lupus syndrome / drug-induced lupus (DIL)	[5]			[14]	[1]		[1]			
Lymphadenopathy	[1]			[1]		[1]				
Lymphoma	[8]	[1]		[9]		[5]	[1]	[1]		✓
Lymphoproliferative disease / lymphoproliferative disorder		[4]	[1]	[1]		[17] (1–5%)				
Maculopapular rash / morbilliform rash						[1]		[1]		
Melanoma	[6]			[1]		[1]		[1]		
Molluscum contagiosum	[1]			[2]		[2]				
Morphea / localized scleroderma	[1]			[1]						
Necrosis (skin necrosis)						[8]	[1]			
Necrotizing fasciitis				[1]		[1]				
Neutrophilic dermatosis	[1]	[4] (76%)								?

Ad Adalimumab; **Az** Azathioprine; **H** Hydroxychloroquine; **I** Infliximab; **L** Leflunomide; **M** Methotrexate; **R** Rituximab; **Toc** Tocilizumab; **Tof** Tofacitinib

	Ad	Az	H	I	L	M	R	Toc	Tof	=
Nevi (naevi)		[3]		[2]						
Nodular eruption					(<10%)	[15]				
Non-Hodgkin's lymphoma	[1]	[1]				[2]				
Palmoplantar pustulosis	[6]			[3]			[4]			
Panniculitis		[1]				[1]				
Papulopustular eruption				[1]				[1]		
Pemphigus			[1]				[1]	[1]		
Peripheral edema	(<5%)			[1]	(<10%)		[1] (14%)	•	[1]	✓
Photosensitivity		[1]	[6]			[9] (5%)		[1]		
Phototoxicity			[3]			[1]				
Pigmentation (Skin) (includes hyperpigmentation)		[1] (37%)	[24] (<10%)		(<10%)	(<10%)				?
Pityriasis lichenoides / pityriasis lichenoides chronica / pityriasis lichenoides et varioliformis acuta	[2]			[3]						
Pruritus (itching)	[6]	[1]	[13] (47%)	[8] (20%)	[3]	[1] (<5%)	[8] (14%)	[1]	•	✓✓
Pseudolymphoma / cutaneous pseudolymphoma	[1]			[2]		[10]				
Psoriasiform dermatitis	[2]			[1]						
Psoriasis	[47] (12%)		[17] (28%)	[57] (19%)		[1]	[4]	[4]	[2] (<6%)	✓
Purpura		[1]	[1]		(<10%)		[1]			
Pustules / pustular eruption	[1]		[1]	[5]						
Pyoderma gangrenosum	[4]	[1]		[2]			[6]	[1]		✓
Rash	[6] (12%)	[11] (<10%)	[5] (<10%)	[13] (25%)	[17] (12%)	[13] (5%)	[13] (58%)	[9]	[3]	✓✓
Raynaud's phenomenon					[1]	[1]				
Rosacea	[1]			[1]						
Sarcoidosis / sarcoid-like reaction (cutaneous sarcoidosis)	[9]			[5]		[1]	[3]	[1]		✓
Scabies		[5]				[1]		[1]		
Scleroderma	[1]	[1]								
SDRIFE				[2]					[2]	
Septic–toxic shock		[1]						[1]		
Serum sickness				[2]			[28] (<20%)			?
Serum sickness-like reaction				[5]			[6] (<17%)			
Skin cancer	[1]			[1]					[1]	
Squamous cell carcinoma	[5]	[11]		[1]		[2]				
Stevens-Johnson syndrome	[2]	[2]	[4]	[3]	[5]	[17]	[6]			✓

Ad Adalimumab; **Az** Azathioprine; **H** Hydroxychloroquine; **I** Infliximab; **L** Leflunomide; **M** Methotrexate; **R** Rituximab; **Toc** Tocilizumab; **Tof** Tofacitinib

	Ad	Az	H	I	L	M	R	Toc	Tof	=
Sweet syndrome	[4]	[19]	[2]	[1]				[1]		✓
Thrombocytopenic purpura	[1]		[2]							
Tinea	[1]	[3]								
Tumors	[1]	[8] (14%)					[1] (11%)			
Ulcerations		[1]		[1]	[3] (<10%)	[14]				
Urticaria / hives	[5]	[5]	[2]	[7] (17%)	•	[4]	[5] (8%)	[2]		✓
Vasculitis (angiitis) / cutaneous vasculitis (angiitis)	[9] (13%)	[5]	[1]	[18] (63%)	[4] (<10%)	[9]	[5]	[1]		✓
Vesiculation	[1]					[1]				
Vitiligo	[10]			[8]						
HAIR										
Alopecia / hair loss	[10]	[14] (54%)	[2]	[8]	[21] (10%)	[28] (10%)	[1]			✓
Alopecia areata	[7]			[4]	[3]					
Alopecia universalis	[4]						[1]			
Follicular mucinosis	[1]			[1]						
Hair pigmentation			[8] (<10%)		(<10%)	[1]				
NAILS										
Discoloration / nails (dyschromia)		[1]	[1]							
Nail pigmentation			[3]			[2]				
Onychocryptosis (ingrowing toe nail)	[1]		[1]							
Onycholysis	[1]					[1]				
Onychomycosis		[2] (5%)		[1] (33%)		[1]				?
MUCOSAL										
Aphthous stomatitis / aphthous ulcer / aphtha (aphthae)		•				[2]		[2]		
Gingivitis					(<10%)	•				
Mucocutaneous reactions						[3] (9%)	[2]			
Mucosal ulceration		[1]				[1]		[2]		
Oral candidiasis				[1]	•	[1] (11%)		[1]		
Oral ulceration		[2]			•	[13] (61%)		[2]		?
Oropharyngeal pain							[1]	[1]	[1] (<6%)	
Stomatitis (oral mucositis)		[3]	[2]	[1]	•	[29] (39–100%)	[2] (69%)	•		✓

Ad Adalimumab; **Az** Azathioprine; **H** Hydroxychloroquine; **I** Infliximab; **L** Leflunomide; **M** Methotrexate; **R** Rituximab; **Toc** Tocilizumab; **Tof** Tofacitinib

EPIDERMAL GROWTH FACTOR RECEPTOR (EGFR) INHIBITORS/ANTAGONISTS

	A	C	D	E	G	L	M	N	O	P	V	=
SKIN												
Acneiform eruption / acneiform dermatitis / acneiform rash	[30] (61–93%)	[69] (97%)	[3] (57%)	[30] (73–80%)	[34] (66–85%)	[4] (90%)	[3] (59%)		[1]	[18] (81%)	[4] (35%)	✓
AGEP		[1]		[3]	[1]							
Anaphylaxis		[7] (13%)		[1] (30%)	[1]					[1]		?
Bullous dermatosis	•			[1]								
Cutaneous adverse reaction		[1] (77%)			[2]				[1]			?
Cutaneous toxicity / skin toxicity	[3]	[22] (63%)	[3] (63%)	[10] (84%)	[12] (68%)	[7] (46%)			[2] (39%)	[26] (95%)	[9] (48–50%)	✓
Dermatitis	[1] (21%)	[4] (80%)	[6] (73%)	[5] (33%)							[1]	?
Desquamation		[3] (89%)		[1]	[2] (39%)					[3] (13%)		?
DRESS syndrome (Drug-induced hypersensitivity syndrome)	[1]			[2]								
Dry skin			[1]				[3] (40%)		[4] (28%)			?
Eczema / eczematous reaction / eczematous eruption		[1]		[1]	[1]					[2]		
Edema / fluid retention				[1]		[1] (29%)	(9%)			[1] (15%)		?
Erosive pustular dermatosis	[2]			[2]	[1]							
Erythema		[3] (14%)		(18%)	[1]	[1]				[5] (65%)		?
Exanthems		[5]		[3] (8%)	[3] (21%)	[1]						?
Exfoliative dermatitis	•				[1]	[1] (14%)				[2] (25%)		
Fissures	[2] (12%)	[4] (14%)	(9%)	[1]				•		[5] (21%)		✓
Folliculitis	[1]	[13] (83%)		[9] (11%)	[4]	[1]				[3]	[5] (49%)	✓
Hand–foot syndrome (palmar–plantar erythrodysesthesia)	[2] (10%)	[5] (6%)	(15%)	[3] (30–60%)	[3] (31%)	[10] (76%)	•	[1] (48%)		[3] (23%)	[4] (36%)	✓
Lupus erythematosus (subacute cutaneous lupus erythematosus (SCLE))				[1]					[1]			

A Afatinib; **C** Cetuximab; **D** Dacomitinib; **E** Erlotinib; **G** Gefitinib; **L** Lapatinib; **M** Mobocertinib; **N** Neratinib; **O** Osimertinib; **P** Panitumumab; **V** Vandetanib

	A	C	D	E	G	L	M	N	O	P	V	=
Maculopapular rash / morbilliform rash			[1]	[1]			[2] (16%)					
Nevi (naevi)		[1]		[1]						[1]		
Papulopustular eruption		[7] (83%)	[1]	[9] (29%)	[3] (21%)					[5] (21–41%)	[1]	✓
Peripheral edema		[1] (40%)			[1] (22%)					[1] (12%)		?
Photosensitivity				[1]							[8] (23%)	?
Pigmentation (Skin) (includes hyperpigmentation)					[1]	[1] (18%)				[1]	[6]	
Pruritus (itching)	[3] (13%)	[9] (40%)	(21%)	[10] (33%)	[6] (61%)	[3] (33%)	[3] (24%)		[1]	[10] (91%)	[2] (11%)	✓
Psoriasis		[1]				[1]						
Purpura				[3]	[1]							
Pustules / pustular eruption		[2]			[1]					[1]		
Radiation recall dermatitis		[4] (32%)		[1]								?
Rash	[54] (61–93%)	[53] (89%)	[15] (90%)	[119] (80%)	[69] (66–85%)	[26] (55%)	[2] (78%)	[1] (18%)	[17] (53%)	[33] (91%)	[35] (67%)	✓✓
Rosacea		[1]		[2]								
SDRIFE	[1]	[1]			[1]				[1]			
Stevens-Johnson syndrome	[8]	[4]			[2]				[6]	[1]	[4]	✓
Telangiectasia		[1]		[1]						[1]		
Ulcerations		[1]			[2]							
Urticaria / hives					[1]				[1]			
Vasculitis (angiitis) / cutaneous vasculitis (angiitis)		[1]		[1]	[1]				[4]			
Xerosis / xeroderma	[8] (36%)	[15] (49%)	[3] (44%)	[13] (56%)	[13] (53%)	[1] (29%)		(6%)	[4] (46%)	[12] (62%)	[3] (15%)	✓
HAIR												
Alopecia / hair loss	[1] (7%)	[2] (5%)	(23%)	[10] (14%)	[6]	[2] (33%)	[1] (19%)	[1] (46%)		[3] (54%)	[1]	✓
Folliculitis decalvans	[1]			[3]								
Hair changes		[3]		[4] (20%)						[2] (9%)	[2]	?
Hypertrichosis		[5]	•	[4]	[2]							
NAILS												
Nail changes	[2] (16%)	[1] (21%)		[3] (25%)	[1] (17%)					[2] (9–29%)		?

A Afatinib; **C** Cetuximab; **D** Dacomitinib; **E** Erlotinib; **G** Gefitinib; **L** Lapatinib; **M** Mobocertinib; **N** Neratinib; **O** Osimertinib; **P** Panitumumab; **V** Vandetanib

	A	C	D	E	G	L	M	N	O	P	V	=
Nail disorder		[3]	[1]			[1] (10%)		(8%)		[1]		✓
Paronychia	[18] (33–85%)	[19] (39%)	[8] (65%)	[14] (23%)	[16] (14–32%)	[4] (27%)	[3] (39%)		[9] (46%)	[14] (85%)	[5] (7%)	✓
Pyogenic granuloma		[1]		[1]	[2]					[1]		
MUCOSAL												
Aphthous stomatitis / aphthous ulcer / aphtha (aphthae)	•	[1]		[1]								
Cheilitis (inflammation of the lips)	[1] (7%)					[1] (14%)						
Epistaxis	[3] (17%)				[1]			(5%)		[1]		
Mucosal inflammation	[7] (69%)		[1] (48%)	[1] (18%)		[1] (15%)				[1] (6%)	[1] (27%)	✓
Mucositis	[10] (50–90%)	[11]	[4] (31%)	[10] (21%)	[4] (6–17%)	[2] (11–35%)		[1] (6%)		[4] (75%)	[2] (14%)	✓
Oral ulceration		[1]	[2] (74%)	[1]	[1]							?
Rhinorrhea	(11%)						[1] (13%)					
Stomatitis (oral mucositis)	[23] (50–90%)	[7] (82%)	[10] (51%)	[12] (26%)	[10] (33%)	[1] (41%)	[3] (46%)	[2] (53%)	[4] (18%)	[4] (100%)	[2] (33%)	✓✓
Xerostomia (dry mouth)	[1] (20%)	(11%)	[1]					•				?

A Afatinib; **C** Cetuximab; **D** Dacomitinib; **E** Erlotinib; **G** Gefitinib; **L** Lapatinib; **M** Mobocertinib; **N** Neratinib; **O** Osimertinib; **P** Panitumumab; **V** Vandetanib

H1 RECEPTOR ANTAGONIST

	As	Az	B	Cet	Chl	Cin	Dex	Dip	F	H	L	Me	Mi	P	T	=
SKIN																
AGEP				[2]				[1]	[1]	[3]						
Anaphylaxis	[1]			[2]	[2]		[1]	[4]		[2]			[2]	[1]		✓
Angioedema (formerly named angioneurotic edema)		•		•	(<10%)		•	[1]		[3]		•		•	[1]	✓
Bullous dermatosis				•										•		
Cutaneous toxicity / skin toxicity								[2]		[1]						
Dermatitis	[1]			•	[4] (<10%)		[1]	[4]		[1]	[1]			[3]		✓
Desquamation				[1]						[1]						
Eczema / eczematous reaction / eczematous eruption								[2]						[1]		
Edema / fluid retention		•					•	•		•						
Erythema multiforme										[2]				[2]		
Exanthems	[1]			[1]				[1]		[3]				[1]	[1]	
Fixed eruption / fixed drug eruption				[7]				[4]		[3]	[3]			[1]	[1]	
Flushing / rubefaction				[1] (60%)						[1]						?
Hypersensitivity										[1]			[1]	[1]		
Lupus erythematosus (subacute cutaneous lupus erythematosus (SCLE))						[1]								[2]	[1]	
Palmar erythema				[1]						[1]						
Photosensitivity	[1]	•		•	(<10%)		•	[3]		•		•		[12]	[3]	✓
Phototoxicity				•				[1]		[1]				[1]		
Pruritus (itching)	[1]			[1]	[1]			[2]								
Psoriasis									[1]						[2]	
Purpura				•				[1]		[1]				[2]		
Rash	[1]	•		•			•	•		•		•		[1]	•	✓
SDRIFE										[1]	[1]					
Stevens-Johnson syndrome	[1]					[1] (5%)		[3]	[2]					[2]		
Urticaria / hives	[2]			[9]					[3]	[4]	[1]			[3]	[1]	
Vasculitis (angiitis) / cutaneous vasculitis (angiitis)		[1]						[1]								

As Astemizole; **Az** Azatadine; **B** Buclizine; **Cet** Cetirizine; **Chl** Chlorpheniramine; **Cin** Cinnarizine; **Dex** Dexchlorpheniramine; **Dip** Diphenhydramine; **F** Fexofenadine; **H** Hydroxyzine; **L** Levocetirizine; **Me** Meclizine; **Mi** Mizolastine; **P** Promethazine; **T** Terfenadine

	As	Az	B	Cet	Chl	Cin	Dex	Dip	F	H	L	Me	Mi	P	T	=
HAIR																
Alopecia / hair loss	[1]			•											[3]	
MUCOSAL																
Oral mucosal eruption	[1]														[1]	
Xerostomia (dry mouth)	[4]	[1] (<10%)		[2] (6%)	(<10%)		(<10%)	[1] (<10%)		[6] (12%)	•	(<10%)	[3]	[2] (<10%)	[1] (<10%)	✓

As Astemizole; **Az** Azatadine; **B** Buclizine; **Cet** Cetirizine; **Chl** Chlorpheniramine; **Cin** Cinnarizine; **Dex** Dexchlorpheniramine; **Dip** Diphenhydramine; **F** Fexofenadine; **H** Hydroxyzine; **L** Levocetirizine; **Me** Meclizine; **Mi** Mizolastine; **P** Promethazine; **T** Terfenadine

HMG-CoA REDUCTASE INHIBITORS/STATINS

	A	F	L	Pi	Pr	R	S	=
SKIN								
Acneiform eruption / acneiform dermatitis / acneiform rash	•						[1] (36%)	?
Angioedema (formerly named angioneurotic edema)	[4]			[1]		[1]	[1]	✓
Bruise / bruising / contusion / ecchymosis (ecchymoses)	•					•		
Cutaneous toxicity / skin toxicity	[2]					[1]	[1]	?
Dermatomyositis	[4]	[1]	[1]		[2]	[1]	[5]	✓
Diaphoresis	•						[1]	
Eczema / eczematous reaction / eczematous eruption	•				[2]		[4] (5%)	
Edema / fluid retention	•		[1] (6%)		•		[2] (30%)	✓
Eosinophilic fasciitis (Shulman syndrome / Shulman disease)	[1]						[2]	
Erythema multiforme					[1]		[2]	
Exanthems			[3] (5%)				[1]	
Flushing / rubefaction			[1] (10%)		[1]		[1] (30%)	?
Herpes zoster	[1]	[1]	[1]		[1]	[1]	[1]	✓
Hypersensitivity	[1]		[1]				[1]	
Jaundice (see also cholestasis / cholestatic jaundice)	[2]						[1]	
Lichenoid eruption / lichenoid reaction	[2]	[1]	[1]		[2]		[2]	✓
Lupus erythematosus (subacute cutaneous lupus erythematosus (SCLE))	[3]	[2]	[4]		[1]		[5]	✓
Peripheral edema						•	[2] (50%)	?
Petechiae	•						[1]	
Photosensitivity	•				[1]		[7]	
Pruritus (itching)	[1]		[2] (5%)		[2]	[1]	[3]	✓
Purpura			[1]		[1]		[3]	
Radiation recall dermatitis						[1]	[1]	
Rash	[2]	•	[3] (5%)		[7] (5–7%)	•	[4] (<10%)	✓
Stevens-Johnson syndrome	[2]		[1]					
Urticaria / hives	[1]						[1]	

A Atorvastatin; **F** Fluvastatin; **L** Lovastatin; **Pi** Pitavastatin; **Pr** Pravastatin; **R** Rosuvastatin; **S** Simvastatin

	A	F	L	Pi	Pr	R	S	=
Vasculitis (angiitis) / cutaneous vasculitis (angiitis)	[1]						[2]	
HAIR								
Alopecia / hair loss	[1]		•					
MUCOSAL								
Cheilitis (inflammation of the lips)	•						[1]	
Oral ulceration	•					[1]		
Stomatitis (oral mucositis)	•						[2] (64%)	?

A Atorvastatin; **F** Fluvastatin; **L** Lovastatin; **Pi** Pitavastatin; **Pr** Pravastatin; **R** Rosuvastatin; **S** Simvastatin

IMMUNE CHECKPOINT INHIBITORS (Incl. PROGRAMMED DEATH-LIGAND (PD-L1) INHIBITORS)

	At	Av	C	D	I	N	P	=
SKIN								
Acneiform eruption / acneiform dermatitis / acneiform rash				•	[1]	[1]		
AGEP	[1]					[1]		
Bullous pemphigoid / pemphigoid	[1]		[2]	[1]		[13]	[21]	✓
Churg-Strauss syndrome					[1]	[1]		
Cutaneous toxicity / skin toxicity				•	[4] (35%)	[7] (7–17%)	[7] (10%)	✓
Dermatitis	[1]			•	[14] (12%)	[3]	[6] (33%)	✓
Dermatomyositis	[1]			[1]	[4]	[7]	[5]	✓
DRESS syndrome (Drug-induced hypersensitivity syndrome)					[3]	[3]		
Eczema / eczematous reaction / eczematous eruption				•	[1]	[2]	[2]	✓
Edema / fluid retention				•		[4] (17%)	[2]	
Eosinophilic fasciitis (Shulman syndrome / Shulman disease)						[6]	[5]	
Erythema		[1]		•	[6]	[5]	[3]	✓
Erythema multiforme		•		•	[2]	[2] (<10%)	[3]	✓
Exanthems				•	[6] (20%)	[3]	[4]	✓
Exfoliative dermatitis		•				(<10%)	•	
Granuloma annulare				[1]	[1]	[2]	[2]	✓
Granulomas					[5]		[1]	
Hand–foot syndrome (palmar–plantar erythrodysesthesia)		[1] (7%)			[1]			
Hidradenitis suppurativa (acne inversa)					[1]	[3]		
Hypersensitivity					[1]	[3]		
Keratoacanthoma (Grzybowski syndrome)			[1]			[3]	[2]	
Lichen planus	[1]			•		[4]	[7]	✓
Lichen planus pemphigoides	[1]					[4]	[7]	
Lichen sclerosus						[4]	[1]	
Lichenoid dermatitis	[2]					[4]	[4]	
Lichenoid eruption / lichenoid reaction		[1]		[1]	[1]	[6]	[7]	✓
Linear IgA	[1]					[1]		
Lipodystrophy / acquired generalized lipodystrophy						[5]	[6]	
Lupus erythematosus (subacute cutaneous lupus erythematosus (SCLE))				[2]	[2]	[5]	[3]	✓

At Atezolizumab; **Av** Avelumab; **C** Cemiplimab; **D** Durvalumab; **I** Ipilimumab; **N** Nivolumab; **P** Pembrolizumab

	At	Av	C	D	I	N	P	=
Lymphadenopathy					[3]	[3]	[1]	
Maculopapular rash / morbilliform rash			[1] (8%)				[2]	
Morphea / localized scleroderma						[4]	[4]	
Pemphigus		•				[1]	[1]	
Peripheral edema	[2] (18%)	(20%)		[1] (26–38%)			[1] (17%)	✓
Pigmentation (Skin) (includes hyperpigmentation)					[1] (23%)	[1]	[1]	?
Pruritus (itching)	[6] (20%)	[1] (10%)	(15%)	[3] (40–60%)	[24] (65%)	[30] (47%)	[21] (33%)	✓✓
Psoriasiform dermatitis						[2]	[3]	
Psoriasiform eruption	[1]			[1]				
Psoriasis	[6]	•		[3]	[2]	[10] (<10%)	[9]	✓
Pustules / pustular eruption				•		[1]		
Rash	[7] (18%)	(22%)	[1] (25%)	[2] (40–60%)	[34] (83%)	[47] (55%)	[26] (50%)	✓✓
Sarcoidosis / sarcoid-like reaction (cutaneous sarcoidosis)	[2]	[1]			[7]	[10]	[12]	✓
Scleroderma		[1]		[1]		[5]	[8]	✓
Skin (dermatological) reaction			•			[1]		
Stevens-Johnson syndrome					[5]	[11]	[19]	
Sweet syndrome					[3]	[1]	[1]	
Thrombocytopenic purpura	[1]			•		[2]		
Thrombotic thrombocytopenic purpura					[3]	[4]	[1]	
Transient acantholytic dermatosis (Grover's disease)					[3]	[2]	[2]	
Ulcerations					[1]	[1]		
Urticaria / hives		[1]			[3]	[2]	[1]	✓
Vasculitis (angiitis) / cutaneous vasculitis (angiitis)					[4]	[3]	[5]	
Vesiculation					[1]	[1]		
Vitiligo					[4]	[15] (5–11%)	[14] (25%)	?
Xerosis / xeroderma				[1] (30–50%)	[1] (13%)			?
HAIR								
Alopecia / hair loss					[3] (19%)	[1]	[2]	
Alopecia areata						[3]	[3]	
Lichen planopilaris						[3]	[2]	
MUCOSAL								
Aphthous stomatitis / aphthous ulcer / aphtha (aphthae)					[1]	[1]		

At Atezolizumab; **Av** Avelumab; **C** Cemiplimab; **D** Durvalumab; **I** Ipilimumab; **N** Nivolumab; **P** Pembrolizumab

	At	Av	C	D	I	N	P	=
Mucositis	[1]				[1]		[2]	
Mucous membrane pemphigoid						[1]	[3]	
Sjögren's syndrome (see also sicca syndrome)	[2]			[1]	[1]	[2]	[3] (6%)	✓
Stomatitis (oral mucositis)						[2] (<10%)	[4] (9%)	
Xerostomia (dry mouth)					[1]	[3]	[2] (10%)	

At Atezolizumab; **Av** Avelumab; **C** Cemiplimab; **D** Durvalumab; **I** Ipilimumab; **N** Nivolumab; **P** Pembrolizumab

MONOCLONAL ANTIBODY

	Ad	An	At	B	D	Ib	In	Ip	N	Pem	Per	R	S	T	U	V	=
SKIN																	
Abscess	[1]			[1]			[4]						[1]				
Acneiform eruption / acneiform dermatitis / acneiform rash	[3]			[6] (83%)			[6]	[1]	[1]							[1]	?
AGEP			[1]		[1]		[2]		[1]					[1]			
Amicrobial pustulosis of the folds	[1]						[1]										
Anaphylaxis	[2]		[4]	[1]		[1]	[11]					[8]		[5]		•	✓
Angioedema (formerly named angioneurotic edema)	[4]			[1]		(5%)	[2] (11%)					[4] (11%)		[1]		[1]	
Basal cell carcinoma							[1]								[1]	[1]	
Bruise / bruising / contusion / ecchymosis (ecchymoses)						(7%)	[1]										
Bullous dermatosis							[1]					[1]			[1]		
Bullous pemphigoid / pemphigoid	[8]		[1]						[13]	[21]			[1]		[5]		
Candidiasis / candidosis	[1]						[4] (5%)						[9] (10%)	[1]			
Cellulitis and pseudocellulitis	[2] (<5%)			[1]	[9]		[5]					[1]		[9]	(<10%)		
Churg-Strauss syndrome								[1]	[1]								
Cutaneous toxicity / skin toxicity	[1]			[9] (16%)		[1]	[2] (75%)	[4] (35%)	[7] (7–17%)	[7] (10%)		[3] (12%)		[1]			✓
Dermatitis	[1]		[1]	[1]	[2] (11%)		[4]	[14] (12%)	[3]	[6] (33%)		[2]					✓
Dermatomyositis	[5]		[1]	[1]				[4]	[7]	[5]							
Diaphoresis						•				[1]		[2] (15%)					
DRESS syndrome (Drug-induced hypersensitivity syndrome)								[3]	[3]					[1]			
Eczema / eczematous reaction / eczematous eruption	[2]				[10] (15%)		[5] (19–30%)	[1]	[2]	[2]			[2]		[1]		✓
Edema / fluid retention				[2] (15%)			[3]		[4] (17%)	[2]	[1] (5–26%)	[1]					?
Eosinophilic cellulitis / Wells' syndrome	[2]						[1]								[2]		

Ad Adalimumab; **An** Anifrolumab; **At** Atezolizumab; **B** Bevacizumab; **D** Denosumab; **Ib** Ibritumomab; **In** Infliximab; **Ip** Ipilimumab; **N** Nivolumab; **Pem** Pembrolizumab; **Per** Pertuzumab; **R** Rituximab; **S** Secukinumab; **T** Tocilizumab; **U** Ustekinumab ; **V** Vedolizumab

	Ad	An	At	B	D	Ib	In	Ip	N	Pem	Per	R	S	T	U	V	=
Eosinophilic fasciitis (Shulman syndrome / Shulman disease)									[6]	[5]							
Epidermolysis bullosa acquisita			[1]									[1]					
Erysipelas	[1] (<5%)				•										[1]		
Erythema	[1]			[1]			[1]	[6]	[5]	[3]	[1]	[2] (16%)					✓
Erythema annulare centrifugum												[1]		[1]	[1]		
Erythema multiforme	[4]						[4]	[2]	[2] (<10%)	[3]			[1]				
Erythema nodosum					[1]				[1]								
Exanthems				[1]	[1]		[4]	[6] (20%)	[3]	[4]		[1]					?
Exfoliative dermatitis									(<10%)	•							
Facial edema							[1]					[1]		[1]			
Fixed eruption / fixed drug eruption	[1]						[1]										
Flushing / rubefaction						(6%)	[2] (39%)					(5%)					?
Folliculitis							[2]	[1] (7%)						[1]			
Granuloma annulare							[1]	[1]	[2]	[2]							
Granulomas	[1]						[1]	[5]		[1]							
Granulomatous reaction	[6]						[1]		[2]								
Hand–foot syndrome (palmar–plantar erythrodysesthesia)				[13] (57%)			[2] (31%)	[1]									?
Hematoma / cutaneous hematoma				[1]						[1]							
Henoch-Schönlein purpura / IgA vasculitis / immunoglobulin A vasculitis	[3]						[5]		[3]			[1]	[3]				
Herpes	[1]						[2]										
Herpes simplex	[1]						[4] (10%)					[2]					
Herpes zoster	[10]	[2] (6%)			•		[11]					[7]		[8]	[2]		
Hidradenitis suppurativa (acne inversa)	[6]						[2]	[1]	[3]			[1]	[3]	[1]			
Hyperhidrosis	[1]			[1] (8%)		(8%)											

Ad Adalimumab; **An** Anifrolumab; **At** Atezolizumab; **B** Bevacizumab; **D** Denosumab; **Ib** Ibritumomab; **In** Infliximab; **Ip** Ipilimumab; **N** Nivolumab; **Pem** Pembrolizumab; **Per** Pertuzumab; **R** Rituximab; **S** Secukinumab; **T** Tocilizumab; **U** Ustekinumab ; **V** Vedolizumab

	Ad	An	At	B	D	Ib	In	Ip	N	Pem	Per	R	S	T	U	V	=
Hypersensitivity	[3]	•			[3] (19%)		[11] (11%)	[1]	[3]		[1] (10%)	[6] (9–11%)		[6]		[1]	✓
Impetigo							[1]						•				
Jaundice (see also cholestasis / cholestatic jaundice)									[1]					[1]			
Kaposi's sarcoma	[1]						[1]					[3]					
Keratoacanthoma (Grzybowski syndrome)							[1]		[3]	[2]							
Leprosy (Hansen disease)	[1]						[1]										
Lesions (includes skin lesions)	[2]						[2]			[1]							
Leukocytoclastic vasculitis (angiitis)	[1]						[6]					[1]	[1]				
Lichen planus			[1]				[4]		[4]	[7]			[1]				
Lichen planus pemphigoides			[1]						[4]	[7]							
Lichen sclerosus							[1]		[4]	[1]							
Lichenoid dermatitis			[2]						[4]	[4]							
Lichenoid eruption / lichenoid reaction	[5]						[4]	[1]	[6]	[7]							
Linear IgA			[1]				[1]		[1]						[1]		
Lipodystrophy / acquired generalized lipodystrophy									[5]	[6]							
Lupus erythematosus (subacute cutaneous lupus erythematosus (SCLE))	[18]			[1]	[1]		[35] (59%)	[2]	[5]	[3]		[1]	[3]		[1]		✓
Lupus syndrome / drug-induced lupus (DIL)	[5]			[1]			[14]	[1]				[1]			[1]		
Lymphadenopathy	[1]						[1]	[3]	[3]	[1]							
Lymphoma	[8]						[9]					[1]		[1]			
Maculopapular rash / morbilliform rash										[2]				[1]			
Melanoma	[6]						[1]							[1]			
Molluscum contagiosum	[1]						[2]										
Morphea / localized scleroderma	[1]						[1]		[4]	[4]							
Necrosis (skin necrosis)				[2]								[1]					
Neutrophilic dermatosis	[1]							[1]									
Nevi (naevi)			[1]				[2]										
Palmoplantar pustulosis	[6]		[1]				[3]					[4]					

Ad Adalimumab; **An** Anifrolumab; **At** Atezolizumab; **B** Bevacizumab; **D** Denosumab; **Ib** Ibritumomab; **In** Infliximab; **Ip** Ipilimumab; **N** Nivolumab; **Pem** Pembrolizumab; **Per** Pertuzumab; **R** Rituximab; **S** Secukinumab; **T** Tocilizumab; **U** Ustekinumab ; **V** Vedolizumab

	Ad	An	At	B	D	Ib	In	Ip	N	Pem	Per	R	S	T	U	V	=
Papulopustular eruption							[1]							[1]			
Pemphigus									[1]	[1]		[1]	[1]	[1]			
Peripheral edema	(<5%)		[2] (18%)	[1] (8%)	(5%)	(8%)	[1]			[1] (17%)	(23%)	[1] (14%)		•			✓
Photosensitivity									[1]					[1]			
Pigmentation (Skin) (includes hyperpigmentation)				[1]				[1] (23%)	[1]	[1]							?
Pigmented purpuric dermatosis / eruption	[1]									[1]							
Pityriasis lichenoides / pityriasis lichenoides chronica / pityriasis lichenoides et varioliformis acuta	[2]						[3]										
Pruritus (itching)	[6]		[6] (20%)	[1] (91%)	•	(7%)	[8] (20%)	[24] (65%)	[30] (47%)	[21] (33%)	(14%)	[8] (14%)	[4]	[1]	(<10%)	[1]	✓
Pseudolymphoma / cutaneous pseudolymphoma	[1]						[2]										
Psoriasiform dermatitis	[2]						[1]		[2]	[3]							
Psoriasiform eruption			[1]				[4]										
Psoriasis	[47] (12%)		[6]				[57] (19%)	[2]	[10] (<10%)	[9]		[4]	[2] (6–16%)	[4]	[3]	[1]	✓
Purpura				[1]		(7%)						[1]					
Pustules / pustular eruption	[1]						[5]		[1]						[2]		
Pyoderma gangrenosum	[4]						[2]			[1]		[6]	[4]	[1]			
Radiation recall dermatitis				[1]						[4]							
Rash	[6] (12%)		[7] (18%)	[18] (91%)	[4]	(7%)	[13] (25%)	[34] (83%)	[47] (55%)	[26] (50%)	[9] (60–70%)	[13] (58%)		[9]		[3]	✓
Rosacea	[1]						[1]	[1]									
Sarcoidosis / sarcoid-like reaction (cutaneous sarcoidosis)	[9]		[2]				[5]	[7]	[10]	[12]		[3]		[1]	[1]		✓
Scleroderma	[1]								[5]	[8]							
Serum sickness							[2]					[28] (<20%)					?
Serum sickness-like reaction						[1]	[5]					[6] (<17%)					
Skin cancer	[1]						[1]						[1]				
Squamous cell carcinoma	[5]						[1]	[1] (7%)							[1]	[1]	

Ad Adalimumab; **An** Anifrolumab; **At** Atezolizumab; **B** Bevacizumab; **D** Denosumab; **Ib** Ibritumomab; **In** Infliximab; **Ip** Ipilimumab; **N** Nivolumab; **Pem** Pembrolizumab; **Per** Pertuzumab; **R** Rituximab; **S** Secukinumab; **T** Tocilizumab; **U** Ustekinumab ; **V** Vedolizumab

	Ad	An	At	B	D	Ib	In	Ip	N	Pem	Per	R	S	T	U	V	=
Stevens-Johnson syndrome	[2]						[3]	[5]	[11]	[20]	[1]	[6]					?
Sweet syndrome	[4]						[1]	[3]	[1]	[1]				[1]			
Thrombocytopenic purpura	[1]		[1]	[2]					[2]						[1]		
Thrombotic thrombocytopenic purpura								[3]	[4]	[1]							
Tinea	[1]												•				
Transient acantholytic dermatosis (Grover's disease)								[3]	[2]	[2]							
Tumors	[1]				[1]							[1] (11%)			[1]	[1]	
Ulcerations				[3]			[1]	[1]	[1]								
Urticaria / hives	[5]					•	[7] (17%)	[3]	[2]	[1]		[5] (8%)	[1]	[2]		[1]	✓
Vasculitis (angiitis) / cutaneous vasculitis (angiitis)	[9] (13%)			[1]			[18] (63%)	[4]	[3]	[5]		[5]	[3]	[1]	[1]		✓
Vesiculation	[1]							[1]	[1]								
Vitiligo	[10]						[8]	[4]	[15] (5–11%)	[14] (25%)			[4]		[1]		?
Xerosis / xeroderma				[1]				[1] (13%)			[1] (11%)						
HAIR																	
Alopecia / hair loss	[10]			[5] (43%)		[1]	[8]	[3] (19%)	[1]	[2]	[1] (61%)	[1]					✓
Alopecia areata	[7]						[4]		[3]	[3]			[4]		[1]		
Alopecia universalis	[4]							[1]				[1]					
Follicular mucinosis	[1]						[1]										
Lichen planopilaris							[2]		[3]	[2]							
NAILS																	
Nail toxicity				[1] (40%)						[1]							?
Onychodystrophy	[1]		[1]														
Onycholysis	[1]								[2]								
Onychomycosis							[1] (33%)						[1]				?
Paronychia				[2] (25%)					[1]		(7%)						

Ad Adalimumab; **An** Anifrolumab; **At** Atezolizumab; **B** Bevacizumab; **D** Denosumab; **Ib** Ibritumomab; **In** Infliximab; **Ip** Ipilimumab; **N** Nivolumab; **Pem** Pembrolizumab; **Per** Pertuzumab; **R** Rituximab; **S** Secukinumab; **T** Tocilizumab; **U** Ustekinumab ; **V** Vedolizumab

	Ad	An	At	B	D	Ib	In	Ip	N	Pem	Per	R	S	T	U	V	=
MUCOSAL																	
Aphthous stomatitis / aphthous ulcer / aphtha (aphthae)								[1]	[1]					[2]		[1]	
Behçet's disease / Behçet's syndrome										[1]			[4]				
Epistaxis				[6] (32%)		(5%)					[1]						?
Mucocutaneous reactions											[1]	[2]					
Mucosal inflammation				[2] (59%)							[1] (28%)						?
Mucositis			[1]	[14] (75%)		[1]		[1]		[2]							?
Mucous membrane pemphigoid									[1]	[3]							
Oral candidiasis							[1]						[2]	[1]			
Oral lichen planus							[1]			[1]			[1]				
Oral ulceration				[2] (18%)							[1] (41–43%)			[2]			?
Oropharyngeal pain												[1]	[1]	[1]	[1]	[1]	
Perianal fistula				[1] (67%)			[1]	[1]									?
Sjögren's syndrome (see also sicca syndrome)			[2]					[1]	[2]	[3] (6%)							
Stomatitis (oral mucositis)				[8] (75%)			[1]		[2] (<10%)	[4] (9%)	[1] (19%)	[2] (69%)		•			?
Xerostomia (dry mouth)								[1]	[3]	[2] (10%)							

Ad Adalimumab; **An** Anifrolumab; **At** Atezolizumab; **B** Bevacizumab; **D** Denosumab; **Ib** Ibritumomab; **In** Infliximab; **Ip** Ipilimumab; **N** Nivolumab; **Pem** Pembrolizumab; **Per** Pertuzumab; **R** Rituximab; **S** Secukinumab; **T** Tocilizumab; **U** Ustekinumab ; **V** Vedolizumab

NON-STEROIDAL ANTI-INFLAMMATORY (NSAIDS)

	Acec	Asp	C	Dexi	Dexk	Dicl	Etod	Etor	I	Ktp	Ktr	Mel	Met	N	S	=
SKIN																
AGEP		[1]	[8]				[1]		[5] (50%)			[1]	[3]			?
Anaphylaxis	[2]	[8] (<10%)	[8]	[1]		[16] (48%)		[1]	[5] (25%)	[4]	[8]	[1]	[12] (9%)	[2]	(<10%)	✓
Angioedema (formerly named angioneurotic edema)		[32] (22%)	[9]			[3]	[1]	[3]	[8]	[1]	[1]	[3]		[5]		✓
Bruise / bruising / contusion / ecchymosis (ecchymoses)		[1]							[1]		•	[1]		•		
Bullous dermatosis		[4]	[1]			[2]			[3]	[1] (29%)		•		[5]		?
Bullous pemphigoid / pemphigoid		[1]	[1]			[1]			[2]							
Contact dermatitis	[2]									[5] (27%)						?
Dermatitis			[2]			[10]			[5]	[29]	•					?
Dermatitis herpetiformis		[1]				[2]			[1]							
Dermatomyositis		[1]				[1]										
Diaphoresis			•			•			[1]	[1]	[2] (<10%)		[1]	[3]		
DRESS syndrome (Drug-induced hypersensitivity syndrome)		[2]	[1]			[2]			[4]				[1]	[4]		
Eczema / eczematous reaction / eczematous eruption						•			[1]	[3]		[1]				
Edema / fluid retention			[5] (6%)						[1]		(<10%)	[1] (6%)		[1] (<9%)		
Embolia cutis medicamentosa (Nicolau syndrome) / livedoid dermatitis						[18]			[2]	[1]						
Erythema			[2] (14%)			[4]		[1]		[4] (21%)	[1]	[2]	[2]	[1]		✓
Erythema multiforme		[9]	[3]			[6]	•	[1]	[12] (13%)	[1]		[1]	[1]	[2]		✓
Erythema nodosum		[9]				•			[1] (<5%)				[1]	[1]		
Erythroderma		[2]											[1]			
Exanthems		[11] (18%)	[7] (49%)			[6] (<5%)	[2]	[1]	[9]	[3]	[1]	[1]	[3]	[9] (14%)		✓
Excoriations									[1] (6%)		[1]					

Acec Aceclofenac; **Asp** Aspirin; **C** Celecoxib; **Dexi** Dexibuprofen; **Dexk** Dexketoprofen; **Dicl** Diclofenac; **Etod** Etodolac; **Etor** Etoricoxib; **I** Ibuprofen; **Ktp** Ketoprofen; **Ktr** Ketorolac; **Mel** Meloxicam; **Met** Metamizole; **N** Naproxen; **S** Salsalate

	Acec	Asp	C	Dexi	Dexk	Dicl	Etod	Etor	I	Ktp	Ktr	Mel	Met	N	S	=
Exfoliative dermatitis		[1]	[1]			[1]			[1]	•	•					
Facial edema			[1]			[1]	[2]			•		[1]				
Fixed eruption / fixed drug eruption	[2]	[22]	[2]			[4] (18%)	[2]	[11]	[17]			[1]	[9] (9%)	[26] (24%)		✓
Flushing / rubefaction		[1]				•	[1]				•					
Hematoma / cutaneous hematoma		[1]									[2]	[3]				
Henoch-Schönlein purpura / IgA vasculitis / immunoglobulin A vasculitis									[1]			[1]				
Herpes simplex		[1]	•											[1]		
Herpes zoster			•						[1]							
Hot flashes / hot flushes			[1]						•	•		•		[1]		
Hypersensitivity	[1]	[5]	[9]			[5]		[1] (10%)	[5]	[1]	[2]	[2] (5%)	[1]	[2]		✓
Jaundice (see also cholestasis / cholestatic jaundice)			[1]								•					
Lichen planus													[1]	[3]		
Lichenoid eruption / lichenoid reaction		[2]												[3]	[1]	
Linear IgA		[2]				[7]				[1]				[1]		
Lupus erythematosus (subacute cutaneous lupus erythematosus (SCLE))			[1]						[5]					[2]		
Necrotizing fasciitis						[1]							[1]			
Pemphigus		[1]				[1]			[1]	[1]			[1]			
Peripheral edema		[1]	[2]			[1]	[1]	[1]	[2] (5%)	•		[1]		[1]		✓
Photoallergic reaction			[1]			[1]				[2]						
Photocontact dermatitis					[5]					[6]						
Photosensitivity	[2]		•			[4]	[1]		[6]	[36] (11%)	•	•		[16]		✓
Pityriasis rosea		[3]												[1]		
Pruritus (itching)		[6]	[6]			[6] (<10%)	[7] (<10%)		[7] (<5%)	[4] (<10%)	[1] (<10%)	[3]		[5] (17%)		✓
Pseudolymphoma / cutaneous pseudolymphoma		[1]				[1]			[1]	[1]				[1]		
Pseudoporphyria		[1]	[1]			[1]			[2]	[2]		[1]		[29]		✓
Psoriasis	[1]	[3]				[1]			[2]	[1]		[1]				
Purpura		[8]	[1]			[2]			[1]	[1]	[1] (<10%)	•		[4]		✓

Acec Aceclofenac; **Asp** Aspirin; **C** Celecoxib; **Dexi** Dexibuprofen; **Dexk** Dexketoprofen; **Dicl** Diclofenac; **Etod** Etodolac; **Etor** Etoricoxib; **I** Ibuprofen; **Ktp** Ketoprofen; **Ktr** Ketorolac; **Mel** Meloxicam; **Met** Metamizole; **N** Naproxen; **S** Salsalate

	Acec	Asp	C	Dexi	Dexk	Dicl	Etod	Etor	I	Ktp	Ktr	Mel	Met	N	S	=
Purpura fulminans						[2]					[1]					
Pustules / pustular eruption			[1]											[2]		
Rash		(<10%)	[11] (40%)			[4] (6%)	[5]		[4]	[1]	[1] (<10%)	[3]		[2]	(<10%)	✓
SDRIFE		[1]	[1]					[1]						[1]		
Serum sickness-like reaction									[1]					[1]		
Stevens-Johnson syndrome	[1]	[14]	[7]			[12] (5%)	•	[8]	[22] (17%)	[1]	•	[1]	[7] (24%)	[5]		✓
Sweet syndrome	[1]		[4]													
Thrombocytopenic purpura						[1]			[1]							
Ulcerations		•											[1]			
Urticaria / hives	[1]	[72] (83%)	[11]			[7]	•	[4]	[10]	[6]	[1]	[4]	[3]	[6] (<5%)	[1]	✓
Vasculitis (angiitis) / cutaneous vasculitis (angiitis)	[3]	[2]	[4]			[3]	[2]		[8]		[1]	•		[9]		✓
Vesiculobullous eruption									[2]					[1]		
Wound complications									[1]		[1]					
Xerosis / xeroderma			•			[3]				[1]						
HAIR																
Alopecia / hair loss		[1]	[3]			•			[2]	[1]	•	•		[3]		✓
NAILS																
Nail changes			•						[1]							
Onycholysis									[1]	[1]						
MUCOSAL																
Aphthous stomatitis / aphthous ulcer / aphtha (aphthae)		[3]				[1]					[1]			[1]		
Epistaxis		[2]									•	[1]				
Oral lesions									[1]	[1]						
Oral mucosal fixed drug eruption								[2]						[1]		
Oral ulceration		[4]				[1]			[1]				[1]	[1]		
Rectal hemorrhage / rectal bleeding											•	[1]				
Stomatitis (oral mucositis)			[4] (8%)			•		[1]		•	(<10%)			•		
Tongue edema						[1]		[1]			•					
Xerostomia (dry mouth)			•		[1]	[2] (26%)			•	[1]	[2]	•	[1]	[2]		✓

Acec Aceclofenac; **Asp** Aspirin; **C** Celecoxib; **Dexi** Dexibuprofen; **Dexk** Dexketoprofen; **Dicl** Diclofenac; **Etod** Etodolac; **Etor** Etoricoxib; **I** Ibuprofen; **Ktp** Ketoprofen; **Ktr** Ketorolac; **Mel** Meloxicam; **Met** Metamizole; **N** Naproxen; **S** Salsalate

PROTON PUMP INHIBITOR (PPI)

	D	E	L	O	P	R	=
SKIN							
Acneiform eruption / acneiform dermatitis / acneiform rash		•	•		•		✓
AGEP			[1]	[2]			
Anaphylaxis		[1]	[7]	[7]	[13]		✓
Angioedema (formerly named angioneurotic edema)		•		[5]	•		✓
Bruise / bruising / contusion / ecchymosis (ecchymoses)					•	•	
Candidiasis / candidosis		•	•				
Dermatitis		•	[1]	[1]	•		✓
Diaphoresis		•	[1]	[1]	[1]	•	✓
Eczema / eczematous reaction / eczematous eruption		[1]		[2]	[1] (9%)		✓
Edema / fluid retention		•	[1]	[2] (<10%)	•		✓
Erythema				[1]			
Erythema dyschromicum perstans / ashy dermatosis		[1]	[1]	[1]			✓
Erythema multiforme			[2]	[1]	•		✓
Erythroderma			[1]	[2]			
Exanthems		•		[1]	•		✓
Exfoliative dermatitis		[1]	[1]	[3]			✓
Facial edema			[2]	[1]	[1]	•	✓
Fixed eruption / fixed drug eruption		[2]		[1]			
Flushing / rubefaction		•	[1]				
Fungal dermatitis		•			•		
Herpes zoster					•	•	
Hypersensitivity			[3]	[2]	[2]	[1]	✓
Lichenoid eruption / lichenoid reaction		[1]	[1]	[2]	[1]		✓
Lupus erythematosus (subacute cutaneous lupus erythematosus (SCLE))		[3]	[3]	[5]	[3]		✓
Peripheral edema		•	[2]	[2]	[2]	•	✓
Photosensitivity		[1]			[1]	•	✓
Pigmentation (Skin) (includes hyperpigmentation)				[1]		•	
Pruritus (itching)		•	[1]	[8] (<10%)	[1]	[2]	✓
Pruritus ani et vulvae		•	[1]				

D Dexlansoprazole; **E** Esomeprazole; **L** Lansoprazole; **O** Omeprazole; **P** Pantoprazole; **R** Rabeprazole

	D	E	L	O	P	R	=
Psoriasis				[1]		•	
Rash		[1]	•	[6]	[3] (9%)	[3]	✓
Rowell syndrome / Rowell's syndrome		[1]		[1]			
SDRIFE				[3]	[2]		
Stevens-Johnson syndrome			[5]	[5]	[1]		✓
Sweet syndrome		[1]		[1]			
Urticaria / hives		[1]	[3]	[9] (<10%)	[2]	•	✓
Vasculitis (angiitis) / cutaneous vasculitis (angiitis)				[2]	[1]		
Xerosis / xeroderma		[1]		[2]	•	•	✓
HAIR							
Alopecia / hair loss			[1]	[2]	•	•	✓
MUCOSAL							
Gingivitis					•	•	
Glossitis (inflammation of the tongue)			[1]		•	•	✓
Oral candidiasis	•			[3]	•		✓
Stomatitis (oral mucositis)			[2]	[1]	•	•	✓
Tongue edema		•			[1]		
Xerostomia (dry mouth)	•		•	[2] (<10%)	•	•	✓

D Dexlansoprazole; **E** Esomeprazole; **L** Lansoprazole; **O** Omeprazole; **P** Pantoprazole; **R** Rabeprazole

TNF INHIBITORS

	A	C	E	G	I	=
SKIN						
Abscess	[1]		[2]		[4]	✓
Acneiform eruption / acneiform dermatitis / acneiform rash	[3]		[1]		[6]	✓
AGEP			[1]		[2]	
Amicrobial pustulosis of the folds	[1]	[1]			[1]	✓
Anaphylaxis	[2]		[2]		[11]	✓
Angioedema (formerly named angioneurotic edema)	[4]	•	[1]		[2] (11%)	✓
Atopic dermatitis			[1]		[1]	
Basal cell carcinoma				[1]	[1]	
Bullous pemphigoid / pemphigoid	[8]		[1]			
Candidiasis / candidosis	[1]				[4] (5%)	
Carcinoma	[2]		[2]			
Cellulitis and pseudocellulitis	[2] (<5%)		[2]		[5]	✓
Cutaneous toxicity / skin toxicity	[1]	[1]		[1]	[2] (75%)	✓
Dermatitis	[1]	•	[3]		[4]	✓
Dermatomyositis	[5]		[4]			
Eczema / eczematous reaction / eczematous eruption	[2]				[5] (19–30%)	?
Eosinophilic cellulitis / Wells' syndrome	[2]		[1]		[1]	✓
Erythema	[1]				[1]	
Erythema multiforme	[4]			[1]	[4]	✓
Erythema nodosum		[1]	[1]			
Exanthems			[2]		[4]	
Fixed eruption / fixed drug eruption	[1]		[1]		[1]	✓
Folliculitis		[1]	[1]		[2]	✓
Granuloma annulare			[1]		[1]	
Granulomas	[1]		[2]		[1]	✓
Granulomatous reaction	[6]		[5]		[1]	✓
Henoch-Schönlein purpura / IgA vasculitis / immunoglobulin A vasculitis	[3]		[3]	[1]	[5]	✓
Herpes	[1]				[2]	

A Adalimumab; **C** Certolizumab; **E** Etanercept; **G** Golimumab; **I** Infliximab

	A	C	E	G	I	=
Herpes simplex	[1]		[1]		[4] (10%)	✓
Herpes zoster	[10]	[3]	[6]		[11]	✓
Hidradenitis suppurativa (acne inversa)	[6]		[2]		[2]	✓
Hypersensitivity	[3]	•	[1]		[11] (11%)	✓
Kaposi's sarcoma	[1]				[1]	
Leprosy (Hansen disease)	[1]		[2]		[1]	✓
Lesions (includes skin lesions)	[2]				[2]	
Leukocytoclastic vasculitis (angiitis)	[1]	[1]		[1]	[6]	✓
Lichen planus		[1]	[2]		[4]	✓
Lichenoid eruption / lichenoid reaction	[5]	[1]	[3]		[4]	✓
Lupus erythematosus (subacute cutaneous lupus erythematosus (SCLE))	[18]		[25]	[3]	[35] (59%)	✓
Lupus syndrome / drug-induced lupus (DIL)	[5]	[1]	[4]		[14]	✓
Lymphadenopathy	[1]				[1]	
Lymphoma	[8]		[3]	[1]	[9]	✓
Lymphoproliferative disease / lymphoproliferative disorder			[1]		[1]	
Melanoma	[6]		[2]	[1]	[1]	✓
Molluscum contagiosum	[1]				[2]	
Morphea / localized scleroderma	[1]		[1]		[1]	✓
Necrotizing fasciitis			[1]		[1]	
Neutrophilic dermatosis	[1]		[1]			
Nevi (naevi)			[1]		[2]	
Non-Hodgkin's lymphoma	[1]		[1]			
Palmoplantar pustulosis	[6]	[1]			[3]	✓
Peripheral edema	(<5%)		[1]		[1]	✓
Pigmented purpuric dermatosis / eruption	[1]	[1]		[1]		✓
Pityriasis lichenoides / pityriasis lichenoides chronica / pityriasis lichenoides et varioliformis acuta	[2]		[1]		[3]	✓
Pruritus (itching)	[6]	[1]	[2] (14%)		[8] (20%)	✓
Pseudolymphoma / cutaneous pseudolymphoma	[1]		[1]		[2]	✓
Psoriasiform dermatitis	[2]				[1]	

A Adalimumab; **C** Certolizumab; **E** Etanercept; **G** Golimumab; **I** Infliximab

	A	C	E	G	I	=
Psoriasiform eruption		[1]			[4]	
Psoriasis	[47] (12%)	[7]	[21]	[2]	[57] (19%)	✓✓
Pustules / pustular eruption	[1]		[2]		[5]	✓
Pyoderma gangrenosum	[4]	[1]	[1]		[2]	✓
Rash	[6] (12%)	[2] (5%)	[8] (15%)	[4]	[13] (25%)	✓✓
Rosacea	[1]		[1]		[1]	✓
Sarcoidosis / sarcoid-like reaction (cutaneous sarcoidosis)	[9]	[1]	[10]		[5]	✓
SDRIFE				[1]	[2]	
Serum sickness		•			[2]	
Skin cancer	[1]		[1]		[1]	✓
Squamous cell carcinoma	[5]		[4]	[1]	[1]	✓
Stevens-Johnson syndrome	[2]				[3]	
Sweet syndrome	[4]				[1]	
Tumors	[1]	[1]				
Urticaria / hives	[5]	•	[3]		[7] (17%)	✓
Vasculitis (angiitis) / cutaneous vasculitis (angiitis)	[9] (13%)	•	[23] (25%)	[1]	[18] (63%)	✓✓
Vitiligo	[10]				[8]	
HAIR						
Alopecia / hair loss	[10]	[1]	[5] (20%)		[8]	✓
Alopecia areata	[7]		[1]	[1]	[4]	✓
Follicular mucinosis	[1]				[1]	
MUCOSAL						
Oral lichen planus		[1]			[1]	

A Adalimumab; **C** Certolizumab; **E** Etanercept; **G** Golimumab; **I** Infliximab

TYROSINE-KINASE INHIBITORS

	A	B	C	D	E	G	I	Lef	Len	O	Pa	Po	R	S	T	=
SKIN																
Acneiform eruption / acneiform dermatitis / acneiform rash	[30] (61–93%)	[1] (<10%)		[2] (<10%)	[30] (73–80%)	[34] (66–85%)	[3]	(<10%)		[1]		[1] (14%)		[1] (<10%)	[4] (5%)	✓
AGEP					[3]	[1]	[7]									
Anaphylaxis		•			[1] (30%)	[1]		•							[1]	?
Bullous dermatosis	•				[1]			[3]						[1] (7%)		
Cellulitis and pseudocellulitis												(<11%)			•	
Cutaneous adverse reaction						[2]	[1] (71%)			[1]			[1]	[1]		?
Cutaneous toxicity / skin toxicity	[3]	[1]	[3]	[8] (36%)	[10] (84%)	[12] (68%)	[9] (30–44%)		[3]	[2] (39%)	[5]	[1]	[5] (73%)	[24] (67%)	[3] (46%)	✓
Dermatitis	[1] (21%)	[1]		[1] (<10%)	[5] (33%)			(<10%)						[1]		?
Dermatomyositis							[1]	[1]							[3]	
Desquamation					[1]	[2] (39%)						[1]	[4] (6%)			?
Diaphoresis							(13%)	(<10%)							[1]	
DRESS syndrome (Drug-induced hypersensitivity syndrome)	[1]				[2]		[5]	[6]								
Eczema / eczematous reaction / eczematous eruption				(<10%)	[1]	[1]		[1]								
Edema / fluid retention		(14%)		[8] (38%)	[1]		[40] (80%)				[1] (6%)	[2] (23%)		[6] (32%)	[1] (5–26%)	✓
Erosive pustular dermatosis	[2]				[2]	[1]										
Erythema		[1]	(11%)	[2]	(18%)	[1]	[5] (<10%)						[1]	[6] (7%)	[2]	✓
Erythema multiforme		•					[2]	[1]					[1]	[1]		
Erythema nodosum				•			[1]					[1]				
Exanthems		[1]			[3] (8%)	[3] (21%)	[9]		(21%)				[1]			?
Exfoliative dermatitis	•	[1]		[1]		[1]	[4]	[1]			[1] (35%)			[1] (10%)		✓
Facial edema					[1]		[3] (<10%)				•			[3] (24%)		?

A Afatinib; **B** Bosutinib; **C** Cabozantinib; **D** Dasatinib; **E** Erlotinib; **G** Gefitinib; **I** Imatinib; **Lef** Leflunomide; **Len** Lenvatinib; **O** Osimertinib; **Pa** Pazopanib; **Po** Ponatinib; **R** Regorafenib; **S** Sunitinib; **T** Trastuzumab

	A	B	C	D	E	G	I	Lef	Len	O	Pa	Po	R	S	T	=
Fissures	[2] (12%)				[1]											
Folliculitis	[1]	[1]			[9] (11%)	[4]	[1]								[1]	
Graft-versus-host reaction				[1]			[1]									
Hand–foot syndrome (palmar–plantar erythrodysesthesia)	[2] (10%)	[1] (31%)	[25] (60%)	[1]	[3] (30–60%)	[3] (31%)	[3]		[16] (57%)		[12] (44%)		[65] (92%)	[78] (67%)	[11] (29%)	✓
Herpes zoster								[1]							•	
Hidradenitis suppurativa (acne inversa)								[1]			[1]					
Hot flashes / hot flushes												[1] (10%)			[1]	
Hyperhidrosis				[1] (<10%)			[1]									
Hyperkeratosis			(7%)						(7%)							
Hypermelanosis														[1]	[1]	
Hypersensitivity		[1] (<10%)		•				[1]							[3]	
Hypomelanosis							[5]							[1]		
Jaundice (see also cholestasis / cholestatic jaundice)			(25%)								[1]			[1]		?
Keratoacanthoma (Grzybowski syndrome)		[1]		[1]									[1]			
Lesions (includes skin lesions)					[1]		[1]							[2] (38%)		?
Leukocytoclastic vasculitis (angiitis)	[1]						[1]				[1]					
Lichen planus							[7]	[1]								
Lichenoid eruption / lichenoid reaction							[15]	[2]		[1]						
Lupus erythematosus (subacute cutaneous lupus erythematosus (SCLE))				[1]	[1]			[9]		[1]						
Maculopapular rash / morbilliform rash					[1]		[1]									
Necrolysis						[1]	[1]									
Necrosis (skin necrosis)					[1]									[1]		
Nevi (naevi)					[1]							[1]	[2]	[2]		
Palmar–plantar hyperkeratosis							[1]							[1]		

A Afatinib; **B** Bosutinib; **C** Cabozantinib; **D** Dasatinib; **E** Erlotinib; **G** Gefitinib; **I** Imatinib; **Lef** Leflunomide; **Len** Lenvatinib; **O** Osimertinib; **Pa** Pazopanib; **Po** Ponatinib; **R** Regorafenib; **S** Sunitinib; **T** Trastuzumab

	A	B	C	D	E	G	I	Lef	Len	O	Pa	Po	R	S	T	=
Panniculitis				[4]			[3]					[1]				
Papulopustular eruption					[9] (29%)	[3] (21%)										?
Peripheral edema		[1] (5%)		[3] (44%)		[1] (22%)	[5] (75%)	(<10%)	[3] (37%)		[1] (16%)	(13–22%)		[1] (17%)	(5–10%)	✓
Photosensitivity				[1]	[1]		[3] (<10%)						[1]		[2]	
Pigmentation (Skin) (includes hyperpigmentation)				[1]		[1]	[14] (60%)	(<10%)			[7] (16%)			[15] (91%)		?
Pityriasis rubra pilaris							[1]					[3]				
Pruritus (itching)	[3] (13%)	[2] (10%)		[5] (18%)	[10] (33%)	[6] (61%)	[3] (10%)	[3]		[1]	[3] (16%)		[1]	[3] (<10%)	•	✓
Psoriasiform eruption							[1]		[1]							
Psoriasis							[3]					[1]				
Purpura					[3]	[1]	[1]	(<10%)								
Pyoderma gangrenosum						[1]	[2]		[1]		[1]			[10]		
Radiation recall dermatitis					[1]				[1]					[1]	[3]	
Rash	[54] (61–93%)	[9] (57%)	[2] (30%)	[12] (34%)	[119] (80%)	[69] (66–85%)	[27] (69%)	[17] (12%)	[1] (23%)	[17] (53%)	[6] (21%)	[10] (54%)	[17] (23–50%)	[17] (31%)	[12] (56%)	✓✓
Rosacea					[2]		[1]									
SDRIFE	[1]					[1]				[1]						
Seborrheic dermatitis				[1]	[1]									[1]		
Squamous cell carcinoma						[1]	[2]						•			
Stevens-Johnson syndrome	[8]	[1]				[2]	[15]	[5]		[6]			[1]	[1]	[1]	✓
Sweet syndrome				[1]	[1]		[4]									
Telangiectasia					[1]		[1]									
Thrombocytopenic purpura													[1]	[4]	[1]	
Ulcerations				[1]		[2]		[3] (<10%)			[1]			[1]	•	
Urticaria / hives		(<10%)		[1] (<10%)		[1]	[3]	•		[1]						
Vasculitis (angiitis) / cutaneous vasculitis (angiitis)					[1]	[1]	[2]	[4] (<10%)		[4]						
Xerosis / xeroderma	[8] (36%)	[1] (6%)	[1] (23%)	[1] (<10%)	[13] (56%)	[13] (53%)	[2] (<10%)	•	[1] (20%)	[4] (46%)	[1]	[6] (42%)	[1]	[3] (17%)	[1]	✓✓

A Afatinib; **B** Bosutinib; **C** Cabozantinib; **D** Dasatinib; **E** Erlotinib; **G** Gefitinib; **I** Imatinib; **Lef** Leflunomide; **Len** Lenvatinib; **O** Osimertinib; **Pa** Pazopanib; **Po** Ponatinib; **R** Regorafenib; **S** Sunitinib; **T** Trastuzumab

	A	B	C	D	E	G	I	Lef	Len	O	Pa	Po	R	S	T	=
HAIR																
Alopecia / hair loss	[1] (7%)		(16%)	[3] (<10%)	[10] (14%)	[6]	[2] (10–15%)	[21] (10%)	(12%)		[2] (23%)		(8%)	[6] (10%)	[6] (33%)	✓
Folliculitis decalvans	[1]				[3]											
Hair changes			(34%)		[4] (20%)						(38%)					?
Hair pigmentation			[2] (34%)	[2]				(<10%)			[9] (58%)		[1]	[8] (38%)		?
Hypertrichosis					[4]	[2]										
NAILS																
Nail changes	[2] (16%)				[3] (25%)	[1] (17%)		[1] (<10%)							[1]	?
Nail disorder				[1]			[1]							[1] (<10%)	[1] (15–40%)	?
Nail dystrophy							[2]								[1]	
Nail pigmentation						[1]	[2]									
Paronychia	[18] (33–85%)				[14] (23%)	[16] (14–32%)				[9] (46%)					[1] (30%)	?
Pyogenic granuloma					[1]	[2]										
MUCOSAL																
Aphthous stomatitis / aphthous ulcer / aphtha (aphthae)	•				[1]		[1]		(41%)							?
Burning Mouth Syndrome / glossodynia / glossalgia / glossopyrosis									(25%)					[1] (15%)		?
Cheilitis (inflammation of the lips)	[1] (7%)						[1]									
Epistaxis	[3] (17%)					[1]			[1] (24%)		[2]		[1]	[2] (13%)	•	✓
Gingivitis								(<10%)	(10%)							
Mucocutaneous eruption				[1]			[1]									
Mucosal inflammation	[7] (69%)	[1] (13%)	[3] (35%)		[1] (18%)				[1] (50%)		[1] (7%)			[4] (54%)	[1]	✓
Mucositis	[10] (50–90%)		[1]	[1] (16%)	[10] (21%)	[4] (6–17%)	[2] (15%)				[1]		[11] (24–36%)	[19] (~60%)	[4] (23%)	✓
Oral ulceration					[1]	[1]	[3] (15%)	•	(41%)							?
Oropharyngeal pain							[1]		(25%)							?

A Afatinib; **B** Bosutinib; **C** Cabozantinib; **D** Dasatinib; **E** Erlotinib; **G** Gefitinib; **I** Imatinib; **Lef** Leflunomide; **Len** Lenvatinib; **O** Osimertinib; **Pa** Pazopanib; **Po** Ponatinib; **R** Regorafenib; **S** Sunitinib; **T** Trastuzumab

	A	B	C	D	E	G	I	Lef	Len	O	Pa	Po	R	S	T	=
Stomatitis (oral mucositis)	[23] (50–90%)		[5] (51%)	[1]	[12] (26%)	[10] (33%)		•	[5] (47%)	[4] (18%)	[5] (16%)	(9–23%)	[5] (27%)	[21] (60%)	[5] (62%)	✓
Xerostomia (dry mouth)	[1] (20%)			[1] (33%)			[1] (44%)	(<10%)	(17%)				(5%)	[2] (~60%)		?

A Afatinib; **B** Bosutinib; **C** Cabozantinib; **D** Dasatinib; **E** Erlotinib; **G** Gefitinib; **I** Imatinib; **Lef** Leflunomide; **Len** Lenvatinib; **O** Osimertinib; **Pa** Pazopanib; **Po** Ponatinib; **R** Regorafenib; **S** Sunitinib; **T** Trastuzumab

GENETIC ASSOCIATIONS

Table 1 – Reported genetic associations with cutaneous adverse drug reactions and other immune-mediated reactions

Elizabeth J. Phillips[1,2] and Neil H. Shear[3]

[1]Vanderbilt University Medical Center, Department of Medicine, Dermatology, Pathology, Microbiology & Immunology, and Vanderbilt University School of Medicine, Department of Pharmacology, Nashville, TN, USA
[2]Institute for Immunology and Infectious Diseases, Murdoch University, Murdoch, WA, Australia
[3]Division of Dermatology, Department of Medicine, Sunnybrook Health Sciences Centre, University of Toronto, Toronto, ON, Canada

Allele	Reaction	Ethnic population	Sensitivity (%)	Specificity (%)	PPV	NPV	Est.	Ref.
ANTI-NEOPLASTIC OR IMMUNOSUPPRESANT								
HLA-DRB1*07:01 HLA-DQB1*02:01 (Asparaginase)	anaphylaxis	Caucasian/European						[110,111]
HLA-DQA1*02:01 HLA-DRB1*07:01 (Azathioprine)	pancreatitis	Caucasian/European			9%			[112]
HLA-C*06:02 (Azathioprine)	Hypersensitivity syndrome	Caucasian/European	33.3%	100%	100%	66.7%		[113]
HLA-DRB1*12:01 (oxaliplatin)	Immediate hypersensitivity, anaphylaxis	Taiwanese						[137]
(Osimertinib, EGFR-Tyrosine kinase inhibitor) HLA-B*51:02 HLA-B*51:01 HLA-B*24:02	 SJS/TEN MPE	Taiwanese	 83.3%	 96.7%	 11.3%	 99.9%		[147]
ANTI-THYROID								
HLA-B*38:02 (*5 SNPS) HLA-B*27:05 (3/5 SNPS) HLA-DRB1*08:03	Agranulocytosis Agranulocytosis Agranulocytosis	Han Chinese European Han Chinese		99.9% >99%	7% 30%			[114,115] [116]
HLA-DRB1*08:03[7] HLA-B*39:01[7]	Agranulocytosis Agranulocytosis	Japanese Japanese						[117]
ANTIBIOTICS, ANTI-INFLAMMATORY								
Dapsone								
HLA-B*13:01	DRESS	Chinese	85.5–90	85.7–93.1	7.8	99.8		[1–4]
HLA-B*13:01	DRESS	Thai						[4,5]
HLA-B*13:01	SJS/TEN	Thai						[4,5]
HLA-B*13:01	DILI	East Indian						[6]
ANTIBIOTICS, BETA-LACTAM								
HLA-B*57:01 (flucloxacillin)	DILI	Caucasian/European			0.12%	99.99%		[19]

Allele	Reaction	Ethnic population	Sensitivity (%)	Specificity (%)	PPV	NPV	Est.	Ref.
HLA-DRB1*15:01 (amoxicillin-clavulanate) HLA-DQB1*06:02 HLA-A*02:01	DILI	Caucasian/European Northern European						[20]
HLA-B*55:01	Self-reported penicillin allergy	Caucasian/European						[21]
HLA-DRB3*02:02	Delayed hypersensitivity to penicillins	Southwestern Europeans						[22]
HLA-DRB1*10:01	Skin test positive immediate penicillin allergy	Caucasian/European	unknown	unknown	unknown	unknown		[23]
HLA-B*55:02 HLA-C*01:02 HLA-DQB1*06:09	Self-reported cephalosporin allergy	Taiwan						[133]
HLA-A*02:01	Cefazolin/ cephalosporin DILI	Over-represented US White (Cefazolin, 95%)						[139]
ANTIBIOTICS, FLUOROQUINOLONE								
Levofloxacin								
HLA-B*13:01 HLA-B*13:02	SJS/TEN SJS/TEN	Chinese	83%	78%				[134]
HLA-DQA1*03:01 HLA-B*57:01	DILI	US White (primarily)						[143]
ANTIBIOTICS, MACROLIDE								
Azithromycin								
HLA-DQA1*03:01	DILI	European						[135]
ANTIBIOTICS, MINOCYCLINE								
HLA-B*35:02	DILI	Caucasian/European						[24]
ANTIBIOTICS, NITROFURANTOIN								
HLA-DRB1*11:04	DILI, autoimmune variant	Caucasian/European (United States)						[25]
HLA-A*33:03	DILI	Caucasian/European						[26]
ANTIBIOTICS, SULFONAMIDES								
Sulfamethoxazole Trimethoprim								
HLA-A*29	SJS/TEN	Caucasian/European						[7]
HLA-A*30	FDE	Turkish						[8]
HLA-A*30-B*13-C*06	FDE	Turkish						[9]
HLA-A*11:01	SJS/DRESS	Japanese						[9]
HLA-B*14:01 HLA-B*35:01	DILI	Caucasian/European African American						[10]
HLA-B12 (HLA-B*44)	SJS/TEN	Caucasian/European						[7]
HLA-B*38	SJS/TEN	Caucasian/European						[11]

Allele	Reaction	Ethnic population	Sensitivity (%)	Specificity (%)	PPV	NPV	Est.	Ref.
HLA-B*13:01[2]	SJS/TEN DRESS	Southeast Asia (Taiwan, Thailand, Malaysia)			3.64 (DRESS)	99.92 (DRESS)		[12]
HLA-B*13:01 HLA-C*08:01	DRESS SJS/TEN SJS/TEN	Thailand HIV co-infected						[13] [14]
HLA-B*07:02/HLA-C*07:02 haplotype[3]	Respiratory Failure	Caucasian/European Children						[15]
HLA-DR*07	SJS/TEN	Caucasian/European						[7]
HLA-B*15:02 HLA-B*38:02	SJS/TEN SJS/TEN	Thai, Taiwanese Thai, Taiwainese, Malaysian, European						[131]
HLA-A*68:01 HLA-B*13:01 HLA-B*39:01	DRESS DRESS DRESS	Overall Malaysian, Taiwanese, Thai Taiwanese, Thai						[131]
HLA-A*11::01 HLA-B*15:02 HLA-C*08:01 HLA-B*38:02	SCAR	Overall/HIV+						[131]
HLA-B*44:03 and binding group HLA-B*38:01 and binding group HLA-C*04:01	SJS/TEN>DRESS	White US Weaker association (underpowered) in South African populations						[140]
ANTIBIOTICS, VANCOMYCIN								
HLA-A*32:01	DRESS	Caucasian/European			20%			[16–18]
HLA-A*32:01	DRESS with DILI	Caucasian/European						[132]
HLA-A*32:01	DRESS	White US						[142]
HLA-A*32:01	Acute generalized exanthematous pustulosis	White US (case)						[144]
ANTICONVULSANTS								
Carbamazepine								
HLA-A*24:02	SJS/TEN	Chinese (Han)						[29]
HLA-A*31	DRESS	Japanese						[30]
HLA-A*31	EM	Japanese						[30]
HLA-A*31	MPE	Japanese						[30]
HLA-A*31	SJS/TEN	Japanese						[30]
HLA-A*31:01	DRESS	Caucasian/European	70	96.1	0.89	99.98		[31,32]
HLA-A*31:01	DRESS	Chinese (Han)	50	95.8	0.59	99.97		[32,33]
HLA-A*31:01	DRESS	Japanese	60.7	87.5			A	[34]
HLA-A*31:01	DRESS	Korean						[35]

Allele	Reaction	Ethnic population	Sensitivity (%)	Specificity (%)	PPV	NPV	Est.	Ref.
HLA-A*31:01	MPE	Caucasian/European						[31]
HLA-A*31:01	MPE	Chinese (Han)						[33,36]
HLA-A*31:01	SJS/TEN	Caucasian/European						[31,37]
HLA-A*31:01	SJS/TEN	Chinese (Han)						[37]
HLA-A*31:01	SJS/TEN	Japanese	60.7	87.5			A	[34,37]
HLA-A*31:01	SJS/TEN	Korean						[37]
HLA-A*31:01	DRESS>SJS/TEN	Japanese + meta-analysis					B	[130]
HLA-B*15:02	MPE	Thai						[38]
HLA-B*15:02	SJS/TEN	Chinese						[39]
HLA-B*15:02	SJS/TEN	Taiwan, Chinese (Han)	72.2–100	86.3–95.8	3.4–9	92–100		[29,32,33,37, 40–48]
HLA-B*15:02	SJS/TEN	Indian						[49]
HLA-B*15:02	SJS/TEN	Korean						[42]
HLA-B*15:02	SJS/TEN	Malaysian	96	88	1.8	100	B	[37,39,42]
HLA-B*15:02	SJS/TEN	Thai	88.1–100	75–88.1	1.92	99.96		[38,42, 50–52]
HLA-B*15:11	SJS/TEN	Chinese (Han)						[29,53]
HLA-B*15:11	SJS/TEN	Japanese						[53]
HLA-B*15:11	SJS/TEN	Korean						[53]
HLA-B*15:11	SJS/TEN	Thai						[53]
HLA-B*15:11	SJS/TEN	Vietnamese						[53]
HLA-B*15:11	SJS/TEN	Japanese + meta-analysis						[130]
HLA-B*15:21	SJS/TEN	Thai						[38]
HLA-B*51:01	DRESS	Chinese (Han)						[53]
HLA-B*51:01	MPE	Chinese (Han)						[53]
HLA-B*58:01	DRESS	Thai						[38]
HLA-B*58:01	MPE	Thai						[38]
HLA-DRB1*14:05	MPE	Chinese (Han)						[54]
HLA-B*38:02	MPE	Chinese (Han)						[136]
Lamotrigine								
HLA-A*02:07	DRESS	Thai						[55]
HLA-A*02:07	MPE	Thai						[55]
HLA-A*02:07	SJS/TEN	Thai						[55]
HLA-A*24:02 / HLA-C*01:02	MPE	Korean						[56]
HLA-A*30:01	MPE	Chinese (Han)						[54]
HLA-A*31:01	DRESS	Korean						[57]
HLA-A*31:01	SJS/TEN	Korean						[57]
HLA-A*33:03	MPE	Thai						[55]

Allele	Reaction	Ethnic population	Sensitivity (%)	Specificity (%)	PPV	NPV	Est.	Ref.
HLA-A*68:01	DRESS	Caucasian/European						[58]
HLA-A*68:01	SJS/TEN	Caucasian/European						[58]
HLA-B*13:02	MPE	Chinese (Han)						[54]
HLA-B*15:02	DRESS	Thai						[55]
HLA-B*15:02	MPE	Thai						[55]
HLA-B*15:02	SJS/TEN	Chinese (Han)	29.4	89.7				[41,45,59]
HLA-B*15:02	SJS/TEN	Thai						[55]
HLA-B*38	SJS/TEN	Caucasian/European						[11]
HLA-B*44:03	MPE	Thai						[55]
HLA-B*58:01	DRESS	Caucasian/European						[58]
HLA-B*58:01	SJS/TEN	Caucasian/European						[58]
HLA-C*07:18	DRESS	Caucasian/European						[58]
HLA-C*07:18	SJS/TEN	Caucasian/European						[58]
HLA-DQB1*06:09	DRESS	Caucasian/European						[58]
HLA-DQB1*06:09	SJS/TEN	Caucasian/European						[58]
HLA-DRB1*13:01	DRESS	Caucasian/European						[58]
HLA-DRB1*13:01	SJS/TEN	Caucasian/European						[58]
HLA-A*31:01 HLA-B*13:01 HLA-B*15:11	DRESS (*eosinophilia) DRESS SJS/TEN	Korean Korean Korean						[148]
Oxcarbazepine								
HLA-B*15:02	MPE	Chinese (Han)						[60]
HLA-B*15:02	SJS/TEN	Chinese (Han)						[36]
HLA-B*38:02	MPE	Chinese (Han)						[61]
Phenobarbital								
CYP2C19*2	DRESS	Thai						[62]
CYP2C19*2	SJS/TEN	Thai						[62]
HLA-B*51:01	SJS/TEN	Japanese						[63]
Phenytoin								
CYP2C9*3	DRESS	Chinese (Han)						[64]
CYP2C9*3	DRESS	Japanese						[64]
CYP2C9*3	DRESS	Malaysian						[64]
CYP2C9*3	SJS/TEN	Chinese (Han)						[64]
CYP2C9*3	SJS/TEN	Japanese						[64]
CYP2C9*3	SJS/TEN	Malaysian						[64]
CYP2C9*3	SJS/TEN	Thai						[65]
HLA-B*13:01	SJS/TEN	Chinese (Han)						[36]
HLA-B*15:02	SJS/TEN	Chinese (Han)	36.6	87.2				[36,41,45]
HLA-B*15:02	SJS/TEN	Malaysian						[66]

Allele	Reaction	Ethnic population	Sensitivity (%)	Specificity (%)	PPV	NPV	Est.	Ref.
HLA-B*15:02	SJS/TEN	Thai						[50]
HLA-B*15:13	DRESS	Malaysian						[67]
HLA-B*15:13	SJS/TEN	Malaysian	53.8	90.6				[66]
HLA-B*56:02	SJS/TEN	Thai						[65]
HLA-B*56:02	DRESS	Australian Aboriginal						[66]
HLA-B*53:01	DRESS & drug-induced liver injury	African Americans	89%	100%	0.6%	100%	A	[129]
HLA-C*08:01	SJS/TEN	Chinese (Han)						[36]
HLA-DRB1*16:02	SJS/TEN	Chinese (Han)						[36]
Zonisamide								
HLA-A*02:07	SJS/TEN	Japanese						[63]
ANTIFUNGAL, TERBINAFINE								
HLA-A*33:01	DILI	Caucasian/European						[23]
ANTIPARASITICS, BENZNIDAZOLE								
HLA*11:01	DRESS	Bolivian			100	70		
HLA*29:02					100	70		
HLA*68					48	84		
HLA-B*35	Moderate to severe morbilliform drug eruption, DRESS, SJS/TEN		64.8%	56.9%	35%	81.9%		[28]
ANTIRETROVIRAL INTEGRASE INHIBITOR								
HLA-B*53:01 (raltegravir)	DRESS	African/African American						[81,82]
ANTIRETROVIRALS								
Nevirapine								
CYP2B6 T983C	SJS/TEN	African (Malawian, Ugandan)						[68]
CYP2B6 T983C	SJS/TEN	African (Mozambique)						[69]
HLA-C*04	DRESS	Chinese (Han)						[70]
HLA-C*04	SJS/TEN	African (Malawian)			2.6	99.2		[70]
HLA-C*04:01 (rs5010528)	SJS/TEN	African (Sub-Saharan)			2.8	42.4		[73]
HLA-C*08	DRESS	Japanese						[72]
HLA-C*08:02 / HLA-B*14:02	DRESS	Caucasian/European (Sardinian)						[74]
HLA-DRB1*01:01	DRESS	Caucasian/European						[75]
ANTIRETROVIRALS, NUCLEOSIDE ANALOG REVERSE TRANSCRIPTASE INHIBITORS								
Abacavir								
HLA-B*57:01	HSS	African/African descent	100	99	50	100	D	[76,77]

Allele	Reaction	Ethnic population	Sensitivity (%)	Specificity (%)	PPV	NPV	Est.	Ref.
HLA-B*57:01	HSS	Caucasian/European	100	96	66	100	D	[76–80]
HLA-B*57:01	HSS	Hispanic	26	99	96	60	D	[77]
CARBONIC ANHYDRASE INHIBITORS								
Acetazolamide								
HLA-B*59	SJS/TEN	Korean						[83]
Methazolamide								
HLA-B*59	SJS/TEN	Japanese						[84]
HLA-B*59:01[4] HLA-B*55:02[4]	SJS/TEN	Han Chinese						[86]
HLA-B*59:01	SJS/TEN	Chinese (Han)	87.5	63.3				[85]
HLA-B*59:01	SJS/TEN	Korean						[87]
HLA-C*01:02	SJS/TEN	Chinese (Han)						[86]
HLA-C*01:02	SJS/TEN	Korean						[87]
CORTICOSTEROIDS								
HLA-DQB1*06:02-HLA-DQA1*01:02 (DILI controls), Intranveous methylprednisolone)	DILI	US populations US White						[145]
DISEASE-MODIFYING ANTIRHEUMATIC DRUGS (DMARDS)								
Sulfasalazine								
HLA-B*13:01	DRESS	Chinese (Han)	66.7	86.7				[88]
DISULFIRAM								
HLA-C*01:01 HLA-DRB1*09:01 (haplotypic in Asian populations)	DILI	US populations US White 81.8% US Asian 18.2% Hispanic 9.1%						[145]
HERBAL DRUGS								
HLA-B*35:01 (Polygonum multiflorum) HLA-B*35:01 (Green Tea Extract)	DILI DILI							[122] [123]
HLA-B*35:01 (Garcinia cambogia and Green Tea)[8]	DILI	European American						[124]
HLA-B*35:01 (Tumeric, Curcumin)	DILI	European American						[125]
HLA-B*35:01 (Kampo medicines)	DILI	Japanese						[126]
IL-1 and IL-6 INHIBITORS								
HLA-DRB1*15:019HLA-DRB1*15 haplotypes9	Delayed hypersensitivity reaction with DRESS features	Caucasian Children with Still's Disease						[127]
NON-STEROIDAL INFLAMMATORY (NSAID)								
Isoxicam, Piroxicam								
HLA-A*02	SJS/TEN	Caucasian/European						[7]

Allele	Reaction	Ethnic population	Sensitivity (%)	Specificity (%)	PPV	NPV	Est.	Ref.
HLA-B*12	SJS/TEN	Caucasian/European						[7]
Oxicams								
HLA-B*73	SJS/TEN	Caucasian/European						[11]
RADIOCONTRAST DYE								
Sulfasalazine								
HLA-DRB1*15:02	Immediate reaction Anaphylaxis	Korean						[138]
STATINS								
DRB1*11:01 DRB1*08:03	Necrotizing autoimmune myopathy	Caucasian/European Japanese						[118] [118]
STRONTIUM RANELATE								
HLA-A*33:03	RESS SJS/TEN	Southeast Asian						[119,120,121]
XANTHINE OXIDASE INHIBITORS								
Allopurinol								
HLA-A*33:03	DRESS	Korean	88	73.7	0.8	99.96	A,C	[89]
HLA-A*33:03	SJS/TEN	Korean	88	73.7	0.8	99.96	A,C	[89]
HLA-B*58:01	DRESS	Caucasian/European						[90–92]
HLA-B*58:01	DRESS	Caucasian/European (Portuguese)						[93]
HLA-B*58:01	DRESS	Chinese (Han)	84–100	82–88.9	1.6–5	100	A	[91,92,94–97]
HLA-B*58:01	DRESS	Japanese						[90,91]
HLA-B*58:01	DRESS	Korean	92–100	89.5–90.7	2.06	99.98	A	[89,91,92,98]
HLA-B*58:01	DRESS	Thai						[91,92]
HLA-B*58:01	MPE	Chinese (Han)	100	88.89			A	[91,92,94]
HLA-B*58:01	MPE	European						[91]
HLA-B*58:01	MPE	Japanese						[91]
HLA-B*58:01	MPE	Korean						[91]
HLA-B*58:01	MPE	Thai						[91]
HLA-B*58:01	SJS/TEN	Asian, East						[99]
HLA-B*58:01	SJS/TEN	Asian, South						[99]
HLA-B*58:01	SJS/TEN	Caucasian/European	50–60		50–60%	95	B,E	[16,91,92,99 100]
HLA-B*58:01	SJS/TEN	Caucasian/European (Portuguese)						[98]
HLA-B*58:01	SJS/TEN	Caucasian/European (Sardinian)						[101]
HLA-B*58:01	SJS/TEN	Chinese (Han)	84–100	82–88.89	1.6–5	100	A	[91,92,94–97,99,100]
HLA-B*58:01	SJS/TEN	Japanese	50–60			99	B	[91,92,99, 100,103]

Allele	Reaction	Ethnic population	Sensitivity (%)	Specificity (%)	PPV	NPV	Est.	Ref.
HLA-B*58:01	SJS/TEN	Korean	92–100	89.5–90.7	2.06	99.98	A	[89,91,92, 98,99]
HLA-B*58:01	SJS/TEN	Thai	100	87	1.52	100		[91,92,99, 103,104]
HLA-B*58:01[5] HLA-C*03:02[5]	SJS/TEN DRESS	Vietnamese Vietnamese						[105]
HLA-B*58:01[6] HLA-A*34:02[6] HLA-B*53:01[6]	DILI	European, African and Hispanic American						[106]
HLA-B*58:01 in presence of HLA-A*24:02 and DRB1*13:02	DRESS	Korean	83.33% 33.33%	89.05% 97.55%	1.62% 2.86%	99.96% 99.85%		[107]
HLA-B*58:01 HLA-A*34:01	SJS/TEN and DRESS	US Black (69%) US White (31%)						[141]
HLA-C*03:02	DRESS	Korean	92	87.7	1.77	99.98	A,C	[89]
HLA-C*03:02	SJS/TEN	Korean	92	87.7	1.77	99.98	A,C	[88]
rs2734583	DRESS	Thai	90.6	86.0			A,C	[108]
rs2734583	SJS/TEN	Thai	90.6	86.0			A,C	[108]
rs2734583 (*BAT1*); rs3094011 (*HCP5*); GA005234 (*MICC*)	SJS/TEN	Japanese					C	[109]
rs3099844	DRESS	Thai	90.6	85.0			A,C	[108]
rs3099844	SJS/TEN	Thai	90.6	85.0			A,C	[108]
rs9263726	DRESS	Thai	90.6	82.4			A,C	[108]
rs9263726	SJS/TEN	Thai	90.6	82.4			A,C	[108]
rs9263726 (*PSORS1C1*)	SJS/TEN	Japanese					C	[109]

A – Sensitivities, specificities, PPVs, and NPVs include or are based on data from studies which analyzed multiple cutaneous reactions (e.g. SJS/TEN, DRESS, MPE, EM, etc.) as a group. If data do not have a range, they are derived from a single study and should be considered as an estimate.
B – Sensitivities, specificities, PPVs, and NPVs include or are based on data from studies which analyzed multiple ethnicities (e.g. Chinese (Han), Japanese, Korean, Thai, Caucasian/European, etc.) as a group. If data do not have a range, they are derived from a single study and should be considered as an estimate.
C – Genes are in linkage with HLA*B*58:01
D – Post-marketing surveillance supports a 100% negative predictive value in all populations including Hispanic and African American
E – 50–60% of African and European ancestry individuals carry HLA-B*58:01 in association with allopurinol SJS/TEN and DRESS [128]
DILI, drug induced liver injury; DRESS, drug reaction with eosinophilia and systemic symptoms; EM, erythema multiforme; FDE, fixed drug eruption; HSS, hypersensitivity syndrome; MPE, maculopapular exanthema; NPV, negative predictive value; PPV, positive predictive value; SJS/TEN, Stevens-Johnson syndrome/toxic epidermal necrolysis; the category DRESS includes drug-induced hypersensitivity syndrome (DIHS) and hypersensitivity syndrome (HSS), excluding abacavir HSS.

References

1. Wang H et al. Association between HLA-B*1301 and Dapsone-Induced Hypersensitivity Reactions among Leprosy Patients in China. J. Invest. Dermatol. 2013;133(11):2642–4.
2. Zhang FR et al. HLA-B*13:01 and the Dapsone Hypersensitivity Syndrome. N. Engl. J. Med. 2013;369(17):1620–8.
3. Chen WT et al. The Function of HLA-B*13:01 Involved in the Pathomechanism of Dapsone-Induced Severe Cutaneous Adverse Reactions. J. Invest. Dermatol; 2018;138(7):1546–1554.

4. Tangamornsuksan W et al. Association between HLA-B*1301 and dapsone-induced cutaneous adverse drug reactions a systematic review and meta-analysis. JAMA Dermatology 2018;154(4):441–6.
5. Tempark T et al. Dapsone-induced severe cutaneous adverse drug reactions are strongly linked with HLA-B 13:01 allele in the Thai population. Pharmacogenet. Genomics 2017;27(12):429–37.
6. Devarbhavi H et al. Association of human leukocyte antigen-B*13:01 with dapsone-induced liver injury. Br J Clin Pharmacol 2022; 88:1369–72.
7. Roujeau JC et al. Genetic susceptibility to toxic epidermal necrolysis. Arch Dermatol. 1987;123(9):1171–1173.
8. Özkaya-Bayazit E et al. Fixed drug eruption induced by trimethoprim-sulfamethoxazole: Evidence for a link to HLA-A30 B13 Cw6 haplotype. J Am Acad Dermatol. 2001;45(5):712–7.
9. Nakamura R et al. Association of HLA-A*11:01 with Sulfonamide-Related Severe Cutaneous Adverse Reactions in Japanese Patients. J Invest Dermatol. 2020;140(8):1659–1662.e6.
10. Li YJ et al. HLA-B*14:01 and HLA-B*35:01 are associated with trimethoprim- sulfamethoxazole induced liver injury. Hepatology. 2021;73(1):268–281.
11. Lonjou C et al. A European study of HLA-B in Stevens-Johnson syndrome and toxic epidermal necrolysis related to five high-risk drugs. Pharmacogenet. Genomics 2008;18(2):99–107.
12. Wang CW et al. Whole genome sequencing identifies genetic variants associated with co-trimoxazole hypersensitivity in Asians. J Allergy Clin Immunol 2021;147:1402–12.
13. Nakkam N et al., Associations of HLA and drug-metabolizing enzyme genes in co-trimoxazole-induced severe cutaneous adverse reactions. Drug Metab Pharmacokinet 2022;47:100480.
14. Sukasem C et al. Genetic Association of Co-Trimoxazole-Induced Severe Cutaneous Adverse Reactions Is Phenotype-Specific: HLA Class I Genotypes and Haplotypes, Clin Pharmacol Ther 2020;108(5):1078–1089.
15. Goldman JL et al. HLA-B*07:02 and HLA-C*07:02 are associated with trimethoprim-sulfamethoxazole respiratory failure. Pharmacogenomics J 2022;22:124–9.
16. Konvinse KC et al. HLA-A*32:01 is strongly associated with vancomycin-induced drug reaction with eosinophilia and systemic symptoms. J Allergy Clin Immunol. 2019;144(1):183–92.
17. Rwandamuriye FX et al. A Rapid Allele-Specific Assay for HLA-A*32:01 to Identify Patients at Risk for Vancomycin-Induced Drug Reaction with Eosinophilia and Systemic Symptoms. J Mol Diagn. 2019;21(5):782–9.
18. Nakkam N et al. Cross-reactivity between vancomycin, teicoplanin and telavancin in HLA-A*32:01 positive vancomycin DRESS patients sharing an HLA-Class II haplotype. J Allergy Clin Immunol. 2021; 147(1): 403–5.
19. Daly AK et al. HLA-B*5701 genotype is a major determinant of drug-induced liver injury due to flucloxacillin. Nat Genet. 2009;41(7):816–9.
20. Lucena MI et al. Susceptibility to amoxicillin-clavulanate-induced liver injury is influenced by multiple HLA class I and II alleles. Gastroenterology. 2011;141(1):338–47.
21. Krebs K et al. Genome-wide Study Identifies Association between HLA-B(*)55:01 and Self-Reported Penicillin Allergy. Am J Hum Genet. 2020;107(4):612–621.
22. Romano A et al. Next-generation sequencing and genotype association studies reveal the association of HLADRB3*02:02 with delayed hypersensitivity to penicillins. Allergy. 2022;77(6):1827–1834.
23. Nicoletti P et al., Beta-lactam-induced immediate hypersensitivity reactions: A genome-wide association study of a deeply phenotyped cohort. J Allergy Clin Immunol. 2021;147(5):1830–1837.e15.
24. Urban TJ et al. Minocycline hepatotoxicity: Clinical characterization and identification of HLA-B *35:02 as a risk factor. J Hepatol. 2017;67(1):137–44.
25. Chalasani N et al., Clinical features, outcomes, and HLA risk factors associated with nitrofurantoin-induced liver injury. J Hepatol. 2023;78(2):293–300.
26. Daly AK et al. Drug-induced liver injury due to nitrofurantoin: Similar clinical features, but different HLA risk alleles in an independent cohort. J Hepatol. 2023;78(5):e165–e166.
27. Fontana RJ et al. The role of HLA-A*33:01 in patients with cholestatic hepatitis attributed to terbinafine. J Hepatol. 2018;69(6):1317–25.
28. Bosch-Nicolau P et al. Association of HLA-B*35 and moderate or severe cutaneous reactions secondary to benznidazole treatment in chronic chagas disease. Clin Microbiol Infect. 2022;28(6):881.e1–881.e5.
29. Shi YW et al. Association between HLA and Stevens-Johnson Syndrome Induced by Carbamazepine in Southern Han Chinese: Genetic Markers besides B*1502? Basic Clin. Pharmacol. Toxicol. 2012;111(1):58–64.
30. Niihara H et al. HLA-A31 strongly associates with carbamazepine-induced adverse drug reactions but not with carbamazepine-induced lymphocyte proliferation in a Japanese population. J. Dermatol. 2012;39(7):594–601.
31. McCormack M et al. HLA-A*3101 and Carbamazepine-Induced Hypersensitivity Reactions in Europeans. N. Engl. J. Med. 2011;364(12): 1134–43.
32. Genin E et al. HLA-A*31:01 and different types of carbamazepine-induced severe cutaneous adverse reactions: an international study and meta-analysis. Pharmacogenomics J. 2014;14(3):281–8.
33. Hsiao YH et al. Genotype-phenotype association between HLA and carbamazepine-induced hypersensitivity reactions: Strength and clinical correlations. J Dermatol Sci; 2014;73(2):101–9.
34. Ozeki T et al. Genome-wide association study identifies HLA-A*3101 allele as a genetic risk factor for carbamazepine-induced cutaneous adverse drug reactions in Japanese population. Hum Mol Genet. 2011;20(5):1034–41.
35. Kim SH et al. Carbamazepine-induced severe cutaneous adverse reactions and HLA genotypes in Koreans. Epilepsy Res; 2011;97(1–2):190–7.
36. Hung S et al. Common risk allele in aromatic antiepileptic-drug induced Stevens-Johnson syndrome and toxic epidermal necrolysis in Han Chinese. Pharmacogenomics 2010;11(3):349–56.
37. Yip VL et al. HLA genotype and carbamazepine-induced cutaneous adverse drug reactions: A systematic review. Clin Pharmacol Ther. 2012; 92(6):757–65.
38. Sukasem C et al. Association between HLA-B Alleles and Carbamazepine-Induced Maculopapular Exanthema and Severe Cutaneous Reactions in Thai Patients. J Immunol Res. 2018;2018.
39. Then S-M et al. Frequency of the HLA-B*1502 allele contributing to carbamazepine-induced hypersensitivity reactions in a cohort of Malaysian epilepsy patients. Asian Pacific J. allergy Immunol. Thailand; 2011;29(3):290–3.
40. Zhang Y et al. Strong association between HLA-B*1502 and carbamazepine-induced Stevens-Johnson syndrome and toxic epidermal necrolysis in mainland Han Chinese patients. Eur J Clin Pharmacol. 2011;67(9):885–7.
41. Cheung YK et al. HLA-B alleles associated with severe cutaneous reactions to antiepileptic drugs in Han Chinese. Epilepsia. 2013;54(7): 1307–14.

42. Tangamornsuksan W et al. Relationship Between the HLA-B*1502 Allele and Carbamazepine-Induced Stevens-Johnson Syndrome and Toxic Epidermal Necrolysis. JAMA Dermatology. 2013;149(9):1025.
43. Chung WH et al. A marker for Stevens-Johnson syndrome. Nature 2004;428(6982):486.
44. Hung SI et al. Genetic susceptibility to carbamazepine-induced cutaneous adverse drug reactions. Pharmacogenet Genomics. 2006;16(4): 297–306.
45. Man CBL et al. Association between HLA-B*1502 allele and antiepileptic drug-induced cutaneous reactions in Han Chinese. Epilepsia 2007;48(5):1015–8.
46. Wu XT et al. Association between carbamazepine-induced cutaneous adverse drug reactions and the HLA-B*1502 allele among patients in central China. Epilepsy Behav. 2010;19(3):405–8.
47. Chen P et al. Carbamazepine-Induced Toxic Effects and HLA-B*1502 Screening in Taiwan. N Engl J Med. 2011;364(12):1126–33.
48. Wang Q et al. Association between HLA-B*1502 allele and carbamazepine-induced severe cutaneous adverse reactions in Han people of southern China mainland. Seizure. 2011;20(6):446–8.
49. Mehta T et al. Association of HLA-BFNx011502 allele and carbamazepine-induced Stevens- Johnson syndrome among Indians. Indian J Dermatol Venereol Leprol. 2009;75(6):579.
50. Locharernkul C et al. Carbamazepine and phenytoin induced Stevens- Johnson syndrome is associated with HLA-B*1502 allele in Thai population. Epilepsia 2008;49(12):2087–91.
51. Tassaneeyakul W et al. Association between HLA-B*1502 and carbamazepine-induced severe cutaneous adverse drug reactions in a Thai population. Epilepsia 2010;51(5):926–30.
52. Kulkantrakorn K et al. HLA-B*1502 Strongly Predicts Carbamazepine-Induced Stevens-Johnson Syndrome and Toxic Epidermal Necrolysis in Thai Patients with Neuropathic Pain. Pain Pract. 2012;12(3):202–8.
53. Wang Q et al. Association between the HLA-B alleles and carbamazepine-induced SJS/TEN: A meta-analysis. Epilepsy Res. 2017;135:19–28.
54. Li LJ et al. Predictive markers for carbamazepine and lamotrigine-induced maculopapular exanthema in Han Chinese. Epilepsy Res; 2013;106(1–2):296–300.
55. Koomdee N et al. Association of HLA-A and HLA-B alleles with lamotrigine-induced cutaneous adverse drug reactions in the Thai population. Front. Pharmacol. 2017;8:1–7.
56. Moon J et al. The HLA-A 2402/Cw 0102 haplotype is associated with lamotrigine-induced maculopapular eruption in the Korean population. Epilepsia 2015;56(10):e161–7.
57. Kim BK et al. HLA-A*31:01 and lamotrigine-induced severe cutaneous adverse drug reactions in a Korean population. Ann. Allergy. Asthma Immunol; 2017 May;118(5):629–30.
58. Kazeem GR et al. High-resolution HLA genotyping and severe cutaneous adverse reactions in lamotrigine-treated patients. Pharmacogenet Genomics 2009;19(9):661–5.
59. Zeng T et al. Association of HLA-B*1502 allele with lamotrigine-induced Stevens-Johnson syndrome and toxic epidermal necrolysis in Han Chinese subjects: A meta-analysis. Int J Dermatol. 2015;54(4):488–93.
60. Hu FY et al. Pilot association study of oxcarbazepine-induced mild cutaneous adverse reactions with HLA-B*1502 allele in Chinese Han population. Seizure. 2011;20(2):160–2.
61. Lv YD et al. The association between oxcarbazepine-induced maculopapular eruption and HLA-B alleles in a Northern Han Chinese population. BMC Neurol. 2013;13.
62. Manuyakorn W et al. Phenobarbital-induced severe cutaneous adverse drug reactions are associated with CYP2C19*2 in Thai children. Pediatr Allergy Immunol. 2013;24(3):299–303.
63. Kaniwa N et al. Specific HLA types are associated with antiepileptic drug-induced Stevens-Johnson syndrome and toxic epidermal necrolysis in Japanese subjects. Pharmacogenomics; 2013;14(15):1821–31.
64. Chung WH et al. Genetic Variants Associated With Phenytoin-Related Severe Cutaneous Adverse Reactions. JAMA 2014;312(5):525.
65. Tassaneeyakul W et al. Associations between HLA class i and cytochrome P450 2C9 genetic polymorphisms and phenytoin-related severe cutaneous adverse reactions in a Thai population. Pharmacogenet Genomics 2016;26(5):225–34.
66. Chang CC et al. Association of HLA-B 15:13 and HLA-B 15:02 with phenytoin-induced severe cutaneous adverse reactions in a Malay population. Pharmacogenomics J. 2017;17(2):170–3.
67. Somogyi AA et al. High and variable population prevalence of HLA-B*56:02 in indigenous Australians and relation to phenytoin-associated drug reaction with eosinophilia and systemic symptoms. Br J Clin Pharmacol. 2019;85(9):2163–9.
68. Carr DF et al. CYP2B6 c.983T>C polymorphism is associated with nevirapine hypersensitivity in Malawian and Ugandan HIV populations. J Antimicrob Chemother. 2014;69(12):3329–34.
69. Ciccacci C et al. Association between CYP2B6 polymorphisms and Nevirapine-induced SJS/TEN: A pharmacogenetics study. Eur J Clin Pharmacol. 2013;69(11):1909–16.
70. Gao S et al. HLA-Dependent Hypersensitivity Reaction to Nevirapine in Chinese Han HIV-Infected Patients. AIDS Res Hum Retroviruses. 2012;28(6):540–3.
71. Carr DF et al. Association of human leukocyte antigen alleles and nevirapine hypersensitivity in a Malawian HIV-infected population. Clin Infect Dis. 2013;56(9):1330–9.
72. Carr DF et al. Genome-wide association study of nevirapine hypersensitivity in a sub-Saharan African HIV-infected population. J Antimicrob Chemother. 2017;72(4):1152–62.
73. Gatanaga H et al. HLA-Cw8 primarily associated with hypersensitivity to nevirapine. AIDS; 2007; 21:264–5.
74. Littera R et al. HLA-dependent hypersensitivity to nevirapine in Sardinian HIV patients. AIDS. 2006;20(12):1621–6.
75. Martin AM et al. Predisposition to nevirapine hypersensitivity associated with HLA-DRB1*0101 and abrogated by low CD4 T-cell counts. AIDS 2005;19(1):97–9.
76. Saag M et al. High Sensitivity of Human Leukocyte Antigen-B*5701 as a Marker for Immunologically Confirmed Abacavir Hypersensitivity in White and Black Patients. Clin Infect Dis. 2008;46(7):1111–8.
77. Sousa-Pinto B et al. Pharmacogenetics of abacavir hypersensitivity: A systematic review and meta-analysis of the association with HLA-B 57:01. J Allergy Clin Immunol. 2015;136(4):1092–1094e3.
78. Hetherington S et al. Genetic variations in HLA-B region and hypersensitivity reactions to abacavir Tamoxifen for breast cancer among hysterectomised women. Lancet. 2002;359:1121–2.
79. Mallal S et al. Association between presence of HLA-B*5701, HLA-DR7, and HLA-DQ3 and hypersensitivity to HIV-1 reverse-transcriptase inhibitor abacavir. Lancet; 2002;359(9308):727–32.
80. Mallal S et al. HLA-B*5701 Screening for Hypersensitivity to Abacavir. N Engl J Med. 2008;358(6):568–79.
81. Thomas M et al. Association of the HLA-B*53:01 Allele With Drug Reaction With Eosinophilia and Systemic Symptoms (DRESS) Syndrome During Treatment of HIV Infection With Raltegravir. Clin Infect Dis. 2017;64(9):1198–203.

82. Lefebvre M et al. Rate of drug reaction with eosinophilia and systemic symptoms (DRESS) syndrome with raltegravir and role of the HLA-B*53: 01 allele. J Acquir Immune Defic Syndr. 2020.
83. Her Y et al. Stevens-Johnson syndrome induced by acetazolamide. J Dermatol. 2011;38(3):272–5.
84. Shirato S et al. S. Stevens-Johnson syndrome induced by methazolamide treatment. Arch. Ophthalmol; 1997;115(4):550–3.
85. Jiang M et al. Unique motif shared by HLA-B*59:01 and HLA-B*55:02 is associated with methazolamide-induced StevensJohnson syndrome and toxic epidermal necrolysis in Han Chinese. J Eur Acad Dermatol Venereol 2022; 36:873–80.
86. Yang F et al. HLA-B 59:01: A marker for Stevens-Johnson syndrome/toxic epidermal necrolysis caused by methazolamide in Han Chinese. Pharmacogenomics J. 2016;16(1):83–7.
87. Kim SH et al. HLA-B*5901 is strongly associated with methazolamide-induced Stevens-Johnson syndrome/toxic epidermal necrolysis. Pharmacogenomics; 2010;11(6):879–84.
88. Yang F et al. HLA-B*13:01 is associated with salazosulfapyridine-induced drug rash with eosinophilia and systemic symptoms in Chinese Han population. Pharmacogenomics; 2014;15(11):1461–9.
89. Kang HR et al. Positive and negative associations of HLA class i alleles with allopurinol-induced SCARs in Koreans. Pharmacogenet. Genomics 2011;21(5):303–7.
90. Lee MH et al. Initiating allopurinol therapy: Do we need to know the patient's human leucocyte antigen status? Intern. Med. J. 2012;42(4):411–6.
91. Jarjour S et al. Genetic markers associated with cutaneous adverse drug reactions to allopurinol: A systematic review. Pharmacogenomics; 2015;16(7):755–67.
92. Ng CY et al. Impact of the HLA-B'58:01 Allele and Renal Impairment on Allopurinol- Induced Cutaneous Adverse Reactions. J. Invest. Dermatol; 2016;136(7):1373–81.
93. Gonçalo Met al. HLA-B*58:01 is a risk factor for allopurinol-induced DRESS and Stevens-Johnson syndrome/toxic epidermal necrolysis in a Portuguese population. Br J Dermatol. 2013;169(3):660–5.
94. Hung SI et al. HLA-B*5801 allele as a genetic marker for severe cutaneous adverse reactions caused by allopurinol. Proc Natl Acad Sci. 2005;102(11):4134–9
95. Cao ZH et al. HLA-B*58:01 allele is associated with augmented risk for both mild and severe cutaneous adverse reactions induced by allopurinol in Han Chinese. Pharmacogenomics 2012;13(10):1193–201.
96. Chiu MLS et al. Association between HLA-B*58:01 allele and severe cutaneous adverse reactions with allopurinol in Han Chinese in Hong Kong. Br J Dermatol. 2012;167(1):44–9.
97. Cheng L et al. HLA-B 58:01 is strongly associated with allopurinol-induced severe cutaneous adverse reactions in Han Chinese patients: A multicentre retrospective case-control clinical study. Br J Dermatol. 2015;173(2):555–8.
98. Ko TM et al. Use of HLA-B 58:01 genotyping to prevent allopurinol induced severe cutaneous adverse reactions in Taiwan: National prospective cohort study. BMJ; 2015;351:h4848.
99. Jung JW et al. HLA-B58 can help the clinical decision on starting allopurinol in patients with chronic renal insufficiency. Nephrol Dial Transplant. 2011;26(11):3567–72.
100. Somkrua Ret al. Association of HLA-B*5801 allele and allopurinol-induced Stevens-Johnson syndrome and toxic epidermal necrolysis: A systematic review and meta-analysis. BMC Med Genet. 2011;12(1):118.
101. Yu KF et al. Diagnostic utility of HLA-B*5801 screening in severe allopurinol hypersensitivity syndrome: an updated systematic review and meta-analysis. Int J Rheum. Dis; 2017;20(9):1057–71.
102. Atzori L et al. Cutaneous adverse drug reactions to allopurinol: 10 year observational survey of the dermatology department – Cagliari University. J Eur Acad Dermatol Venereol. 2012;26(11):1424–30.
103. Kaniwa N et al. HLA-B locus in Japanese patients with anti-epileptics and allopurinol-related Stevens-Johnson syndrome and toxic epidermal necrolysis. Pharmacogenomics; 2008;9(11):1617–22.
104. Tassaneeyakul W et al. Strong association between HLA-B*5801 and allopurinol-induced Stevens-Johnson syndrome and toxic epidermal necrolysis in a Thai population. Pharmacogenet Genomics 2009;19(9):704–9.
105. Ha Pham TT et al. Allopurinol-induced severe cutaneous adverse reactions in Vietnamese: the role of HLA alleles and other risk factors. Pharmacogenomics 2022; 23:303–13.
106. Fontana RJ et al. Allopurinol hepatotoxicity is associated with human leukocyte antigen Class I alleles. Liver Int 2021; 41:1884–93.
107. Kim MY et al. HLA-A*24:02 increase the risk of allopurinol-induced drug reaction with eosinophilia and systemic symptoms in HLA-B*58:01 carriers in a Korean population; a multicenter cross-sectional case-control study. Clin Transl Allergy. 2022;12(9):e12193.
108. Saksit N et al. Comparison between the HLA-B 58: 01 Allele and Single-Nucleotide Polymorphisms in Chromosome 6 for Prediction of Allopurinol-Induced Severe Cutaneous Adverse Reactions. J Immunol Res. 2017;2017.
109. Tohkin M et al. A whole-genome association study of major determinants for allopurinol-related Stevens-Johnson syndrome and toxic epidermal necrolysis in Japanese patients. Pharmacogenomics J; 2013;13(1):60–9.
110. Fernandez CA et al. HLA-DRB1*07:01 is associated with a higher risk of asparaginase allergies. Blood. 2014;124(8):1266–76.
111. Gagne V et al. HLA alleles associated with asparaginase hypersensitivity in childhood ALL: a report from the DFCI Consortium. Pharmacogenomics. 2020;21(8):541–7.
112. Heap GA et al. HLA-DQA1-HLA-DRB1 variants confer susceptibility to pancreatitis induced by thiopurine immunosuppressants. Nat Genet. 2014;46(10):1131–4.
113. Salehi T et al. Human leukocyte antigen association with azathioprine-induced drug hypersensitivity reactions in patients with anti-neutrophil cytoplasmic antibody associated vasculitis. Hum Immunol. 2023;84(3):196–198.
114. Cheung CL et al. HLA-B*38:02:01 predicts carbimazole/methimazole-induced agranulocytosis. Clin Pharmacol Ther. 2016;99(5):555–61.
115. Chen WT et al. Associations of HLA genotypes with antithyroid drug-induced agranulocytosis: A systematic review and meta-analysis of pharmacogenomics studies. Br J Clin Pharmacol. 2019;85(9):1878–87.
116. Hallberg P et al. Genetic variants associated with antithyroid drug-induced agranulocytosis: a genome-wide association study in a European population. Lancet Diabetes Endocrinol. 2016;4(6):507–16.
117. Nakakura S et al. HLA-B*39:01:01 is a novel risk factor for antithyroid drug-induced agranulocytosis in Japanese population. Pharmacogenomics J 2021; 21:94–101.
118. Ohnuki Y et al. HLA-DRB1 alleles in immune-mediated necrotizing myopathy. Neurology. 2016;87(18):1954–5.
119. Lee HY et al. Increased risk of strontium ranelate-related SJS/TEN is associated with HLA. Osteoporos Int. 2016;27(8):2577–83.
120. Wang YHet al. The Medication Risk of Stevens-Johnson Syndrome and Toxic Epidermal Necrolysis in Asians: The Major Drug Causality and Comparison With the US FDA Label. Clin Pharmacol Ther. 2019;105(1):112– 20.
121. Chen CB et al. The risk of anti-osteoporotic agent-induced severe cutaneous adverse drug reactions and their association with HLA. J Eur Acad Dermatol Venereol. 2021;35(3):712–720.

122. Li C et al. HLA-B*35:01 Allele Is a Potential Biomarker for Predicting Polygonum multiflorum-Induced Liver Injury in Humans. Hepatology. 2019;70(1):346–57.
123. Hoofnagle JH et al. HLA-B*35:01 and Green Tea Induced Liver Injury. Hepatology. 2021;73(6):2484–2493.
124. Vuppalanchi R et al. Garcinia cambogia, Either Alone or in Combination With Green Tea, Causes Moderate to Severe Liver Injury. Clin Gastroenterol Hepatol 2022; 20:e1416–e25.
125. Halegoua-DeMarzio D et al. Liver Injury Associated with Turmeric-a Growing Problem: Nine Cases from the Drug-Induced Liver Injury Network [DILIN]. Digestive Disease Week. 2022. EP1206.
126. Nakamura R et al. Significant association between HLA-B*35:01 and onset of drug-induced liver injury caused by Kampo medicines in Japanese patients. Hepatol Res. 2023;53(5):440–449.
127. Saper VE et al. Severe delayed hypersensitivity reactions to IL-1 and IL-6 inhibitors link to common HLADRB1*15 alleles. Ann Rheum Dis 2022; 81:406–15.
128. Lonjou C et al. A marker for Stevens-Johnson syndrome ...: ethnicity matters. Pharmacogenomics J. 2006;6(4):265–8.
129. Nicoletti P et al. Drug Induced Liver Injury Network (DILIN) investigators. HLA-B*53:01 Is a Significant Risk Factor of Liver Injury due to Phenytoin and Other Antiepileptic Drugs in African Americans. Am J Gastroenterol. 2024;119(1):200–202.
130. Fukunaga K et al. Differential Effects of HLA-B*15:11 and HLA-A*31:01 on Carbamazepine-Induced Cutaneous Adverse Reactions. J Invest Dermatol. 2024;144(4):908–911.e7.
131. Wu PC et al. Human Leukocyte Antigens and Sulfamethoxazole/Cotrimoxazole-Induced Severe Cutaneous Adverse Reactions: A Systematic Review and Meta-Analysis. JAMA Dermatol. 2024;160(5):525–534.
132. Asif BA et al. Drug Induced Liver Injury Network (DILIN). Vancomycin-Induced Liver Injury, DRESS, and HLA-A*32:01. J Allergy Clin Immunol Pract. 2024;12(1):168–174.e2.
133. Wang CC et al. Association of HLA alleles with cephalosporin allergy in the Taiwanese population. Sci Rep. 2024;14(1):17167.
134. Jiang M et al. An association study of HLA with levofloxacin-induced severe cutaneous adverse drug reactions in Han Chinese. iScience. 2023;26(8):107391.
135. Conlon C et al. Drug-Induced Liver Injury Network (DILIN). Clinical characteristics and HLA associations of azithromycin-induced liver injury.Aliment Pharmacol Ther. 2024.
136. Meng Q et al. Carbamazepine cutaneous adverse reactions and HLA gene variation in the Chinese population: a systematic review and meta-analysis. Pharmacogenomics. 2023;24(8):459–474.
137. Hsu HC, Chung WH, Lin YC, et al. Clinical characteristics and genetic HLA marker for patients with oxaliplatin-induced adverse drug reactions. Allergol Int. 2024:S1323–8930(24)00041–8.
138. Chung SJ et al. HLA-DRB1*15: 02 Is Associated With Iodinated Contrast Media-Related Anaphylaxis. Invest Radiol. 2020;55(5):304–309.
139. Vuppalanchi R et al., Clinical and Genetic Associations in Cephalosporin-Induced Liver, .Aliment Pharmacol Ther. 2025;apt.70284.
140. Li Y et al., HLA-B Alleles with Shared Peptide Binding Specificities Define Global Risk of Cotrimoxazole-induced SCAR. 2025:25328237.
141. Campbell CN et al. SJS Survivor Study. HLA-B*58:01 is an Incomplete Predictor of Allopurinol-Induced Severe Cutaneous adverse reactions. medRxiv. 2025;25328236.
142. Krantz MS et al. Specific clinical features define HLA-A*32:01-positive vancomycin drug Reaction with eosinophilia and systemic symptoms: A multi-institution crosssectional study. J Allergy Clin Immunol Pract. 2025:S2213-2198(25)00492-1.
143. Ahmad J et al. Clinical and HLA Associations of Fluoroquinolone-Induced Liver Injury: Results From the Drug-Induced Liver Injury Network. Am J Gastroenterol. 2025;0000000000003457.
144. Mukherjee EM et al. Single-cell immunopathology of recurrent acute generalized Exanthematous pustulosis associated with vancomycin. J Allergy Clin Immunol Glob. 2025;4(2):100426.
145. Ahmad J et al. Liver Injury due to Intravenous Methylprednisolone in the Drug-Induced Liver Injury Network. Liver Int. 2025;45(2):e16242.
146. Gopalakrishna H et al. Drug-induced Liver Injury Due to Medications for Alcohol Use Disorder:Results From the DILIN Prospective Study. J Addict Med. 2025;19(3):314-321.
147. Chen CB et al. Class I HLA Alleles Are Associated With an Increased Risk of Osimertinib-Induced Hypersensitivity. J Allergy Clin Immunol Pract. 2025;13(1):143-154.e10.
148. Kim HJ et al. Association of HLA-B*13:01 with DRESS and HLA-A*31:01 with eosinophilia in SJS/TEN induced by carbamazepine. J Allergy Clin Immunol Pract. 2024;12(12):3436-3438.e3.

The table of recommendations from various sources regarding genetic screening to prevent cutaneous adverse drug reactions is now available on the Litt database at https://www.drugeruptiondata.com/about_book.

Concordance of Synonyms and Trade Names with Generic Names

Synonym/Trade name	Generic
3,4-methylenedioxymethamphetamine	MDMA
3TC	lamivudine
4-aminopyridine	dalfampridine
4-AP	dalfampridine
4-demethoxydaunorubicin	idarubicin
4-DMDR	idarubicin
5-Aminolevulinic acid	aminolevulinic acid
5-aminosalicylic acid	mesalamine
5-ASA	mesalamine
5-aza-2'-deoxycytidine	decitabine
5-fluorouracil	fluorouracil
6-mercaptopurine	mercaptopurine
6-MP	mercaptopurine
13-cis-retinoic acid	isotretinoin
17-α-propionate	clascoterone

A

Synonym/Trade name	Generic
Abbokinase	urokinase
Abelcet	amphotericin B
Abilify	aripiprazole
Abreva	docosanol
Accolate	zafirlukast
Accrufer	ferric maltol
AccuNeb	albuterol
Accupril	quinapril
Accupro	quinapril
Accuretic	hydrochlorothiazide, quinapril
Accutane	isotretinoin
acemetacine	acemetacin
acemetacinum	acemetacin
Aceon	perindopril
acetylsalicylic acid	aspirin
aciclovir	acyclovir
Aciphex	rabeprazole
Aclasta	zoledronate
Aclovate	alclometasone
Acomplia	rimonabant
Acova	argatroban
ACT	dactinomycin
Actemra	tocilizumab
ActHIB	Hemophilus B vaccine
Actidose-Aqua	charcoal
Actifen	dexibuprofen
Actigall	ursodiol
Actimmune	interferon gamma
actinomycin-D	dactinomycin
Actiq	fentanyl
Activase	alteplase
activated carbon	charcoal
activated charcoal	charcoal
Actonel	risedronate
Actos	pioglitazone
Acular	ketorolac
ACV	acyclovir
acycloguanosine	acyclovir
Aczone	dapsone
Adalat	nifedipine
Adapin	doxepin
Adasuve	loxapine
Adcetris	brentuximab vedotin
Adcirca	tadalafil
Adderall	dextroamphetamine
Addyi	flibanserin
Adempas	riociguat
adenine arabinoside	vidarabine
Adenocard	adenosine
Adenocur	adenosine
Adipex-P	phentermine
Adlyxin	lixisenatide
Adoxa	doxycycline
Adrenaclick	epinephrine
Adrenalin	epinephrine
adrenaline	epinephrine
AdreView	iobenguane
Adriamycin	doxorubicin
Advair	fluticasone propionate, salmeterol
Advantan	methylprednisolone
Advicor	lovastatin, niacin
Advil	ibuprofen
Aerobid	flunisolide
Afinitor	everolimus
Afluria	influenza vaccine
Agenerase	amprenavir
Aggrastat	tirofiban
Aggrenox	aspirin, dipyridamole
Agrippal	influenza vaccine
Agrylin	anagrelide
Ajovy	fremanezumab
Akineton	biperiden
Aklief	trifarotene
Aknemycin Plus	tretinoin
Akynzeo	netupitant & palonosetron
ALA	alpha-lipoic acid
Ala-Cort	hydrocortisone
Alamast	pemirolast
Alavert	loratadine
Albalon	naphazoline
Albenza	albendazole
Aldactazide	hydrochlorothiazide, spironolactone
Aldactone	spironolactone
Aldara	imiquimod
Aldoclor	chlorothiazide, methyldopa
Aldoril	hydrochlorothiazide
Aldurazyme	laronidase
Alecensa	alectinib
Alesse	oral contraceptives
Aleve	naproxen
Alfenta	alfentanil
Alimta	pemetrexed

Alinia	nitazoxanide
Aliqopa	copanlisib
Alkeran	melphalan
all-trans-retinoic acid	tretinoin
Allegra-D	pseudoephedrine
Allegra	fexofenadine
Alli	orlistat
Almogran	almotriptan
Alocril	nedocromil
Alora	estradiol
Aloxi	palonosetron
alpha tocopherol	vitamin E
Alphadrol	fluprednisolone
Alphagan P	brimonidine
Alphanate	factor VIII - von Willebrand factor
Alprolix	coagulation factor IX (recombinant)
Alrex	loteprednol
Alsuma	sumatriptan
Altace	ramipril
Altoprev	lovastatin
Alunbrig	brigatinib
Alurate	aprobarbital
Alvesco	ciclesonide
Amaryl	glimepiride
Ambi	hydroquinone
Ambien	zolpidem
AmBisome	amphotericin B
Ameluz	aminolevulinic acid
Amerge	naratriptan
amethopterin	methotrexate
Amevive	alefacept
amfepramone	diethylpropion
Amgevita	adalimumab
Amicar	aminocaproic acid
Amikacin sulfate	amikacin
Amitiza	lubiprostone
Amjevita	adalimumab
Amnesteem	isotretinoin
Amoxapine	amoxapine
Amoxil	amoxicillin
amoxycillin	amoxicillin
Amphocin	amphotericin B
Amphotec	amphotericin B
Ampyra	dalfampridine
amrinone	inamrinone
Amyvid	florbetapir F18
Anacin-3	acetaminophen
Anacin	aspirin
Anafranil	clomipramine
Analgin	metamizole
Anamantle HC	lidocaine
Anandron	nilutamide
Ancef	cefazolin
Ancobon	flucytosine
Androcur	cyproterone
Androderm	testosterone
AndroGel	testosterone
Android	methyltestosterone
Anectine	succinylcholine
Angiomax	bivalirudin
Ansaid	flurbiprofen
Antabuse	disulfiram

antegren	natalizumab
Antivert	meclizine
Antizol	fomepizole
Anturane	sulfinpyrazone
Anzemet	dolasetron
APAP	acetaminophen
Aphthasol	amlexanox
Aphtheal	amlexanox
Apidra	insulin glulisine
Apokyn	apomorphine
Apresazide	hydralazine
Apresoline	hydralazine
Aprovel	irbesartan
Aptiom	eslicarbazepine
Aptivus	tipranavir
Aquasol A	vitamin A
Aquasol E	vitamin E
ara-A	vidarabine
ara-C	cytarabine
Aralen	chloroquine
Aranesp	darbepoetin alfa
Arava	leflunomide
Arcalyst	rilonacept
Arcapta Neohaler	indacaterol
Arcoxia	etoricoxib
Arduan	pipecuronium
Aredia	pamidronate
Aricept Evess	donepezil
Aricept	donepezil
Arimidex	anastrozole
Aristada	aripiprazole
Aristospan	triamcinolone
Arixtra	fondaparinux
Arnuity	fluticasone furoate
Aromasin	exemestane
Arpraziquantel	praziquantel
Arranon	nelarabine
Arsenic trioxide (Trisenox)	arsenic
Arthro-Aid	glucosamine
Arthrotec	diclofenac
Arzerra	ofatumumab
ASA	aspirin
Asacol	mesalamine
Ascriptin	aspirin
Asmanex	mometasone
Astelin	azelastine
Atabrine	quinacrine
Atacand HCT	hydrochlorothiazide
Atacand	candesartan
Atarax	hydroxyzine
Atelvia	risedronate
Atgam	anti-thymocyte globulin (equine)
Athimil	mianserin
Ativan	lorazepam
ATP	adenosine
ATRA	tretinoin
Atripla	efavirenz, emtricitabine, tenofovir disoproxil
Atromid-S	clofibrate
Atrovent	ipratropium
Aubagio	teriflunomide
Augmentin	amoxicillin
auranofin	gold & gold compounds

Aurorix	moclobemide
aurothioglucose	gold & gold compounds
Austedo	deutetrabenazine
Auvi-Q	epinephrine
Avage	tazarotene
Avalide	hydrochlorothiazide, irbesartan
Avandamet	metformin, rosiglitazone
Avandaryl	glimepiride, rosiglitazone
Avandia	rosiglitazone
Avapro	irbesartan
Avastin	bevacizumab
Avelox	moxifloxacin
Aventyl	nortriptyline
Aviane	oral contraceptives
Avinza	morphine
Avodart	dutasteride
Avonex	interferon beta
Avycaz	ceftazidime & avibactam
Axert	almotriptan
Axid	nizatidine
Aygestin	progestins
Ayvakit	avapritinib
Azactam	aztreonam
Azacytidine	azacitidine
Azasan	azathioprine
AzaSite	azithromycin
AZD9291	osimertinib
azidothymidine	zidovudine
Azilect	rasagiline
Azmacort	triamcinolone
Azopt	brinzolamide
AZT	zidovudine
Azulfidine	sulfasalazine
Azzalure	botulinum toxin (A & B)

B

Baciguent	bacitracin
Baciim	bacitracin
Bacille Calmette-Guerin	BCG vaccine
Baclofen	baclofen
Bactrim	co-trimoxazole, sulfamethoxazole, trimethoprim
BAL5788	ceftobiprole
BAL	dimercaprol
Balversa	erdafitinib
Banflex	orphenadrine
Banzel	rufinamide
Baraclude	entecavir
Baratol	indoramin
Barhemsys	amisulpride
Basaglar	insulin glargine
Bavencio	avelumab
Beconase AQ	beclomethasone
Beleodaq	belinostat
Bellafill	collagen (bovine)
Belviq	lorcaserin
Benadryl	diphenhydramine, pseudoephedrine
BeneFIX	coagulation factor IX (recombinant)
Benicar	olmesartan
Benlysta	belimumab
Bentyl	dicyclomine
Benzaclin	clindamycin
bepotastine besilate	bepotastine
Bepreve	bepotastine
Berinert	C1-esterase inhibitor
Beromun	tasonermin
Besivance	besifloxacin
Besponsa	inotuzumab ozogamicin
Beta-Adalat	atenolol
Beta-Val	betamethasone
Betaferon	interferon beta
Betagan	levobunolol
Betapace	sotalol
Betaseron	interferon beta
Betatrex	betamethasone
Betaxon	levobetaxolol
Betoptic [Ophthalmic]	betaxolol
Bevyxxa	betrixaban
Bexsero	meningococcal group B vaccine
Bextra	valdecoxib
Bexxar	tositumomab & iodine^{131}
Bezalip	bezafibrate
BG-12	dimethyl fumarate
Biaxin	clarithromycin
Biaxsig	roxithromycin
BiCNU	carmustine
Bifril	zofenopril
Biktarvy	bictegravir/emtricitabine/tenofovir alafenamide
Biltricide	praziquantel
Binosto	alendronate
Bio-Active Selenium	selenium
BioThrax	anthrax vaccine
Blenoxane	bleomycin
bleo	bleomycin
Blephamide	prednisolone, sulfacetamide
BLM	bleomycin
Blocadren	timolol
BNT162b2	covid-19 vaccine, mrna
Bocouture	botulinum toxin (A & B)
Bolvidon	mianserin
Bondronat	ibandronate
Boniva	ibandronate
Bontril	phendimetrazine
Bosulif	bosutinib
Botox	botulinum toxin (A & B)
Braftovi	encorafenib
Bredinin	mizoribine
Breo	fluticasone furoate
Brethine	terbutaline
Brevibloc	esmolol
Brevicon	oral contraceptives
Brevital	methohexital
Brexafemme	ibrexafungerp
Bricanyl	terbutaline
Bridion	sugammadex
Brilinta	ticagrelor
Brisdelle	paroxetine mesylate
British anti-Lewisite	dimercaprol
BritLofex	lofexidine
Briviact	brivaracetam
Bromfed	brompheniramine, pseudoephedrine
BromSite	bromfenac
Brovana	arformoterol
Brukinsa	zanubrutinib
Bumex	bumetanide

BuSpar	buspirone
Butisol	butabarbital
Bydureon	exenatide
Byetta	exenatide
Byfavo	remimazolam
Bystolic	nebivolol
Byvalson	nebivolol, valsartan

C

C7E3	abciximab
Caduet	amlodipine, atorvastatin
Calan	verapamil
calcidiol	calcifediol
Calcimar	calcitonin
calcipotriene	calcipotriol
Calquence	acalabrutinib
Camoquin	amodiaquine
Campath	alemtuzumab
Campral	acamprosate
Camptosar	irinotecan
Canasa	mesalamine
Cancidas	caspofungin
Canesten	clotrimazole
cannabis	marihuana
Capastat	capreomycin
Capex	fluocinolone
Caplyta	lumateperone
Capmatinib hydrochloride	capmatinib
Capoten	captopril
Capozide	captopril, hydrochlorothiazide
Caprelsa	vandetanib
Carac	fluorouracil
Carafate	sucralfate
carampicillin	bacampicillin
Carbastat Ophthalmic	carbachol
carbidopa	levodopa
Carbocaine	mepivacaine
Carbometyx	cabozantinib
Carbomix	charcoal
Cardase	ethoxzolamide
Cardene	nicardipine
Cardicor	bisoprolol
Cardizem	diltiazem
Cardura	doxazosin
Casodex	bicalutamide
Cataflam	diclofenac
Catapres	clonidine
Catena	idebenone
Caverject	alprostadil
Cayston	aztreonam
CDDP	cisplatin
Ceclor	cefaclor
Cedax	ceftibuten
CeeNU	lomustine
cefalexin	cephalexin
Cefizox	ceftizoxime
Cefobid	cefoperazone
cefradine	cephradine
Ceftin	cefuroxime
Celebrex	celecoxib
Celectol	celiprolol
Celestone	betamethasone
Celexa	citalopram
CellCept	mycophenolate
Celol	celiprolol
Celontin	methsuximide
Celsentri	maraviroc
Ceptaz	ceftazidime
Cerdelga	eliglustat
Cerebyx	fosphenytoin
Certican	everolimus
Certolizumab pegol	certolizumab
Cervidel	dinoprostone
Champix	varenicline
Chantix	varenicline
Chemet	succimer
Chibroxin	norfloxacin
Chirocaine	levobupivacaine
Chlor-Trimeton	chlorpheniramine
chloroiodoquin	clioquinol
chlorphenamine	chlorpheniramine
chlortalidone	chlorthalidone
Cholbam	cholic acid
Choledyl SA	oxtriphylline
Choledyl	oxtriphylline
Cholestagel	colesevelam
Cialis	tadalafil
Cibinqo	abrocitinib
Ciloxan Ophthalmic	ciprofloxacin
Cimzia	certolizumab
Cinryze	C1-esterase inhibitor
Cipramil	citalopram
Cipro	ciprofloxacin
Ciproxin	ciprofloxacin
Citanest	prilocaine
citrovorum factor	leucovorin
Claforan	cefotaxime
Claravis	isotretinoin
Clarinex	desloratadine
Claritin-D	loratadine
Claritin	loratadine
Clavulin	amoxicillin
Cleocin	clindamycin
Cleocin-T	clindamycin
Cleviprex	clevidipine
Clexane	enoxaparin
Climara	estradiol
Clindagel	clindamycin
Clindets	clindamycin
Clinoril	sulindac
Clomid	clomiphene
Clopixol Depot	zuclopenthixol decanoate
Clopixol	zuclopenthixol
Cloxapen	cloxacillin
Clozaril	clozapine
club drug	MDMA
Coartem	artemether/lumefantrine
Cogentin	benztropine
Cognex	tacrine
Colase	docusate
Colazal	balsalazide
Colazide	balsalazide
Cold-Eeze	zinc
Colestid	colestipol

Colofac	mebeverine
Colomycin	colistin
Combivent	albuterol, ipratropium
Combivir	lamivudine, zidovudine
Cometriq	cabozantinib
Comirnaty	covid-19 vaccine, mrna
Compazine	prochlorperazine
Complera	emtricitabine, rilpivirine, tenofovir disoproxil
Comtan	entacapone
Comtess	entacapone
Comvax	Hemophilus B vaccine, influenza vaccine
Concerta	methylphenidate
Concor	bisoprolol
Contrave	naltrexone
Copaxone	glatiramer
Copegus	ribavirin
copolymer-1	glatiramer
Coracten	nifedipine
Cordarone	amiodarone
Coreg	carvedilol
Corflo	nicorandil
Corlanor	ivabradine
Corlopam	fenoldopam
Cortef	hydrocortisone
Cortenema	hydrocortisone
Cortexolone 17&#x03B1	clascoterone
Cortisporin	bacitracin
Cortone	cortisone
Corvert	ibutilide
Corzide	bendroflumethiazide, nadolol
Cosela	trilaciclib
Cosentyx	secukinumab
Cosmegen	dactinomycin
Cosopt	dorzolamide, timolol
Cotazym	pancrelipase
Cotellic	cobimetinib
Cotrimoxazole	co-trimoxazole
Coumadin	warfarin
Covera-HS	verapamil
Cozaar	losartan
CPM	cyclophosphamide
Creon	pancrelipase
Cresemba	isavuconazonium sulfate
Crestor	rosuvastatin
Crixivan	indinavir
cromolyn sodium	cromolyn
Crystapen	penicillin G
CsA	cyclosporine
CT-P13 is biosimilar infliximab	infliximab
CTX	cyclophosphamide
Cubicin	daptomycin
Cufence	trientine
Cuprior	trientine
Cutivate	fluticasone propionate
Cuvposa	glycopyrrolate
Cuvrior	trientine
CyA	cyclosporine
Cyclosporine-A	cyclosporine
Cyklokapron	tranexamic acid
Cylert	pemoline
Cymbalta	duloxetine
Cyramza	ramucirumab
Cystagon	cysteamine
Cystrin	oxybutynin
CYT	cyclophosphamide
Cytadren	aminoglutethimide
Cytomel	liothyronine
Cytosar-U	cytarabine
Cytovene	ganciclovir
Cytoxan	cyclophosphamide

D

D4T	stavudine
D-cycloserine	cycloserine
D.H.E. 45	dihydroergotamine
Dacogen	decitabine
Daklinza	daclatasvir
Daliresp	roflumilast
Dalmane	flurazepam
Dalvance	dalbavancin
Daraprim	pyrimethamine
Darvocet-N	acetaminophen, propoxyphene
Darvon Compound	aspirin, propoxyphene
Darvon	propoxyphene
Darzalex	daratumumab
daunomycin	daunorubicin
DaunoXome	daunorubicin
Daxas	roflumilast
Daypro	oxaprozin
Dayvigo	lemborexant
DDAVP	desmopressin
Deca-Durabolin	nandrolone
Decadron	dexamethasone
Decapeptyl	triptorelin
Decentan	perphenazine
Declomycin	demeclocycline
Defitelio	defibrotide
Delatestryl	testosterone
Delstrigo	doravirine/lamiduvine/tenofovir disoproxil
Delta-Cortef	prednisolone
Deltaran	dexibuprofen
Deltasone	prednisone
Demadex	torsemide
Demerol	meperidine
Demulen	oral contraceptives
Deniban	amisulpride
Denzapine	clozapine
deoxycoformycin	pentostatin
Depacon	valproic acid
Depade	naltrexone
Depakene	valproic acid
Depakote	valproic acid
Depen	penicillamine
Depo-Provera	medroxyprogesterone
DepoCyt	cytarabine
deprenyl	selegiline
Derma-Smoothe	fluocinolone
Descovy	emtricitabine, tenofovir alafenamide
Desferal	deferoxamine
Desogen	oral contraceptives
Desoxyn	methamphetamine
Destolit	ursodiol
Desyrel	trazodone
Detrol	tolterodine

Dexedrine	dextroamphetamine
Dexilant	dexlansoprazole
Dexone	dexamethasone
Dexoptifen	dexibuprofen
DHT	dihydrotachysterol
Diabeta	glyburide
Diabinese	chlorpropamide
Diamicron MR	gliclazide
Diamicron	gliclazide
Diamox	acetazolamide
Diastat	diazepam
Dibenzyline	phenoxybenzamine
DIC	dacarbazine
Dicolmax	diclofenac
Dicynene	etamsylate
Didrex	benzphetamine
Didronel	etidronate
Differin	adapalene
Difflam	benzydamine
Diflucan	fluconazole
diiodohydroxyquin	iodoquinol
Dilacor XR	diltiazem
Dilantin	phenytoin
Dilatrate-SR	isosorbide dinitrate
Dilaudid	hydromorphone
dimethyl (E) butenedioate	dimethyl fumarate
Diovan HCT	hydrochlorothiazide, valsartan
Diovan	valsartan
Dipentum	olsalazine
diphenylhydantoin	phenytoin
Diprivan	propofol
Diprolene	betamethasone
dipyrone	metamizole
disodium cromoglycate	cromolyn
Ditropan	oxybutynin
Diurexan	xipamide
Diuril	chlorothiazide
divalproate	valproic acid
divalproex	valproic acid
Divigel	estradiol
DMSA	succimer
DNR	daunorubicin
Dobutrex	dobutamine
Dolmatil	sulpiride / levosulpiride
Dolobid	diflunisal
Dolophine	methadone
Doptelet	avatrombopag
Doral	quazepam
Doralese Tiltab	indoramin
Doribax	doripenem
Doryx	doxycycline
Dostinex	cabergoline
Dovonex	calcipotriol
Doxil	doxorubicin
DPH	phenytoin
Dramamine	dimenhydrinate
Drisdol	ergocalciferol
Droxia	hydroxyurea
DRSP (drospirenone)	drospirenone/estetrol
DTIC-Dome	dacarbazine
Duexis	famotidine
Dulcolax	bisacodyl
Dulera	formoterol, mometasone
Duoneb	albuterol, ipratropium
Duopa	levodopa
Dupixent	dupilumab
Duragesic	fentanyl
Duramorph	morphine
Duratuss	hydrocodone
Duricef	cefadroxil
Durlaza	aspirin
Duzallo	allopurinol, lesinurad
Dyazide	hydrochlorothiazide, triamterene
Dycill	dicloxacillin
Dymelor	acetohexamide
Dynabac	dirithromycin
Dynacin	minocycline
DynaCirc	isradipine
Dyrenium	triamterene
Dysport	botulinum toxin (A & B)

E

E4 (estetrol)	drospirenone/estetrol
E	MDMA
Ebixa	memantine
Ecalta	anidulafungin
Ecotrin	aspirin
ecstasy	MDMA
Edarbi	azilsartan
Edecrin	ethacrynic acid
Edex	alprostadil
Edronax	reboxetine
Edurant	rilpivirine
Effexor XL	venlafaxine
Effexor	venlafaxine
Effient	prasugrel
Efudex	fluorouracil
ELA-Max	lidocaine
Elavil	amitriptyline
Eldepryl	selegiline
Elepsia XR	levetiracetam
Elestat	epinastine
Elestrin	estradiol
Elidel	pimecrolimus
Eligard	leuprolide
Eliquis	apixaban
Elitek	rasburicase
Elixophyllin	aminophylline
ella	ulipristal
ellaOne	ulipristal
Ellence	epirubicin
Elmiron	pentosan
Elocon	mometasone
Eloxatin	oxaliplatin
Elspar	asparaginase
Emcor	bisoprolol
Emcyt	estramustine
Emend	aprepitant
Emflaza	deflazacort
Emflex	acemetacin
EMLA	lidocaine
Emsam	selegiline
Emselex	darifenacin
Emtriva	emtricitabine

F

folacin	folic acid
folate	folic acid
FOLFOXIRI	folfirinox
folinic acid	leucovorin
Folotyn	pralatrexate
Foradil	formoterol
Forane	isoflurane
Fortamet	metformin
Fortaz	ceftazidime
Forteo	teriparatide
Fortesta	testosterone
Fosamax	alendronate
Foscavir	foscarnet
Fosrenol	lanthanum
Fostemsavir tromethamine	fostemsavir
FP	fluticasone propionate
Fragmin	dalteparin
Frisium	clobazam
Frova	frovatriptan
Fucidin	fusidic acid
Fucithalmic	fusidic acid
Fulvicin	griseofulvin
Fumaderm	dimethyl fumarate
Furadantin	nitrofurantoin
Fusilev	levoleucovorin
Fuzeon	enfuvirtide
Fycompa	perampanel

G

Gabitril	tiagabine
Gablofen	baclofen
gadobenate dimeglumine	gadobenate
Gadovist	gadobutrol
Galvus	vildagliptin
Gamifant	emapalumab
Gamimune	immune globulin IV
Gammagard	immune globulin IV
gammaphos	amifostine
Gammar PIV	immune globulin IV
Gamunex	immune globulin IV
Gantrisin	sulfisoxazole
Garamycin	gentamicin
Gastrocrom	cromolyn
Gastrografin	diatrizoate
Gazyva	obinutuzumab
Gemtesa	vibegron
Gemzar	gemcitabine
GenESA	arbutamine
Genoptic	gentamicin
Genotropin	somatropin
Genvoya	cobicistat/elvitegravir/emtricitabine/tenofovir alafenamide
Geocillin	carbenicillin
Geodon	ziprasidone
Geref	sermorelin
GHB	sodium oxybate
Gilenya	fingolimod
Gilotrif	afatinib
Glatopa	glatiramer
Gleevec	imatinib
Gliadel Wafer	carmustine
glibenclamide	glyburide
Glucagon Emergency Kit	glucagon
Glucobay	acarbose
Glucophage	metformin
Glucosamine sulfate	glucosamine
Glucotrol	glipizide
Glucovance	glyburide, metformin
glybenclamide	glyburide
glyceryl trinitrate	nitroglycerin
glycopyrronium bromide, glycopyrronium tosylate	glycopyrrolate
Glynase	glyburide
Glypressin	terlipressin
Glyset	miglitol
Glyxambi	empagliflozin, linagliptin
Gocovri	amantadine
Granix	granulocyte colony-stimulating factor (G-CSF)
grass	marihuana
Grifulvin V	griseofulvin
Gris-PEG	griseofulvin
GS-5734	remdesivir
Gyno-Pervaryl	econazole
Gynodiol	estradiol

H

Habitrol Patch	nicotine
Haemate	factor VIII - von Willebrand factor
Halaven	eribulin
Halcion	triazolam
Haldol	haloperidol
Halfan	halofantrine
Halotestin	fluoxymesterone
Halotussin	codeine
Harvoni	ledipasvir & sofosbuvir
hashish	marihuana
Head & Shoulders Shampoo	selenium
Hectorol	doxercalciferol
Helidac	bismuth, tetracycline
Hemangeol	propranolol
Hep-Flush	heparin
Hepsera	adefovir
Herceptin	trastuzumab
Hetlioz	tasimelteon
Hexalen	altretamine
hexamethylmelamine	altretamine
Hibiclens	chlorhexidine
HibTITER	Hemophilus B vaccine
Hiprex	methenamine
Histeamen	astemizole
Histex	carbinoxamine
Horizant	gabapentin
Humatin	paromomycin
Humatrope	somatropin
Humira	adalimumab
Humulin	insulin
Hyalgan	hyaluronic acid
Hyaluronan	hyaluronic acid
Hycamtin	topotecan
Hycotuss	hydrocodone
Hydeltrasol	prednisolone
Hydrea	hydroxyurea
Hydrocortone	hydrocortisone
Hydromet	hydrocodone
hydroxycarbamide	hydroxyurea

hydroxydaunomycin	doxorubicin
Hygroton	chlorthalidone
Hylan G-F 20	hyaluronic acid
hyoscine	scopolamine
Hyperstat	diazoxide
Hypnomidate	etomidate
Hysingla ER	hydrocodone
Hytakerol	dihydrotachysterol
Hytone	hydrocortisone
Hytrin	terazosin
Hyzaar	hydrochlorothiazide, losartan

I

IB-Stat	hyoscyamine
ibandronic acid	ibandronate
Ibrance	palbociclib
Iclusig	ponatinib
Idamycin	idarubicin
Idelvion	coagulation factor IX (recombinant)
Ifex	ifosfamide
IFN	interferon alfa
IGIV	immune globulin IV
IL-2	aldesleukin
Ilaris	canakinumab
Iletin Lente	insulin
Ilumya	tildrakizumab
Imbruvica	ibrutinib
Imdur	isosorbide mononitrate
Imfinzi	durvalumab
Imigran	sumatriptan
imipemide	imipenem/cilastatin
Imitrex	sumatriptan
Imodium	loperamide
Imovane	eszopiclone
IMOVAX Polio	inactivated polio vaccine
Impavido	miltefosine
Imuran	azathioprine
Inapsine	droperidol
Incivek	telaprevir
Incruse	umeclidinium
Inderal	propranolol
Inderide	hydrochlorothiazide
indometacin	indomethacin
Inegy	simvastatin
INF	interferon alfa
Infergen	interferon alfa
Inflamase	prednisolone
Inflectra	infliximab
Inflexal V	influenza vaccine
Infumorph	morphine
Ingrezza	valbenazine
INH	isoniazid
Inhibase	cilazapril
Injectafer	ferric carboxymaltose (injection)
Inlyta	axitinib
Innofem	estradiol
Innohep	tinzaparin
Innovace	enalapril
Inovelon	rufinamide
Inrebic	fedratinib hydrochloride
Inspra	eplerenone
Intal	cromolyn
Integrilin	eptifibatide
Intelence	etravirine
interleukin-2	aldesleukin
intravenous immunoglobulin (IVIg)	immune globulin IV
Intron A	interferon alfa
Intropin	dopamine
Invanz	ertapenem
Invega	paliperidone
Invirase	saquinavir
Invivac	influenza vaccine
Invokamet	canagliflozin, metformin
Invokana	canagliflozin
Iodine^{131} I-Tositumomab	tositumomab & iodine^{131}
iodochlorhydroxyquin	clioquinol
Iomeron	iomeprol
Ionamin	phentermine
Iopidine	apraclonidine
Ipratropium Steri-Neb	ipratropium
IPV	inactivated polio vaccine
Iquix	levofloxacin
Iressa	gefitinib
Isavuconazole	isavuconazonium sulfate
Isentress	raltegravir
Ismelin	guanethidine
isonicotinic acid hydrazide	isoniazid
Isopredon	fluprednisolone
Isoptin	verapamil
Isordil	isosorbide dinitrate
Isovorin	levoleucovorin
Istin	amlodipine
Istodax	romidepsin
Isturisa	osilodrostat
Isuprel	isoproterenol
Iveegam	immune globulin IV
IVIG	immune globulin IV
Ixempra	ixabepilone

J

Jadenu	deferasirox
Jakafi	ruxolitinib
Jalyn	dutasteride, tamsulosin
Janumet	metformin, sitagliptin
Januvia	sitagliptin
Jardiance	empagliflozin
Jemperli	dostarlimab
Jevtana	cabazitaxel
Joicela	lumiracoxib
Jublia	efinaconazole
Juluca	dolutegravir, rilpivirine
Jurnista	hydromorphone
Juvederm	hyaluronic acid
Juxtapid	lomitapide

K

Kabikinase	streptokinase
Kadcyla	trastuzumab emtansine / ado-trastuzumab emtansine
Kadian	morphine
Kalbitor	ecallantide
Kaletra	lopinavir, ritonavir
Kalten	atenolol
Kalydeco	ivacaftor

Kanuma sebelipase alfa
Keflex cephalexin
Keftab cephalexin
Kemadrin procyclidine
Kenalog triamcinolone
Kengreal cangrelor
Keppra levetiracetam
Keral dexketoprofen
Kerendia finerenone
Kerlone betaxolol
Ketalar ketamine
Ketek telithromycin
Ketesse dexketoprofen
Keveyis dichlorphenamide
Kevzara sarilumab
Keytruda pembrolizumab
KI potassium iodide
Kidrolase asparaginase
Kineret anakinra
Kisqali ribociclib
Klaron sulfacetamide
Klonopin clonazepam
Korandil nicorandil
Korlym mifepristone
Kovanaze tetracaine & oxymetazoline
Krintafel tafenoquine
Kuvan sapropterin
Kwells scopolamine
Kyleena levonorgestrel
Kynapid vernakalant
Kytril granisetron

L

L-asparaginase asparaginase
L-Cysteine acetylcysteine
L-deprenyl selegiline
L-dopa levodopa
L-thyroxine sodium levothyroxine
Lambrolizumab pembrolizumab
Lamictal lamotrigine
Lamisil terbinafine
Lamprene clofazimine
Lanoxin digoxin
Lantanon mianserin
Lantus insulin glargine
Lariam mefloquine
Lasix furosemide
Lastacaft alcaftadine
Latisse bimatoprost
Latuda lurasidone
laViv azficel-t
Lenvima lenvatinib
Leponex clozapine
Lerivon mianserin
Lescol fluvastatin
Letairis ambrisentan
Leukeran chlorambucil
Leukine granulocyte colony-stimulating factor (G-CSF)
leuprorelin leuprolide
Leustatin cladribine
Levamlodipine (levoamlodipine) amlodipine
Levaquin levofloxacin
Levatol penbutolol
Levbid hyoscyamine
Levemir insulin detemir
Levitra vardenafil
Levlen oral contraceptives
Levlite oral contraceptives
Levora oral contraceptives
Levosulpiride sulpiride / levosulpiride
Levothyroid levothyroxine
Levoxyl levothyroxine
Levsin/SL hyoscyamine
Levsin hyoscyamine
Levsinex hyoscyamine
Levulan Kerastick aminolevulinic acid
Lexapro escitalopram
Lexiscan regadenoson
Lexiva fosamprenavir
Lexxel enalapril, felodipine
Lialda mesalamine
Librax clidinium
Libritabs chlordiazepoxide
Librium chlordiazepoxide
Libtayo cemiplimab
Lidoderm lidocaine
lignocaine lidocaine
Limbitrol amitriptyline, chlordiazepoxide
Lincocin lincomycin
Linzess linaclotide
Lioresal baclofen
Lipitor atorvastatin
Lipostat pravastatin
Liptruzet atorvastatin, ezetimibe
liquid antidote charcoal
Lithobid lithium
Livalo pitavastatin
Livial tibolone
Lo/Ovral oral contraceptives
Lodine etodolac
Loestrin oral contraceptives
Lomaira phentermine
Lomotil atropine sulfate, diphenoxylate
Loniten minoxidil
Lonsurf trifluridine & tipiracil
Lopid gemfibrozil
Lopressor hydrochlorothiazide, metoprolol
Loprox ciclopirox
Lorabid loracarbef
Lorbrena lorlatinib
Lorcet acetaminophen
Lortab hydrocodone
Lotemax loteprednol
Lotensin HCT benazepril, hydrochlorothiazide
Lotensin benazepril, hydrochlorothiazide
Lotrel amlodipine, benazepril
Lotronex alosetron
Lovenox enoxaparin
Loxitane loxapine
Lozol indapamide
Lucemyra lofexidine
Lucentis ranibizumab
Lugol's solution potassium iodide
Lumakras sotorasib

Brand / name	Drug
Lumigan	bimatoprost
Luminal	phenobarbital
Lunelle	medroxyprogesterone, oral contraceptives
Lunesta	eszopiclone
Lupkynis	voclosporin
Lupron Depot-Ped	leuprolide
Lupron	leuprolide
Lustra	hydroquinone
Luvox	fluvoxamine
Luxiq	betamethasone
Lynparza	olaparib
Lyrica	pregabalin
Lyrinel	oxybutynin
Lyxumia	lixisenatide

M

Brand / name	Drug
Maalox	loperamide
MabCampath	alemtuzumab
MabThera	rituximab
Macrobid	nitrofurantoin
Macrodantin	nitrofurantoin
Macugen	pegaptanib
Malarone	atovaquone/proguanil
Manerix	moclobemide
Marcaine	bupivacaine
marijuana	marihuana
Marinol	dronabinol
Marplan	isocarboxazid
Matulane	procarbazine
Mavik	trandolapril
Mavyret	glecaprevir & pibrentasvir
Maxair	pirbuterol
Maxalt	rizatriptan
Maxidone	hydrocodone
Maxipime	cefepime
Maxitrol	neomycin
Mayzent	siponimod
mecapegfilgrastim (pegfilgrastim biosimilar)	granulocyte colony-stimulating factor (G-CSF)
Medrol	methylprednisolone
Megace	progestins
Mekinist	trametinib
Melflufen	melphalan flufenamide
Mellaril	thioridazine
Menadione	menadione
Menest	estrogens
Menostar	estradiol
mepacrine	quinacrine
Mephyton	phytonadione
Mepron	atovaquone
Meptid	meptazinol
mercaptamine	cysteamine
mereletinib	osimertinib
Meridia	sibutramine
Meronem	meropenem
mesalazine	mesalamine
Mesantoin	mephenytoin
Mestinon	pyridostigmine
Metadate CD	methylphenidate
Metaglip	glipizide
metaiodobenzylguanidine	iobenguane
Methadose	methadone

Brand / name	Drug
Methergine	methylergonovine
Methohexitone	methohexital
methotrimeprazine	levomepromazine
Methylin	methylphenidate
methylmorphine	codeine
Meticorten	prednisone
Metrocream	metronidazole
MetroGel	metronidazole
Metrolotion	metronidazole
Mevacor	lovastatin
Mexitil	mexiletine
mFOLFOX6	folfox
Miacalcin	calcitonin
Miaxan	mianserin
MIBG	iobenguane
Micardis	hydrochlorothiazide, telmisartan
Micronase	glyburide
Micronor	progestins
Microzide	hydrochlorothiazide
Midamor	amiloride
Mifeprex	mifepristone
Migard	frovatriptan
Migradon	propyphenazone
Migranal	dihydroergotamine
Miltown	meprobamate
Mimpara	cinacalcet
Minipress	prazosin
Minirin	desmopressin
Minitran	nitroglycerin
Minizide	polythiazide, prazosin
Minocin	minocycline
Miochol	acetylcholine
Miradon	anisindione
Mirapex	pramipexole
Mircette	oral contraceptives
Mirena	levonorgestrel
Mirvaso	brimonidine
Mithramycin	plicamycin
mitomycin-C	mitomycin
Mivacron	mivacurium
Mizollen	mizolastine
Mnesis	idebenone
Moban	molindone
Mobic	meloxicam
Mobiflex	tenoxicam
Modalim	ciprofibrate
Moderna Covid-19 Vaccine, mRNA	covid-19 vaccine, mrna
Modicon	oral contraceptives
Modrasone	alclometasone
Moduretic	amiloride, hydrochlorothiazide
Mogadon	nitrazepam
molly	MDMA
Monistat	miconazole
Mono-Gesic	salsalate
Monoket	isosorbide mononitrate
Monopril	fosinopril
Monurol	fosfomycin
Morphabond	morphine
Motegrity	prucalopride
Motifene	diclofenac
Motilium	domperidone
Motrin	ibuprofen

Movantik	naloxegol
Moxeza	moxifloxacin
MS Contin	morphine
MSIR Oral	morphine
MTC	mitomycin
MTX	methotrexate
Multaq	dronedarone
Multihance	gadobenate
Muse	alprostadil
mustine	mechlorethamine
Mutamycin	mitomycin
Myambutol	ethambutol
Mycamine	micafungin
Mycelex	clotrimazole
Mycobax	BCG vaccine
Mycobutin	rifabutin
mycophenolate mofetil, mycophenolate sodium, mycophenolic acid	mycophenolate
Mydayis	dextroamphetamine
Myfortic	mycophenolate
Myleran	busulfan
Mylotarg	gemtuzumab
Myobloc	botulinum toxin (A & B)
Myochrysine	gold & gold compounds
Myocrisin	gold & gold compounds
Myozyme	alglucosidase alfa
Myrbetriq	mirabegron
Mysoline	primidone

N

N/A	androstenedione
N-acetylcysteine	acetylcysteine
NAC	acetylcysteine
Nafcil	nafcillin
Nalorex	naltrexone
Namenda	memantine
Naprosyn	naproxen
Naramig	naratriptan
Nardil	phenelzine
Naropin	ropivacaine
Nasacort	triamcinolone
Nasalcrom	cromolyn
Nasalide	flunisolide
Nasarel	flunisolide
Nascobal	cyanocobalamin
Nasonex	mometasone
Natesto	testosterone
Naturetin	bendroflumethiazide
Navelbine	vinorelbine
Navidrex	cyclopenthiazide
Nebilet	nebivolol
NebuPent	pentamidine
Necon	oral contraceptives
NeoMercazole	carbimazole
Neoral	cyclosporine
Neosar	cyclophosphamide
Neosporin	bacitracin, neomycin
Neotigason	acitretin
NEPA	netupitant & palonosetron
Nerlynx	neratinib
Nesina	alogliptin
Neulactil	pericyazine
Neulasta	granulocyte colony-stimulating factor (G-CSF)
Neupogen	granulocyte colony-stimulating factor (G-CSF)
Neupro	rotigotine
Neurobloc	botulinum toxin (A & B)
Neurontin	gabapentin
Nexavar	sorafenib
Nexium	esomeprazole
Nexletol	bempedoic acid
Nextstellis	drospirenone/estetrol
Niacor	niacin
Niaspan	niacin
Nicoderm	nicotine
Nicoran	nicorandil
Nicorette	nicotine
nicotinamide	niacinamide
nicotinic acid	niacin
Nicotrol	nicotine
Nilandron	nilutamide
Nimbex	cisatracurium
Nimotop	nimodipine
Ninlaro	ixazomib
Nipent	pentostatin
Nipride	nitroprusside
Nitoman	tetrabenazine
Nitrodur	nitroglycerin
nitrogen mustard	mechlorethamine
nitroglycerol	nitroglycerin
Nitrolingual	nitroglycerin
Nitropress	nitroprusside
Nitrostat	nitroglycerin
Nizoral	ketoconazole
Noctiva	desmopressin
Nolvadex	tamoxifen
Nootropil	piracetam
Norco	hydrocodone
Nordette	oral contraceptives
Norditropin SimpleXx	somatropin
Norditropin	somatropin
Norflex	orphenadrine
Norgesic	aspirin
Norinyl	oral contraceptives
Noritate	metronidazole
Noroxin	norfloxacin
Norpace	disopyramide
Norpramin	desipramine
Norprolac	quinagolide
Norval	mianserin
Norvasc	amlodipine
Norvir	ritonavir
Nourianz	istradefylline
Novantrone	mitoxantrone
Novolin R	insulin
NovoLog	insulin aspart
NovoRapid	insulin aspart
Noxafil	posaconazole
Nozinan	levomepromazine
NTG	nitroglycerin
Nubain	nalbuphine
Nubeqa	darolutamide
Nucala	mepolizumab
Nucofed	codeine
Nucynta ER	tapentadol

Nucynta	tapentadol
Nulev	hyoscyamine
Nulojix	belatacept
Nuplazid	pimavanserin
Nuromax	doxacurium
Nurtec ODT	rimegepant
Nutropin	somatropin
NutropinAq	somatropin

O

Ocaliva	obeticholic acid
Ocrevus	ocrelizumab
Octagam	immune globulin IV
Ocuflox	ofloxacin
Ocupress (ophthalmic)	carteolol
Ocusert Pilo	pilocarpine
Odefsey	emtricitabine/rilpivirine/tenofovir alafenamide
ODM-201	darolutamide
Odomzo	sonidegib
Ofev	nintedanib
Oforta	fludarabine
Ogen	estrogens
Oil of Wintergreen	methyl salicylate
Oleptro	trazodone
Olinvyk	oliceridine
Olmetec	olmesartan
Olumiant	baricitinib
Olysio	simeprevir
Omnaris	ciclesonide
Omnicef	cefdinir
OmniHIB	Hemophilus B vaccine
Omnipaque	iohexol
Omontys	peginesatide
OnabotulinumtoxinA	botulinum toxin (A & B)
Onbrez Breezhaler	indacaterol
oncovin	vincristine
Onfi	clobazam
Ongentys	opicapone
Onglyza	saxagliptin
Onivyde	irinotecan
Onmel	itraconazole
Onpattro	patisiran
Ontak	denileukin
Onzetra Xsail	sumatriptan
Opana	oxymorphone
Opdivo	nivolumab
Opilon	moxisylyte
Opivate	factor VIII - von Willebrand factor
Opizone	naltrexone
Opsumit	macitentan
Opticrom	cromolyn
Optimine	azatadine
OptiPranolol	metipranolol
Optivar	azelastine
Orabloc	articaine
Oracea	doxycycline
OraDisc	amlexanox
Orap	pimozide
Oravig	miconazole
Orbactiv	oritavancin
Orencia	abatacept
Orgaran	danaparoid
Orgovyx	relugolix
Orilissa	elagolix sodium
Orinase	tolbutamide
Orkambi	lumacaftor/ivacaftor
Orladeyo	berotralstat
Ortho Tri-Cyclen	oral contraceptives
Ortho-Cept	oral contraceptives
Ortho-Cyclen	oral contraceptives
Ortho-Novum	oral contraceptives
Orudis	ketoprofen
Oruvail	ketoprofen
Osphena	ospemifene
Otezla	apremilast
Otrivine	xylometazoline
Ovace	sulfacetamide
Ovcon	oral contraceptives
Ovral	oral contraceptives
Ovrette	progestins
Oxbryta	voxelotor
Oxsoralen	methoxsalen, psoralens
Oxtellar XR	oxcarbazepine
OxyContin	oxycodone
OxyIR	oxycodone
Ozempic	semaglutide
Ozurdex	dexamethasone

P

PA-824	pretomanid
Pabal	carbetocin
Pacerone	amiodarone
Palexia	tapentadol
Palladone	hydromorphone
Pamelor	nortriptyline
Panadol	acetaminophen
Panretin	alitretinoin
Panzyga	immune globulin IV
para-aminosalicylate sodium	aminosalicylate sodium
paracetamol	acetaminophen
Paraflex	chlorzoxazone
Parafon Forte DSC	chlorzoxazone
Paraplatin	carboplatin
Parlodel	bromocriptine
Parnate	tranylcypromine
Paroven	oxerutins
PAS	aminosalicylate sodium
Paser Granules	aminosalicylate sodium
Pataday	olopatadine
Patanol	olopatadine
Paxil CR	paroxetine hydrochloride
Paxil	paroxetine hydrochloride
PBZ	tripelennamine
PCE	erythromycin
PDGF	becaplermin
Pediapred	prednisolone
PedivaxHIB	Hemophilus B vaccine
Peganone	ethotoin
pegfilgrastim	granulocyte colony-stimulating factor (G-CSF)
PegIntron	PEG-interferon
Pemazyre	pemigatinib
Penetrex	enoxacin
Penlac	ciclopirox
Pennsaid	diclofenac

Pentacarinat	pentamidine
Pentam 300	pentamidine
Pentasa	mesalamine
Penthrane	methoxyflurane
Pentoxil	pentoxifylline
Pepaxto	melphalan flufenamide
Pepcid	famotidine
Pepto-Bismol	bismuth
Percocet	acetaminophen, oxycodone
Perforomist	formoterol
Peri-Colase	docusate
Perjeta	pertuzumab
Perlane	hyaluronic acid
Persantine	dipyridamole
pethidine	meperidine
Pfizer-BioNTech Covid-19 mRNA Vaccine	covid-19 vaccine, mrna
PGE	alprostadil
Phenergan	promethazine
phenobarbitone	phenobarbital
Phenurone	phenacemide
phenylethylmalonylurea	phenobarbital
phenytoin sodium	phenytoin
Phyllocontin	aminophylline
Physiotens	moxonidine
Pico-Salax	sodium picosulfate
Pifeltro	doravirine
Pilopine	pilocarpine
Pipracil	piperacillin
Piqray	alpelisib
Pitocin	oxytocin
Plan B	levonorgestrel
Plaquenil	hydroxychloroquine
Platinol	cisplatin
Plavix	clopidogrel
Plegridy	interferon beta
Plenaxis	abarelix
Plendil	felodipine
Pletal	cilostazol
Plexion	sulfacetamide
Polocaine	mepivacaine
Polymyxin E	colistin
Pomalyst	pomalidomide
Ponvory	ponesimod
pot	marihuana
Potassium arsenite solution (Fowler's solution)	arsenic
Potiga	ezogabine
PPA	phenylpropanolamine
PPS	pentosan
Pradaxa	dabigatran
Praluent	alirocumab
Prandin	repaglinide
Pravachol	pravastatin
Precedex	dexmedetomidine
Precose	acarbose
Prelay	troglitazone
Prelone	prednisolone
Premarin	estrogens
Premphase	medroxyprogesterone
Prempro	medroxyprogesterone
Prepidil	dinoprostone
Prepopik	sodium picosulfate
Preservex	aceclofenac
Prestalia	amlodipine, perindopril
Prevacid	lansoprazole
Prevpac	amoxicillin
Prevymis	letermovir
Prexige	lumiracoxib
Prezcobix	darunavir
Prezista	darunavir
Prialt	ziconotide
Priftin	rifapentine
Prilosec	omeprazole
Primacor	milrinone
Primaquine	primaquine
Primaxin	imipenem/cilastatin
Primovist	gadoxetate
Prinivil	lisinopril
Prinzide	hydrochlorothiazide, lisinopril
Pristiq	desvenlafaxine
Proamatine	midodrine
Probuphine	buprenorphine
Procan	procainamide
Procanbid	procainamide
Procardia	nifedipine
Procoralan	ivabradine
Procrit	epoetin alfa
Procysbi	cysteamine
Prograf	tacrolimus
ProHIBIT	Hemophilus B vaccine
Prolensa	bromfenac
Proleukin	aldesleukin
Prolia	denosumab
Prolixin	fluphenazine
Promacta	eltrombopag
Propecia	finasteride
Propyl-Thyracil	propylthiouracil
Proscar	finasteride
prostaglandin E_1	alprostadil
Prostigmin	neostigmine
Prostin VR	alprostadil
Protelos	strontium ranelate
Protium	pantoprazole
Protonix	pantoprazole
Protopic	tacrolimus
Proventil	albuterol
Provera	medroxyprogesterone, progestins
Provigil	modafinil
Prozac	fluoxetine
Pulmicort Turbuhaler	budesonide
Purinethol	mercaptopurine
Pyostacine	pristinamycin
Pyrazinamide	pyrazinamide
Pyridium	phenazopyridine
Pyrukynd	mitapivat

Q

Qelbree	viloxazine
Qnasl	beclomethasone
Qsymia	phentermine, topiramate
Qtern	dapagliflozin, saxagliptin
Qualaquin	quinine
Qudexy	topiramate
Questran	cholestyramine
Quibron	aminophylline

Quixin	levofloxacin
Qulipta	atogepant
Quvivo	daridorexant
Qvar	beclomethasone

R

Radicava	edaravone
Radiesse	calcium hydroxylapatite
Ranexa	ranolazine
Rapaflo	silodosin
Rapamune	sirolimus
rapamycin	sirolimus
Rapivab	peramivir
Rasilez	aliskiren
Rasuvo	methotrexate
Rayaldee	calcifediol
Razadyne	galantamine
Rebetol	ribavirin
Rebetron	interferon alfa, ribavirin
Rebif	interferon beta
Reclast	zoledronate
Refludan	lepirudin
Regitine	phentolamine
Reglan	metoclopramide
REGN2810	cemiplimab
Regonol	pyridostigmine
Regranex	becaplermin
Relafen	nabumetone
relastat	epinastine
Relistor	methylnaltrexone
Relpax	eletriptan
Remeron	mirtazapine
Remicade	infliximab
Remimazolam besylate	remimazolam
Reminyl	galantamine
Remodulin	treprostinil
Remsima	infliximab
Renagel	sevelamer
Renese	polythiazide
Renflexis	infliximab
Renova	tretinoin
Renvela	sevelamer
ReoPro	abciximab
Repatha	evolocumab
Requip	ropinirole
Rescriptor	delavirdine
Restasis	cyclosporine
Restoril	temazepam
Restylane Fine Lines	hyaluronic acid
Retavase	reteplase
Retevmo	selpercatinib
retigabine	ezogabine
Retin-A Micro	tretinoin
Retisert	fluocinolone
Retrovir	zidovudine
Revatio	sildenafil
Revex	nalmefene
ReVia	naltrexone
Revlimid	lenalidomide
Revolade	eltrombopag
Rexulti	brexpiprazole
Reyataz	atazanavir
Reyvow	lasmiditan
Rezulin	troglitazone
Rheumatrex	methotrexate
Rhinocort	budesonide
Rhopressa	netarsudil
Ribomustin	bendamustine
Ridaura	gold & gold compounds
Rifadin	rifampin
Rifamate	isoniazid
rifampicin	rifampin
Rifater	isoniazid, pyrazinamide
Rilutek	riluzole
Rimactane	rifampin
Rimatil	bucillamine
Rinatec	ipratropium
Rinvoq	upadacitinib hemihydrate
Risperdal Consta	risperidone
Risperdal	risperidone
Ritalin	methylphenidate
Rituxan	rituximab
Rixubis	coagulation factor IX (recombinant)
Roaccutane	isotretinoin
RoActemra	tocilizumab
Robaxin	methocarbamol
Robinul	glycopyrrolate
Robitussin AC	codeine
Robitussin-CF	pseudoephedrine
Robitussin	dextromethorphan
Rocephin	ceftriaxone
Roferon-A	interferon alfa
Rogaine	minoxidil
Romazicon	flumazenil
Romicin	roxithromycin
Rondec	brompheniramine
Rosula	sulfacetamide
Rowasa	mesalamine
Roxanol	morphine
Roxicodone	oxycodone
Roxit	roxatidine
Rozerem	ramelteon
Rozlytrek	entrectinib
Rtsun	artesunate
Rubex	doxorubicin
rubidomycin	daunorubicin
Rukobia	fostemsavir
Rulid	roxithromycin
Rupafin	rupatadine
Rybix ODT	tramadol
Rydapt	midostaurin
Rynatan	phenylephrine
Rynatuss	ephedrine
Rytary	levodopa
Rythmol	propafenone
Ryzodeg	insulin aspart, insulin degludec

S

S-1	tegafur/gimeracil/oteracil
(S)-amlodipine	amlodipine
Sabril	vigabatrin
Saizen	somatropin
Salagen	pilocarpine
salazopyrin	sulfasalazine

salazosulfapyridine	sulfasalazine
salbutamol	albuterol
salicylazosulfapyridine	sulfasalazine
Salonpas	methyl salicylate
Samsca	tolvaptan
Sanctura	trospium
Sancuso	granisetron
Sandimmune	cyclosporine
Sandostatin	octreotide
Sanomigran	pizotifen
Sansert	methysergide
Saphnelo	anifrolumab
Saphris	asenapine
Sarafem	fluoxetine
sargramostim	granulocyte colony-stimulating factor (G-CSF)
Saridon	propyphenazone
Savaysa	edoxaban
Savella	milnacipran
Saxenda	liraglutide
Scemblix	asciminib
Scitropin A	somatropin
Scopoderm-TTS	scopolamine
Sebvio	telbivudine
Seconal	secobarbital
Secretin-Ferring	secretin
Sectral	acebutolol
Seebri Neohaler	glycopyrrolate
Selectol	celiprolol
Selectren	fluprednisolone
SelenoMax	selenium
Selsun Blue	selenium
Selsun Shampoo	selenium
Selzentry	maraviroc
Sensipar	cinacalcet
Sensorcaine	bupivacaine
Septanest	articaine
Septocaine	articaine
Septra	co-trimoxazole, sulfamethoxazole, trimethoprim
Ser-Ap-Es	hydralazine, reserpine
Seractil	dexibuprofen
Serax	oxazepam
Serdolect	sertindole
Serentil	mesoridazine
Serevent	salmeterol
Sernivo	betamethasone
Seromycin	cycloserine
Serophene	clomiphene
Seroquel	quetiapine
Serostim	somatropin
Seroxat	paroxetine hydrochloride
Serpasil	reserpine
Serzone	nefazodone
Seysara	sarecycline
Signifor	pasireotide
Silenor	doxepin
Siliq	brodalumab
Simcor	niacin, simvastatin
Simponi	golimumab
Simulect	basiliximab
Sinemet	levodopa
Singulair	montelukast
Sinquan	doxepin
Sinthrome	acenocoumarol
Sintrom	acenocoumarol
Sirturo	bedaquiline
Sitavig	acyclovir
sitaxsentan	sitaxentan
Skelaxin	metaxalone
Skelid	tiludronate
Sklice	ivermectin
Skyrizi	risankizumab
Slo-Niacin	niacin
SMX-TMP	co-trimoxazole
SMZ-TMP	co-trimoxazole
Solage	tretinoin
Solaraze Gel	diclofenac
Solatene	beta-carotene
Solfa	amlexanox
Solganal	gold & gold compounds
Solian	amisulpride
Soliqua	insulin glargine, lixisenatide
Soliris	eculizumab
Solodyn	minocycline
Solu-Cortef	hydrocortisone
Solu-Medrol	methylprednisolone
Soluspan	betamethasone
Soma Compound	aspirin
Soma	carisoprodol
somatostatin	somatropin
Somatuline Autogel	lanreotide
Somatuline Depot	lanreotide
Somatuline LA	lanreotide
Somavert	pegvisomant
Sonata	zaleplon
Soolantra	ivermectin
Sorbitrate	isosorbide dinitrate
Soriatane	acitretin
Sovaldi	sofosbuvir
Spectracef	cefditoren
Spikevax	covid-19 vaccine, mrna
Spiriva	tiotropium
Splenda	sucralose
Sporanox	itraconazole
Spravato (S-isomer)	ketamine
Sprycel	dasatinib
SSKI	potassium iodide
St. Joseph Aspirin-Free Cold Tablets	phenylpropanolamine
Stablon	tianeptine
Stadol	butorphanol
Stalevo	entacapone, levodopa
Stamaril	yellow fever vaccine
Stelara	ustekinumab
Stendra	avanafil
Stimate	desmopressin
Stiolto Respimat	olodaterol, tiotropium
Stivarga	regorafenib
Strattera	atomoxetine
Streptase	streptokinase
Streptomycin	streptomycin
Stribild	cobicistat/elvitegravir/emtricitabine/tenofovir disoproxil
Striverdi Respimat	olodaterol
Stromectol	ivermectin
Stugeron	cinnarizine

Suboxone	buprenorphine, naloxone
Subutex	buprenorphine
Sucaryl	cyclamate
Sudafed	pseudoephedrine
Sufenta	sufentanil
Sular	nisoldipine
Sulfacet Sodium	sulfacetamide
Sulfacet-R	sulfacetamide
sulfamethoxazole-trimethoprim	co-trimoxazole
Sulide	nimesulide
Sumavel DosePro	sumatriptan
Sumycin	tetracycline
Sunosi	solriamfetol
Suprane	desflurane
Suprax	cefixime
Surfak	docusate
Surmontil	trimipramine
Survanta	beractant
Sustiva	efavirenz
Sustol	granisetron
Sutent	sunitinib
suxamethonium	succinylcholine
Sylatron	PEG-interferon
Symbicort	budesonide, formoterol
Symbyax	fluoxetine, olanzapine
Symdeko	tezacaftor/ivacaftor
Symlin	pramlintide
Symmetrel	amantadine
Symproic	naldemedine
Synalar	fluocinolone
Syndros	dronabinol
Synflex	naproxen
Synjardy	empagliflozin, metformin
Synkavite	menadione
Synthroid	levothyroxine
Syprine	trientine

T

T_3 sodium	liothyronine
T_4	levothyroxine
T-DM1	trastuzumab emtansine / ado-trastuzumab emtansine
Tabrecta	capmatinib
Tafinlar	dabrafenib
Tagamet	cimetidine
Tagrisso	osimertinib
Taltz	ixekizumab
Talwin Compound	aspirin
Talwin-NX	naloxone
Talwin	pentazocine
Talzenna	talazoparib
Tambocor	flecainide
Tamiflu	oseltamivir
Tanafed	dexchlorpheniramine
Tanzeum	albiglutide
TAO	troleandomycin
Tapazole	methimazole
Taravid	ofloxacin
Tarceva	erlotinib
Targiniq	naloxone, oxycodone
Targocid	teicoplanin
Targretin	bexarotene
Tarka	trandolapril, verapamil
Tasigna	nilotinib
Tavanic	levofloxacin
Tavist	clemastine
Taxol	paclitaxel
Taxotere	docetaxel
Tazicef	ceftazidime
Tazorac	tazarotene
Tecentriq	atezolizumab
Tecfidera	dimethyl fumarate
Technivie	ombitasvir/paritaprevir/ritonavir
Teczem	diltiazem, enalapril
Teflaro	ceftaroline fosamil
Tegretol	carbamazepine
Tegsedi	inotersen
Tekamlo	aliskiren, amlodipine
Tekturna HCT	aliskiren, hydrochlorothiazide
Tekturna	aliskiren
Temodar	temozolomide
Tenex	guanfacine
Tenif	atenolol, nifedipine
Tenoret 50	atenolol
Tenoretic	atenolol, chlorthalidone
Tenormin	atenolol
Tensilon	edrophonium
Tensipine MR	nifedipine
Tenuate	diethylpropion
Tequin	gatifloxacin
Terlipressin acetate	terlipressin
Terlipressin	terlipressin
Terramycin	oxytetracycline
Tessalon	benzonatate
Testim	testosterone
Testred	methyltestosterone
tetrahydrocannabinol	dronabinol
Tetralysal	lymecycline
Tetramide	mianserin
TEV-48125	fremanezumab
Tev-Tropin	somatropin
Teveten HCT	hydrochlorothiazide
Teveten	eprosartan
Teysuno	tegafur/gimeracil/oteracil
Thalitone	chlorthalidone
Thalomid	thalidomide
THC	dronabinol
Thelin	sitaxentan
theophylline ethylenediamine	aminophylline
thiamazole	methimazole
Thiopental	thiopental
Thioplex	thiotepa
Thorazine	chlorpromazine
Thymoxamine (British Approved Name)	moxisylyte
Tiazac	diltiazem
Ticar	ticarcillin
TICE BCG	BCG vaccine
Ticlid	ticlopidine
Tikosyn	dofetilide
Tilade	nedocromil
Timentin	ticarcillin
Timolide	timolol
Timoptic	timolol
Tindamax	tinidazole

Tivicay	dolutegravir
TMP-SMX	co-trimoxazole
TMP-SMZ	co-trimoxazole
TOBI	tobramycin
TobraDex	tobramycin
Tofranil	imipramine
Tolak	fluorouracil
Tolectin	tolmetin
Tolvon	mianserin
Topamax	topiramate
Toprol XL	metoprolol
Toradol	ketorolac
Torasemide	torsemide
Torem	torsemide
Torisel	temsirolimus
Totacillin	ampicillin
Toviaz	fesoterodine
Tozinameran	covid-19 vaccine, mrna
tPA	alteplase
Tracleer	bosentan
Tracrium	atracurium
Tradjenta	linagliptin
Trandate	labetalol
Transderm-Scop Patch	scopolamine
Transtec	buprenorphine
Tranxene	clorazepate
Trasicor	oxprenolol
Trasylol	aprotinin
Treanda	bendamustine
Trecator-SC	ethionamide
Trelstar	triptorelin
Tremfya	guselkumab
Trental	pentoxifylline
Treprostinil palmitil (an ester prodrug)	treprostinil
Tresiba	insulin degludec
Tri-Levlen	oral contraceptives
Tri-Norinyl	oral contraceptives
Triacet	triamcinolone
Triaminic	chlorpheniramine
Tricor	fenofibrate
triethylenetetramine	trientine
Trilafon	perphenazine
Trileptal	oxcarbazepine
Trilipix	choline fenofibrate
Trimox	amoxicillin
Trinalin	azatadine, pseudoephedrine
Trintellix (formerly Brintellix)	vortioxetine
Triostat	liothyronine
Triphasil	oral contraceptives
Trisenox	arsenic
Trisoralen	psoralens
Tritace	ramipril
Triumeq	abacavir, dolutegravir, lamivudine
Trivora	oral contraceptives
Trizivir	abacavir, lamivudine, zidovudine
Trobalt	ezogabine
Trobicin	spectinomycin
Trokendi XR	topiramate
Troxyca	naltrexone, oxycodone
Trulicity	dulaglutide
Trumenba	meningococcal group B vaccine
Truseltiq	infigratinib
Trusopt	dorzolamide
Truvada	emtricitabine, tenofovir disoproxil
TS-1	tegafur/gimeracil/oteracil
Tudorza Pressair	aclidinium
Tukysa	tucatinib
Tussi-12D	phenylephrine
Tussi-Organidin	codeine
Tussionex	hydrocodone
Tygacil	tigecycline
Tykerb	lapatinib
Tylenol	acetaminophen
Tylox	oxycodone
Tymlos	abaloparatide
Typherix	typhoid vaccine
Typhim Vi	typhoid vaccine
Tysabri	natalizumab
Tyvaso	treprostinil
Tyzeka	telbivudine

U

Ubrelvy	ubrogepant
Ubretid	distigmine
UDCA	ursodiol
Uftoral	uracil/tegafur
Uloric	febuxostat
Ultane	sevoflurane
Ultracet	tramadol
Ultram	tramadol
Ultrasa	pancrelipase
Unasyn	ampicillin/sulbactam
Uniretic	hydrochlorothiazide
Unithroid	levothyroxine
Uprima	apomorphine
Uptravi	selexipag
Urdox	ursodiol
Urief	silodosin
Urispas	flavoxate
Uroxatral	alfuzosin
Urso 250	ursodiol
Urso Forte	ursodiol
ursodeoxycholic acid	ursodiol
Ursogal	ursodiol
Utibron Neohaler	glycopyrrolate, indacaterol

V

V-cillin K	penicillin V
Vabomere	meropenem & vaborbactam
Vabysmo	faricimab
Vagifem	estradiol
Valcyte	valganciclovir
Valium	diazepam
Valni XL	nifedipine
valproate sodium	valproic acid
Valtrex	valacyclovir
Valturna	aliskiren, valsartan
Vanceril	beclomethasone
Vancocin	vancomycin
Vandazole	metronidazole
Vaniqa	eflornithine
Vantin	cefpodoxime
Vaprisol	conivaptan
Varubi	rolapitant

Vascace	cilazapril
Vaseretic	enalapril, hydrochlorothiazide
Vasocidin	sulfacetamide
Vasosulf	sulfacetamide
Vasotec	enalapril
Vaxchora	cholera vaccine
Vaxigrip	influenza vaccine
Vectibix	panitumumab
Veklury	remdesivir
Velban	vinblastine
Velbe	vinblastine
Velcade	bortezomib
Veletri	epoprostenol
Velosef	cephradine
Velosulin	insulin
Velsar	vinblastine
Veltin	clindamycin/tretinoin
Vemlidy	tenofovir alafenamide
Venclexta	venetoclax
Venoglobulin	immune globulin IV
Ventavis	iloprost
Ventolin	albuterol
VePesid	etoposide
Verelan	verapamil
Vermox	mebendazole
Versed	midazolam
Vertizin	cinnarizine
Verzenio	abemaciclib
Vesanoid	tretinoin
Vesicare	solifenacin
Vfend	voriconazole
Viadur	leuprolide
Viaflex	heparin
Viagra	sildenafil
Vibativ	telavancin
Viberzi	eluxadoline
Vibra-Tabs	doxycycline
Vibramycin-D	doxycycline
Vicks Formula 44	dextromethorphan
Vicks Vatronol	ephedrine
Vicodin	acetaminophen, hydrocodone
Vicoprofen	hydrocodone, ibuprofen
Victoza	liraglutide
Victrelis	boceprevir
Vidaza	azacitidine
Videx	didanosine
Viekira Pak	ombitasvir/paritaprevir/ritonavir
Viekira XR	ombitasvir/paritaprevir/ritonavir and dasabuvir
Viekirax	ombitasvir/paritaprevir/ritonavir
Viibryd	vilazodone
Vimpat	lacosamide
Vincasar	vincristine
Vioform	clioquinol
Viokace	pancrelipase
viosterol	ergocalciferol
Vioxx	rofecoxib
Vira-A Ophthalmic	vidarabine
Viracept	nelfinavir
Viramune	nevirapine
Virazole	ribavirin
Viread	tenofovir disoproxil
Visipaque	iodixanol
Visken	pindolol
Vistabel	botulinum toxin (A & B)
Vistaril	hydroxyzine
Vistide	cidofovir
Vitamin B_{12}	cyanocobalamin
vitamin B_1	thiamine
vitamin B_3	niacin, niacinamide
vitamin B_6	pyridoxine
vitamin B_9	folic acid
Vitamin C	ascorbic acid
vitamin D_2	ergocalciferol
vitamin K_1	phytonadione
vitamin K_3	menadione
Vitamin K	phytonadione
Vitrase	hyaluronic acid
Vivactil	protriptyline
Vivelle-Dot	estradiol
Vivelle	estradiol
Vivitrex	naltrexone
Vivitrol	naltrexone
Vivotif	typhoid vaccine
Vizimpro	dacomitinib
Volibris	ambrisentan
Volmax	albuterol
Voltaren	diclofenac
Voltarol	diclofenac
Vonjo	pacritinib
Vosevi	sofosbuvir/velpatasvir/voxilaprevir
Votrient	pazopanib
Vraylar	cariprazine
Vumon	teniposide
Vyleesi	bremelanotide
Vyndaqel	tafamidis meglumine
Vytorin	ezetimibe, simvastatin
Vyvanse	lisdexamfetamine

W

Wakix	pitolisant hydrochloride
Welchol	colesevelam
Wellbutrin	bupropion
Wellvone	atovaquone
Wigrettes	ergotamine
Winlevi	clascoterone
Winstrol	stanozolol

X

X	MDMA
Xadago	safinamide
Xagrid	anagrelide
Xalatan	latanoprost
Xalkori	crizotinib
Xanax	alprazolam
Xarelto	rivaroxaban
Xatral	alfuzosin
Xcopri	cenobamate
Xeglyze	abametapir
Xeljanz	tofacitinib
Xeloda	capecitabine
Xenazine	tetrabenazine
Xenical	orlistat
Xeomin	botulinum toxin (A & B)
Xgeva	denosumab

Xifaxan	rifaximin
Xifaxanta	rifaximin
Xigduo XR	dapagliflozin, metformin
Xigris	drotrecogin alfa
Xofluza	baloxavir marboxil
Xolair	omalizumab
Xomolix	droperidol
Xopenex	levalbuterol
Xospata	gilteritinib
Xtampza ER	oxycodone
Xtandi	enzalutamide
Xultophy	insulin degludec, liraglutide
xylocaine	lidocaine
Xyrem	sodium oxybate
Xyzal	levocetirizine

Y

Yasmin	oral contraceptives
Yaz	oral contraceptives
Yentreve	duloxetine
Yervoy	ipilimumab
YF-VAX	yellow fever vaccine
Yondelis	trabectedin
Yosprala	aspirin, omeprazole

Z

Zaditor	ketotifen
Zadiva	dimethyl fumarate
Zagam	sparfloxacin
Zaltrap	aflibercept
Zanaflex	tizanidine
Zanosar	streptozocin
Zantac	ranitidine
Zantipres	zofenopril
Zaponex	clozapine
Zarontin	ethosuximide
Zaroxolyn	metolazone
Zarxio	granulocyte colony-stimulating factor (G-CSF)
Zavesca	miglustat
Zebeta	bisoprolol
Zebinix	eslicarbazepine
Zecuity	sumatriptan
Zeftera	ceftobiprole
Zejula	niraparib
Zelapar	selegiline
Zelboraf	vemurafenib
Zelnorm	tegaserod
Zemdri	plazomicin
Zemplar	paricalcitol
Zemuron	rocuronium
Zenapax	daclizumab
Zenpep	pancrelipase
Zepatier	elbasvir & grazoprevir
Zephrex	benzalkonium
Zeposia	ozanimod
Zerbaxa	ceftolozane & tazobactam
Zerit	stavudine
Zestoretic	hydrochlorothiazide, lisinopril
Zestril	lisinopril
Zetia	ezetimibe
Zevalin	ibritumomab
Ziac	bisoprolol, hydrochlorothiazide
Ziagen	abacavir
Ziana	clindamycin/tretinoin
Zimovane	eszopiclone
Zinacef	cefuroxime
Zinbryta	daclizumab
Zipsor	diclofenac
Zithromax	azithromycin
ziv-aflibercept	aflibercept
Zocor	simvastatin
Zofenil	zofenopril
Zofepril	zofenopril
Zofil	zofenopril
Zofran	ondansetron
Zohydro ER	hydrocodone
Zokinvy	lonafarnib
Zoladex	goserelin
zoledronic acid	zoledronate
Zolinza	vorinostat
Zoloft	sertraline
Zomacton	somatropin
ZoMaxx Drug-Eluting Coronary Stent	zotarolimus
Zometa	zoledronate
Zomig	zolmitriptan
Zonegran	zonisamide
Zontivity	vorapaxar
Zopranol	zofenopril
Zorac	tazarotene
Zorbtive	somatropin
Zortress	everolimus
Zosyn	piperacillin, piperacillin/tazobactam
Zovia	oral contraceptives
Zovirax	acyclovir
Zulresso	brexanolone
Zuplenz	ondansetron
Zurampic	lesinurad
Zyban	bupropion
Zyclara	imiquimod
Zydelig	idelalisib
Zyderm	collagen (bovine)
Zydone	hydrocodone
Zyflo	zileuton
Zykadia	ceritinib
Zyloprim	allopurinol
Zymar	gatifloxacin
Zymaxid	gatifloxacin
Zynicor	nicorandil
Zynlonta	loncastuximab tesirine
Zyplast	collagen (bovine)
Zyprexa Relprevv	olanzapine
Zyprexa	olanzapine
Zyrtec	cetirizine
Zytiga	abiraterone
Zyvox	linezolid

www.ingramcontent.com/pod-product-compliance
Lightning Source LLC
LaVergne TN
LVHW080114011026
849160LV00013B/1104
* 9 7 8 1 0 4 1 2 0 2 2 8 8 *